NEURONAL NETWORKS IN BRAIN FUNCTION, CNS DISORDERS, AND THERAPEUTICS

NEURONAL NETWORKS IN BRAIN FUNCTION, CNS DISORDERS, AND THERAPEUTICS

Edited by

CARL L. FAINGOLD
Southern Illinois University School of Medicine, Springfield, IL, USA

HAL BLUMENFELD
Yale University School of Medicine, New Haven, CT, USA

ELSEVIER

AMSTERDAM • BOSTON • HEIDELBERG • LONDON
NEW YORK • OXFORD • PARIS • SAN DIEGO
SAN FRANCISCO • SINGAPORE • SYDNEY • TOKYO

Academic Press is an imprint of Elsevier

Academic Press is an imprint of Elsevier
32 Jamestown Road, London NW1 7BY, UK
225 Wyman Street, Waltham, MA 02451, USA
525 B Street, Suite 1800, San Diego, CA 92101-4495, USA

British Library Cataloguing-in-Publication Data
A catalogue record for this book is available from the British Library

Library of Congress Cataloging-in-Publication Data
A catalog record for this book is available from the Library of Congress

ISBN : 978-0-12-415804-7

For information on all Academic Press publications visit our website at elsevierdirect.com

Typeset by TNQ Books and Journals Pvt. Ltd.
www.tnq.co.in

14 15 16 17 18 10 9 8 7 6 5 4 3 2 1

Dedications

I would like to express my profound appreciation and love to my wife, Carol Faingold, for her caring and unwavering support throughout my career, and especially during this project, which has been an impossible dream and a true exercise in tilting at windmills of the mind. The graduate students, post doctoral fellows, and colleagues who participated in the research from my laboratory deserve much of the credit for our work, but we all ultimately recognize that nature is the true professor and we are all but students. I want to thank the National Institutes of Health (NINDS and NIAAA), Citizens United for Research in Epilepsy, and Epilepsy Foundation for funding our research, and the Southern Illinois University School of Medicine for providing the scientific home, where all our research was carried out. This project would not have been completed without the assistance of my current and former secretaries, Gayle Stauffer and Diana Smith, who labored with me and our coeditor as well as all the authors to make this book a reality. I would also like to thank my family, my sons Scott, Rob, and Chuck; my daughter-in-law Trisha; and my grandkids, Noah, Samantha, Ryan, and Manny for their support. I would also like to thank my late parents, Charles and Anne Faingold, for starting me on the path of my three score and ten year journey to *tikkun olam*. As a life-long sufferer from a neurological disorder, I can only hope that application of the ideas expressed in this book can help advance the treatment of serious brain disorders that plague so many other patients.

Carl L. Faingold, PhD

I would like to dedicate this book to my family—the wonderful love of my life Michelle, our children Eva, Jesse, and Lev who keep a smile on my face, my parents who continue to make me proud, sister who is always there for me, loving in-laws, and all the other family members sharing our journey through life.

Hal Blumenfeld, MD, PhD

Contents

8. Volume Transmission and the Russian-Doll Organization of Brain Cell Networks: Aspects of Their Integrative Actions

L.F. AGNATI, S. GENEDANI, P.F. SPANO, D. GUIDOLIN, K. FUXE

9. Electrophysiological Mechanisms of Network Control: Bursting in the Brain—From Cells to Networks

TAUFIK A. VALIANTE, PETER L. CARLEN

10. Network Control Mechanisms—Cellular Milieu

VICTOR V. UTESHEV, ALEXANDER G. GUSEV, EVGENY A. SAMETSKY

11. Neuronal Network Mechanisms—Sex and Development

ARISTEA S. GALANOPOULOU, SOLOMON L. MOSHÉ

12. Astrocytic Regulation of Synapses, Neuronal Networks, and Behavior

MICHAEL M. HALASSA, MARCELLO D'ASCENZO, ANNA BOCCACCIO, TOMMASO FELLIN

13. The Fear Memory Network

GLENN E. SCHAFE

14. Orchestration of the Circadian Clock Network by the Suprachiasmatic Nucleus

SHELLEY A. TISCHKAU, STACEY L. KRAGER

15. mTOR Signaling in Cortical Network Development

TIFFANY V. LIN, ANGELIQUE BORDEY

16. Network Control Mechanisms—Synaptogenesis and Epilepsy Development

KEVIN STALEY, JONAS DYHRFJELD-JOHNSEN, WALDEMAR SWIERCZ, F. EDWARD DUDEK

17. The Brain and Spinal Cord Networks Controlling Locomotion

LARRY M. JORDAN, URSZULA SŁAWIŃSKA

18. The Brainstem Respiratory Network

TARA G. BAUTISTA, TERESA E. PITTS, PAUL M. PILOWSKY, KENDALL F. MORRIS

19. Visual Network

MORAN FURMAN

20. Auditory Neuronal Networks and Chronic Tinnitus

THOMAS J. BROZOSKI, CAROL A. BAUER

21. Consciousness and Subcortical Arousal Systems

JOSHUA MOTELOW, HAL BLUMENFELD

22. Networks of Normal and Disordered Sleep

PIERRE-HERVÉ LUPPI, PATRICE FORT

23. Networks for the Modulation of Acute and Chronic Pain

INNA SUKHOTINSKY, MARSHALL DEVOR

24. Networks in Mood and Anxiety Disorders

HAMADA HAMID

25. Neuronal Networks and Therapeutics in Neurodegenerative Disorders

AMANDA-AMRITA D. LAKRAJ, BAHMAN JABBARI, DUARTE G. MACHADO

26. Neuronal Networks in Epilepsy: Comparative Audiogenic Seizure Networks

CARL L. FAINGOLD, MANISH RAISINGHANI, PROSPER N'GOUEMO

27. Physiological and Pathophysiological Expansion of Neuronal Networks

PROSPER N'GOUEMO, NORBERTO GARCIA-CAIRASCO, CARL L. FAINGOLD

28. Neuronal Network Plasticity and Network Interactions are Critically Dependent on Conditional Multireceptive (CMR) Brain Regions

CARL L. FAINGOLD, AWAIS RIAZ, JAMES D. STITTSWORTH, JR.

29. Neuronal Network Interactions in the Startle Reflex, Learning Mechanisms, and CNS Disorders, Including Sudden Unexpected Death in Epilepsy

CARL L. FAINGOLD, SRINIVASAN TUPAL

30. Emergent Properties of Neuronal Networks

CARL L. FAINGOLD

31. Neuronal Network Involvement in Stimulation Therapies for CNS Disorders

CARL L. FAINGOLD, HUA-JUN FENG

32. Neuronal Network Effects of Drug Therapies for CNS Disorders

CARL L. FAINGOLD

33. Future Trends in Neuronal Networks—Selective and Combined Targeting of Network Hubs

CARL L. FAINGOLD, HAL BLUMENFELD

List of Contributors

L.F. Agnati Fondazione IRCCS San Camillo, Venezia Lido, Venice, Italy

Carol A. Bauer Division of Otolaryngology, Head and Neck Surgery, Southern Illinois University School of Medicine, Springfield, IL, USA

Tara G. Bautista The Florey Institute of Neuroscience and Mental Health, Melbourne, VIC, Australia

Hal Blumenfeld Department of Neurology, Yale University School of Medicine, New Haven, CT, USA; Department of Neurosurgery, Yale University School of Medicine, New Haven, CT, USA; Department of Neurobiology, Yale University School of Medicine, New Haven, CT, USA

Anna Boccaccio Department of Neuroscience and Brain Technologies, Istituto Italiano di Tecnologia, Genova, Italy

Angelique Bordey Departments of Neurosurgery and Cellular and Molecular Physiology, Yale University School of Medicine, New Haven, CT, USA

Thomas J. Brozoski Division of Otolaryngology, Head and Neck Surgery, Southern Illinois University School of Medicine, Springfield, IL, USA

Peter L. Carlen Department of Surgery, Division of Neurosurgery, Toronto, Ontario, Canada; Division of Fundamental Neurobiology, Toronto Western Hospital Research Institute, Toronto Western Hospital, Ontario, Canada; Krembil Neuroscience Center, University Health Network, Toronto, Ontario, Canada

Marcello D'Ascenzo Institute of Human Physiology, Medical School, Università Cattolica, Rome, Italy

Alain Destexhe Unité de Neurosciences, Information et Complexité (UNIC), Centre National de la Recherche Scientifique (CNRS), France

Marshall Devor Department of Cell and Developmental Biology, Silberman Institute of Life Sciences and the Center for Research on Pain, The Hebrew University of Jerusalem, Jerusalem, Israel

F. Edward Dudek Department of Neurosurgery, University of Utah, Salt Lake City, UT, USA

Jonas Dyhrfjeld-Johnsen Sensorion, Montpellier, France

Carl L. Faingold Departments of Pharmacology and Neurology, Division of Neurosurgery, Southern Illinois University School of Medicine, Springfield, IL, USA

Tommaso Fellin Department of Neuroscience and Brain Technologies, Istituto Italiano di Tecnologia, Genova, Italy

Hua-Jun Feng Department of Anesthesia, Critical Care and Pain Medicine, Massachusetts General Hospital and Harvard Medical School, Boston, MA, USA

Craig F. Ferris Center for Translational NeuroImaging, Northeastern University, Boston, MA, USA

Patrice Fort INSERM, U1028, CNRS, UMR5292, Lyon Neuroscience Research Center, Team "Physiopathologie des réseaux neuronaux responsables du cycle veille-sommeil", Lyon, France and University Lyon 1, Lyon, France

Moran Furman Department of Neurology, Yale University School of Medicine, New Haven, CT, USA

K. Fuxe Department of Neuroscience, Karolinska Institutet, Stockholm, Sweden

Aristea S. Galanopoulou Saul R. Korey Department of Neurology, Dominick P. Purpura Department of Neuroscience and Comprehensive Einstein/Montefiore Epilepsy Center, Albert Einstein College of Medicine, Bronx, NY, USA

Norberto Garcia-Cairasco Department of Physiology, School of Medicine of Ribeirão Preto, University of São Paulo Ribeirão Preto, São Paulo, Brazil

S. Genedani Department of Biomedical Sciences, University of Modena and Reggio Emilia, Modena, Italy

D. Guidolin Department of Molecular Medicine, University of Padova, Padova, Italy

Jennifer N. Guo Department of Neurology, Yale University School of Medicine, New Haven, CT, USA

Alexander G. Gusev Department of Pharmacology, Southern Illinois University School of Medicine, Springfield, IL, USA; Institute of Neuroscience, University of Oregon, Eugene, OR, USA

Michael M. Halassa Department of Psychiatry, Massachusetts General Hospital, Boston, MA, USA

Hamada Hamid Departments of Psychiatry and Neurology, Yale University, New Haven, CT, USA; Connecticut Veterans Administration Health Care System, West Haven, CT, USA; Yale Concussion Center, New Haven, CT, USA; Connecticut Veterans Administration Epilepsy Center of Excellence, West Haven, CT, USA

Bahman Jabbari Department of Neurology, Yale University School of Medicine, New Haven, CT, USA

Larry M. Jordan Department of Physiology, Spinal Cord Research Centre, University of Manitoba, Winnipeg, MB, Canada

Stacey L. Krager Department of Internal Medicine, Southern Illinois University School of Medicine, Springfield, IL, USA

Amanda-Amrita D. Lakraj Department of Neurology, Yale University School of Medicine, New Haven, CT, USA

Tiffany V. Lin Departments of Neurosurgery and Cellular and Molecular Physiology, Yale University School of Medicine, New Haven, CT, USA

Pierre-Hervé Luppi INSERM, U1028, CNRS, UMR5292, Lyon Neuroscience Research Center, Team "Physiopathologie des réseaux neuronaux responsables du cycle veille-sommeil", Lyon, France and University Lyon 1, Lyon, France

Duarte G. Machado Department of Neurology, Yale University School of Medicine, New Haven, CT, USA

Kendall F. Morris Department of Molecular Pharmacology and Physiology, University of South Florida College of Medicine, Tampa, FL, USA

Solomon L. Moshé Saul R. Korey Department of Neurology, Dominick P. Purpura Department of Neuroscience and Comprehensive Einstein/Montefiore Epilepsy Center, Albert Einstein College of Medicine, Bronx, NY, USA; Department of Pediatrics, Albert Einstein College of Medicine, Bronx, NY, USA

Joshua Motelow Department of Neurology, Yale University School of Medicine, New Haven, CT, USA

Prosper N'Gouemo Department of Pediatrics, Georgetown University Medical Center, Washington, DC, USA

Paul M. Pilowsky Macquarie University, Sydney, NSW, Australia

Teresa E. Pitts Department of Physiological Sciences, University of Florida, Gainesville, FL, USA

Manish Raisinghani P2ALS Foundation, Columbia University Medical Center, New York, NY, USA

Awais Riaz Department of Neurology, University of Utah School of Medicine, Salt Lake City, UT, USA

Evgeny A. Sametsky Department of Pharmacology, Southern Illinois University School of Medicine, Springfield, IL, USA

Glenn E. Schafe Department of Psychology and Center for Study of Gene Structure and Function, Hunter College, The City University of New York, New York, NY, USA

Urszula Sławińska Department of Neurophysiology, Nencki Institute of Experimental Biology PAS, Warsaw, Poland

P.F. Spano Fondazione IRCCS San Camillo, Venezia Lido, Venice, Italy; Department of Biomedical Sciences and Biotechnology, University of Brescia, Brescia, Italy

Kevin Staley Department of Neurology, Massachusetts General Hospital, Harvard Medical School, Boston, MA, USA

James D. Stittsworth, Jr. Florida State College at Jacksonville, Kent Campus, Jacksonville, FL, USA

Inna Sukhotinsky Gonda Multidisciplinary Brain Research Center, Bar-Ilan University, Ramat-Gan, Israel

Waldemar Swiercz Department of Neurology, Massachusetts General Hospital, Boston, MA, USA

Jeffrey Tenney Department of Pediatrics, Division of Neurology, Cincinnati Children's Hospital Medical Center, Cincinnati, OH, USA

Shelley A. Tischkau Department of Pharmacology, Southern Illinois University School of Medicine, Springfield, IL, USA

Srinivasan Tupal Department of Anatomy and Neurobiology, Washington University, St. Louis, MO, USA

Victor V. Uteshev Department of Pharmacology and Neuroscience, University of North Texas Health Science Center, Fort Worth, TX, USA; Department of Pharmacology, Southern Illinois University School of Medicine, Springfield, IL, USA

Taufik A. Valiante Department of Surgery, Division of Neurosurgery, Toronto, Ontario, Canada; Division of Fundamental Neurobiology, Toronto Western Hospital Research Institute, Toronto Western Hospital, Ontario, Canada; Krembil Neuroscience Center, University Health Network, Toronto, Ontario, Canada

CHAPTER

1

Introduction to Neuronal Networks of the Brain

Carl L. Faingold[1], *Hal Blumenfeld*[2]

[1]Departments of Pharmacology and Neurology, Division of Neurosurgery, Southern Illinois University School of Medicine, Springfield, IL, USA, [2]Departments of Neurology, Neurobiology, and Neurosurgery, Yale University School of Medicine, New Haven, CT, USA

INTRODUCTION

In recent years, it has become clear that an understanding of the brain's neuronal networks is a critical requirement for understanding normal brain function. In addition, an understanding of how neuronal networks are altered in central nervous system (CNS) disorders is yielding improved insights on the mechanisms of these disorders. Finally, knowledge of the properties of neuronal networks has a significant potential to improve the targeting of therapies for these CNS disorders, as discussed in Chapters 31 and 32.

"SILOS" IN CNS NETWORK RESEARCH

Much of recent brain-related research has emphasized molecular, genetic, and single-channel recording techniques. As valuable as these approaches are, it has become clear that research at the network and the network interaction levels are also vitally important to understanding brain function. However, much of the network-related research that does occur has involved evaluating "single-function" networks, such as the visual or auditory systems. No one can deny the importance of these approaches and the need for further research in these specific functional areas, some of which are covered in several of the chapters in this book. Unfortunately, this approach can yield a "silo" effect, where one area of research rarely considers the *interaction* of the specific network with other brain networks. A possible critique of the network interaction idea is that the level of knowledge of each single network is still incomplete, so it is premature to try to connect them, which may explain why potentially important "cross-silo" research is relatively uncommon. However, it is a major thrust of this volume that a better understanding of brain function, brain disorders, and therapy of these disorders is needed now to alleviate human suffering from the disorders, many of which involve cross-silo network interactions.

TYPES OF NETWORK INTERACTIONS

Network interactions can take several different forms and occur to varying degrees (Chapter 29). The main types of interactions are positive and negative interactions, as shown in the simplified diagram in Figure 1.1. Positive network interactions can involve the projection of an individual network, which can activate another network. In the example in Figure 1.1, Network 1 is shown as not undergoing a significant degree of self-organization, and Network 2 is depicted as capable of self-organization. The degree of self-organization is a critical network property, which can lead to an important network characteristic—an emergent property—which is discussed in this chapter and in detail in Chapter 30. Activation of Input 1 activates Net 1 and leads to Function 1. An example of Input 1 might be a simple acoustic stimulus to the auditory network (Net 1) and results in Function 1, perception of the acoustic stimulus. Net 2 could be the network that controls locomotion, which is subject to a considerable degree of self-organization and in nonexigent states maintains postural control or mediates ambulation (Function 2). Self-organization, which is a major feature of many neuronal networks, can lead to nonlinear amplification of network function (see Chapters 28 and 32). Net 1 and Net 2 can interact in a positive or negative way. Thus, an intense sensory stimulus, which is potentially exigent for the organism, can cause a major motor response by activating the locomotion network. An example of this is the acoustic startle

Neuronal Networks in Brain Function, CNS Disorders, and Therapeutics
http://dx.doi.org/10.1016/B978-0-12-415804-7.00001-0

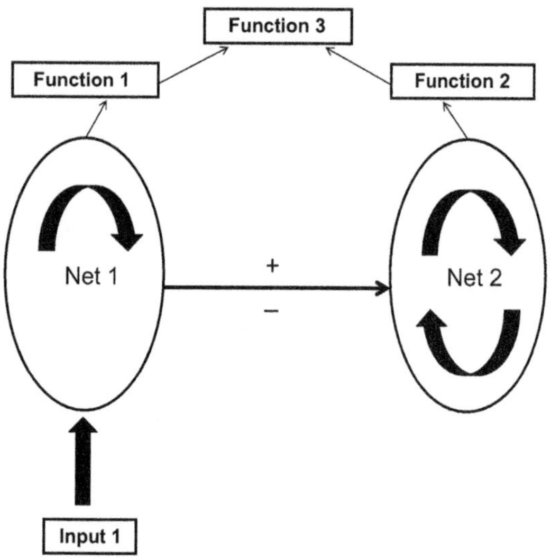

FIGURE 1.1 Simplified diagram of potential network interactions and mechanisms. Both positive (+) and negative (−) interactions can occur, as indicated by the signs above and below the arrow. The two networks are symbolized by the ovals (Net 1 and Net 2). Net 1 has an exogenous and/or endogenous input (Input 1). For simplicity, the input to Network 2 is omitted, but it may be spontaneously active. Each network is considered to have a function and behavior that it controls (Function 1 and Function 2). Net 1 is shown as not undergoing a significant degree of self-organization, as illustrated by the convention of a single semicircular arrow, and Net 2 has paired semicircular arrows and readily undergoes self-organization. Positive network interactions can involve the activation of one individual network, which then activates the second network. For example, Net 1 could be the auditory network, which is responsible for the organism's ability to perceive acoustic stimuli, and Net 2 could be the locomotor network responsible for the organism's ability to move. An example of the interaction of these networks is the acoustic startle response, in which an intense or unexpected auditory stimulus results in projection from the auditory network to the locomotor network that results in a rapid motor movement (jump or flinch), which would be Function 3. A second major form of network interaction that occurs is a negative interaction. This is where the activation of one network can interfere with the function of a second network. An example of a negative network interaction between these same networks would occur if the acoustic stimulus were a creaking noise underfoot when the organism is walking that causes it to stop moving, because it may indicate an unsteady walking surface and a cessation of Function 2–mediated ambulation. Sometimes, two networks can be activated at overlapping times without apparent behavioral consequences.

response, in which an intense or unexpected acoustic stimulus induces a motor movement (jump or flinch) (Function 3). This is an example of a positive interaction of elements of the auditory network with elements of the locomotor network. A second form of network interaction that occurs is a negative interaction. This is where the activation of one network can interfere with the function of a second network. An example of a negative network interaction between these same networks would occur if the acoustic stimulus were a creaking noise underfoot when the organism is walking that causes it to stop moving, because it may indicate an unsteady walking surface and a cessation of Function 2–mediated ambulation. Interactions of different stimuli within the same network can also occur and lead to changes in function. An early prototype of a negative network interaction is the "gate theory of pain" at the spinal cord level[1] (see Chapter 23). Network interactions can exert a beneficial or harmful effect for the individual, depending on the situation. Sometimes, two networks can be activated at overlapping times, but there are no apparent behavioral consequences for the individual. For example, innocuous auditory and visual events can often occur in close temporal proximity, but, unless this sequence of events is repeated or one of the stimuli is not innocuous, no effect on the individual's behavior is observable.

EPILEPSY AS A TEMPLATE FOR NETWORK STUDIES

Some of the most prominent examples of network interactions are seen in the group of CNS disorders called the epilepsies, and these diseases will be emphasized in this book. The question that could be raised is "Why emphasize epilepsy?" Epilepsy has long been considered an important research window into brain mechanisms.[2] Modern human brain research started in earnest with the original studies of Berger, who discovered the human electroencephalogram (EEG),[3] which was followed by pioneering research on the EEG of epileptic patients,[4] elucidating both normal and abnormal EEG patterns. Invasive studies have proven critical to evaluating brain function; these were pioneered by the eminent neurosurgeon Wilder Penfield,[5] who was the first to successfully map the cortical surface in awake patients. This exploration could be done ethically because these patients had intractable epilepsy that potentially required neurosurgery, which can be curative. The leading role of epilepsy studies in neuroscience research and particularly in neuronal network research[6] has extended from the 1950s to today. The recording of single neuronal firing in the awake brain, which is highly instructive of brain function and dysfunction,[7,8] has been done almost exclusively in epilepsy patients. For ethical reasons, the use of neuronal recording is possible in patients in few other CNS disorders. However, this recording technique can greatly facilitate subsequent epilepsy surgery, which remains an important treatment modality for seizure control in intractable epilepsy cases. Finally, the nature of essentially all forms of epilepsy involves disordered network function,[6] often on such a pervasive scale that the epilepsy-related changes are relatively easy to identify. However, as it will hopefully become clear, the common and normal network interactions and changes in other situations, from the simple acoustic startle response to more complex learning paradigms, involve smaller, more localized, and often transient network interactions in medium-sized (mesoscopic) networks. These mesoscopic networks have been considerably more difficult to investigate as easily and thoroughly. The types of network changes that are being identified in the various forms of epilepsy are yielding an extensive classification of many of the types of changes that can occur in CNS networks generally, which may be applicable to the networks that mediate other CNS disorders. However, the network changes in the other CNS disorders are likely to be of a smaller scale, since most of these other disorders do not have the pervasive and even life-threatening effects on the organism that are seen in epilepsy (Chapter 29). Thus, the explication of the types of network changes discovered through epilepsy research will hopefully be instructive for understanding these other CNS disorder networks as well.

NETWORK TECHNICAL APPROACHES

Neuronal networks of the brain are being explored using a wide variety of experimental techniques, as listed in Table 1.1 and expanded upon in several subsequent chapters in this book. Computational approaches are integrated throughout this volume, especially in Chapters 2 and 6, and some recent advances in computationally based studies of network theory are discussed here.

TABLE 1.1 Experimental Approaches to Network Research

1. Anatomical studies (e.g. c-fos and 2-DG imaging) (Chapter 3)
2. Neuroimaging (Chapters 3 and 6)
   a. Anatomical MRI and diffusion techniques
   b. Functional MRI, PET, SPECT, and NIRS
   c. MR spectroscopy
3. Focal inactivation (reversible blockade or lesion) (Chapters 4 and 7)
   a. Lesion
   b. Focal neurotransmission changes
      – Excitatory neurotransmission block
      – Inhibitory neurotransmission increase
4. Focal stimulation: mimicry (electrical, chemical, and/or light) in vivo (Chapter 4)
5. Electrophysiology (Chapters 4–6, 9, and 22)
   a. Electroencephalogram oscillations and magnetoencephalogram
   b. Neuronal electrophysiology in vivo
   c. Combined stimulation and neuronal recording in net sites in vivo
   d. In vitro patch or sharp intracellular recordings
6. Computational techniques
7. Genetic mutation techniques (Chapters 4, 11, 14, 15, and 22)

Abbreviations: 2-DG: 2-deoxyglucose; MRI: magnetic resonance imaging; NIRS: Near-infrared spectroscopy; PET: positron emission tomography; SPECT: single-photon emission computed tomography.

COMPUTATIONAL APPROACHES TO NEURONAL NETWORKS

Network-related studies are used in a number of fields from weather to sociology, as well as in neuroscience. A computational approach to the study of the many forms of networks has been developed based on graph theory.[5,9,10] Using this theory, three major network categories were established: regular, small-world, and random. The consensus in this field is that neuronal networks of the brain fall into the small-world category, which is a network with many local connections and a few longer connections as well.[9] This approach is based on different types of biological data, including neuroanatomy, brain imaging, and electrophysiological techniques, including the EEG.[5,9,11] Graph theory also evaluates networks based on the connectivity between elements (nodes) of the network, and brain networks are considered to be "broad scale" or not "scale free", which means that all network elements are not completely connected, but connectivity is constrained presumably by anatomical pathways and specific projections. Hub nodes, or "hubs", have a large number of connections and are critical for the function of these brain networks[11–13] but are not always found in other, nonneurological fields of study.[9]

Changes in network configuration have also been observed in aging, Alzheimer's disease, and schizophrenia by applying graph theory analysis to human-functional magnetic resonance imaging, EEG, and magnetoencephalographic data.[13,14] Graph theory analysis has been applied to specific brain regions, including the brainstem reticular formation,[15] which is discussed in more detail in Chapter 28. It is not clear if the changes that occur as a result of network expansion (Chapters 27 and 29) have been evaluated using this computational approach, but a broader scale and increase in connectivity would be expected for these network changes. In contrast, in degenerative disorders such as Parkinson's disease (Chapter 25) and stroke, which result in network disconnections, it is suggested there is a breakdown of small-world structure, and these networks may actually become more random.[16,17]

Complex network theory, combining graph theory and complex systems, has been advanced recently as a framework to interpret structure–function relationships in neuronal networks, particularly during development.[11,18] Hierarchical structure and function are also dealt with in the computational approach, and a few hierarchical studies have been performed using biological techniques. For example, a clear hierarchical process is seen in audiogenic seizure studies, which show dynamic changes in the hierarchy within a network, with dominance changes that occur during and potentially mediate the sequential behaviors that occur in this phenomenon (see Chapter 26).

Genetic studies are also important to the study of neuronal networks in several ways. Thus, genetic abnormalities are known to occur in CNS disorders, including channelopathies (disorders in the function of ion channels) and other protein mutations, which have emerged as important genetic causes of network malfunctions that lead to human and animal models of CNS disorders.[19] Such abnormal channels can also become targets for therapy of those disorders.[20,21] In addition, experimental genetic manipulation of various CNS proteins, using knock-in and knock-out strategies, is also widely used in network explorations to explore the role of a particular protein in control of a given network (e.g. Chapters 11, 14, 15, and 22). It must always be taken into account that compensation mechanisms for the deleted gene often develop, since the protein is missing during the animal's entire developmental period. The conditional knock-out technique, wherein the knock-out or mutation is induced in the genetically engineered organism only when a specific treatment of the animal is initiated, can be used to offset the issues associated with compensation. The conditional knock-out can be induced in a population of cells and at a defined point in time, allowing the modification to be restricted spatially and temporally and allowing only a specific nucleus in a network to display the genetic modification.[22] The knock-down technique involving the use of small interfering RNA is also used to silence their target genes through enzymatic cleavage of target mRNA. In addition, genetic manipulation is also used to explore networks using the technique of optogenetics (see Chapter 4).

NETWORK EXPLORATION PROCESS: AN OVERVIEW

Establishing the nature of neuronal networks has been a major area of neuroscience research in both animals and humans. Approaches based on specific electrographic oscillation frequency characteristics or imaging techniques are being used[23] (see Chapters 6 and 9). For example, specific patterns, such as the theta oscillations (4–11 Hz), can exert control on particular local networks in the hippocampus, while other local networks in the same structure do not show this effect, which was demonstrated by focal blockade studies[24] (see Chapter 4). Thus, oscillation and imaging studies need to be followed with specific intracranial approaches, including lesions and focal blockade of specific network sites if possible (see Chapter 4). Once a putative network is established, it is vital to probe the network to understand how it works. In addition, it must also be kept in mind that important neuronal network connectivity changes occur during development and maturation, which must be considered, depending on the age of the organism being evaluated[25] (see Chapter 11).

Brain disorders that involve changes in established networks need to be evaluated for pathophysiological mechanisms and to determine which specific brain structures are critical in mediating the disorder. Recording neuronal firing patterns in these sites (see Chapter 4) is vital to establish mechanisms that drive the function of the network and to establish the validity of the findings of the noninvasive network techniques mentioned here. This is important, since some disagreements between neuronal firing and the noninvasive techniques, such as imaging, have been shown to occur (see Chapter 6). The next step is to evaluate therapeutic measures, such as drugs or electrical stimulation (Chapters 31 and 32), to target specific sites within the network for treatment of brain disorders that may be due to network malfunctions. When drug administration and a network probe are combined, such an electrical or sensory stimulus can determine if a specific part of the network is critical to the therapeutic action of the drug at the dose that is effective in the disorder (Chapter 32). The issue of drug dosage is an extremely important factor, since supertherapeutic doses of a drug can exert actions on network sites that may not be relevant to the therapeutic action of the drug in the intact organism, but it is often overlooked. Thus, a number of the earlier studies on the mechanisms of action of the oldest drug known, ethanol, were done in in vitro studies with concentrations of ethanol that would be toxic to the intact organism.[26–28]

NEURONAL NETWORK VERSUS NEUROANATOMY

It is obvious that a neuronal network is based on the anatomical connections that exist between neurons within the nuclei of the network, which constitute the *structural* organizational element of the network. However, anatomical connectivity often does not accurately reflect functional involvement, and function can actually be subject to changes due to network intensification, expansion, or degeneration (Chapters 7, 25, and 27). In addition, anatomical connections can often be inhibitory, which could fine-tune, dampen, or disrupt network function. Even for sites with excitatory connections, the degree of activation of a neuron or group of neurons that is anatomically connected within a neuronal network is often variable, with few exceptions. In many brain sites, especially in conditional multireceptive (CMR) brain regions, neurons can undergo both positive and negative extremes of involvement in network function (see Chapter 28). Therefore, the neuronal components of the neuronal network that are active during the operation of the network constitute the *functional* organizational elements.[29] One of the major reasons for the variability of neuronal responses within a network nucleus is thought to be due to the fact that many synaptic events in neurons are subthreshold (see Chapter 28). However, when a perturbation due to external stimuli or changes in the internal milieu affects elements of the network, a certain number of these events can exceed threshold, leading to enlargement of the functionally active circuit[30] (see Chapter 27). This could also involve a loss of efficacy of inhibitory connections.[31] Occasionally, the activity of a critical mass of these neural elements reaches a threshold, causing dramatic changes and emergent properties of dormant or nascent networks[30] (see Chapters 28 and 30). Thus, the subthreshold nature of the interactions between many CNS neurons in a given network provides the basis for the *functional* connections between neurons within a network to change in strength such that latent pathways that are not normally active can become operative (see Chapter 28). An example of such a functional change is seen in the physiological control of sleep by the interaction of several brainstem nuclei (Chapter 21). Thus, for example, cholinergic neurons that are normally inactive during non–rapid eye movement (NREM) sleep can become very active when the inhibition mediated by serotonin and norepinephrine is reduced, which is associated with the onset of REM sleep (Chapter 21).

The network approach is based on the ubiquitous finding that neuronal connections are modifiable via both short- and long-term plasticity (Chapter 28). This modifiability introduces a degree of uncertainty into the process of network function, which makes exclusive reliance on commonly used reductionist approaches to brain research potentially problematic (see Chapter 5). Studying a single neuron or receptor system in ex vivo and in vitro conditions or under anesthesia isolates these neurons from many of their normal connections and in vivo influences, which can significantly modify the properties normally expressed in an intact brain. However, when isolated spinal cord neurons were placed in culture, they spontaneously formed networks that exhibited synchronized bursting, although the relationship of these networks to those spinal cord networks that occur in vivo has not been established.[32] Self-organization has also been observed recently in hippocampal cultures,[33] which exhibit the emergent functional properties of neuronal networks, as discussed in the "Emergent Properties" section.

EMERGENT PROPERTIES OF NEURONAL NETWORKS

The brain is estimated to contain 50–100 billion neurons and trillions of synapses, and in order to better understand the mechanisms of brain function in health and disease, nonlinear dynamical systems theory and its correlate, complexity theory, have been invoked.[30] In complexity theory, nonlinearity can lead to self-organization that results in a sudden and unpredictable spectrum of outputs,[29,34] and this leads to new and unexpected forms of organization called "emergent" properties. These emergent properties are not a priori predictable based on the properties of the individual elements. Emergent properties can result from a change in a host of elements within a network[30] or can involve the functional interaction of otherwise independent networks (see Chapter 30). The emergent properties that result can transcend the function of the networks that create them and be beneficial to the organism, as occurs in learning, or harmful to it, as seen in CNS disorders. Thus, emergent properties are network characteristics that are not originally predictably based on the properties of individual member neurons. However, once these emergent properties have been observed, they can become a relatively predictable property of the brain that expresses them. This allows identification of a consistent brain property that can become a potential target for therapy (see Chapter 32). Emergent properties are discussed in greater detail in Chapter 30. Approaches to simplify some of the complexity implicit in the emergent properties of networks in control of behaviors are the concepts of central program generators and cellular automata, which contain variable neuronal elements and exist to perform specific functions[35–38] (see Chapter 17). Larger networks are made up of several subnetworks, which can be viewed as a collection of interacting cellular automata.[39,40] Analysis of brain organization based on the modularity and hierarchical modularity of networks has been applied to human neuroimaging and EEG data to provide further insights into changes in function in normal and dysfunctional networks[41] (see Chapters 6 and 9). These types of simplification appear to be necessary to deal with the sheer volume of information about membrane properties and ligand- and voltage-gated channels that affect the multitude of neurons and their synaptic interactions within a network, which are discussed in the "Mechanisms" section.

MECHANISMS RESPONSIBLE FOR NETWORK CONTROL

A number of mechanisms are responsible for control of neuronal networks. The structural organization of a network is obviously based on the neuroanatomy of the pathway. As described in detail in many chapters of this book, the scope and function of a network can be controlled by the action of many elements (Table 1.2). These include neurophysiological mechanisms, such as burst firing (Chapter 9), which is a temporal firing pattern change that involves brief, recurring periods of rapid firing that is highly activating. The function of a network can also be controlled by the action of neuroactive agents, which are active via both synaptic transmission and volume transmission (Chapter 8). Endogenous neuroactive agents include monoamines, such as serotonin, which can activate inactive networks (see Chapter 7). Exogenous neuroactive agents, including drugs such as anesthetics and stimulants, can also exert profound effects on network function, which may actually be a critical mechanism for how the drugs act to exert their therapeutic effects (Chapter 32). The neuronal milieu, including levels of oxygen, can also alter network function significantly (see Chapter 10). Network connections, including interneurons, astrocytes, other nonneuronal cells, as well as external inputs, and the multiplicity of synaptic inputs can strongly modulate network function (see Chapters 7, 8, and 12). Cyclical conditions are often critical in network function on a short-term basis, such as circadian rhythms (Chapter 14) and sleep state (Chapter 21). These conditions can also exert long-term effects, contributing to synaptic plasticity changes and neurogenesis associated with learning and aging, as well as neuronal degeneration of CNS diseases, which are discussed in Chapters 7, 15, and 25. Some of these influences on neuronal network function are illustrated diagrammatically in Figure 1.2 and are listed in more detail in Table 1.2.

We have categorized these in vivo influences into five general categories—neuronal properties, neuroactive agents, neuronal milieu, network connections, and neuronal "life cycle" events (development and aging)—and they encompass 17 specific identified influences. It is important to note that when neurons from a network nucleus are isolated, using ex vivo or in vitro approaches, many of these influences are lost, which greatly modifies the properties of these neurons. For example, the high oxygen level commonly used in brain slice studies can actually cause hyperexcitability of neurons in the slice[42] (see Chapters 5 and 10).

Two major thrusts of this book are that knowledge of neuronal networks is extremely important to the therapy of CNS disorders and that emergent properties of elements within a network can be targets for drug action in the intact network (see Chapter 32). However, this site selectivity can be significantly altered in isolated elements of the network when studied using ex vivo and in vitro techniques (Chapter 5).

TABLE 1.2 Elements that Control Network Function and Interaction

1. Neuronal properties (Chapter 9)
   a. Burst firing
   b. Gap junctions
   c. Electrical field effects (ephaptic interactions)
2. Neuroactive agent (endogenous and exogenous, e.g. CNS drugs) (Chapters 7, 8, and 32)
   d. Excitatory or inhibitory
   e. Endogenous or exogenous
   f. Synaptic or volume transmission
   g. Tonic or phasic
3. Neuronal milieu (Chapter 10)
   h. Extracellular ions and gases (O_2)
   i. Temperature
   j. Buffering capacity (pH)
4. Network connections (Chapters 7, 12, 28, and 29)
   k. Interneuron activity
   l. Astrocytic integration
   m. External stimuli
   n. Multiplicity of synaptic inputs
5. Cyclic and "life cycle" events (Chapters 7, 11, 14–16, 21–23, and 25) (development, experience, degeneration, aging, and repair)
   o. Brain state (circadian, sleep, and coma)
   p. Synaptic plasticity (strength changes and synaptogenesis)
   q. Neurogenesis
   r. Neurodegeneration

NEUROPLASTICITY

One of the key elements that govern changes in brain function is the ability of the brain and behavior to undergo major degrees of plasticity, which can involve a number of short-term and long-term processes, including synaptogenesis and neurogenesis (see Chapters 7 and 16). Neuroplastic changes in brain function, whether beneficial or harmful, can take many forms (Chapter 28), and research on brain mechanisms for learning does often actually involve cross-network interactions (Chapter 13). Interaction among brain networks is also very common in other forms of neuroplasticity, including that seen in many CNS disorders (see Chapter 29). Long-lasting changes in the function of neuronal networks and even in their structure can take place as a result of single (or, more commonly, repetitive) experiences. Thus, behavioral-conditioning paradigms can produce long-lasting changes in the way neurons respond to stimuli in several parts of the brain. Thus, neurons that were minimally responsive to a stimulus before conditioning can become extensively responsive after the conditioning process[43–45] (see Chapter 28). Thus, behavioral-conditioning methods allowed the stimulus to expand the network membership to neurons that were connected to the circuit but not initially actively involved in the network. Neuroplasticity can also be associated with harmful outcomes for the

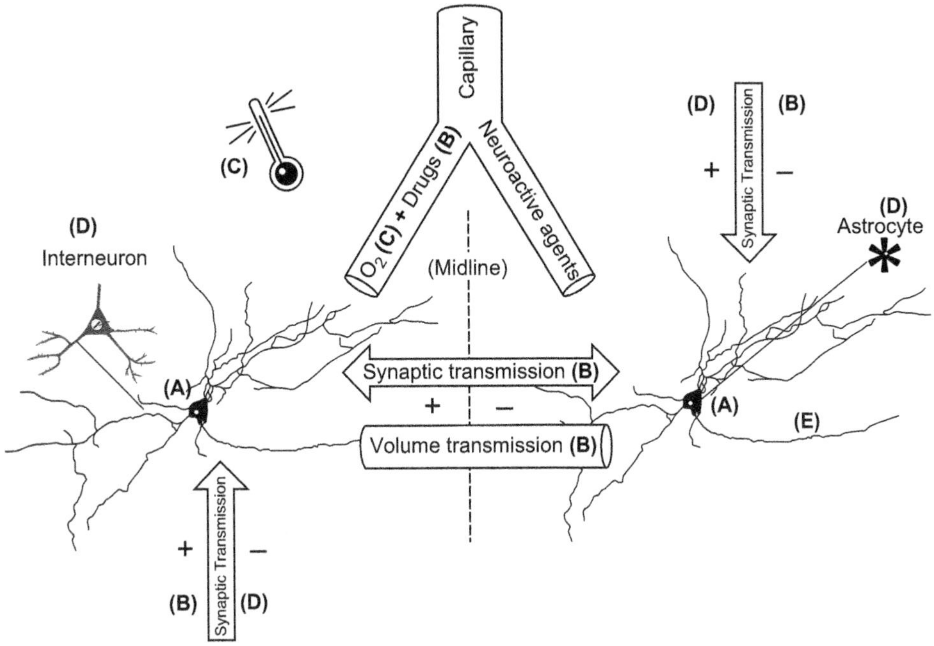

FIGURE 1.2 Diagram of a number of the types of influences that control network function. In this example, two neurons of a bilateral structure are shown, which are connected synaptically across the midline. The influences on these neurons include (A) neurophysiological mechanisms, such as ion channels, which mediate specific neuronal firing patterns, such as burst firing. The function of a network can also be controlled by (B) the action of neuroactive agents, which exert effects via both synaptic transmission and volume transmission (Chapter 8). Endogenous neuroactive agents include monoamines, which can activate inactive networks or direct excitatory transmitters, such as glutamate. Exogenous neuroactive agents delivered via capillaries and volume transmission, including drugs such as anesthetics and stimulants, can also exert profound effects on network function. (C) The neuronal milieu includes levels of oxygen and temperature, and it can also alter network function significantly. (D) Network connections include interneurons, astrocytes, external inputs, and the multiplicity of synaptic inputs. Other elements (E) include neuronal cyclical events, such as circadian rhythms and sleep states; synaptic plasticity; neurogenesis associated with learning and aging; and neuronal degeneration of certain CNS disorders. (For color version of this figure, the reader is referred to the online version of this book.)

organism. Thus, intense or repetitive occurrence of seizures can induce neurogenesis in susceptible brain sites, particularly in the hippocampus.[46–48] Such structural changes include mossy fiber reorganization, which may contribute to an increasing severity of seizures induced by seizure repetition.[49–51] The molecular effectors that contribute to neuroplasticity include brain-derived neurotrophic factor (BDNF), which has been implicated in mechanisms for network expansion in epilepsy induced by seizure repetition[52,53] (see Chapter 7).

EMERGENT PROPERTIES OF NETWORKS AS THERAPEUTIC TARGETS

As mentioned in this chapter, emergent properties of neuronal ensembles may be critically important to the function of neuronal networks. Various behaviors, including seizures, can be considered to be emergent properties at the macroscopic level. However, emergent network properties can occur based on the confluence of influences that impinge on neuronal ensembles in a specific network nucleus, as exemplified in Figure 1.2 (also see Chapter 30). We suggest that these emergent properties of neuronal networks in the brain may, in fact, be a critical therapeutic target on which neuroactive agents, including exogenously administered centrally acting drugs, exert their pharmacological effect[26] (see Chapter 32). Thus, CNS drug therapy is proposed to be directed at these emergent properties. This could involve an intensified reactivity of a specific intrinsic property of a particular type of neuron in a specific brain site and/or a compilation of all the actions exerted by the drug on various receptive elements (channels and receptors) within the affected network site(s) (Chapter 32). The data that are being generated on this issue suggest that the emergent properties that are critical to the expression of seizures can be the target of anticonvulsant drug action in epilepsy, as discussed in this section. When the cells in a well-defined invertebrate network were isolated in cell culture, a loss of emergent properties occurred, suggesting that most features of the functional network in vivo were determined primarily by interactions within the network.[54] Another example was observed in the mammalian brainstem network for respiration, where a particular ionic current (persistent sodium current) was thought to govern respiratory rhythm in a nucleus of this network.[55,56] However, a neuroactive agent (riluzole) that blocks this current did not alter respiratory-related motor output, suggesting that respiratory rhythm is an emergent property of the network.[57] Thalamic rhythmicity was once thought to be generated by the "pacemaker" properties of thalamic neurons, but this activity has also been found to be an emergent property of the thalamic relay-nucleus (reticularis) network. The network "controlled" by these neurons is activated and deactivated by the endogenous release of neuroactive substances.[58,59] Drug effects have helped to establish the function of specific network components in the overall function of the network by the use of *therapeutically effective* doses that selectively affect neurons in one nucleus of a network, while not affecting neurons elsewhere in the network (see Chapter 32). This approach can help determine the most sensitive therapeutic targets and lead to improvements in drug therapy. However, such drug effect data may suggest agents to avoid in certain CNS disorders. Finally, drugs including depressant and convulsant agents may be used as tools to probe networks and provide information on putative network control mechanisms (Chapters 28 and 32). Certain drugs that exert stimulatory effects on neurons have been shown to induce extensive short-term plastic neuronal response changes, particularly in areas of the brain that are highly changeable in their response patterns, which we have termed CMR brain regions (Chapter 28). Thus, dramatic increases of the sensory responses of CMR neurons were induced by administration of drugs that block inhibitory neurotransmission (see Chapter 28). Focal microinjection of excitatory substances into specific network nuclei can also lead to short-term or long-term changes in network function[60,61] (see Chapter 4). Neuronal network function is also greatly influenced by substances that inhibit neuronal firing, including general anesthetics, sedatives, and anticonvulsant drugs, which can potentially be useful in therapy of CNS disorders. However, network research done in the presence of these agents can totally alter network function and yield erroneous information (Chapters 28 and 32). Drugs used primarily in psychiatric disorders have also been shown to exert both short- and long-term effects on network function that may be very important to their therapeutic effects.[62,63] Nondrug therapeutic approaches, including electrical stimulation and acupuncture (Chapter 31), can also be useful in understanding networks and treating CNS disorders by modifying network function, and these effects may be critical to the therapeutic effects of these treatments.[64]

One of the main goals of this book is to advance the understanding of how the brain carries out important tasks by acting via neuronal networks, how these networks interact during normal brain functions, and how brain disorders can result from aberrant interactions between neuronal networks.[65] We provide evidence that illustrates how therapy of these disorders could be advanced through this network approach. We will emphasize that the interactions of different normal networks with one another facilitate major changes in brain function. One of the major principles of this interaction is that they commonly involve the considerable pool of CMR neurons in specific brain regions that receive major inputs from and project to many other networks. The brain regions that contain large populations of CMR neurons have the ability to undergo major functional changes that are mediated by long-term and/or short-term plasticity (Chapter 28) and result in major changes in brain function from learning to epilepsy. These regions may correspond to "hubs" uncovered through computational approaches, as discussed in this chapter. Only by understanding small and mesoscopic brain networks, using multidisciplinary approaches and techniques, can the common mechanisms of normal and abnormal brain function be better understood, leading to novel advances in uncovering basic brain mechanisms and improving the therapy of brain disorders.

This book is not intended to cover all the known normal networks, and there are many other brain networks for normal function as well as psychiatric and neurological disorders in addition to the ones included. However, to try to increase the coverage to these other networks would require a series of books. The chapter topics that are included in this volume often have a degree of data and conceptual overlap, because a chapter on a network for a specific function, such as respiration, must deal with the general concepts, such as emergent properties, which comprise the topic of another chapter. Likewise, the chapter on glial involvement in network control overlaps to some degree with the chapter on neuroactive substances, since astroglia (Chapter 12) play an important role in the uptake, release, and metabolism of many neuroactive substances (Chapter 7). The book is intended to be a snapshot and overview of the neuronal network field, including techniques, influences, and mechanisms that control network function. This volume includes specific sensory and motor networks and network interactions as well as network changes associated with learning and psychiatric and neurological disorders. The book also looks at the therapeutic implications of network function and how emergent properties of these disordered networks can be selective targets for therapeutic interventions. The reader may notice a certain amount of redundancy among the information covered in the different chapters, which was in some cases intentional. However, in other cases the redundancy is due to the fact that in such a broad undertaking, as this volume is, the editors needed to utilize their own experimental experiences to illustrate a number of general network issues.

Acknowledgments

The authors gratefully acknowledge support by NIH NINDS, CURE, and NIAAA during the experiments from our labs discussed in this chapter and the critical comments of Professor Walter J. Freeman, University of California, Berkeley. We also are grateful for the assistance of Gayle Stauffer in preparing this manuscript.

References

1. Melzack R, Wall PD. Pain mechanisms: a new theory. *Science.* 1965;150(3699):971–979.
2. Lockard JS, Ward AA. *Epilepsy: A Window to Brain Mechanisms.* New York: Raven Press; 1980.
3. Berger H. Elektrenkephalogramm des menschen. *Arch F Psychiat.* 1929;87:527–570.
4. Lennox WG, Lennox MA. *Epilepsy and Related Disorders.* Boston, MA: Little, Brown; 1960.
5. Reijneveld JC, Ponten SC, Berendse HW, Stam CJ. The application of graph theoretical analysis to complex networks in the brain. *Clin Neurophysiol.* 2007;118:2317–2331.
6. Faingold CL, Fromm GH. *Drugs for Control of Epilepsy: Actions on Neuronal Networks Involved in Seizure Disorders.* Boca Raton, FL: CRC Press; 1992.
7. Colder BW, Frysinger RC, Wilson CL, Harper RM, Engel Jr J. Decreased neuronal burst discharge near site of seizure onset in epileptic human temporal lobes. *Epilepsia.* 1996;37:113–121.
8. Truccolo W, Donoghue JA, Hochberg LR, et al. Single-neuron dynamics in human focal epilepsy. *Nat Neurosci.* 2011;14:635–641.
9. Bullmore E, Sporns O. Complex brain networks: graph theoretical analysis of structural and functional systems. *Nat Rev Neurosci.* 2009;10:186–198.
10. Watts DJ, Strogatz SH. Collective dynamics of 'small-world' networks. *Nature.* 1998;393(6684):440–442.
11. van den Heuvel MP, Stam CJ, Boersma M, Hulshoff Pol HE. Small-world and scale-free organization of voxel-based resting-state functional connectivity in the human brain. *Neuroimage.* 2008;43(3):528–539.
12. Salvador R, Suckling J, Schwarzbauer C, Bullmore E. Undirected graphs of frequency-dependent functional connectivity in whole brain networks. *Philos Trans R Soc Lond B Biol Sci.* 2005;360(1457):937–946.
13. Tomasi D, Volkow ND. Functional connectivity hubs in the human brain. *Neuroimage.* 2011;57:908–917.
14. Bassett DS, Bullmore ET. Human brain networks in health and disease. *Curr Opin Neurol.* 2009;22:340–347.
15. Humphries MD, Gurney K, Prescott TJ. The brainstem reticular formation is a small-world, not scale-free, network. *Proc Biol Sci.* 2006;273:503–511.
16. Nomura EM, Gratton C, Visser RM, Kayser A, Perez F, D'Esposito M. Double dissociation of two cognitive control networks in patients with focal brain lesions. *Proc Natl Acad Sci USA.* 2010;107:12017–12022.
17. Wu T, Wang L, Chen Y, Zhao C, Li K, Chan P. Changes of functional connectivity of the motor network in the resting state in Parkinson's disease. *Neurosci Lett.* 2009;460:6–10.
18. Feldt S, Bonifazi P, Cossart R. Dissecting functional connectivity of neuronal microcircuits: experimental and theoretical insights. *Trends Neurosci.* 2011;34:225–236.
19. Olivetti PR, Noebels JL. Interneuron, interrupted: molecular pathogenesis of ARX mutations and X-linked infantile spasms. *Curr Opin Neurobiol.* 2012;22(5):859–865.
20. Glasscock E, Yoo JW, Chen TT, Klassen TL, Noebels JL. Kv1.1 potassium channel deficiency reveals brain-driven cardiac dysfunction as a candidate mechanism for sudden unexplained death in epilepsy. *J Neurosci.* 2010;30(15):5167–5175.
21. Brenner R, Wilcox KS. Potassium channelopathies of epilepsy. In: Noebels JL, Avoli M, Rogawski MA, Olsen RW, Delgado-Escueta AV, eds. *Jasper's Basic Mechanisms of the Epilepsies [Internet].* 4th ed. Bethesda, MD: National Center for Biotechnology Information (US); 2012.
22. Morozov A, Kellendonk C, Simpson E, Tronche F. Using conditional mutagenesis to study the brain. *Biol Psychiatry.* 2003; 54(11):1125–1133.
23. Holscher C. Functional roles of Theta and Gamma oscillations in the association and dissociation of neuronal networks in primates and rodents. In: Holscher C, Munk M, eds. *Information Processing by Neuronal Populations.* Cambridge, UK: Cambridge University Press; 2008:151–173.
24. Koenig J, Linder AN, Leutgeb JK, Leutgeb S. The spatial periodicity of grid cells is not sustained during reduced theta oscillations. *Science.* 2011;332(6029):592–595.
25. Joseph JE, Swearingen JE, Clark JD, et al. The changing landscape of functional brain networks for face processing in typical development. *Neuroimage.* 2012;63:1223–1236.
26. Faingold CL. Emergent properties of CNS neuronal networks as targets for pharmacology: application to anticonvulsant drug action. *Prog Neurobiol.* 2004;72:55–85.
27. Faingold CL, N'Gouemo P, Riaz A. Ethanol and neurotransmitter interactions—from molecular to integrative effects. *Prog Neurobiol.* 1998;55:509–535.
28. Olsen RW, Hanchar HJ, Meera P, Wallner M. $GABA_A$ receptor subtypes: the "one glass of wine" receptors. *Alcohol.* 2007;41: 201–209.
29. Mikulecky DC. Complexity, communication between cells, and identifying the functional components of living systems: some observations. *Acta Biotheor.* 1996;44:179–208.
30. Freeman WJ, Kozma R, Werbos PJ. Biocomplexity: adaptive behavior in complex stochastic dynamical systems. *Biosystems.* 2001;59:109–123.
31. Vogels TP, Sprekeler H, Zenke F, Clopath C, Gerstner W. Inhibitory plasticity balances excitation and inhibition in sensory pathways and memory networks. *Science.* 2011;334(6062): 1569–1573.
32. Zhang HM, Robinson N, Gomez-Curet I, Wang W, Harrington MA. Neuronal and network activity in networks of cultured spinal motor neurons. *Neuroreport.* 2009;20:849–854.
33. Marconi E, Nieus T, Maccione A, et al. Emergent functional properties of neuronal networks with controlled topology. *PLoS One.* 2012;7(4):e34648. http://dx.doi.org/10.1371/journal.pone.0034648.
34. Reilly DL, Cooper LN. An overview of neuronal networks: early models to real world systems. In: Zorngetzer SF, Davis JL, Lau C, eds. *An Introduction to Neural and Electronic Networks.* San Diego: Academic Press; 1990:227–245.
35. Grillner S, Parker D, el Manira A. Vertebrate locomotion—a lamprey perspective. *Ann N Y Acad Sci.* 1998;860:1–18.
36. Grillner S, Markram H, De Schutter E, Silberberg G, LeBeau FE. Microcircuits in action—from CPGs to neocortex. *Trends Neurosci.* 2005;28:525–533.
37. Harris-Warrick RM. Neuromodulation and flexibility in Central Pattern Generator networks. *Curr Opin Neurobiol.* 2011;21:685–692.
38. Jordan LM. Initiation of locomotion in mammals. *Ann N Y Acad Sci.* 1998;860:83–93.

39. Manchanda K, Yadav AC, Ramaswamy R. Scaling behavior in probabilistic neuronal cellular automata. *Phys Rev E Stat Nonlin Soft Matter Phys*. 2013;87(1):012704.
40. Traub RD, Schmitz D, Jefferys JG, Draguhn A. High-frequency population oscillations are predicted to occur in hippocampal pyramidal neuronal networks interconnected by axoaxonal gap junctions. *Neuroscience*. 1999;92:407–426.
41. Meunier D, Lambiotte R, Bullmore ET. Modular and hierarchically modular organization of brain networks. *Front Neurosci*. 2010;4:200.
42. Garcia III AJ, Putnam RW, Dean JB. Hyperbaric hyperoxia and normobaric reoxygenation increase excitability and activate oxygen-induced potentiation in CA1 hippocampal neurons. *J Appl Physiol*. 2010;109:804–819.
43. Freeman JH, Steinmetz AB. Neural circuitry and plasticity mechanisms underlying delay eyeblink conditioning. *Learn Mem*. 2011;18:666–677.
44. Woody CD, Zotova E, Gruen E. Multiple representations of information in the primary auditory cortex of cats. I. Stability and change in slow components of unit activity after conditioning with a click conditioned stimulus. *Brain Res*. 2000;868:56–65.
45. Zellner MR, Ranaldi R. How conditioned stimuli acquire the ability to activate VTA dopamine cells: a proposed neurobiological component of reward-related learning. *Neurosci Biobehav Rev*. 2010;34:769–780.
46. Kuruba R, Hattiangady B, Shetty AK. Hippocampal neurogenesis and neural stem cells in temporal lobe epilepsy. *Epilepsy Behav*. 2009;14:65–73.
47. Parent JM, Murphy GG. Mechanisms and functional significance of aberrant seizure-induced hippocampal neurogenesis. *Epilepsia*. 2008;49:19–25.
48. Schneider-Mizell CM, Parent JM, Ben-Jacob E, Zochowski MR, Sander LM. From network structure to network reorganization: implications for adult neurogenesis. *Phys Biol*. 2010;7:046008.
49. Dudek FE, Sutula TP. Epileptogenesis in the dentate gyrus: a critical perspective. *Prog Brain Res*. 2007;163:755–773.
50. Lynch M, Sutula T. Recurrent excitatory connectivity in the dentate gyrus of kindled and kainic acid-treated rats. *J Neurophysiol*. 2000;83:693–704.
51. Rakhade SN, Jensen FE. Epileptogenesis in the immature brain: emerging mechanisms. *Nat Rev Neurol*. 2009;5:380–391.
52. McNamara JO, Scharfman HE. Temporal lobe epilepsy and the BDNF receptor, TrkB. In: Noebels JL, Avoid M, Rogawski MA, Olsen RW, Delgado-Escueta AV, eds. *Jasper's Basic Mechanisms of the Epilepsies (Internet)*. 4th ed. Bethesda: National Center for Biotechnology Information (US); 2012.
53. Simonato M, Zucchini S. Are the neurotrophic factors a suitable therapeutic target for the prevention of epileptogenesis? *Epilepsia*. 2010;51:48–51.
54. Straub VA, Staras K, Kemenes G, Benjamin PR. Endogenous and network properties of lymnaea feeding central pattern generator interneurons. *J Neurophysiol*. 2002;88:1569–1583.
55. Onimaru H, Homma I. A novel functional neuron group for respiratory rhythm generation in the ventral medulla. *J Neurosci*. 2003;23:1478–1486.
56. Ramirez JM, Zuperku EJ, Alheid GF, Lieske SP, Ptak K, McCrimmon DR. Respiratory rhythm generation: converging concepts from in vitro and in vivo approaches? *Respir Physiol Neurobiol*. 2002;131:43–56.
57. Del Negro CA, Morgado-Valle C, Feldman JL. Respiratory rhythm: an emergent network property? *Neuron*. 2002;34: 821–830.
58. Beenhakker MP, Huguenard JR. Neurons that fire together also conspire together: is normal sleep circuitry hijacked to generate epilepsy? *Neuron*. 2009;62:612–632.
59. Buzsaki G. The thalamic clock: emergent network properties. *Neuroscience*. 1991;41:351–364.
60. Raisinghani M, Feng H-J, Faingold CL. Glutamatergic activation of the amygdala differentially mimics the effects of audiogenic seizure kindling in two sub-strains of genetically epilepsy-prone rats. *Exp Neurol*. 2003;183:516–522.
61. Tupal S, Faingold CL. Inhibition of adenylyl cyclase in amygdale blocks the effect of audiogenic seizure kindling in genetically epilepsy-prone rats. *Neuropharmacology*. 2010;59:107–111.
62. Hanson ND, Owens MJ, Nemeroff CB. Depression, antidepressants, and neurogenesis: a critical reappraisal. *Neuropsychopharmacology*. 2011;36:2589–2602.
63. Samuels BA, Hen R. Neurogenesis and affective disorders. *Eur J Neurosci*. 2011;33:1152–1159.
64. Faingold CL. Electrical stimulation therapies for CNS disorders and pain are mediated by competition between different neuronal networks in the brain. *Med Hypotheses*. 2008;71: 668–681.
65. Shew WL, Yang H, Yu S, Roy R, Plenz D. Information capacity and transmission are maximized in balanced cortical networks with neuronal avalanches. *J Neurosci*. 2011;31:55–63.

CHAPTER

2

Network Models of Absence Seizures

Alain Destexhe

Unité de Neurosciences, Information et Complexité (UNIC), Centre National de la Recherche Scientifique (CNRS), France

INTRODUCTION

Absence epilepsy is a very common disorder in young children and consists of seizures that are characterized by the sudden onset of ~3 Hz large-amplitude oscillations in the electroencephalogram (EEG) (Figure 2.1). These generalized seizures terminate as suddenly as they appear, and brain activity almost immediately reverts back to normal activity. The typical pattern of the oscillation consists of one or several sharp deflections ("spikes") followed by a surface-positive "wave". Spike-and-wave patterns of similar characteristics are also seen in a number of experimental models in cats, rats, mice, and monkeys, as well as in many other types of epilepsies.

Similar to other pathologies, absence epilepsy can result from the disturbance of mechanisms of synaptic transmission (reviewed in Refs. 1,2). In particular, disturbing inhibitory interactions have been found to be extremely effective for generating seizures, sometimes with contrasting effects (reviewed in Ref. 3). In the thalamus and cortex, inhibitory transmission essentially uses γ-aminobutyric acid (GABA) as a transmitter, and operates through two main receptor types, called $GABA_A$ and $GABA_B$. These two receptors mediate fast and slow inhibition, respectively. Both types of receptor are of primary importance in seizure mechanisms, as overviewed in detail here.

In this chapter, we review experimental evidence for a respective thalamic and cortical contribution to the genesis of absence seizures (in the "Experimental Characterization" section), and how computational models can be used to test mechanisms and formulate possible explanations for the sometimes contrasting experimental results. We first consider thalamic networks and how they can generate hypersynchronized oscillations at ~3 Hz (in the "Network Models of Thalamic Hypersynchronized Oscillations" section), then how cortical networks can generate spike-and-wave patterns (in the "Network Models of Cortical Spike-and-Wave Seizures" section), and, finally, we review how thalamocortical networks can display generalized spike-and-wave seizures under certain conditions (in the "Network Model of ~3 Hz Spike-and-Wave Oscillations in the Thalamocortical System" section). In the "Intact Thalamic Circuits can be Forced into ~3 Hz Oscillations" section, we will show that computational models predicted that a key ingredient in seizure generation is the effect of the feedback connections from cortex to thalamus. We will review experiments that successfully tested this corticothalamic feedback mechanism for absence seizure generation (in the "Testing the Predictions of the Models" section). We terminate with a summary of possible mechanisms to account for why seizures occur at ~3 Hz in cats, monkeys, and humans, but at 5–10 Hz in rodents.

EXPERIMENTAL CHARACTERIZATION OF GENERALIZED SPIKE-AND-WAVE SEIZURES

Experimental Evidence for Thalamic Participation in Absence Seizures

As suggested more than 60 years ago,[5] the thalamus is a possible source of generalized seizures because of its central position and the fact that it projects widely to all of the cerebral cortex. This "centrencephalic" view is now supported by several findings. (1) Simultaneous thalamic and cortical recordings in humans during absence seizures demonstrated a clear thalamic participation during the seizure.[6] The same study also showed that the oscillations usually started in the thalamus before signs of seizure appeared in the EEG. (2) A

Neuronal Networks in Brain Function, CNS Disorders, and Therapeutics
http://dx.doi.org/10.1016/B978-0-12-415804-7.00002-2

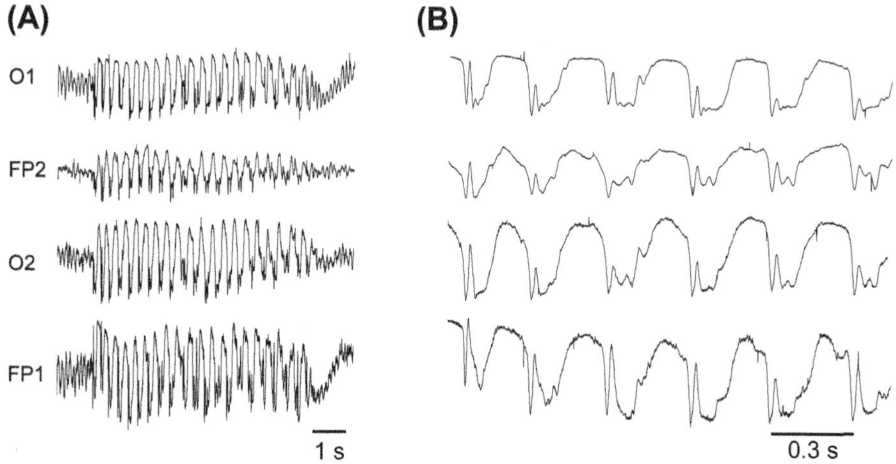

FIGURE 2.1 Electroencephalogram (EEG) recording during an absence seizure in a human subject. (A) Absence seizure in different EEG leads; FP1 and FP2 measure the potential difference between the frontal and parietal regions of the scalp, whereas O1 and O2 correspond to the measures between occipital regions. The seizure lasted approximately 5 s and consisted of an oscillation at around ~3 Hz, which appeared nearly simultaneously in all EEG leads. (B) Same seizure at higher temporal resolution, which reveals the "spike-and-wave" patterns during each cycle of the oscillation. *Modified from Ref. 4.*

thalamic participation in human absence seizures was also shown by positron emission tomography (PET).[7] (3) In some experimental models, spike-and-wave seizures disappear following thalamic lesions or by inactivating the thalamus.[8–10] (4) Electrophysiological recordings in experimental models of spike-and-wave seizures show that cortical and thalamic cells fire prolonged discharges in phase with the "spike" component, while the "wave" is characterized by a silence in all cell types.[11–20] Electrophysiological recordings also indicate that spindle oscillations, which are generated by thalamic circuits,[21,22] can be gradually transformed into spike-and-wave discharges, and all manipulations that promote or antagonize spindles have the same effect on spike-and-wave seizures.[15,23,24]

More recent investigations have shed light into the ionic channels implicated in seizure generation in the thalamus. Knockout mice lacking the gene for the T-type calcium current in thalamic relay cells display a resistance to absence seizures,[25] which strongly suggests that the T-type current, which mediates bursting in thalamic cells, is involved in this type of seizure activity. Pharmacological manipulations suggest that some synaptic receptor types are also involved in thalamic hypersynchronized oscillations, and in particular the $GABA_B$ receptors. In rats, $GABA_B$ agonists exacerbate seizures, while $GABA_B$ antagonists suppress them.[26–29] More specifically, antagonizing thalamic $GABA_B$ receptors leads to the suppression of spike-and-wave discharges,[30] which is another indication for a critical role of the thalamus.

The two thalamic cell types mainly involved in generating oscillations are the thalamocortical (TC) cells, also called relay cells, and the inhibitory neurons of the thalamic reticular (RE) nucleus. In some area of the thalamus and in some species, RE cells provide the sole source of inhibition to relay cells. The connections from RE to TC cells contain both $GABA_A$ and $GABA_B$ receptors, and there is evidence that $GABA_B$ receptors are critical to generate hypersynchronized oscillations. In particular, clonazepam, a known anti-absence drug ($GABA_A$ antagonist), was shown to indirectly diminish $GABA_B$-mediated inhibitory postsynaptic potentials (IPSPs) in TC cells, reducing their tendency to burst in synchrony.[31,32] The action of clonazepam appears to reinforce $GABA_A$ receptors within the RE nucleus.[31,33] Indeed, there is a diminished frequency of seizures following reinforcement of $GABA_A$ receptors in the RE nucleus.[34]

Further evidence for the involvement of the thalamus was that in ferret thalamic slices, spindle oscillations can be transformed into slower and more synchronized oscillations at ~3 Hz following blockade of $GABA_A$ receptors (Figure 2.2; and see Ref. 35). This behavior is similar to the transformation of spindles to spike-and-wave discharges in cats following the systemic administration of penicillin, which acts as a weak $GABA_A$ receptor antagonist.[23,24] Moreover, like spike-and-wave seizures in rats, the ~3 Hz paroxysmal oscillations in thalamic slices are suppressed by $GABA_B$ receptor antagonists (Figure 2.2; and see Ref. 35).

Taken together, these experiments suggest that thalamic neurons are actively involved in the genesis of spike-and-wave seizures, and that both $GABA_A$ and $GABA_B$ receptors play a critical role. It is important to note, however, that although such results clearly suggest

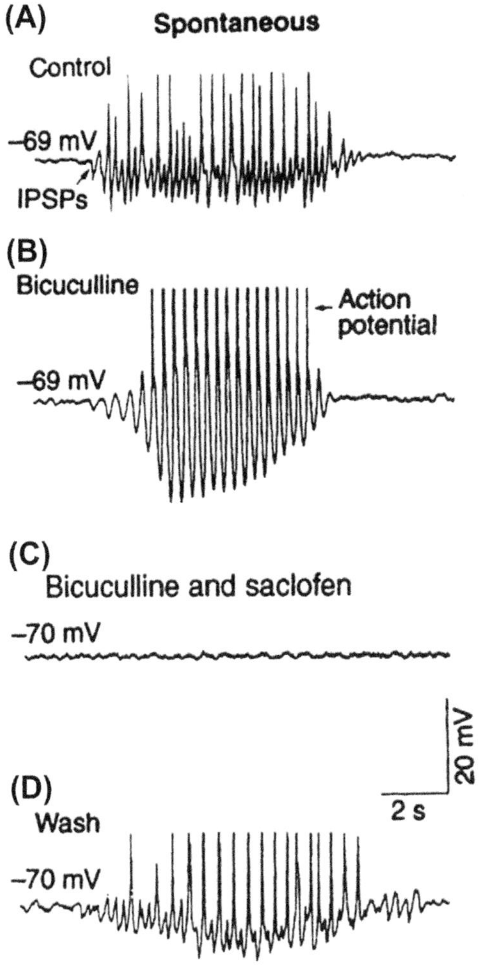

FIGURE 2.2 Bicuculline-induced 3 Hz oscillation in thalamic slices. (A) Control spindle sequence (~10 Hz) started spontaneously by an IPSP (arrow). (B) Slow oscillation (~3 Hz) following block of $GABA_A$ receptors by bicuculline. (C) Suppression of the slow oscillation in the presence of the $GABA_B$ antagonist baclofen. (D) Recovery after wash. *Modified from Ref. 35.*

that the thalamus is important in seizure generation, there is also considerable evidence that the cortex plays a primary role, as reviewed in the "Experimental Evidence for a Decisive Role of the Cerebral Cortex in Spike-and-Wave Generation" section.

Experimental Evidence for a Decisive Role of the Cerebral Cortex in Spike-and-Wave Generation

A number of experiments demonstrated that the thalamus is necessary, but not sufficient, to explain spike-and-wave seizures, and that the cortex plays a key role. Thalamic injections of high doses of $GABA_A$ antagonists, such as penicillin[36,37] or bicuculline,[38] led to 3–4 Hz oscillations with no sign of spike-and-wave discharge. This suggests that the action of these drugs may explain the slow oscillation frequency, but it is insufficient to explain the full spike-and-wave patterns expressed during seizures. In contrast, injection of the same drugs to the cortex, with no change in the thalamus, resulted in seizure activity with spike-and-wave patterns.[37–39] In addition, the threshold for epileptogenesis was much lower in the cortex compared to the thalamus.[38] Finally, it was shown that a diffuse application of a dilute solution of penicillin to the cortex resulted in spike-and-wave seizures, although the thalamus was intact.[37]

As we have seen, spike-and-wave seizures disappear following thalamic lesions or by inactivating the thalamus.[8–10] In some experiments, however, a purely cortical spike-and-wave activity was observed in the isolated cortex or athalamic preparations in cats.[8,38,40] These experiments revealed a slow type of spike-and-wave activity (1–2 Hz), with a less prominent "spike" component. In contrast, such intracortical spike-and-wave activity does not occur in rats[10] and has never been reported in neocortical slices. Nevertheless, the experiments in cats show that at least some cortical structures are capable of endogenously generating spike-and-wave activity, and further confirm the importance of the cortex in generating seizures, although the typical spike-and-wave patterns of generalized seizures require both cortex and thalamus.

In addition, it was shown more recently that absence seizures in rats seem to start in a focus located in the somatosensory cortex,[41] again suggesting a cortical origin. The same study[41] also demonstrated that interhemispheric synchrony is larger than intrahemispheric synchrony during the seizure, which would argue for an important role of callosal fibers in the synchrony and generalized aspects of the seizure.

Intracortically generated spike-and-wave seizures were described experimentally in cats under barbiturate anesthesia using multisite field potential recordings[38,42] (see the scheme in Figure 2.3(A)). In control conditions, the local field potentials (LFPs) displayed 7–14 Hz spindle oscillations, typical of barbiturate anesthesia (Figure 2.3(B)). After application of the $GABA_A$ antagonist bicuculline to the cortex, this activity developed into seizures with spike-and-wave complexes, at a frequency of 2–4 Hz (Figure 2.3(C)). Experiments were also realized in athalamic cats, where a complete thalamectomy was performed (histological controls are described in Ref. 38). Similar to above, the application of bicuculline to the cerebral cortex after thalamectomy led to the development of seizures with spike-and-wave patterns (Figure 2.3(D)). In this case, however, the morphology of the spike–wave complexes was different as the negative "spike" was less pronounced (compare (C) and (D) in Figure 2.3) and the oscillation frequency was slower (about 1.8 Hz in Figure 2.3(D); range 1.8–2.5 Hz).

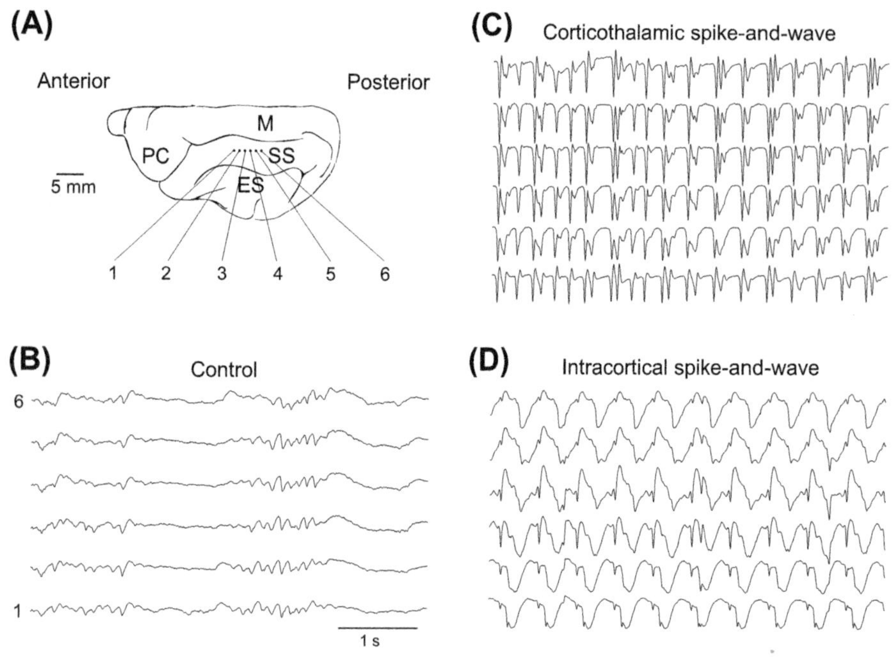

FIGURE 2.3 Multisite field potential recordings in cat suprasylvian cortex. (A) Scheme illustrating the disposition of recording electrodes (SS: suprasylvian gyrus; PC: postcruciate gyrus; ES: ectosylvian gyrus; and M: marginal gyrus). (B) "Control" spindle oscillations during barbiturate anesthesia. (C) Spike-and-wave paroxysms in the same animal after injection of bicuculline in the cortex (between electrodes 3 and 4). (D) Spike-and-wave oscillation in the same brain area after a complete thalamectomy (different animal as in (A)–(B)). *Modified from Ref. 42.*

Experimental Evidence for Thalamocortical Mechanisms in Spike-and-Wave Seizures

We have seen in the "Experimental Evidence for Thalamic Participation in Absence Seizures" section that thalamic circuits can generate hypersynchronized oscillations at Hz, resembling the typical oscillation frequency during absence seizures. However, there is ample evidence that the thalamus is not sufficient to explain seizure generation. $GABA_A$-receptor antagonists induce spike-and-wave seizures when applied to the cerebral cortex,[37–39] while they fail to generate such paroxysms when injected to the thalamus.[36–38] A majority of thalamic neurons are steadily hyperpolarized and completely silent during cortical seizures.[43–45] Finally, seizure activity can be observed in the cortex following thalamic inactivation or thalamectomy.[8,38,40] Several features of such intracortical seizures can be accounted for by computational models[42] (see the "Network Models of Cortical Spike-and-Wave Seizures" section).

Although such data may suggest that seizures could be generated intracortically, the thalamus appears to be necessary, as reviewed in the "Experimental Evidence for Thalamic Participation in Absence Seizures" section. The main argument is that spike-and-wave seizures disappear following thalamic lesions or by inactivating the thalamus.[8–10] Blocking thalamic $GABA_B$ receptors also leads to the suppression of spike-and-wave seizures.[30] Finally, it was shown that a diffuse application of a dilute solution of penicillin to the cortex resulted in spike-and-wave seizures, although the thalamus needed to be intact.[37]

In conclusion, the experiments clearly point to key roles of both the thalamus and cerebral cortex in generating seizures. The thalamus can generate ~3 Hz hypersynchronized oscillations, while the cortex can generate a form of spike-and-wave seizure. In the cat feline generalized penicillin epilepsy (FGPE) model, a diffuse increase of cortical excitability was shown to be sufficient to generate seizures, but an intact thalamus was necessary. These experiments raised the important question of how an excitable cortex connected to an intact thalamus could generate 3 Hz spike-and-wave oscillations. To attempt to answer this question, we consider in the "Network Models" section computational models in three steps: thalamic models, cortical models, and the fully connected thalamocortical network.

NETWORK MODELS OF SPIKE-AND-WAVE SEIZURES

In the "Experimental Characterization" section, we reviewed data suggesting that *both* the cortex and thalamus are necessary for absence seizures (reviewed in Ref. 1,46). In this section, we review computational models that addressed mechanisms for seizure generation based on thalamocortical loops, where the thalamus acts as the generator of the ~3 Hz oscillation (or 5–10 Hz in rodents) while the cortex generates the spike-and-wave patterns.[47,48] We will show that a single mechanism can be consistent with all of the experiments reviewed in the "Experimental Characterization" section (for details, see Refs 49–51).

A General Introduction to Biophysical Network Models

Which Type of Modeling Approach should be Used to Model Epilepsy?

As shown in this chapter, and as reviewed previously,[49,52,53] the genesis of epileptic behavior depends on a number of brain structures, such as the cortex and the thalamus, their interconnectivity, and a number of important biophysical properties. For example, it is important to take into account the intrinsic neuronal properties such as the bursting behavior of thalamic neurons to account for the genesis of oscillations—this behavior requires modeling the appropriate ionic conductances in thalamic cells.[52] Another factor that is of primary importance is the type of postsynaptic receptor present in the circuits, taking into account the correct time course of receptors such as the glutamate α-amino-3-hydroxy-5-methyl-4-isoxazolepropionic acid (AMPA) and N-methyl-D-aspartate (NMDA) receptors, or the $GABA_A$ and $GABA_B$ receptors, which have been found to mediate synaptic transmission at most synapses in the thalamocortical system.[54] The data reviewed in this chapter emphasize the important role of $GABA_A$ and $GABA_B$ receptors to explain epileptic discharges in various places in the thalamocortical network and in different preparations. It is therefore important to accurately model the activation of these receptors to account for the basic features of epileptogenesis.

In agreement with this, several modeling studies (reviewed in Refs 49,52) demonstrated that modeling the correct frequency of oscillations, the correct phase relations between cells, and their main intracellular features requires precisely modeling the ionic conductances implicated. This precise modeling should capture the kinetics and activation properties of the corresponding ionic channels, and this task can be quite challenging in some cases.

In the present work, we review a particular class of models where the main concern is to model precisely the dynamics of ionic channels and conductances, the cellular intrinsic properties, as well as the different types of postsynaptic receptors present in the circuits. These so-called *biophysical models* are based on a formalism close to that originally developed by Hodgkin and Huxley[55] to model the genesis of action potentials. It is interesting to see that more than 60 years later, this formalism is still heavily used today.

General Structure of the Models

In all models reviewed in this chapter, the neurons were described by the generic membrane equation:

$$C_m \frac{dV}{dt} = -g_L(V_i - E_L) - \sum_j I_{int}^{ji} - \sum_k I_{syn}^{ki} \tag{2.1}$$

where V_i is the membrane potential, $C_m = 1\ \mu F/cm^2$ is the specific capacity of the membrane, g_L (in mS/cm^2) is the leakage conductance density, and E_L (in mV) is the leakage reversal potential. Intrinsic and synaptic currents are, respectively, represented by I_{int}^{ji} and I_{syn}^{ki}(in $\mu A/cm^2$).

Intrinsic voltage-dependent or calcium-dependent currents were modeled using kinetic models of the Hodgkin–Huxley[55] type. These intrinsic membrane currents were described by the following generic equation:

$$I_{int} = \bar{g}_{int} m^N h^M (V - E_{int}) \tag{2.2}$$

$$\frac{dm}{dt} = \alpha_m(1 - m) - \beta_m m \tag{2.3}$$

$$\frac{dh}{dt} = \alpha_h(1 - h) - \beta_h h \tag{2.4}$$

where I_{int} is the intrinsic membrane current, $\bar{g}_{int}$ (in mS/cm^2) is the maximal conductance density, and E_{int} is the reversal potential. The gating properties of the current depend on N activation gates and M inactivation gates, with m and h representing the fraction of gates in open form, with respective rate constants α_m, β_m, α_h, and β_h. Rate constants were dependent on either membrane voltage (V) or intracellular calcium concentration.

Synaptic interactions were mediated by glutamatergic and GABAergic receptors using kinetic models of postsynaptic receptors.[56,57]

$$I_{syn} = \bar{g}_{syn} m (V - E_{syn}) \tag{2.5}$$

$$\frac{dm}{dt} = \alpha[T](1 - m) - \beta_m \tag{2.6}$$

where I_{syn} is the postsynaptic current, $\bar{g}_{syn}$ is the maximal conductance, m is the fraction of open receptors, E_{syn} is the reversal potential, $[T]$ is the transmitter concentration in the cleft, and α and β are forward and backward binding rate constants of T to open the receptors. This scheme was used to simulate AMPA, NMDA, and $GABA_A$ types of receptors (see Ref. 57 for parameters).

Network Models of Thalamic Hypersynchronized Oscillations

Early Models

The introduction of an experimental model for thalamic oscillations in ferret thalamic slices demonstrated the spontaneous occurrence of spindle oscillations.[35] It was also demonstrated that spindles can be transformed into ~3 Hz oscillations by blocking $GABA_A$ receptors (Figure 2.2). It was further shown that this oscillation is sensitive to blockade of $GABA_B$ receptors by saclofen (Figure 2.2) and is also suppressed by glutamate AMPA receptor antagonists.[35] These in vitro experiments thus suggested that ~3 Hz paroxysmal thalamic oscillations are mediated by a reciprocal interaction between TC and RE cells, with $GABA_B$ IPSPs (RE→TC) and AMPA excitatory postsynaptic potentials (EPSPs) (TC→RE).

This mechanism was first investigated with computational models using a simple TC–RE circuit consisting of a single TC cell reciprocally connected to a single RE cell.[58] In this model, the intrinsic firing behavior of the TC cell was determined by I_T and I_h; these currents were modeled using the Hodgkin–Huxley[55] type of models based on voltage-clamp data in TC cells. Calcium regulation of I_h accounted for the waxing and waning of oscillations, as described in Ref. 59. The intrinsic firing properties of the RE cell were determined by I_T, $I_{K[Ca]}$, and I_{CAN} using Hodgkin–Huxley-type[55] kinetics and calcium-activated schemes, as described in Ref. 60. The two cell types also included the fast I_{Na} and I_{Kd} currents necessary to generate action potentials, with kinetics taken from Ref. 61.

A simple circuit of interconnected TC and RE cells endowed with such properties displayed waxing-and-waning spindle oscillations at a frequency of 8–10 Hz.[58] The circuit also displayed a transformation to ~3 Hz oscillations when the kinetics of the GABAergic current were slowed.[58] The decay of inhibition greatly affected the frequency of the spindle oscillations, with slow decay corresponding to low frequencies. When the decay was adjusted to match experimental recordings of $GABA_B$-mediated currents (obtained from Ref. 62), the circuit oscillated at around 3 Hz.[58]

Although this simple model could simulate the essential features of the slow thalamic oscillation, it was not satisfactory because the slowing down of GABA currents from a 10 to 200 ms decay time constant is not plausible biophysically. Therefore, more realistic mechanisms must be considered for the transformation of normal spindles to slow hypersynchronized oscillations. It is also critical to correctly capture this mechanism to explain the emergence of pathologies such as absence seizures.

Model Prediction of Cooperative $GABA_B$ Responses

To explain this transformation to hypersynchrony, computational models made an essential prediction: it is necessary that the $GABA_B$ responses are strongly nonlinear, or "cooperative". A detailed biophysical modeling of synaptic transmission on GABAergic receptors[63] explored the idea that single-synapse postsynaptic mechanisms could explain the nonlinear stimulus dependence observed for $GABA_B$ responses. We hypothesized that this nonlinearity arises from the transduction mechanisms underlying $GABA_B$ responses, in particular at the level of the activation of K^+ channels by G-proteins. The assumption that K^+ channels must bind to four G-proteins to open provides the nonlinearity required to account for $GABA_B$ responses[63]; this is consistent with the tetrameric structure of K^+ channels.[64] With these assumptions, the $GABA_B$ model reproduced the typical nonlinearity of $GABA_B$ responses: intense release conditions (such as high-frequency bursts) are necessary to activate significant $GABA_B$ currents. This effect arises locally at the synapse and should be detectable using dual recordings, a prediction that was later confirmed experimentally.[65,66]

The activation properties of $GABA_B$ receptors were based on the following steps (Figure 2.4(A)): (1) the binding of GABA on the $GABA_B$ receptor, leading to an activated receptor; (2) the activated $GABA_B$ receptor catalyzes the activation of G-proteins in the intracellular side; and (3) the binding of activated G-proteins to open a K^+ channel. These steps are described by the following equations:

$$I_{GABA_B} = \bar{g}_{GABA_B} \frac{s^n}{s^n + K_d}(V - E_K) \tag{2.7}$$

$$\frac{dr}{dt} = K_1[T](1 - r) - K_2 r \tag{2.8}$$

$$\frac{ds}{dt} = K_3 r - K_4 s \tag{2.9}$$

where $[T]$ is the GABA concentration in the synaptic cleft, r is the fraction of $GABA_B$ receptors in the activated form, s is the normalized G-protein concentration in activated form, $\bar{g}_{GABA_B}$ is the maximal postsynaptic conductance of K^+ channels, K_d is the dissociation constant of G-protein binding on K^+ channels, V is the postsynaptic membrane potential, and E_K is the equilibrium potential for K^+. Fitting of this model to experimental $GABA_B$ responses led to the following values of parameters[57]: $K_d = 100$, $K_1 = 9 \times 10^4\ M^{-1}\ s^{-1}$, $K_2 = 1.2\ s^{-1}$, $K_3 = 180\ s^{-1}$, and $K_4 = 34\ s^{-1}$, with $n = 4$ binding sites.

This mechanism constitutes the basis of the nonlinear behavior of $GABA_B$-mediated responses. A single presynaptic spike induced relatively low amplitudes of

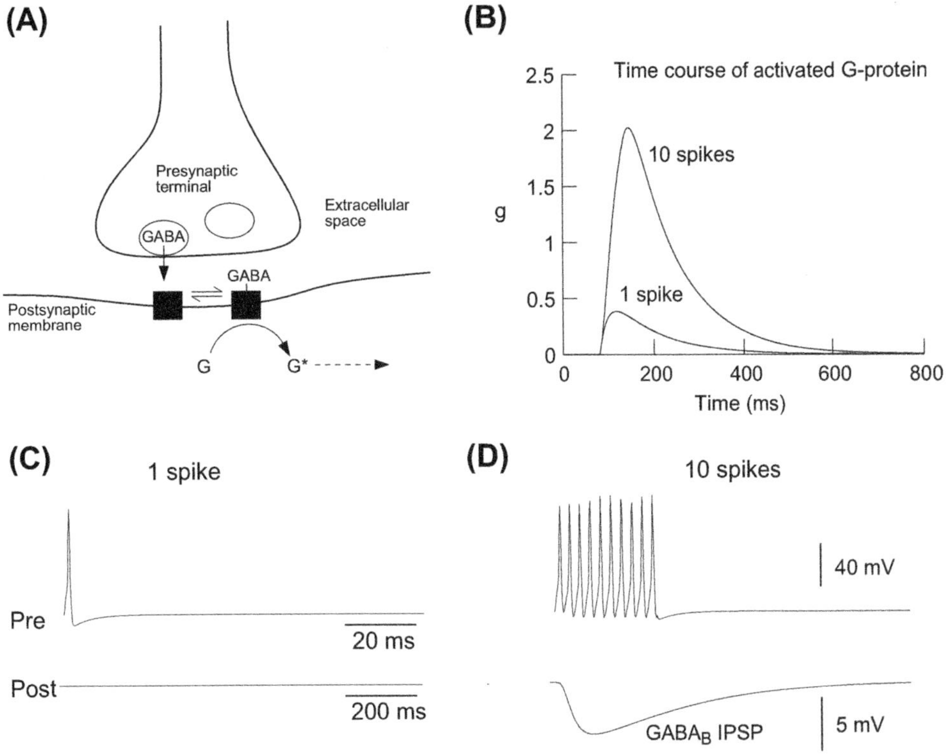

FIGURE 2.4 Modeling nonlinear GABA$_B$-mediated responses. (A) Scheme of the release of GABA, activation of the receptor by binding of GABA, and catalysis of G-proteins into activated form (G*) by the bound receptor. Subsequently, activated G-proteins may affect the gating of ion channels and participate in other biochemical mechanisms, or be degraded into an inactive form (dashed arrow). To yield responses in agreement with experiments, the binding of four G-proteins was needed to activate the K^+ channels.[63] (B) Typical slow time course of G-protein concentration following one or 10 presynaptic spikes at 200 Hz. (C) Simulation of GABA$_B$-mediated responses with a single presynaptic spike. No detectable GABA$_B$ IPSP is observed. (D) Same simulation as in (C), but with 10 presynaptic spikes at high frequency. In this case, the stimulus recruited a strong GABA$_B$-mediated IPSP. (A)–(B) modified from Thomson and Destexhe (1998). (C)–(D) modified from Ref. 47. *Model from Ref. 63.*

G-protein (Figure 2.4(B)), and no GABA$_B$-mediated IPSP in the postsynaptic cell (Figure 2.4(C)). In contrast, a burst of high-frequency spikes evoked a strong GABA$_B$-mediated IPSP (Figure 2.4(D)). The main hypothesis of this model is that the typical nonlinearity observed in GABA$_B$ responses is explainable by transduction kinetics at the level of a single GABAergic synapse (for details, see Ref. 63). We will see in the "Network Models of Cortical Spike-and-Wave Seizures" section that this property enables one to explain several important experimental observations relevant to absence seizures.

Cooperative GABA$_B$ Responses Can Explain the Effect of Clonazepam in the Thalamus

As a first step toward explaining the genesis of hypersynchronized oscillations, the cooperative model of GABA$_B$ responses was checked in the context of the effect of the anti-absence drug clonazepam. Experiments showed that clonazepam reduces GABA$_B$-mediated IPSPs in TC cells,[31,32] but the action of clonazepam was not on TC cells, but was to reinforce GABA$_A$ receptors in the RE nucleus.[31] To explain this effect, we constructed a circuit comprising model RE cells, including a low-threshold calcium current and lateral GABA$_A$-mediated synaptic interactions within the RE nucleus.[63] Under normal conditions, stimulation in the RE nucleus evoked biphasic IPSPs in TC cells, with a rather small GABA$_B$ component. We mimicked an increase of intensity by increasing the number of RE cells discharging. The ratio between GABA$_A$ and GABA$_B$ IPSPs was independent of the intensity of stimulation in the model,[63] as observed experimentally.[67] However, this ratio could be changed by blocking GABA$_A$ receptors locally in the RE nucleus, leading to enhanced burst discharge in RE cells and a more prominent GABA$_B$ component in TC cells. This is consistent with the effect of clonazepam in reinforcing the GABA$_A$ IPSPs in the RE nucleus, resulting in diminished GABA$_B$ IPSPs in TC cells.[31] The reduction of the GABA$_B$ component was a direct consequence of the cooperativity of GABA$_B$ responses.

Cooperative $GABA_B$ Responses Can Explain the Genesis of Thalamic Hypersynchronized Oscillations

This cooperative model of $GABA_B$ responses was integrated in a circuit comprising TC and RE cells and the different receptor types mediating their interactions ($GABA_A$ and $GABA_B$ receptors from RE to TC, and AMPA receptors from TC to RE; see the scheme in Figure 2.5).[68] In control conditions (Figure 2.5(A)), the circuit generated spindle oscillations with characteristics consistent with electrophysiological recordings. Suppression of $GABA_A$ receptors led to slower oscillations (Figure 2.5(B)). These oscillations were a consequence of the properties of $GABA_B$ responses as described in Figure 2.4. Following removal of $GABA_A$-mediated inhibition, the RE cells could produce prolonged bursts that evoked strong $GABA_B$ currents in TC cells. These prolonged IPSPs evoked robust rebound bursts in TC cells, and TC bursts in turn elicited bursting in RE cells through EPSPs. These mutual TC–RE interactions recruited the system into a 3–4 Hz oscillation, with characteristics similar to those of bicuculline-induced paroxysmal oscillations in ferret thalamic slices. The mechanisms responsible for these oscillations were similar to those that give rise to normal spindle oscillations, but the shift in the balance of inhibition leads to

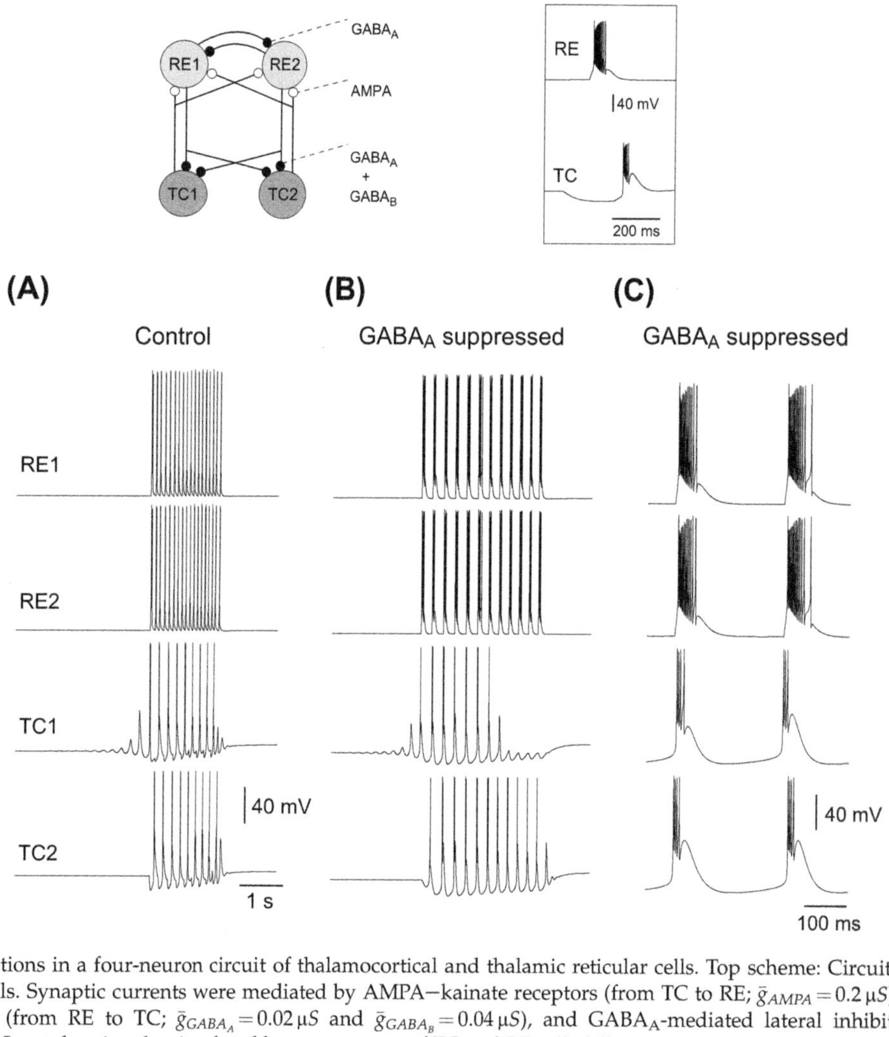

FIGURE 2.5 Oscillations in a four-neuron circuit of thalamocortical and thalamic reticular cells. Top scheme: Circuit diagram consisting of two TC and two RE cells. Synaptic currents were mediated by AMPA–kainate receptors (from TC to RE; $\bar{g}_{AMPA} = 0.2\,\mu S$), a mixture of $GABA_A$ and $GABA_B$ receptors (from RE to TC; $\bar{g}_{GABA_A} = 0.02\,\mu S$ and $\bar{g}_{GABA_B} = 0.04\,\mu S$), and $GABA_A$-mediated lateral inhibition between RE cells ($\bar{g}_{GABA_A} = 0.2\,\mu S$). Right: Inset showing the simulated burst responses of TC and RE cells following current injection (pulse of 0.3 nA during 10 ms for RE and −0.1 nA during 200 ms for TC). (A) Spindle oscillations arose as the first TC cell (TC1) started to oscillate, recruiting the two RE cells, which in turn recruited the second TC cell. The oscillation was maintained for a few cycles and repeated with silent periods of 15–25 s. (B) Slow 3–4 Hz oscillation obtained when $GABA_A$ receptors were suppressed, mimicking the effect of bicuculline. The first TC cell (TC1) started to oscillate, recruiting the two RE cells, which in turn recruited the second TC cell. The mechanism of recruitment between cells was identical to spindle oscillations, but the oscillations were more synchronized, were of slower frequency, and had a 15% longer silent period. The burst discharges were prolonged due to the loss of lateral inhibition in the RE. (C) Magnification of one cycle of the oscillation from B, showing the high synchrony of the slow oscillation. *Modified from Ref. 68.*

oscillations that were slower and more synchronized (Figure 2.5(C); see details in Ref. 68).

Other mechanisms have been proposed to account for the effects of blocking of $GABA_A$ receptors in thalamic circuits.[69–71] The model of Ref. 69 tested the proposition that disinhibition of interneurons projecting to TC cells with $GABA_B$ receptors may result in stronger discharges when $GABA_A$ receptors are antagonized.[72] A model including TC, RE, and interneurons[69] reproduced the stronger discharges in TC cells following application of bicuculline. Although it is possible that this mechanism plays a role in thalamically generated epileptic discharges, it does not account for experiments showing the decisive influence of the RE nucleus in preparations devoid of interneurons (in this case, the sole source of inhibition is the RE nucleus; see Refs 31,67). Increased synchrony and stronger discharges were also reported in the model of Ref. 70, but the synchronous state coexisted with a desynchronized state of the network, which has never been observed experimentally. The cooperative activation proposed for $GABA_B$ receptors[63] produced robust synchronized oscillations and traveling waves at the network level,[68,71] similar to those observed in thalamic slices.[73] This property also led to the transformation of spindles to ~3 Hz paroxysmal oscillations following block of $GABA_A$ receptors.[68] The latter study remains so far the only one consistent with the largest body of experimental data, including the effect of clonazepam, the characteristic nonlinearity of $GABA_B$ responses, and network effects such as traveling oscillations.

In conclusion, biophysical models incorporating the known intrinsic properties of thalamic neurons, together with the properties of their receptor types, account for the genesis of hypersynchronized oscillations. Several ingredients are essential to this mechanism. First, the presence of lateral inhibitory ($GABA_A$-mediated) connections in the RE nucleus normally prevents RE cells from producing excessive burst discharges. Diminishing the efficacy of these connections enables RE cells to produce prolonged bursts. Second, due to the nonlinear properties of $GABA_B$ responses discussed in this chapter, significant $GABA_B$-mediated IPSPs are seen only when presynaptic cells produce prolonged discharges. Therefore, if for some reason (e.g. diminishing the efficacy of $GABA_A$ receptors) RE burst discharges become stronger, they activate significant $GABA_B$-mediated responses in TC cells and entrain the entire thalamic circuits into slow synchronized oscillations. The $GABA_A$-mediated interactions between RE cells therefore act as a powerful means of avoiding hypersynchrony.[74,75]

Network Models of Cortical Spike-and-Wave Seizures

Model of Cooperative $GABA_B$ Responses Can Explain the Genesis of Spike-and-Wave Patterns in LFPs

As a necessary step to studying the genesis of spike-and-wave patterns, one must determine the conditions of activity to generate the typical "spike" and "wave" patterns in LFPs. To this end, a single-compartment model was simulated with postsynaptic currents generated by 100 excitatory synapses (AMPA and NMDA receptors) and 100 inhibitory synapses ($GABA_A$ and $GABA_B$ receptors; see the scheme in Figure 2.6(A)). Extracellular field potentials were calculated from postsynaptic currents in single-compartment models, according to a simple model essentially based on Coulomb's law (see Ref. 76):

$$V_{ext} = \frac{R_e}{4\pi} \sum_j \frac{I_j}{r_j} \tag{2.10}$$

where V_{ext} is the electrical potential at a given extracellular site, $R_e = 230\ \Omega\text{cm}$ is the extracellular resistivity, I_j are the total membrane currents (spikes excluded) and r_j is the distance between the site of generation of I_j and the extracellular site.

The field potentials generated by this model for different stimulus conditions are shown in Figure 2.6(B)–(C). With presynaptic trains consisting of single spikes, the voltage showed mixed EPSP–IPSP sequences and the field potential was dominated by negative deflections (Figure 2.6(B)). In contrast, bursts of high-frequency presynaptic spikes produced mixed EPSPs and IPSPs followed by large $GABA_B$-mediated IPSPs in the cell (Figure 2.6(C)). In the latter case, the fast EPSPs and IPSPs generated spiky field potentials, followed by a slow positive wave due to $GABA_B$ currents (intrinsic slow K^+-mediated conductances responsible for spike-frequency adaptation also contributed to the "wave"). This simple model shows that synchronous high-frequency discharges of excitatory and inhibitory cells in the presence of $GABA_B$ receptors are sufficient to generate field potential waveforms resembling interleaved "spikes" and "waves".

Thus, this simple model shows that the hypersynchronized release of excitatory and inhibitory synapses, every 300 ms, is sufficient to explain the spike-and-wave patterns, where the "wave" is due to the activation of slow K^+ conductances due to $GABA_B$ receptors and voltage-dependent currents. Whichever of these two contributions dominates will depend on their relative conductance.

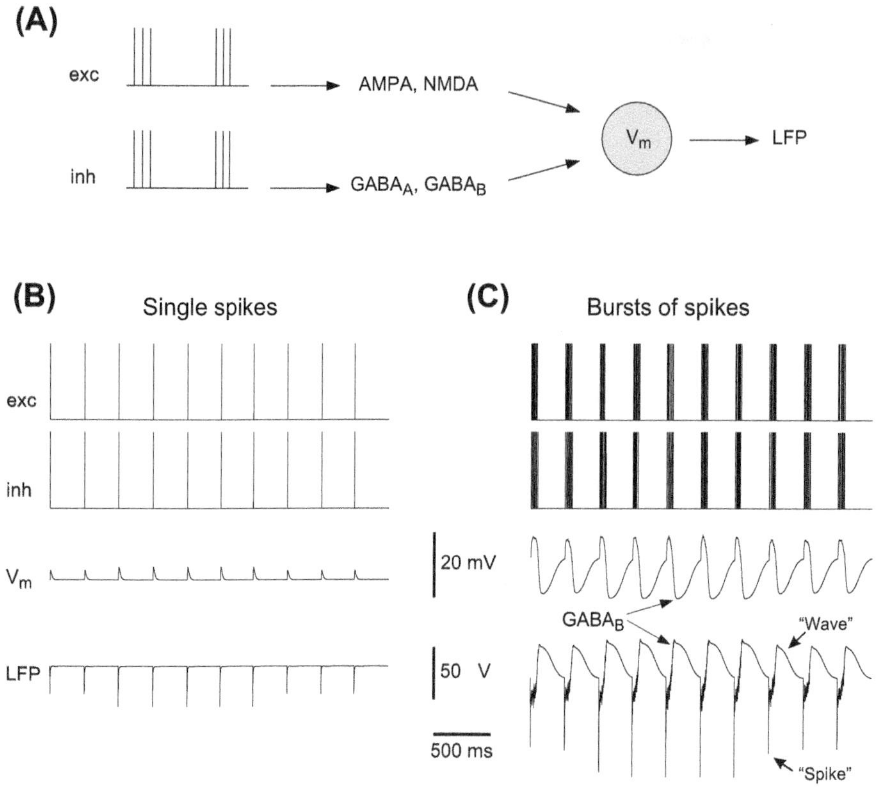

FIGURE 2.6 Simulation of spike-and-wave field potentials based on the properties of $GABA_B$ receptors. (A) Scheme for the model of local field potentials. Excitatory and inhibitory presynaptic trains of action potentials stimulated AMPA, NMDA, $GABA_A$, and $GABA_B$ postsynaptic receptors at 100 synapses of each type on a single compartment model, and they were used to calculate the extracellular field potential at a distance of 5 μm from the simulated neuron. (B) Field potentials generated by single presynaptic spikes. The mixed EPSP–IPSP sequence in the cell led to negative deflections in the field potentials (bottom trace). (C) Same simulation as in (B), but using bursts of presynaptic spikes. In this case, fast spiky components ("spikes") alternate with slow positive deflections ("waves"), similar to spike-and-wave patterns. These slow positive waves were due to the activation of $GABA_B$-mediated currents (arrows). Conductance values were 4 nS, 1 nS, 1.5 nS, and 4 nS for individual AMPA, NMDA, $GABA_A$, and $GABA_B$ synapses, respectively. *Modified from Ref. 47.*

Network Models of Intracortically Generated Spike-and-Wave Oscillations

In a second step, we consider network models of the cerebral cortex and determine how to generate spike-and-wave LFPs from network activity.

A network model was built, and the main hypothesis explored was that the rebound bursting properties observed in a subset of cortical cells, combined with $GABA_B$ IPSPs, could generate this intracortical form of spike-and-wave seizures.[42] In vivo intracellular recordings were performed in the same area of neocortex from which the intracortical seizures were recorded. Low-threshold spike (LTS) activity was observed in a significant fraction (about 10%) of intracellularly recorded cells.[42] These LTS neurons generate adapting trains of action potentials in response to depolarizing current injection, similar to the classic "regular-spiking" response of cortical neurons (as in Ref. 77). In addition, they can generate a burst of action potentials in response to injection of hyperpolarizing current pulses.[42] This property was also identified in deep layers of guinea pig cerebral cortex in vitro[78] and was shown to be due to the presence of the T-type (low-threshold) calcium current I_T.

Models could reproduce these intrinsic firing properties based on single-compartment representations of pyramidal neurons. To generate the classic "regular-spiking" behavior, the model included three voltage-dependent currents represented by Hodgkin–Huxley-type[55] kinetics: a slow voltage-dependent K^+ current termed I_M (kinetics from Ref. 79), as well as the I_{Na} and I_K currents for action potential generation (kinetics from Ref. 61). In addition, to generate rebound bursting behavior, the T-type calcium current was included (kinetics from Ref. 80), and its peak amplitude was adjusted to match voltage-clamp recordings of this current in pyramidal neurons.[78] A density of T-channels of 0.8 mS/cm^2 was needed to match the relatively small amplitude of this current measured in pyramidal neurons. Note that the peak amplitude of I_T in pyramidal neurons (0.4–0.8 nA in guinea pig cerebral cortex[78]) is much smaller than in TC neurons (5.8 ± 1.7 nA[80]). Using this relatively moderate T-current density, the model generated weak rebound bursts at the offset of hyperpolarizing current. From hyperpolarized levels, this model generated an initial burst followed by an adapting train of action potentials, which is a feature commonly observed in neocortical neurons.[77]

These cell types were included in a network model to investigate the genesis of cortical spike-and-wave seizures. The network consisted of excitatory (pyramidal) neurons and interneurons, whose connectivity was mediated by AMPA, $GABA_A$, and $GABA_B$ receptors (Figure 2.7(A)). In control conditions, no oscillatory behavior could be observed if a significant proportion of pyramidal neurons (up to 20%) had LTS properties similar to experimental observations.[42] This is due to the fact that in control conditions, all cells in the network generate brief discharge patterns, which lead to the activation of IPSPs that are dominated by the $GABA_A$ component, with negligible $GABA_B$ activation. Because of the relatively weak conductance of I_T in LTS cortical cells, $GABA_A$-mediated IPSPs were not sufficient to activate any rebound burst in these neurons.

In contrast, when $GABA_B$-mediated inhibition was suppressed, mimicking the effect of bicuculline, the disinhibited network generated self-sustained oscillations (Figure 2.7(B)). Due to the removal of fast inhibition, all cells in the network produced prolonged discharge patterns. The prolonged discharge of interneurons was optimal to activate $GABA_B$-mediated inhibition in pyramidal cells, in agreement with the highly nonlinear activation properties of these receptors (see the "Model Prediction of Cooperative $GABA_B$ Responses" section). If the $GABA_B$ conductance was sufficiently large (0.05–0.1 μS), $GABA_B$-mediated IPSPs could activate a

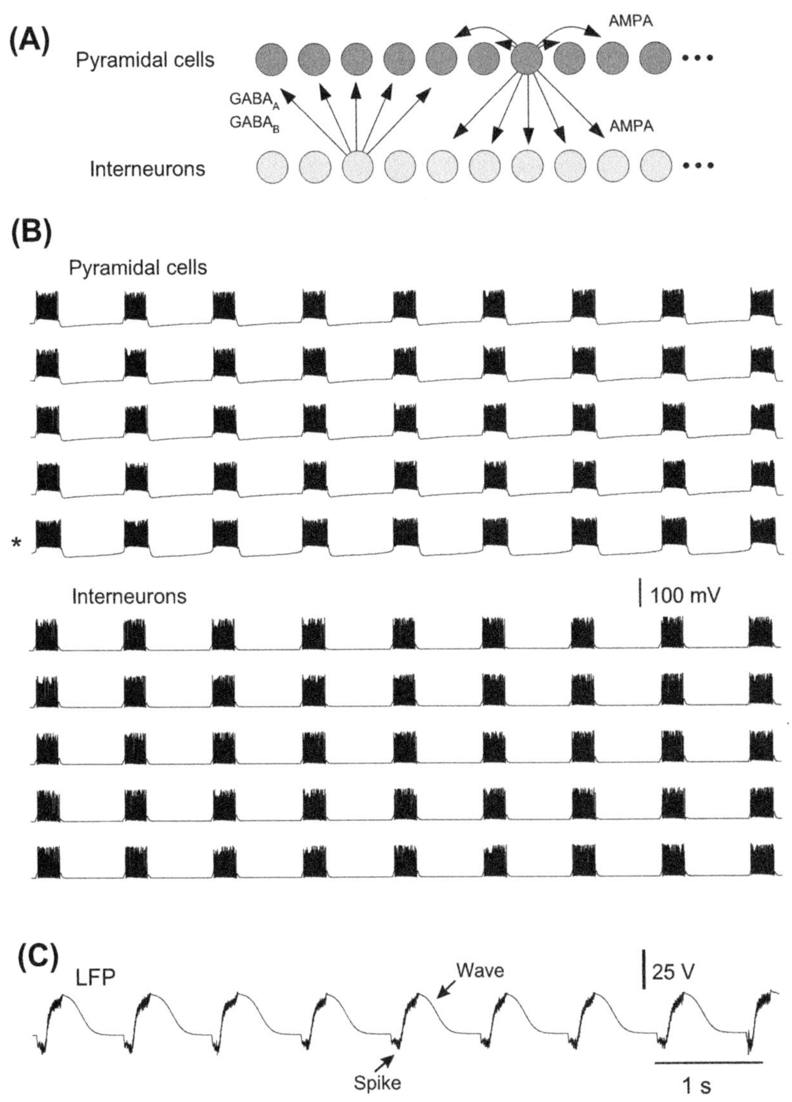

FIGURE 2.7 Simulation of intracortically generated spike-and-wave oscillations. (A) Scheme of the network: All pyramidal cells had I_{Na}, I_K, and I_M currents, and 5% of pyramidal neurons were rebound bursting cells containing an additional weak density of T-current (model taken from Ref. 42). (B) Oscillatory activity after removing $GABA_A$ connections. All cells displayed prolonged discharges in phase, separated by periods of silence dominated by K^+ currents, at a frequency of ~1.3 Hz. * indicates a rebound bursting pyramidal cell. No thalamic cells were included in this simulation. (C) Field potentials calculated from the same simulation showed spike-and-wave complexes. *Modified from Ref. 42.*

rebound burst in the pyramidal neurons that contained I_T, similar to experiments with current injection.[42] The oscillation therefore consisted of $GABA_B$ IPSP-rebound sequences, in which the rebound of the entire network was triggered by a minority of pyramidal neurons containing I_T. A small proportion of LTS pyramidal cells (as small as 5%, depending on the connectivity used) was sufficient to generate slow oscillations in the disinhibited network.

In calculated extracellular field potentials, this slow oscillation generated spike-and-wave patterns. Similar to what was discussed in the "Model of Cooperative $GABA_B$ Responses" section, the synchronized discharge of all cells in the network generated a negative "spike" component (Figure 2.7(C)). The subsequent activation of $GABA_B$ IPSPs induced a period of silence in the network, during which pyramidal neurons were hyperpolarized by K^+ currents (a mixture of $GABA_B$-mediated IPSPs and voltage-dependent K^+ currents). These outward currents generated a slow positive "wave" in the field potentials (Figure 2.7(C)). Therefore, the disinhibited cortical network can generate a form of spike-and-wave oscillation on its own.

Similar findings were also reported in a model of cortex consisting of interconnected pyramidal neurons and interneurons.[81] This model included an I_h current in pyramidal neurons and the elevated extracellular K^+ concentration in the epileptic focus, leading to particularly strong rebound properties of I_h-containing pyramidal neurons, entraining the network in slow hypersynchronized oscillations.

As a conclusion to this section, we presented a network model of cerebral cortical neurons that can generate a form of spike-and-wave activity whose mechanisms are based on the following sequence of events: (1) due to suppressed $GABA_A$-mediated inhibition, the disinhibited cortical network generated prolonged discharges. These events generated a negative "spike" in simulated field potentials. (2) Due to the prolonged firing of interneurons, powerful $GABA_B$-mediated IPSPs hyperpolarized pyramidal cells, stopping their discharge. These slow IPSPs, as well as other slow K^+ currents maximally activated due to the prolonged firing, generated a slow positive "wave" in field potentials. (3) At the offset of $GABA_B$ IPSPs, a fraction of pyramidal cells generated a rebound burst, entraining the entire network in prolonged discharges and restarting the oscillation cycle.

Thus, we see that some form of spike-and-wave activity, with a relatively slow frequency, can be generated autonomously by cortical circuits. How to reconcile this type of activity with the thalamic synchronized oscillation, and build a unified model, is examined in the "Network Model of ~3 Hz Spike-and-Wave Oscillations" section.

Network Model of ~3 Hz Spike-and-Wave Oscillations in the Thalamocortical System

As we have seen in this chapter, experiments point to a thalamocortical mechanism where seizures are due to an augmented cortical excitability but an intact thalamus is necessary. To understand such a mechanism, we proceed here in two steps. We first show how an excessive corticothalamic feedback can change the frequency and synchrony of oscillations in the thalamus. Second, we integrate these properties in a full thalamocortical network model and investigate how it can generate spike-and-wave seizures.

Intact Thalamic Circuits can be Forced into ~3 Hz Oscillations Due to $GABA_B$ Receptor Cooperativity

To understand these thalamocortical interactions, the first question to be addressed is how thalamic circuits are controlled by the cortex. Thalamic networks have a propensity to generate oscillations on their own, such as the 7–14 Hz spindle oscillations.[22,35] Although these oscillations are generated in the thalamus, the neocortex can trigger them,[82–84] and, more generally, corticothalamic feedback exerts a decisive control over thalamic oscillations.[85]

To reproduce these observations, computational models made a strong prediction: the cortical action on the thalamus needed to be inhibitory on thalamic relay cells.[86] Because corticothalamic synapses are excitatory, the only way to obtain a net inhibitory action is with very strong corticothalamic excitation on RE cells, which mediate strong feedforward IPSPs onto TC cells. This "dominant inhibition" in thalamic relay cells was indeed observed experimentally in many instances.[87–89] It was later shown experimentally that, indeed, the quantal conductance of cortical EPSPs is about twice as large in RE neurons compared to TC cells (266 ± 48 pS versus 103 ± 25 pS, respectively; see Ref. 90). Moreover, RE cells are exquisitely sensitive to cortical EPSPs (see Ref. 91 for experiments and Refs 92,93 for models), probably due to powerful T-current in their dendrites.[94] In addition, cortical synapses contact only the distal dendrites of TC cells[95] and are likely to be further attenuated for this reason. Taken together, these data suggest that corticothalamic feedback operates mainly by eliciting bursts in RE cells, which in turn evoke powerful IPSPs on TC cells that largely overwhelm the direct cortical EPSPs.

This "dominant inhibition" effect of the corticothalamic feedback on the thalamic circuit was investigated with the thalamic model (Figure 2.8; and see Ref. 47). Simulated cortical EPSPs evoked bursts in RE cells (Figure 2.8(B), arrow), which recruited TC cells through IPSPs, and triggered a ~10 Hz oscillation in the circuit.

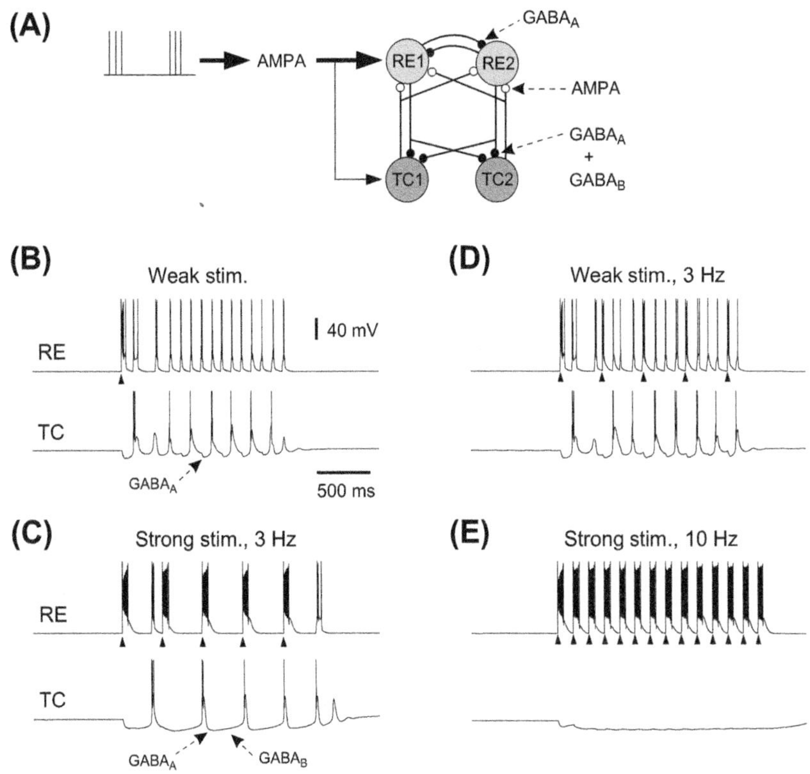

FIGURE 2.8 Corticothalamic feedback can force thalamic circuits into ~3 Hz oscillations due to the properties of $GABA_B$ receptors. (A) Connectivity and receptor types in a circuit of thalamocortical (TC) and thalamic reticular (RE) neurons. Corticothalamic feedback was simulated through AMPA-mediated synaptic inputs (shown on the left of the connectivity diagram; total conductance of 1.2 μS to RE cells and 0.01 μS to TC cells). (B) A single stimulation of corticothalamic feedback (arrow) entrained the circuit into a 10 Hz mode similar to spindle oscillations. (C) With a strong-intensity stimulation at ~3 Hz (arrows; 14 spikes per stimulus), RE cells were recruited into large bursts, which evoked IPSPs onto TC cells dominated by $GABA_B$-mediated inhibition. In this case, the circuit could be entrained into a different oscillatory mode, with all cells firing in synchrony. (D) Weak stimulation at ~3 Hz (arrows) entrained the circuit into spindle oscillations (identical intensity as in B). (E) Strong stimulation at 10 Hz (arrows) led to quiescent TC cells due to sustained $GABA_B$ current (identical intensity as in C). *Modified from Ref. 47.*

During the oscillation, TC cells rebound once every two cycles following $GABA_A$-mediated IPSPs, and RE cells discharged only a few spikes, evoking $GABA_A$-mediated IPSPs in TC cells with no significant $GABA_B$ currents (Figure 2.8(B)). These features are typical of spindle oscillations.[22,35]

The most interesting observation was that a different type of oscillatory behavior could be elicited from the circuit by repetitive stimulation at ~3 Hz with high intensity (14 spikes every 333 ms; Figure 2.8(C)). All cell types were entrained to discharge in synchrony at Hz. In other words, *strong cortical stimulation can switch intact thalamic circuits to oscillate at ~3 Hz.*[47] If the stimulation is at low intensity, it produces spindle oscillations (Figure 2.8(D)) similar to those seen in Figure 2.8(A). High-intensity stimulation at 10 Hz led to quiescence in TC cells (Figure 2.8(E)) due to sustained $GABA_B$ currents, similar to findings in a previous analysis (see Figure 2.12 in Ref. 44).

By which mechanisms can strong corticothalamic feedback at ~3 Hz force thalamic circuits in a ~3 Hz oscillation? Cortical EPSPs force RE cells to fire large bursts (Figure 2.8(C), arrows), fulfilling the conditions needed to activate $GABA_B$ responses. The consequence was that TC cells were "clamped" at hyperpolarized levels by $GABA_B$ IPSPs during ~300 ms before they could rebound. The nonlinear properties of $GABA_B$ responses are therefore responsible here for the coexistence between two types of oscillations in the same circuit: moderate corticothalamic feedback recruited the circuit in ~10 Hz spindle oscillations, while strong feedback could force the intact circuit at a ~3 Hz frequency due to the nonlinear activation properties of intrathalamic $GABA_B$ responses.

This finding—or prediction—that *intact* thalamic circuits can be forced into a hypersynchronized ~3 Hz mode is fundamental to explain spike-and-wave seizures, as explained in the "Full Thalamocortical Network Model of ~3 Hz Spike-and-Wave Oscillations" section.

Full Thalamocortical Network Model of ~3 Hz Spike-and-Wave Oscillations

All of the ingredients described in this chapter were assembled into a thalamocortical network model. The model consists of different layers of cortical and

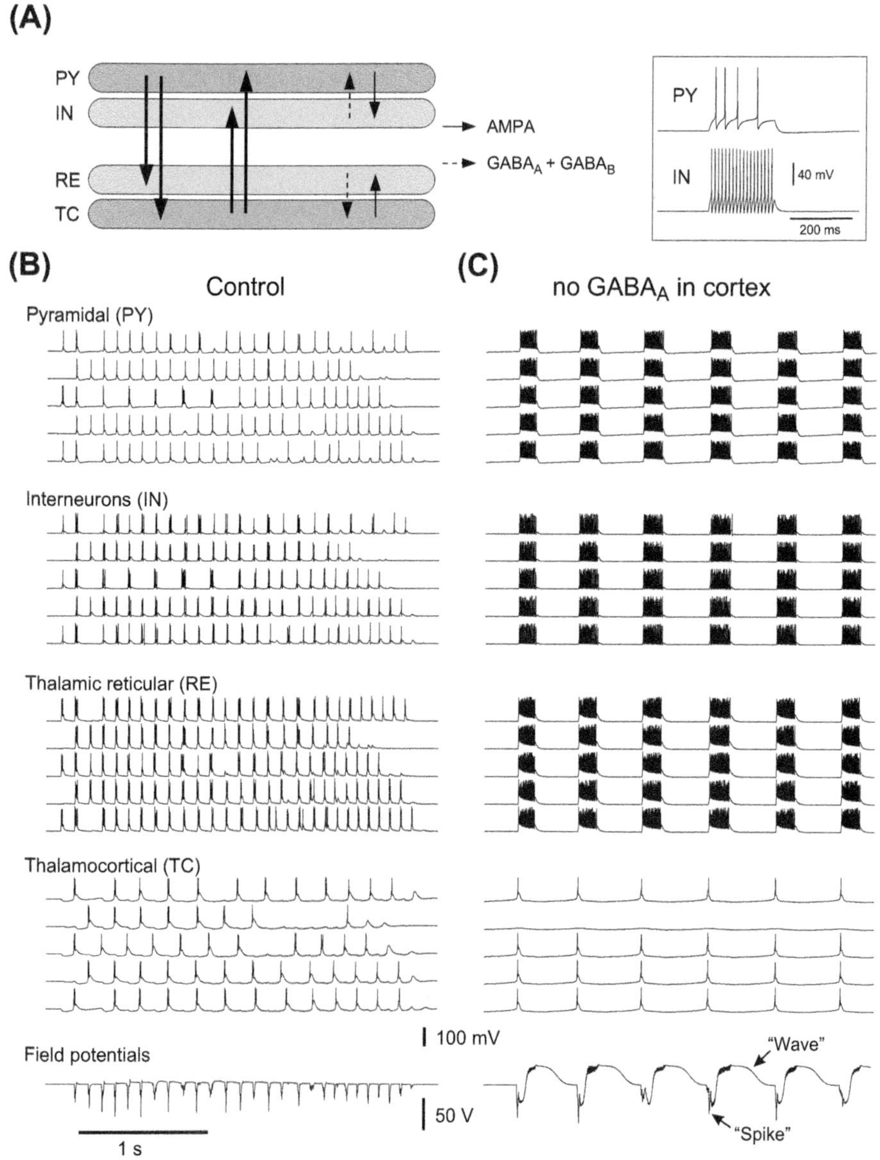

FIGURE 2.9 Transformation of spindle oscillations into ~3 Hz spike-and-wave oscillations by reducing cortical inhibition in a thalamocortical network model. (A) Connectivity between different cell types: 100 cells of each type were simulated, including TC and RE cells, cortical pyramidal (PY) cells, and cortical interneurons (IN). The connectivity is shown by continuous arrows, representing AMPA-mediated excitation, and dashed arrows, representing mixed $GABA_A$ and $GABA_B$ inhibition. In addition, PY cells were interconnected using AMPA receptors, and RE cells were interconnected using $GABA_A$ receptors. The inset shows the repetitive firing properties of PY cells and IN following depolarizing current injection (0.75 nA during 200 ms; −70 mV rest). (B) Spindle oscillations in the thalamocortical network in control conditions. Five cells of each type, equally spaced in the network, are shown (0.5 ms time resolution). The field potentials, consisting of successive negative deflections at ~10 Hz, are shown at the bottom. (C) Oscillations following the suppression of $GABA_A$-mediated inhibition in cortical cells with thalamic inhibition intact. All cells displayed prolonged discharges in phase, separated by long periods of silence, at a frequency of ~2 Hz. $GABA_B$ currents were maximally activated in TC and PY cells during the periods of silence. Field potentials (bottom) displayed spike-and-wave complexes. Thalamic inhibition was intact in B and C. *Modified from Ref. 47.*

thalamic cells, including thalamic TC and RE cells, and a simplified representation of the deep layers of the cortex, in which pyramidal (PY) cells constitute the major source of corticothalamic fibers. As corticothalamic PY cells receive a significant proportion of their excitatory synapses from ascending thalamic axons,[96,97] these cells mediate a monosynaptic excitatory feedback loop (thalamus–cortex–thalamus), which was modeled here. The structure of the network, with TC, RE, and PY cells and cortical interneurons (IN), is schematized in Figure 2.9(A). Each cell type contained the minimal set of calcium- and voltage-dependent currents necessary to account for their intrinsic properties: TC cells contained I_T, I_h, and a calcium-dependent upregulation of I_h; RE cells contained I_{Ts}; and PY cells had a slow voltage-dependent K^+ current I_M responsible for spike-frequency adaptation similar to "regular-spiking" pyramidal cells.[77] All cell types had the I_{Na} and I_{Kd} currents necessary to generate action potentials. All currents were modeled using Hodgkin–Huxley-type[55] kinetics based on voltage-clamp data. Synaptic interactions were mediated by glutamate AMPA and NMDA receptors, as well as GABAergic $GABA_A$ and $GABA_B$ receptors, and were simulated using kinetic models of postsynaptic receptors.[56,57] All excitatory connections (TC → RE, TC → IN, TC → PY, PY → PY, PY → IN, PY → RE, and PY → TC) were mediated by AMPA receptors, some inhibitory connections (RE → TC and IN → PY) were mediated by a mixture of $GABA_A$ and $GABA_B$ receptors, while intra-RE connections were mediated by $GABA_A$ receptors. Simulations were also performed using NMDA receptors added to all excitatory connections (with maximal conductance set to 25% of the AMPA conductance), and no appreciable difference was observed. They were not included in the present model. Extracellular field potentials were calculated from postsynaptic currents in PY cells according to the model described in the "Model of Cooperative $GABA_B$ Responses" section, assuming that all cells were arranged equidistantly in a one-dimensional layer (see details in Ref. 47).

In control conditions (Figure 2.9(B)), this thalamocortical network was set to generate synchronized spindle oscillations with cellular discharges in phase between all cell types, as observed experimentally.[84] TC cells discharged on average once every two cycles following $GABA_B$-mediated IPSPs, while all other cell types discharged roughly at every cycle at ~10 Hz, consistent with the typical features of spindle oscillations observed intracellularly.[21,35] The simulated field potentials displayed successive negative deflections at ~10 Hz (Figure 2.9(B)), in agreement with the pattern of field potentials during spindle oscillations.[21] This pattern of field potentials was generated by the limited discharge in PY cells, which fired roughly one spike per oscillation cycle.

As seen in this chapter, a key experiment is that a diffuse application of the $GABA_A$ antagonist penicillin to the cortex, with no change in thalamus, leads to spike-and-wave oscillations in cats.[37] In the model, this situation was simulated by decreasing $GABA_B$ conductances in cortical cells, while the thalamus was left intact. Alteration of $GABA_B$ receptors in the cortex had a considerable impact in generating spike-and-wave activity. Under these conditions, the spindle oscillations transformed into 2–3 Hz oscillations (Figure 2.9(C); and see Ref. 47). The field potentials generated by these oscillations reflected a pattern of spikes and waves (Figure 2.9(C), bottom).

In this network model, there was a progressive transformation of spindle oscillations into spike-and-wave discharges, similar to the experiments in the FGPE model. Reducing the intracortical fast inhibition from 100% to 50% increased the occurrences of prolonged high-frequency discharges during spindle oscillations (Figure 2.10; and see Ref. 47). Further decreases in intracortical fast inhibition led to fully developed spike-and-wave patterns similar to those in Figure 2.9(C).[47] Field potentials displayed one or several negative–positive sharp deflections, followed by a slowly developing positive wave (Figure 2.9(C), bottom). During the "spike", all cells fired prolonged high-frequency discharges in synchrony, while the "wave" was associated with neuronal silence in all cell types. This portrait is typical of experimental recordings of cortical and thalamic cells during spike-and-wave patterns.[11,12,14–17,19] Some TC cells stayed hyperpolarized during the entire oscillation (second TC cell in Figure 2.9(C)), as also observed experimentally.[43] A similar oscillation arose if $GABA_B$ receptors were suppressed in the entire network (not shown in Figure 2.9).

This network model suggests that spindles can be transformed into an oscillation with field potentials displaying spike-and-wave activity, and that this transformation can occur by alteration of cortical inhibition with no change in the thalamus, in agreement with spike-and-wave discharges obtained experimentally by diffuse application of diluted penicillin onto the cortex.[37] The mechanism of the ~3 Hz oscillation of this model depends on a thalamocortical loop where both cortex and thalamus are necessary, but none of them generates the 3 Hz rhythmicity alone (see details in Ref. 47).

The network model can also be used to simulate other experiments. Removing intrathalamic $GABA_A$-mediated inhibition also affected the oscillation frequency, but it did not generate spike-and-wave activity, because pyramidal cells were still under the strict control of cortical fast inhibition.[47] This is in agreement with in vivo injections of bicuculline into the thalamus, which exhibited slow oscillations with increased thalamic synchrony, but no spike-and-wave patterns in the field potentials.[36,38]

Note that in this network model, spike-and-wave oscillations may follow a similar waxing-and-waning envelope as spindles, and they were a network consequence of the properties of a single ion channel (I_h) in TC cells.[47] A calcium-dependent upregulation of I_h was included in TC cells, similar to previous models.[59,68] The possibility that I_h upregulation underlies the waxing and waning of spindles at the level of thalamic networks has been demonstrated in vitro[98–100] and predicted by models.[58,68] This mechanism may also underlie the waxing and waning of spindles at the level of

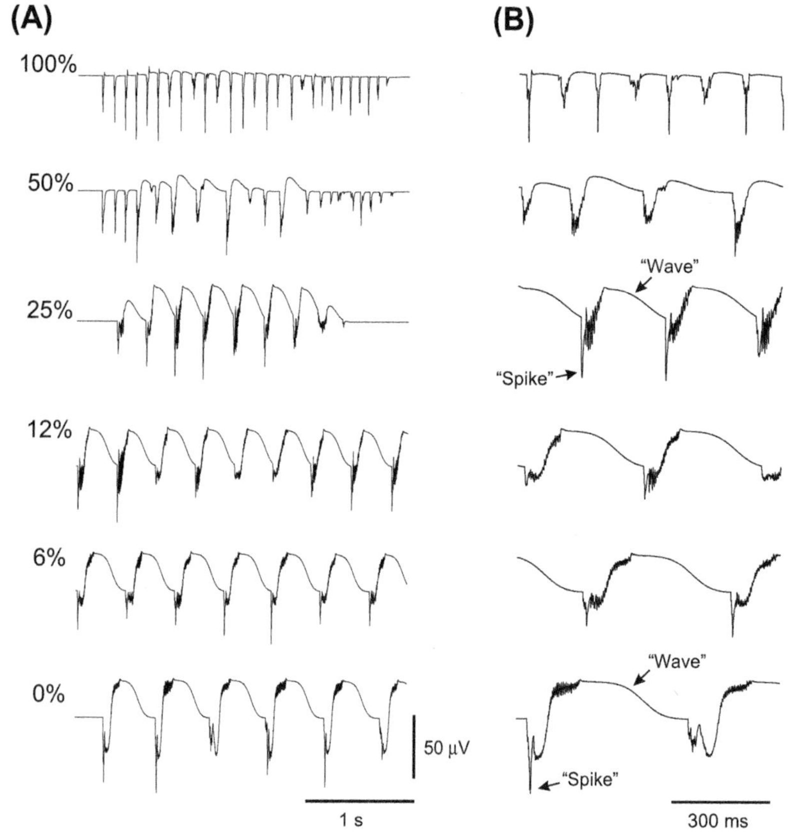

FIGURE 2.10 Gradual transformation of spindles to spike-and-wave complexes. (A) Field potentials obtained from simulations similar to those in Figure 2.9 for different levels of cortical $GABA_A$-mediated inhibition. The conditions were identical except that intracortical $GABA_A$-mediated inhibition (IN → PY) was reduced, with total conductance values of 0.15 μS (100%), 0.075 μS (50%), 0.0375 μS (25%), 0.018 μS (12%), and 0.009 μS (6%). At 100% $GABA_A$ intracortical inhibition there was a spindle sequence (as in Figure 2.9(B)), and at 0% there were fully developed spike-and-wave complexes (as in Figure 2.9(C)); intrathalamic inhibition was intact in all cases. (B) Same simulations at higher temporal resolution. *Modified from Ref. 47.*

thalamocortical networks.[86] The present model suggests that the upregulation of I_h in TC cells is responsible for temporal modulation of spike-and-wave oscillations and may evoke several cycles of spike-and-wave oscillations, interleaved with long periods of silence (~20 s), as is observed experimentally in sleep spindles and spike-and-wave epilepsy, thus emphasizing further the resemblance between the two types of oscillation.

Model of "Fast" (5–10 Hz) Spike-and-Wave Oscillations in the Thalamocortical System

The network model shown here can simulate experiments on the cat penicillin model of spike-and-wave activity, which displays ~3 Hz oscillations. However, other experimental models in rats and mice display a "fast" type of spike-and-wave seizure, where the oscillation frequency is around 5–10 Hz.[10,101] Can the same mechanism as described in this chapter explain these "fast" seizures?

As the 3 Hz frequency was due to the activation of $GABA_B$ receptors, it is possible that faster oscillation frequencies reflect smaller involvement of these receptors in some experimental models.[48] Indeed, intracellular recordings from the thalamus in the "generalized absence epilepsy rat from Strasbourg" (GAERS) reported that, during 5–10 Hz spike-and-wave discharges, TC cells are paced by $GABA_A$ IPSPs.[45] This raises the question of whether the 3 Hz mechanism also applies to rodents, or if the fast spike-and-wave seizures observed in these species stem from a fundamentally different mechanism.

This question was investigated using computational models, which explored the hypothesis that a different balance of GABAergic conductances in TC cells might explain both the fast (5–10 Hz) and slow (2–3 Hz) type of spike-and-wave oscillations based on similar thalamocortical mechanisms.[48] The same thalamocortical network model of spike-and-wave activity as given in this chapter was used, with three differences: (1) TC cells had a depolarized resting membrane potential of −56 mV, as observed experimentally in GAERS[45]; (2) the $GABA_B$ conductance from RE → TC was smaller than in the previous model (0.015 μS versus 0.04 μS); and (3) the $GABA_A$ conductance from RE → TC was larger than in the previous model (0.03 μS versus 0.02 μS).

In "control" conditions, this thalamocortical network generated 8–12 Hz spindle oscillations, in which all cell types produced moderate rates of discharge approximately in phase, while the field potentials displayed successive negative deflections (Figure 2.11(A)). These features are in agreement with experimental

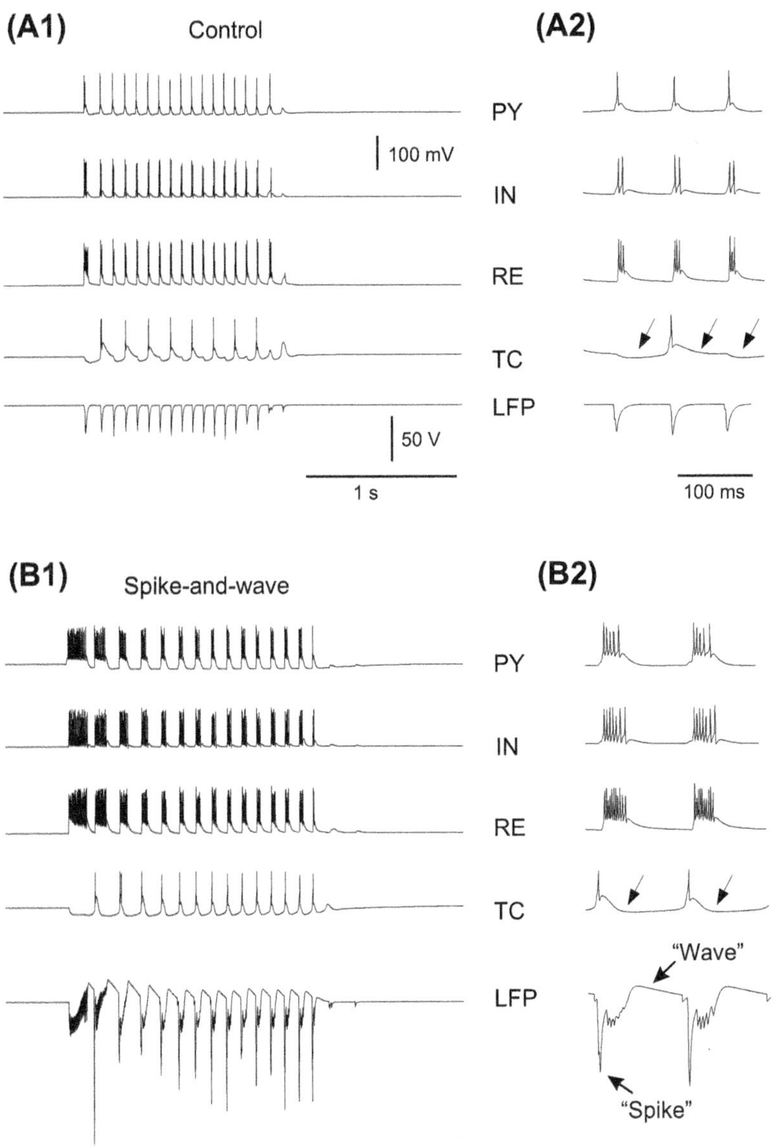

FIGURE 2.11 Fast spike-and-wave oscillations with stronger $GABA_A$ conductances in TC cells. (A1) Control spindle oscillations elicited by injection of depolarizing current into PY cells (1 nA during 20 ms). All cell types displayed moderate discharges at 10–12 Hz accompanied by negative deflections in the local field potential (LFP). (B1) Spike-and-wave oscillations following increase of cortical excitability (same simulation as in A, with intracortical $GABA_A$ conductances decreased from 0.15 to 0.04 μS). All cell types displayed synchronized discharges at 5–10 Hz, and the field potentials consisted of spike-and-wave patterns. The right panels ((A2) and (B2)) show two oscillation cycles at higher temporal resolution. Arrows indicate $GABA_A$ IPSPs in TC cells. *Modified from Ref. 48.*

observations in thalamic and cortical neurons during sleep spindles.[21] In the model, these oscillations were not critically dependent on the strengths of $GABA_A$ and $GABA_B$ conductances in TC cells, as shown in Figure 2.11(A).

The excitability of the cortical network was increased by decreasing the effectiveness of $GABA_A$-mediated intracortical inhibition, as in the previous model, but the network generated a different type of oscillation (Figure 2.11(B)) in which cortical (PY and IN) and thalamic RE cells fired prolonged discharge patterns in synchrony, interleaved with periods of silence that occurred simultaneously in all cell types. This cellular pattern generated spike-and-wave field potentials: the "spike" component was generated by fast EPSPs followed immediately by $GABA_A$-mediated IPSPs in PY cells, while the positive "wave" was due to activation of slow K^+ currents ($GABA_B$-mediated and voltage-dependent I_M) in PY cells.

The oscillatory pattern of discharge depended on the positive feedback in the corticothalamic loop, which was also essential here, as in the 3 Hz spike-and-wave model. The 5–10 Hz oscillation shown in Figure 2.11(B) differed, however, from the 2–4 Hz frequency in Figure 2.9(B). The fast oscillation frequency of the discharge of TC cells was shaped by $GABA_A$-mediated IPSPs (arrows in Figure 2.11(B2)). $GABA_B$ receptors also contributed to the oscillation but produced a sustained hyperpolarization in TC and PY cells, a feature that has also been observed experimentally.[45,102] This sustained hyperpolarization contributed to maintaining the oscillations, since smaller $GABA_B$ conductances led to a markedly reduced tendency to oscillate, and larger $GABA_B$ conductances led to a slower, 2–3 Hz spike-and-wave oscillation.[48] Reducing the conductance of the $GABA_A$ IPSPs markedly reduced oscillatory sequences, and increasing them led to prolonged oscillations; thus, the spike-and-wave seizures in this model critically depend on a balance between both types of IPSPs (see details in Ref. 48).

TESTING THE PREDICTIONS OF THE MODELS

The different models reviewed in the "Network Models" section account for the main features of the experimental data about absence seizures in different experimental models. A series of predictions were generated by these models, which we discuss in this section.

Corticothalamic Feedback

As outlined in this chapter, it is necessary to reconcile the data suggesting thalamic participation on one hand, and cortical participation on the other hand. This apparent paradox can be explained by the fact that *physiologically intact* thalamic circuits can be forced to oscillate at a frequency of ~3 Hz by the action of corticothalamic feedback, as depicted in the "Intact Thalamic Circuits can be Forced into ~3 Hz Oscillations" section (Figure 2.8; and see Ref. 47). This model makes a very strong prediction: it should be possible to force intact thalamic circuits at a slow hypersynchronized frequency of ~3 Hz, and this forcing should depend on $GABA_B$ receptors.

Two independent groups realized an experiment to test these predictions in thalamic slices.[103,104] In this experiment, the activity of thalamic relay cells was used to trigger the electrical stimulation of corticothalamic fibers (Figure 2.12(A)). With this feedback, the activity in the slice depended on the stimulus strength. For mild feedback, the slice generated normal spindle oscillations (Figure 2.12(B)). However, for strong stimulation of corticothalamic fibers, the activity switched to slow synchronized oscillations at ~3 Hz (Figure 2.12(C)). This behavior was dependent on $GABA_B$ receptors, as shown by its sensitivity to $GABA_B$ antagonists.[103,104] These results suggest that strong corticothalamic feedback can force physiologically intact thalamic circuits to oscillate synchronously at ~3 Hz.

Further experiments[103,104] revealed that this forcing of intact thalamic circuits was accompanied by (1) a strong synchronization of the discharges of TC cells, and (2) an enhancement of the burst discharges of RE

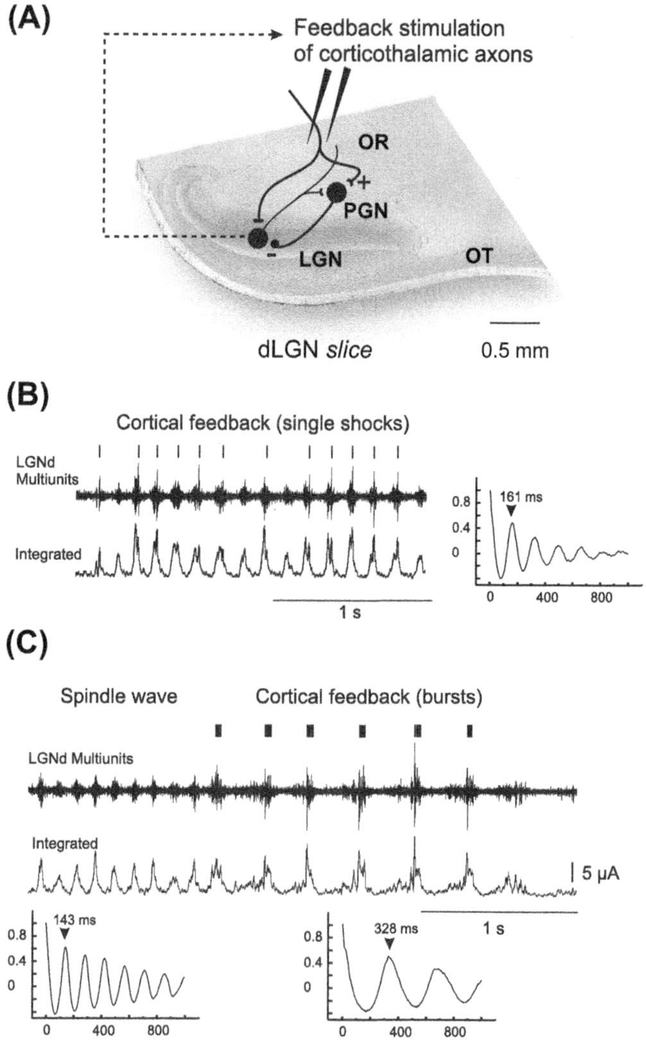

FIGURE 2.12 Control of thalamic oscillations by corticothalamic feedback in ferret thalamic slices. (A) Schematic thalamic slice. Corticothalamic axons run in the optic radiation (OR), and they connect thalamocortical cells in the lateral geniculate nucleus layers and GABAergic interneurons in the perigeniculate nucleus (PGN). Bipolar stimulating electrodes were placed in the OR (OT: optic tract). (B) Weak (single-shock) stimulation at a latency of 20 ms after the detection of multiunit bursts of activity (upper trace). Lower trace: Smooth integration of the multiunit signal. (C) A 7 Hz control spindle is robustly slowed to 3 Hz oscillation by the feedback stimulation (5 shocks; 100 Hz; 20 ms delay). *Modified from Ref. 103.* (For color version of this figure, the reader is referred to the online version of this book.)

cells. The latter is in agreement with the fact that prolonged discharge patterns underlie the emergence of a dominant $GABA_B$ IPSP, as also predicted by the model.

Thus, it seems that this fundamental ingredient of the model is confirmed experimentally: an exceedingly strong corticothalamic feedback can switch intact thalamic circuits into a different oscillatory mode, which is slow, hypersynchronized, and implies the activation of $GABA_B$-mediated currents in TC cells. This oscillation is similar to the slow oscillation observed in the presence of bicuculline (see the "Experimental Evidence for Thalamic Participation in Absence Seizures" section). This oscillation arises because of prolonged discharges in RE cells, which can be caused either by pharmacologically suppressing $GABA_A$-mediated lateral inhibition between RE cells, or by providing a strong excitatory input to RE cells via corticothalamic synapses. Large burst discharges were indeed observed in RE cells during seizures in GAERS.[105]

Cooperative Properties of $GABA_B$ Receptors

As discussed in the "Model Prediction of Cooperative $GABA_B$ Responses" section, one of the essential biophysical ingredients in the mechanisms for absence seizures is the nonlinear properties of $GABA_B$ responses. Such responses appear only under intense release conditions, and it was hypothesized that this property arises from the activation characteristics of $GABA_B$-mediated currents.[63]

This hypothesis was tested experimentally using dual intracellular recordings of pairs of connected thalamic[65] or cortical neurons.[66] In the thalamus, it was shown that evoking single spikes in RE cells does not evoke any detectable $GABA_B$ component in the IPSP of the target TC cell, whereas evoking large burst discharges evokes strong $GABA_B$-mediated IPSPs,[65] exactly like the model prediction. In the neocortex, the same paradigm was observed in single-axon inhibitory connections that contained $GABA_B$ receptors.[66] In this case, the cortical interneuron had to discharge at least three spikes at high frequency (around 100 Hz) in order to evoke a detectable $GABA_B$ component in the target pyramidal cell, and the response saturates for more than 10 presynaptic spikes, exactly as predicted by the model.

This property was also seen in more sophisticated models of $GABA_B$ responses. A computational model of GABA release, diffusion in extracellular space, and uptake by glial cells, similar to that of Ref. 63, was investigated based on data from the neocortex.[66] As in the thalamic model, extracellular accumulation of GABA alone could not account for the nonlinear relationship between spike number and IPSP amplitude (see details in Ref. 66). Different kinetic models were considered for how G-proteins activate K^+ channels, including a kinetic model using four G-protein binding sites, and an allosteric model.[66] All models were fit to experimental data and predicted an optimum of $n = 4$ G-protein binding sites on K^+ channels, consistent with the tetrameric structure of K^+ channels.[64]

Finally, it was found recently that the antiepileptic drug vigabatrin strongly affects spike-and-wave discharges in rats.[106] This drug increases GABA concentrations by inhibiting GABA transaminase, one of the major enzymes implicated in GABA degradation. In particular, Ref. 106 demonstrated that vigabatrin decreases the frequency of spike-and-wave discharges (from 7.5 to 5.6 Hz), as well as prolongs the duration of seizures (from 1.04 to 1.52 s). This effect occurs presumably through boosting of both $GABA_A$ and $GABA_B$ responses, and it is in agreement with predictions of the model (see Figure 2.3 in Ref. 48).

Open Questions for Future Studies

A first experimental observation that is not consistent with the present model is the fact that an apparent intact cortical inhibition was reported in cats treated with penicillin.[107] This contrasts with the fact that intracortical inhibition is decreased in the present model. However, this experimental study did not distinguish between $GABA_A$- and $GABA_B$-mediated inhibition. In the present model, even when $GABA_A$ was antagonized, IPSPs remained approximately the same size because cortical interneurons fired stronger discharges (Figure 2.9(C)) and led to stronger $GABA_B$ currents. There was a compensation effect between $GABA_A$- and $GABA_B$-mediated IPSPs (not shown), which may lead to an apparent preservation of cortical inhibition. Indeed, an impaired intracortical inhibition was reported in the WAG–Rij genetic model of absence epilepsy in rats.[108]

A second inconsistency is that some $GABA_A$ agonists, like barbiturates, may increase the frequency of seizures,[109] possibly through interactions with $GABA_A$ receptors in TC cells.[33] A similar effect was seen in the model,[47] but this effect was weak. More accurate simulation of these data would require modeling the variants of $GABA_A$ receptor types in different cells to address how the threshold for spike-and-wave discharges is affected by various types of GABAergic conductances.

Another effect that was not incorporated here is the possible presence of GABA receptors in presynaptic terminals.[3,110] Such inhibition of synaptic release could mediate various effects, such as disinhibition at GABAergic terminals or presynaptic inhibition of excitatory transmission (assuming that GABA could act on presynaptic excitatory terminals via spillover). Although all of the evidence discussed here points to postsynaptic mechanisms, a presynaptic contribution cannot be ruled out and should be examined by future models.

Finally, it was shown that in the Wag–Rij rat genetic model of absence epilepsy, the seizure seems to start in a focus located in the somatosensory cortex.[41] This observation is consistent with the present thalamocortical model. More recent experiments found that deep (layer 5–6) cortical neurons are hyperexcitable and seem to lead the discharges during ictal activity.[111] As layer 6 neurons project to the thalamus, this finding is consistent with the idea that an excessive corticothalamic feedback may be a primary cause of seizure initiation. However, although this is consistent with the thalamocortical mechanism explored here, it is less clear how the epileptic activity invades "nonepileptic" regions of the thalamocortical system. Is there a bistability between normal and epileptic activity even in a normal cortex? These important questions should be considered by future models.

CONCLUSIONS: A CORTICOTHALAMIC MECHANISM FOR ABSENCE SEIZURES

A Thalamocortical Loop Mechanism for Absence Seizures

The mechanism proposed for absence seizures can be summarized as follows. During sleep spindles, the oscillation is generated by intrathalamic interactions (TC–RE loops) and is reinforced by thalamocortical loops, as suggested in a previous model.[86] The combined action of intrathalamic and thalamocortical loops provides RE cells with moderate excitation, which evokes $GABA_B$-mediated IPSPs in TC cells and sets the frequency to ~10 Hz. During spike-and-wave seizures, due to increased cortical excitability, corticothalamic feedback becomes strong enough to force prolonged burst discharges in RE cells, which in turn evoke IPSPs in TC cells dominated by the $GABA_B$ component. In this case, the prolonged inhibition sets the frequency to ~3 Hz and the oscillation is generated by a thalamocortical loop in which the thalamus is intact (see details in Ref. 47). Therefore, if the cortex is inactivated during spike-and-wave activity, this model predicts that the thalamus should resume generating spindle oscillations, as observed experimentally in cats treated with penicillin.[112]

This corticothalamic model of spike-and-wave seizures also predicts specific phase relations between the different cell types. High-frequency discharges generated "spike" components in the field potentials, whereas the hyperpolarization of PY cells during the "wave" was generated by K^+ currents (adaptation currents and $GABA_B$ IPSPs) in PY cells. Adaptation currents were due to the strong discharge of PY cells during the "spike", while $GABA_B$-mediated currents were due to the prolonged firing of cortical IN. The relative contribution of each current to the "wave" depends on their respective conductance values (see details in Ref. 47).

The "spike" component was generated by a concerted prolonged discharge of all cell types. However, the discharges were not perfectly in phase. There was a significant phase advance of TC cells, as observed experimentally.[17,19] This phase advance was responsible for the initial negative spike in the field potentials, which coincided with the first spike in the TC cells. Thalamic EPSPs may also trigger an initial avalanche of discharges due to pyramidal cell firing, before IPSPs arise, which would also result in a pronounced negative spike component in field potentials. These EPSP–IPSP sequences in PY cells generate one or several successive "spikes" in the simulated spike-and-wave complexes.[47]

Cortical versus Thalamocortical Seizures

The models investigated here displayed oscillations with spike-and-wave field potentials arising either from intracortical mechanisms (see the "Network Models of Cortical Spike-and-Wave Seizures" section) or from thalamocortical loops (see the "Network Model of ~3 Hz Spike-and-Wave Oscillations in the Thalamocortical System" section). As outlined in this chapter, the two types of seizures display fundamental differences. First, the oscillation frequency is slower in intracortical seizures compared to thalamocortical seizures (1.8–2.5 Hz compared to 2–4 Hz; see Ref. 38; Figure 2.13). The same was observed in the models (1.3 Hz in Figure 2.7 compared to 2–4 Hz in Figure 2.9; see Figure 2.13(C) and details in Refs 42,47). This effect was due in the intracortical model to the relatively small conductance of I_T in pyramidal cells, which gave rise to a significant delay before rebound and consequently a slower oscillation frequency. Second, the "spike" component is less prominent in intracortical spike-and-wave complexes (compare (C) and (D) in Figure 2.3), and this was also reproduced by the models (Figure 2.13(C)). In the thalamocortical model, the pronounced negative "spike" was due to thalamic EPSPs that preceded other EPSPs in pyramidal cells (see Figure 2.8B in Ref. 47). These events were, of course, absent in the intracortical model, leading to a less prominent negative "spike" component, in agreement with Figure 2.3(C).

In both cases, the negative "spike" component was due to the EPSPs from the initial discharge of excitatory neurons (and thalamic EPSPs, if applicable). The slow positive "wave" was mediated by $GABA_B$ IPSPs and voltage-dependent K^+ currents. In both cases, the oscillation was generated by similar mechanisms based on rebound firing following K^+-mediated hyperpolarizing events (see the "A Thalamocortical Loop Mechanism for Absence Seizures" section).

The coexistence of two different seizure mechanisms (intracortical versus corticothalamic) should be investigated by future models and experimental studies. No intracellular recording has been made so far during intracortical spike-and-wave seizures, and this may bring important information regarding the possible similarities—or differences—with thalamocortical seizures. The two models of intracortical and thalamocortical seizures should also be integrated into the same network,

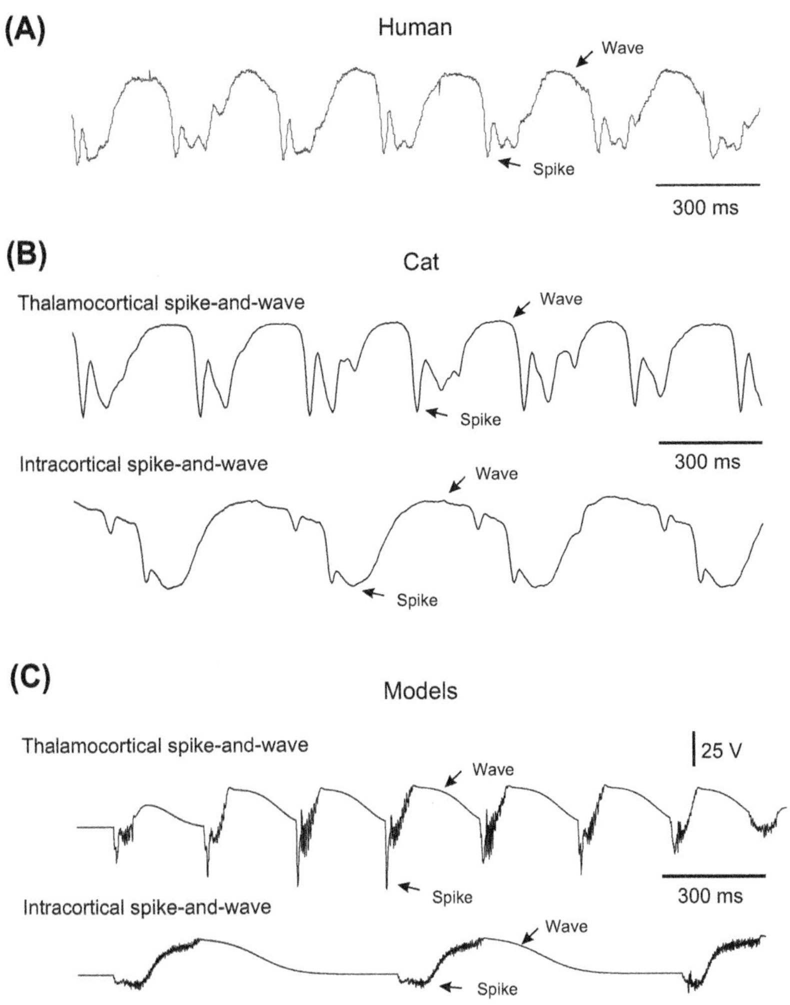

FIGURE 2.13 Comparison of the morphology of spike-and-wave complexes in experiments and models. (A) EEG during a human absence seizure. Same data as in Figure 2.1, replotted at higher resolution. (B) Local field potential (LFP) measurements in cats in two different experimental models of spike-and-wave seizures following cortical injection of bicuculline. Top: Seizure obtained in the intact thalamocortical system. Bottom: Seizure in athalamic cat (data replotted from Figure 2.3(B) and (C), respectively). (C) Simulated LFPs in models of spike-and-wave seizures. Top: Thalamocortical model (replotted from Figure 2.9). Bottom: Intracortical model (replotted from Figure 2.7). In each case, the spikes and the waves are indicated (see figures for references).

to study under which conditions intracortical loops prevail over corticothalamic loops, which may help to explain the rich variety of paroxysmal patterns observed experimentally.

Conclusions

In conclusion, we have presented here a corticothalamic mechanism for absence seizure generation,[47,49–51] and described the essential biophysical and functional ingredients implicated in this mechanism. Such a corticothalamic scheme differs from previous proposals. Similarly to Gloor's "corticoreticular" scheme,[113] this mechanism postulates an increased cortical excitability. However, instead of considering that spike-and-wave activity arises from an abnormal cortical response to normal afferent thalamocortical inputs,[113] the present mechanism points to the reverse pathway, corticothalamic feedback. An exceedingly strong action of the cortex to the thalamus can switch thalamic circuits into a hypersynchronized oscillatory mode and entrain the whole thalamocortical system into a slow spike-and-wave oscillation. Thus, the primary deficit is cortical, which is consistent with the finding that absence seizures in rats start in the cortex.[41] In a corticothalamic mechanism, however, cortical excitability need not be uniform across all layers, but it may be local to deep layers (those projecting to the thalamus). Indeed, it was shown recently that in a rat model of absence seizures, deep (layer 5–6) cortical neurons are hyperexcitable and seem to lead the discharges during ictal activity.[111] This finding is consistent with the fact that increased cortical activity "forces" the thalamus to generate excessive discharges, which entrains the entire thalamocortical system into hypersynchronized oscillatory activity.

Models can be most useful in predicting targets for suppressing seizures. For example, it was shown that reducing the conductance of glutamateric receptors from cortical synapses in RE cells could suppress absence seizures.[47] Other possible targets are also possible, and the search for such targets constitutes a very promising field where computational models may make significant contributions.

At present, the corticothalamic mechanism reviewed here seems the most consistent with all the available data. It differs from Gloor's mechanism, which would primarily postulate an increased excitability of superficial layers, and the hyperexcitable cortex "responds" to a normal thalamic input by generating spike-and-wave patterns. The present mechanism predicts increased excitability in deep layers, and predicts that thalamic discharges are modified during seizures. These differences constitute strong predictions that should be tested by future experiments.

Acknowledgments

Part of this research was supported by the MRC of Canada, the FRSQ of Quebec, the European Community, the HFSP program, and CNRS (France). All simulations were performed using NEURON.[114] Supplementary information, such as program codes and computer-generated animations of network activity, are available at http://cns.iaf.cnrs-gif.fr.

References

1. Gloor P, Fariello RG. Generalized epilepsy: some of its cellular mechanisms differ from those of focal epilepsy. *Trends Neurosci.* 1988;11:63–68.
2. Crunelli V, Leresche N. Childhood absence epilepsy: genes, channels, neurons and networks. *Nat Rev Neurosci.* 2002;3: 371–382.
3. Sperk G, Furtinger S, Schwarzer C, Pirker S. GABA and its receptors in epilepsy. *Adv Exp Med Biol.* 2004;548:92–103.
4. Destexhe A. Nonlinear Dynamics of the Rhythmical Activity of the Brain. 1992, PhD dissertation, Universite Libre de Bruxelles, Brussels, Belgium.
5. Jasper H, Kershman J. Electroencephalographic classification of the epilepsies. *Arch Neurol Physchiatry.* 1941;45:903–943.
6. Williams D. A study of thalamic and cortical rhythms in petit mal. *Brain.* 1953;76:50–69.
7. Prevett MC, Duncan JS, Jones T, Fish DR, Brooks DJ. Demonstration of thalamic activation during typical absence seizures during $H_2^{15}O$ and PET. *Neurology.* 1995;45:1396–1402.
8. Pellegrini A, Musgrave J, Gloor P. Role of afferent input of subcortical origin in the genesis of bilaterally synchronous epileptic discharges of feline generalized epilepsy. *Exp Neurol.* 1979;64:155–173.
9. Avoli M, Gloor P. The effect of transient functional depression of the thalamus on spindles and bilateral synchronous epileptic discharges of feline generalized penicillin epilepsy. *Epilepsia.* 1981;22:443–452.
10. Vergnes M, Marescaux C. Cortical and thalamic lesions in rats with genetic absence epilepsy. *J Neural Transm.* 1992;35(Suppl.): 71–83.
11. Pollen DA. Intracellular studies of cortical neurons during thalamic induced wave and spike. *Electroencephalogr Clin Neurophysiol.* 1964;17:398–404.
12. Steriade M. Interneuronal epileptic discharges related to spike-and-wave cortical seizures in behaving monkeys. *Electroencephalogr Clin Neurophysiol.* 1974;37:247–263.
13. Fisher RS, Prince DA. Spike-wave rhythms in cat cortex induced by parenteral penicillin. II. Cellular features. *Electroencephalogr Clin Neurophysiol.* 1977;42:625–639.
14. Avoli M, Gloor P, Kostopoulos G, Gotman J. An analysis of penicillin-induced generalized spike and wave discharges using simultaneous recordings of cortical and thalamic single neurons. *J Neurophysiol.* 1983;50:819–837.
15. McLachlan RS, Avoli M, Gloor P. Transition from spindles to generalized spike and wave discharges in the cat: simultaneous single-cell recordings in the cortex and thalamus. *Exp Neurol.* 1984;85:413–425.
16. Buzsaki G, Bickford RG, Ponomareff G, Thal LJ, Mandel R, Gage FH. Nucleus basalis and thalamic control of neocortical activity in the freely moving rat. *J Neurosci.* 1988;8:4007–4026.
17. Inoue M, Duysens J, Vossen JMH, Coenen AML. Thalamic multiple-unit activity underlying spike-wave discharges in anesthetized rats. *Brain Res.* 1993;612:35–40.
18. McCormick DA, Hashemiyoon R. Thalamocortical neurons actively participate in the generation of spike-and-wave seizures in rodents. *Abstr Soc Neurosci.* 1998;24:129.
19. Seidenbecher T, Staak R, Pape HC. Relations between cortical and thalamic cellular activities during absence seizures in rats. *Eur J Neurosci.* 1998;10:1103–1112.
20. Staak R, Pape HC. Contribution of GABA(A) and GABA(B) receptors to thalamic neuronal activity during spontaneous absence seizures in rats. *J Neurosci.* 2001;21:1378–1384.
21. Steriade M, Jones EG, Llinas RR. *Thalamic Oscillations and Signalling.* New York: John Wiley & Sons; 1990.
22. Steriade M, McCormick DA, Sejnowski TJ. Thalamocortical oscillations in the sleeping and aroused brain. *Science.* 1993; 262:679–685.
23. Kostopoulos G, Gloor P, Pellegrini A, Gotman J. A study of the transition from spindles to spike and wave discharge in feline generalized penicillin epilepsy: microphysiological features. *Exp Neurol.* 1981;73:55–77.
24. Kostopoulos G, Gloor P, Pellegrini A, Siatitsas I. A study of the transition from spindles to spike and wave discharge in feline generalized penicillin epilepsy: EEG features. *Exp Neurol.* 1981; 73:43–54.
25. Kim D, Song U, Keum S, et al. Lack of the burst firing of thalamocortical relay neurons and resistance to absence seizures in mice lacking the a_{1G} T-type Ca^{2+} channels. *Neuron.* 2001;31: 35–45.
26. Hosford DA, Clark S, Cao Z, et al. The role of $GABA_B$ receptor activation in absence seizures of lethargic (lh/lh) mice. *Science.* 1992;257:398–401.
27. Snead OC. Evidence for $GABA_B$-mediated mechanisms in experimental generalized absence seizures. *Eur J Pharmacol.* 1992;213:343–349.
28. Puigcerver A, Van Luijtenaar EJLM, Drinkenburg WHIM, Coenen ALM. Effects of the $GABA_B$ antagonist CGP-35348 on sleep-wake states, behaviour and spike-wave discharges in old rats. *Brain Res Bull.* 1996;40:157–162.
29. Smith KA, Fisher RS. The selective $GABA_B$ antagonist CGP-35348 blocks spike-wave bursts in the cholesterol synthesis rat absence epilepsy model. *Brain Res.* 1996;729:147–150.
30. Liu Z, Vergnes M, Depaulis A, Marescaux C. Involvement of intrathalamic $GABA_B$ neurotransmission in the control of absence seizures in the rat. *Neuroscience.* 1992;48:87–93.
31. Huguenard JR, Prince DA. Clonazepam suppresses $GABA_B$-mediated inhibition in thalamic relay neurons through effects in nucleus reticularis. *J Neurophysiol.* 1994;71:2576–2581.
32. Gibbs JW, Berkow-Schroeder G, Coulter DA. $GABA_A$ receptor function in developing rat thalamic reticular neurons: whole cell

recordings of GABA-mediated currents and modulation by clonazepam. *J Neurophysiol.* 1996;76:2568–2579.
33. Hosford DA, Wang Y, Cao Z. Differential effects mediated by $GABA_A$ receptors in thalamic nuclei of lh/lh model of absence seizures. *Epilepsy Res.* 1997;27:55–65.
34. Liu Z, Vergnes M, Depaulis A, Marescaux C. Evidence for a critical role of GABAergic transmission within the thalamus in the genesis and control of absence seizures in the rat. *Brain Res.* 1991;545:1–7.
35. von Krosigk M, Bal T, McCormick DA. Cellular mechanisms of a synchronized oscillation in the thalamus. *Science.* 1993;261: 361–364.
36. Ralston B, Ajmone-Marsan C. Thalamic control of certain normal and abnormal cortical rhythms. *Electroencephalogr Clin Neurophysiol.* 1956;8:559–582.
37. Gloor P, Quesney LF, Zumstein H. Pathophysiology of generalized penicillin epilepsy in the cat: the role of cortical and subcortical structures. II. Topical application of penicillin to the cerebral cortex and subcortical structures. *Electroencephalogr Clin Neurophysiol.* 1977;43:79–94.
38. Steriade M, Contreras D. Spike-wave complexes and fast components of cortically generated seizures. I. Role of neocortex and thalamus. *J Neurophysiol.* 1998;80:1439–1455.
39. Fisher RS, Prince DA. Spike-wave rhythms in cat cortex induced by parenteral penicillin. I. Electroencephalographic features. *Electroencephalogr Clin Neurophysiol.* 1977;42:608–624.
40. Marcus EM, Watson CW. Bilateral synchronous spike wave electrographic patterns in the cat: interaction of bilateral cortical foci in the intact, the bilateral cortical-callosal and adiencephalic preparations. *Arch Neurol.* 1966;14:601–610.
41. Meeren HK, Pijn JP, Van Luijtelaar EL, Coenen AM, Lopes da Silva FH. Cortical focus drives widespread corticothalamic networks during spontaneous absence seizures in rats. *J Neurosci.* 2002;22:1480–1495.
42. Destexhe A, Contreras D, Steriade M. LTS cells in cerebral cortex and their role in generating spike-and-wave oscillations. *Neurocomputing.* 2001;38:555–563.
43. Steriade M, Contreras D. Relations between cortical and thalamic cellular events during transition from sleep patterns to paroxysmal activity. *J Neurosci.* 1995;15:623–642.
44. Lytton WW, Contreras D, Destexhe A, Steriade M. Dynamic interactions determine partial thalamic quiescence in a computer network model of spike-and-wave seizures. *J Neurophysiol.* 1997;77:1679–1696.
45. Pinault D, Leresche N, Charpier S, et al. Intracellular recordings in thalamic neurones during spontaneous spike and wave discharges in rats with absence epilepsy. *J Physiol.* 1998;509: 449–456.
46. Danober L, Deransart C, Depaulis A, Vergnes M, Marescaux C. Pathophysiological mechanisms of genetic absence epilepsy in the rat. *Progr Neurobiol.* 1998;55:27–57.
47. Destexhe A. Spike-and-wave oscillations based on the properties of $GABA_B$ receptors. *J Neurosci.* 1998;18:9099–9111.
48. Destexhe A. Can $GABA_A$ conductances explain the fast oscillation frequency of absence seizures in rodents? *Eur J Neurosci.* 1999;11:2175–2181.
49. Destexhe A, Sejnowski TJ. *Thalamocortical Assemblies.* Oxford UK: Oxford University Press; 2001.
50. Destexhe A. Spike-and-wave oscillations. *Scholarpedia.* 2007;2(2):1402. http://www.scholarpedia.org/article/Spike-and-Wave_Oscillations.
51. Destexhe A. Cortico-thalamic feedback: a key to explain absence seizures. In: Soltesz I, Staley K, eds. *Computational Neuroscience in Epilepsy.* Amsterdam: Elsevier; 2008:184–214.
52. Destexhe A, Sejnowski TJ. Interactions between membrane conductances underlying thalamocortical slow-wave oscillations. *Physiol Rev.* 2003;83:1401–1453.
53. Steriade M. *Neuronal Substrates of Sleep and Epilepsy.* Cambridge, UK: Cambridge University Press; 2003.
54. McCormick DA. Neurotransmitter actions in the thalamus and cerebral cortex and their role in neuromodulation of thalamocortical activity. *Prog Neurobiol.* 1992;39:337–388.
55. Hodgkin AL, Huxley AF. A quantitative description of membrane current and its application to conduction and excitation in nerve. *J Physiol.* 1952;117:500–544.
56. Destexhe A, Mainen ZF, Sejnowski TJ. An efficient method for computing synaptic conductances based on a kinetic model of receptor binding. *Neural Comput.* 1994;6:14–18.
57. Destexhe A, Mainen ZF, Sejnowski TJ. Kinetic models of synaptic transmission. In: Koch C, Segev I, eds. *Methods in Neuronal Modeling.* 2nd ed. Cambridge, MA: MIT Press; 1998:1–26.
58. Destexhe A, McCormick DA, Sejnowski TJ. A model for 8–10 Hz spindling in interconnected thalamic relay and reticularis neurons. *Biophys J.* 1993;65:2474–2478.
59. Destexhe A, Babloyantz A, Sejnowski TJ. Ionic mechanisms for intrinsic slow oscillations in thalamic relay neurons. *Biophys J.* 1993;65:1538–1552.
60. Destexhe A, Contreras D, Sejnowski TJ, Steriade M. A model of spindle rhythmicity in the isolated thalamic reticular nucleus. *J Neurophysiol.* 1994;72:803–818.
61. Traub RD, Miles R. *Neuronal Networks of the Hippocampus.* Cambridge, UK: Cambridge University Press; 1991.
62. Otis TS, Dekoninck Y, Mody I. Characterization of synaptically elicited $GABA_B$ responses using patch-clamp recordings in rat hippocampal slices. *J Physiol.* 1993;463:391–407.
63. Destexhe A, Sejnowski TJ. G-protein activation kinetics and spillover of GABA may account for differences between inhibitory responses in the hippocampus and thalamus. *Proc Natl Acad Sci USA.* 1995;92:9515–9519.
64. Hille B. *Ionic Channels of Excitable Membranes.* 3rd ed. Sunderland, MA: Sinauer Associates; 2001.
65. Kim U, Sanchez-Vives MV, McCormick DA. Functional dynamics of GABAergic inhibition in the thalamus. *Science.* 1997;278: 130–134.
66. Thomson AM, Destexhe A. Dual intracellular recordings and computational models of slow IPSPs in rat neocortical and hippocampal slices. *Neuroscience.* 1999;92:1193–1215.
67. Huguenard JR, Prince DA. Intrathalamic rhythmicity studied in vitro, nominal T-current modulation causes robust antioscillatory effects. *J Neurosci.* 1994;14:5485–5502.
68. Destexhe A, Bal T, McCormick DA, Sejnowski TJ. Ionic mechanisms underlying synchronized oscillations and propagating waves in a model of ferret thalamic slices. *J Neurophysiol.* 1996;76:2049–2070.
69. Wallenstein GV. The role of thalamic $IGABA_B$ in generating spike-wave discharges during petit mal seizures. *Neuroreport.* 1994;5:1409–1412.
70. Wang XJ, Golomb D, Rinzel J. Emergent spindle oscillations and intermittent burst firing in a thalamic model: specific neuronal mechanisms. *Proc Natl Acad Sci USA.* 1995;92:5577–5581.
71. Golomb D, Wang XJ, Rinzel J. Propagation of spindle waves in a thalamic slice model. *J Neurophysiol.* 1996;75:750–769.
72. Soltesz I, Crunelli V. $GABA_A$ and pre- and post-synaptic $GABA_B$ receptor-mediated responses in the lateral geniculate nucleus. *Progr Brain Res.* 1992;90:151–169.
73. Kim U, Bal T, McCormick DA. Spindle waves are propagating synchronized oscillations in the ferret LGNd in vitro. *J Neurophysiol.* 1995;74:1301–1323.

74. Sanchez-Vives MV, McCormick DA. Functional properties of perigeniculate inhibition of dorsal lateral geniculate nucleus thalamocortical neurons in vitro. *J Neurosci.* 1997;17:8880–8893.
75. Huntsman MM, Porcello DM, Homanics GE, DeLorey TM, Huguenard JR. Reciprocal inhibitory connections and network synchrony in the mammalian thalamus. *Science.* 1999;283: 541–543.
76. Nunez PL. *Electric Fields of the Brain: The Neurophysics of EEG.* Oxford, UK: Oxford University Press; 1981.
77. Connors BW, Gutnick MJ. Intrinsic firing patterns of diverse neocortical neurons. *Trends Neurosci.* 1990;13:99–104.
78. de la Peña E, Geijo-Barrientos E. Laminar organization, morphology and physiological properties of pyramidal neurons that have the low-threshold calcium current in the guinea-pig frontal cortex. *J Neurosci.* 1996;16:5301–5311.
79. McCormick DA, Wang Z, Huguenard J. Neurotransmitter control of neocortical neuronal activity and excitability. *Cereb Cortex.* 1993;3:387–398.
80. Destexhe A, Neubig M, Ulrich D, Huguenard JR. Dendritic low-threshold calcium currents in thalamic relay cells. *J Neurosci.* 1998;18:3574–3588.
81. Timofeev I, Bazhenov M, Sejnowski TJ, Steriade M. Cortical hyperpolarization-activated depolarizing current takes part in the generation of focal paroxysmal activities. *Proc Natl Acad Sci USA.* 2002;99:9533–9537.
82. Steriade M, Wyzinski P, Apostol V. Corticofugal projections governing rhythmic thalamic activity. In: Frigyesi TL, Rinvik E, Yahr MD, eds. *Corticothalamic Projections and Sensorimotor Activities.* New York: Raven Press; 1972:221–272.
83. Roy JP, Clercq M, Steriade M, Deschenes M. Electrophysiology of neurons in lateral thalamic nuclei in cat: mechanisms of long-lasting hyperpolarizations. *J Neurophysiol.* 1984;51:1220–1235.
84. Contreras D, Steriade M. Spindle oscillation in cats: the role of corticothalamic feedback in a thalamically-generated rhythm. *J Physiol.* 1996;490:159–179.
85. Contreras D, Destexhe A, Sejnowski TJ, Steriade M. Control of spatiotemporal coherence of a thalamic oscillation by corticothalamic feedback. *Science.* 1996;274:771–774.
86. Destexhe A, Contreras D, Steriade M. Mechanisms underlying the synchronizing action of corticothalamic feedback through inhibition of thalamic relay cells. *J Neurophysiol.* 1998;79: 999–1016.
87. Burke W, Sefton AJ. Inhibitory mechanisms in lateral geniculate nucleus of rat. *J Physiol.* 1966;187:231–246.
88. Deschênes M, Hu B. Electrophysiology and pharmacology of the corticothalamic input to lateral thalamic nuclei: an intracellular study in the cat. *Eur J Neurosci.* 1990;2:140–152.
89. Contreras D, Destexhe A, Steriade M. Intracellular and computational characterization of the intracortical inhibitory control of synchronized thalamic inputs in vivo. *J Neurophysiol.* 1997;78: 335–350.
90. Golshani P, Liu XB, Jones EG. Differences in quantal amplitude reflect GluR4-subunit number at corticothalamic synapses on two populations of thalamic neurons. *Proc Natl Acad Sci USA.* 2001;98:4172–4177.
91. Contreras D, Curró Dossi R, Steriade M. Electrophysiological properties of cat reticular thalamic neurones in vivo. *J Physiol.* 1993;470:273–294.
92. Destexhe A. Modeling corticothalamic feedback and the gating of the thalamus by the cerebral cortex. *J Physiol (Paris).* 2000;94: 391–410.
93. Destexhe A, Sejnowski TJ. The initiation of bursts in thalamic neurons and the cortical control of thalamic sensitivity. *Philos Trans R Soc Lond B Biol Sci.* 2002;357:1649–1657.
94. Destexhe A, Contreras D, Steriade M, Sejnowski TJ, Huguenard JR. In vivo, in vitro and computational analysis of dendritic calcium currents in thalamic reticular neurons. *J Neurosci.* 1996;16:169–185.
95. Liu XB, Honda CN, Jones EG. Distribution of four types of synapse on physiologically identified relay neurons in the ventral posterior thalamic nucleus of the cat. *J Comp Neurol.* 1995; 352:69–91.
96. Hersch SM, White EL. Thalamocortical synapses on corticothalamic projections neurons in mouse SmI cortex: electron microscopic demonstration of a monosynaptic feedback loop. *Neurosci Lett.* 1981;24:207–210.
97. White EL, Hersch SM. A quantitative study of thalamocortical and other synapses involving the apical dendrites of corticothalamic cells in mouse SmI cortex. *J Neurocytol.* 1982;11: 137–157.
98. Bal T, McCormick DA. What stops synchronized thalamocortical oscillations? *Neuron.* 1996;17:297–308.
99. Luthi A, McCormick DA. Periodicity of thalamic synchronized oscillations: the role of Ca^{2+}-mediated upregulation of I_h. *Neuron.* 1998;20:553–563.
100. Luthi A, McCormick DA. Modulation of a pacemaker current through Ca^{2+}-induced stimulation of cAMP production. *Nat Neurosci.* 1999;2:634–641.
101. Coenen AM, Van Luijtelaar EL. Genetic animal models for absence epilepsy: a review of the WAG/Rij strain of rats. *Behav Genet.* 2003;33:635–655.
102. Charpier S, Leresche N, Deniau JM, Mahon S, Hughes SW, Crunelli V. On the putative contribution of GABA(B) receptors to the electrical events occurring during spontaneous spike and wave discharges. *Neuropharmacology.* 1999;38:1699–1706.
103. Bal T, Debay D, Destexhe A. Cortical feedback controls the frequency and synchrony of oscillations in the visual thalamus. *J Neurosci.* 2000;20:7478–7488.
104. Blumenfeld H, McCormick DA. Corticothalamic inputs control the pattern of activity generated in thalamocortical networks. *J Neurosci.* 2000;20:5153–5162.
105. Slaght SJ, Leresche N, Deniau J-M, Crunelli V, Charpier S. Activity of thalamic reticular neurons during spontaneous genetically determined spike and wave discharges. *J Neurosci.* 2002; 22:2323–2334.
106. Bouwman BM, van den Broek PL, van Luijtelaar G, van Rijn CM. The effects of vigabatrin on type II spike wave discharges in rats. *Neurosci Lett.* 2003;338:177–180.
107. Kostopoulos G, Avoli M, Gloor P. Participation of cortical recurrent inhibition in the genesis of spike and wave discharges in feline generalized epilepsy. *Brain Res.* 1983;267:101–112.
108. Luhmann HJ, Mittmann T, van Luijtelaar G, Heinemann U. Impairment of intracortical GABAergic inhibition in a rat model of absence epilepsy. *Epilepsy Res.* 1995;22:43–51.
109. Vergnes M, Marescaux C, Micheletti G, Depaulis A, Rumbach L, Warter JM. Enhancement of spike and wave discharges by GABAmimetic drugs in rats with spontaneous petit-mal-like epilepsy. *Neurosci Lett.* 1984;44:91–94.
110. Waldmeier PC, Baumann PA. Presynaptic GABA receptors. *Ann N Y Acad Sci.* 1990;604:136–151.
111. Polack PO, Guillemain I, Hu E, Deransart C, Depaulis A, Charpier S. Deep layer somatosensory cortical neurons initiate spike-and-wave discharges in a genetic model of absence seizures. *J Neurosci.* 2007;27:6590–6599.
112. Gloor P, Pellegrini A, Kostopoulos GK. Effects of changes in cortical excitability upon the epileptic bursts in generalized penicillin epilepsy of the cat. *Electroencephalogr Clin Neurophysiol.* 1979;46:274–289.

113. Gloor P. Generalized cortico-reticular epilepsies: some considerations on the pathophysiology of generalized bilaterally synchronous spike and wave discharge. *Epilepsia*. 1968;9:249–263.
114. Hines ML, Carnevale NT. The NEURON simulation environment. *Neural Comput*. 1997;9:1179–1209.

Further Reading

1. Avoli M, Gloor P. Role of the thalamus in generalized penicillin epilepsy: observations on decorticated cats. *Exp Neurol*. 1982;77:386–402.
2. Bal T, von Krosigk M, McCormick DA. Synaptic and membrane mechanisms underlying synchronized oscillations in the ferret LGNd in vitro. *J Physiol*. 1995;483:641–663.
3. Contreras D, Steriade M. Cellular basis of EEG slow rhythms: a study of dynamic corticothalamic relationships. *J Neurosci*. 1995;15:604–622.
4. Davies CH, Davies SN, Collingridge GL. Paired-pulse depression of monosynaptic GABA- mediated inhibitory postsynaptic responses in rat hippocampus. *J Physiol*. 1990;424:513–531.
5. Dutar P, Nicoll RA. A physiological role for $GABA_B$ receptors in the central nervous system. *Nature*. 1988;332:156–158.
6. Foehring RC, Lorenzon NM, Herron P, Wilson CJ. Correlation of physiologically and morphologically identified neuronal types in human association cortex in vitro. *J Neurophysiol*. 1991;66: 1825–1837.
7. Friedman A, Gutnick MJ. Low-threshold calcium electrogenesis in neocortical neurons. *Neurosci Lett*. 1987;81:117–122.
8. Hamill OP, Huguenard JR, Prince DA. Patch-clamp studies of voltage-gated currents in identified neurons of the rat cerebral cortex. *Cereb Cortex*. 1991;1:48–61.
9. Liu XB, Warren RA, Jones EG. Synaptic distribution of afferents from reticular nucleus in ventroposterior nucleus of the cat thalamus. *J Comp Neurol*. 1995;352:187–202.
10. Suffczynski P, Kalitzin S, Lopes Da Silva FH. Dynamics of non-convulsive epileptic phenomena modeled by a bistable neuronal network. *Neuroscience*. 2004;126:467–484.
11. Tsakiridou E, Bertollini L, de Curtis M, Avanzini G, Pape HC. Selective increase in T-type calcium conductance of reticular thalamic neurons in a rat model of absence epilepsy. *J Neurosci*. 1995;15:3110–3117.

CHAPTER

3

Functional Magnetic Resonance Imaging in Epilepsy: Methods and Applications Using Awake Animals

Craig F. Ferris [1], *Jeffrey Tenney* [2]

[1]Center for Translational NeuroImaging, Northeastern University, Boston, MA, USA,
[2]Department of Pediatrics, Division of Neurology, Cincinnati Children's Hospital Medical Center, Cincinnati, OH, USA

INTRODUCTION

Awake-animal imaging has become an important tool in behavioral neuroscience and preclinical drug discovery. Noninvasive, ultra-high-field, functional magnetic resonance imaging (fMRI) provides a window to the mind, making it possible to image changes in brain activity across distributed, integrated neural circuits with high temporal and spatial resolution. The power of magnetic resonance imaging (MRI) enables one to observe changes in brain function, anatomy, and chemistry in the same animal from early life into old age under stable or changing environmental conditions. This prospective capability of animal imaging to follow changes in brain neurobiology following genetic or environmental insult has great value in the field of epilepsy as one can follow the etiology and pathophysiology of disease progression. In addition, awake-animal imaging offers the ability to record signal changes across the entire brain in seconds. When combined with the use of three-dimensional (3D) segmented, annotated brain atlases and computational analysis, it is possible to reconstruct distributed, integrated neural circuits of seizure activity.

In the context of understanding epilepsy, what advantages does awake-animal imaging bring that are not already realized in human imaging? We argue that animal MRI provides greater detailed understanding of the neurobiology of brain function and integrated neural circuits that cannot be achieved in human imaging. Obvious advantages are found in higher magnetic field strengths, intraspecies homogeneity, 3D segmented atlases, greater experimental latitude, and prospective experimental designs. For example, in the field of epilepsy, one can study the functional consequences of epileptogenic insults on the naïve brain that can include an interaction between different developmental periods, environments, and genetic phenotypes. With the advent of optogenetics, different areas in the neural circuitry of a seizure can be turned on and off to assess their contribution to the functional connectivity of the integrated neural circuit. These studies would be unethical and disallowed in humans. Indeed, any prospective study on the brain that follows the functional and neurobiological consequences of an insult or genetic manipulation (e.g. traumatic brain injury, traumatic stress, exposure to neurotoxins and drugs of abuse, transgenic mutations for Parkinson's, and Alzheimer's diseases) can be done only in animals. In these areas, noninvasive animal imaging is an indispensable tool.

Other methods for mapping brain networks may be complementary to fMRI and are mentioned as network mapping techniques in other chapters in this book. These techniques for identifying regional changes in brain activity include 2-deoxyglucose autoradiography[1,2] and immunohistochemistry for changes in expression of immediate-early genes such as c-fos and c-jun.[3–5] While such methods have higher spatial resolution than current neuroimaging methods and allow the identification of individual neuronal cell types, they lack the dynamic temporal resolution of fMRI.

Our laboratory pioneered the field of awake-animal imaging, with our first publication in 1998 looking at changes in brain activity in rats in response to foot shock.[6] Since then, we have published over 50 writings

Neuronal Networks in Brain Function, CNS Disorders, and Therapeutics
http://dx.doi.org/10.1016/B978-0-12-415804-7.00003-4

on using fMRI in awake animals. These studies include a variety of behavioral and neurological models ranging from sexual arousal in monkeys[7] to pup suckling in rat dams,[8,9] generalized absence seizures in rats and monkeys,[10–12] aggressive and sexual motivation in rats,[13] and nongenomic effects of stress hormone.[14] In this chapter, we describe the methods used to image awake animals and the recent advances in radiofrequency (RF) electronics, pulse sequences, and the development of 3D segmented atlases and software for image analysis. Results from earlier studies using chemicals to induce absence seizures and generalized clonic-tonic seizures in awake animals are discussed, along with the application of more advanced hardware and software in seizure research.

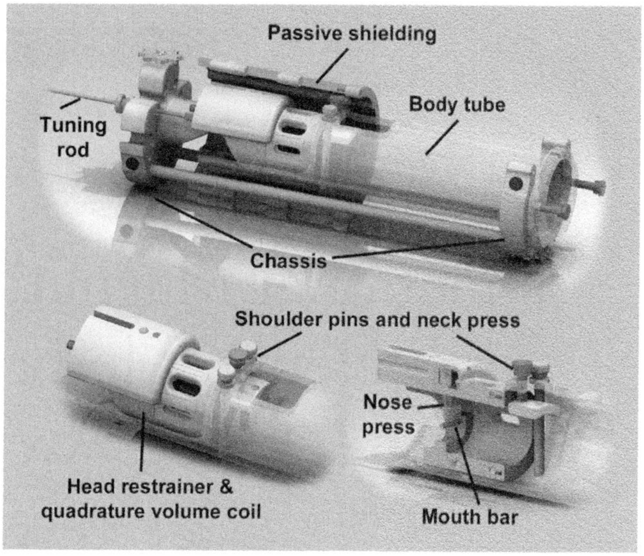

FIGURE 3.1 **Rat-imaging system.** Shown are the different components of the system designed for awake-rat imaging. (For color version of this figure, the reader is referred to the online version of this book.)

SETTING UP AND IMAGING AWAKE ANIMALS

Designing Restrainers to Minimize Motion Artifact

There are multiple technical and methodological issues to overcome in order to perform awake-animal imaging. The first and foremost is the issue of head restraint and motion artifact. Any minor head movement distorts the image and may also create a change in signal intensity that can be mistaken for stimulus-associated changes in brain activity.[15] In addition to head movement, motion outside the field of view (FOV) caused by respiration, swallowing, and muscle contractions in the face and neck are other major sources of motion artifact and can alter field homogeneity.[16–18] To minimize motion artifacts, studies are performed using one of several different restrainers that are custom designed to fit a variety of rodents (e.g. mice, voles, and rats) or nonhuman primates (e.g. the common marmoset, squirrel monkey, cynomolgus monkey, and Rhesus macaque). An example of a rat-imaging system is shown in Figure 3.1.

The setup for an experienced user takes less than 5 min. In brief, just prior to the imaging session, animals are placed into a small airtight anesthesia box connected to a vaporizer set to deliver 2–3% isoflurane. Anesthesia is sustained with a nose cone and 1% isoflurane when the animal is removed from the box for fitting in the MR-compatible restrainer. A topical anesthetic of 10% lidocaine gel is applied to the skin around the ears and over the bridge of the nose. A plastic semicircular headpiece with blunted ear plugs is designed to fit into the auditory meatus of the temporal bone (i.e. the ear canals). The ear plugs do not fit directly into the ear canals; rather, they press into the overlying skin and nestle into the depression of the temporal bone. Presumably, sound would be muffled and attenuated by the ear plugs and the overlying layer of compressed skin and fur, although we have no experimental evidence to confirm this notion. This standard method of preparing the head for immobilization would probably preclude any studies using auditory stimuli to evoke changes in brain activity, although it does not prevent one from recording sounds made by the animal being imaged. Once the ear plugs are positioned, the head is placed into a cylindrical head holder with a built-in quadrature transmit or receive coil. The coil design limits the FOV to the head, reducing physiological noise coming from the thoracic cavity. The rat's canines are secured over a bite bar, and adjustable screws fitted into lateral sleeves on the head holder are used to lock down the ear plugs and stabilize the head. The body of the animal is placed into a body restrainer, and the shoulders stabilized by two vertical posts and a shoulder plate pressed down on the back of the neck. The body restrainer "floats" down the center of the chassis connecting at the front and rear end-plates. The headpiece locks into a mounting post on the front of the chassis. This design isolates all of the body movements from the head restrainer and minimizes motion artifact. The design of the head restraint prevents little to no motion in the Z and X planes (Figure 3.2(A)), while some motion still persists in the Y plan from shoulder movement. Data stability, as estimated by a 3D rigid body model with six degrees of freedom for translational and rotational movement over a 15 min imaging session, is shown in Figure 3.2(B).

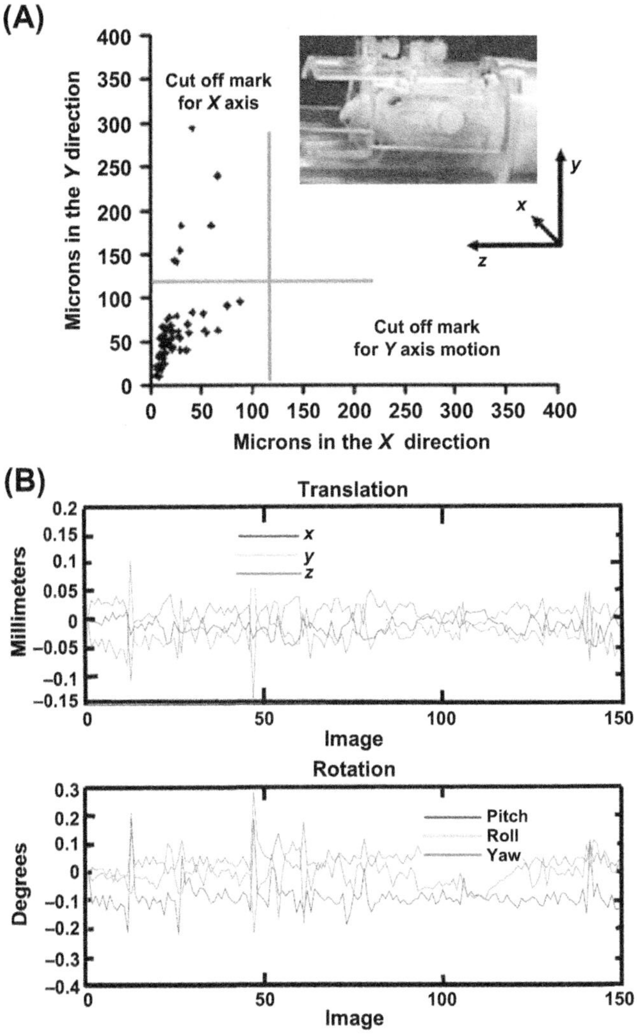

FIGURE 3.2 **Plotting voxel movement to assess motion artifact.** Shown in (A) above are motion data in the X and Y directions for 71 animals. Data points within the gray cross-hairs marked at 120 μm were judged to be acceptable. Note that unacceptable motion was limited to the Y direction (movement of the head up and down near the neck). The insert shows a rat positioned in the head restrainer.[13] Shown in (B) are data stability as estimated by a 3D rigid body model with six degrees of freedom for translational and rotational movement.

Assessing Motion Artifact

Subject motion is an important issue in fMRI data analysis; even the slightest movement during the scan can displace voxel location corresponding to a distinct physical area. Unlike human fMRI, this issue is more prevalent in small animals like rats as voxel size is much larger than the physical (anatomical) area in the brain. The change in signal intensity due to motion can be (and usually is) greater than the blood oxygen level–dependent (BOLD) signal, especially at the edge of the brain and tissue boundaries, which essentially leads to artifact in the activation map. To avoid this, "motion correction" has become a common preprocessing step in fMRI data analysis. Commonly used motion correction tools include automatic image registration,[18–22] analysis of functional neuroimages,[23] and statistical parametric mapping (SPM) realign tools.[24]

However, it has been reported that motion correction may induce spurious activation in motion-free fMRI data.[25] This artifact stems from the fact that activated areas behave like biasing outliers for the difference of square-based measures usually driving such registration methods. This problem is amplified in the case of small animals where the BOLD signal change can be 10% or greater over baseline. Indeed, if motion parameters are included in the general linear model for event-related data, it makes little difference if motion correction is actually applied to the data.[26] So, one should be judicious in the use of motion correction in preprocessing data. Consequently, we developed a method to obtain unbiased measures of motion that cause false-negative and false-positive signal changes.[13] From these measures, we identify data sets requiring motion correction. We set conservative criteria of 120 μm standard deviation of motion in any direction as acceptance criteria (Figure 3.2). Motion in the Z and X direction is usually small as compared to the Y direction. In an example provided in Figure 3.2(A), animals showing an average displacement exceeding 25% of the total in-plane (X–Y) voxel resolution (>120 μm out of 468 μm) or more than 25% displacement in the slice (Z) direction (>300 μm out of 1200 μm slice thickness) were identified for preprocessing for motion correction. Most of the motion was in the Y direction (64 ± 42 μm). Data are corrected for drift and motion with SPM8 software (Statistical Parametric Mapping (SPM), Wellcome Trust Centre for Neuroimaging, London, UK). Despite these postprocessing steps to correct for data stability, experiments with motion artifact exceeding our exclusion criteria are usually not usable.

Animal Acclimation Procedure

The stress associated with head restraint, restricted movement in the body tube, noise from the gradient coil, and the duration of the imaging session are all concerns when imaging awake animals. To address these problems, protocols have been developed for acclimating animals to the environment of the MR scanner and imaging procedure, leading to a reduction in stress hormone levels and measures of autonomic activity regulated by the sympathetic nervous system.[27,28] Acclimation protocols have been used to prepare awake animals for a range of behavioral, neurological, and pharmacological imaging studies, including sexual arousal in monkeys,[7] generalized seizures in rats and monkeys,[10,11] and exposure to psychostimulants like cocaine,[9,29,30] nicotine,[31] and apomorphine,[28,32] and monkeys conditioned to respond to visual stimuli.[33] In all cases, acclimation to the scanning session is achieved by putting subjects through several simulated imaging studies. To reduce the stress associated with head restraint, rats are acclimated to the holding device shown in Figure 3.1. On each day of acclimation, animals are anesthetized with 2–3% isoflurane while being secured into the imaging system. When fully conscious, the imaging system is placed into a black opaque box "mock scanner" for 60 min with a tape recording of an MRI pulse sequence to simulate the bore of the magnet and an imaging protocol. A significant decline in respiration, heart rate, motor movements, and plasma corticosterone has been measured when the first and last acclimation periods are compared[27] (Figure 3.3). The reduction in autonomic and somatic measures of arousal and stress improves the signal resolution and quality of the MR images. Critical in this acclimation study was the demonstration that unacclimated and acclimated animals show no difference in baseline cerebral blood flow (CBF) (Figure 3.3). This finding is critical in light of the fact that BOLD signal changes are affected by baseline CBF and that the level of stress in awake animals does not alter autoregulation of CBF and baseline blood flow. Animals are studied within 1 week after their final acclimation session.

More recently, we have looked at other behavioral parameters to assess the effectiveness of acclimation. Long Evans rats show reduced ultrasonic vocalizations over the course of a 5-day acclimation procedure (Figure 3.4(A)). When observed in a forced-swim test, acclimated animals show significantly less inclination to climb the walls of the pool as opposed to swimming (Figure 3.4(B)). In an interesting study using functional connectivity to validate the effectiveness of acclimation in awake-animal imaging, Upadhyay and coworkers

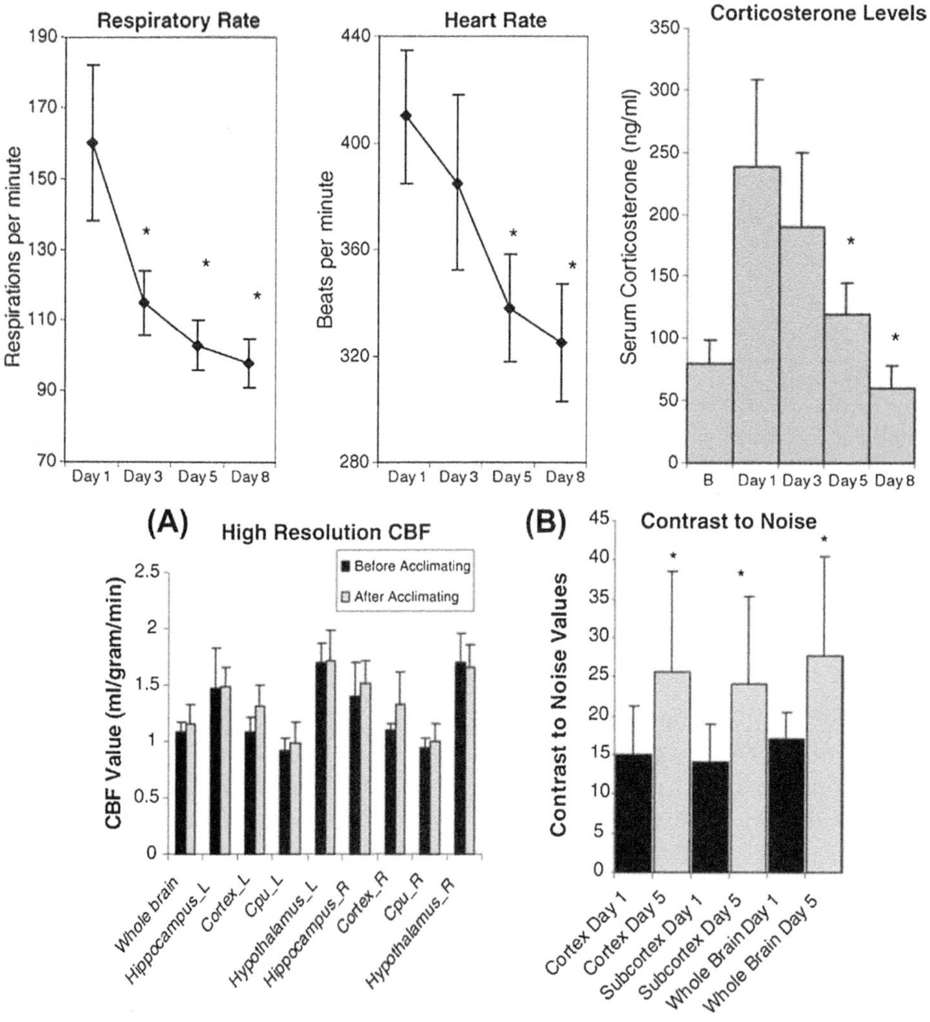

FIGURE 3.3 **Acclimation.** Shown in the upper panels are data on autonomic arousal (i.e. respiratory rate, heart rate, and stress hormone) over 4 days of acclimation. The lower-left panel shows cerebral blood flow values in the same rats in different brain areas prior to and following acclimation. The bottom-right panel shows contrast to noise values prior to and following acclimation[27] *$p < 0.05$.

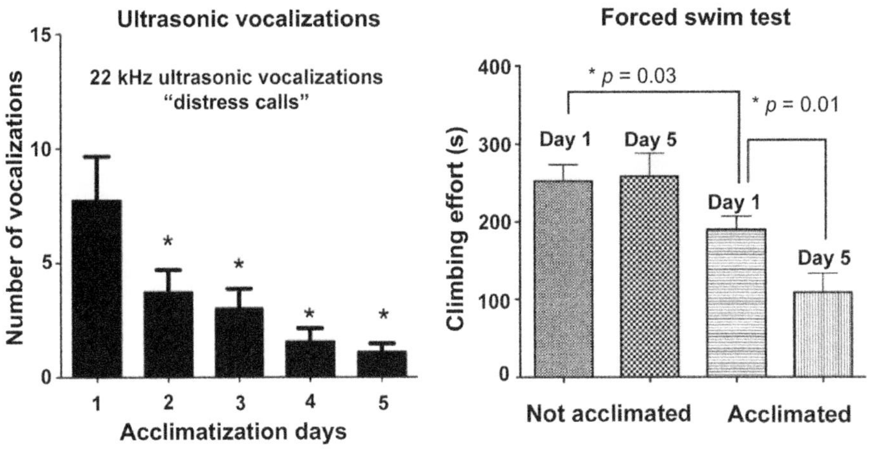

FIGURE 3.4 **Ultrasound.** Shown in the left panel are the mean number of ultrasonic vocalizations over 5 consecutive days of acclimation to the imaging procedure. The panel on the right shows the mean number of seconds that animals spent trying to climb the walls of a water bath when tested on day 1 and day 5 with and without acclimation. Vertical lines denote SEM.

demonstrated the presence of a default-mode network in rats only after the habituation of anxiety to restrain stress.[34]

SPATIAL RESOLUTION AND NEUROANATOMICAL FIDELITY

RF Electronics

Choosing an RF coil or "probe" is critical to any brain-imaging study. The goal is to optimize the signal-to-noise ratio (SNR) with maximum brain coverage. A majority of past and present studies have been performed with a two-coil system composed of a single surface coil for receiving and a larger volume coil for transmitting. The positioning of the surface coil immediately above or in direct contact with the dorsal surface of the head ensures high SNR because of the proximity of the coil to the brain. The volume coil transmits an RF signal, creating a homogeneous B_1 field perpendicular to the main, static magnetic field B_0. Protons spinning in this transverse plane give off an RF signal that is received by the surface coil and used to create images. The obvious advantage to this coil arrangement is high SNR in dorsal brain areas like the cerebral cortex. However, there are two major drawbacks to the single receiving coil: first, there is a drop-off in SNR going from the dorsal to the ventral surface of the brain. This causes the activity at the bottom of the brain, in areas like the amygdala, ventral tegmental area, substantia nigra, and ventral hippocampus, to be "underrepresented" as compared to activity in areas closer to the surface of the brain. The drop-off in SNR may be as high as 15–20%. Second is the limited brain coverage by a single surface coil. The major advantage to limiting the area of coverage is a reduction in noise caused by electromagnetic interference, which is usually motion associated with muscle movement, particularly respiration, outside the FOV. While images have less motion artifact, they are confined to the rostral areas of the brain.

To circumvent the limitations posed by a single surface coil, we have designed a quadrature transmit-receive volume coil. The quadrature coil design allows signal acquisition from proton spins that are both perpendicular and parallel to the receiving element or a full 360°, improving SNR by a factor of 1.4. The volume coil, a modified bird-cage design, provides excellent field homogeneity in the *X*, *Y*, and *Z* planes and coverage of the entire rat brain extending over 2 cm in the rostral-caudal direction (Figure 3.5). To optimize space filling and reduce the drop-off of signal due to the distance between signal source and the receive element, the coil was built into the head holder. With an appropriately large rat head, the fit approximates the distance of a surface coil, giving exceptional SNR and homogeneity over the entire brain.

Pulse Sequence

Our functional MRI studies are designed to image the entire brain with high enough spatial and temporal resolution to enable the identification of distributed, integrated neural networks (Figure 3.6). A typical segmented atlas of the rat based on cytoarchitecture and immunohistochemistry of cell markers and neurotransmitters displays several hundred brain areas.[36] Understanding the cellular and molecular activity of these brain areas and their interconnections forms the foundation of years of neurobiological research on the brain. If the study of brain activity with fMRI is going to make a meaningful contribution to this knowledge base, then localizing signal changes to discrete brain areas within a subject and across subjects is paramount. To do so requires high image resolution and neuroanatomical fidelity. Many brain areas in a segmented rat atlas have in-plane boundaries of less than 400 μm^2

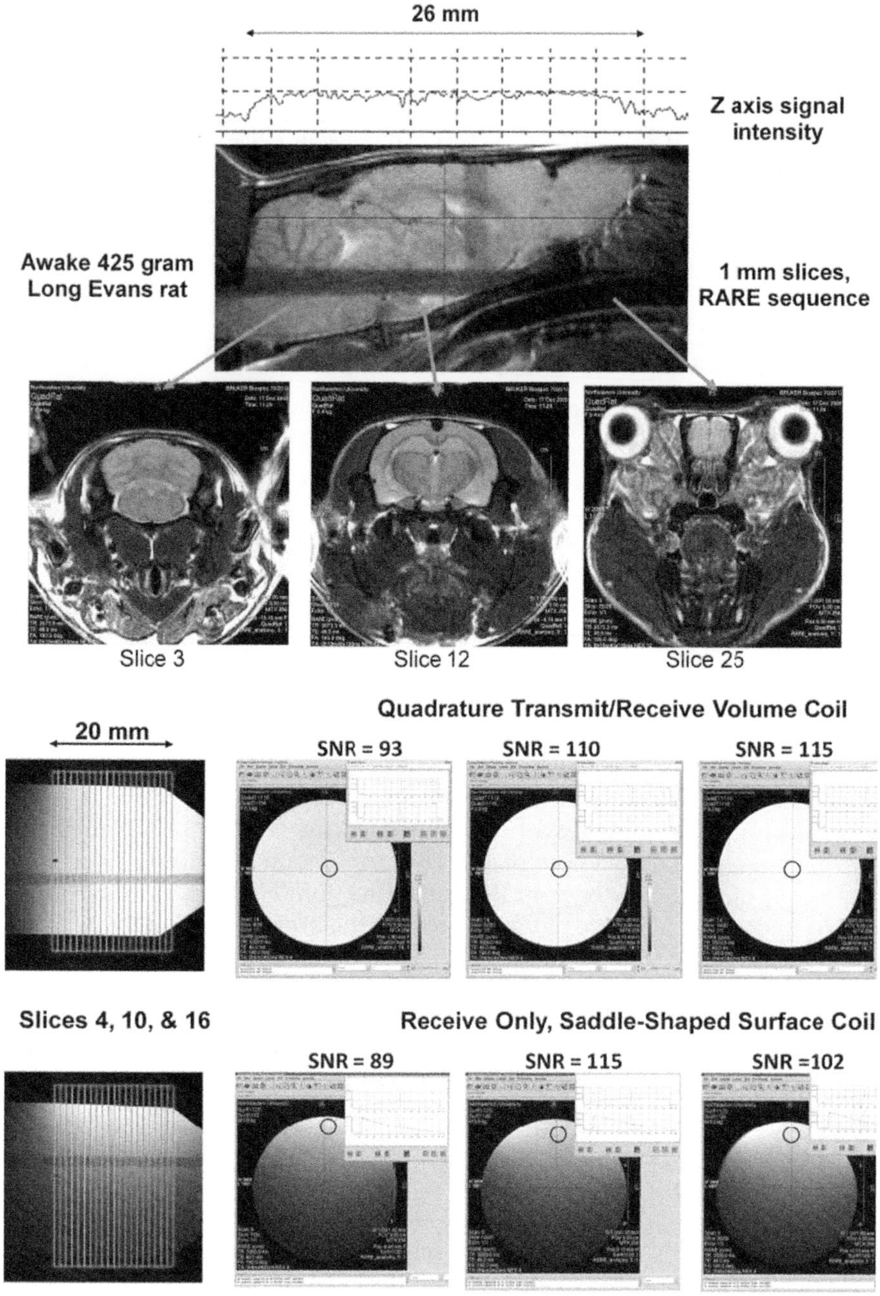

FIGURE 3.5 **Brain coverage and homogeneity.** The top image provides a sagittal view of a rat brain. Note the linearity along the *Z* axis. The three axial images from a 26-slice spin echo sequence (1 mm thickness) demonstrate complete brain coverage from the olfactory bulbs to the brainstem. The bottom panels compare image homogeneity using a quadrature transmit and receive volume coil (top) versus a surface coil (bottom).

and may extend for over 1000 μm in the rostral-caudal plane. With the advent of segmented, annotated 3D MRI atlases for rodents, it is now possible to localize functional imaging data to precise 3D "volumes of interest" in clearly delineated brain areas. Therefore, it is critical that the images are a very accurate reconstruction of the original brain.

While there are many things that contribute to image fidelity, one of the most important is the choice of pulse sequence. Choosing a pulse sequence that reflects the time course of the hemodynamic changes characteristic of the BOLD signal (Figure 3.6) together with high neuroanatomical fidelity and spatial resolution is key to a successful imaging study. There are two basic pulse sequences used in fMRI: gradient-echo echo planar imaging (EPI) and fast spin echo. The major advantages to a gradient-echo EPI are rapid image acquisition, a low specific absorption ratio (SAR), a measure of heat deposition, and high sensitivity to magnetic susceptibility with T_2* weighting contributing to an enhanced BOLD signal at low field strengths ($\leq$200 MHz). However, the major drawback to a

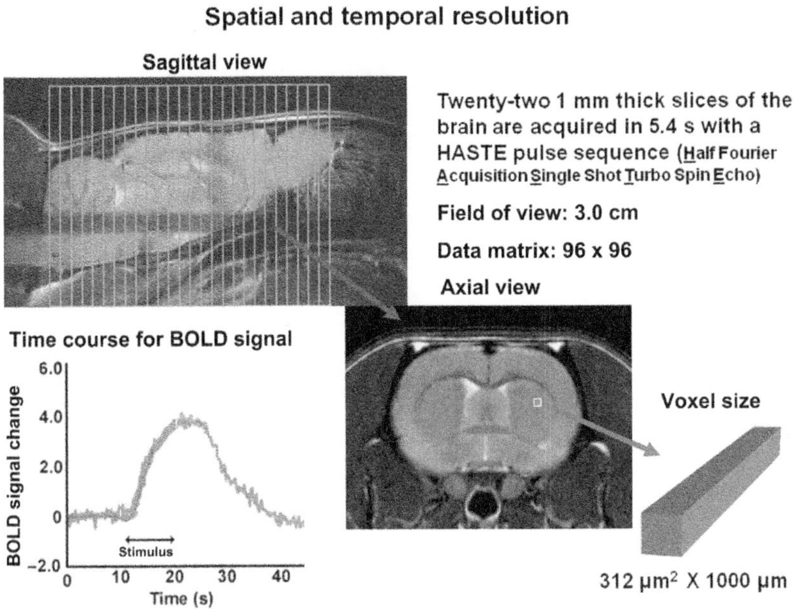

FIGURE 3.6 **Spatial and temporal resolution.** Shown in the top panel is a slice selection array on a sagittal view of the brain. Twenty-two slices of 1 mm thickness can be acquired in less than 6 s. A FOV of 3.0 cm and data matrix of 96 × 96 give an in-plane voxel dimension of 312 × 312 μm. With these parameters, there are approximately 17,000 voxels in the brain volume. Shown is an insert of BOLD signal change occurring over a 40 s time course.[35] These hemodynamic changes are within the temporal window of the image acquisition.

gradient-echo sequence is image distortion around the air-filled sinuses (Figure 3.7) and geometric distortion and in-plane susceptibility artifacts due to long EPI readouts. Spin echo EPI can reduce many of the issues associated with field inhomogeneity and susceptibility artifacts, but cannot provide the needed neuroanatomical fidelity over the entire brain needed to co-register data sets from multiple subjects for group statistics on hundreds of 3D brain areas.

The major advantage to a spin echo pulse sequence is its tolerance to magnetic susceptibility and motion artifact (Figure 3.7). The 180° RF refocusing pulse corrects for the lack of field homogeneity, chemical shift, tissue artifacts, and magnetic susceptibility from static dephasing in BOLD imaging. The disadvantage is loss of signal contrast and high SAR. The problem of sensitivity can be addressed with higher field strengths where the BOLD signal becomes a function of dynamic dephasing from the diffusion of water at the level of the capillaries.[38,39] Using multislice, fast spin echo sequences, the signal contrast with BOLD imaging is a function of T_2 and not T_2* at high field strengths. The extravascular signal surrounding capillary beds and small vessels is more reflective of the metabolic changes in brain parenchyma than a signal from large draining veins in helping to improve the localization of the signal changes.[22] The BOLD signal is linear and reproducible at stimulus intervals of 1 s.[40]

To achieve these goals, we developed a multislice, single-shot, fast spin echo pulse sequence using a partial

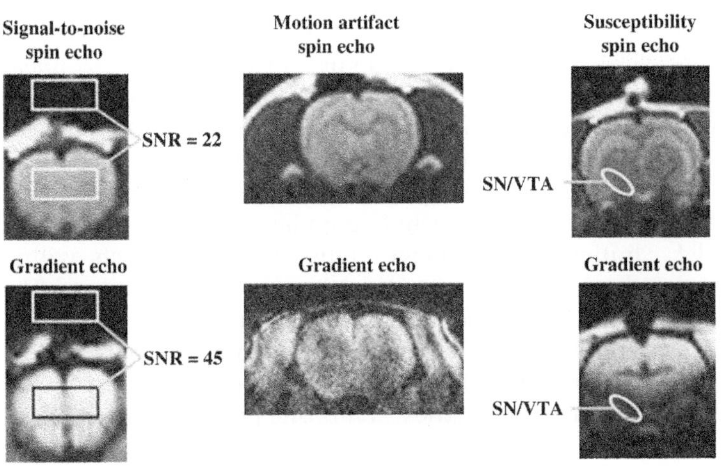

FIGURE 3.7 **Spin echo versus gradient echo.** Shown are magnetic resonance images highlighting the advantages and disadvantages of spin echo and gradient echo pulse sequences. All images were collected from the same animal over the same imaging session. Susceptibility artifact is very pronounced in the substantia nigra (SN) and ventral tegmental area (VTA). SNR: signal-to-noise ratio.[37]

Fourier acquisition with a 9/16 ratio. Sequences of this type are given the name HASTE (half-Fourier acquisition, single-shot, turbo spin echo). With this sequence, it is possible to collect 22 axial slices that are 1 mm thick in less than 6 s. With a FOV of 3.0 cm and a data matrix of 96 × 96, the in-plane pixel resolution is 312 μm^2 (Figure 3.6).

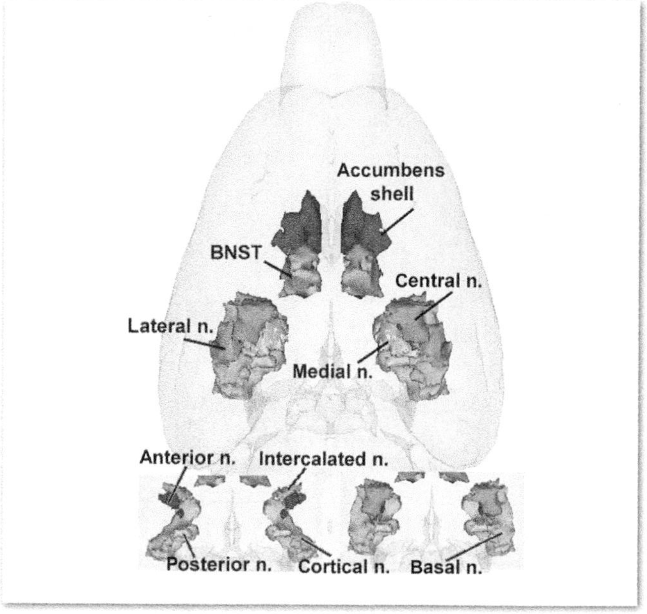

FIGURE 3.8 **Amygdala in 3D.** The image shows a translucent shell of the brain with the location of different subregions of the amygdala depicted in color as 3D volumes. (The figure is reproduced in color section.)

DATA ANALYSIS

Within-Group Statistics

Region of interest–based statistical analyses are done using medical image visualization and analysis software. Anatomy images for each subject are obtained at a resolution of $256^2 \times 22$ slices and a FOV of 3.0 cm with a slice thickness of 1.0 mm. Subsequent functional imaging is performed at a resolution of $96^2 \times 22$ slices with the same FOV and slice thickness. Each subject is registered to a segmented and annotated 3D MRI rat brain atlas. Details of the alignment of scans to the rat brain atlas have been published elsewhere.[9]

The fully segmented 3D rat brain atlas has the potential to delineate and analyze 152 distinct anatomical volumes within the brain. Because the in-plane spatial resolution of our functional scans (data matrix: 96 × 96; FOV: 3.0 cm) is 312 μm^2 with a depth of 1000 μm, many small brain areas (e.g. the nucleus of the lateral olfactory tract) cannot be resolved; or, if they could be resolved, they would be represented by one or two voxels only. Consequently, small detailed regions are not included in the analysis or are grouped into larger "minor volumes" of similar anatomical classification. For example, we list the basal nucleus of the amygdala as a minor volume (Figure 3.8). This area is a composition of the anterior and posterior basomedial amygdala and the anterior and posterior basolateral amygdala. In addition, we group brain areas into "major volumes" (e.g. the amygdala, hippocampus, hypothalamus, and cerebrum) (Figure 3.8). The volume of activation (number of significant voxels) can be visualized in these 3D major and minor anatomical groupings. We also combined minor volumes to form functional neuroanatomical pathways such as the habenular system as shown in Figure 3.9.

Scanning sessions can last from 10 min to over an hour. The control window is usually the first 5 min with 50 scan repetitions (6 s/acquisition). Statistical t tests are performed on each voxel (c. 15,000 in number) of each subject within their original coordinate system. The baseline threshold is set at 2% based on data showing that BOLD signal changes above this threshold are reliably above noise levels for awake rat imaging.[41] The t test statistics use a 95% confidence level, two-tailed distributions, and heteroscedastic variance assumptions. As a result of the multiple t test analyses performed, a false-positive detection controlling mechanism is introduced.[42] This subsequent filter guarantees that, on average, the false-positive detection rate is below our cutoff of 0.05. These analysis settings provided conservative estimates for significance. Those pixels deemed statistically significant retain their percentage change values (stimulation mean minus control mean) relative to the control mean. All other pixel values are set to zero.

A statistical composite is created for each group of subjects. The individual analyses are summed within groups. The composite statistics are built using the inverse transformation matrices. Each composite pixel location (i.e. row, column, and slice), premultiplied by $[Ti]^{-1}$, maps it within a voxel of subject (i). A tri-linear interpolation of the subject's voxel values (percentage change) determined the statistical contribution of subject (i) to the composite (row, column, and slice) location. The use of $[Ti]^{-1}$ ensured that the full volume set of the composite is populated with subject contributions. The average value from all subjects within the group determines the composite value. The BOLD response maps of the composite are somewhat broader in their spatial coverage than in an individual subject, so only the average number of activated pixels that have the highest composite percent change values in a particular ROI is displayed in the composite map.

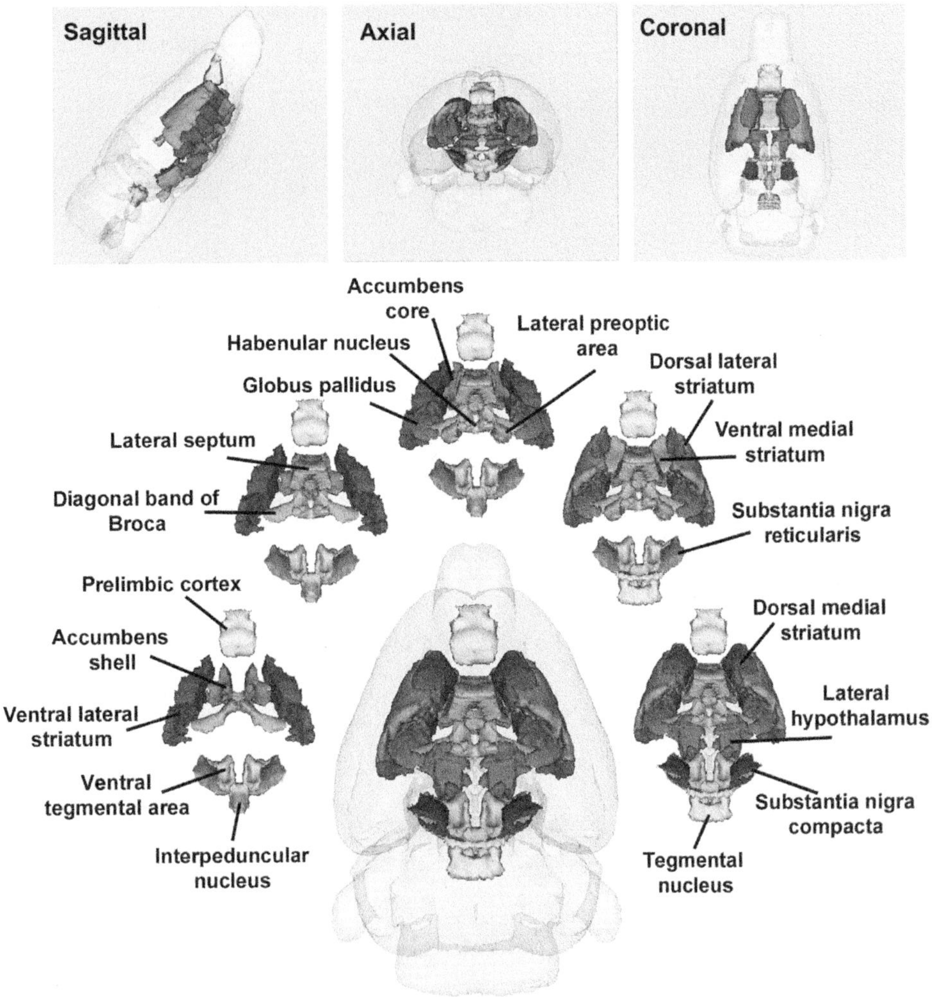

FIGURE 3.9 **Habenular system.** The central image is a coronal view of a translucent shell of the brain, showing the total composite and location of different subregions of the habenular system depicted in color as 3D volumes. Surrounding this are different layers of the habenular system showing a caudal (deepest)-to-dorsal perspective to enable identification of all subregions. The panels on the top show the habenular system in different orthogonal directions. (The figure is reproduced in color section.)

The composite percent change for the time history graphs for each region is based on the weighted average of each subject, as follows:

$$\text{Composite Percent Change} = \frac{\sum_{i=1}^{N} \text{Activated Pixel Subject}(i) \times \text{Percent Change}(i)}{\text{Activated Composite Pixels}}$$

where N is the number of subjects.

Between-Group Statistics

For the first stage of the fMRI analyses (described in this chapter), summary statistics per ROI for each individual functional scan are calculated independently. Activation maps are created for subjects and, as noted here, each map contributes to the composite maps shown in Figure 3.17. The initial analysis provides values of percent change in the BOLD signal for each of 152 ROIs and activated voxel numbers (representative of the volume of activity) (Figure 3.10). Although the number of animals per group are usually equal, we assumed that the data were nonnormally distributed or heteroscedastic and therefore used nonparametric statistical testing. Statistical differences between drug doses or experimental conditions are determined using Newman–Keuls multiple comparisons test (alpha value was set at 5%) (Figure 3.10). Tests are done separately for each ROI. Significant differences for the multiple comparisons tests are summarized in the bar graphs. BOLD signal changes over time (Figure 3.10) are compared between experimental groups using a repeated ANOVA followed by a Bonferroni test.

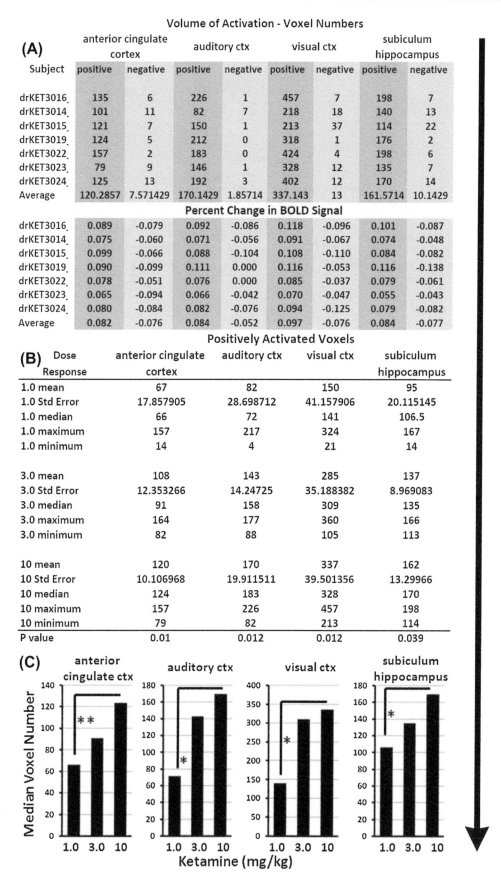

(A) Volume of Activation - Voxel Numbers

Subject	anterior cingulate cortex positive	anterior cingulate cortex negative	auditory ctx positive	auditory ctx negative	visual ctx positive	visual ctx negative	subiculum hippocampus positive	subiculum hippocampus negative
drKET3016_	135	6	226	1	457	7	198	7
drKET3014_	101	11	82	7	218	18	140	13
drKET3015_	121	7	150	1	213	37	114	22
drKET3019_	124	5	212	0	318	1	176	2
drKET3022_	157	2	183	0	424	4	198	6
drKET3023_	79	9	146	1	328	12	135	7
drKET3024_	125	13	192	3	402	12	170	14
Average	120.2857	7.571429	170.1429	1.85714	337.143	13	161.5714	10.1429

Percent Change in BOLD Signal

Subject	anterior cingulate cortex positive	anterior cingulate cortex negative	auditory ctx positive	auditory ctx negative	visual ctx positive	visual ctx negative	subiculum hippocampus positive	subiculum hippocampus negative
drKET3016_	0.089	-0.079	0.092	-0.086	0.118	-0.096	0.101	-0.087
drKET3014_	0.075	-0.060	0.071	-0.056	0.091	-0.067	0.074	-0.048
drKET3015_	0.099	-0.066	0.088	-0.104	0.108	-0.110	0.084	-0.082
drKET3019_	0.090	-0.099	0.111	0.000	0.116	-0.053	0.116	-0.138
drKET3022_	0.078	-0.051	0.076	0.000	0.085	-0.037	0.079	-0.061
drKET3023_	0.065	-0.094	0.066	-0.042	0.070	-0.047	0.055	-0.043
drKET3024_	0.080	-0.084	0.082	-0.076	0.094	-0.125	0.079	-0.082
Average	0.082	-0.076	0.084	-0.052	0.097	-0.076	0.084	-0.077

(B) Positively Activated Voxels

Dose Response	anterior cingulate cortex	auditory ctx	visual ctx	subiculum hippocampus
1.0 mean	67	82	150	95
1.0 Std Error	17.857905	28.698712	41.157906	20.115145
1.0 median	66	72	141	106.5
1.0 maximum	157	217	324	167
1.0 minimum	14	4	21	14
3.0 mean	108	143	285	137
3.0 Std Error	12.353266	14.24725	35.188382	8.969083
3.0 median	91	158	309	135
3.0 maximum	164	177	360	166
3.0 minimum	82	88	105	113
10 mean	120	170	337	162
10 Std Error	10.106968	19.911511	39.501356	13.29966
10 median	124	183	328	170
10 maximum	157	226	457	198
10 minimum	79	82	213	114
P value	0.01	0.012	0.012	0.039

(C)

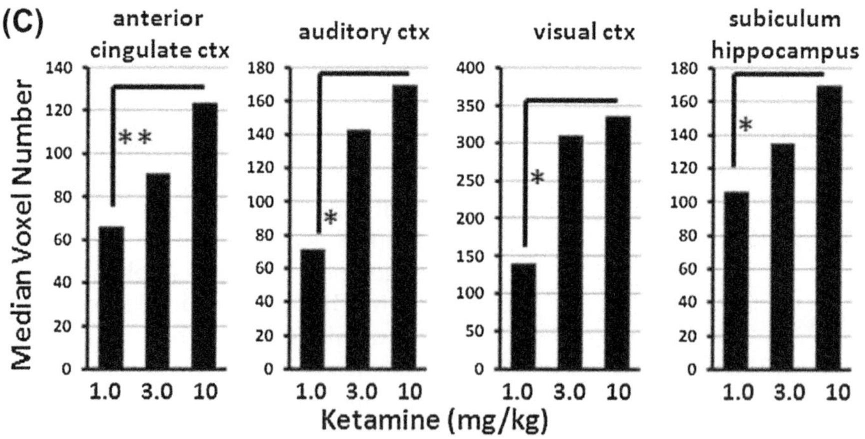

FIGURE 3.10 **Analysis.** Shown is an example of the data generated for each subject in a study (A), the results from a multiple comparisons test (B), and the presentation of these results as bar graphs (C). The top of panel A lists the different subjects in a study (far-left column), and this is followed by the volume of activation (i.e. a significant number of positive and negative voxels in four of 152 regions of interest that have been identified in the 3D, segmented, rat atlas). The bottom of panel A again lists the same subjects followed by their significant percent change in BOLD signal intensity, both positive and negative. Panel B shows both parametric (mean and standard error) and nonparametric (medium,

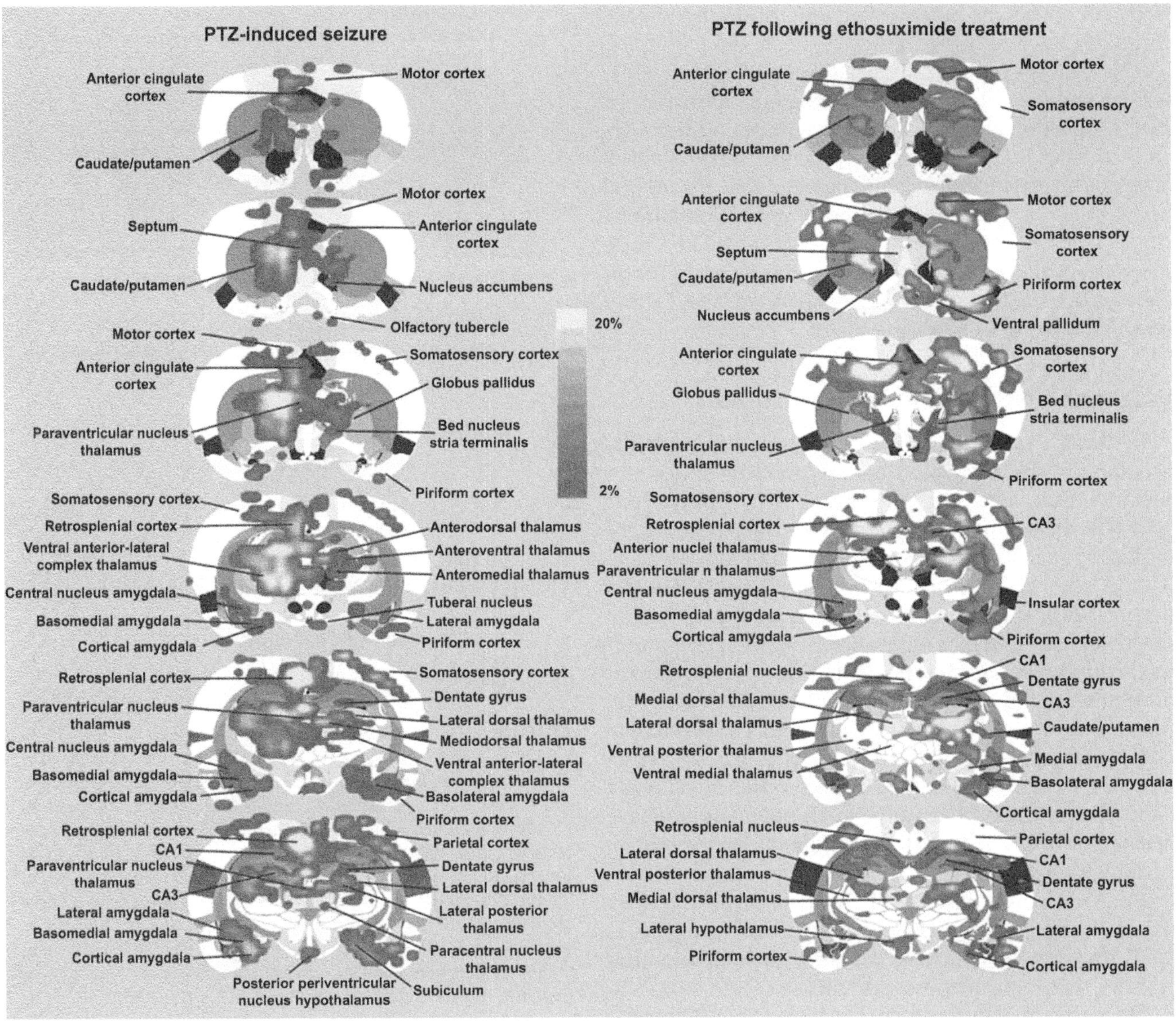

FIGURE 3.11 **Pentylenetetrazol-induced seizure.** Shown in the left column is the pattern of PTZ-induced changes in BOLD signal before seizure onset (first 30 s after PTZ injection). The right column is the pattern of PTZ-induced activity in the presence of ethosuximide (ESM). The composite map of all subjects ($n = 5$ in each group) is shown registered to six contiguous coronal sections of the segmented atlas. The scale bar shows the percentage change in BOLD signal intensity. *Source: Adapted from Ref. 43.* (The figure is reproduced in color section.)

AWAKE SEIZURE STUDIES

Pentylenetetrazol-Induced Seizure

Pentylenetetrazol (PTZ)-induced seizure in rats, a relevant model of human absence epilepsy and of generalized tonic-clonic epilepsy, can be used to stimulate seizure activity within 30 s of administration while collecting continuous, high-resolution, multislice images at subsecond intervals. In these studies, we developed a model giving PTZ directly into the lateral cerebroventricle to stimulate seizure activity in awake rats while collecting images from the forebrain at 4.7 T.[43] Ethosuximide (ESM), a commonly used antiepileptic, was used to block seizure activity (Figure 3.11).

Within 2–4 s of PTZ administration, a rapid increase in BOLD signal intensity is noted in the thalamus, especially the anterior thalamic nuclei. Activity in the anterior thalamus peaks c. 15 s before seizure onset and is more than twofold greater than that in all other individual thalamic areas. The retrosplenial cortex shows a twofold greater increase in activity as compared with other cortical areas, also peaking at c. 15 s. The dentate gyrus is twice as active as other hippocampal areas but peaks just before seizure onset. Treatment with ESM blocks seizures, decreasing PTZ-induced activation in most

minimum, and maximum) results of a multiple comparisons test of three different doses of a drug plus vehicle for volume of activation in four of 152 brain regions. The data from three of these brain areas (medial dorsal striatum, medial dorsal thalamus, and ventral CA1 of the hippocampus) are shown in panel C as bar graphs of the medium number of voxels. The numbers in parentheses above each bar are the minimum and maximum voxel number with significant differences between doses as noted. $^*p < 0.05$; $^{**}p < 0.01$. (For color version of this figure, the reader is referred to the online version of this book.)

forebrain areas. The anterior thalamus and retrosplenial cortex are essentially blocked by pretreatment with ESM.

This study on PTZ-induced general clonic-tonic seizure shows that the anterior thalamus, retrosplenial cortex, and dentate gyrus present with the greatest increases in BOLD signal activity before seizure onset. Neurons in these areas may contribute to the neural network controlling the initiation of generalized tonic-clonic seizure. While this model was useful to study the genesis of seizure activity, the accompanying motor convulsions after seizure onset precluded any further imaging because of motion artifact.

γ-Butyrolactone-Induced Seizure in Rats

In these experiments, we examined the feasibility of studying the integrated neural circuitry of absence seizures using fMRI in awake rats.[11] γ-hydroxybutyric acid (GHB) is a naturally occurring metabolite of the inhibitory neurotransmitter γ-aminobutyric acid (GABA). Normal rats given an intraperitoneal (IP) injection of GHB will show all the behavioral and electrophysiological signs of generalized absence seizure.[44] Interestingly, γ-butyrolactone (GBL), the precursor molecule to GHB, can induce absence seizure with better reproducibility, predictability, and rapidity of onset than GHB itself. Whereas it might take as much as 20 min after IP injection of GHB to induce absence seizures, GBL can produce bilaterally synchronous spike-wave discharges (SWDs) within 2–5 min of its peripheral administration (see Figure 3.12), along with behavioral arrest, facial myoclonus, and vibrissal twitching (39). Again, these experiments involved BOLD imaging at 4.7 T. Imaging was performed before, during, and after absence seizure induction with GBL.

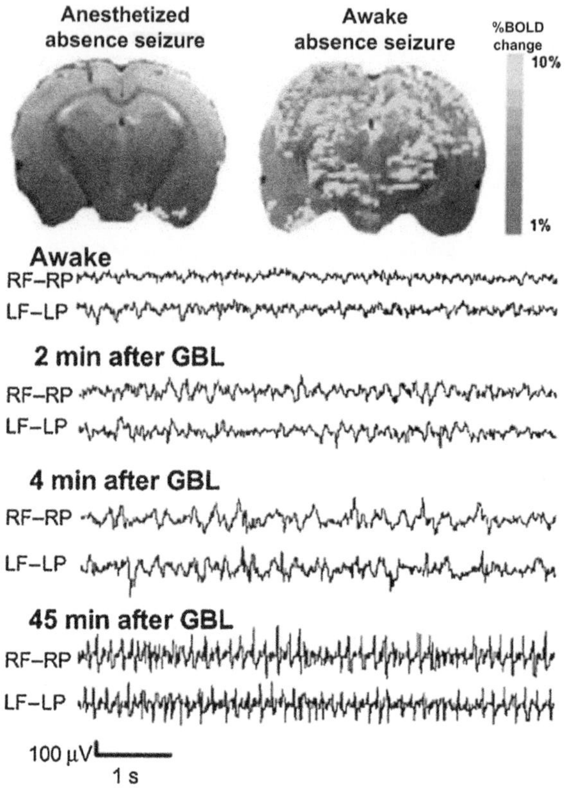

FIGURE 3.12 **γ-Butyrolactone-induced seizure in rats.** The top left image shows BOLD signal changes in a rat experiencing an absence seizure while continuously anesthetized with 2% isoflurane. The top right image shows BOLD signal changes in a rat experiencing an absence seizure but not anesthetized. The bottom traces show representative data from an EEG recording collected during the functional magnetic resonance imaging experiment. Nonmagnetic epidural electrodes were placed in the frontal and parietal cortices to monitor seizure activity during the imaging session. Placement of electrode leads is labeled. RF: right frontal cortex; RP: right parietal cortex; LF: left frontal cortex; LP: left parietal cortex. *Source: Adapted from Ref. 11.* (The figure is reproduced in color section.)

The corticothalamic circuitry, critical for SWD formation in absence seizure, shows robust BOLD signal changes after GBL administration, consistent with electroencephalographic (EEG) recordings in the same animals. Predominantly positive BOLD changes occur in the thalamus. Sensory and parietal cortices show mixed positive and negative BOLD changes, whereas temporal and motor cortices show only negative BOLD changes.

Genetic Model of Absence Seizures

Genetic rat models of absence epilepsy have been studied for many years and are thought to mimic more accurately the spontaneous seizures of human epilepsy than do drug-induced animal models as demonstrated in our GBL studies. How dissimilar are the patterns of brain activation between the chemical and genetic models? This, in part, was our motivation for these experiments.[10] We studied a strain of rats named WAG/Rij that are inbred for absence-like characteristics and exhibit spontaneous SWDs that have a frequency of 7–11 Hz, which is not unlike that induced by GBL treatment.[45] In these experiments, we used EEG-triggered BOLD fMRI to study the pattern of brain activation during spontaneous SWDs. We continuously monitored the EEG of WAG/Rij while in the magnet and manually triggered image acquisition on identifying seizure-related EEG changes. This procedure is possible because of the delay between the change in metabolic activity associated with neuronal activity and the increase in blood flow.[35] Again, BOLD imaging was done on a 4.7 T scanner.

Significant positive BOLD activation was found in the thalamus, including the nucleus reticularis, ventral posteromedial and posterolateral nuclei, posterior nuclei, and mediodorsal nuclei. Significant positive BOLD also was found throughout the cortex, including the sensory, parietal, and temporal cortices. The pattern of brain activation was very similar to that observed in the GBH model, with a predominant change in the thalamic and cortical areas reflecting the underlying functional connectivity that is characteristic of absence seizures (Figure 3.13).

GBL-Induced Seizure in Monkeys

The key diagnostic feature of an absence seizure in humans is a 3 Hz SWD. Unfortunately, in our chemical and genetic models of absence seizure, the SWD was 11–12 Hz. This raises the possibility that the neural mechanisms of absence across mammalian species are different, thus reducing the translational significance of rodent imaging. This was the key motivation behind our efforts to develop an absence seizure model in nonhuman primates. To this end, we treated adult male marmoset monkeys (*Callithrix jacchus*) with GBL to induce prolonged absence seizures, and the resulting SWDs were analyzed to determine their similarity to the 3 Hz SWDs that characterize the disorder in humans.[12] Again, BOLD fMRI at 4.7 T was used for these studies.

EEG recordings during imaging showed 3 Hz SWDs typical of human absence seizures (Figure 3.14). This synchronized EEG pattern started within 15–20 min of drug administration and persisted for >60 min. In addition, pretreatment with the antiepileptic drug ESM blocked the behavioral and EEG changes caused by GBL. Changes in BOLD signal intensity in the thalamus and sensorimotor cortex correlated with the onset of 3 Hz SWDs (Figure 3.15). The change in BOLD signal intensity was bilateral but heterogeneous, affecting some brain areas more than others. Because typical absence seizures last seconds, the current model is more applicable to absence status epilepticus. Whereas positive BOLD activation in the corticothalamic circuit correlates with electrophysiologic recordings of structures contributing to SWD formation, the hippocampus, a structure where SWDs have not previously been recorded, showed positive BOLD signal in this study.

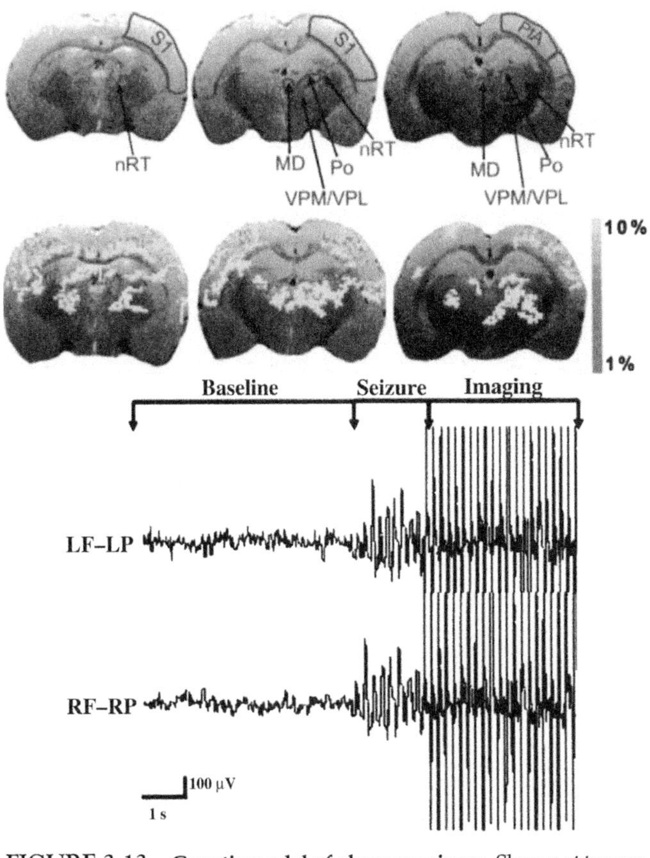

FIGURE 3.13 **Genetic model of absence seizure.** Shown at top are representative BOLD activation maps of three consecutive axial sections of the rat brain during spontaneous spike-and-wave discharges from a single subject. The top row shows the regions of interest used for analysis. MD: mediodorsal thalamic nuclei; nRT: nucleus reticularis thalami; Po: posterior thalamic nuclear group; PtA: parietal association cortex; S1: sensory cortex; Te: temporal cortex; VPM and VPL: ventral posteromedial and posterolateral thalamic nucleus. At the bottom are representative EEG recordings collected during the imaging session. Nonmagnetic epidural electrodes were placed in the frontal and parietal cortices to monitor seizure activity during the imaging session. Normal, awake EEG was present during baseline imaging. Imaging was triggered after the formation of epileptiform activity similar to that shown during the seizure period. Artifact due to image acquisition can be seen with a delay of ~2 s after seizure activity. RF: right frontal cortex; RP: right parietal cortex; LF: left frontal cortex; LP: left parietal cortex. *Source: Adapted from Ref. 10.* (The figure is reproduced in color section.)

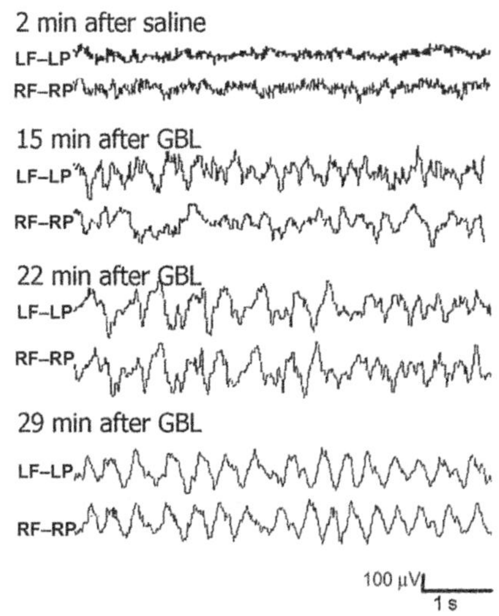

FIGURE 3.14 **γ-Butyrolactone-induced 3 Hz SWD in monkeys.** Shown is a representative EEG recording collected during an imaging session. Nonmagnetic subdermal needle electrodes were placed in the scalp over the frontal and parietal cortices to monitor seizure activity during the imaging session. Placement of electrode leads is labeled. RF: right frontal cortex; RP: right parietal cortex; LF: left frontal cortex; LP: left parietal cortex. *Source: Adapted from Ref. 12.*

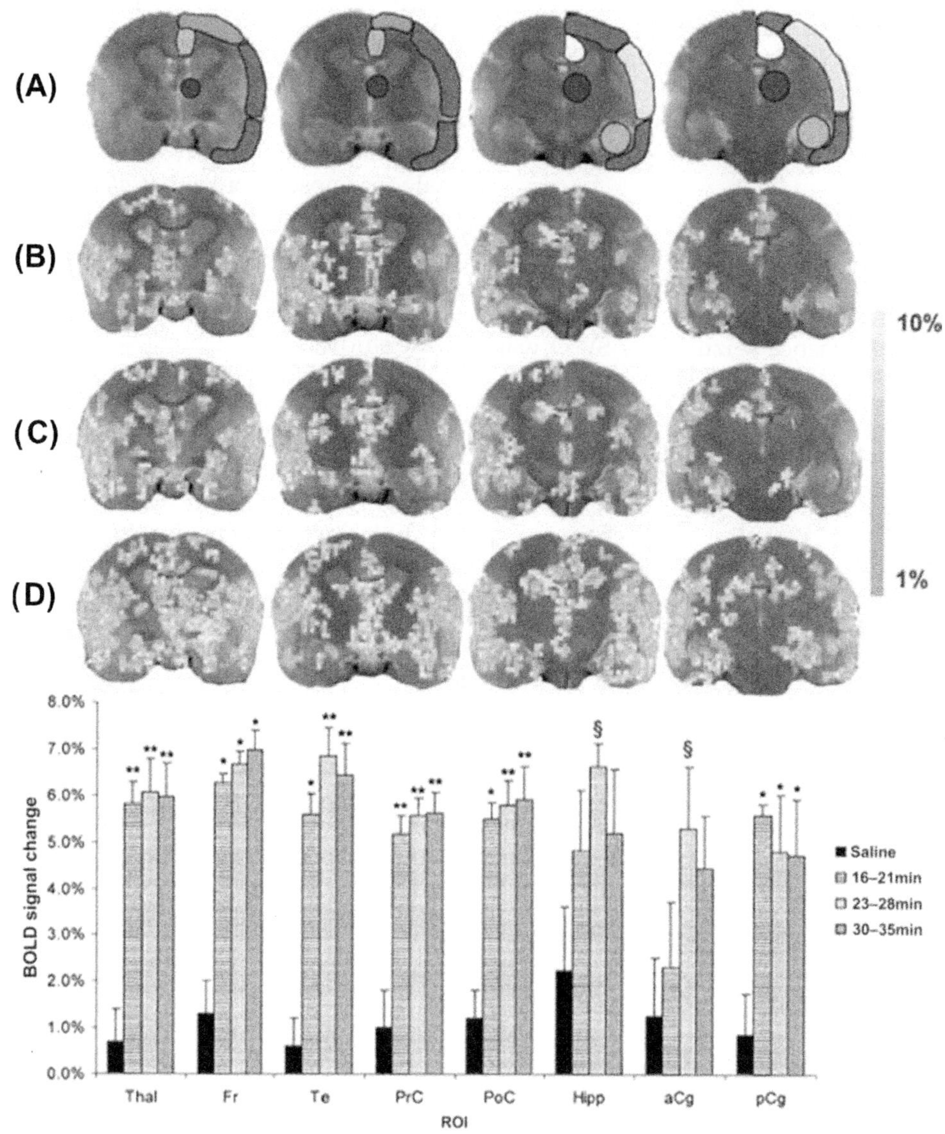

FIGURE 3.15 **γ-Butyrolactone-induced seizure activity in monkeys.** Activation maps of blood oxygenation level–dependent (BOLD) signal responses during absence seizure. The colored pixels indicate the statistically significant ($p < 0.05$) pixels, which are determined by t test analysis and overlaid onto the corresponding anatomy. Four consecutive slices through the brain are shown for an individual marmoset. (A) Anatomic images, with regions of interest used for analysis outlined according to the following color code: thalamus (blue), hippocampus (orange), frontal cortex (red), temporal cortex (purple), precentral cortex (green), postcentral cortex (yellow), anterior cingulate cortex (light blue), and posterior cingulate cortex (white). (B–D) Activation corresponding to images collected 16–21 min, 23–28 min, and 30–35 min after γ-butyrolactone injection, respectively. Change in blood-oxygen-level–dependent (BOLD) signal intensity for each region of interest (ROI). The BOLD signal intensity change during 3 Hz spike-wave discharges is shown for cortical and subcortical ROIs (mean ± SEM, $N = 5$ marmosets). Signal changes after the control injection of saline are shown, along with signal changes occurring 16–21 min, 23–28 min, and 30–35 min after the γ-butyrolactone injection. Time blocks with significantly different signal changes from the control injection are noted (§$p < 0.05$, *$p < 0.01$, **$p < 0.001$). All ROIs are bilateral structures, so the signal changes from each hemisphere were combined. Thal: thalamus; Fr: frontal cortex; Te: temporal cortex; PrC: precentral cortex; PoC: postcentral cortex; Hipp: hippocampus; aCg: anterior cingulate cortex; pCg: posterior cingulate cortex. *Source: Adapted from Ref. 12.* (The figure is reproduced in color section.)

GBL-Induced Seizure in Rats: Tract Tracing with Manganese Chloride

To better elucidate the neuroanatomy responsible for the behavioral and EEG effects of the GBL-induced seizures, we undertook manganese-enhanced MRI (data unpublished). Mn^{2+} is a calcium analog and MR contrast agent that has been used to noninvasively visualize calcium-dependent neural activities. A unique property of Mn^{2+} is that, once internalized, it is transported transynaptically via functional connections of neurons. We hypothesize that a cortical microinjection

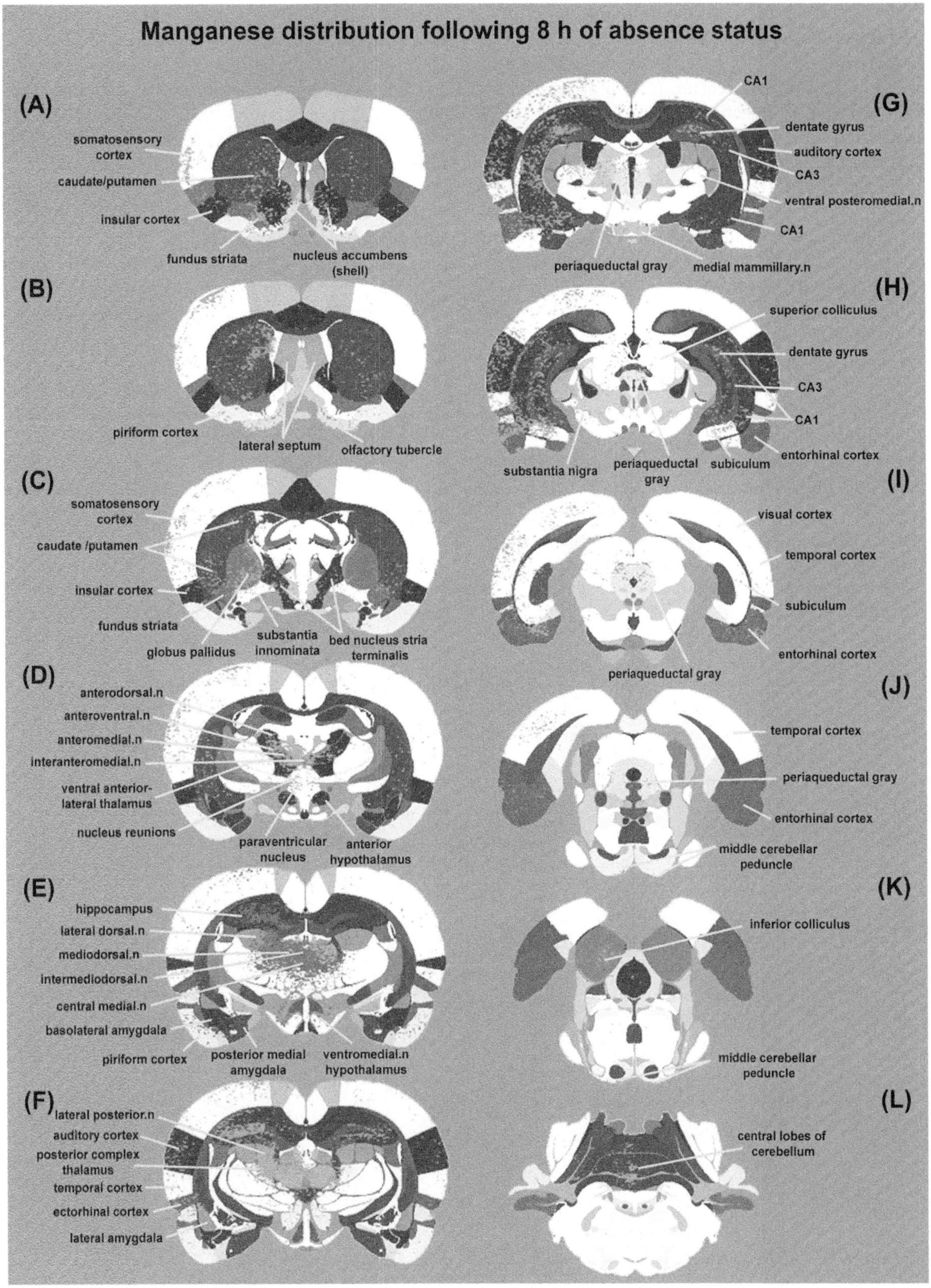

FIGURE 3.16 **Manganese distribution with absence status epilepticus.** Areas with increased signal intensity due to the presence of manganese are shown above as red dots. The serial brain sections are taken from a single rat and are representative of the distribution pattern observed in all animals studied. (The figure is reproduced in color section.)

of Mn^{2+} in rats, during an absence seizure, will "highlight" the neurons in this circuit.

Male rats were stereotaxically implanted with a cannula in the somatosensory cortex (peri-oral area). Rats were then given an IP injection of vehicle or 200 mg/kg GBL (used to induce the absence seizure). Five minutes after GBL or vehicle administration, rats were microinjected with 100 nl of 100 mM $MnCl_2$ into the somatosensory cortex. The SWDs characterizing the seizure were maintained for 8 h by repeated injections of GBL to allow sufficient transport of the Mn^{2+}. Rats were then transcardially perfused with formaldehyde, and brains were removed for imaging. All images were acquired using a 9.4 T small-bore magnet. T_1-weighted images were acquired using a spin echo sequence (TR = 150 ms; TE = 4.5 ms; 256 × 512; FOV = 22 × 22 mm; slice thickness = 0.75 mm, averages = 46). Images were registered to the 3D segmented rat atlas.

The anticipated cortical-thalamic loop critical in the generation and maintenance of the 3 Hz SWDs characteristic of absence seizures is labeled (Figure 3.16). Much of the activity was lateralized to the site of the Mn^{2+} injection. One of the most interesting observations is the paucity of labeling in the reticular nucleus of the thalamus. This area is critical in the neural circuitry of absence seizures, having a reciprocal relationship with most dorsal thalamic nuclei but not the cortex. Instead, areas like the nucleus accumbens, bed nucleus of the stria terminalis, olfactory tubercles, septum, hypothalamic nuclei, periaqueductal gray, and hippocampus showed high levels of labeling. Indeed, the most compelling concentration of Mn^{2+} outside the thalamus was in the hippocampus. The anterior thalamic nuclei and medial dorsal (MD) and lateral dorsal (LD) thalamic areas are considered principle limbic nuclei because of their connections with the hippocampus and amygdala.

To complement these manganese studies, we repeated our earlier work with BOLD imaging but with a more detailed 3D segmented rat atlas and advanced RF electronics that enabled us to better image the distributed integrated neural circuits by including the brainstem and cerebellum as shown in Figure 3.17. These data are not unlike those generated with manganese labeling, even though the manganese is several hours of absence status, while the BOLD images were acquired 30 min post GBL administration. The reticular nucleus did show some activation, as seen in Figure 3.17(D). Interestingly, the somatosensory cortex showed high activation, but the labeling was in deeper cortical layers and not along the

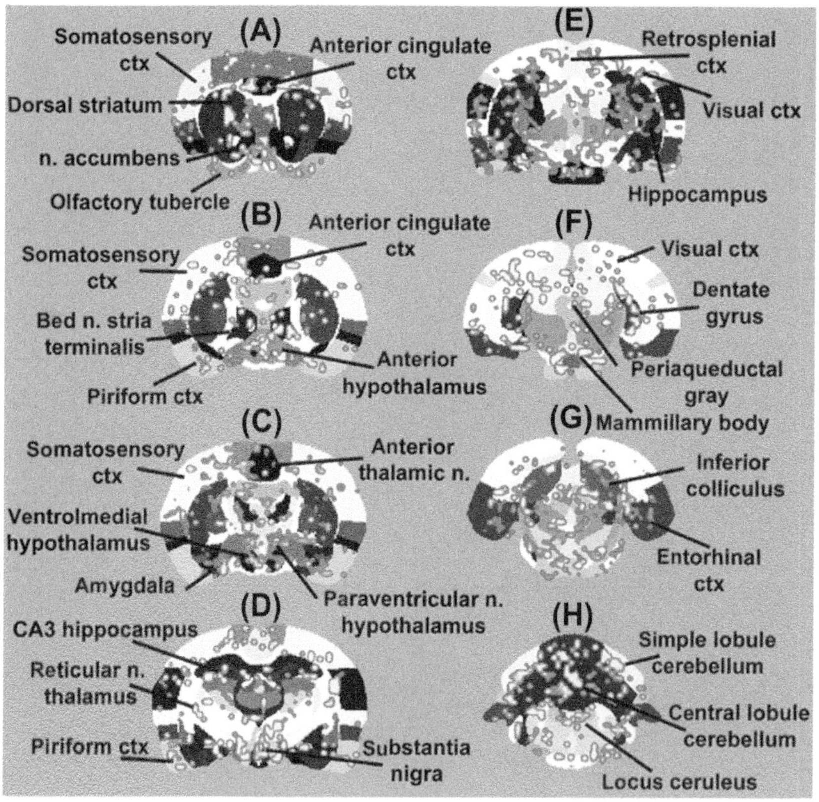

FIGURE 3.17 **BOLD imaging following γ-butyrolactone.** Shown are activation maps of positive BOLD signal registered to axial sections of the 3D MRI rat atlas. The red-yellow depicts the localization of significantly activated and interpolated voxels that exceed a 2% threshold above baseline. The data are the significant change over baseline as an average of five animals. (The figure is reproduced in color section.)

most superficial cortex, as shown with manganese. The cerebellum showed high levels of BOLD activation.

SUMMARY

Advances in the development of RF electronics, pulse sequences, 3D MRI atlases, data analysis tools, and provocation paradigms are helping to make awake-animal imaging an important method in neuroscience research. Although fMRI does not have the cellular or spatial resolution of immunostaining for immediate early genes, or the millisecond temporal resolution of electrophysiology, it does provide a global perspective of changing brain function that fits the temporal window of hemodynamic coupling to areas of enhanced metabolism. The neuroanatomical fidelity within and across animals makes it possible to reconstruct distributed, integrated neural circuits or fingerprints that are characteristic of seizure activity. Thus, fMRI in awake animals provides a systems approach to the study of the brain, complementing and building on other neurobiological techniques to understand how neural circuits are organized and integrated across multiple brain regions.

Abbreviations

fMRI functional magnetic resonance imaging
FOV field of view
SPM statistical parametric mapping
AIR automatic image registration
AFNI analysis of functional neuroimages
CBF cerebral blood flow
RF radiofrequency
SNR signal-to-noise ratio
B_1 magnetic field associated with radiofrequency pulse
B_0 main static magnetic field
BOLD blood oxygen level dependent
EPI echo planar imaging
SAR specific absorption ratio
T_2^* time constant for apparent transverse relaxation
T_2 time constant for transverse relaxation
ROI region of interest
ANOVA analysis of variance
HASTE half-Fourier acquisition, single-shot, turbo spin echo
MIVA medical image visualization and analysis

References

1. Lothman EW, Hatlelid JM, Zorumski CF. Functional mapping of limbic seizures originating in the hippocampus: a combined 2-deoxyglucose and electrophysiologic study. *Brain Res.* 1985; 360(1–2):92–100.
2. McIntyre DC, Gilby KL. Mapping seizure pathways in the temporal lobe. *Epilepsia.* 2008;49(Suppl. 3):23–30.
3. Akiyama K, Ishikawa M, Saito A. mRNA expression of activity-regulated cytoskeleton-associated protein (arc) in the amygdala-kindled rats. *Brain Res.* 2008;1189:236–246.
4. Peng Z, Houser CR. Temporal patterns of fos expression in the dentate gyrus after spontaneous seizures in a mouse model of temporal lobe epilepsy. *J Neurosci.* 2005;25(31):7210–7220.
5. Storey TW, et al. Age-dependent differences in flurothyl-induced c-fos and c-jun mRNA expression in the mouse brain. *Dev Neurosci.* 2002;24(4):294–299.
6. Lahti KM, et al. Imaging brain activity in conscious animals using functional MRI. *J Neurosci Methods.* 1998;82(1):75–83.
7. Ferris CF, et al. Activation of neural pathways associated with sexual arousal in non-human primates. *J Magn Reson Imaging.* 2004;19(2):168–175.
8. Febo M, Numan M, Ferris CF. Functional magnetic resonance imaging shows oxytocin activates brain regions associated with mother-pup bonding during suckling. *J Neurosci.* 2005;25(50): 11637–11644.
9. Ferris CF, et al. Pup suckling is more rewarding than cocaine: evidence from functional magnetic resonance imaging and three-dimensional computational analysis. *J Neurosci.* 2005; 25(1):149–156.
10. Tenney JR, et al. fMRI of brain activation in a genetic rat model of absence seizures. *Epilepsia.* 2004;45(6):576–582.
11. Tenney JR, et al. Corticothalamic modulation during absence seizures in rats: a functional MRI assessment. *Epilepsia.* 2003; 44(9):1133–1140.
12. Tenney JR, et al. fMRI of generalized absence status epilepticus in conscious marmoset monkeys reveals corticothalamic activation. *Epilepsia.* 2004;45(10):1240–1247.
13. Ferris CF, et al. Imaging the neural circuitry and chemical control of aggressive motivation. *BMC Neurosci.* 2008;9:111.
14. Ferris CF, Stolberg T. Imaging the immediate non-genomic effects of stress hormone on brain activity. *Psychoneuroendocrinology.* 2010;35(1):5–14.
15. Hajnal JV, et al. Artifacts due to stimulus correlated motion in functional imaging of the brain. *Magn Reson Med.* 1994; 31(3):283–291.
16. Birn RM, et al. Magnetic field changes in the human brain due to swallowing or speaking. *Magn Reson Med.* 1998;40(1):55–60.
17. Raj D, Anderson AW, Gore JC. Respiratory effects in human functional magnetic resonance imaging due to bulk susceptibility changes. *Phys Med Biol.* 2001;46(12):3331–3340.
18. Yetkin FZ, et al. Effect of motion outside the field of view on functional MR. *AJNR Am J Neuroradiol.* 1996;17(6):1005–1009.
19. Woods RP, Cherry SR, Mazziotta JC. Rapid automated algorithm for aligning and reslicing PET images. *J Comput Assist Tomogr.* 1992;16(4):620–633.
20. Woods RP, et al. Automated image registration: I. General methods and intrasubject, intramodality validation. *J Comput Assist Tomogr.* 1998;22(1):139–152.
21. Woods RP, et al. Automated image registration: II. Intersubject validation of linear and nonlinear models. *J Comput Assist Tomogr.* 1998;22(1):153–165.
22. Yacoub E, et al. Robust detection of ocular dominance columns in humans using Hahn Spin Echo BOLD functional MRI at 7 Tesla. *Neuroimage.* 2007;37(4):1161–1177.
23. Cox RW. AFNI: software for analysis and visualization of functional magnetic resonance neuroimages. *Comput Biomed Res.* 1996;29(3):162–173.
24. Friston KJ, et al. Movement-related effects in fMRI time-series. *Magn Reson Med.* 1996;35(3):346–355.
25. Freire L, Mangin JF. Motion correction algorithms may create spurious brain activations in the absence of subject motion. *Neuroimage.* 2001;14(3):709–722.
26. Johnstone T, et al. Motion correction and the use of motion covariates in multiple-subject fMRI analysis. *Hum Brain Mapp.* 2006;27(10):779–788.

27. King JA, et al. Procedure for minimizing stress for fMRI studies in conscious rats. *J Neurosci Methods.* 2005;148(2):154–160.
28. Zhang Z, et al. Functional MRI of apomorphine activation of the basal ganglia in awake rhesus monkeys. *Brain Res.* 2000; 852(2):290–296.
29. Febo M, et al. The neural consequences of repeated cocaine exposure revealed by functional MRI in awake rats. *Neuropsychopharmacology.* 2005;30(5):936–943.
30. Febo M, et al. Imaging cocaine-induced changes in the mesocorticolimbic dopaminergic system of conscious rats. *J Neurosci Methods.* 2004;139(2):167–176.
31. Skoubis PD, et al. Mapping brain activity following administration of a nicotinic acetylcholine receptor agonist, ABT-594, using functional magnetic resonance imaging in awake rats. *Neuroscience.* 2006;137(2):583–591.
32. Chin CL, et al. Pharmacological MRI in awake rats reveals neural activity in area postrema and nucleus tractus solitarius: relevance as a potential biomarker for detecting drug-induced emesis. *Neuroimage.* 2006;33(4):1152–1160.
33. Chen G, et al. Functional magnetic resonance imaging of awake monkeys: some approaches for improving imaging quality. *Magn Reson Imaging.* 2012;30(1):36–47.
34. Upadhyay J, et al. Default-mode-like network activation in awake rodents. *PLoS One.* 2011;6(11):e27839.
35. Logothetis NK, et al. Neurophysiological investigation of the basis of the fMRI signal. *Nature.* 2001;412(6843):150–157.
36. Paxinos GWC. *The Rat Brain in Stereotaxic Coordinates.* Academic Press; 1986.
37. Ludwig R, et al. A dual RF resonator system for high-field functional magnetic resonance imaging of small animals. *J Neurosci Methods.* 2004;132(2):125–135.
38. Duong TQ, et al. Microvascular BOLD contribution at 4 and 7 T in the human brain: gradient-echo and spin-echo fMRI with suppression of blood effects. *Magn Reson Med.* 2003;49(6):1019–1027.
39. Norris DG. Principles of magnetic resonance assessment of brain function. *J Magn Reson Imaging.* 2006;23(6):794–807.
40. Zhang N, et al. Linearity of blood-oxygenation-level dependent signal at microvasculature. *Neuroimage.* 2009;48(2):313–318.
41. Brevard ME, et al. Changes in MRI signal intensity during hypercapnic challenge under conscious and anesthetized conditions. *Magn Reson Imaging.* 2003;21(9):995–1001.
42. Genovese CR, Lazar NA, Nichols T. Thresholding of statistical maps in functional neuroimaging using the false discovery rate. *Neuroimage.* 2002;15(4):870–878.
43. Brevard ME, et al. Imaging the neural substrates involved in the genesis of pentylenetetrazol-induced seizures. *Epilepsia.* 2006;47(4):745–754.
44. Snead 3rd OC. Basic mechanisms of generalized absence seizures. *Ann Neurol.* 1995;37(2):146–157.
45. Coenen AM, et al. Genetic models of absence epilepsy, with emphasis on the WAG/Rij strain of rats. *Epilepsy Res.* 1992;12(2):75–86.

CHAPTER

4

Network Experimental Approaches: Inactivation, Microinjection, Neuronal Stimulation, and Recording

Hua-Jun Feng[1], *Carl L. Faingold*[2]

[1]Department of Anesthesia, Critical Care and Pain Medicine, Massachusetts General Hospital and Harvard Medical School, Boston, MA, USA

[2]Departments of Pharmacology and Neurology, and Division of Neurosurgery, Southern Illinois University School of Medicine, Springfield, IL, USA

INTRODUCTION

In order to define a neuronal network for a given behavior or CNS disorder, a number of techniques are utilized as mentioned in Chapter 1. Once anatomical mapping methods such as c-fos or 2-deoxyglucose (see Chapter 3) and/or brain imaging (see Chapters 3 and 6) have provided suggestive evidence for putative brain sites that are involved in the network, other techniques are needed to confirm and extend the anatomical data and determine if the sites are truly requisite for the generation of the function or behavior which are carried out in animal models almost exclusively. These techniques include inactivation via lesion or microinjection; stimulation via electrical, chemical, or light stimuli; and neuronal recording. Most of these techniques are best performed in awake, behaving animals without the use of anesthetic agents, since anesthetics and related drugs greatly modify normal network function (see Chapters 28 and 32). If the data from the inactivation and stimulation techniques support the involvement of a specific site, recording of neuronal firing in awake, behaving animals can help to determine detailed information on how the patterns of neuronal firing change in that site and contribute to generation of the behavior.

INACTIVATION TECHNIQUES

Various approaches have been utilized to inactivate brain structures that the anatomical techniques have implicated in the neuronal network under investigation. These include electrolytic, chemical, and physical lesions as well as reversible focal microinjection techniques, which are a major focus in this chapter. Each of these approaches utilizes stereotaxic brain surgery, using a standard brain atlas (e.g. Paxinos and Watson[1]) (in rats) unless the structure under evaluation is at or near the cortical surface.

Lesions

The earliest inactivation techniques involved making physical electrolytic or heat lesions of the site[2–4] and determining whether this resulted in a change in function or behavior. Mechanical lesioning was also shown to be useful in some studies.[5] Problems that have arisen with these lesioning approaches include considerable tissue damage, lack of specificity, and the fact that both the cell bodies of the neurons in the site and the fibers of neurons that are only passing through the site are both damaged by these techniques.[6] All of these lesioning techniques have the additional drawback that they are more or less permanent, and the animals do not recover from them; or, if some recovery does occur, it is unpredictable. To circumvent this drawback, more transient and "recoverable" lesioning techniques were developed. Freezing inactivation and lesions with cryoprobes have been used in animal studies and to treat brain diseases in patients,[7–9] but fibers of passage are also affected by this technique. The concerns with lesioning and freezing have led to the widespread utilization of focal

Neuronal Networks in Brain Function, CNS Disorders, and Therapeutics
http://dx.doi.org/10.1016/B978-0-12-415804-7.00004-6

microinjection to alter the activation of brain structures in neuronal network studies.

Microinjection

The focal microinjection approach into specific brain network sites involves using a very small cannula to apply a very small volume of a substance that either damages the site with a toxin or blocks neuronal firing. Thus, focal microinjection through an implanted cannula of a small volume has been used to inactivate a structure; this uses a relatively selective toxic substance, such as ibotenic acid or 6-hydroxydopamine, both of which are thought to be toxic to neurons without affecting fibers of passage.[10–12] However, like the physical lesions, these chemical disruptions do not allow the observation of recovery. The use of microinjection of local anesthetics or other sodium channel blockers can temporarily and reversibly inactivate brain structures.[13,14] Although this approach is functionally reversible, the problems with this technique lie in that the blockade is not specific and the fibers of passage are also affected. These problems led to the microinjection of agents that selectively affect neurotransmitter action as a means of inactivating a structure to determine its role in neuronal network function. Commonly used agents include substances that block excitant amino acid receptors or activate inhibitory amino acid receptors, especially those for the inhibitory amino acid gamma aminobutyric acid (GABA).[14–17] These techniques have provided effective and selective inactivation of neurons in a brain site that is temporary, allowing recovery of the behavior to be observed, usually within a 24 h period.[18–20]

These techniques have been used, for example, in studying the neuronal network for a common rodent pathophysiological phenomenon called audiogenic seizures (AGS). In AGS, an intense acoustic stimulus evokes generalized seizures in rodents with certain genetic deficits, such as the severe seizure strain of genetically epilepsy-prone rats (GEPR-9s) and DBA mice, as well as in rodents withdrawn from certain drugs after repeated administration, including those experiencing ethanol withdrawal (ETX).[21–26] These animal models of seizure share similar seizure behaviors, including wild running followed by clonus and/or tonus, suggesting that the neuronal networks mediating these seizures may share common brain structures[15,19] (Chapter 26). The ventrolateral periaqueductal gray (PAG) has been established as a requisite component of the AGS network for one of these forms of AGS in GEPR-9s.[27] An example of using the microinjection technique in ETX rats involved examination of whether the PAG is also implicated in the neuronal network for AGS in these rats. Thus, an excitant amino acid antagonist (2-amino-7-phosphonoheptanoate, or AP7), acting at the *N*-methyl-D-aspartate (NMDA) glutamate receptor, was bilaterally microinjected into the PAG of rats during ETX, and its effect on ETX seizures was examined (see Figure 4.1). The microinjection of AP7 into the PAG significantly suppressed seizures in ETX rats, but microinjection of the vehicle into the PAG had no effect. The blockade of AGS occurred 30 min after infusion, and susceptibility to AGS recovered by 5 h after microinjection.[28] These data indicated that the PAG is also a requisite component of the neuronal network for AGS during ETX, since inactivation of this structure temporarily prevented the seizure from occurring. The lack of effect of microinjection of vehicle and the recovery

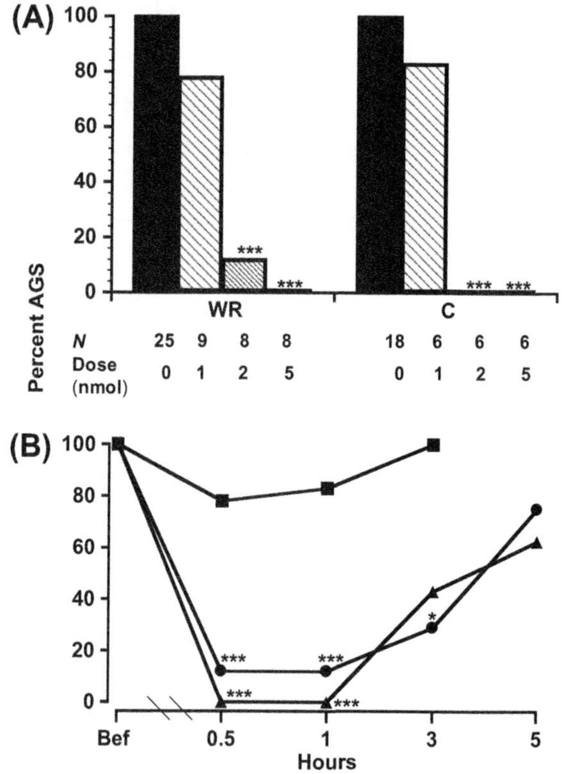

FIGURE 4.1 Example of using microinjection to explore the involvement of periaqueductal gray (PAG) in the neuronal network for audiogenic seizures (AGS) induced by ethanol withdrawal (ETX). One week after guide cannula implantation, ethanol dependence was induced in normal Sprague-Dawley rats by intragastric intubation of ethanol for 4 days.[22] These animals became susceptible to AGS after ETX, which consisted of wild running (WR) and clonus (C) behaviors. (A) The incidence of specific AGS behaviors. Infusion of vehicle (saline: dose 0) into PAG had no effect on AGS. However, microinjection of an NMDA glutamate receptor antagonist (2-amino-7-phosphonoheptanoate, or AP7) significantly reduced ETX seizures at doses of 2 and 5 nmol/side, but not a dose of 1 nmol/side. (B) The time course of effects of microinjection of AP7 on AGS susceptibility. The maximal suppression of AGS was observed at 0.5–1 h after infusion of AP7 at doses of 2 and 5 nmol/side. The suppressing effect of AP7 disappeared at 5 h after infusion. The zero dose represents the vehicle controls. *N*: number of animals. Bef: before microinjection; squares: 1 nmol; circles: 2 nmol; triangles: 5 nmol; $^{*}p < 0.05$; $^{***}p < 0.001$ (paired *t*-test). *Source: From Yang and coworkers[28] with permission.*

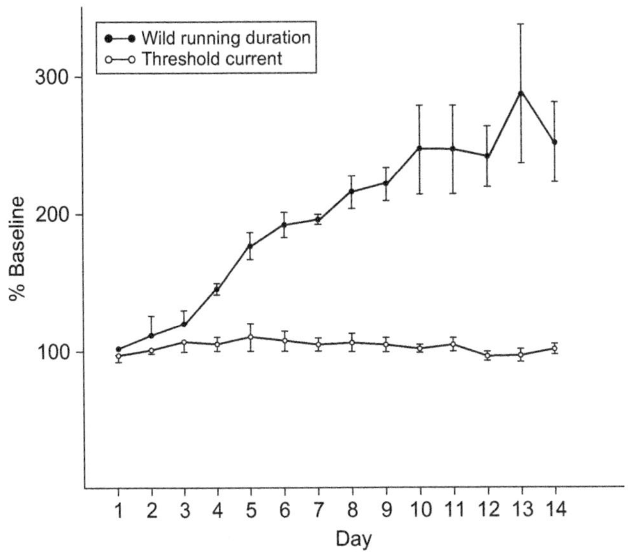

FIGURE 4.2 Example of the use of electrical stimulation to evaluate the involvement of a specific proposed structure in the neuronal network for seizures. Previous evidence had suggested the involvement of the inferior colliculus (IC) in the neuronal network for audiogenic seizures (AGS). Chronic electrical stimulation (twice a day for 14 days) in the IC of normal rats evoked wild-running seizure behaviors mimicking the initial behavior seen in AGS, which provided additional evidence of the involvement of this structure in the neuronal network for AGS. The current intensity required to trigger wild-running behavior did not change during the stimulation course, and the wild running always occurred in the first 2–4 s of the threshold current stimulation. However, the duration of wild running progressively increased during the stimulation period. In addition, more severe seizure behaviors, including forelimb extension or myoclonic jerks, were evoked following the wild-running episode at later stages of stimulation (resembling the severity increase seen with rats that are genetically susceptible to AGS). *Source: From McCown and coworkers[44] with permission.*

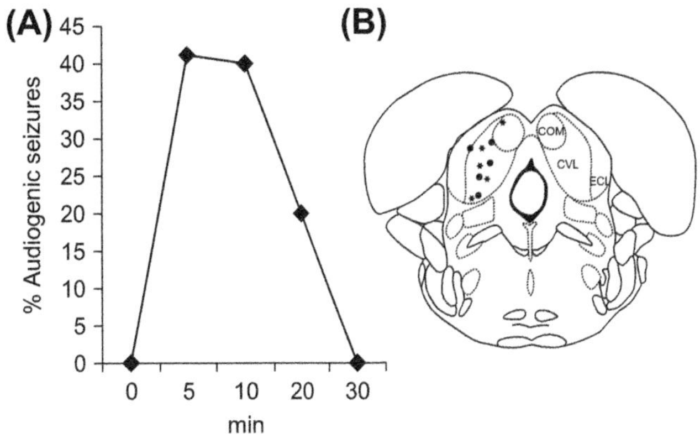

FIGURE 4.3 Example of the use of focal bilateral chemical stimulation to explore the neuronal network that mediates audiogenic seizures (AGS). This involved an attempt to induce susceptibility to AGS in a putatively important network site in the inferior colliculus (IC) in normal Sprague-Dawley rats. Using chronically implanted guide cannulae, a small volume (0.5 μl) of the $GABA_A$ antagonist bicuculline (15–30 pmol/side) was microinjected at a rate of 0.1 μl/min into the IC of awake, behaving normal rats. The rats were then subjected to an acoustic stimulus (a 109 dB electrical bell) at 5 min intervals for 30 min. This resulted in a 41% susceptibility to AGS alone, and an additional 41% of rats exhibited AGS plus spontaneous seizures (for a total of 82%; data not shown). Neither AGS nor spontaneous seizures were seen in rats receiving microinjections of the saline vehicle. The percentage of rats that exhibited seizures decreased over time, and at 30 min the animals were no longer susceptible (A). This result verified the importance of the IC in initiating AGS in genetically susceptible rats and also supported the importance of $GABA_A$ receptors in this brain site in the network for AGS. The representative microinjection sites were illustrated in (B). *Source: Data based on experiments in Millan and coworkers[30] with permission.*

from the blockade of the PAG indicated that no permanent lesion was involved, and the block of neurotransmitter receptors indicated that drug effects on fibers of passage did not make a major contribution to the effect produced. These results also suggest that NMDA receptors in the PAG are critically involved in AGS during ETX. Thus, this study provides an example of the use of the microinjection technique in exploring the role of a brain structure in a neuronal network.

Histological verification: When using stereotaxic techniques in microinjection or any of the other techniques in this chapter, it is critical to verify that the probe is actually placed in the target structure, which requires histological confirmation after the experiment is completed using dye injection or electrolytic lesion in the deeply anesthetized animal and subsequent sectioning of the brain. It is extremely important to verify the sites of microinjection, according to a standard stereotaxic atlas such as Paxinos and Watson[1] (see Figure 4.3). Examples of experimental procedures for the microinjection technique can be found in References 29,30.

Advantages and limitations: Microinjection is very useful for testing the drug effect in behaving animals. Most implantations of cannulae are done on a chronic basis, often with a guide cannula that does not penetrate deeply into the brain. This approach is utilized to reduce tissue reactivity in the target site to sustained cannula placement, which is known to induce such changes. Following a multiday recovery from the implant surgery, the animals are not constrained or anesthetized during the microinjection experiments. In addition, the drug effect is reversible so that the animal behaviors often recover over a short time course.

However, like many other neuroscience approaches, some limitations exist for this technique. Microinjection can cause tissue damage in the brain, especially when the target structure is located more ventrally, since the infusion cannula needs to travel a longer distance through upper levels of brain tissues to reach the target structure. To reduce tissue damage, investigators have used glass micropipettes (5–25 μm tip diameter)[13] instead of stainless-steel or plastic infusion cannulae (~400 μm in diameter) for drug delivery. Although drug delivery using glass micropipettes can minimize tissue damage, they are more useful in anesthetized animals. It is a challenge to perform drug delivery on awake animals due to the fragility of the glass pipettes.[13] While most receptor agonists and antagonists only exert effects on neuronal cell bodies, local anesthetics and sodium channel blockers such as tetrodotoxin affect both cell bodies and fibers.[14] As noted here, another problem exists if a local anesthetic or tetrodotoxin is infused into a structure: it can interrupt the conduction of the fibers of passage,[13,14] which may potentially confound the experimental results. Another limitation is the degree of localization achievable with microinjection, since it has been shown that the diameter of diffusion after microinjection of a chemical is often ~1 mm, depending on the volume of the microinjection.[31–33] When drugs are microinjected into a small nucleus, the concentration of the drug that diffuses out of the target nucleus may be sufficient to affect adjacent structures.[31] So, for small nuclei, it is best to use infusion cannulae with smaller diameters and/or reduced infusion volume to better localize the effects. Finally, if the dose of the microinjected substance is relatively high (compared to effective doses of the same substance at other sites in the same network), you cannot be sure that the effect achieved is localized to the specific site, since the volume transmission system of the brain (Chapter 8) can potentially allow the substance to exert effects at distant sites.

NEURONAL STIMULATION

Another important experimental approach that has been utilized to explore the nature and function of neuronal networks is neurostimulation. Neurostimulation can be achieved by different means, such as electrical, light, and chemical stimuli.[34–37] In early neuroscience experiments, relatively large electrodes, as compared to the microwire recording electrodes discussed in this chapter, were utilized to deliver patterns of stimulation into specific brain sites to help evaluate the role that structure played in a given behavior. This approach continues to this day and is becoming increasingly used in human conditions to treat a variety of neurological and psychiatric disorders, as discussed extensively in Chapters 13 and 24–27 (Chapter 31).

Electrical Stimulation

Electrical stimulation has been widely used to study synaptic plasticity.[34] Brief high-frequency electrical stimulation can lead to long-term potentiation, and prolonged low-frequency stimulation results in long-term depression (see Chapter 27).[34,38] Electrical stimuli can also be used to simulate a disease process and, under certain conditions, can deactivate a brain structure or change its pattern of firing.[39] Kindling is a widely used animal model to simulate epileptogenesis, and it can be produced by repetitive and intermittent electrical or chemical stimulation of limbic structures of the brain, including the amygdala.[40–42] Electrically-kindled animals exhibit stimulus-evoked generalized motor seizures as well as spontaneous seizures, which are similar to temporal lobe epilepsy in humans.[43] Another example of the use of this technique can be found in exploring neuronal networks in AGS. Thus, low-current electrical stimulation of the inferior colliculus (IC) induces seizures in normal rats, including wild running,[44,45] that resemble seizure behaviors seen in AGS-susceptible rodents as described here. Thus, in Figure 4.2, electrical stimulation in the IC of normal rats evoked the wild-running seizure behavior, closely paralleling the initial behavior seen in AGS, which provided additional evidence of the involvement of this structure in the neuronal network for AGS. This finding is consistent with studies using microinjection that found that the IC is the initiation site for AGS[20,30,46–48] (discussed in the "Chemical Stimulation via Microinjection" section). Acute electrical stimulation of the IC induces seizure activity that does not involve forebrain structures, such as the amygdala, in normal rats. However, repeated electrical stimulation of the IC generated postictal epileptiform electrographic activity in the amygdala, similar to that seen in amygdala kindling.[49] With twice-daily repetition of the electrical stimulus, the duration of the wild running increased and the more severe seizure behaviors, including limb extension, were evoked, resembling the severity increase seen with rats genetically susceptible to AGS.52. This is an example of how electrical stimulation within the putative seizure network provided further evidence of the involvement of a specific structure in the AGS network. These results are consistent with the repetitive induction of AGS (audiogenic kindling), which causes the neuronal network for AGS to expand from brainstem to forebrain structures, including the amygdala (see Chapter 27).[35,50,51]

Chemical Stimulation via Microinjection

Microinjection, as described in the "Microinjection" section, has also been utilized for the purpose of stimulation. Microinjection of agents that block the action of inhibitory transmitters (e.g. $GABA_A$ receptor antagonists) or increase the activation of excitatory neurotransmitters (e.g. glutamate agonists) into brain structures enhances neuronal firing, which can modify the function of the neuronal network.[53] In the example in Figure 4.3, the neuronal network that mediates AGS was explored using focal chemical stimulation to attempt to induce susceptibility to AGS in normal rats in a putatively important network site in the IC. A small volume of a low concentration of a $GABA_A$ antagonist was bilaterally microinjected into the IC in awake, behaving normal rats. When the rats were subjected to an intense acoustic stimulus, this resulted in a significant degree of susceptibility to AGS, which was never seen in rats receiving the vehicle.[30] AGS susceptibility declined with time, and at 30 min post infusion, the animals were no longer susceptible. This approach corroborated the important role of the IC in initiating AGS in the various seizure models that exhibit this seizure type, which anatomical lesion and electrical stimulation studies had suggested. These results also supported the importance of $GABA_A$ receptors in this brain site in the AGS network.[30] Subsequent work employing focal blockade, neuronal recording, and other techniques further supported these conclusions that the IC is an important element in the networks for AGS (see Chapter 26).

In other stimulation studies, repetitive administration of low concentrations of excitatory substances, including GABA antagonists and glutamate agonists, leads to the gradual development of a fully kindled state (chemical kindling),[54,55] which may share a similar neuronal network to that of the electrical kindling.[55] As seen in Figure 4.3, the effect achieved with a single microinjection of most excitatory substances is generally transient, which allows recovery of function to be observed. However, certain substances that work at targets beyond the receptor level in the molecular cascade can mimic the effect triggered by frequent and repetitive transmitter release (Chapter 27). These molecular mechanisms have been strongly implicated in neuroplastic changes that neuronal networks can often exhibit. Microinjection of substances that activate these molecular mechanisms can then result in long-lasting effects that mimic those seen in neuroplastic changes in the networks that occur in learning or dysfunctional changes that occur in brain disorders, including epilepsy. In addition, in a model of anxiety disorders called fear conditioning, as discussed in Chapter 13, neuroplastic changes in circuitry between the auditory network (the medial geniculate body) and the anxiety–mood network (Chapter 24) result in the establishment of learning (fear conditioning), which can be enhanced or inhibited by agents that alter molecular mechanisms, including those involved in cyclic adenosine monophosphate (cAMP) synthesis.[56,57] Interestingly, the same pathway is involved in audiogenic kindling, induced by repetitive AGS. Thus, microinjection of a cAMP-enhancing agent into the amygdala of nonkindled GEPR-9s produces a long-lasting mimicry of audiogenic kindling,[58] but acute activation of NMDA receptors in the amygdala evokes only a temporary mimicry of the audiogenic kindling effect.[59]

Advantages and limitations: Electrical stimulation has been used as a gold standard for neural stimulation in basic research and clinical treatment for over a century. By varying electrical parameters, a variety of stimulation paradigms can be used to manipulate the neuronal activities.[60] However, several limitations of this technique are observed.[36,61] For example, electrical energy is delivered through the electrode–tissue interface, which can cause tissue damage. Furthermore, the current spreads beyond the electrode, and thus the spatial selectivity is low. In addition, electrical stimulation always produces a "stimulus artifact", which interferes with recordings adjacent to the stimulating site.

The advantages and limitations of chemical stimulation using microinjection have been described in the "Microinjection" section. It is noted that most excitatory substances affect neuronal excitability by interacting with corresponding receptors, which are mainly localized on the soma and dendrites.

Light Stimulation

To resolve many limitations of electrical stimulation, alternative stimulation approaches, including light stimulation, were developed. It was reported that optical stimulation using pulsed, low-energy infrared laser light induces physiological responses from peripheral nerve–muscle preparations, and these responses are similar to those elicited by electrical stimulation.[61,62] Infrared light stimulation has been shown to alter GABAergic neurotransmission.[36] The optical stimulation exhibits several advantages over electrical stimulation. First, it does not require an electrode–tissue interface (i.e. it is contact-free and damage-free). Second, it does not produce a stimulus artifact (i.e. it is artifact-free), allowing for recordings close to the stimulating site. And, finally, it can stimulate specific target nerve fibers without affecting adjacent fibers, thus providing high spatial selectivity.[36]

Recently, optogenetics has been developed to study neuronal circuitry function with a high temporal and spatial resolution.[63–65] Channelrhodopsins (ChR2), blue light-activated nonspecific cation channels, are expressed on neurons by transfection or transgenic approaches. Light-evoked cation influx can depolarize neuronal membrane and facilitate the firing of action potentials (APs) on a temporal scale that is comparable to physiological rates.[64] More importantly, ChR2 genes can be expressed in different cell types targeted by appropriate promoters,[66] allowing for precise, cell type-specific control. These approaches provide useful alternatives to electrical stimulation to dissect the function of neuronal networks.

Figure 4.4 demonstrated the neuronal responses evoked by photostimulation of the neurons in the cortex of transgenic ChR2–YFP mice.[67] ChR2–YFP was specifically expressed on neurons using the *Thy1* promoter. Extracellular recordings were performed as photostimulation was applied on the neurons in layer 5 of the

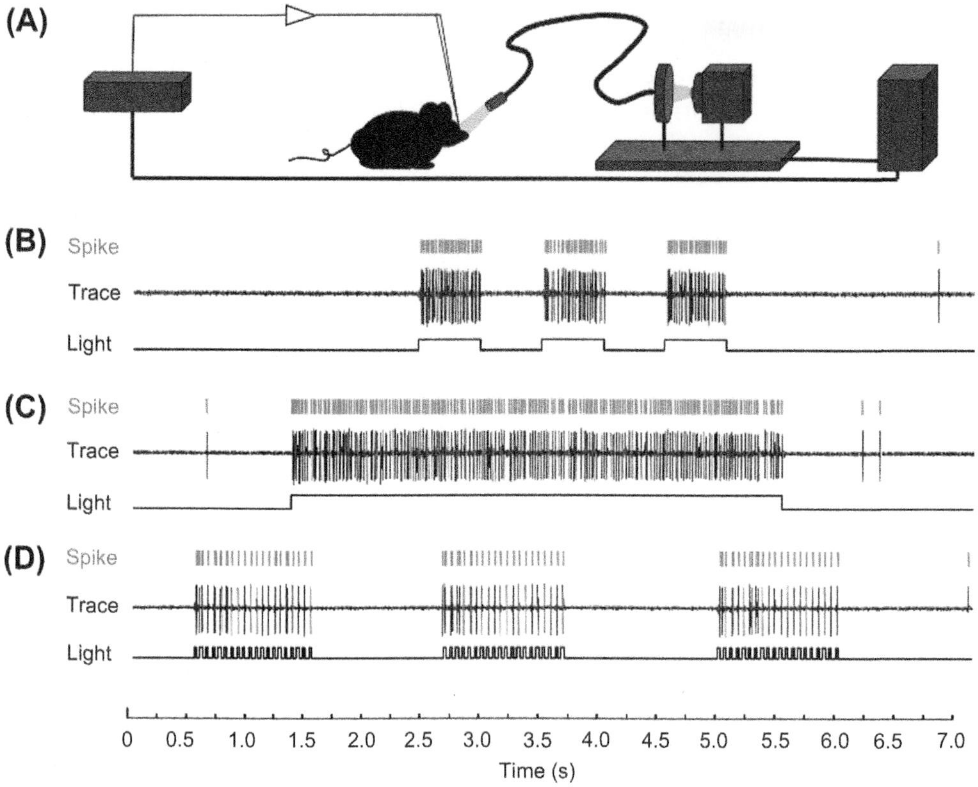

FIGURE 4.4 Example of the use of the light stimulation technique. Extracellular recordings of single-unit activity in response to photostimulation of layer 5 cortical neurons expressing ChR2 in transgenic ChR2–YFP mice. (A) A cartoon to illustrate the in vivo light delivery and electrophysiology system for recording of the extracellular single-unit activity evoked by light stimulation in anesthetized mice. The dorsal surface of the brain was exposed for photostimulation by small-window craniotomy. A silica optical fiber, which was connected to a 100 W mercury light source gated using a mechanical shutter, was used for light delivery. Note that photostimulation evoked a strong and time-locked single-unit response from cortical neurons that expressed ChR2. (B–D) Examples of recording traces demonstrating reliable temporal resolution of spike activity from a unit in response to different light stimulus paradigms. (B) Single-unit responses to three 500 ms exposures spaced 500 ms apart; (C) neuronal responses to a single 4 s light exposure; and (D) neuronal responses to three 20 Hz stimulations. *Source: From Arenkiel and coworkers[67] with permission.* (For color version of this figure, the reader is referred to the online version of this book.)

cortex. Each photostimulation reliably evoked a single-unit response from the neuron. Photostimulation using different light stimulus paradigms could evoke strong and reliable time-locked neuronal responses, allowing for precise manipulation of the neuronal network activity. Thus, photostimulation of the mitral cells, the principal excitatory neurons of the olfactory bulb, showed that the level of the excitatory input to the piriform cortex is dependent on the number of activated mitral cells. These data support the existing model of the olfactory-processing network in which multiple mitral cells act as an integrative input for action potential initiation and propagation in the piriform cortex and also illustrate another important technique, neuronal recording.[67] Several other molecular and optical techniques for selective control of neuronal networks have also been developed in recent years, such as RNAi (RNA interference),[68] DREADD (designer receptors exclusively activated by designer drugs),[69,70] and optogenetic inhibition using halorhodopsin or archaerhodopsin.[71–73]

NEURONAL RECORDING

Neuronal recordings in awake, behaving animals have been utilized to record extracellular APs in network sites in a number of brain areas. This allows the study of neuronal firing correlates of specific behavior, providing further information on the actual neuronal mechanisms that control network function. Originally, neuronal recording was done in anesthetized animals until it was realized that all anesthetics, even in low doses, exerted profound effects on network function, such that the neurons often fired very differently in the absence of anesthesia (see Chapter 32). This is particularly true in areas of the brain that are known to undergo major neuroplastic changes during network operation (see Chapter 28). For example, amygdala neurons exhibit several types of firing patterns in behaving GEPR-9s, but these firing patterns are greatly altered in the presence of ketamine, a dissociative anesthetic, since it almost completely suppresses amygdala neuronal firing, even at low, subanesthetic dosage.[74,75]

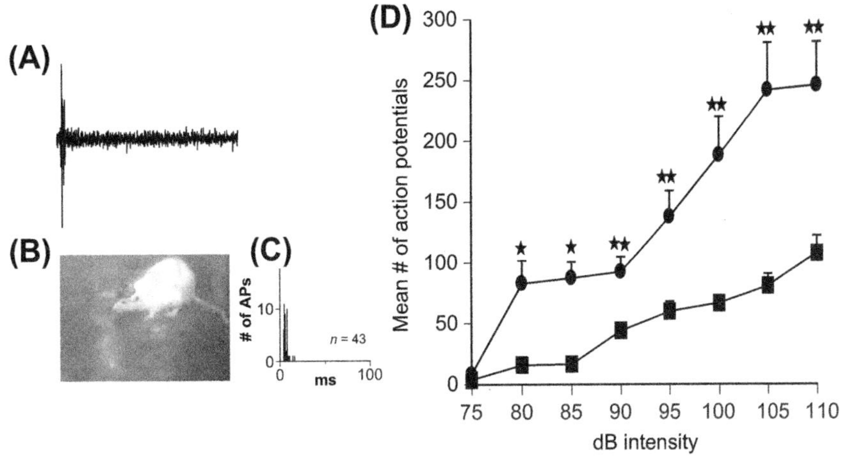

FIGURE 4.5 Example of the use of a neuronal recording technique in awake, behaving animals. Microwire single-unit recording of the neuron from the lateral nucleus of the amygdala (LAMG) prior to and after audiogenic kindling in GEPR-3s. Representative example of a digital oscilloscope trace, demonstrating LAMG neuronal firing (A) and video frame of the awake, behaving GEPR-3 (B), from which the neuron was recorded. The poststimulus time histogram (PSTH; 100 ms scan length, 1 ms bin width, and 50 stimulus presentations) is shown in (C). Action potential amplitude: 400 μV; *n*: number of action potentials (APs) in the PSTH. (Acoustic stimulus parameters: 12 kHz tone burst, 100 ms duration, 5 ms rise-fall, 95 dB SPL, 0.5 Hz rate, and 50 presentations.) (D) Comparison of mean (±S.E.M.) LAMG neuronal responses between nonkindled ($n = 12$; squares) and AGS-kindled ($n = 12$; circles) GEPR-3s to increasing intensity of acoustic stimulus. A significantly greater number of LAMG action potentials (APs) were evoked in kindled as compared to nonkindled GEPR-3s at 80 and 85 dB SPL ($p < 0.01$, ANOVA with repeated measures) and at 90–110 dB SPL ($p < 0.005$, ANOVA with repeated measures). *Source: Modified from Raisinghani and Faingold*[103] *with permission.*

Furthermore, amygdala neurons only display one type of firing pattern in anesthetized rats when afferent fibers are stimulated from another structure.[35] After the obfuscating effects of anesthetics and related agents were realized, other approaches were used, including pharmacologically induced paralysis or decortication in which the animals' respiration was supported.[76–79] However, these approaches were largely abandoned because of ethical issues. Recording of neuronal firing in awake, behaving animals was eventually developed,[80–83] and it is particularly useful for studies of sleep, as discussed in Chapters 21 and 22. Many other neuronal networks have also been explored using this technique.[74,84–88] This technique has been utilized in a variety of species, such as mice,[89] rats,[81,90] guinea pigs,[91] cats,[92,93] nonhuman primates,[94,95] as well as humans.[96] Electrodes were developed that were flexible enough and small enough to isolate "single units" or extracellular APs in animals that had the ability to move. With the help of hardware and software detection techniques, it is possible to assure that single rather than multiple units are being analyzed.[94,97] These techniques also allowed multiple electrodes to be implanted in the same areas at the same time to get a population of single units simultaneously.[98–100] These arrays of electrodes have progressed to ever larger numbers up to hundreds of neuronal recordings simultaneously,[101,102] which is applicable for larger volume brain sites, especially the cerebral cortex.

We utilized this technique to explore the neuronal firing changes in the amygdala in the moderate-seizure strain of genetically epilepsy-prone rats (GEPR-3s) that underwent audiogenic kindling (frequent AGS repetition), since this structure has been shown to be a component of the neuronal network subserving audiogenic kindling in other AGS models (see Chapter 27).[50,51] Microwire single-unit recording was utilized to evaluate neuronal firing in the lateral nucleus of the amygdala (LAMG) prior to and after audiogenic kindling in GEPR-3s (Figure 4.5).[103] This technique allowed evaluation of the role of the LAMG in the neuronal network for seizures in the GEPR-3 model of AGS and the firing increases induced by the AGS kindling in these animals.[103] An illustration of the use of the microwire technique shows a typical example of the recording of evoked LAMG extracellular APs in an awake, behaving GEPR-3 and a photo of the rat from which the neuron was recorded (Figure 4.5, left panel). This LAMG neuron responded consistently to acoustic stimuli, as shown by the poststimulus time histogram [Figure 4.5(C)]. A comparison of the mean LAMG neuronal responses between nonkindled and AGS-kindled GEPR-3s (Figure 4.5(D)) showed that a significantly greater number of APs was evoked in the LAMG of kindled as compared to nonkindled GEPR-3s at all intensities of the acoustic stimulus. The microwire technique provided dynamic mechanistic data on the operation of the neuronal network once the imaging functional techniques described in this chapter and in Chapters 3 and 6 had provided evidence for the importance of this structure in the neuronal network for this behavior.

Thus, anatomical, microinjection, and stimulation techniques can strongly implicate a specific brain structure as a critical component of the neuronal network for a specific behavior, such as AGS. However, these latter techniques are not adequate to determine the nature of the mechanisms that subserve real-time operation of the network. The use of neuronal recording in awake, unanesthetized animals allows determination of the precise nature of the contribution of a network component to a specific behavior and allows a temporal evaluation of how and when the nucleus contributes to the behavior being evaluated, including AGS.[104,105] In the case of AGS, microwire single-unit recordings allow the pursuit of these questions since the preictal neuronal activity undergoes dynamic changes in each nucleus of the neuronal network for seizures. Thus, by using microwire neuronal recording, we can detect the neuronal firing changes prior to or around the time of the seizures in the nuclei of the AGS network.[104] This information can be used to predict the occurrence of an ictal event and also to map the extent of a focus in human epilepsy.[106] Neuronal network explorations often couple microwire recording with behavioral analysis. For example, we have evaluated which component of the AGS network contributes most importantly to the wild running and clonic or tonic seizure seen in AGS.[104] Experimental procedures for microwire recording can be found in References 74,81.

Sometimes, it is helpful to assess the role of a specific pathway in a neuronal network by combining the neuronal recording technique with focal electrical or chemical stimulation or inhibition within the network in the same animal. For example, a pathway from the medial geniculate body (MGB) in the thalamus to the amygdala has been identified,[107] and both of these brain structures were reported to be involved in audiogenic kindling in one model of AGS.[51] We evaluated whether audiogenic kindling led to synaptic changes in the pathway from the MGB to the amygdala to alter the efficacy of the thalamo-amygdala component of this network.[35] Electrical stimuli were delivered to the MGB, and neuronal responses were recorded in the LAMG. We observed several changes, indicating that the excitability of the thalamo-amygdala pathway was enhanced after audiogenic kindling. The threshold of neuronal response was reduced in kindled GEPR-9s as compared with nonkindled GEPR-9s. In addition, for each stimulus intensity, the LAMG neuronal response was larger in kindled GEPR-9s than in controls (Figure 4.6), which suggested that a significant neuroplastic change had occurred in this component of the AGS network as a result of audiogenic kindling. These

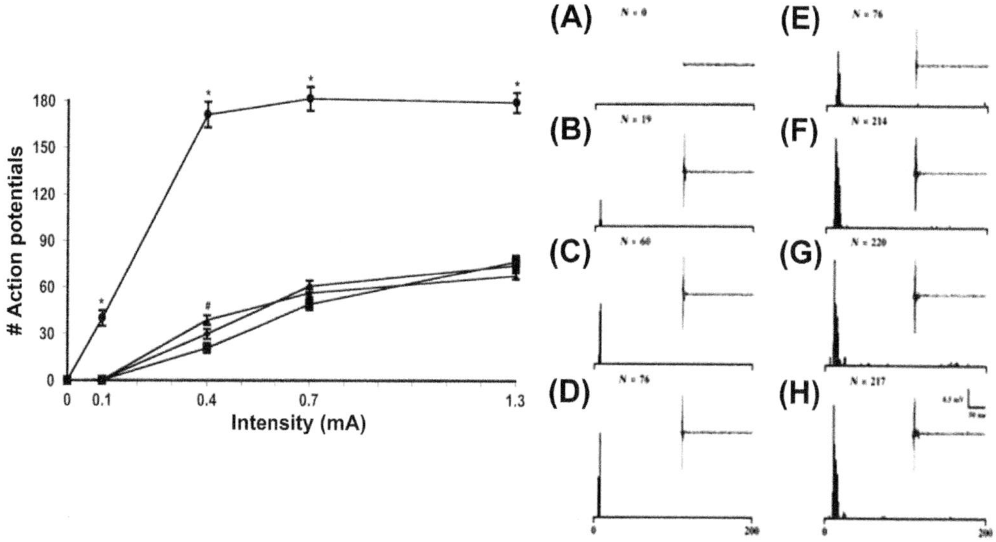

FIGURE 4.6 Example of the use of electrical stimulation and neuronal recording simultaneously in awake, behaving animals. Amygdala neuronal firing in response to electrical stimulation in the medial geniculate body (MGB) was evaluated. A bipolar concentric electrode was inserted stereotaxically into the medial division of the MGB, and a tungsten microelectrode was placed into the lateral nucleus of the amygdala (LAMG). Left panel: Mean number of action potentials (APs) recorded in the LAMG of AGS-kindled GEPR-9s (K-GEPR-9s), nonkindled GEPR-9s (NK-GEPR-9s), sham-kindled Sprague-Dawley rats (SK-SD) and nonkindled Sprague-Dawley rats (NK-SD) in response to electrical stimulation of the MGB at different stimulus intensities. The mean number of APs at 0.1 mA was significantly greater in K-GEPR-9s than in NK-GEPR-9s, SK-SD, and NK-SD, indicating that the neuronal response threshold was lowered in K-GEPR-9s. For each stimulus intensity, LAMG neurons in K-GEPR-9s fired a larger number of APs than those in the other groups of animals. The number of APs recorded at 0.4 mA was greater in SK-SD than in NK-SD. Circles: K-GEPR-9s; diamonds: NK-GEPR-9s; triangles: SK-SD; squares: NK-SD. *$p < 0.05$ compared with NK-GEPR-9s, SK-SD, and NK-SD; #$p < 0.05$ compared with NK-SD (ANOVA of repeated measures, Tukey's test). Right panel: Examples showing the number of APs evaluated using a poststimulus time histogram (PSTH) (200 ms scan length, 1 ms bin width, and 50 stimuli) evoked by electrical stimulation at 0.1, 0.4, 0.7, and 1.3 mA in SK-SD (A–D) and K-GEPR-9s (E–H). The corresponding digital oscilloscope trace of neuronal activity is shown above each PSTH. For each intensity from 0.1 to 1.3 mA, the number of APs was elevated in K-GEPR-9s as compared with SK-SD. *N* represents total APs/PSTH. *Source: Modified from Feng and Faingold[35] with permission.*

results, which were obtained using electrical stimulation, suggest that audiogenic kindling leads to neuronal network expansion from brainstem to forebrain structures, at least in part, via the thalamo-amygdala pathway (see Chapter 27). This approach allowed the relationship between different nuclei in the seizure network to be evaluated separately and showed evidence of a neuroplastic change in this pathway that was induced by the treatment (audiogenic kindling).

Advantages and limitations: Microwire neuronal recording is a widely used neuroscience technique to examine neuronal firing in free, behaving animals. One major advantage of this technique is that neuronal firing recording can be performed for long-term experimentation (up to months or years) with chronically implanted electrodes.[95,97] There are several potential limitations for this technique. Neuronal recordings often detect the neuronal firing changes in an experimental paradigm, but the mechanisms underlying neuronal firing changes are not detectable, and ex vivo techniques are needed (Chapter 5). For example, a decrease in neuronal firing may be caused by enhancement of an inhibitory system such as GABAergic inhibition and/or reduction of an excitatory system such as glutamatergic excitation. For long-term experiments, the microwire electrode viability may be compromised by corrosion of the tungsten wires.[108] Also, a microwire electrode, as a foreign body, can potentially trigger a tissue reaction in the brain structures. However, recent studies show that, although persistent inflammation and enhanced blood–brain barrier permeability can occur around the electrode, the overall tissue reactivity is very mild.[109] No reactive gliosis increasing over time or progressive neuronal loss was observed at the electrode brain–tissue interface over months of an indwelling period.[109,110] These histological studies are consistent with the recording data from our laboratory and other research groups, showing that stable neuronal recordings can last for months to years.[95,97] It was reported that using polypyrrole microwire electrode instead of metal or silicon electrode could reduce inflammation.[111] Finally, loss of the electrode implant may occur, especially during long-term experiments.

CONCLUSIONS

As discussed in Chapter 1, many techniques are required to explore the structure and function of neuronal networks in the intact mammalian brain. Once the neuroanatomical-based approaches, discussed in Chapters 3 and 6, are utilized to identify possible network structures, additional approaches are needed to understand network function in intact animals, because these anatomical techniques do not define the nature of the contribution to the network or if the changes may be compensatory, as indicated in Chapter 6. The contemporary use of the various experimental approaches discussed in this chapter involves using intact and behaving animals to observe modifications and/or operating mechanisms of network function that result from these experimental manipulations. Blockade of a network site using a reversible method that affects only those neurons in the presumptive network nucleus, such as focal microinjection of a compound that enhances an inhibitory transmitter action (e.g. a GABA agonist), will allow evaluation of the network function change that results. If this microinjection results in prevention of network function, it would support the importance of the specific structure in the network and designate the site as a "requisite" site for network function. Likewise, if stimulation of a presumptive network site results in activation or increased sensitivity to activation of network function, this would further support the importance of that site in the function of the network. Furthermore, after both stimulation and blockade of a network site implicate a structure as a requisite network site, recording of extracellular APs in that site before, during, and after the network becomes activated in the intact animal will allow an understanding of how the neurons in this site actually participate in the physiology or pathophysiology of the network function. Finally, ex vivo brain slice studies of the cellular mechanisms (Chapter 5) responsible for these extracellular firing changes would be performed to fully understand the physiological process underlying network function. To illustrate this process, we have used data on the role of the IC in AGS, which is discussed extensively in Chapter 26. Anatomical studies strongly implicated the IC as an important structure in AGS, and IC blockade studies showed block of AGS, reversibly. Electrical or chemical stimulation of the IC mimicked AGS. Neuronal recording in the IC indicated a major increase in firing only at the onset of AGS. These findings indicated that IC neurons played a major role in initiation of AGS, but that other structures were more important in the propagation of these seizures, which were then evaluated in efferent nuclei in the AGS network (Chapter 26). Finally, subsequent ex vivo studies[112] provided further evidence on intracellular mechanisms in the IC that mediate the changes observed in vivo, revealing a more complete understanding of the role of this most critical structure in the operation of the network.

Acknowledgments

We thank Gayle Stauffer for assistance with the manuscript. H-JF Support: NINDS and Citizens United for Research in Epilepsy (CURE). CLF Support: NINDS, NIAAA, Excellence in Academic Medicine, Southern Illinois University School of Medicine.

References

1. Paxinos G, Watson C. *The Rat Brain in Stereotaxic Coordinates*. Sydney: Academic Press; 2005.
2. Agid Y, Javoy F, Glowimski J. Chemical or electrolytic lesion of the substantia nigra: early effects on neostriatal dopamine metabolism. *Brain Res*. 1974;74:41–49.
3. Billingsley ML, Straw JA, Mandel HG. Glial DNA synthesis and cell proliferation in the lesioned frontal cortex of the rat. *Brain Res*. 1982;247:325–334.
4. So KF. Development of abnormal recrossing retinotectal projections after superior colliculus lesions in newborn Syrian hamsters. *J Comp Neurol*. 1979;186:241–257.
5. Browning RA, Nelson DK, Mogharreban N, Jobe PC, Laird II HE. Effect of midbrain and pontine tegmental lesions on audiogenic seizures in genetically epilepsy-prone rats. *Epilepsia*. 1985;26:175–183.
6. Sawynok J. The 1988 Merck Frosst Award. The role of ascending and descending noradrenergic and serotonergic pathways in opioid and non-opioid antinociception as revealed by lesion studies. *Can J Physiol Pharmacol*. 1989;67:975–988.
7. Faingold CL, Hoffmann WE, Caspary DM. On the site of pentylenetetrazol-induced enhancement of auditory responses of the reticular formation: localized cooling and electrical stimulation studies. *Neuropharmacology*. 1983;22:961–970.
8. Rand RW. Role of cryosurgery and MRI for Parkinson's disease. *Stereotact Funct Neurosurg*. 1995;65:18–22.
9. Skinner JE. A cryoprobe and cryoplate for reversible functional blockade in the brains of chronic animal preparations. *Electroencephalogr Clin Neurophysiol*. 1970;29:204–205.
10. Castellan-Baldan L, da Costa Kawasaki M, Ribeiro SJ, Calvo F, Correa VM, Coimbra NC. Topographic and functional neuroanatomical study of GABAergic disinhibitory striatum-nigral inputs and inhibitory nigrocollicular pathways: neural hodology recruiting the substantia nigra, pars reticulate, for the modulation of the neural activity in the inferior colliculus involved with panic-like emotions. *J Chem Neuroanat*. 2006;32:1–27.
11. Jarrard LE. Use of excitotoxins to lesion the hippocampus: update. *Hippocampus*. 2002;12:405–414.
12. Piallat B, Benazzouz A, Benabid AL. Neuroprotective effect of chronic inactivation of the subthalamic nucleus in a rat model of Parkinson's disease. *J Neural Transm Suppl*. 1999;55:71–77.
13. Malpeli JG. Reversible inactivation of subcortical sites by drug injection. *J Neurosci Methods*. 1999;86:119–128.
14. Martin JH, Ghez C. Pharmacological inactivation in the analysis of the central control of movement. *J Neurosci Methods*. 1999;86: 145–159.
15. Faingold CL, N'Gouemo P, Riaz A. Ethanol and neurotransmitter interactions-from molecular to integrative effects. *Prog Neurobiol*. 1998;55:509–535.
16. Feng HJ. Allosteric modulation of αβδ $GABA_A$ receptors. *Pharmaceuticals*. 2010;3:3461–3477. http://dx.doi.org/10.3390/ph3113461.
17. Schousboe A, Drejer J, Hansen GH, Meier E. Cultured neurons as model systems for biochemical and pharmacological studies on receptors for neurotransmitter amino acids. *Dev Neurosci*. 1985;7: 252–262.
18. Faingold CL, Randall ME, Naritoku DK, Boersma Anderson CA. Noncompetitive and competitive NMDA antagonists exert anticonvulsant effects by actions on different sites within the neuronal network for audiogenic seizures. *Exp Neurol*. 1993;119: 198–204.
19. Feng HJ, Yang L, Faingold CL. Role of the amygdala in ethanol withdrawal seizures. *Brain Res*. 2007;1141:65–73.
20. Frye GD, McCown TJ, Breese GR. Characterization of susceptibility to audiogenic seizures in ethanol-dependent rats after microinjection of γ-aminobutyric acid (GABA) agonists into the inferior colliculus, substantia nigra or medial septum. *J Pharmacol Exp Ther*. 1983;227:663–670.
21. Faingold CL. Neuronal networks in the genetically epilepsy-prone rat. *Adv Neurol*. 1999;79:311–321.
22. Faingold CL. The Majchrowicz binge alcohol protocol: an intubation technique to study alcohol dependence in rats. *Curr Protoc Neurosci*. 2008;44:9.28.1–9.28.12. http://dx.doi.org/10.1002/0471142301.ns0928s44.
23. Faingold CL, Randall M, Tupal S. DBA/1 mice exhibit chronic susceptibility to audiogenic seizures followed by sudden death associated with respiratory arrest. *Epilepsy Behav*. 2010;17: 436–440.
24. Garcia-Cairasco N. A critical review on the participation of inferior colliculus in acoustic-motor and acoustic-limbic networks involved in the expression of acute and kindled audiogenic seizures. *Hear Res*. 2002;168:208–222.
25. Tupal S, Faingold CL. Evidence supporting a role of serotonin in modulation of sudden death induced by seizures in DBA/2 mice. *Epilepsia*. 2006;47:21–26.
26. Venit EL, Shepard BD, Seyfried TN. Oxygenation prevents sudden death in seizure-prone mice. *Epilepsia*. 2004;45:993–996.
27. N'Gouemo P, Faingold CL. The periaqueductal grey is a critical site in the neuronal network for audiogenic seizures: modulation by $GABA_A$, NMDA and opioid receptors. *Epilepsy Res*. 1999;35: 39–46.
28. Yang L, Long C, Randall ME, Faingold CL. Neurons in the periaqueductal gray are critically involved in the neuronal network for audiogenic seizures during ethanol withdrawal. *Neuropharmacology*. 2003;44:275–281.
29. Feng HJ, Faingold CL. Modulation of audiogenic seizures by histamine and adenosine receptors in the inferior colliculus. *Exp Neurol*. 2000;163:264–270.
30. Millan MH, Meldrum BS, Faingold CL. Induction of audiogenic seizure susceptibility by focal infusion of excitant amino acid or bicuculline into the inferior colliculus of normal rats. *Exp Neurol*. 1986;91:634–639.
31. Lohman RJ, Liu L, Morris M, O'Brien TJ. Validation of a method for localised microinjection of drugs into thalamic subregions in rats for epilepsy pharmacological studies. *J Neurosci Methods*. 2005;146:191–197.
32. Malpeli JG, Schiller PH, Colby CL. Response properties of single cells in monkey striate cortex during reversible inactivation of individual lateral geniculate laminae. *J Neurophysiol*. 1981;46: 1102–1119.
33. Millan MH, Patel S, Mello LM, Meldrum BS. Focal injection of 2-amino-7-phosphonoheptanoic acid into prepiriform cortex protects against pilocarpine-induced limbic seizures in rats. *Neurosci Lett*. 1986;70:69–74.
34. Albensi BC, Oliver DR, Toupin J, Odero G. Electrical stimulation protocols for hippocampal synaptic plasticity and neuronal hyper-excitability: are they effective or relevant? *Exp Neurol*. 2007;204:1–13.
35. Feng HJ, Faingold CL. Synaptic plasticity in the pathway from the medial geniculate body to the lateral amygdala is induced by seizure repetition. *Brain Res*. 2002;946:198–205.
36. Feng HJ, Kao C, Gallagher MJ, et al. Alteration of GABAergic neurotransmission by pulsed infrared laser stimulation. *J Neurosci Methods*. 2010;192:110–114.
37. Zhang F, Gradinaru V, Adamantidis AR, et al. Optogenetic interrogation of neural circuits: technology for probing mammalian brain structures. *Nat Protoc*. 2010;5:439–456.
38. Luscher C, Nicoll RA, Malenka RC, Muller D. Synaptic plasticity and dynamic modulation of the postsynaptic membrane. *Nat Neurosci*. 2000;3:545–550.

39. Vitek JL. Deep brain stimulation: how does it work? *Cleve Clin J Med*. 2008;75:S59–S65.
40. Goddard GV. Development of epileptic seizures through brain stimulation at low intensity. *Nature*. 1967;214:1020–1021.
41. Loscher W, Kohling R. Functional, metabolic, and synaptic changes after seizures as potential targets for antiepileptic therapy. *Epilepsy Behav.* 2010;19:105–113.
42. Racine RJ. Modification of seizure activity by electrical stimulation. II. Motor seizure. *Electroencephalogr Clin Neurophysiol.* 1972; 32:281–294.
43. Coulter DA, McIntyre DC, Loscher W. Animal models of limbic epilepsies: what can they tell us? *Brain Pathol.* 2002;12: 240–256.
44. McCown TJ, Greenwood RS, Frye GD, Breese GR. Electrically elicited seizures from the inferior colliculus: a potential site for the genesis of epilepsy. *Exp Neurol*. 1984;86:527–542.
45. McCown TJ, Givens BS, Breese GR. Amino acid influences on seizures elicited within the inferior colliculus. *J Pharmacol Exp Ther.* 1987;243:603–608.
46. Bagri A, Di Scala G, Sandner G. Wild running elicited by microinjection of bicuculline or morphine into the inferior colliculus of rats: lack of effect of periaqueductal gray lesions. *Pharmacol Biochem Behav.* 1992;41:727–732.
47. Bagri A, Di Scala G, Sandner G. Myoclonic and tonic seizures elicited by microinjection of cholinergic drugs into the inferior colliculus. *Therapie*. 1999;54:589–594.
48. Faingold CL, Naritoku DK, Copley CA, et al. Glutamate in the inferior colliculus plays a critical role in audiogenic seizure initiation. *Epilepsy Res*. 1992;13:95–105.
49. McCown TJ, Greenwood RS, Breese GR. Inferior colliculus interactions with limbic seizure activity. *Epilepsia*. 1987;28:234–241.
50. Feng HJ, Naritoku DK, Randall ME, Faingold CL. Modulation of audiogenically kindled seizures by γ-aminobutyric acid-related mechanisms in the amygdala. *Exp Neurol*. 2001;172:477–481.
51. Hirsch E, Danober L, Simler S, et al. The amygdala is critical for seizure propagation from brainstem to forebrain. *Neuroscience*. 1997;77:975–984.
52. Dailey JW, Jobe PC. Anticonvulsant drugs and the genetically epilepsy-prone rat. *Fed Proc*. 1985;44:2640–2644.
53. Faingold CL. Electrical stimulation therapies for CNS disorders and pain are mediated by competition between different neuronal networks in the brain. *Med Hypotheses*. 2008;71:668–681.
54. Bradford HF. Glutamate, GABA and epilepsy. *Prog Neurobiol*. 1995;47:477–511.
55. Gilbert ME. Does the kindling model of epilepsy contribute to our understanding of multiple chemical sensitivity? *Ann N Y Acad Sci*. 2001;933:68–91.
56. Johansen JP, Cain CK, Ostroff LE, LeDoux JE. Molecular mechanisms of fear learning and memory. *Cell*. 2011;147:509–524.
57. Monfils MH, Cowansage KK, LeDoux JE. Brain-derived neurotrophic factor: linking fear learning to memory consolidation. *Mol Pharmacol*. 2007;72:235–237.
58. Tupal S, Faingold CL. Precipitous induction of audiogenic kindling by activation of adenylyl cyclase in the amygdala. *Epilepsia*. 2010;51:354–361.
59. Raisinghani M, Feng HJ, Faingold CL. Glutamatergic activation of the amygdala differentially mimics the effects of audiogenic seizure kindling in two substrains of genetically epilepsy-prone rats. *Exp Neurol*. 2003;183:516–522.
60. Merrill DR, Bikson M, Jefferys JG. Electrical stimulation of excitable tissue: design of efficacious and safe protocols. *J Neurosci Methods*. 2005;141:171–198.
61. Wells J, Konrad P, Kao C, Jansen ED, Mahadevan-Jansen A. Pulsed laser versus electrical energy for peripheral nerve stimulation. *J Neurosci Methods*. 2007;163:326–337.
62. Wells J, Kao C, Jansen ED, Konrad P, Mahadevan-Jansen A. Application of infrared light for in vivo neural stimulation. *J Biomed Opt*. 2005;10:064003.
63. Boyden ES, Zhang F, Bamberg E, Nagel G, Deisseroth K. Millisecond-timescale, genetically targeted optical control of neural activity. *Nat Neurosci*. 2005;8:1263–1268.
64. Fenno L, Yizhar O, Deisseroth K. The development and application of optogenetics. *Annu Rev Neurosci*. 2011;34:389–412.
65. Gradinaru V, Zhang F, Ramakrishnan C, et al. Molecular and cellular approaches for diversifying and extending optogenetics. *Cell*. 2010;141:154–165.
66. Gradinaru V, Thompson KR, Zhang F, et al. Targeting and readout strategies for fast optical neural control in vitro and in vivo. *J Neurosci*. 2007;27:14231–14238.
67. Arenkiel BR, Peca J, Davison IG, et al. In vivo light-induced activation of neural circuitry in transgenic mice expressing channelrhodopsin-2. *Neuron*. 2007;54:205–218.
68. Dann CT. New technology for an old favorite: lentiviral transgenesis and RNAi in rats. *Transgenic Res*. 2007;16:571–580.
69. Sasaki K, Suzuki M, Mieda M, Tsujino N, Roth B, Sakurai T. Pharmacogenetic modulation of orexin neurons alters sleep/wakefulness states in mice. *PLoS One*. 2011;6:e20360.
70. Nair SG, Strand NS, Neumaier JF. DREADDing the lateral habenula: a review of methodological approaches for studying lateral habenula function. *Brain Res*. 2013;1511:93–101.
71. Krook-Magnuson E, Armstrong C, Oijala M, Soltesz I. On-demand optogenetic control of spontaneous seizures in temporal lobe epilepsy. *Nat Commun*. 2013;4:1376.
72. Paz JT, Davidson TJ, Frechette ES, et al. Closed-loop optogenetic control of thalamus as a tool for interrupting seizures after cortical injury. *Nat Neurosci*. 2013;16:64–70.
73. Tsunematsu T, Tabuchi S, Tanaka KF, Boyden ES, Tominaga M, Yamanaka A. Long-lasting silencing of orexin/hypocretin neurons using archaerhodopsin induces slow-wave sleep in mice. *Behav Brain Res*. 2013. http://dx.doi.org/10.1016/j.bbr.2013.05.021. pii: S0166–4328.
74. Feng HJ, Faingold CL. Repeated generalized audiogenic seizures induce plastic changes on acoustically evoked neuronal firing in the amygdala. *Brain Res*. 2002;932:61–69.
75. Feng HJ, Faingold CL. Ketamine in mood disorders and epilepsy. In: Costa A, Villalba E, eds. *Horizons in Neuroscience Research*. 2013; vol. 10. New York, NY: Nova Science Publishers; 2013:103–122.
76. Clark D, Engberg G, Pileblad E, et al. An electrophysiological analysis of the actions of the 3-PPP enantiomers on the nigrostriatal dopamine system. *Naunyn Schmiedebergs Arch Pharmacol*. 1985;329:344–354.
77. Kita H, Chang HT, Kitai ST. Pallidal inputs to subthalamus: intracellular analysis. *Brain Res*. 1983;264:255–265.
78. Morrell F, Hoeppner TJ, de Toledo-Morrell L. Conditioning of single units in visual association cortex: cell-specific behavior within a small population. *Exp Neurol*. 1983;80:111–146.
79. Scarnati E, Proia A, Di Loreto S, Pacitti C. The reciprocal electrophysiological influence between the nucleus tegmenti pedunculopontinus and the substantia nigra in normal and decorticated rats. *Brain Res*. 1987;423:116–124.
80. Bonhaus DW, Russell RD, McNamara JO. Activation of substantia nigra pars reticulata neurons: role in the initiation and behavioral expression of kindled seizures. *Brain Res*. 1991;545:41–48.
81. Faingold CL, Anderson CA. Loss of intensity-induced inhibition in inferior colliculus neurons leads to audiogenic seizure susceptibility in behaving genetically epilepsy-prone rats. *Exp Neurol*. 1991;113:354–363.
82. Sasaki K, Ono T, Nishino H, Fukuda M, Muramoto KI. A method for long-term artifact-free recording of single unit activity in

freely moving, eating and drinking animals. *J Neurosci Methods.* 1983;7:43–47.

83. Szymusiak R, Nitz D. Chronic recording of extracellular neuronal activity in behaving animals. *Curr Protoc Neurosci.* 2003: 6.16.1–6.16.24.
84. Green JT, Arenos JD. Hippocampal and cerebellar single-unit activity during delay and trace eyeblink conditioning in the rat. *Neurobiol Learn Mem.* 2007;87:269–284.
85. Wang JY, Luo F, Chang JY, Woodward DJ, Han JS. Parallel pain processing in freely moving rats revealed by distributed neuron recording. *Brain Res.* 2003;992:263–271.
86. Wang CM, Yang L, Lu D, et al. Simultaneous multisite recordings of neural ensemble responses in the motor cortex of behaving rats to peripheral noxious heat and chemical stimuli. *Behav Brain Res.* 2011;223:192–202.
87. Yang G, Lobarinas E, Zhang L, et al. Salicylate induced tinnitus: behavioral measures and neural activity in auditory cortex of awake rats. *Hear Res.* 2007;226:244–253.
88. Zhang X, Zhang RL, Zhang ZG, Chopp M. Measurement of neuronal activity of individual neurons after stroke in the rat using a microwire electrode array. *J Neurosci Methods.* 2007;162: 91–100.
89. Dzirasa K, Fuentes R, Kumar S, Potes JM, Nicolelis MA. Chronic in vivo multi-circuit neurophysiological recordings in mice. *J Neurosci Methods.* 2011;195:36–46.
90. Tseng WT, Yen CT, Tsai ML. A bundled microwire array for long-term chronic single-unit recording in deep brain regions of behaving rats. *J Neurosci Methods.* 2011;201:368–376.
91. Chang FC, Scott TR, Harper RM. Methods of single unit recording from medullary neural substrates in awake, behaving guinea pigs. *Brain Res Bull.* 1988;21:749–756.
92. Banks D, Kuriakose M, Matthews B. A technique for recording the activity of brain-stem neurones in awake, unrestrained cats using microwires and an implantable micromanipulator. *J Neurosci Methods.* 1993;46:83–88.
93. Palmer C. A microwire technique for recording single neurons in unrestrained animals. *Brain Res Bull.* 1978;3:285–289.
94. Jackson A, Fetz EE. Compact movable microwire array for long-term chronic unit recording in cerebral cortex of primates. *J Neurophysiol.* 2007;98:3109–3118.
95. Nicolelis MA, Dimitrov D, Carmena JM, et al. Chronic, multisite, multielectrode recordings in macaque monkeys. *Proc Natl Acad Sci USA.* 2003;100:11041–11046.
96. Thorp CK, Steinmetz PN. Interference and noise in human intracranial microwire recordings. *IEEE Trans Biomed Eng.* 2009;56:30–36.
97. Feng HJ, Faingold CL. The effects of chronic ethanol administration on amygdala neuronal firing and ethanol withdrawal seizures. *Neuropharmacology.* 2008;55:648–653.
98. Borroni A, Chen FM, LeCursi N, Grover LM, Teyler TJ. An integrated multielectrode electrophysiology system. *J Neurosci Methods.* 1991;36:177–184.
99. Kralik JD, Dimitrov DF, Krupa DJ, Katz DB, Cohen D, Nicolelis MA. Techniques for long-term multisite neuronal ensemble recordings in behaving animals. *Methods.* 2001;25:121–150.
100. Vos BP, Wijnants M, Taeymans S, De Schutter E. Miniature carrier with six independently movable electrodes for recording of multiple single-units in the cerebellar cortex of awake rats. *J Neurosci Methods.* 1999;94:19–26.
101. Dick TE, Morris KF. Quantitative analysis of cardiovascular modulation in respiratory neural activity. *J Physiol.* 2004;556: 959–970.
102. Nicolelis MA, Ghazanfar AA, Faggin BM, Votaw S, Oliveira LM. Reconstructing the engram: simultaneous, multisite, many single neuron recordings. *Neuron.* 1997;18:529–537.
103. Raisinghani M, Faingold CL. Neurons in the amygdala play an important role in the neuronal network mediating a clonic form of audiogenic seizures both before and after audiogenic kindling. *Brain Res.* 2005;1032:131–140.
104. Faingold CL. Brainstem networks: reticulo-cortical synchronization in generalized convulsive seizures. In: Noebels JL, Avoli M, Rogawski MA, Olsen RW, Delgado-Escueta AV, eds. *Jasper's Basic Mechanisms of the Epilepsies.* 4th ed. New York, NY: Oxford University Press; 2012:257–271.
105. Mishra M, Jones B, Simonotto JD, et al. Pre-ictal entropy analysis of microwire data from an animal model of limbic epilepsy. *Conf Proc IEEE Eng Med Biol Soc.* 2006;1:1605–1607.
106. Truccolo W, Donoghue JA, Hochberg LR, et al. Single-neuron dynamics in human focal epilepsy. *Nat Neurosci.* 2011;14:635–641.
107. Ottersen OP, Ben-Ari Y. Afferent connections to the amygdaloid complex of the rat and cat. I. Projections from the thalamus. *J Comp Neurol.* 1979;187:401–424.
108. Patrick E, Orazem ME, Sanchez JC, Nishida T. Corrosion of tungsten microelectrodes used in neural recording applications. *J Neurosci Methods.* 2011;198:158–171.
109. Winslow BD, Tresco PA. Quantitative analysis of the tissue response to chronically implanted microwire electrodes in rat cortex. *Biomaterials.* 2010;31:1558–1567.
110. Winslow BD, Christensen MB, Yang WK, Solzbacher F, Tresco PA. A comparison of the tissue response to chronically implanted Parylene-C-coated and uncoated planar silicon microelectrode arrays in rat cortex. *Biomaterials.* 2010;31:9163–9172.
111. Bae WJ, Ruddy BP, Richardson AG, Hunter IW, Bizzi E. Cortical recording with polypyrrole microwire electrodes. *Conf Proc IEEE Eng Med Biol Soc.* 2008:5794–5797.
112. Li Y, Evans MS, Faingold CL. Inferior colliculus neuronal membrane and synaptic properties in genetically epilepsy-prone rats. *Brain Res.* 1994;660:232–240.

CHAPTER

5

Network Experimental Approaches: Ex vivo Recording

Victor V. Uteshev

Department of Pharmacology and Neuroscience, University of North Texas Health Science Center, Fort Worth, TX, USA

INTRODUCTION

In a functional brain, contributions of individual neurons can often be most effective if the neuronal activity is synchronized. Synchronization can be achieved either by a direct communication among neurons or by inhibition of asynchrony (i.e. reducing the chances of individual neurons to act differently from the rest of the group). For example, in the olfactory bulb, a direct communication among neurons via synaptic connections and gap junctions[1] prevents external tufted (ET) cells of the same glomerulus from behaving asynchronously with the rest of the neuronal population, while natural pacemaker neurons of the hypothalamic histaminergic tuberomammillary (TM) nucleus that are electrically independent from one another (as discussed in this chapter) can be synchronously shut off during sleep by GABAergic inputs from the ventrolateral preoptic nucleus.[2] Therefore, in some cases, the impact of individual neurons on the network status can be deduced either from understanding of the network structure as well as synaptic and/or gap junction connections, or from knowledge of pharmacology and kinetics of the external inputs and neuronal receptors involved in signaling. Neurons, on the other hand, may define the level of sustained excitability of neuronal networks, network stability, and sensitivity to the action of endogenous and exogenous compounds.

Although "in vitro" is a term that has been often applied to brain slice work, it is perhaps more accurate to label acute slice work as "ex vivo", which is done in this chapter. The term "in vitro" is used to refer to cultured neurons and cell lines.

DIRECT SYNCHRONIZATION VIA CHEMICAL AND ELECTRICAL SYNAPSES IN THE OLFACTORY BULB

The olfactory bulb is a complex and intriguing brain structure involved in encoding, transfer, processing, and decoding of odorant-evoked sensory information. It has a multifaceted network of interneuronal connections that include dendrodendritic chemical synapses and electrical synapses, also known as gap junctions.[3] Organization and properties of neuronal and synaptic connections facilitate neuronal synchronization, which may be critical for effective odor discrimination.[4–6] Moreover, optimal neuronal synchronization may enhance transmission of information from sensory receptors to higher order brain structures.[7,8]

Integration and processing of sensory olfactory information at the level of the olfactory bulb involve stimulation of a complex neuronal circuitry, specific patterns of activation of chemical and electrical synapses, and coordination of activity of multiple glomeruli. The glomeruli of the olfactory bulb serve as the sites of the first synapse for olfactory sensory inputs, which are processed by three types of glomerular juxtaglomerular (JG) neurons: ET, periglomerular (PG), and short axon (SA) cells. Olfactory bulb output neurons exhibit highly synchronized activity in acute ex vivo preparation of brain slices despite deprivation of their normal sensory inputs. Synchronous activity is common among output neurons whose tufted dendrites belong to the same glomerulus. Such synchronization was found among mitral cells,[9] ET cells,[1] tufted cells,[10] and mitral cells.[11] Furthermore, additional interactions among neurons within the same glomerulus or different glomeruli arise from

Neuronal Networks in Brain Function, CNS Disorders, and Therapeutics
http://dx.doi.org/10.1016/B978-0-12-415804-7.00005-8

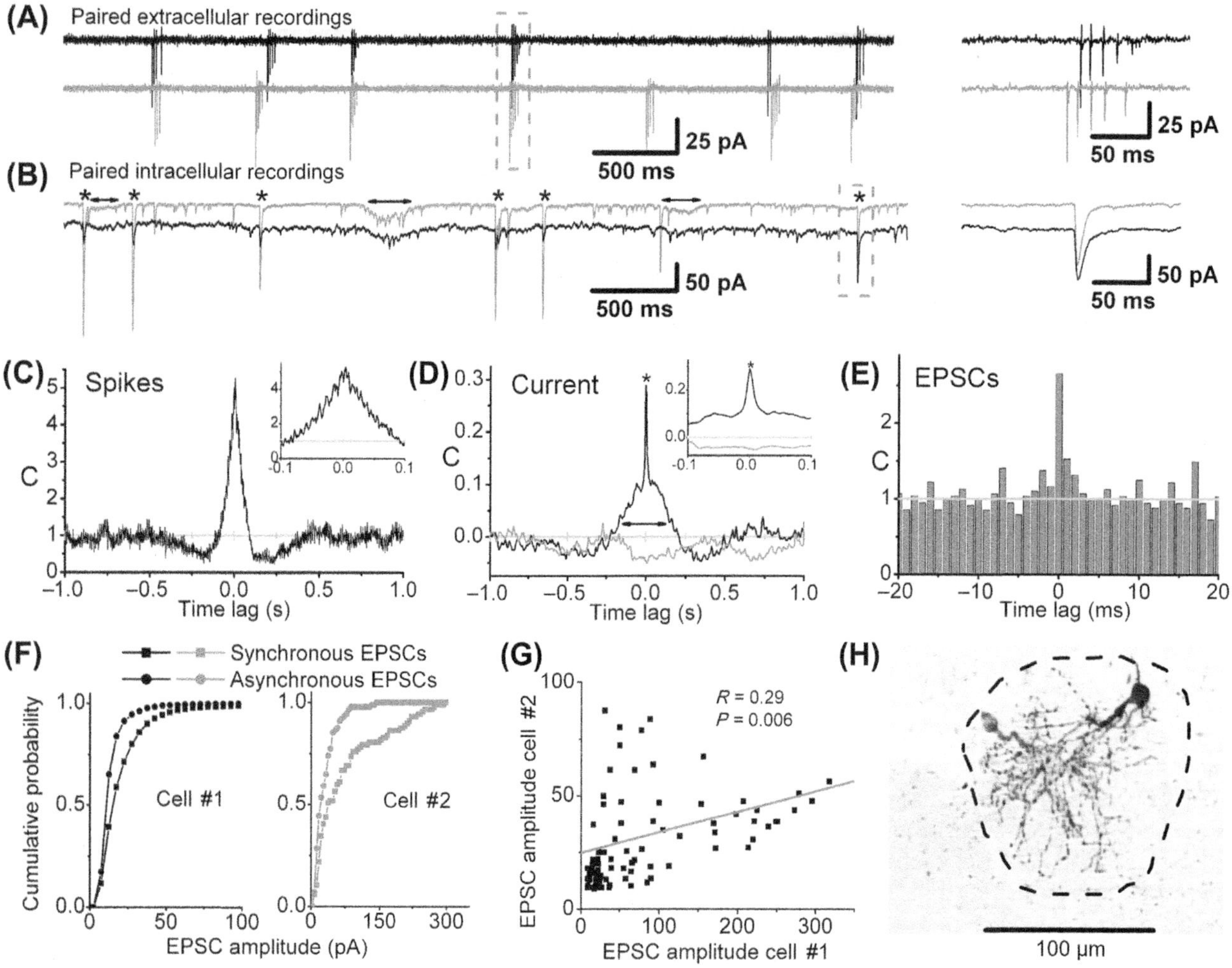

FIGURE 5.1 **Synchronous slow and fast Excitatory Post-Synaptic Currents (EPSCs) in ET cells of the same glomerulus.** All data presented in this figure were obtained from the same ET cell pair. (A) Simultaneous extracellular recordings from two ET cells with correlated spike bursting (correlated spikes shown in the inset at right). (B) The same two cells were then recorded in whole-cell configuration in voltage clamp (HP of −60 mV) using electrodes (containing $CsMeSO_3$ and QX-314). Note the synchronous slow (horizontal lines with arrows on both sides) and fast (asterisks; example shown at right) EPSCs. (C) Cross-correlogram of the spike trains (5 min recording sample, 1 ms bins) shows a significant correlation with a peak near zero lag time (see inset). (D) The cross-correlogram of the membrane current (50 s of intracellular recording sample, 2 ms bins) shows both a broad (small lines with arrows on both sides) and narrow (asterisk; see inset) correlation that peaked at zero time lag. The gray trace is the cross-correlogram of the membrane current traces after shifting the second trace by 5 s (to determine significance, see "Materials and Methods" in Ref. 1). (E) Cross-correlogram of the EPSC trains (5 min recording sample, 1 ms bins) shows a significant peak only in the bin at zero time lag, indicating synchronous EPSCs in the two recorded cells. The vertical axes in (C–E) demonstrate a cross-correlation value, C. (F) Cumulative probability histograms of the EPSC amplitudes of synchronous and asynchronous EPSCs recorded in both cells (during 5 min). The synchronous EPSCs exhibited significantly larger amplitude than asynchronous EPSCs ($p < 0.0001$, K–S test). (G) Scatterplot of the amplitude of synchronous EPSCs in cell 2 versus cell 1 and a linear regression fit showing a significant positive correlation. (H) Photograph of the two recorded cells after biocytin staining showing the overlap of dendrites in the same glomerulus (dashed line). *Source: From Hayar et al., 2005,*[1] *with permission from the Society for Neuroscience.*

extensive lateral dendrites found in output neurons that establish dendrodendritic connections with interneurons.[12] For example, a highly correlated activity was found among ET cells, SA cells, and PG cells[13,14] and among mitral cells and granule cells.[15]

Using an ex vivo olfactory bulb slice preparation and dual patch-clamp recordings from the JG circuitry (Figure 5.1), it has been determined that ET cells spontaneously fire rhythmic spike bursts in the theta frequency range and receive monosynaptic olfactory nerve input.[1,16] By contrast, SA and most PG cells do not receive monosynaptic olfactory input, but receive instead monosynaptic excitatory inputs from ET cells. These observations demonstrated that ET cells serve as a major excitatory link between olfactory nerve input and other JG cells. Intriguingly, within the same glomerulus, spontaneous bursts among ET cells are highly correlated even in the absence of activity of fast chemical

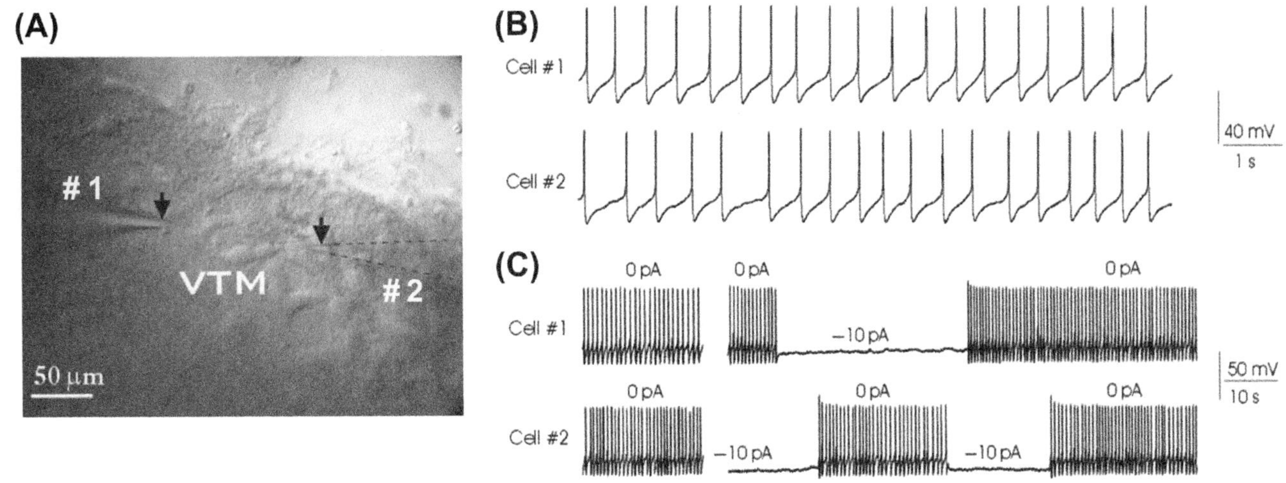

FIGURE 5.2 **Simultaneous recordings from pairs of ventral TM (VTM) neurons in acute hypothalamic brain slices.** Neighboring TM neurons (arrows) located within 200 μm from one another (A) were selected for simultaneous recordings of spontaneous action potentials (APs) in current-clamp patch-clamp experiments (B–C). The results obtained from analyzing nine pairs of TM neurons demonstrated random uncorrelated patterns of spontaneous APs of neighboring TM neurons. In each pair, spontaneous APs fired in one TM neuron were not detectable in the other TM neuron inhibited by injection of small (10 pA) hyperpolarizing currents (C).

synapses (i.e. when activity of GABAergic and glutamatergic fast synapses is blocked).[1] Analysis of experimental data indicated that the synchronized spontaneous bursting of ET cells within the same glomerulus is coordinated by synaptic transmission and gap junction coupling among ET cells (Figure 5.1). Therefore, the synchronous bursting of ET cells and, thus, synchronized odor-evoked glomerular output may function to amplify transient sensory inputs and coordinate glomerular outputs to ensure that the high fidelity of the specific odorant profile information is relayed to higher order brain structures. Moreover, the bursting activity of ET cells is readily entrained by patterns of odor-evoked sensory inputs at sniffing frequencies.[13] These results suggest that amplification of the sensory input by ET cells may help enhance synchronization of the glomerular network tuned to the sniffing of the animal and, thus, enhance its functionality. The presence of highly multifaceted neuronal interactions in the olfactory bulb circuitry may reflect a need of olfactory bulb neurons to tune their activity to the animal's respiratory cycle[17–19].

INHIBITION OF ASYNCHRONY IN SPONTANEOUS ACTIVITY OF HYPOTHALAMIC HISTAMINERGIC TM NEURONS

The TM nucleus of the posterior hypothalamus represents the sole source of brain histamine and contributes to regulation of normal cognition, sleep–wakefulness cycles, food and water consumption, and energy metabolism (see Chapter 21).[20,21] Histamine, a "waking substance", regulates sleep and wakefulness, while blood–brain barrier permeable histamine H1 receptor antagonists cause sedation. TM neurons are typical, natural pacemakers and demonstrate spontaneous firing in the absence of synaptic inputs in vivo,[22,23] in vitro,[24–26] and after acute dissociation.[27,28] The firing pattern of TM neurons as well as the histamine concentration in cerebrospinal fluid follow a circadian rhythm (see Chapter 14) and depend on the state of arousal.[29,30] The highest frequency of TM neuronal spontaneous firing (6–8 Hz) corresponds to wakefulness in vivo. The activity of TM neurons decreases during non–rapid eye movement (non-REM) sleep and ceases completely during rapid eye movement (REM) sleep.[22,23] Blocking spontaneous firing by hypothalamic perfusion with tetrodotoxin inhibits histamine release,[31,32] which has been shown to require extracellular Ca^{2+} in vivo[33] and in vitro.[31,34] The presence of both inactivating and non-inactivating voltage-gated calcium channels in TM neurons[35] produces a dynamic equilibrium supportive of sustained spontaneous firing via associated Ca^{2+} signaling.[36,37]

In contrast to olfactory ET cells, TM neurons do not communicate with their TM neighbors via chemical or electrical synapses (Figure 5.2). Instead, TM neurons fire action potentials independently and within a relatively narrow range (1–6 Hz) of frequencies unless inhibited, for instance, via GABAergic inputs from the ventrolateral preoptic nucleus.[2]

A strong relationship between the frequency of spontaneous firing and the corresponding Ca^{2+} influx in TM neurons has been established in ex vivo experiments

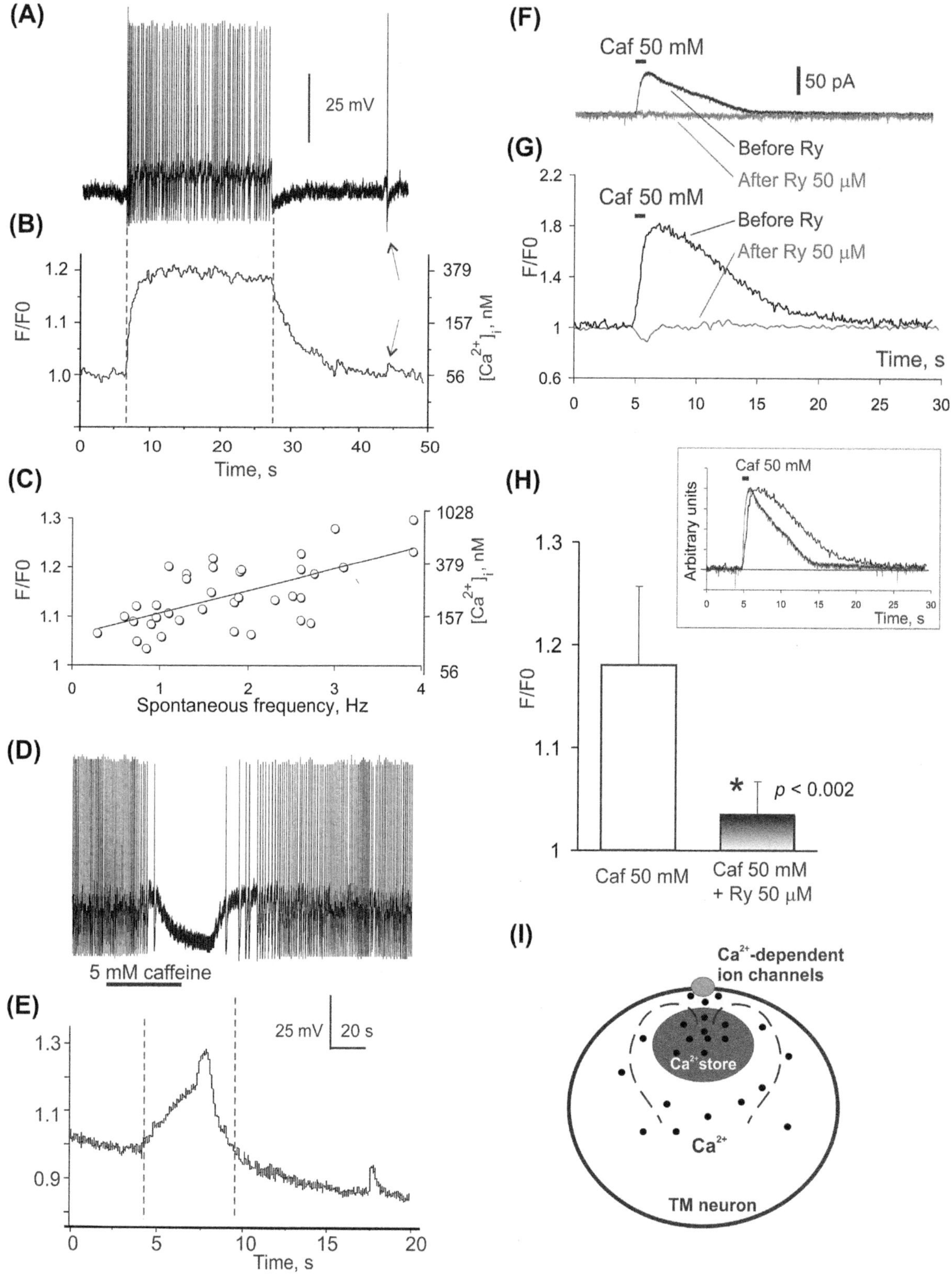

FIGURE 5.3 **Correlation among neuronal properties and function.** (A–B) A typical example of simultaneous current-clamp (A) and Ca^{2+} (B) recordings from the same TM neuron. Spontaneous firing of TM neurons (A) correlates with elevation in $[Ca^{2+}]_i$ (B) measured using Ca^{2+} Green-1 dye included into the intracellular pipette solution. A graphic relationship between the frequency of spontaneous firing and Ca^{2+} influx (in μM and as a ratio of F/F0) is shown in (C). Firing frequencies (1–4 Hz) that are observed in vivo during wakefulness correspond to $[Ca^{2+}]_i \sim 0.2$–1 μM and may support histamine release. (D–E) Caffeine inhibits spontaneous firing of TM neurons (D) by stimulating Ca^{2+} release from Ca^{2+} stores (E) and activation of Ca^{2+}-dependent potassium conductance (K_{Ca}). Both an outward conductance measured in

utilizing simultaneous Ca^{2+} imaging and electrophysiological patch-clamp recordings from TM neurons in acute brains slices.[25] As the firing pattern of TM neurons defines the rate of histamine release and arousal state in mammals,[22,23,31,32] this correlation between spontaneous firing and $[Ca^{2+}]_i$ predicts the levels of cytosolic Ca^{2+} that correspond to specific behavioral states (e.g. sleep or wakefulness) (Figure 5.3(A)–(C)). In particular, the maximum firing frequency observed in these ex vivo experiments was ~4 Hz.[25] This frequency corresponds to wakefulness in vivo[22,23] and elevates $[Ca^{2+}]_i$ to over 1 μM ex vivo.[25] Therefore, one could expect cytosolic levels of Ca^{2+} in TM neurons to reach 1 μM during wakefulness and drop to the baseline near 60 nM during sleep.[25] Accordingly, intermediate firing frequencies (i.e. 1–2 Hz) would be expected to correspond to intermediate phases of sleep–wakefulness (e.g. non-REM sleep) and generated intermediate levels of $[Ca^{2+}]_i$ in the range of ~300 nM (Figure 5.3(C)). The observed changes in $[Ca^{2+}]_i$ were rapid and fully reversible. These results demonstrate a prolonged presence of high levels of $[Ca^{2+}]_i$ (i.e. >300 nM) in TM neurons during phases of activity that could correspond to TM firing during wakefulness. These high levels of $[Ca^{2+}]_i$ may be essential for controlling histamine release, a Ca^{2+}-dependent process, while several sources of Ca^{2+} may contribute to this regulation, including high-threshold voltage-activated Ca^{2+} ion channels (HVACCs),[25] Ca^{2+} stores (Figure 5.3), and Na^+–Ca^{2+} exchangers.[38] Interestingly, transient elevations of Ca^{2+} levels elicited by Ca^{2+} release from cytosolic stores inhibited spontaneous firing of TM neurons and, thus, would be expected to inhibit histamine release due to activation of Ca^{2+}-dependent K^+ ion channels (K_{Ca}) (Figure 5.3(D)–(E)). These results suggest intimate links between Ca^{2+} stores and K_{Ca} within the TM cytoplasm and the ability of Ca^{2+} stores to modulate neuronal excitability of TM neurons. Given the role of TM neurons in circadian rhythms regulation, Ca^{2+} stores may participate in the maintenance of the sleep–wakefulness cycle.

The involvement of K_{Ca} in the inhibition of TM spontaneous firing elicited by Ca^{2+} release from internal stores is supported by the sensitivity of caffeine-mediated responses to the external concentration of K^+ ions ($[K^+]_o$) (Figure 5.4) and ryanodine (Ry) (an irreversible agonist of Ry receptors, RyRs) (Figure 5.3(F)–(G)), as well as 50 μM cyclopiazonic acid (CPA, a blocker of Ca^{2+}-ATPase) (not shown). These results are summarized in Figures 5.3(H) and 5.4. The presence of intimate links between Ca^{2+} stores and K_{Ca} is supported by the similarity in the rates of onsets of $[Ca^{2+}]_i$ elevation and K_{Ca} current (Figure 5.3(H), *insert*). However, the duration of elevated $[Ca^{2+}]_i$ is clearly extended past the duration of K_{Ca} current, pointing to limitations in the potency of Ca^{2+} release for inhibition of TM firing.

The presented data argue that elevation in TM $[Ca^{2+}]_i$ can significantly affect the firing patterns and behavior of TM neurons and, thus, modulate histamine release. However, although stimulation of Ca^{2+} stores can produce robust effects on TM firing (Figure 5.3(D)–(E)), the membrane voltage is likely to be the main player in integration of cytosolic Ca^{2+} signals in TM neurons[25,37] as Ca^{2+} currents can be activated during afterhyperpolaryzation (AHP) with a strong dependence of the Ca^{2+} net charge on the membrane voltage where an equilibrium between activation and inactivation of multiple types of Ca^{2+} currents and AHP currents near the threshold of firing may support the physiological need in histamine. The HVACCs are expected to be especially important for regulation of spontaneous firing and histamine metabolism in the TM because of their noninactivating nature and control over the amount of Ca^{2+} influx during the action potential.[35,37]

STOCHASTIC ENHANCEMENT OF NEURONAL EXCITABILITY: CAN A SINGLE ION CHANNEL EXCITE THE ENTIRE NEURON?

Nicotinic α7 acetylcholine receptors (α7 nAChRs) are widely expressed in the central nervous system. Under normal physiological conditions, the duration of α7 channel openings are extremely short (~0.1 ms[39]), but in the presence of type II positive allosteric modulators (α7-PAMs) such as PNU-120596, the duration of α7 open channels can be substantially increased (~1 s[40]). In the absence of PNU-120596, the generation of whole-cell α7 responses requires high synchrony of

voltage-clamp patch-clamp recordings (F) and the corresponding elevation in $[Ca^{2+}]_i$ (G) are blocked by 50 μM ryanodine (Ry) (F–G) added to Artificial Cerebrospinal Fluid (ACSF), supporting the involvement of Ca^{2+} stores and K_{Ca}. Traces shown in (F) and (G) share the same time scale shown in (G). (H) A summary of results obtained from $n = 9$ TM neurons. Significance is defined by the p-value evaluated using an unpaired two-tail Student test. The *insert* illustrates the kinetics of K_{Ca} outward current versus elevation in $[Ca^{2+}]_i$ obtained from the same pressure application of 50 mM caffeine (Caf) to a TM neuron as shown in (F–G). Although the rates of onset of both processes are similar, the duration of elevated $[Ca^{2+}]_i$ is clearly extended past the duration of K_{Ca} current. (I) A simplified model of a TM neuron illustrating functional links between Ca^{2+} stores and K_{Ca} channels. Although normal TM spontaneous firing can elevate $[Ca^{2+}]_i$ to ~1 μM, it is the release of Ca^{2+} from Ca^{2+} stores that activates K_{Ca} channels and inhibits spontaneous firing supporting these links. *Source: Panels (A–C) are from Uteshev and Knot, 2005,[25] with permission from Elsevier.* (For color version of this figure, the reader is referred to the online version of this book.)

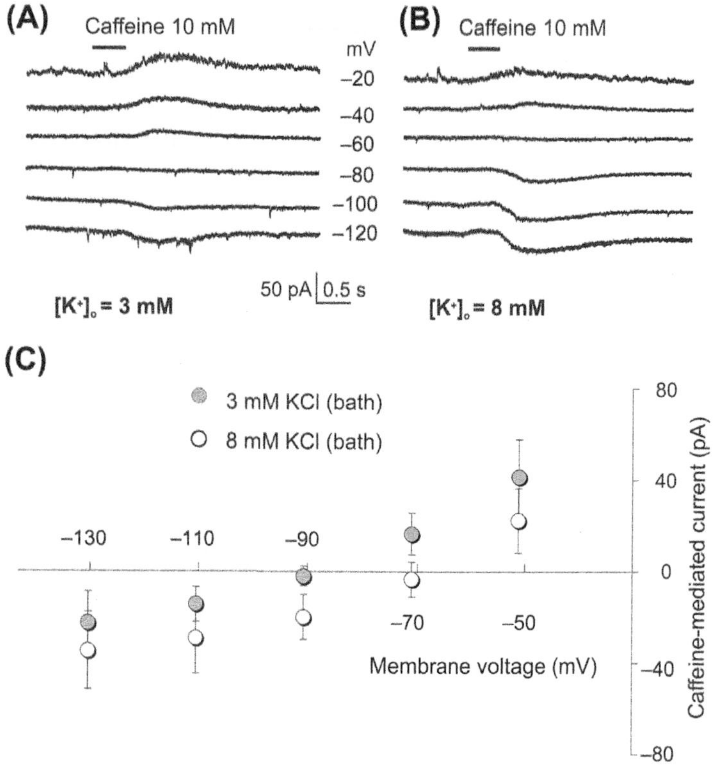

FIGURE 5.4 The current–voltage relationship and sensitivity to $[K^+]_o$ of caffeine-induced K_{Ca} currents. (A–B) Typical current traces obtained from TM neurons held at various membrane voltages (indicated in the center) by brief pressure application of 10 mM caffeine. ACSF contained either 3 mM (A) or 8 mM (B) K^+. (C) The current–voltage dependence obtained from $n = 5$ TM neurons. A clear depolarizing shift in the reversal potential is seen, reflecting an increase in $[K^+]_o$. This shift and the responsiveness to caffeine support the involvement of Ca^{2+}-dependent K^+ ion channels triggered by Ca^{2+} release from Ca^{2+} stores.

activation of many α7 channels. For instance, given the mean α7 open channel duration in the absence of PNU-120596 (i.e. ~0.1 ms), theoretically, up to 10,000 α7 channels can open each second without considerable overlay and thus not result in detectable whole-cell responses. By contrast, the same 10,000 channels opened for an average duration of ~1 s in the presence of PNU-120596 would be expected to generate a 50–80 nA response. This example illustrates a strong synchronizing action of PNU-120596 on α7 nAChR-mediated ion channel activity.

In the presence of PNU-120596 and physiological levels of choline (i.e. ~5–20 μM), a weak persistent level of α7 nAChR activation can be achieved[41,42] that is sufficient for triggering action potentials, thus enhancing the excitation of CA1 pyramidal neurons.[43] The physiological importance of these effects at physiological temperatures has been recently questioned due to observations that the responsiveness of heterologously expressed α7 nAChRs to nicotinic agonists in the presence of PNU-120596 is significantly reduced at near-physiological temperatures.[44] However, PNU-120596 is effective in vivo (thus at physiological temperatures),[45–49] and thus, although activation of α7 nAChRs in the presence of PNU-120596 is reduced at physiological temperatures, it can still be therapeutically beneficial. Alternatively, only the agonist binding and activation of α7 nAChRs, but not ionic influx and activation of α7 nAChR-mediated ion channels, may be neuroprotective. In that event, a decrease in α7-mediated ionic influx at physiological temperatures may in fact be neuroprotective in at least two ways: by preserving agonist-receptor binding (which may be directly neuroprotective) and reducing ionic influx (which may be directly neurotoxic).

At least at room temperatures, multiple simultaneous openings of α7 channels may alter neuronal behavior. This is illustrated in Figure 5.5, where synchronous openings of at least four α7 ion channels send hippocampal CA1 interneurons to prolonged bursts of action potentials, sometimes lasting for over a minute. CA1 interneurons may directly inhibit CA1 pyramidal neurons via GABAergic synaptic inputs,[50] or they may excite CA1 pyramidal neurons by inhibiting other CA1 interneurons (i.e. via disinhibition).[51] Although PNU-120596 would be expected to enhance activation of α7 nAChRs in pyramidal neurons and interneurons proportionally, the net effect of this activation remains unknown and is likely to be concentration dependent. Moreover, in the presence of PNU-120596, the activation of α7 nAChRs by ACh would be expected to be substantially enhanced, while the activation of non-α7 nAChRs should remain unchanged. Therefore, in the presence of PNU-120596, the net effect on the hippocampal output

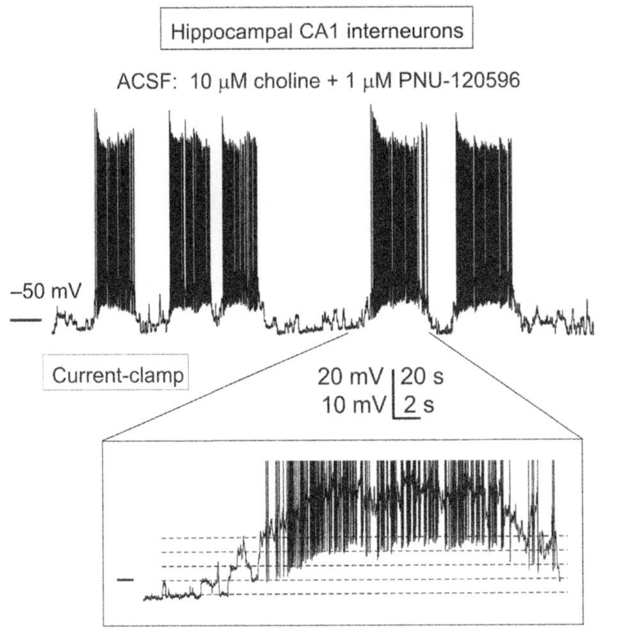

FIGURE 5.5 Excitability of hippocampal CA1 interneurons can be enhanced by stochastic summation of α7 single ion channel openings in the presence of physiological choline and PNU-120596. A weak persistent activation of individual α7 nAChRs in hippocampal CA1 interneurons can be achieved by adding 10 μM choline and 1 μM PNU-120596 to ACSF. These α7 nAChR-mediated single-channel openings can be observed in whole-cell current-clamp recordings as step-like voltage deviations. A typical example of current-clamp recordings from a hippocampal CA1 interneuron is shown where simultaneous activation of four or more α7 nAChRs triggers prolonged bursts of action potentials. Recordings were done at room temperature. This enhanced excitability of inhibitory GABAergic interneurons would be expected to cause a prolonged inhibition of CA1 pyramidal neurons and, thus, the hippocampal output. A typical example of PNU-120596-induced bursts of action potentials recorded in whole-cell current-clamp mode is amplified and shown in the *insert*. Horizontal dashed lines indicate amplitudes of step-like voltage deviations that correspond to individual α7 single ion channel openings. A solid horizontal bar in front of traces indicates the membrane voltage of −50 mV.

of activation of CA1 α7 nAChRs will likely depend on the strength, timing, and location of cholinergic terminals and the relative densities of expression of pre- and postsynaptic α7 and non-α7 subtypes of nAChRs, as discussed.[51,52] Nevertheless, since CA1 GABAergic interneurons act as the prime inhibitory source for CA1 pyramidal neurons, it is likely that enhanced bursting activity evoked by simultaneous activation of several α7 ion channels in the presence of PNU-120596 and physiological choline will inhibit some pyramidal neurons while disinhibiting others and, thus, alter the hippocampal output.[51,52] Therefore, additional research is essential to determine whether an optimal range of α7 activation exists in the hippocampus that would allow preserving the hippocampal output while enhancing the resistance of hippocampal principal neurons and interneurons to injury and various insults.[42]

CONCLUSION

This chapter illustrates the effectiveness of ex vivo techniques in supplementing in vivo approaches and providing a detailed understanding of ion channel and neurotransmitter receptor mechanisms in some network functions. Properties of individual neurons and synaptic connections shape the outputs of neuronal networks that are often synchronized and amplified by sensory inputs and their derivatives. Neuronal networks that are able to interpret patterns of sensory inputs are referred to as cognitive to distinguish them from autonomic networks that relay sensory inputs to higher brain regions or generate uninterpreted (i.e. unconscious) motor responses. However, there is a possibility that the interpretation of sensory information itself is input driven and may not be sustainable in the absence of a continuous sensory drive or its derivatives. In that event, the corresponding cognitive network signaling can be viewed as a sensory-driven reflex that initiates and supports its own interpretation by the network. This view supports a notion that links between cognitive and autonomic homeostases may be more intimate than currently appreciated.

References

1. Hayar A, Shipley MT, Ennis M. Olfactory bulb external tufted cells are synchronized by multiple intraglomerular mechanisms. *J Neurosci.* 2005;25(36):8197–8208.
2. Sherin JE, Elmquist JK, Torrealba F, Saper CB. Innervation of histaminergic tuberomammillary neurons by GABAergic and galaninergic neurons in the ventrolateral preoptic nucleus of the rat. *J Neurosci.* 1998;18(12):4705–4721.
3. Karpuk N, Hayar A. Activation of postsynaptic GABAB receptors modulates the bursting pattern and synaptic activity of olfactory bulb juxtaglomerular neurons. *J Neurophysiol.* 2008;99(1):308–319.
4. Laurent G, Stopfer M, Friedrich RW, Rabinovich MI, Volkovskii A, Abarbanel HD. Odor encoding as an active, dynamical process: experiments, computation, and theory. *Annu Rev Neurosci.* 2001;24:263–297.
5. Linster C, Cleland TA. How spike synchronization among olfactory neurons can contribute to sensory discrimination. *J Comput Neurosci.* 2001;10(2):187–193.
6. Stopfer M, Bhagavan S, Smith BH, Laurent G. Impaired odour discrimination on desynchronization of odour-encoding neural assemblies. *Nature.* 1997;390(6655):70–74.
7. Lisman JE. Bursts as a unit of neural information: making unreliable synapses reliable. *Trends Neurosci.* 1997;20(1):38–43.
8. Roy SA, Alloway KD. Coincidence detection or temporal integration? What the neurons in somatosensory cortex are doing. *J Neurosci.* 2001;21(7):2462–2473.

9. Carlson GC, Shipley MT, Keller A. Long-lasting depolarizations in mitral cells of the rat olfactory bulb. *J Neurosci.* 2000;20(5):2011–2021.
10. Ma J, Lowe G. Correlated firing in tufted cells of mouse olfactory bulb. *Neuroscience.* 2010;169(4):1715–1738.
11. De Saint Jan D, Hirnet D, Westbrook GL, Charpak S. External tufted cells drive the output of olfactory bulb glomeruli. *J Neurosci.* 2009;29(7):2043–2052.
12. Aungst JL, Heyward PM, Puche AC, et al. Centre-surround inhibition among olfactory bulb glomeruli. *Nature.* 2003; 426(6967):623–629.
13. Hayar A, Karnup S, Shipley MT, Ennis M. Olfactory bulb glomeruli: external tufted cells intrinsically burst at theta frequency and are entrained by patterned olfactory input. *J Neurosci.* 2004;24(5):1190–1199.
14. Murphy GJ, Darcy DP, Isaacson JS. Intraglomerular inhibition: signaling mechanisms of an olfactory microcircuit. *Nat Neurosci.* 2005;8(3):354–364.
15. Dietz SB, Murthy VN. Contrasting short-term plasticity at two sides of the mitral-granule reciprocal synapse in the mammalian olfactory bulb. *J Physiol.* 2005;569(Pt 2):475–488.
16. Hayar A, Karnup S, Ennis M, Shipley MT. External tufted cells: a major excitatory element that coordinates glomerular activity. *J Neurosci.* 2004;24(30):6676–6685.
17. Philpot BD, Lyders EM, Brunjes PC. The NMDA receptor participates in respiration-related mitral cell synchrony. *Exp Brain Res.* 1998;118(2):205–209.
18. Spors H, Grinvald A. Spatio-temporal dynamics of odor representations in the mammalian olfactory bulb. *Neuron.* 2002;34(2):301–315.
19. Wachowiak M. All in a sniff: olfaction as a model for active sensing. *Neuron.* 2011;71(6):962–973.
20. Brown RE, Stevens DR, Haas HL. The physiology of brain histamine. *Prog Neurobiol.* 2001;63(6):637–672.
21. Haas H, Panula P. The role of histamine and the tuberomammillary nucleus in the nervous system. *Nat Rev Neurosci.* 2003;4(2):121–130.
22. Steininger TL, Alam MN, Gong H, Szymusiak R, McGinty D. Sleep-waking discharge of neurons in the posterior lateral hypothalamus of the albino rat. *Brain Res.* 1999;840(1–2): 138–147.
23. Vanni-Mercier G, Sakai K, Jouvet M. Specific neurons for wakefulness in the posterior hypothalamus in the cat. *C R Acad Sci III.* 1984;298(7):195–200.
24. Haas HL, Reiner PB. Membrane-properties of histaminergic tuberomammillary neurons of the rat hypothalamus in vitro. *J Physiol-London.* 1988;399:633–646.
25. Uteshev VV, Knot HJ. Somatic Ca^{2+} dynamics in response to choline-mediated excitation in histaminergic tuberomammillary neurons. *Neuroscience.* 2005;134(1):133–143.
26. Uteshev VV, Meyer EM, Papke RL. Regulation of neuronal function by choline and 4OH-GTS-21 through α7 nicotinic receptors. *J Neurophysiol.* 2003;89(4):1797–1806.
27. Taddese A, Bean BP. Subthreshold sodium current from rapidly inactivating sodium channels drives spontaneous firing of tuberomammillary neurons. *Neuron.* 2002;33(4):587–600.
28. Uteshev V, Stevens DR, Haas HL. A persistent sodium current in acutely isolated histaminergic neurons from rat hypothalamus. *Neuroscience.* 1995;66(1):143–149.
29. Mochizuki T, Yamatodani A, Okakura K, Horii A, Inagaki N, Wada H. Circadian rhythm of histamine release from the hypothalamus of freely moving rats. *Physiol Behav.* 1992;51(2): 391–394.
30. Prast H, Saxer A, Philippu A. Pattern of in vivo release of endogenous histamine in the mammillary body and the amygdala. *Naunyn Schmiedebergs Arch Pharmacol.* 1988;337(1): 53–57.
31. Nishibori M, Oishi R, Itoh Y, Saeki K. Glucose modulates the release of histamine from the mouse hypothalamus in vitro. *J Neurochem.* 1986;47(6):1761–1767.
32. Okakura K, Yamatodani A, Mochizuki T, Horii A, Wada H. Glutamatergic regulation of histamine release from rat hypothalamus. *Eur J Pharmacol.* 1992;213(2):189–192.
33. Mochizuki T, Yamatodani A, Okakura K, Takemura M, Inagaki N, Wada H. In vivo release of neuronal histamine in the hypothalamus of rats measured by microdialysis. *Naunyn Schmiedebergs Arch Pharmacol.* 1991;343(2):190–195.
34. Arrang JM, Garbarg M, Schwartz JC. Autoregulation of histamine release in brain by presynaptic H3-receptors. *Neuroscience.* 1985;15(2):553–562.
35. Ishibashi H, Rhee JS, Akaike N. Regional difference of high voltage-activated Ca^{2+} channels in rat CNS neurones. *Neuroreport.* 1995;6(12):1621–1624.
36. Stevens DR, Haas HL. Calcium-dependent prepotentials contribute to spontaneous activity in rat tuberomammillary neurons. *J Physiol-London.* 1996;493(3):747–754.
37. Stevens DR, Eriksson KS, Brown RE, Haas HL. The mechanism of spontaneous firing in histamine neurons. *Behav Brain Res.* 2001;124(2):105–112.
38. Eriksson KS, Stevens DR, Haas HL. Serotonin excites tuberomammillary neurons by activation of Na^+/Ca^{2+}-exchange. *Neuropharmacology.* 2001;40(3):345–351.
39. Mike A, Castro NG, Albuquerque EX. Choline and acetylcholine have similar kinetic properties of activation and desensitization on the α7 nicotinic receptors in rat hippocampal neurons. *Brain Res.* 2000;882(1–2):155–168.
40. Gusev AG, Uteshev VV. Physiological concentrations of choline activate native α7-containing nicotinic acetylcholine receptors in the presence of PNU-120596 [1-(5-chloro-2,4-dimethoxyphenyl)-3-(5-methylisoxazol-3-yl)-urea]. *J Pharmacol Exp Ther.* 2010; 332(2):588–598.
41. Li Y, Papke RL, He YJ, Millard WJ, Meyer EM. Characterization of the neuroprotective and toxic effects of α7 nicotinic receptor activation in PC12 cells. *Brain Res.* 1999;830(2): 218–225.
42. Uteshev VV. Somatic integration of single ion channel responses of α7 nicotinic acetylcholine receptors enhanced by PNU-120596. *PloS One.* 2012;7(3):e32951.
43. Kalappa BI, Gusev AG, Uteshev VV. Activation of functional α7-containing nAChRs in hippocampal CA1 pyramidal neurons by physiological levels of choline in the presence of PNU-120596. *PloS One.* 2010;5(11):e13964.
44. Sitzia F, Brown JT, Randall AD, Dunlop J. Voltage- and temperature-dependent allosteric modulation of α7 nicotinic receptors by PNU120596. *Front Pharmacol.* 2011;2:81.
45. Freitas K, Carroll FI, Damaj MI. The antinociceptive effects of nicotinic receptors α7-positive allosteric modulators in murine acute and tonic pain models. *J Pharmacol Exp Ther.* 2012; 344(1):264–275.
46. Freitas K, Negus SS, Carroll FI, Damaj MI. In vivo pharmacological interactions between a type II positive allosteric modulator of α7 nicotinic acetylcholine receptors and nicotinic agonists in a murine tonic pain model. *Br J Pharmacol.* 2013;169(3):567–79.
47. Hurst RS, Hajos M, Raggenbass M, et al. A novel positive allosteric modulator of the α7 neuronal nicotinic acetylcholine receptor: in vitro and in vivo characterization. *J Neurosci.* 2005; 25(17):4396–4405.
48. Kalappa BI, Sun F, Johnson SR, Jin K, Uteshev VV. A positive allosteric modulator of α7 nAChRs augments neuroprotective effects of

endogenous nicotinic agonists in cerebral ischemia. *Br J Pharmacol.* 2013; In Press. doi: 10.1111/bph.12247 (PMID: 23713819).

49. McLean SL, Idris N, Grayson B, et al. PNU-120596, a positive allosteric modulator of α7 nicotinic acetylcholine receptors, reverses a sub-chronic phencyclidine-induced cognitive deficit in the attentional set-shifting task in female rats. *J Psychopharmacol.* 2012; 26(9):1265–70.
50. Alkondon M, Pereira EF, Barbosa CT, Albuquerque EX. Neuronal nicotinic acetylcholine receptor activation modulates gamma-aminobutyric acid release from CA1 neurons of rat hippocampal slices. *J Pharmacol Exp Ther.* 1997;283(3): 1396–1411.
51. Ji D, Dani JA. Inhibition and disinhibition of pyramidal neurons by activation of nicotinic receptors on hippocampal interneurons. *J Neurophysiol.* 2000;83(5):2682–2690.
52. Ji D, Lape R, Dani JA. Timing and location of nicotinic activity enhances or depresses hippocampal synaptic plasticity. *Neuron.* 2001;31(1):131–141.

CHAPTER

6

Network Imaging

Jennifer N. Guo [1], *Hal Blumenfeld* [1,2]

[1]Department of Neurology, Yale University School of Medicine, New Haven, CT, USA,
[2]Departments of Neurobiology and Neurosurgery, Yale University School of Medicine, New Haven, CT, USA

INTRODUCTION

One of the fundamental debates in neuroscience has been the contrasting ideas of localized versus distributed functioning within the brain.[1,2] The modular paradigm can be traced from the earliest debates between Golgi and Cajal on a cellular level to modern cognitive neuropsychology, which makes inferences about normal cognitive function through selective cognitive deficits. Cognitive modularity has been substantiated through the identification of anatomical units within the brain based on cytoarchitecture.[3–5] Additionally, a confluence of studies using a variety of methods based on both anatomical and functional parcellation has clearly demonstrated specialization within the brain in primary sensory and association cortices.[6–8] Tremendous discoveries within neuroscience have been made within this modular viewpoint. Yet newer methods have demonstrated considerable interactions between brain regions in cognitive processes and have given rise to the emerging view of the brain as a network. For example, even within the well-described visual system, top-down directed attention has been shown to modulate activity as early as V1.[9,10]

Neuronal networks have been explored at various scales—from cells to local circuits to large-scale networks across the entire brain.[11] While many different techniques are used to describe brain networks, the connections within these networks may, broadly speaking, be broken down to anatomical and functional connectivity. Anatomical connectivity consists of physical connections via single axons or white matter tracts between physically defined units within the brain. In living humans, these connections can now be described by parcellation of gray matter from structural magnetic resonance imaging (MRI) or direct measurements of white matter tracts by diffusion tensor imaging (DTI),[12] diffusion spectrum imaging,[13] and diffusion-weighted MRI (Figure 6.1).[14]

In contrast to anatomical connectivity, functional connectivity can exist between interacting areas to give rise to cognitive functions even in the absence of direct physical connections. Functional connectivity is also more dynamic and can change on time scales ranging from seconds to hours at varying levels of consciousness, while both functional and anatomical connectivity can change at longer time scales through learning, development, or disease. Of course, functional connectivity typically reflects anatomical connectivity, but "connectivity" that is mediated by volume transmission is a major exception to this rule (Chapter 8). Functional brain networks in humans have been constructed from functional magnetic resonance imaging (fMRI) and, to a lesser extent, electroencephalography (EEG) and magnetoencephalography (MEG). The fundamental principle underlying functional connectivity is that individual nodes within the network have temporally covarying activity that allows for emergent functions (see Chapter 30) and cognitive processing. This statistical interdependence is assumed to reflect processing of mutual information. The recruitment of functional units for a given cognitive process may be constrained by intrinsic properties such as cellular architecture or connectivity patterns to other brain regions. Unit boundaries may be defined via common patterns of connectivity to other brain areas.[15,16]

The present chapter will focus on underlying principles of network theory, recent developments in understanding large-scale neural networks, how normal cognitive functions emerge from these networks, and how these networks are altered in disease. Particular emphasis will be given to evidence from fMRI. fMRI

Neuronal Networks in Brain Function, CNS Disorders, and Therapeutics
http://dx.doi.org/10.1016/B978-0-12-415804-7.00006-X

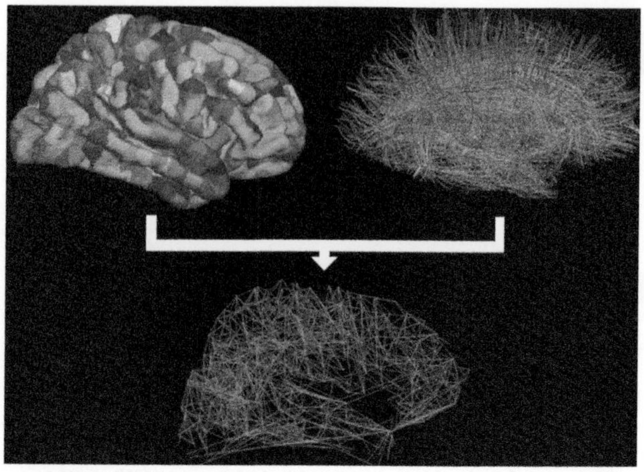

FIGURE 6.1 Identification of networks in the human brain by anatomical parcellation into 1000 regions (top left) and tractography using diffusion spectrum imaging (top right). The two methods are combined to form a whole-brain anatomical network composed of neural regions and their white matter connections (bottom). (*Source: Reproduced with permission from Ref. 13.*) (The figure is reproduced in color section.)

is well suited to imaging networks given its good spatial coverage and fair temporal resolution to capture dynamic cognitive processes. Though fMRI indirectly measures brain activity via blood oxygenation level–dependent (BOLD) signals rather than direct electrical activity, evidence from animal models and simultaneous EEG–fMRI in humans has demonstrated a generally positive correlation between electrical activity and BOLD signal changes.

Evidence from EEG and MEG, which directly measure electrical neuronal activity from the brain with higher temporal resolution (although with worse spatial resolution than fMRI), will also be discussed.

THE RELATIONSHIP BETWEEN ANATOMICAL AND FUNCTIONAL CONNECTIVITY

Anatomy constrains functional connectivity. One possible mechanism is that dynamic ongoing signals travel through white matter fiber tracks. Conversely, functional connectivity may also drive growth or pruning of anatomical connections over the course of development, possibly due to modulation of synaptic activity and long-term structural modifications to neuronal morphology. Callosal agenesis in several patients has been related to decreased functional connectivity,[17] while complete bisection of the corpus callosum in humans has been shown to lead to loss of interhemispheric connectivity.[18] DTI and fMRI in normal subjects have shown that areas within commonly found functional networks, including primary sensory networks and the default mode network (DMN), are connected via well-known white matter tracts.[19] Skudlarski and colleagues directly compared anatomical connectivity measured with DTI with functional connectivity between regions of interest, and then divided resting connectivity values for the whole connectivity matrix into 25 bins. Anatomical and functional connectivity showed a strong linear relationship.[20] In another study, a high degree of anatomical connectivity between regions in diffusion spectrum imaging was quantitatively predictive of greater functional connectivity, with a correlation coefficient of $r^2 = 0.62$.[13] Regions with a greater number and strength of connections were typically in the medial cortex (closer to the corpus callosum), including the cuneus and precuneus, the anterior and posterior cingulate cortex, and the superior temporal cortex.[13,21] However, indirect connections may also partially account for variance in functional connectivity. Using fMRI and diffusion spectrum tracking in the same subjects, Honey and colleagues found a strong relationship between functional and anatomical connectivity independent of the length of connection fibers, although fiber length strongly affected the degree of functional connectivity.[22] Furthermore, significant functional connectivity was found between regions lacking direct white matter connections, which is likely due to polysynaptic pathways between these regions. Another possibility is that enhanced intrinsic excitability or enhanced synaptic efficacy could lead to increased functional connectivity between regions even when structural connectivity is diminished, as can be seen in pathological conditions such as epilepsy.[21] Although volume conduction can theoretically lead to false measurements of functional connectivity, particularly in EEG and MEG,[23] metrics insensitive to volume conduction such as the phase lag index rather than phase coherence can be used to compute connectivity.[11,24] Computational modeling used to examine the effect of particular connection architectures on functional connectivity patterns has shown that systematically varying connection architectures can directly influence patterns of neuronal activity.[25]

NETWORK PROPERTIES AND MEASURES

The brain has been increasingly viewed as a small-world network, with topology that allows for a functionally optimal balance of integration and segregation. Neural networks maintain an intermediate topography in between regular lattices, on one hand, and random connections, on the other.[26] A number of biologically relevant measures have been proposed for

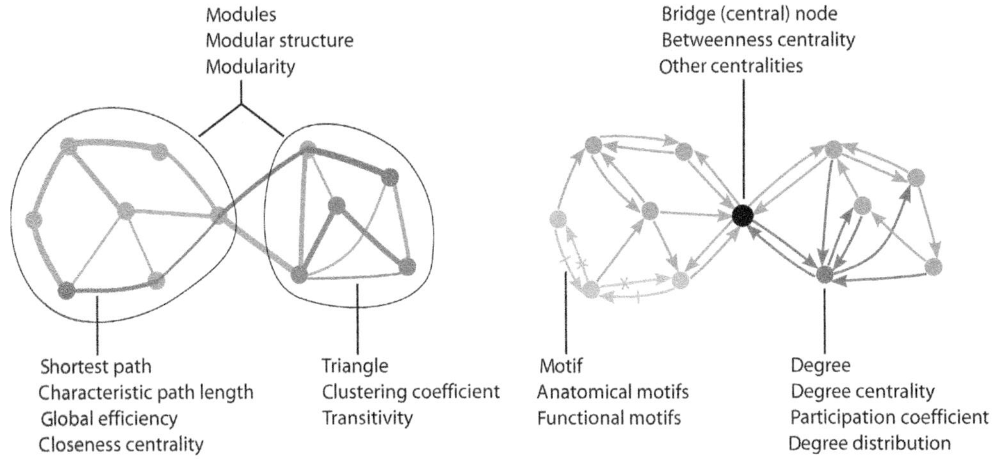

FIGURE 6.2 Common graph theoretical metrics for network-level analysis. Measures of integration are in green, while measures of segregation are in blue. Measures of node degree are in red, and patterns of local connectivity as measured by motifs are in yellow. An example of a node with high centrality and short path length is marked in black. See text of this chapter for further details on each metric. (*Source: Reproduced with permission from Rubinov, Sporns. Neuroimage. 2010.*) (For interpretation of the references to color in this figure legend, the reader is referred to the online version of this book.)

network-level analysis (see Figure 6.2 for examples of these metrics in a representative network). A fundamental feature of networks is the concept of nodes, which within a neuroimaging framework typically are composed of brain regions. Edges are links between nodes and may represent either anatomical or functional connections between nodes. Nodes of interest are often based on distinguishing anatomical features, function, or data-driven parcellations of the cortex based on time courses of activity. Edges are then calculated between them, with significance set at some arbitrary threshold to discard spurious connections. Links between nodes are often calculated as binary, unweighted connections for simplicity of analysis or can be weighed by connection strength. Causal relationships between nodes can also be measured as directed connectivity. A more detailed discussion of causal analyses will follow in this chapter. Degree is another basic measure of connectivity and is calculated as the number of edges per node. The average degree of a network is a measure of the density of an interconnected network.

Neural functions ranging from basic computations to consciousness have been postulated to necessarily require a balance between integrative versus segregative functions within subsets of a network.[27] Functional segregation is a measure of specialization within a larger group of connected regions and may be quantified by the absolute number of triangles within a network. The number of triangles, or two mutually connected nodes that are both connected to a third node, can be a measure of segregation in the network (Figure 6.2). For a single node, the percentage of the number of triangles around that node divided by the number of triangles in the whole network is known as the clustering coefficient, and it is a measure of the proportion of the node's connections that are also connected to each other. This metric, normalized for the number of nodes within networks, is the transitivity. Finally, optimization algorithms may be used to reorganize random nodes within a network into a modular structure, by which groups of nodes may form subnetworks with a high degree of interconnectivity.

Functional integration within a network allows for transmission of information across distributed brain areas. Greater efficiency is achieved via fewer relays along the path from any node to another. This can be measured by the characteristic path length, the average shortest path length between all node pairs in a network. Local connectivity within a network may be organized into motifs. These patterns of connectivity may be anatomical or functional, although motifs such as feedforward or feedback loops are typically used only in the analysis of directed networks. Finally, the brain or a network of the brain may be quantified as a whole based on the repertoire of possible neural states.[27] Phi (Φ) is a measurement of discriminable states within a system that, when functionally integrated, carry information beyond that represented by the larger network from which the subnetworks are drawn. Tononi has hypothesized that the level of consciousness available to a system at any given point in time is determined by Φ.[27] However, this measurement may also be applicable to various functions of consciousness (i.e. the contents of consciousness). While Φ has realistically been measured only for simulated systems thus far, it may be possible to develop empirical measures of Φ based on data from EEG, fMRI, or other modalities.

THE NEUROENERGETIC BASIS FOR SMALL-WORLD NETWORK FUNCTIONS

Energy maximization places a fundamental constraint upon biological organization and function. A network with parallel, recurrent interactions minimizes the costs of information processing by lowering wiring costs.[28,29] Computational modeling suggests that the biological distribution of cortical regions in humans, compared to artificial distributed cortical networks, is optimal in minimizing wiring costs by reducing axonal volume.[30,31] Small-world topology, with dense local connections and sparse long-range connections, also allows for a greater speed and extent of information transfer.[26] Furthermore, estimates of energy usage predict that distributed coding with a small percentage of simultaneously active neurons, rather than optimizing the number of state representations, allows for maximization of computation power at a given level of energy consumption.[32,33] Parallel and distributed processing within the brain is well established[2,34,35] in realms including audition[36] (see Chapter 20) and pain perception[37] (see Chapter 23), and it has been hypothesized to allow for emergent properties (Chapter 30), such as memory formation.[38] Of note, a recent study using model-free approaches suggests that BOLD–fMRI changes may be seen in a widely distributed network of regions even when subjects performed a simple visual attention task.[39] By averaging over 100 runs per subject to minimize noise and contributions from spontaneous fluctuations, the authors showed fMRI changes time locked to the stimulus in >95% of the brain.

METHODS FOR EXTRACTING NETWORK ACTIVITY

The first network analysis of mammalian cortex was compiled from prior tract-tracing literature in the macaque visual cortex.[34] Most of the 305 axonal connections were shown to be reciprocal, with sparse connectivity between local clusters of regions and parallel processing pathways. Most efforts to extract neuronal networks have been based on noninvasive measures, including fMRI, EEG, or MEG. One of the most common methods for analyzing imaging data in fMRI has been statistical parametric mapping based on general linear modeling.[40] This method allows for extraction of brain maps using a linear combination of regressors of interest by minimizing a residual error term. Defining these regressors allows for the estimation and removal of, for example, the effects of fixation from the effects of more complex visual attention tasks. These subtraction-based analyses have typically been used to isolate areas within the brain that are associated with an experimentally controlled variable. However, this approach assumes that cognitive processes add linearly and modularly. General linear models also tend to assume some standard hemodynamic response function that is uniform throughout the brain, although this assumption has been shown to be false.[41–43] Functional network analyses can also take time into consideration by plotting the percentage of change of fMRI–BOLD activity from baseline over time. This method is free of assumptions about the hemodynamic response function and provides moving maps of functional activity over the entire duration of the event rather than a snapshot of activity at one time. This method has been used successfully to show a dynamic change in activity in response to seizure activity, with varying hemodynamic response functions in various areas of the cortex.[41]

More recently, functional connectivity has been used to extract network activity. Correlations in slow fluctuations (<0.1 Hz) of fMRI signals during rest were first discovered by Biswal and colleagues in the motor network.[44] Using a seed region in the left somatosensory cortex, they found a covarying time course of activation in the contralateral cortex. Resting-state networks often have similar patterns as task-based networks. Evidence for this comes from the discovery of well-known cortical networks using resting-state data as well as direct comparisons between networks found in resting versus task-based studies. Networks activated during a visual processing task have been found to be similar to areas that covary in the resting state (Figure 6.3(A)).[45] Similarly, a high degree of correlation has been found for voxels activated during a semantic categorization task compared to fixation (Figure 6.3(B)).[46] Lowe and colleagues also showed that areas activated during a working memory task were similar to areas found with a resting functional connectivity analysis.[47] Together, these studies indicate that cortical hubs seem to persist even across task states. Resting-state data have the benefit of being amenable to averaging without needing to account for minor differences in tasks, and they may capture a functional network more fully than data from any specific task.

Furthermore, most of the brain's energy consumption is used for spontaneous, ongoing activity rather than task-related activity.[48] Because of this, functional connectivity is often, although not necessarily, calculated using spontaneous fluctuations in neural activity rather than evoked responses to external stimuli. The role of spontaneous activity has also been explored through more direct measurements of neuronal activity. Optical imaging of cat visual cortex has shown that spontaneous activity recapitulates evoked activity as well as affects firing patterns at the single neuron level.[49–51]

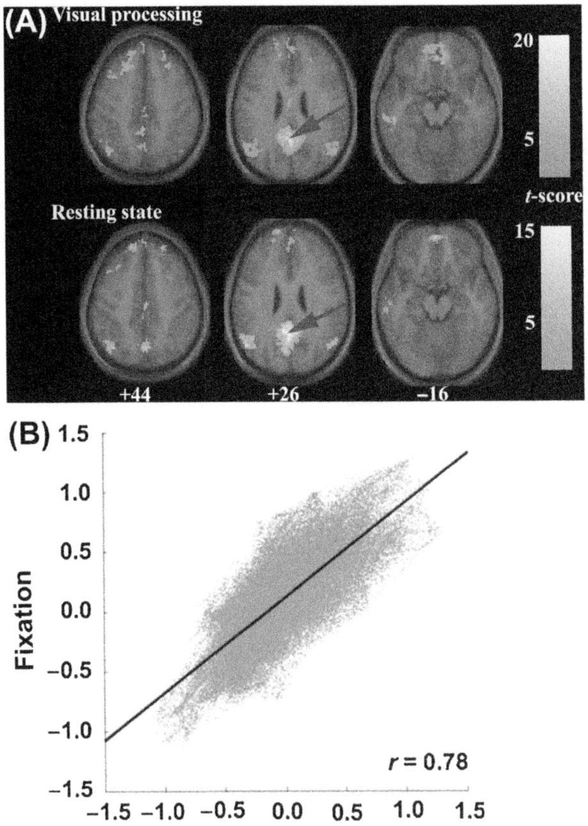

FIGURE 6.3 Resting state networks recapitulate task-based networks. (A) Connectivity maps for the posterior cingulate cortex. Networks found during a visual processing task (top) and resting state (bottom) are similar. *(Source: Reproduced with permission from Ref. 45. Copyright © 2003 National Academy of Sciences USA.)* (The figure is reproduced in color section.) (B) Voxel-by-voxel correlations in cortical hubs across a semantic categorization task and fixation. Hubs persist across task states with a correlation coefficient $r = 0.78$. *(Source: Reproduced with permission from Ref. 46.)* (For color version of this figure, the reader is referred to the online version of this book.)

Additionally, while spontaneous neuronal activity is dynamic, the cortex has been shown to have "preferred cortical states".[49,50] These findings are significant because they demonstrate that behaviorally relevant, dynamic cortical states are embedded in spontaneous fluctuations in neural activity, and imply that networks may be extracted from this spontaneous activity without a task. Why the brain cycles through these functional cortical states remains to be determined. It is possible that this activity is necessary to maintain useful network connections, although this hypothesis remains to be tested through learning or developmental paradigms.

In contrast to functional connectivity, which measures covariance in brain activity and is a measure of how two brain regions may be functionally related, effective connectivity is a measure of the direct influence that one brain region may have on another.[52] While these two concepts are closely related, functional and effective connectivity are not necessarily the same. For example, two regions that are functional connected may be mediated by a third common region without direct connections to each other. In addition, effective connectivity may be mediated by a series of polysynaptic connections, but with a low level of functional connectivity between the start and end regions. Causality is determined by temporal delays in signal fluctuations between areas, and several mathematical methods exist to determine causal relationships in brain signals. In addition, there are several methods for measuring effective connectivity to determine causal relationships between nodes of a network. Dynamic causal modeling is based on bilinear dynamic models and compares the probabilities of competing network-based changes in observed signals in response to experimentally applied perturbations to nodes or edges.[53] Granger causality, in contrast, does not require a priori modeling of networks, and it infers directional relationships based on how well temporal changes in one brain area can predict changes in another area.[54] One caveat to the calculation of causal relationships in fMRI data is that the temporal delay of the BOLD signal limits detection of directed connectivity. In one study, BOLD signals from simulated local field potentials (LFPs) with no causal relationship have demonstrated spurious effective connectivity.[54] However, careful experimental manipulations may be able to nonetheless tease out causal relationships between predefined networks. For example, structural equation modeling has been used to show the effect of light on the visual system in rats[55] and the effect of attentional modulation on an occipito-parieto-frontal network in humans.[56]

ELECTROPHYSIOLOGICAL ACTIVITY IS RELATED TO RESTING FUNCTIONAL CONNECTIVITY

BOLD signals in fMRI measure blood oxygenation responses and, therefore, are not a direct measure of neuronal activity. However, much work has been done to determine the neuronal underpinnings of the fMRI signal. Animal and human ^{13}C nuclear magnetic resonance (NMR) measurements show a direct relationship between energy metabolism and neuronal activity mediated by the neurotransmitter glutamate.[48,57,58] Total neurotransmitter cycling can be resolved into individual glutamatergic and GABAergic components, with GABAergic neurons accounting for approximately 20% of total glucose flux in rats.[59] Furthermore, glucose oxidation for both components was found to increase with neuronal activity. NMR spectroscopy has also shown a positive relationship between the glutamate cycling rate and the cerebral metabolic rate of oxygen consumption ($CMRO_2$), cerebral blood flow (CBF), and cerebral blood volume over a wide range of neuronal activity.[60] In contrast, the biophysics of electrical contributions from cortical areas to generate potentials is better understood. Cortical potentials arise mainly from extracellular current flow that is mostly due to synaptic activity.[61] These potentials form an electric field that can be measured with temporal resolution on the order of milliseconds using a variety of methods in humans, including EEG recorded from the scalp, electrocorticogram (ECoG) recorded by subdural electrodes, or LFP recorded by depth electrodes inserted into cortical tissue. EEG signals are integrated from 6 to 10 cm^2 of cortex, are poor at distinguishing between signals from superficial versus deeper layers of cortex, and attenuate signals from higher frequencies due to low-pass filtering from bone and scalp tissues. LFPs are the most invasive and measure signals from much smaller cortical volumes, although estimates of the exact spatial extent of the LFP range from ~250 μm up to 12 mm.[62] Finally, MEG can be used to measure the magnetic fields induced by the same underlying electrical activity as measured by EEG. Because measured signals are orthogonal to those induced by EEG, they are also less susceptible to attenuation of signal from deeper sources.[62,63] Additionally, MEG signals are not affected by heterogeneous head conductivity across skin, bone, and neural tissue.

Logothetis and colleagues performed one of the first direct investigations of the relationship between fMRI signals and electrical correlates using simultaneous LFP, single- and multiunit recordings, and BOLD responses from monkey visual cortex.[64] These relationships have also been investigated by parallel measurements in the rat.[65,66] fMRI BOLD signals were found to be correlated to both LFPs, a measure of summed synaptic currents flowing through similarly oriented neurons in the cortex, and multiunit activity, a measure of neuronal firing. However, important exceptions to this relationship have been found. Recordings from the basal ganglia during spike-wave discharges in a rat model of absence epilepsy have demonstrated increases in multiunit activity and LFP with simultaneous decreases in the BOLD signal.[67] LFP signals have also found to be positively and linearly related to the BOLD signal in the cortex, but not in the brainstem of rats undergoing sensory stimulation.[68] These variations in the BOLD–electrophysiology relationship may be due to regional differences in vascularization patterns, mediators of neuromuscular coupling, or the rate of change in CBF in response to the local $CMRO_2$.

Regional CBF and oxidative metabolism contribute to the fMRI signal, and oxidative metabolism is necessary to restore membrane potentials following neuronal firing. While glutamatergic activity accounts for the vast majority of energy utilization in the brain,[59] the effect of inhibitory GABAergic activity cannot be discounted and may also cause changes in the fMRI signal. For example, electrophysiological recordings of spontaneous network activity during slow oscillations in ferrets have been shown to be well balanced between excitation and inhibition due to recurrent excitation and feedback inhibitions within local networks.[69] Simultaneous measurements of local CBF and spiking activity in Purkinje neurons showed increases in CBF with stimulation of both excitatory and inhibitory pathways.[70] In contrast, autoradiography studies in rats and humans with GABA agonists have shown decreases in energy metabolism.[71–73] Computational modeling has suggested that these contradictory relationships may be due to the direct versus polysynaptic inhibitory connections measured, the amount of excitation a region receives from external sources, as well as the level of excitatory recurrence within a circuit, which could affect whether metabolism and CBF reflect mostly local or afferent synaptic activity.[74]

Relationships between resting fMRI connectivity and electrophysiology have also been investigated. Simultaneous LFP and fMRI recordings in monkeys showed correlations between the BOLD signal in the <0.1 Hz range with widespread, coherent LFP power, particularly in the gamma band.[75] Using similar methods, Schölvinck and colleagues found that fluctuations during rest of the LFP signal were positively correlated with fMRI signals over widespread areas of the cortex, with the highest correlations in the gamma band range, although a positive correlation was also observed between 2 and 15 Hz (Figure 6.4).[76] Finally, Magri and colleagues further explored the relationship between LFP power at different frequency bands to both the timing and amplitude of the hemodynamic response function in anesthetized macaques. They found that gamma power was most predictive of BOLD amplitude, although alpha power also carried complementary information in predicting signal amplitude.[68] Furthermore, the relationship between beta and gamma power correlated with the latency of the BOLD response.

OSCILLATORY NETWORKS CAN BE MEASURED BY EEG AND MEG

While most studies of brain networks have come from measures of BOLD changes, EEG and MEG have also been used to more directly measure how the brain coordinates large-scale networks that are spatially distributed. Some evidence exists that neuronal oscillations can synchronize these distributed processes to

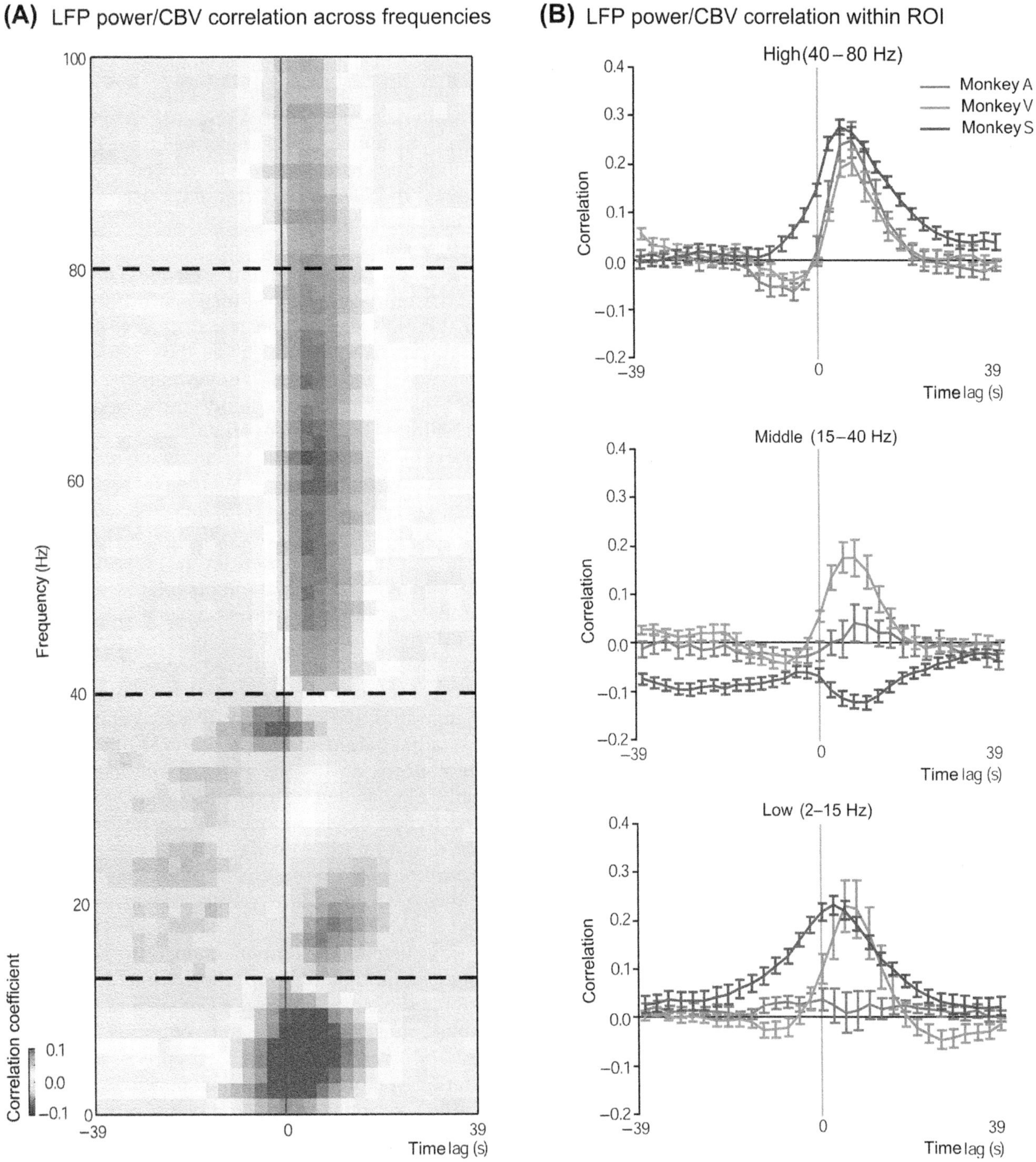

FIGURE 6.4 In simultaneous fMRI and electrophysiological recordings in macaque V1, resting state fMRI signals are related to local field potentials. (A) Correlations between fMRI and LFP power during the resting state show distinct relationships across frequency bands. (B) For three monkeys, correlation is consistently positive in the 40–80 Hz range, has a variable and slightly negative correlation in the 15–40 Hz range, and is generally positive in the 2–15 Hz range. (*Source: Reproduced with permission from Ref. 76.*) (The figure is reproduced in color section.)

perform cognitive operations, particularly in the gamma range, where spike synchronization has been shown to be associated with sensory awareness.[77,78] Rhythmic oscillations arise from rhythmic fluctuations in membrane potentials and can have within-frequency phase–phase interactions or cross-frequency phase–amplitude interactions. These synchronizations give rise to a favored neural signal via temporally coincident oscillations and allow for downstream propagation of that signal. Synchrony across

EEG electrodes or MEG sensors has been with object recognition,[79] attention,[80,81] and conscious perception.[82]

MEG measures magnetic field changes associated with electrophysiological brain activity. Independent component analysis and seed-based analysis of source-localized MEG data have demonstrated resting-state networks with spatial similarity as compared to those found by fMRI.[83] Network analyses have also been applied to resting MEG data, in which connectivity between different sensors was determined for common frequency bands.[84] Interestingly, the low-frequency band (8–13 Hz) and β band (13–30 Hz) had regular, lattice-like topology, whereas graphs from low- and high-frequency bands (δ, $\theta < 8$ Hz or $\gamma > 30$ Hz) showed small-world properties.

NETWORKS IN COGNITION AND CONSCIOUSNESS

Converging evidence from task-related imaging paradigms has distinguished between the dorsal and ventral attentional systems.[85] The dorsal system consists of the intraparietal sulcus and superior frontal cortex, and is thought to be responsible for goal-directed, top-down attention. In contrast, the ventral system, consisting of the right temporoparietal and inferior frontal cortices, detects behavioral-relevant bottom-up inputs and acts as a circuit breaker to appropriately redirect attention. Slow fluctuations in activity detected using resting functional connectivity have successfully recaptured these same networks, demonstrating that attentional networks not only emerge as a response to external perturbations but also are an intrinsic component of neuronal brain states.[86]

One of the best studied networks consists of a set of regions found to be deactivated during tasks but activated during rest in positron emission tomography (PET) and fMRI,[87,88] and later validated using resting functional connectivity analysis.[45] These so-called DMN regions include the posterior cingulate cortex and precuneus, the medial prefrontal cortex, and the lateral parietal cortex, and they have been shown to be anticorrelated with task-positive regions.[89] The DMN is thought to be activated during self-referential thought or introspection, and is deactivated when the brain is engaged in external, sensory-driven tasks.[88,90] However, the DMN has also been shown to be conserved in anesthetized states in primates, indicating that it is a feature of neural organization independent of levels of consciousness.[91] While debate remains regarding the precise function of the DMN,[92] it has been consistently shown to be activated during the resting state[93] and is preferentially affected in disease states such as Alzheimer's and epilepsy.[46,94]

Network connectivity can change dynamically due to development, learning, and changes in levels of consciousness. Development in rodents has been linked to systematic changes in BOLD responses as well as interhemispheric connectivity in response to forepaw stimulation.[95] In humans, the transition from childhood to adulthood is characterized by reduced functional connectivity on EEG via decreased clustering of nodes and increased characteristic path length.[96] Network connectivity can also change on a shorter time scale in response to task-dependent demands on the brain. Data-driven clustering of functional fMRI during a visual attention task demonstrated grouping of functionally disparate areas, such as the high-order visual cortex and motor cortex, suggesting that task performance can dynamically bind areas from otherwise differentiated resting networks.[39]

Dynamic changes in connectivity are also evident in changes to connectivity patterns in normal subjects through variable levels of consciousness such as in moving from wakefulness to sleep (Chapters 21 and 22). This transition is marked by neurotransmitter-mediated hyperpolarization of membrane potentials and decreased neuronal excitability, with a concomitant slowing of cortical rhythms on EEG to bistable up and down states.[97] Massimini and colleagues directly measured efficiency of information transmission during the wakeful and nonrapid eye movement (NREM) states by using transcranial magnetic stimulation (TMS) to activate the premotor area during sleep and wakefulness and high-density EEG to measure resulting changes in effective connectivity.[98] They found that the response to TMS broke down rapidly during NREM sleep compared to wakefulness, suggesting decreased effective connectivity during sleep. These results converge with those found in fMRI data during NREM sleep. Using a data-driven independent component analysis, Boly and colleagues found that the proportion of interactions within assemblies increased relative to interactions between assemblies during NREM sleep compared to wakefulness.[99] In other words, NREM sleep is associated with clustering of large-scale neuronal networks into smaller modules. Information integration in any system has been thought to involve a balance of functional segregation and integration.[27] Thus, increased modularity during NREM sleep decreases the brain's capacity for information integration and may constitute the mechanism for loss of consciousness during sleep.

Loss of consciousness during anesthesia has been found to be associated with decreases in CBF in the frontal cortex, posterior cingulate cortex, and precuneus.[100] In examining connections between areas, John and colleagues described decreased gamma coherence on EEG in long-range connections between the anterior and posterior cortices in patients with induced loss of consciousness via general anesthesia.[101] This result has been validated in a separate study using incremental doses of isoflurane, although the authors also demonstrated preservation of local coherence.[102] Similarly, propofol-induced anesthesia also has been associated with a reduction of network connections, most prominently in the gamma range, although a basic organization was found to be preserved across consciousness states, particularly in the default mode area.[103] Lee and colleagues constructed moving windows of connection matrices and demonstrated changes in coherence as subjects lost, then regained, consciousness.[103] In particular, isoflurane-induced loss of consciousness in an animal model caused an initial decrease in feedback information rather than feedforward information in the gamma range.[104] Functional and effective connectivity within the thalamocortical and corticocortical networks has been shown to decrease in response to anesthesia in humans.[105] The authors suggest that this loss of effective connectivity was due to increases in low-frequency oscillations at the cost of high-frequency rhythms due to neuronal hyperpolarization. Subsequent studies have also demonstrated stepwise responses in connectivity levels to sevoflurane.[106] Furthermore, graph theoretical analysis of fMRI data for propofol-sedated humans has shown a decrease in thalamic centrality but an increase in brainstem centrality, suggesting increased influence of the brainstem in decreased arousal states such as sedation.[107] The role of the brainstem in mediating anesthesia-induced loss of cortical connectivity has been supported by animal studies. For example, several anesthetics had a generally depressive effect on the spontaneous activity of mesencephalic reticular neurons.[108] Finally, selective lesions of brainstem nuclei have been shown to decrease the minimum alveolar concentration of halothane in rats.[109]

NETWORK DISRUPTIONS IN DISEASE

Functional connectivity via coherent cortical oscillations has been used to investigate networks in both normal and diseased states. Buckner and colleagues have shown good spatial correlation between areas of high amyloid beta (Aβ) deposition seen on PET in Alzheimer's patients and cortical hubs with a high degree of connectivity across the brain in controls. These hubs also show a striking resemblance with DMN areas.[46] The authors hypothesize that Aβ deposition may disproportionally affect these areas due to intrinsic stable properties such as glycolytic metabolism. Measurements of lactate levels by in vivo microdialysis have shown that neuronal activity due to sensory stimulation is directly linked to interstitial Aβ levels within minutes to hours[110] and reveal region-specific vulnerabilities to Aβ deposition over development.[111] Targeted loss of connectivity has also been demonstrated by small-world analysis of MEG data in Alzheimer's patients.[24] At the network level, the cognitive decline of Alzheimer's disease has been hypothesized to be due to loss of connectivity between long-range cortical hubs. Graph theoretical analysis of EEG and MEG data in patients has shown lower alpha- and beta-band synchronization, with higher characteristic path lengths but preserved local clustering, indicating decreased global efficiency.[24,112]

Altered resting functional connectivity also has been found in multiple sclerosis, an autoimmune disease characterized by demyelination of white matter tracts. Patients with multiple sclerosis showed decreases in low-frequency BOLD fluctuations between bilateral primary sensorimotor cortices, and an inverse correlation between fractional anisotropy on DTI of the transcallosal motor pathway and functional connectivity between sensorimotor areas of the brain.[113,114]

Similar disruptions in network properties have been shown in schizophrenia. Weighted EEG networks in schizophrenic patients under resting conditions showed lower clustering, shorter average path lengths, and lower centrality of major cortical hubs compared to controls, leading to the intriguing hypothesis that inappropriate linkages between disparate clusters of nodes may contribute to the pathology of schizophrenia.[115] Similar patterns of disruptions in small-world properties were found during a working memory task in schizophrenic patients.[116]

Finally, network changes have also been noted in epilepsy across multiple seizure types, including complex partial, tonic-clonic, and absence epilepsy.[117] While the specific mechanisms of onset and propagation differ across these seizure types, loss of consciousness in seizures always seems to be correlated with inhibition of subcortical arousal systems that normally maintain activity in the default mode and other cortical networks. These observations have led to the network inhibition hypothesis, whereby seizures cause loss of consciousness via active inhibition of subcortical arousal systems, which in turn leads to deactivation of cortical areas normally responsible for sustaining consciousness.[118] For example, limbic seizures in animal models and humans have been shown to cause activation in subcortical structures, including the septum and thalamus, but deactivation in neocortical areas such as the frontoparietal association cortices,[119,120] while electrically induced tonic-clonic seizures have also been shown to preferentially affect the consciousness system.[121] Interestingly, simple partial seizures that do not cause loss of consciousness do not show these network changes but are constrained to their site of origin in the temporal

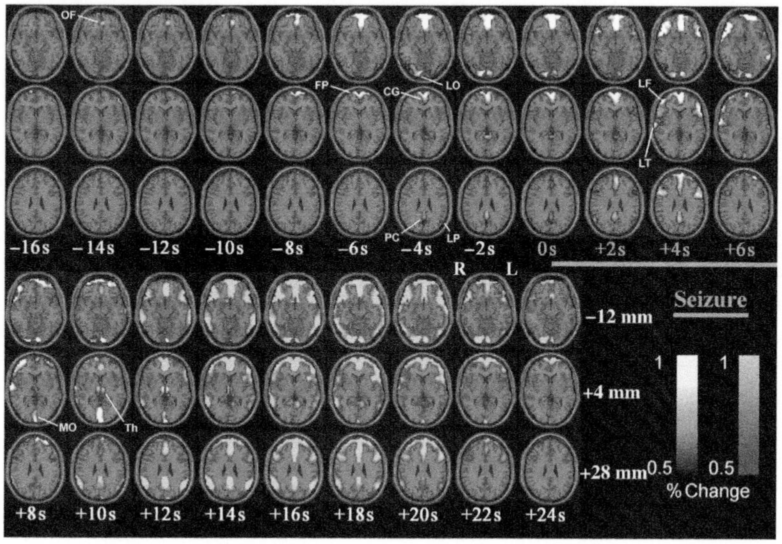

FIGURE 6.5 Dynamic changes in network activation before, during, and after absence seizures. Time course maps of percentage change from baseline show early increases (red) even before seizure onset in the frontal cortex, then progress to include a frontoparietal network and the thalamus. Profound widespread decreases (blue) are seen after end of seizure. (*Source: Reproduced with permission from Ref. 41.*) (The figure is reproduced in color section.)

cortex.[122] Specific behavioral impairments during seizures have also been linked to focal disruptions of neuronal networks.[123,124] Absence seizures, which are characterized by 3−4 Hz spike-and-wave discharges on EEG, disrupt select bilateral cortical and subcortical networks to cause brief impairments of consciousness.[125−127] Interictal changes have also been noted in absence epilepsy, with abnormally increased resting functional connectivity in the bilateral orbitofrontal cortex[21] and decreased functional connectivity between areas of the attention network.[128]

Graph theoretical analysis of interictal data in temporal lobe epilepsy has shown that patients demonstrate increased cortical path lengths and cluster coefficients compared to controls, as well as changes in distribution of highly connected cortical hubs.[129] These changes have been correlated with surgical outcome[129] and duration of disease history.[130] Evolving changes in network properties on EEG have been found in seizure activity, with an increase (then decrease) in characteristic path length and cluster coefficient over the course of seizures.[131] Finally, time-course analysis of fMRI during absence seizures has also shown dynamic changes within a frontoparietal network, with initial decreases followed by profound decreases well after the end of the seizure (Figure 6.5).[41]

CONCLUSION

The brain is composed of a complex structural network that allows for emergent functional connections (Chapter 30) spanning across cortical areas. The emerging view of the brain as a network of hubs has led to advances in characterizing network dynamics underlying normal cognition and disease. Additionally, graph-theoretical approaches provide a framework to precisely quantify topological changes of complex small-world networks. These techniques have been increasingly used in the analysis of EEG, MEG, and fMRI data and provide a powerful tool to the understanding of the brain as a structural and functional network in humans. Future research using network-based analysis of neuroimaging data may allow for better understanding of normal cognition, behavior, and disease.

Acknowledgments

This work was supported by NIH F31NS077540 (to JNG) and by NIH R01NS055829, R01NS066974, R01MH67528, R01HL059619, P30NS052519, U01NS045911, a Donaghue Foundation Investigator Award, and the Betsy and Jonathan Blattmachr Family.

References

1. Phillips CG, Zeki S, Barlow HB. Localization of function in the cerebral cortex. Past, present and future. *Brain*. 1984;107:327−361.
2. Young MP. Objective analysis of the topological organization of the primate cortical visual system. *Nature*. 1992;358:152−155.
3. Brodmann K. *Vergleichende Lokalisationslehre der Grosshirnrinde*. Leipzig: Johann Ambrosius Bart; 1909.
4. Schleicher A, Amunts K, Geyer S, Morosan P, Zilles K. Observer-independent method for microstructural parcellation of cerebral cortex: a quantitative approach to cytoarchitectonics. *Neuroimage*. 1999;9:165−177.
5. Amunts K, Zilles K. Advances in cytoarchitectonic mapping of the human cerebral cortex. *Neuroimaging Clin N Am*. 2001;11:151−169.
6. Rajkowska G, Goldman-Rakic PS. Cytoarchitectonic definition of prefrontal areas in the normal human cortex: I. Remapping of areas 9 and 46 using quantitative criteria. *Cereb Cortex*. 1995;5:307−322.
7. Geyer S, Schleicher A, Zilles K. The somatosensory cortex of human: cytoarchitecture and regional distributions of receptor-binding sites. *Neuroimage*. 1997;6:27−45.

8. Amunts K, Malikovic A, Mohlberg H, Schormann T, Zilles K. Brodmann's areas 17 and 18 brought into stereotaxic space-where and how variable? *Neuroimage*. 2000;11:66–84.
9. Gandhi SP, Heeger DJ, Boynton GM. Spatial attention affects brain activity in human primary visual cortex. *Proc Natl Acad Sci USA*. 1999;96:3314–3319.
10. Martínez A, Anllo-Vento L, Sereno MI, et al. Involvement of striate and extrastriate visual cortical areas in spatial attention. *Nat Neurosci*. 1999;2:364–369.
11. Aertsen AM, Gerstein GL, Habib MK, Palm G. Dynamics of neuronal firing correlation: modulation of "effective connectivity". *J Neurophysiol*. 1989;61:900–917.
12. Gong G, He Y, Concha L, et al. Mapping anatomical connectivity patterns of human cerebral cortex using in vivo diffusion tensor imaging tractography. *Cereb Cortex*. 2009;13:524–536.
13. Hagmann P, Cammoun L, Gigandet X, et al. Mapping the structural core of human cerebral cortex. *PLoS Biol*. 2008;6:e159.
14. Iturria-Medinaa Y, Soterob RC, Canales-Rodrígueza EJ, Alemán-Gómeza Y, Melie-Garcíaa L. Studying the human brain anatomical network via diffusion-weighted MRI and Graph Theory. *Neuroimage*. 2007;40:1064–1076.
15. Johansen-Berg H, Behrens TEJ, Robson MD, et al. Changes in connectivity profiles define functionally distinct regions in human medial frontal cortex. *Proc Natl Acad Sci USA*. 2004;101:13335–13340.
16. Johansen-Berg H, Rushworth MFS. Using diffusion imaging to study human connectional anatomy. *Annu Rev Neurosci*. 2009;32:75–94.
17. Quigley M, Cordes D, Turski P, et al. Role of the corpus callosum in functional connectivity. *AJNR Am J Neuroradiol*. 2003;24:208–212.
18. Johnston JM, Vaishnavi SN, Smyth MD, et al. Loss of resting interhemispheric functional connectivity after complete section of the corpus callosum. *J Neurosci*. 2008;28:6453–6458.
19. Van Den Heuvel MP, Mandl RCW, Kahn RS, Hulshoff Pol HE. Functionally linked resting-state networks reflect the underlying structural connectivity architecture of the human brain. *Hum Brain Mapp*. 2009;30:3127–3141.
20. Skudlarski P, Jagannathan K, Calhoun V, Hampson M, Skularska B, Pearlson G. Measuring brain connectivity: diffusion tensor imaging validates resting state temporal correlations. *Neuroimage*. 2008;43:554.
21. Bai X, Guo JN, Killory B, et al. Resting functional connectivity between the hemispheres in childhood absence epilepsy. *Neurology*. 2011;76:1960–1967.
22. Honey CJ, Sporns O, Cammoun L, et al. Predicting human resting-state functional connectivity from structural connectivity. *Proc Natl Acad Sci USA*. 2009;106:2035–2040.
23. Srinivasan R, Winter WR, Ding J, Nunez PL. EEG and MEG coherence: measures of functional connectivity at distinct spatial scales of neocortical dynamics. *J Neurosci Methods*. 2007;166:41–52.
24. Stam C, De Haan W, Daffertshofer A, et al. Graph theoretical analysis of magnetoencephalographic functional connectivity in Alzheimer's disease. *Brain*. 2009;132:213–224.
25. Sporns O, Chialvo DR, Kaiser M, Hilgetag CC. Organization, development and function of complex brain networks. *Trends Cogn Sci*. 2004;8:418–425.
26. Watts DJ, Strogatz SH. Collective dynamics of 'small-world' networks. *Nature*. 1998;393:440–442.
27. Tononi G. An information integration theory of consciousness. *BMC Neurosci*. 2004;5:42.
28. Bassett DS, Bullmore E. Small-world brain networks. *Neuroscientist*. 2006;12:512–523.
29. Petermann T, Rios PDL. Spatial small-world networks: a wiring-cost perspective. *Arxiv preprint cond-mat/0501420*. 2005.
30. Chklovskii D, Schikorski T, Stevens C. Wiring optimization in cortical circuits. *Neuron*. 2002;34:341–347.
31. Klyachko V, Stevens C. Connectivity optimization and the positioning of cortical areas. *Proc Natl Acad Sci USA*. 2003;100:7937–7941.
32. Levy WB, Baxter RA. Energy efficient neural codes. *Neural Comput*. 1996;8:531–543.
33. Attwell D, Laughlin SB. An energy budget for signaling in the grey matter of the brain. *J Cereb Blood Flow Metab*. 2001;21:1133–1145.
34. Felleman D, Van Essen D. Distributed hierarchical processing in the primate cerebral cortex. *Cereb Cortex*. 1991;1:1–47.
35. Haxby JV, Gobbini M, Furey ML, Ishai A, Schouten JL, Pietrini P. Distributed and overlapping representations of faces and objects in ventral temporal cortex. *Science*. 2001;293:2425–2430.
36. Rauschecker JP. Parallel processing in the auditory cortex of primates. *Audiol Neurootol*. 1998;3:86–103.
37. Coghill RC, Sang CN, Maisog JM, Iadarola MJ. Pain intensity processing within the human brain: a bilateral, distributed mechanism. *J Neurophysiol*. 1999;82:1934–1943.
38. Hopfield JJ. Neural networks and physical systems with emergent collective computational abilities. *Proc Natl Acad Sci USA*. 1982;79:2554–2558.
39. Gonzalez-Castillo J, Saad ZS, Handwerker DA, Inati SJ, Brenowitz N, Bandettini PA. Whole-brain, time-locked activation with simple tasks revealed using massive averaging and model-free analysis. *Proc Natl Acad Sci USA*. 2012;109:5487–5492.
40. Friston K, Holmes A, Worsley K, Poline J, Frith C, Frackowiak R. Statistical parametric maps in functional imaging: a general linear approach. *Hum Brain Mapp*. 1994;2:189–210.
41. Bai X, Vestal M, Berman R, et al. Dynamic timecourse of typical childhood absence seizures: EEG, behavior and fMRI. *J Neurosci*. 2010;30:5884–5893.
42. Meltzer J, Negishi M, Constable R. Biphasic hemodynamic responses influence deactivation and may mask activation in block-design fMRI paradigms. *Hum Brain Mapp*. 2008;29:385–399.
43. Handwerker DA, Ollinger J, D'Esposito M. Variation of BOLD hemodynamic responses across subjects and brain regions and their effects on statistical analyses. *Neuroimage*. 2004;21:1639–1651.
44. Biswal B, Yetkin FZ, Haughton VM, Hyde JS. Functional connectivity in the motor cortex of resting human brain using echo-planar MRI. *Magn Reson Med*. 1995;34:537–541.
45. Greicius MD, Krasnow B, Reiss AL, Menon V. Functional connectivity in the resting brain: a network analysis of the default mode hypothesis. *Proc Natl Acad Sci USA*. 2003;100:253–258.
46. Buckner RL, Sepulcre J, Talukdar T, et al. Cortical hubs revealed by intrinsic functional connectivity: mapping, assessment of stability, and relation to Alzheimer's disease. *J Neurosci*. 2009;29:1860–1873.
47. Lowe MJ, Dzemidzic M, Lurito JT, Mathews VP, Phillips MD. Correlations in low-frequency BOLD fluctuations reflect cortico-cortical connections. *Neuroimage*. 2000;12:582–587.
48. Shulman RG, Rothman DL. Interpreting functional imaging studies in terms of neurotransmitter cycling. *Proc Natl Acad Sci USA*. 1998;95:11993–11998.
49. Arieli A, Sterkin A, Grinvald A, Aertsen A. Dynamics of ongoing activity: explanation of the large variability in evoked cortical responses. *Science*. 1996;273:1868–1871.
50. Tsodyks M, Kenet T, Grinvald A, Arieli A. Linking spontaneous activity of single cortical neurons and the underlying functional architecture. *Science*. 1999;286:1943–1946.
51. Kenet T, Bibitchkov D, Tsodyks M, Grinvald A, Arieli A. Spontaneously emerging cortical representations of visual attributes. *Nature*. 2003;425:954–956.
52. Friston KJ. Functional and effective connectivity in neuroimaging: a synthesis. *Hum Brain Mapp*. 1994;2:56–78.

53. Friston K, Harrison L, Penny W. Dynamic causal modelling. *Neuroimage*. 2003;19:1273–1302.
54. Roebroeck A, Formisano E, Goebel R. Mapping directed influence over the brain using Granger causality and fMRI. *Neuroimage*. 2005;25:230–242.
55. McIntosh A, Gonzalez-Lima F. Structural equation modeling and its application to network analysis in functional brain imaging. *Hum Brain Mapp*. 1994;2:2–22.
56. Büchel C, Friston K. Modulation of connectivity in visual pathways by attention: cortical interactions evaluated with structural equation modelling and fMRI. *Cereb Cortex*. 1997;7:768–788.
57. Rothman DL, Sibson NR, Hyder F, Shen J, Behar KL, Shulman RG. In vivo nuclear magnetic resonance spectroscopy studies of the relationship between the glutamate–glutamine neurotransmitter cycle and functional neuroenergetics. *Philos Trans R Soc Lond B Biol Sci*. 1999;354:1165–1177.
58. Magistretti PJ, Pellerin L, Rothman DL, Shulman RG. Energy on demand. *Science*. 1999;283:496–497.
59. Patel AB, de Graaf RA, Mason GF, Rothman DL, Shulman RG, Behar KL. The contribution of GABA to glutamate/glutamine cycling and energy metabolism in the rat cortex in vivo. *Proc Natl Acad Sci USA*. 2005;102:5588–5593.
60. Hyder F, Patel AB, Gjedde A, Rothman DL, Behar KL, Shulman RG. Neuronal–glial glucose oxidation and glutamatergic–GABAergic function. *J Cereb Blood Flow Metab*. 2006;26:865–877.
61. Buzsáki G, Anastassiou C, Koch C. The origin of extracellular fields and currents—EEG, ECoG, LFP and spikes. *Nat Rev Neurosci*. 2012;13:407–420.
62. Kajikawa Y, Schroeder C. How local is the local field potential? *Neuron*. 2011;72:847–858.
63. Katzner S, Nauhaus I, Benucci A, Bonin V, Ringach D, Carandini M. Local origin of field potentials in visual cortex. *Neuron*. 2009;61:35–41.
64. Logothetis NK, Pauls J, Augath M, Trinath T, Oeltermann A. Neurophysiological investigation of the basis of the fMRI signal. *Nature*. 2001;412:150–157.
65. Smith A, Blumenfeld H, Behar K, Rothman DL, Shulman GL, Hyder F. Cerebral energetics and spiking frequency: the neurophysiological basis of fMRI. *Proc Natl Acad Sci USA*. 2002;99:10765–10770.
66. Hyder F, Sanganahalli B, Herman P, et al. Neurovascular and neurometabolic couplings in dynamic calibrated fMRI: transient oxidative neuroenergetics for block-design and event-related paradigms. *Front Neuroenergetics*. 2010;2:1–11.
67. Mishra A, Ellens D, Schridde U, et al. Where fMRI and electrophysiology agree to disagree: corticothalamic and striatal activity patterns in the WAG/Rij rat. *J Neurosci*. 2012;31:15053–15064.
68. Devonshire IM, Papadakis NG, Port M, et al. Neurovascular coupling is brain region-dependent. *Neuroimage*. 2012;59:1997–2006.
69. Haider B, Duque A, Hasenstaub AR, McCormick DA. Neocortical network activity in vivo is generated through a dynamic balance of excitation and inhibition. *J Neurosci*. 2006;26:4535–4545.
70. Mathieson C, Caesar K, Akgören N, Lauritzen M. Modification of activity-dependent increases of cerebral blood flow by excitatory synaptic activity and spikes in rat cerebellar cortex. *J Physiol*. 1998;512:555–566.
71. Kelly P, Ford I, McCulloch J. The effect of diazepam upon local cerebral glucose use in the conscious rat. *Neuroscience*. 1986;19:257–265.
72. Kelly P, McCulloch J. Effects of the putatitve GABAergic agonists, muscimol and THIP, upon local cerebral glucose utilisation. *J Neurochem*. 1982;39.
73. Roland P, Friberg L. The effect of GABA-A agonist THIP on regional cortical blood flow in humans. A new test of hemispheric dominance. *J Cereb Blood Flow Metab*. 1988:314–323.
74. Tagamets M, Horwitz B. Interpreting PET and fMRI measures of functional neural activity: the effects of synaptic inhibition on cortical activation in human imaging studies. *Brain Res Bull*. 2001;54:267–273.
75. Shmuel A, Leopold DA. Neuronal correlates of spontaneous fluctuations in fMRI signals in monkey visual cortex: implications for functional connectivity at rest. *Hum Brain Mapp*. 2008;29:751–761.
76. Schölvinck ML, Maier A, Ye FQ, Duyn JH, Leopold DA. Neural basis of global resting-state fMRI activity. *Proc Natl Acad Sci USA*. 2010;107:10238–10243.
77. Fries P, Reynolds J, Rorie A, Desimone R. Modulation of oscillatory neuronal synchronization by selective visual attention. *Science*. 2001;291:1560–1563.
78. Womelsdorf T, Schoffelen J, Oostenveld R, et al. Modulation of neuronal interactions through neuronal synchronization. *Science*. 2007;316:1609–1612.
79. Freunberger R, Klimesch W, Griesmayr B, Sauseng P, Gruber W. Alpha phase coupling reflects object recognition. *Neuroimage*. 2008;42:928–935.
80. Gross J, Schmitz F, Schnitzler I, et al. Modulation of long-range neural synchrony reflects temporal limitations of visual attention in humans. *Proc Natl Acad Sci USA*. 2004;101:13050–13055.
81. Siegel M, Donner T, Oostenveld R, Fries P, Engel A. Neuronal synchronization along the dorsal visual pathway reflects the focus of spatial attention. *Neuron*. 2008;60:709–719.
82. Melloni L, Molina C, Pena M, Torres D, Singer W, Rodriguez E. Synchronization of neural activity across cortical areas correlates with conscious perception. *J Neurosci*. 2007;27:2858–2865.
83. Brookes MJ, Woolrich M, Luckhoo H, et al. Investigating the electrophysiological basis of resting state networks using magnetoencephalography. *Proc Natl Acad Sci USA*. 2011;108: 16783–16788.
84. Stam C. Functional connectivity patterns of human magnetoencephalographic recordings: a small-world network? *Neurosci Lett*. 2004;355:25–28.
85. Corbetta M, Shulman GL. Control of goal-directed and stimulus-driven attention in the brain. *Nat Rev Neurosci*. 2002;3:201–215.
86. Fox MD, Corbetta M, Snyder AZ, Vincent JL, Raichle ME. Spontaneous neuronal activity distinguishes human dorsal and ventral attention systems. *Proc Natl Acad Sci USA*. 2006;103:10046–10051.
87. Binder JR, Frost JA, Hammeke TA, Bellgowan PS, Rao SM, Cox RW. Conceptual processing during the conscious resting state. A functional MRI study. *J Cogn Neurosci*. 1999;11:80–95.
88. Raichle ME, MacLeod AM, Snyder AZ, Powers WJ, Gusnard DA, Shulman GL. A default mode of brain function. *Proc Natl Acad Sci USA*. 2001;98:676–682.
89. Fox MD, Snyder AZ, Vincent JL, Corbetta M, Essen DCV, Raichle ME. The human brain is intrinsically organized into dynamic, anticorrelated functional networks. *Proc Natl Acad Sci USA*. 2005;102:9673–9678.
90. Buckner RL, Carroll DC. Self-projection and the brain. *Trends Cogn Sci*. 2007;11:49–57.
91. Vincent JL, Patel GH, Fox MD, et al. Intrinsic functional architecture in the anaesthetized monkey brain. *Nature*. 2007;447:83–86.
92. Hampson M, Driesen NR, Skudlarski P, Gore JC, Constable RT. Brain connectivity related to working memory performance. *J Neurosci*. 2006;26:13338–13343.

93. Meindl T, Teipel S, Elmouden R, et al. Test-retest reproducibility of the default-mode network in healthy individuals. *Hum Brain Mapp*. 2009;31:237–246.
94. Danielson NB, Guo JN, Blumenfeld H. The default mode network and altered consciousness in epilepsy. *Behav Neurol*. 2011;24:55–65.
95. Colonnese MT, Phillips MA, Constantine-Paton M, Kaila K, Jasanoff A. Development of hemodynamic responses and functional connectivity in rat somatosensory cortex. *Nat Neurosci*. 2008;11:72–79.
96. Micheloyannis S, Vourkas M, Tsirka V, Karakonstantaki E, Kanatsouli K, Stam C. The influence of ageing on complex brain networks: a graph theoretical analysis. *Hum Brain Mapp*. 2009;30:200–208.
97. McCormick D, Bal T. Sleep and arousal: thalamocortical mechanisms. *Annu Rev Neurosci*. 1997;20:185–215.
98. Massimini M, Ferrarelli F, Huber R, Esser SK, Singh H, Tononi G. Breakdown of cortical effective connectivity during sleep. *Science*. 2005;309:2228–2232.
99. Boly M, Perlbarg V, Marrelec G, et al. Hierarchical clustering of brain activity during human nonrapid eye movement sleep. *Proc Natl Acad Sci USA*. 2012;109:5856–5861.
100. Kaisti K, Metsähonkala L, Teräs M, et al. Effects of surgical levels of propofol and sevoflurane anesthesia on cerebral blood flow in healthy subjects studied with positron emission tomography. *Anesthesiology*. 2002;96:1358–1370.
101. John ER, Prichep LS, Kox W, et al. Invariant reversible QEEG effects of anesthetics. *Conscious Cogn*. 2001;10:165–183.
102. Imas OA, Ropella KM, Wood JD, Hudetz AG. Isoflurane disrupts anterio-posterior phase synchronization of flash-induced field potentials in the rat. *Neurosci Lett*. 2006;402:216–221.
103. Lee UC, Oh GJ, Kim S, Noh GJ, Choi BM, Mashour GA. Brain networks maintain a scale-free organization across consciousness, anesthesia, and recovery: evidence for adaptive reconfiguration. *Anesthesiology*. 2010;113:1081–1091.
104. Imas OA, Ropella KM, Ward BD, Wood JD, Hudetz AG. Volatile anesthetics disrupt frontal-posterior recurrent information transfer at gamma frequencies in rat. *Neurosci Lett*. 2005;387:145–150.
105. White NS, Alkire MT. Impaired thalamocortical connectivity in humans during general-anesthetic-induced unconsciousness. *Neuroimage*. 2003;19:402–411.
106. Peltier SJ, Kerssens C, Hamann SB, et al. Functional connectivity changes with concentration of sevoflurane anesthesia. *Neuroreport*. 2005;16:285–288.
107. Gili T, Saxena N, Diukova A, Murphy K, Hall JE, Wise RG. The thalamus and brainstem act as key hubs in alterations of human brain network connectivity induced by mild propofol sedation. *J Neurosci*. 2013;33:4024–4031.
108. Shimoji K, Bickford R. Differential effects of anesthetics on mesencephalic reticular neurons. I. Spontaneous firing patters. *Anesthesiology*. 1971;35:151–155.
109. Roizen M, White P, Eger EI, Brownstein M. Effects of ablation of serotonin or norepinephrine brain-stem areas on halothane and cyclopropane MACs in rats. *Anesthesiology*. 1978;49:252–255.
110. Cirrito J, Yamada K, Finn M, et al. Synaptic activity regulates interstitial fluid amyloid-beta levels in vivo. *Neuron*. 2005;48:913–922.
111. Bero A, Yan P, Roh J, et al. Neuronal activity regulates the regional vulnerability to amyloid-beta deposition. *Nat Neurosci*. 2011;14:750–756.
112. Stam C, Jones B, Nolte G, Breakspear M, Scheltens P. Small-world networks and functional connectivity in Alzheimer's disease. *Cereb Cortex*. 2007;17:92–99.
113. Lowe M, Phillips M, Lurito J, Mattson D, Dzemidzic M, Mathews V. Multiple sclerosis: low-frequency temporal blood oxygen level–dependent fluctuations indicate reduced functional connectivity—initial results. *Radiology*. 2002;224:184–192.
114. Lowe M, Beall E, Sakaie K, et al. Resting state sensorimotor functional connectivity in multiple sclerosis inversely correlates with transcallosal motor pathway transverse diffusivity. *Hum Brain Mapp*. 2008;29:818–827.
115. Rubinov M, Knock SA, Stam CJ, et al. Small-world properties of nonlinear brain activity in schizophrenia. *Hum Brain Mapp*. 2009;30:403–416.
116. Micheloyannis S, Pachou E, Stam C, et al. Small-world networks and disturbed functional connectivity in schizophrenia. *Schizophr Res*. 2006;87:60–66.
117. Blumenfeld H. Impaired consciousness in epilepsy. *Lancet Neurol*. 2012;11:814–826.
118. Norden AD, Blumenfeld H. The role of subcortical structures in human epilepsy. *Epilepsy Behav*. 2002;3:219–231.
119. Englot D, Modi B, Mishra A, DeSalvo M, Hyder F, Blumenfeld H. Cortical deactivation induced by subcortical network dysfunction in limbic seizures. *J Neurosci*. 2009;29:13006–13018.
120. Englot D, Yang L, Hamid H, et al. Impaired consciousness in temporal lobe seizures: role of cortical slow activity. *Brain*. 2010;133:3764–3777.
121. Enev M, McNally K, Varghese G, Zubal I, Ostroff R, Blumenfeld H. Imaging onset and propagation of ECT-induced seizures. *Epilepsia*. 2007;48:238–244.
122. Blumenfeld H, McNally K, Vanderhill S, et al. Positive and negative network correlations in temporal lobe epilepsy. *Cereb Cortex*. 2004;14:892–902.
123. Blumenfeld H. Consciousness and epilepsy: why are patients with absence seizures absent? *Prog Brain Res*. 2005;150: 271–603.
124. Kostopoulos G. Involvement of the thalamocortical system in epileptic loss of consciousness. *Epilepsia*. 2001;42:13–19.
125. Meeren H, van Luijtelaar G, Lopes da Silva F, Coenen A. Evolving concepts on the pathophysiology of absence seizures: the cortical focus theory. *Arch Neurol*. 2005;62:371–376.
126. Blumenfeld H. Cellular and network mechanisms of spike-wave seizures. *Epilepsia*. 2005;46:271–286.
127. Berman R, Negishi M, Vestal M, et al. Simultaneous EEG, fMRI, and behavior in typical childhood absence seizures. *Epilepsia*. 2010;51:2011–2022.
128. Killory B, Bai X, Negishi M, et al. Impaired attention and network connectivity in childhood absence epilepsy. *Neuroimage*. 2011;56:2209–2217.
129. Bernhardt BC, Chen Z, He Y, Evans AC, Bernasconi N. Graph-theoretical analysis reveals disrupted small-world organization of cortical thickness correlation networks in temporal lobe epilepsy. *Cereb Cortex*. 2011;21:2147–2157.
130. Van Dellen E, Douw L, Baayen J, et al. Long-term effects of temporal lobe epilepsy on local neural networks: a graph theoretical analysis of corticography recordings. *PLoS One*. 2009;4:e8081.
131. Schindler KA, Bialonski S, Horstmann MT, Elger CE, Lehnertz K. Evolving functional network properties and synchronizability during human epileptic seizures. *Chaos*. 2008;18:033119.

CHAPTER

7

Network Control Mechanisms: Cellular Inputs, Neuroactive Substances, and Synaptic Changes

Carl L. Faingold

Departments of Pharmacology, Neurology and Division of Neurosurgery, Southern Illinois University School of Medicine, Springfield, IL, USA

INTRODUCTION

As noted in Chapter 1, cellular inputs are key elements of network connections, which are a critical determinant of network control and function. The main function of principal neurons in a physiological network in the brain, which contains multiple nuclei, is to receive input and project output to the next nucleus (or effector) of the network. However, nuclei in essentially all neuronal networks in the brain receive multiple inputs, and the principal neurons in the nucleus must integrate these inputs with its intrinsic "spontaneous" activity into an output or a pattern of outputs. The outputs range from a simple increase or decrease in firing to a complex sequential firing pattern, such as burst firing (Chapter 9). The specific principal cells that provide the output of a given nucleus in most brain sites is determined by processing a complex set of both excitatory and inhibitory inputs from the connections to these cells (see Figure 7.1). These inputs include local interneurons and astrocytic networks within the nucleus, as well as inputs from other network nuclei and also, directly or indirectly, from external inputs such as sensory stimuli. Integration of this multiplicity of inputs among the principal neurons within each network nucleus, impinging on the other nuclei of the network, will ultimately determine the activity and function of the network. Commonly, the effect of an input on neurons within the network involves the action of one or more neuroactive substances released upon principal neurons and other cellular elements of the network nucleus, and it results in release by these cells of a neuroactive substance that affects cells in the subsequent network nuclei, as discussed in this chapter. The released neuroactive substance can result in changes in synaptic function, especially with repetition of the input. These processes can result in short- and long-term changes in network function, which have the potential to induce changes in synaptic efficacy within the network.

Two major categories of stimulus-evoked network change include stimulus-induced network activation and stimulus-induced changes in network oscillations.[1] Stimulus-locked network oscillations depend on the continuing presentation of the stimulus, and they are seen commonly in sensory networks, including neurons in the primary auditory system (see Chapter 20). As mentioned in this section, principal neurons within a specific nucleus of a network often exhibit spontaneous activity due to their intrinsic properties. These properties include pacemaker activity in certain nuclei (e.g. in the respiratory network and circadian networks; see Chapters 14 and 18), which can be observed when these neurons are removed from the network in ex vivo and in vitro electrophysiological studies (see Chapter 5).

The principal neurons in a network nucleus in the intact brain receive important influences from within the nucleus from local interneurons and glia. These local connections, coupled with the ascending and descending inputs from neurons in other network nuclei, determine the output of the nucleus and its role in the overall function of the entire network. This is often modeled in ex vivo (brain slice) studies by electrical stimulation of nearby network sites within the slice or the incoming fiber pathways that remain in the slice (e.g. Reference 2). However, obtaining a physiologically relevant balance with these electrical stimuli in a slice can be problematic, because preparation of the slice necessitates the removal of the sources of many inputs. Evaluations of the role of inputs in vivo is also done using electrical stimuli, comparing responses before and after paradigms

Neuronal Networks in Brain Function, CNS Disorders, and Therapeutics
http://dx.doi.org/10.1016/B978-0-12-415804-7.00007-1

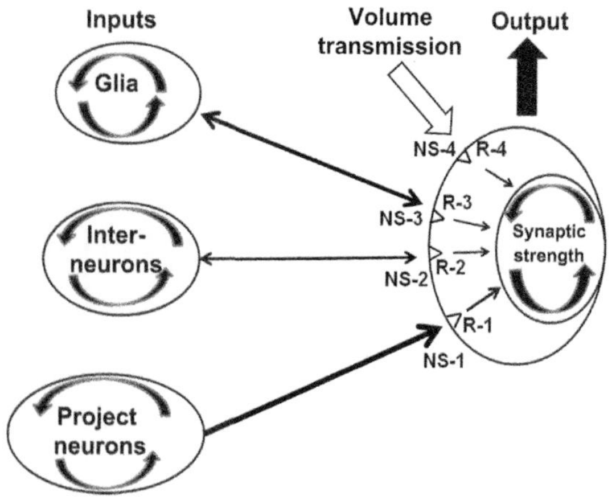

FIGURE 7.1 Diagram depicting a simplified scheme for the effects of inputs and neuroactive substances (NS-1–4) on their respective receptors (R-1–4) and the resulting changes in synaptic strength of principal neurons of a major network nucleus (large oval on right). The oval on the bottom left symbolizes the projection (Project) neurons from a major input nucleus that releases a neuroactive substance (NS-1) onto receptors (R-1) of the principal cells of the target major network nucleus (large oval on the right). The middle oval on the left symbolizes the interneurons within the major nucleus that provide another important input by releasing a neuroactive substance (NS-2) onto receptors (R-2) of the principal cells. The top oval on the left symbolizes the input from glia within the major nucleus on the principal cells that release a neuroactive substance (NS-3) onto receptors (R-3) of the principal cells. The hollow downward arrow in the top middle of the diagram symbolizes a neuroactive substance (NS-4) that is conducted via volume transmission (see Chapter 8) and acts on its receptors (R-4) on the principal cells. All of the receptors (R-1–4), when repetitively activated, can potentially result in changes in synaptic strength by affecting intracellular events (see Figure 7.3), which can greatly modify the output (large filled arrow) of the principal cells of this network nucleus. Note: paired semicircular arrows indicate that the networks readily undergo self-organization. (For color version of this figure, the reader is referred to the online version of this book.)

designed to modify the network (e.g. Reference 3), but if anesthesia is utilized certain inputs can be greatly diminished[4] (see Chapter 32).

Thus, in the normal networks discussed in several chapters of this book, the function of the network—be it motor, as in the locomotor network (see Chapter 17), or sensory, as in the auditory network (see Chapter 20)—is clearly dependent on the inputs from neurons in one nucleus, which project to the neurons in the next nucleus (in hierarchical networks) within that network and govern the pattern of motor movement or auditory perception, respectively, that results. For example, plastic changes in the organization of the sensorimotor cortex network are induced by exogenous stimulation.[5] Stimuli that originate from the external milieu via the sensory networks obviously play a major role in controlling primary sensory neuronal networks, but sensory stimuli can also play important roles in the control of networks that subserve totally different functions, such as locomotion or emotional states. Thus, an acoustic stimulus obviously exerts major control of the primary auditory network, but it can also activate the locomotion network in the case of the acoustic startle response[6] (see Chapter 28).

PROJECTION NEURON INPUTS

An example of how input, in the form of an acoustic stimulus, acts on the primary auditory network is seen in the inferior colliculus (IC), which is a midbrain primary auditory nucleus that is required for normal hearing (see Chapter 20). The central nucleus of the IC is the major input of the ascending auditory pathway to the thalamus [the medial geniculate body (MGB)], and from there to the auditory cortex. The characteristics of the acoustic stimulus determine the output of the IC in a complex way, since the input connections to IC principal neurons consist of an extensive array of ascending auditory nuclei that exert different and sometimes competing influences on IC neurons.

IC principal cells appear to possess some intrinsic activity, since they are spontaneously active in brain slice.[2,7] The main excitatory input to the principal IC projection neurons ascends from the superior olivary complex and is mediated by the excitatory neurotransmitter, glutamate (GLU).[8,9] However, several other inputs to the principal IC neurons are inhibitory, mediated by the neurotransmitter γ-aminobutyric acid (GABA), and these can also be activated simultaneously or sequentially by the same acoustic stimuli. These inhibitory inputs onto IC principal cells emanate from local interneurons,[10] as well as ascending projections from more caudal brainstem auditory nuclei, including the dorsal nucleus of the lateral lemniscus (DNLL)[11,12] and superior periolivary nucleus.[13,14] Inputs from each of these different sources result in distinctly different patterns of GABA-mediated inhibition, which include binaural (simultaneous to both ears), intensity-induced (nonmonotonic rate-intensity function), and offset forms of inhibition in response to acoustic stimuli.[15]

When the same acoustic stimulus is presented binaurally, a significant reduction of IC central neuronal responses, called binaural inhibition, is evoked in many IC principal neurons. As noted in this section, the DNLL is one major source of GABAergic input to the IC, and modification of this input selectively alters this form of acoustically evoked inhibition. Stimulation of the DNLL (electrical or chemical) simulates binaural inhibition in most contralateral IC neurons. Focal blockade of the DNLL, by microinjecting a local anesthetic (lidocaine) or a $GABA_A$ agonist, reversibly blocked acoustically evoked binaural inhibition and increased

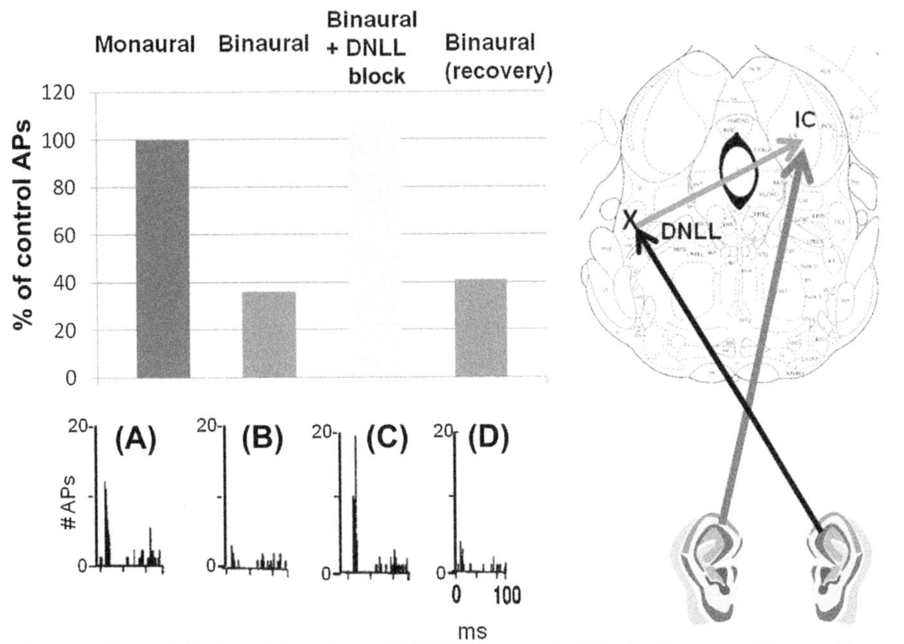

FIGURE 7.2 An example of the effects of blockade of a major inhibitory input on the activity of the principal cells of the inferior colliculus (central nucleus, IC) excitatory activity evoked by its major excitatory input as a result of an auditory stimulus. In the diagram on the right, acoustic stimuli are presented to the left ear (monaural), ascend via the brainstem auditory network (see Chapter 20) to the contralateral IC, and evoke a major increase in firing mediated by glutamate.[8] This is illustrated by the time-locked peak in the poststimulus-time histogram (PSTH) in A, which represents 100% (control) and is represented in the bar graph above A (stimulus onset is at 0 ms in each PSTH). The PSTH in B shows the IC neuronal response when the same stimulus is repetitively presented to both ears, as indicated by the decreased time-locked peak. This significant decrease in evoked action potentials, called binaural inhibition, is represented by the bar graph above B. The dorsal nucleus of the lateral lemniscus (DNLL) is also part of the brainstem auditory pathway. DNLL neurons provide input to the principal neurons of IC and release GABA onto these neurons,[15] which greatly reduces the response when the stimulus is presented to both ears. When a local anesthetic or other inhibitory substance is focally microinjected (X) into DNLL, this blocks the inhibitory input from DNLL and causes the same binaural stimulus to evoke increased neuronal firing (PSTH in C), which actually exceeds control (illustrated by the bar above C). The effect of the DNLL block dissipated due to diffusion and metabolism of the microinjected substance and, 5–20 min later (in different examples), the response to presentation of the stimulus to both ears (D), resulting in recovery of the binaural inhibition, as illustrated by the bar above D (stimuli: 39 dB; SPL, 50 presentations PSTH at 2/sec, 13.8 kHz in Sprague–Dawley rat). See References 11,16 (for neuroanatomy). APs = action potentials. (For color version of this figure, the reader is referred to the online version of this book.)

spontaneous firing in most contralateral IC neurons (Figure 7.2).[11] This is an example of the major impact that one of many inputs to the IC can exert that greatly alters the function of the normal auditory network.

This variety of connections governs the role of the IC in the normal auditory network, but it also leads to the role of this structure in the pathophysiological network that mediates audiogenic seizures (AGS) (see Chapter 26). AGS is mediated, in part, by a deficit of acoustically evoked GABAergic inhibition, involving loss of several forms of inhibition, including intensity-induced inhibition, which results in excessive firing of IC neurons at the high stimulus intensities required to induce AGS. The excessive output from the IC provides excessive input to the brainstem locomotor network (see Chapter 17), triggering the motor manifestations of the generalized convulsive seizure (see Chapter 26). Thus, the auditory network performs, along with its primary role of providing sensory input to higher centers, an additional role of triggering motor output to the spinal cord via the locomotor network. Another example of how variations in input can alter neuronal output is seen in the primary visual system. When different temporal and intensity patterns of visual stimuli are presented, the neuronal responsiveness in the primary visual cortex can be diminished.[17]

MULTIPLE INPUTS

Inputs from multiple sensory modalities are constantly impinging on the awake, behaving organism, and multisensory integration can produce even more complex effects on neuronal network function in the brain. Thus, inputs from more than one network can result in both negative and positive effects on network function. An example of this is seen in fear conditioning (see Chapter 13). Limbic system networks are involved in the generation of normal emotions, and dysfunctions in these networks are associated with certain psychiatric disorders, including depression and anxiety (see Chapter 24). Inputs from outside the limbic network can have a major impact on the function of these emotional networks. Thus, as noted here, connections with the auditory network can result in major functional changes of these limbic networks, particularly in the amygdala. An example is fear conditioning (see Chapter 13), which is a behavioral conditioning paradigm that involves repetitive pairing of an acoustic stimulus input transmitted via the auditory network (up to the MGB) that is temporally coupled with an aversive foot shock transmitted via the somatosensory network. This classical conditioning paradigm results in a lasting change in network function and behavior[18] (see Chapter 13).

Unprovoked external inputs from other networks can also give rise to major changes in the function of a given network. Thus, input from the dorsal raphe nucleus provides an important excitatory influence that alters the intrinsic pacemaker activity of the respiratory network.[19] Somatosensory and other sensory inputs onto the locomotor network can greatly affect the ongoing function of this network as well.[20] In addition, external inputs to a neuronal network engaged in an ongoing state can exert major effects on that state. Thus, an "up state", which is a robust network-wide state of subthreshold depolarizations (see Chapter 32), can be terminated by electrical stimulation at a distant site that is not part of the network.[21]

Network-wide activity in the form of oscillations in specific frequency bands is detectable in humans, using electroencephalography or magnetoencephalography, and these oscillations are also subject to significant alterations when external stimuli are presented.[22] Based on neuroimaging data, an intrinsic resting-state activity of the brain networks characterized as the "default mode network" has been proposed[23] (see Chapter 6), and this default mode is also subject to modification in response to external input.[24]

An example of the effect of multiple inputs from separate neuronal networks that modify the function of a third network is seen in the kindling of audiogenic seizures (AGS kindling) paradigm, discussed in Chapter 27. In this example, the brainstem locomotor network that produces the symmetrical locomotor behaviors of wild running and generalized tonic convulsion is triggered by input from the auditory network. After AGS kindling (frequent repetitive seizures), an additional locomotor pattern called generalized (all-limb) clonus is expressed immediately following the tonic convulsive motor behavior. This "new" locomotor pattern change is triggered by a different network, the limbic network, since stimulation or blockade in that network (in the amygdala) specifically controls only this new locomotor output but does not affect the original locomotor pattern (see Chapters 26 and 27). There is evidence that a specific part of the network, the periaqueductal gray, may be the nexus for the input of both auditory and limbic projections to the locomotor network.[3]

ELECTROPHYSIOLOGICAL MECHANISMS

A number of different electrophysiological events are known to mediate the effects of the inputs to neurons in network nuclei, and these events play key roles in network function. A key electrophysiological event is the pattern of neuronal firing, including single action potentials, tonic firing, and "burst firing", as discussed in Chapters 8 and 9. Gap junctions, field effects, and ephaptic connections can also make major contributions to the control of network functions. The nature of these electrophysiological events is a critical determinant of the effect of the inputs to a specific nucleus on the output of that nucleus, which in most cases involves the release of one or more neuroactive substances that affects subsequent site(s) in the network.

NEUROACTIVE SUBSTANCES

Neuroactive substances include a broad range of agents, which act on an array of targets e.g., (receptors) via both synaptic and volume transmission (see Chapter 8). Neuroactive substances exert their actions on neuronal networks over time scales ranging from milliseconds to months or even years. Ionic substances such as extracellular Ca^{2+} can exert profound effects on the milieu of cellular elements of a neuronal network and typically exert their initial influences rapidly over a few milliseconds, as discussed in Chapter 10. Classical neurotransmitters are a major type of neuroactive substance and include amino acids, such as GABA and GLU, which act on ligand-gated receptors. These neurotransmitters act rapidly over milliseconds, but effects of these transmitters can also be persistent, as seen with GABA-mediated tonic inhibition. Slower and more diffusely acting classical neurotransmitters, such as 5-hydroxytryptamine (5-HT) and norepinephrine, act largely on metabotropic G-protein coupled receptors. Neuromodulators, such as adenosine, also act on metabotropic receptors with a long course of action. Cytokines, such as tumor necrosis factor alpha (TNF-α), and neurotropic factors, such as brain-derived neurotropic factor (BDNF), can also exert significant long-term influences on network function, as discussed in this chapter. Central nervous system (CNS) drugs are another major class of neuroactive agent, which modify network function largely by interacting with the endogenous targets mentioned here, as discussed in Chapter 32. The influences of any of these neuroactive substances can be prolonged, especially when they are released into the extracellular fluid and/or the cerebrospinal fluid (see Chapter 8). In a number of cases, a single neuroactive substance can exert effects in more than one temporal domain due to its downstream effects, which may include changes in expression of immediate early genes (IEGs). Such actions can lead to increased synthesis of neurotropic factors such as BDNF that can produce long-term changes in network function and even structure. Thus, the actions of neuroactive substances on neuronal networks can result in transient changes (gain or loss) of function as well as exert beneficial or harmful effects on the organism and result in changes in network function that can last indefinitely.

Neuroactive substances include endogenous neurotransmitters, neuromodulators, and exogenously administered pharmacological agents, and these substances can exert significant control over neuronal network function. In addition to their normal "simple" role in neurohumoral transmission, these substances can exert control over a neuronal network and even lead to formation or activation of a network that was not functionally active before the substance was introduced, as seen in ex vivo and in vitro preparations.[25–30] Neuroactive substances can act via network-wide effects even more prominently in large networks operating in vivo (e.g. in neuronal networks controlling sleep or mood) (see Chapters 21, 22, and 24), as discussed in this chapter. Neurons in an invertebrate network that exhibit rhythmic properties in vivo lose this property when the cells are isolated in culture, but rhythmic activity in these isolated neurons could be restored in the presence of a specific neuroactive substance.[31,32] Actions of certain neuroactive substances may be less effectively studied in vitro because of cumulative threshold effects that are only seen with larger networks in vivo. This difference causes the effects of these neuroactive agents to occur at considerably lower concentrations in the intact organism than are required to induce an effect in vitro or ex vivo.[33,34] Endogenous and exogenous neuroactive substances can also exert their actions on emergent properties of neurons in a network nucleus, which is often seen only in intact networks of unanesthetized animals, as discussed in Chapters 28, 30, and 32.

Channelopathies, involving mutations in receptors for neuroactive substances, are known to occur in animal models and human CNS disorders. These channelopathies can alter the sensitivity of the receptors and the response of the organism to neuroactive substances. Such a genetic mutation can be a key event that predisposes individuals to these CNS disorders by altering the normal balance of excitation and inhibition in the networks controlled by this neuroactive substance. Neuroactive substances can also exert major effects on networks through actions on synaptic strength and/or neurogenesis, as discussed in this chapter.

In addition to the effects of neuroactive substances on local synaptic receptors, these agents exert "spillover" effects on nearby synapses and exert actions on extrasynaptic receptors that are involved in sustained low-level activities, such as tonic inhibition[35–39] (see Chapter 8). Neuroactive substances can also exert effects on neuronal networks at a distance via volume transmission carried by the "circulation system" of the brain, that is, diffusion of a neuroactive substance three-dimensionally within extracellular and cerebrospinal fluids of the CNS[40–42] (see Chapter 6). Neuroactive substances exert their effects in different temporal domains with very different time courses. Even those neuroactive substances that initially act within milliseconds can also trigger longer term events mediated by second messengers, IEGs, and neurotropic factors, as discussed in this chapter. The field of neurotransmitters and neuromodulators is vast and extensive and has been the subject of many reviews and monographs. Therefore, this chapter will only briefly consider a few examples of the network-wide effects exerted by these endogenous neuroactive substances.

γ-Aminobutyric Acid

GABA is a major inhibitory neurotransmitter in the brain, and it mediates much of the synaptic inhibition of brain neurons via synaptic and extrasynaptic $GABA_A$, $GABA_B$, and $GABA_C$ receptors. GABAergic projection neurons are also known to play a critical role in the temporal coordination of neuronal activity in distant brain areas.[43] An example of the synaptic effects of GABA is shown in this chapter in the discussion of the effects of GABAergic auditory inputs to the IC, which mediate synaptic inhibition by projections from several different nuclei in the auditory network. Network-wide effects of GABA have also been shown that involve extrasynaptic $GABA_A$ receptors, which mediate tonic inhibition in many brain sites. An example of how GABA extrasynaptically mediated tonic inhibition affecting the olfactory network has been demonstrated on the final output from the olfactory bulb to the piriform cortex by controlling the occurrence of suprathreshold responses during olfactory stimulation.[44] GABA can also produce network-wide inhibition by acting via astrocytic activation of extrasynaptic $GABA_A$ receptors.[45] These network-modifying effects mirror what GABA does during development, when GABAergic interneurons exert major effects on cortical network function, including trophic and neuronal pacing effects as the networks mature.[46] GABA-mediated disruptions in network dynamics are proposed to occur in several CNS disorders, including schizophrenia, epilepsy, and Parkinson's disease, due to alterations of extrasynaptic $GABA_A$ tonic inhibition.[47]

Glutamate

GLU is the major excitatory neurotransmitter in the brain. GLU mediates much of the synaptically driven excitation in brain neurons, acting on the many receptors for this neurotransmitter, including alpha-amino-3-hydroxy-5-methyl-4-isoxazole propionic acid (AMPA), kainate, and *N*-methyl-D-aspartate (NMDA), as well as a variety of metabotropic glutamate (mGLU) receptors. A number of network-wide effects of GLU have been observed. These effects can involve both synaptic and extrasynaptic NMDA receptors that are associated with axonal and glial contacts, as well as spillover effects.[36,37] An example of network-wide effects has been observed in the perigenual anterior cingulate cortex, which is considered part of the default-mode network, as mentioned in this chapter. A combined functional magnetic resonance imaging and magnetic resonance spectroscopy study indicated that the concentration of GLU is directly related to the level of resting-state activity in the same region, but this relationship did not occur in certain other brain networks.[48] Network-wide GLU effects have also been observed in the respiratory network, where it controls the firing of pacemaker neurons in this network. This involves an effect of excitatory transmission mediated by AMPA receptors as well as other neuroactive substance interactions with Ca^{2+}-activated nonspecific cation currents to alter the function of these pacemaker neurons and exert major changes in respiratory network function.[49–52] GLU, acting at NMDA receptors, can also control the locomotor rhythms generated in the central-pattern-generator circuit for locomotion in the spinal cord by exerting major influences on the pacemaker properties of the neurons in this network (see Chapter 17).[53] mGLU receptors are also reported to modulate excitatory transmission within a specific region of the hippocampus and contribute importantly to the strength and timing of network activity within this region.[54]

5-Hydroxytryptamine

5-HT, also known as serotonin, is a major neurotransmitter in the brain. 5-HT acts on over a dozen different receptor subtypes, is involved in the network that controls sleep states (see Chapters 21 and 22), and makes important contributions to neuronal networks that mediate emotional states (e.g. depression). 5-HT exerts major actions emanating from a central set of brainstem nuclei, the raphe nuclei in the pons and midbrain, which project widely throughout much of the brain. The diffuse distribution of 5-HT projections from the raphe nuclei in the pons and midbrain to a wide variety of sites provides a rich substrate for the network-wide effects of 5-HT that have been observed in networks that control respiration, sleep, epilepsy, and mood.[55] Thus, a function of 5-HT neurons in the respiratory network involves the detection of changes in pH and CO_2 and control of ventilation due to the critical role of 5-HT in the excitatory drive to this network (see Chapter 18).[19] 5-HT also plays a major role in control of state transitions in the sleep cycle in concord with several other neuroactive substances[56–58] (Chapters 21 and 22). It has been proposed that the organization of the sleep-waking cycle is an emergent property of forebrain and brainstem local neuronal networks, involving 5-HT as a major neuroactive substance that causes the brain to undergo state transitions; failure of this organization leads to several different sleep pathologies[59,60] (Chapter 22). Networks involved in mood and anxiety disorders are widely studied (see Chapter 24), and 5-HT dysfunction plays an important role in control of these networks. Drugs that enhance 5-HT receptor activation have important therapeutic roles in the treatment of these disorders as well as epilepsy-related disorders[61,62] (see Chapter 29).

Adenosine

Adenosine is an important neuromodulator that is produced metabolically and plays a key role in astrocytic networks of the brain. Adenosine is a purine, which has been identified as a transmitter or co-transmitter in many peripheral and CNS sites, and it plays a major role in glial function and neuronglial interactions[63] (Chapter 12). Endogenous extracellular adenosine is generated by the metabolic breakdown of adenosine triphosphate and is proposed to set a global inhibitory tone in brain networks via volume transmission[64] (Chapter 8). Adenosine in the brain exerts its action by activating G-protein coupled receptors, including A1, $A2_A$, $A2_B$, and A3 receptor subtypes. A1R and A3R inhibit, whereas $A2_AR$ and $A2_BR$ stimulate, production of the second messenger, cyclic adenosine monophosphate (cAMP). A1R and $A2_AR$ are activated by nanomolar concentrations of adenosine, whereas $A2_BR$ and A3R become activated only when adenosine levels rise into the micromolar range during inflammation, hypoxia, ischemia, or seizures.[65] Adenosine is able to modulate excitatory transmission through the activation of widespread inhibitory A1 receptors and synaptically located $A2_A$ receptors. It is proposed that high-frequency firing in a network induces widespread A1 receptor–mediated inhibition in the network along with the local synaptic activation of $A2_A$ receptors.[64] There are differential distributions of adenosine levels, metabolic enzyme activity, receptors, and transporters, depending on brain region, age, and gender.[66] Astrocytic networks exist in many brain regions and are uniquely connected together and to neurons, allowing them to exert network-wide effects (Chapter 12). Astrocytic networks are also an important interface between the brain's blood vessels and neurons, and these glial networks function to integrate within and among CNS neuronal networks. This integrative role is mediated by release of neuroactive substances, among which adenosine is critically important.[67] It has been proposed that these astrocytic networks play a role in the detection of changes in chemical or physical properties of both brain microcirculation and neuropil and transmission of this information to the neuronal networks that control vital behaviors, including chemosensory control of respiration.[67] Astrocytic networks have been implicated in mechanisms governing perception and learning.

These actions involve their role as local hubs that integrate information from neuronal and glial networks as well as integrating the action of several brain networks to exert a major controlling influence on global states of consciousness.[68] Thus, adenosine and related nucleosides are also proposed to participate in the regulation of sleep, cognition, memory, and nociception, and the control of seizure susceptibility (see Chapter 29). Adenosine is also suggested to play a role in the pathophysiology of neurodegenerative and neuropsychiatric diseases.[66] Adenosine is also proposed to act in concert with cytokines, such as TNF-α, and interleukin-1β, in exerting network-wide control of brain states, including sleep states and chronic pain syndromes, by altering neuronal and glial transmission.[59]

CYTOKINE INVOLVEMENT IN NETWORK CONTROL

As noted in this chapter, network-wide function is also affected by the actions of cytokines, such as TNF-α. These cytokines are most abundant in pathological CNS states, such as stroke.[69,70] Neurodegeneration and neurotoxicity induce inflammatory responses and activate microglia, which release potentially cytotoxic substances, including cytokines.[71] Cytokine increases in the brain, associated with the activation of microglia, have been proposed to be a mediator of normal fatigue because of effects on structures in the arousal, sleep, and circadian networks.[72] Cytokines in the healthy brain can also have other important roles in controlling synaptic transmission and plasticity, including control of AMPA receptor trafficking and GLU release from astrocytes.[73–75]

SYNAPTIC STRENGTH CHANGES, SYNAPTOGENESIS, AND NEUROGENESIS

As a result of activating their receptors, endogenous neuroactive substances can lead to altered expression of IEGs, especially if receptor activation is sustained or repetitive. This occurs with neuroactive substances that act via ionotropic or metabotropic receptors. Thus, for example, glutamatergic activation of ionotropic NMDA receptors can activate several IEGs, including c-fos and c-jun.[76,77] Likewise, 5-HT acting at specific metabotropic 5-HT receptor subtypes activates c-fos and tis1, among other IEGs, and these effects vary, depending on the brain area studied.[78]

Repetitive activation of NMDA receptors can lead to long-term synaptic plasticity changes in brain networks, including long-term potentiation (LTP) (see Chapter 27). The early phase of LTP is mediated, in part, by activation of kinases, including calcium-calmodulin-dependent

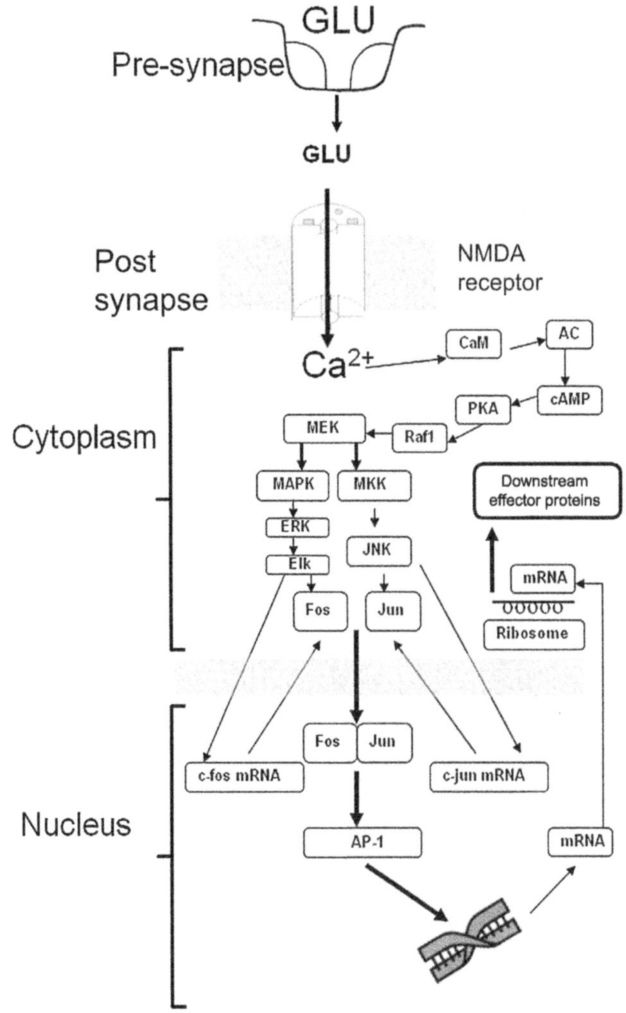

FIGURE 7.3 Diagram depicting putative processes and targets for affecting changes in synaptic strength. Binding of glutamate (GLU) to the *N*-methyl-D-aspartate (NMDA) receptor mediates increases in intracellular Ca^{2+} that can lead to changes in synaptic function via calmodulin (CaM), which activates adenylyl cyclase (AC), leading to increased synthesis of cyclic adenosine monophosphate (cAMP), which then activates protein kinase A (PKA), which activates Raf1, leading to phosphorylation of mitogen-activated protein–extracellular signal-regulated kinase (MEK) and mitogen-activated protein kinase (MKK). MKK activates jun N-terminal kinase (JNK), leading to Jun activation. MEK also activates mitogen-activated protein kinase (MAPK) by phosphorylation, and MKK activates ERK, leading to activation of Elk that activates Fos. Fos and Jun combine in a key process in the intracellular pathways cascade, leading to activation of the activator protein 1 (AP-1) transcription factor. The resulting increase in AP-1 activity increases the transcription of target genes to increase mRNA. This can lead to increased translation of downstream effector proteins and finally synaptic remodeling (increases in synaptic strength, changes in dendritic spines, synaptogenesis, and/or axonal sprouting), which can mediate long-term structural changes in the brain, including neurogenesis (based, in part, on Refs 79–81). (For color version of this figure, the reader is referred to the online version of this book.)

kinase II (CAMKII), protein kinase C, and mitogen-activated protein kinase (MAPK) (Figure 7.3). This results in molecular changes, while the late phase of LTP is associated with protein synthesis, including synthesis of IEGs such as c-fos, which can lead to increases in BDNF and structural changes.[82] Increased IEG expression leads to activation of the intracellular cascades that result in activation of cAMP-response element-binding protein (CREB) via MAPK signaling to the nucleus.[76] These events can lead to changes in synaptic strength, dendritic spines, synaptogenesis, axonal sprouting, and neurogenesis, which result in major changes in network function and even structure.

As noted in this chapter, synaptic strength is an important phenomenon in the control of the function of neuronal networks. There are many mechanisms involved in altering synaptic strength. Changes in synaptic plasticity can occur over a broad range of time from milliseconds for short-term plasticity to months-years for long-term plasticity, depending on these mechanisms. Short-term plasticity dynamically alters the strength of synaptic events in response to periods of repeated activity that occur during the normal functioning of neurons. Enhancement or depression of transmission across the synapses involved can lead to regulation of synaptic strength due to the action of neuroactive substances and plays a role in information processing by the network.[83] Long-term plastic events involve processes such as LTP and long-term depression, as discussed here.

NEUROTROPIC FACTORS

Synaptogenesis is a key process involved in the original formation of neuronal networks during development, but these mature synaptic relationships remain potentially subject to a variable degree of plasticity due to experience with either beneficial or harmful consequences, as noted in this chapter.[84] Thus, changes in synaptic morphology, strength, and synaptic partner choice are hypothesized to be involved in plasticity in neuronal networks.[85] Neuronal activity can regulate neuronal circuits through activity-regulated genes and their downstream effectors, including BDNF. Thus, activity-dependent transcription of BDNF is proposed to promote the development of GABAergic synapses in the cortex.[86] BDNF also plays a role in the enhanced adaptability of mood networks (see Chapter 24) when treated with antidepressants, which is proposed to involve neurogenesis and synaptic plasticity.[87] Synaptic strength is proposed to be determined, in part, by postsynaptic influx of Ca^{2+}, leading to changes in dendritic spine size,[88] and, if these changes are sustained, this can result in long-term synaptic plasticity.[89] "Weak" synapses, such as those found in "conditional multireceptive" brain regions (see Chapter 28), can undergo a much greater degree of increase than synapses that are more stable, such as those seen in primary sensory and motor networks.[90]

AXONAL SPROUTING

Axonal sprouting is a key process during development, but it can also occur in mature animals. Axonal sprouting was observed in the rat hippocampus in a spatial learning paradigm, and in the visual cortex during recovery from retinal lesions[91,92] (see Chapter 16). Maladaptive axonal sprouting is also seen in neuronal network remodeling in many epilepsy models[93] (see Chapter 27). A single neuroactive substance, such as serotonin, can exert both short- and long-term plastic effects initially by acting synaptically and subsequently lead to changes in IEGs and BDNF. The effect of these factors can lead to significant alterations of synaptic strength and network architecture.[94] Thus, effects of neuroactive substances on networks can result in transient changes (gain or loss) of function as well as exert beneficial or harmful effects for the individual that can result in changes in network function that last indefinitely. An example that results in increases in synaptic strength is the phenomenon of fear conditioning discussed in this chapter[18] (see also Chapter 13).

As mentioned in the "Multiple Inputs" section, the AGS kindling paradigm involves periodic repetition of AGS in rodents that are susceptible to these seizures, which expands the neuronal network that mediates these convulsive behaviors (see Chapter 27). In one audiogenic seizure model (GEPR-9s), the requisite neuronal network resides exclusively in the brainstem[95] (see Chapter 26). AGS kindling results in expansion of the network to the forebrain, including the MGB and amygdala, and this pathway is also implicated in fear conditioning, as noted here.[18] A significant increase in synaptic strength in the MGB-to-amygdala pathway, as indicated by elevated responsiveness of lateral amygdala neurons to electrical stimuli in the MGB, occurs in AGS-kindled animals.[96] GLU released by MGB neurons, acting at NMDA receptors on lateral amygdala neurons, appears to be the proximate cause for these events. Evidence for this includes the effect of focal microinjection of NMDA into the amygdala of the animals (prior to AGS kindling), which will temporarily mimic the overt behavioral change induced by AGS kindling.[97] If the molecular cascade triggered by the activation of the NMDA receptors is activated by enhancing the cAMP step by microinjection into the amygdala of a forskolin derivative in an animal prior to AGS kindling, this also mimics the behavioral effects of AGS kindling. However, this is a long-term rather than short-term effect.[98] The effect of AGS kindling can also be reversed by focal microinjection of an antagonist of cAMP.[99] This example illustrates the steps in the process outlined in this chapter. Thus, AGS kindling causes MGB neurons to show long-lasting increases in firing, including burst firing, a major network-synchronizing mechanism (Chapter 9) that provides intensified input to the lateral amygdala.[100] This increased MGB input leads to repetitive activation of NMDA receptors in the amygdala, which triggers a molecular cascade, such as in the scheme illustrated in Figure 7.3. Thus, as noted here, NMDA receptors are known to activate c-fos, which can trigger the cascade that leads to cAMP activation. This cascade can lead to long-lasting increases in synaptic strength due to changes in gene expression, as illustrated in Figure 7.3, resulting in a permanent change in this brain network. NMDA receptors can also trigger cascades that involve mTOR (mammalian target of rapamycin) that lead to long-lasting network changes (see Chapter 15).

NEUROGENESIS

Neuroactive substances can exert profound effects on networks in the mature brain through actions on neurogenesis (see Chapter 15). G-protein coupled receptors are implicated in adult neurogenesis since they are expressed in adult neural stem cells and their progenitors.[101] Adult neurogenesis has been suggested to play a major role in the self-repair of neuronal networks in neuropathologic conditions, as well as in the action of certain exogenous neuroactive substances.[102] Neurogenesis has also been seen with 5-HT in a drug-induced epilepsy network.[103] Thus, neuronal networks have the potential to undergo major functional changes due to influences that lead to alterations of synaptic strength. These changes include dendritic spine changes, synaptogenesis, axonal sprouting, and neurogenesis, which can exert positive or negative effects on the physiological function of the networks as well as on the neuronal network pathology involved in CNS disorders.

CONCLUSIONS

Control of neuronal network function involves many different elements (see Chapter 1). The role of each nucleus in the network is affected by its cellular inputs, the neuroactive substances released by these inputs, and the synaptic changes that can result from the repetitive release of these substances. The principal neurons in a network nucleus are the key elements in network function, but their intrinsic activity is largely altered by the cellular inputs from projection neurons, local interneurons, and glial elements that greatly modify and organize the output of these principal cells. In addition to the normal synaptic role played by neuroactive substances, network-wide actions have also been observed, many of which involve volume transmission of these agents via the extracellular and cerebrospinal fluid (see Chapter 8). Repetitive actions of these substances can lead to major changes in network function through changes in synaptic strength, dendritic spine changes, axonal sprouting, synaptogenesis, and neurogenesis. A complex integration of all of these network control elements and the other control mechanisms, discussed in other chapters of this book, determines the output of a given network nucleus within the hierarchy of the network. This process determines the dynamic function of the network and whether it operates normally or pathologically in CNS disorders. Knowledge of normal and pathological network function will potentially lead to the development of network-based approaches to improve the therapy of these disorders.

Acknowledgments

The authors acknowledge the input and advice of Drs. Ronald Browning and Vickram Ramkumar on this chapter. The authors gratefully acknowledge the manuscript assistance of Gayle Stauffer and Diana Smith in preparing this manuscript.

References

1. Quill U, Worgotter F. Investigations on emergent spatio-temporal neural response characteristics in a small network model. *Biol Cybern*. 2000;83(5):461–470.
2. Li Y, Evans MS, Faingold CL. In vitro electrophysiology of neurons in subnuclei of rat inferior colliculus. *Hear Res*. 1998; 121(1–2):1–10.
3. Tupal S, Faingold CL. The amygdala to periaqueductal gray pathway: plastic changes induced by audiogenic kindling and reversal by gabapentin. *Brain Res*. 2012;1475:71–79.
4. Feng HJ, Faingold CL. Repeated generalized audiogenic seizures induce plastic changes on acoustically evoked neuronal firing in the amygdala. *Brain Res*. 2002;932(1–2):61–69.
5. Rebesco JM, Stevenson IH, Körding KP, Solla SA, Miller LE. Rewiring neural interactions by micro-stimulation. *Front Syst Neurosci*. 2010;4. Article 39:1–15.
6. Davis M, Antoniadis EA, Amaral DG, Winslow JT. Acoustic startle reflex in rhesus monkeys: a review. *Rev Neurosci*. 2008;19(2–3):171–185.
7. Sivaramakrishnan S, Oliver DL. Neuronal responses to lemniscal stimulation in laminar brain slices of the inferior colliculus. *J Assoc Res Otolaryngol*. 2006;7(1):1–14.
8. Faingold CL, Hoffmann WE, Caspary DM. Effects of excitant amino acids on acoustic responses of inferior colliculus neurons. *Hear Res*. 1989;40(1–2):127–136.
9. Kelly JB, Zhang H. Contribution of AMPA and NMDA receptors to excitatory responses in the inferior colliculus. *Hear Res*. 2002;168(1–2):35–42.
10. Mayko ZM, Roberts PD, Portfors CV. Inhibition shapes selectivity to vocalizations in the inferior colliculus of awake mice. *Front Neural Circuits*. 2012;6:73.
11. Faingold CL, Anderson CA, Randall ME. Stimulation or blockade of the dorsal nucleus of the lateral lemniscus alters binaural and tonic inhibition in contralateral inferior colliculus neurons. *Hear Res*. 1993;69(1–2):98–106.

12. Loftus WC, Bishop DC, Oliver DL. Differential patterns of inputs create functional zones in central nucleus of inferior colliculus. *J Neurosci.* 2010;30(40):13396–13408.
13. Kulesza Jr RJ, Spirou GA, Berrebi AS. Physiological response properties of neurons in the superior paraolivary nucleus of the rat. *J Neurophysiol.* 2003;89(4):2299–2312.
14. Saldaña E, Aparicio MA, Fuentes-Santamaría V, Berrebi AS. Connections of the superior paraolivary nucleus of the rat: projections to the inferior colliculus. *Neuroscience.* 2009;163(1):372–387.
15. Faingold CL. Role of GABA abnormalities in the inferior colliculus pathophysiology – audiogenic seizures. *Hear Res.* 2002; 168(1–2):223–237.
16. Paxinos G, Watson C. *The Rat Brain in Stereotaxic Coordinates.* Sydney: Elsevier Academic Press; 2005.
17. Ohshiro T, Angelaki DE, DeAngelis GC. A normalization model of multisensory integration. *Nat Neurosci.* 2011;14(6):775–782.
18. Johansen JP, Cain CK, Ostroff LE, Ledoux JE. Molecular mechanisms of fear learning and memory. *Cell.* 2011;147(3):509–524.
19. Hodges MR, Richerson GB. The role of medullary serotonin (5-HT) neurons in respiratory control: contributions to eupneic ventilation, CO_2 chemoreception, and thermoregulation. *J Appl Physiol.* 2010;108(5):1425–1432.
20. Kyriakatos A, Mahmood R, Ausborn J, Porres CP, Buschges A, El Manira A. Initiation of locomotion in adult zebrafish. *J Neurosci.* 2011;31(23):8422–8431.
21. Kasanetz F, Riquelme LA, O'Donnell P, Murer MG. Turning off cortical ensembles stops striatal Up states and elicits phase perturbations in cortical and striatal slow oscillations in rat in vivo. *J Physiol.* 2006;577(Pt 1):97–113.
22. Ross B, Herdman AT, Pantev C. Stimulus induced desynchronization of human auditory 40-Hz steady-state responses. *J Neurophysiol.* 2005;94(6):4082–4093.
23. Raichle ME, Snyder AZ. A default mode of brain function: a brief history of an evolving idea. *Neuroimage.* 2007;37(4):1083–1090.
24. Northoff G, Qin P, Nakao T. Rest-stimulus interaction in the brain: a review. *Trends Neurosci.* 2010;33(6):277–284.
25. Brezina V. Beyond the wiring diagram: signaling through complex neuromodulator networks. *Philos Trans R Soc Lond B Biol Sci.* 2010;365(1551):2363–2374.
26. Brezina V, Weiss KR. Analyzing the functional consequences of transmitter complexity. *Trends Neurosci.* 1997;20(11):538–543.
27. Fellous JM, Linster C. Computational models of neuromodulation. *Neural Comput.* 1998;10(4):771–805.
28. Marder E. Neuromodulation of neuronal circuits: back to the future. *Neuron.* 2012;76(1):1–11.
29. Whittington MA, Traub RD, Kopell N, Ermentrout B, Buhl EH. Inhibition-based rhythms: experimental and mathematical observations on network dynamics. *Int J Psychophysiol.* 2000;38(3): 315–336.
30. Wu JS, Vilim FS, Hatcher NG, et al. Composite modulatory feed forward loop contributes to the establishment of a network state. *J Neurophysiol.* 2010;103:2174–2184.
31. Selverston AI. Invertebrate central pattern generator circuits. *Philos Trans R Soc Lond B Biol Sci.* 2010;365(1551):2329–2345.
32. Straub VA, Staras K, Kemenes G, Benjamin PR. Endogenous and network properties of lymnaea feeding central pattern generator interneurons. *J Neurophysiol.* 2005;88:1569–1583.
33. Narahashi T. Chemical modulation of sodium channels and $GABA_A$ receptor channel. *Adv Neurol.* 1999;79:457–480.
34. Song JH, Narahashi T. Modulation of sodium channels of rat cerebellar Purkinje neurons by the pyrethroid tetramethrin. *J Pharmacol Exp Ther.* 1996;277(1):445–453.
35. Bright DP, Renzi M, Bartram J, et al. Profound desensitization by ambient GABA limits activation of delta-containing $GABA_A$ receptors during spillover. *J Neurosci.* 2011;31(2):753–763.
36. Okubo Y, Lino M. Visualization of glutamate as a volume transmitter. *J Physiol.* 2011;589(Pt 3):481–488.
37. Petralia RS. Distribution of extrasynaptic NMDA receptors on neurons. *Scientific World Journal.* 2012;2012:267120.
38. Stanchev D, Sargent PB. α7-containing and non-α7-containing nicotinic receptors respond differently to spillover of acetylcholine. *J Neurosci.* 2011;31(42):14920–14930.
39. Tang ZQ, Lu Y. Two $GABA_A$ responses with distinct kinetics in a sound localization circuit. *J Physiol.* 2012;590(Pt 16): 3787–3805.
40. Agnati LF, Fuxe K. Volume transmission as a key feature of information handling in the central nervous system possible new interpretative value of the Turing's B-type machine. *Prog Brain Res.* 2000;125:3–19.
41. Agnati LF, Zoli M, Stromberg I, Fuxe K. Intercellular communication in the brain: wiring versus volume transmission. *Neuroscience.* 1995;69(3):711–726.
42. Bach-y-Rita P, Aiello GL. Nerve length and volume in synaptic vs diffusion neurotransmission: a model. *Neuroreport.* 1996;7(9): 1502–1504.
43. Caputi A, Melzer S, Michael M, Monyer H. The long and short of GABAergic neurons. *Curr Opin Neurobiol.* 2013;23(2):179–186.
44. Labarrera C, London M, Angelo K. Tonic inhibition sets the state of excitability in olfactory bulb granule cells. *J Physiol.* 2013; 591(Pt 7):1841–1850.
45. Héja L, Nyitrai G, Kékesi O, et al. Astrocytes convert network excitation to tonic inhibition of neurons. *BMC Biol.* 2012;10:26.
46. Le Magueresse C, Monyer H. GABAergic interneurons shape the functional maturation of the cortex. *Neuron.* 2013;77(3): 388–405.
47. Brickly G, Mody I. Extrasynaptic $GABA_A$ receptors: their function in the CNS and implications for disease. *Neuron.* 2012;73(1): 23–34.
48. Enzi B, Duncan NW, Kaufmann J, Tempelmann C, Wiebking C, Northoff G. Glutamate modulates resting state activity in the perigenual anterior cingulate cortex – a combined fMRI–MRS study. *Neuroscience.* 2012;227C:102–109.
49. Mironov S. Respiratory circuits: function, mechanisms, topology, and pathology. *Neuroscientist.* 2009;15(2):194–208.
50. Mutolo D, Bongianni F, Cinelli E, Pantaleo T. Role of neurokinin receptors and ionic mechanisms within the respiratory network of the lamprey. *Neuroscience.* 2010;169(3):1136–1149.
51. Pace RW, Del Negro CA. AMPA and metabotropic glutamate receptors cooperatively generate inspiratory-like depolarization in mouse respiratory neurons in vitro. *Eur J Neurosci.* 2008;28(12): 2434–2442.
52. Viemari JC, Ramirez JM. Norepinephrine differentially modulates different types of respiratory pacemaker and nonpacemaker neurons. *J Neurophysiol.* 2006;95(4):2070–2082.
53. Li WC. Generation of locomotion rhythms without inhibition in vertebrates: the search for pacemaker neurons. *Integr Comp Biol.* 2011;51:879–889.
54. Cosgrove KE, Galván EJ, Barrionuevo G, Meriney SD. mGluRs modulate strength and timing of excitatory transmission in hippocampal area CA3. *Mol Neurobiol.* 2011;44(1):93–101.
55. Richerson GB, Buchanan GF. The serotonin axis: shared mechanisms in seizures, depression, and SUDEP. *Epilepsia.* 2011; 52(Suppl 1):28–38.
56. Espana RA, Scammell TE. Sleep neurobiology from a clinical perspective. *Sleep.* 2011;34(7):845–858.
57. Monti JM. Serotonin control of sleep-wake behavior. *Sleep Med Rev.* 2011;15(4):269–281.
58. Saper CB, Chou TC, Scammell TE. The sleep switch: hypothalamic control of sleep and wakefulness. *Trends Neurosci.* 2001; 24(12):726–731.

59. Clinton JM, Davis CJ, Zielinski MR, Jewett KA, Krueger JM. Biochemical regulation of sleep and sleep biomarkers. *J Clin Sleep Med.* 2011;7(Suppl 5):S38–S42.
60. Vetrugno R, Montagna P. From REM sleep behaviour disorder to status dissociatus: insights into the maze of states of being. *Sleep Med.* 2011;12(Suppl. 2):S68–S71.
61. Dominguez-Lopez S, Howell R, Gobbi G. Characterization of serotonin neurotransmission in knockout mice: implications for major depression. *Rev Neurosci.* 2012;23(4):429–443.
62. Hale MW, Shekhar A, Lowry CA. Stress-related serotonergic systems: implications for symptomatology of anxiety and affective disorders. *Cell Mol Neurobiol.* 2012;32(5):695–708.
63. Burnstock G. Introduction to purinergic signaling in the brain. *Adv Exp Med Biol.* 2013;986:1–12.
64. Cunha RA. Different cellular sources and different roles of adenosine: A_1 receptor-mediated inhibition through astrocytic-driven volume transmission and synapse-restricted A_{2A} receptor-mediated facilitation of plasticity. *Neurochem Int.* 2008;52(1–2): 65–72.
65. Paul S, Elsinga PH, Ishiwata K, Dierckx RA, van Waarde A. Adenosine A_1 receptors in the central nervous system: their functions in health and disease, and possible elucidation by PET imaging. *Curr Med Chem.* 2011;18(31):4820–4835.
66. Kovács Z, Juhász G, Palkovits M, Dobolyi A, Kékesi KA. Area, age and gender dependence of the nucleoside system in the brain: a review of current literature. *Curr Top Med Chem.* 2011;11(8):1012–1033.
67. Gourine AV, Kasparov S. Astrocytes as brain interoceptors. *Exp Physiol.* 2011;96(4):411–416.
68. Pereira Jr A, Furlan FA. Astrocytes and human cognition: modeling information integration and modulation of neuronal activity. *Prog Neurobiol.* 2010;92(3):405–420.
69. Tobinick E, Kim M, Rezin G, Rodriguez-Romanacce H, DePuy V. Selective TNF inhibition for chronic stroke and traumatic brain injury: an observational study involving 629 consecutive patients treated with perispinal etanercept. *CNS Drugs.* 2012;26(12): 1051–1070.
70. Wang L, Lu Y, Guan H, et al. Tumor necrosis factor receptor-associated factor 5 is an essential mediator of ischemic brain infarction. *J Neurochem*; Feb 16, 2013. (Epub ahead of print).
71. Kraft AD, Harry GJ. Features of microglia and neuroinflammation relevant to environmental exposure and neurotoxicity. *Int J Environ Res Public Health.* 2011;8(7):2980–3018.
72. Harrington ME. Neurobiological studies of fatigue. *Prog Neurobiol.* 2012;99(2):93–105.
73. Boulanger LM. Immune proteins in brain development and synaptic plasticity. *Neuron.* 2009;64:93–109.
74. Pickering M, Cumiskey D, O'Connor JJ. Actions of TNF-alpha on glutamatergic synaptic transmission in the central nervous system. *Exp Physiol.* 2005;90(5):663–670.
75. Santello M, Volterra A. TNF-alpha in synaptic function: switching gears. *Trends Neurosci.* 2012;35(10):638–647.
76. Platenik J, Kuramoto N, Yoneda Y. Molecular mechanisms associated with long-term consolidation of the NMDA signals. *Life Sci.* 2000;67(4):335–364.
77. Shan Y, Carlock LR, Walker PD. NMDA receptor overstimulation triggers a prolonged wave of immediate early gene expression: relationship to excitotoxicity. *Exp Neurol.* 1997;144(2):406–415.
78. Tilakaratne N, Friedman E. Genomic responses to 5-HT_{1A} or $5\text{-HT}_{2A/2C}$ receptor activation is differentially regulated in four regions of rat brain. *Eur J Pharmacol.* 1996;307(2):211–217.
79. Clayton DF. The genomic action potential. *Neurobiol Learn Mem.* 2000;74(3):185–216.
80. Meng Q, Xia Y. c-Jun, at the crossroad of the signaling network. *Protein Cell.* 2011;2(11):889–898.
81. Waltereit R, Weller M. Signaling from cAMP/PKA to MAPK and synaptic plasticity. *Mol Neurobiol.* 2003;27(1):99–106.
82. Steward O, Huang F, Guzowski JF. A form of perforant path LTP can occur without ERK1/2 phosphorylation or immediate early gene induction. *Learn Mem.* 2007;14(6):433–445.
83. Klug A, Borst JG, Carlson BA, Kopp-Scheinpflug C, Klyachko VA, Xu-Friedman MA. How do short-term changes at synapses fine-tune information processing? *J Neurosci.* 2012;32(41):14058–14063.
84. Margeta MA, Shen K. Molecular mechanisms of synaptic specificity. *Mol Cell Neurosci.* 2010;43(3):261–267.
85. Procko C, Shaham S. Synaptogenesis: new roles for an old player. *Curr Biol.* 2009;19(24):R1114–R1115.
86. Lu B, Wang KH, Nose A. Molecular mechanisms underlying neural circuit formation. *Curr Opin Neurobiol.* 2009;19(2):162–167.
87. Castren E, Hen R. Neuronal plasticity and antidepressant actions. *Trends Neurosci.* 2013;36(5):259–267.
88. Okabe S. Molecular dynamics of the excitatory synapse. *Adv Exp Med Biol.* 2012;970:131–152.
89. O'Donnell C, Nolan III MF, van Rossum MC. Dendritic spine dynamics regulate the long-term stability of synaptic plasticity. *J Neurosci.* 2011;31(45):16142–16156.
90. Yasumatsu N, Matsuzaki M, Miyazaki T, Noguchi J, Kasai H. Principles of long-term dynamics of dendritic spines. *J Neurosci.* 2008;28:13592–13608.
91. Chen J, Yamahachi H, Gilbert CD. Experience-dependent gene expression in adult visual cortex. *Cereb Cortex.* 2010;20(3):650–660.
92. Su B, Pan S, He X, Li P, Liang Y. Sprouting of nervous fibers and upregulation of C-X-C chemokine receptor type 4 expression in hippocampal formation of rats with enhanced spatial learning and memory. *Anat Rec (Hoboken).* 2012;295(1):121–126.
93. Dudek FE, Sutula TP. Epileptogenesis in the dentate gyrus: a critical perspective. *Prog Brain Res.* 2007;163:755–773.
94. Neto FL, Borges G, Torres-Sanchez S, Mico JA, Berrocoso E. Neurotrophins role in depression neurobiology: a review of basic and clinical evidence. *Curr Neuropharmacol.* 2011;9(4):530–552.
95. Faingold CL. Brainstem networks: reticulo-cortical synchronization in generalized convulsive seizures. In: Noebels JL, Avoli M, Rogawski MA, Olsen RW, Delgado-Escueta AV, eds. *Jasper's Basic Mechanisms of the Epilepsies.* 4th ed. New York, NY: Oxford University Press; 2012:257–271.
96. Feng HJ, Faingold CL. Synaptic plasticity in the pathway from the medial geniculate body to the lateral amygdala is induced by seizure repetition. *Brain Res.* 2002;946(2):198–205.
97. Raisinghani M, Feng HJ, Faingold CL. Glutamatergic activation of the amygdala differentially mimics the effects of audiogenic seizure kindling in two substrains of genetically epilepsy-prone rats. *Exp Neurol.* 2003;183(2):516–522.
98. Tupal S, Faingold CL. Precipitous induction of audiogenic kindling by activation of adenylyl cyclase in the amygdala. *Epilepsia.* 2010;51(3):354–361.
99. Tupal S, Faingold C. Inhibition of adenylyl cyclase in amygdala blocks the effect of audiogenic seizure kindling in genetically epilepsy-prone rats. *Neuropharmacology.* 2010;59(1–2):107–111.
100. N'Gouemo P, Faingold CL. Audiogenic kindling increases neuronal responses to acoustic stimuli in neurons of the medial geniculate body of the genetically epilepsy-prone rat. *Brain Res.* 1997;761(2):217–224.
101. Doze VA, Perez DM. G-protein-coupled receptors in adult neurogenesis. *Pharmacol Rev.* 2012;64(3):645–675.
102. Surget A, Tanti A, Leonardo ED, et al. Antidepressants recruit new neurons to improve stress response regulation. *Mol Psychiatry.* 2011;16(12):1177–1188.
103. Radley JJ, Jacobs BL. Pilocarpine-induced status epilepticus increases cell proliferation in the dentate gyrus of adult rats via a 5-HT_{1A} receptor-dependent mechanism. *Brain Res.* 2003;966(1):1–12.

CHAPTER

8

Volume Transmission and the Russian-Doll Organization of Brain Cell Networks: Aspects of Their Integrative Actions

Luigi Francesco Agnati[1], *Susanna Genedani*[2], *PierFranco Spano*[1,3], *Diego Guidolin*[4], *Kjell Fuxe*[5]

[1]Fondazione IRCCS San Camillo, Venezia Lido, Venice, Italy, [2]Department of Biomedical Sciences, University of Modena and Reggio Emilia, Modena, Italy, [3]Department of Biomedical Sciences and Biotechnology, University of Brescia, Brescia, Italy, [4]Department of Molecular Medicine, University of Padova, Padova, Italy, [5]Department of Neuroscience, Karolinska Institutet, Stockholm, Sweden

GENERAL PREMISES

Some concepts deduced from studies on evolution (e.g. of the various apparatuses in mammals) can also be applied for the most complex human organ: the central nervous system (CNS). In particular, the exaptation concept[1] and the Russian-doll organization concept of living beings[2] will be used.

Let us briefly introduce these concepts:

- Exaptation: With regard to their roles in evolution, a subtle but important distinction should be made between "adaptation" and "exaptation". While adaptation refers to a feature produced by natural selection for its current function (e.g. echolocation in bats), exaptation has been defined as a feature that performs a function but was not produced by natural selection for its current use (e.g. feathers that might have originally arisen in the context of selection for insulation; see e.g. Ref. 3). Thus, exaptation indicates a feature that performs a function that was not developed for its current use by natural selection, although natural selection may subsequently operate upon such a new function. Related to this concept and focused on the brain function is Anderson's concept of redeployment (or reuse) of a neural structure for a new function.[4,5] There are obvious evolutionary advantages to the redeployment of brain areas, and Anderson analyzes this phenomenon in relation to cognition. In this chapter, the concept is also applied at the network level, considering different time courses besides the evolutionary time scale (see this chapter's discussion on "polymorphic networks").
- According to Jacob,[2] from a structural standpoint, the living organism is organized as a complex of "Russian Matryoshka Dolls". According to this concept, smaller structures are contained within larger ones in multiple layers. Our group has proposed that computational elements of the CNS are organized according to a "nested" hierarchic criterion.[6–9] It should be noted that the hierarchic organization and the identity of the elements at each level are interconnected to carry out a computational task (i.e. the "building of the Russian doll"). This organization is not permanent, but the complex computational system is organized as the need arises and can change dynamically from moment to moment.[10]

These concepts are utilized to propose a new model of the cellular networks in the brain and to explore their integrative actions.

INTRODUCTION

In the outstanding contributions of Cajal and Sherrington,[11,12] which are still largely accepted, the schematic representation of neuronal networks in the

Neuronal Networks in Brain Function, CNS Disorders, and Therapeutics
http://dx.doi.org/10.1016/B978-0-12-415804-7.00008-3

CNS is as a collection of neurons connected via regions of discontinuity, the so-called synaptic gap.[13]

After a century, this model is still useful in most instances, but it should be pointed out that it is basically an oversimplification.[14–16] The extraordinary intuition of Cajal and Sherrington (preceded by Tanzi[17]) that there is a crucial region of structural and functional discontinuity, the synapse, where complex integrative actions (leading e.g. to learning[11,12,17]) could occur is well established and is still an incessant source of new information.

However, in the last three decades, our group as well as other groups[14,18] have provided new data on the communication modes in the CNS that, while not dismissing the fundamental relevance of synaptic contacts, have broadened the field. Furthermore, a modern model of the organization of cellular networks in the CNS[6,19–23] has been proposed by suggesting that cellular networks should be viewed not in a two-dimensional frame but rather in a three-dimensional space in which all the resident cells contained in a brain region together with microvessels and the extracellular matrix (ECM) that fills the extracellular space (ECS) should be considered as participants in the function of a network.

To deal with such a complex set of elements and communication modes involved in information handling by the CNS, the following concepts have been introduced:

1. Complex cellular networks (CCNs; see Ref. 24) are formed by neurons, glial cells, endothelial cells, pericytes, mast cells, and ECM that, by interacting with each other within a certain brain volume, give each other a trophic reciprocal support forming plastic trophic units (TUs; see Ref. 25). These elements also produce information that participates in the integrative actions of the brain (see the "functional module" list item here). It should be noted that the concept of TUs has similarities and differences with the concept of neurovascular units (NVUs), which has been defined as the result of *interactions between circulating blood elements and the blood vessel wall, ECM, glia, and neurons.*[26] The main difference is that interactions at the TU level are considered more on the brain side than NVUs, which are more on the blood side.[27] It has been suggested that alterations in the proper functions of NVUs may be the initiating trigger not only for vascular dementias but also for other neurodegenerative diseases such as Alzheimer's disease (AD).[27] It may also be surmised that the main pathogenic trigger can be located on the brain side, hence in the cells of TUs that only indirectly affect blood–brain interaction.
2. Functional modules (FMs)[28]: it should be noted that the concept of a "column" at the cortical level has been proposed by the pioneering work of Lorente de No[29] and Mountcastle.[30] The existence of such integrative structures is proven to a certain extent.[31–33] However, as Rockland[34] points out, the simple question "What is a column?" is not yet easy to answer, since columns are not anatomical structures but are part of locally interdigitizing functional systems. Hence, any delimited column also participates in a widely distributed network. Furthermore, Rockland underlines that columns are not only a cortical feature, since columns (as "modules") occur widely in the brain in noncortical structures.[34] However, the concept of FMs is different from that of columns because FMs are based not on a volume of brain tissue but, rather, on a computing device organized as a "Russian doll" (as discussed in this chapter).

As far as communication modes are concerned, and on the basis of theoretical speculations and experimental data, the following concepts have been introduced:

1. The dichotomy between wiring transmission (WT) and volume transmission (VT);
2. The further distinction between "classical WT" (mainly synaptic contacts) and the tunneling nanotube WT (TNT-WT); and
3. The further distinction between "classical VT" (diffusion of chemical and physical signals) and "roamer-type VT" (diffusion of microvesicles) in the brain mass, in the ECS pathways, and in the cerebrospinal fluid (CSF).

These are the main topics of the present chapter, and on this basis some comments will be made on their possible physiological and pathological implications (see the "Conclusions" section).

ON THE STRUCTURAL ORGANIZATION OF THE CNS

Complex Cellular Networks

Brain integrative action mainly depends on neuronal networks and on the plasticity of synaptic transmission.[12] This signaling backbone, however, is significantly complemented by astrocytes, microglial cells, oligodendroglial cells, ependymal cells, macrophages, pericytes, and mast cells. Hence, the concept of "complex cellular networks" has been introduced as the set of cells of any type that exchange signals in a certain volume of brain tissue and, thanks to this cross-talk, are capable not only of integrating multiple inputs to give out appropriate outputs but also of supporting each other's survival.[18] Some of these cells (especially astrocytes and neurons)[35–38] produce the ECM, which is a three-dimensional organized molecular net.[39–42] Astrocytes also act as liaisons for endothelial-neuronal coupling since perivascular neuronal boutons abut astrocytic endfeet surrounding cerebral microvessel walls.[27]

An interesting topic to be investigated is the multifaceted role of pericytes and mast cells in the CCN's integrative actions.[43–47] These cells are deeply involved *inter alia* in releasing many different VT signals, and they likely represent a basic functional connection between neuronal network needs (e.g. blood supply) and certain peripheral inputs (e.g. steroid hormones). Hence, they likely play a role as CCN cells at the body–brain interface.

As far as pericytes are concerned, they not only are integral cellular components of the blood–brain barrier but also, together with other cells (endothelial cells, astrocytes, and neurons), make fine-tuned regulatory adjustments and adaptations to promote tissue survival.[48] It should be noted that these highly complex regulatory cells communicate with endothelial cells, astrocytes, and neurons by direct physical contact and through autocrine and paracrine signals. Under conditions of stress or injury, the pericytes undergo phenotypic and functional changes that may include migration, proliferation, or differentiation.[48–51]

As far as mast cells are concerned, they are resident cells in the brain with the ability to migrate. Mast cells act via autocrine and paracrine mechanisms and operate as "single-cell glands" by delivering mediators, including neurotransmitters, cytokines, and chemokines, that are released in response to a variety of natural triggers; their secretions can reach large brain volumes. Their granule remnants can even be acquired by neurons through endocytosis.[52,53] The residence of mast cells in the meninges and perivascular locations on the brain side of the blood–brain barrier, primarily in the thalamic and hippocampal regions, indicates that they are strategically situated to initiate neural and vascular responses.

As mentioned in this chapter, the number of mast cells in the brain fluctuates with stress and various behavioral and endocrine states. These properties suggest that mast cells are poised to influence neural systems underlying behavior. It is interesting to note that mast cell–deficient mice had a greater anxiety-like phenotype than wild-type and heterozygote littermate control animals in the open field arena and in an elevated-plus-maze setting.[54] Nautiyal and collaborators have also demonstrated that blockade of brain (but not peripheral) mast cell activation increased anxiety-like behavior.[54] These data implicate an important role of brain mast cells in the modulation of CCNs involved in the control of anxiety-like behavior, and, hence, they play a role as a link between behavior and neuro-immune responses.

On this basis, we proposed that the integrative tasks of the CNS should be studied by considering not only neuronal networks but also whole compartments of brain tissue where different cell types and the ECM work as an integrated computational unit.[25] It has also been proposed that, in addition to the CCNs, the molecular networks formed by organized elements of the ECM should be considered. These molecular networks, mainly made up of proteins and carbohydrates, interact with the cell membrane molecular networks to form a global molecular network (GMN), which enmeshes the entire CNS.[23,24,55,56] Thus, according to our hypothesis, the CNS is a system with computational capabilities in which computing nets, the CCN and the GMN, work sometimes as parallel circuits, sometimes as serial circuits, and overlap with each other at the cell membrane level.

It should be noted that the integrative mechanisms of a CCN depend on the special characteristics of the communication modes in operation in a particular moment among its cells. Several of these characteristics are as follows:

- Rapidity of the message transmission from the source to the target cell.
- Safety of the message transfer (i.e. its probability of reaching unaltered the appropriate target cell).
- Number of targets of the message: "private" versus "public (broadcast)" message.
- Complexity of the action of the message on the target. In fact, the message can act in several different ways, and including on-off action on metabotropic or ionotropic receptors, transfer of receptors (e.g. G protein-coupled receptors, or GPCRs), transfer of proteins and/or lipids, transfer of mRNA, transfer of mitochondrial (mt) DNA, and transfer of organelles.[57–59]
- Plasticity, which is the facility of forming, removing, or changing shapes and/or characteristics of cell networks (see e.g. plastic changes in dendritic spines in Ref. 60).

Obviously, most of these characteristics are influenced not only by astrocytes but also by the ECM composition and/or geometry.[40,55]

Functional Modules

This point will be discussed in the framework of our proposed "Russian doll" organization of brain integrative networks.[6] It should be underlined that the term "functional module" is different from the module metaphor that is largely used in functional magnetic resonance imaging. In this chapter, FMs are used not as a metaphor but as real structural and functional units endowed with the basic aspects pointed out by Bassett and collaborators.[61] Thus, it is proposed that FMs are aggregates of computational elements without well-delimited anatomical borders similar to cortical columns[62] that can perform basic operations providing both compartmentalization and redundancy, which reduces the interdependence of components, enhances robustness, and facilitates behavioral adaptation. Modular organization also confers evolvability to a system by reducing constraints on change. Indeed, a putative relationship between modularity and adaptability in the context of human neuroscience has recently been posited.[63]

According to our group's previous proposal, the brain is organized as a system of FMs formed by CCNs that contain computational networks of different degrees of miniaturization nested within each other from the cell network level down to the molecular network level. Hence, each FM has a Russian-doll structural organization, and at each miniaturization level the involved computing elements (e.g. cells, dendritic spines, or proteins) form a "mosaic".[19,64,65] The term "mosaic" has been introduced in order to convey the concept of topology that may have a potentially great impact on the integrative functions of the assembly, since it underlines the possibility that within the same set of "tesserae" (i.e. computational elements), markedly different mosaics can be assembled at a certain level of miniaturization, and these become capable of handling information differently. A schematic representation of an FM is illustrated in Figure 8.1, distinguishing a horizontal organization (mosaic pattern) and a vertical (hierarchical) organization of computational elements.

Elaboration of the information can occur simultaneously at different miniaturization levels but sometimes in different temporal domains. The highest level of a "horizontal elaboration" is formed by mosaics of FMs, while the lowest level occurs at the molecular level (e.g. within multimeric protein complexes).[10]

In line with the classical Hebb hypothesis on the possible existence of cell assemblies interconnected via reverberating circuits,[66,67] it has been suggested that different FMs can be transiently interconnected to form a higher order mosaic, and, as indicated in this chapter, a "three-dimensional elaboration of the information" is in operation in the CNS.[7] So-called synaptic clusters (SCs) likely play particularly important roles, since SCs were shown to be very plastic entities from both the structural[60] and the functional[68] points of view. In fact,

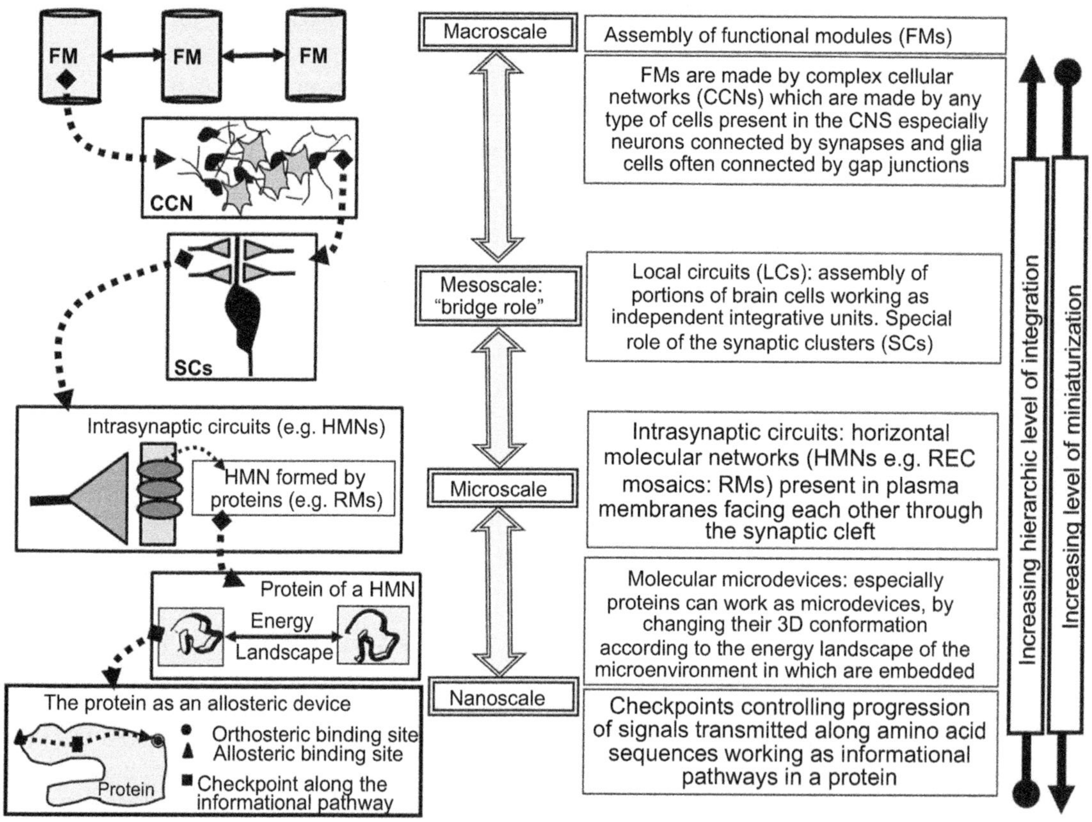

FIGURE 8.1 Schematic representation of computational mosaics, at different degrees of miniaturization, that are encased within each other as a "Russian Matryoshka Doll". As indicated in the scheme, within each functional module (FM) forming the mosaic of the highest hierarchical level, smaller and smaller computational structures are buried within each other down to the allosteric protein level. It should be noted that, as the scheme indicates, horizontal and vertical elaborations of the information take place. For further details, see the text.

it has been reported that plastic changes induced by long-term potentiation (LTP) at one synaptic contact lower the threshold for the induction of LTP at neighboring synapses at a stimulation strength that did not cause any plastic changes under control conditions.

The extent of this sensitized plasticity zone spans about 10 μm of dendrite and lasts for 10 min, affecting neighboring spines.[69] These characteristics allow the SC to act as a sort of "intelligent layer" between the activity at the cellular level and the integrative functions performed at the molecular level by supramolecular complexes, such as those formed at the cell membrane by GPCRs, due to direct receptor–receptor interactions (see Refs 21,70,71 for reviews). The relevance of SCs can also be deduced by the possibility of reverberating microcircuits formed by the synaptic contacts belonging to an SC. As pointed out in Ref. 7, a crucial quantitative difference in neuronal density (neurons/mm^3 in layers I–VI) distinguishes the human brain from those of other species. Neuronal density in the cerebral cortex is lower in humans (24,186/mm^3) than in rats (54,483/mm^3) and mice (120,315/mm^3), whereas the number of synapses per neuron is higher in humans (29,807) than in rats (18,018) and mice (21,133).[72] The number of dendritic spines of basal dendrites of layer III pyramidal neurons also differs in the mouse and human temporal cortex. The mean number (±standard error) of spines per 10 μm segment is 10.9 ± 0.5 for cells in the temporal cortex of mice and 14.2 ± 0.4 for those in the temporal cortex of humans.[73]

It should be noted that a high density of synaptic contacts per neuron allows several alternative pathways in the high-density local circuits of the human brain. This, in turn, allows recirculation of the information that may be of basic importance for further integrations,[72,74] which are likely also involved in memory processes[67,75–77] and may play a role in the so-called internal theater in human consciousness as represented by classical metaphor.[7,78]

THE DICHOTOMY DISTINCTION BETWEEN WIRING AND VOLUME TRANSMISSION

In 1986, we published our original proposal on the existence of two main modes of intercellular communication in the CNS, the WT and the VT[14]; this aimed to complement Cajal's and Sherrington's view of the CNS as a computational apparatus basically formed by neurons interacting via specialized sites of "contiguity", namely, the synaptic contacts.[11,12] Our proposal was influenced by others' important contributions on communication in the CNS[79–87]; and it was based on a number of observations, especially on the central monoamine neurons (for reviews, see Refs 18,88,89). The concept of VT introduced the ECS and the ventricular system as important channels for chemical transmission in the CNS that are complementary to synaptic transmission, and are basically due to the diffusion and flow of transmitters, ions, and trophic factors in the extracellular fluid (ECF) and CSF. Furthermore, our proposal in 1986 considered that the VT signals could interconnect not only neurons in neuronal networks but also any cells of CCNs of the brain.[18] The basic dichotomous classification of intercellular communication in the brain that was proposed more than two decades ago is still valid. However, evidence on the existence of new specialized structures for intercellular communication, such as microvesicles[90] and TNT,[91–93] called for an updating of our original conceptual model.[15]

The criteria that can be applied to characterize WT and VT and their subclasses have been deduced not only from structural and neurochemical findings, but also from concepts and from the lexicon offered by informatics.[94] Our presentation, after a condensed summary of the main features of the "classical" modes of WT and VT,[18] will deal with TNT and microvesicles as novel types of WT and VT, respectively.

In this respect, it has to be observed that the main criteria that allow the differentiation of WT from VT are the characteristics of the communication channel and, more precisely, the physical boundaries of the channel, which are well delimited for WT but not for VT.

The classification can be further detailed by taking into account the other signal features, some of them briefly mentioned here:

Signal privacy: a signal is characterized by high privacy (i.e. a "reserved signal") if it is decrypted only by cells endowed with a specific recognition–decoding apparatus (e.g. specific receptors) for the signal in WT. In contrast to VT, with WT we are dealing with a low-privacy signal (i.e. a "broadcast signal") in which any cell reached by the signal can have access to it.

Signal safety: as far as safety is concerned, we are dealing with a "safe signal" if it is not altered during its conduction from the source to the target cell, and with an "unsafe signal" if it can be altered during its pathway. This occurs, for instance, with some VT signals that can be broken down or modified (e.g. by enzymes) or be trapped in a cul-de-sac in the ECS pathways.

Connectivity: if the connections between cells can be rapidly formed or removed, they provide a "dynamic network". In contrast, the structure of a communication network is "static" when the pattern of connections is mostly stable in time.

Thus, based on these concepts, a unitary scheme could be devised for a more detailed characterization of WT and VT and of their subtypes (see Table 8.1).

TABLE 8.1 Different Types of WT and VT Forming the Communication Networks of the Brain and their Main Features[15]

Communication mode	Channel type	Signal privacy	Signal safety	Connectivity
Synaptic transmission	Private (WT)	Reserved	Safe	Static and/or dynamic
Gap junctions	Private (WT)	Broadcast	Safe	Dynamic
Tunneling nano-tubes	Private (WT)	Broadcast	Safe	Dynamic
Extrasynaptic transmission	Diffuse (VT)	Reserved	Unsafe	Dynamic
Classical VT	Diffuse (VT)	Reserved (common) or broadcast (rare)	Unsafe	Dynamic
Roamer-type VT	Diffuse (VT)	Reserved or broadcast	Safe	Dynamic

Communication features	Types	Description
Channel	Private	Physically delimited pathway between two nodes of the network. This type of channel characterizes WT.
	Diffuse	The whole available space between the network nodes is potentially used to exchange signals. This type of channel characterizes VT.
Signal privacy	Reserved	Signal needs a specific "decoder" to be decrypted. Neurotransmitters and, more generally, signals using specific receptor systems are of this type.
	Broadcast	"Public" signal (i.e. interpreted by all the involved elements). Physical quantities or membrane-permeable molecules are of this type.
Signal safety	Safe	The signal comes to the destination without alteration.
	Unsafe	The signal can be altered during its travel from the source to the target.
Connectivity	Static	The communication network structure does not change with time.
	Dynamic	The communication network has a time-varying structure as a consequence of dynamic processes (plasticity).

Wiring Transmission

Chemical Synapses

These represent the prototype of the WT, characterized by a virtually continuous wire connecting the cell source of the electrical message with its target cells. Actually, a small gap (with a synaptic cleft smaller than 50 nm) in the channel is present between the site of release of the transmitter (presynaptic terminal) and the site where the receptors capable of detecting and transducing the signal are located (postsynaptic target cells). However, in "classical synaptic transmission", it is assumed that this gap does not interfere with the continuity of the channel[95] and with the "safety" of the message. The signal can be classified as "reserved" since specific receptors are needed to decode the message (Table 8.1). A detailed description of chemical synapses can be found in some excellent recent articles,[96,97] and the reader is referred to these important reviews.

Electrical Synapses (Gap Junctions)

Connexins (Cxs) are a large family of homologous membrane proteins in vertebrates; they form gap junction (GJ) channels that provide a direct pathway for electrical and metabolic signaling between cells, especially astrocytes.[98–100] Each GJ channel, which has an inner pore diameter of 10–12 Å, is composed of two hemi-channels (connexons), which in turn are composed of six Cx subunits. Connexons can be coupled with a hemi-channel of an adjacent cell to form a GJ. At least 20 distinct Cx isoforms have been cloned with possible different functions, and they vary in permeability selectivity from being nonselective to being preferentially selective for cations or anions.[101] GJs are also found between activated microglia, between many types of neurons, between astrocytes[102,103] and oligodendrocytes,[104] and in a few somewhat controversial instances between astrocytes and neurons.[105]

The function of GJs between astrocytes is to minimize the differences for substrates such as glucose and in dissipating extracellular K^+ or glutamate, whose extracellular accumulation can be detrimental for proper neuronal functions.

It should be underlined that recent evidence demonstrates the astrocyte's important role in the functional organization of the cerebral cortex, from specific interactions with single synaptic contacts to modulatory interactions with entire neuronal networks.[106,107]

Mixed Synapses

GJs can also be observed in chemical synapses. Hence, "mixed synapses" are possible, which may have a significant modulatory role on the neural networks, imparting fundamental alterations to their properties. Thus, mixed synapses provide the structural and functional components that are required for both chemical and electrical transmission within a single synaptic contact on an individual postsynaptic element.[108,109] The presence of both types of synaptic communications allows a more subtle and complex neuronal computation than might occur with only one type of synaptic contact. It has been surmised that in the mixed synapse, direct physical interactions between receptors and connexins could play an important role.[110] It has to be pointed out, however, that in the mammalian CNS, the physiological roles and distributions of mixed synapses are still to be clearly established.[109,110]

Tunneling Nano-Tube WT

Tunneling nano-tubes are structures involved in intercellular communication, and they have been discovered by means of in vitro studies.[93] In a transient way, they connect two cells, forming a "private" direct channel that has no gaps and resembles the plasmodesmata of plant cells. As far as animal cells are concerned, they have been identified in a variety of cultured cell systems, including cells of the immune system, kidney cells, PC12 cells, and human glioblastoma cells.[57,93]

TNTs have a diameter of 50–200 nm and a length of up to several cell diameters. These transcellular channels could lead to the formation of syncytial cellular networks.[93,111–113] As mentioned here, they are transient structures with variable lifetimes ranging from less than 60 min (T cells) up to several hours (PC12 cells).[114]

Several in vitro studies demonstrated that these structures make possible the exchange of molecules, proteins, and whole organelles between cells. Thus, mitochondrial DNA as well as RNA can migrate along TNTs from one cell to neighboring cells.[57,93,112,115,116] Furthermore, it has been shown that membrane proteins can be exchanged unidirectionally between cells either along the membrane of TNTs or during phases of their transient contacts.[93,112,117–120] Mitochondria can also migrate unidirectionally along TNTs from one cell to neighboring cells either inside or along their surface.[57,93,112,114,118,121,122] It has also been demonstrated that membrane receptors can move from one cell to the plasma membrane of another cell, which, through this mechanism, can acquire for a transient period of time the capability to recognize and transduce signals otherwise not recognized.[28,59] Thus, this mechanism could represent an interesting and significant type of WT, provided this mode of communication is really used in vivo by neurons and/or by other cell types in CCNs.

Volume Transmission

Classical VT

The functional assumption of a diffuse mode of intercellular communication affecting and modulating the activity of entire brain regions has gained support from studies on monoaminergic and peptidergic neurons[123–127] and led to the definition of VT.[14,18]

VT is characterized by the absence of any "wire-like" channel connecting the source of the signal with its own targets, and this feature usually leads to reduced safety, since the VT signal migrates in the ECF (Table 8.1). VT is primarily mediated by diffusion but also by pressure waves due to the arterial pulses in the cerebral arteries and the thermal and electrical gradients.[128–131]

This communication mode uses several often spatially divergent tortuous channels (diffusion pathways) that are made by the clefts (about 20 nm in diameter; see Ref. 132) between cells and filled with ECF and ECM. The ECS also fulfills active tasks in the elaboration of the information, since it may address the diffusion of electrochemical messages in an anisotropic fashion favoring or preventing the communication between two brain areas. This may be due, in part, to the fact that the ECM is not an amorphous filling and can also differ among the various cell types of the CNS.[18] Furthermore, the ECM may affect the messages released by the CNS cells. For example, this can lead to the formation of different sets of fragments from the same parent peptide and, thus, result in interactions with different chemical networks that can modulate various CCNs eliciting different types of integrated responses.[24,64,70,133] Thus, the ECS may be imagined as a system of interconnected channels demarcated by cellular membranes and filled with an ionic solution, primarily sodium chloride, along with macromolecules of the ECM (especially negatively charged proteoglycans and glycosaminoglycans). It should be noted that the ECS forms a reservoir of ions that establishes the resting potentials of cells and mediates fluxes across the membranes.[134]

Diffusion is significantly hindered and the volume of the ECS is reduced in many neuropathological states that are associated with cellular edema and ischemia.[135–137] As mentioned here, signals migrate in the ECS and may be stopped if they reach a blind alley (a cul-de-sac),[138] are inactivated by enzymes or cleared over the brain capillaries,[139] or are taken up into cells via transporters.[140] VT signals can be released from any type of brain cells. They can be released from neurons (in particular from dendrites), from soma and axon terminals (varicosities) entirely lacking synaptic membrane specializations,[141] and from astroglial, microglial, oligodendroglial, mast, and ependymal cells as well as pericytes.

Type of VT Signals and Their Intercellular Transfer

Available evidence supports the original assumption that VT can also employ the same set of signals as WT, namely, transmitters and ions. Other types of signals, however, were suggested to be exchanged by VT.[20,22,128,130,131] A list of the VT signals includes the following:

1. Classical and nonclassical intercellular chemical mediators: neurotransmitters, neuromodulators, growth factors, ions (e.g. Ca^{2+}), and gases (NO, CO_2, and CO). Moreover, it is important to distinguish lipophilic from hydrophilic VT signals, since while the former can also diffuse across membranes (i.e. they have a large space of diffusion), the latter are practically confined to the ECS (i.e. about 20% of the brain volume).
2. Physical signals: electrochemical signals and thermal and pressure waves have been considered as important VT signals.[15,24,128,130,142] Their main characteristics in brief:
   a. Field potentials: it should be mentioned that the ephaptic transmission (or electrical VT) was the first type of VT to be proposed to exist in the CNS.[143] This form of VT is the main one that inspired us to propose the VT mode as a significant communication mode in the brain in view of its self-evident existence deriving from physical concepts already well established by Volta two centuries ago.[144] As a matter of fact, Golgi postulated it by stating that material contact between neurons is not a necessary condition for their communication by electrical signals. Golgi based his bold statement on Volta's studies on the second class of conductors (i.e. the so-called volume conductors), which are electrolytic solutions, such as body fluids.
   b. Thermal waves: temperature macrogradients (i.e. between a brain active region and a brain inactive region)[145] and microgradients via uncoupling protein have been described. Hence, thermal waves can diffuse in the brain mass, affecting especially neurons endowed with high Q10 values (i.e. sensitivity to temperature elevation), such as those present in particular hypothalamic regions.[130,142,146,147]
   c. Pressure waves: these result from cyclic rhythmic cardiac activity, and they pervade and deform the entire mass of the brain, affecting the stretch-sensitive ion channels present in some neurons and astrocytes[148–150] and also *N*-methyl-D-aspartate (NMDA) channels, which respond to membrane tension.[151]

In general, the signals (released by any type of cells) involved in VT are driven toward the target cells (any type of cells) by the following energy gradients: concentration gradients (diffusion of uncharged signals), gradients of electrical potentials (for charged signals), thermal gradients, and pressure gradients (vector-mediated migration for charged and uncharged signals).

It should be noted that electrical, thermal, and pressure gradients can operate both as VT signals producing "waves" in ECS, which can affect brain cell function, and as energy gradients favoring other VT signal migration (as discussed in this chapter).

An important basic VT characteristic needs to be emphasized: it occurs with much lower space filling in comparison to WT, since it does not need a dedicated channel but takes advantage of the ECS.[130,152]

Summing up, intercellular communication occurs via both WT and VT for most of the CCNs, with some of them using mainly (or even only) one of the two modes. In the case of neurons, the ratio between WT and VT can vary from one neuron system to the other and with the structural and functional state of each neuron of the CCNs. Thus, sometimes the two modes occur together, allowing more subtle modulations of intercellular communications, as in the case of the "extrasynaptic VT".

In view of the potential importance of the subject, some aspects will be briefly discussed, focusing especially on neurons.

Extrasynaptic VT

This can be considered as a mixed WT–VT mode since it is linked to synaptic transmission, and likely VT takes place to a varying degree as a consequence of the type of transmitter released at the synaptic level and to the degree of incompleteness of diffusion barriers. The synaptic transmitter reaches the perisynaptic domains of the pre- and postsynaptic membrane, the astroglia, and even adjacent synapses, especially in the case of SCs. Thus, modulation of the volume of brain tissue affected by the extrasynaptic VT depends on glial sheaths around the synapse and the ECM, forming perineuronal nets[153] that act as diffusion barriers. The volume of brain tissue is also affected by the fate of the escaping transmitter molecules, which is determined by the activity of the transmitter transporters and/or the inactivating enzymes.

However, even in the classical synapse where signaling occurs through the "private" synaptic cleft, the insulation of the synapses is often insufficient to prevent extrasynaptic VT,[86,87,154,155] with the diffusion of mediators from the synaptic cleft reaching perisynaptic regions and astroglia rich in receptors[156,157] and finally leading to "synaptic spill-over" to other synapses.[158,159] This important field was investigated in the mid-1990s, mainly by Gonon and Kullmann, who proposed neurotransmitter spill-over as one mechanism for intersynaptic crosstalk.[160,161] For example, glutamate released during synaptic events could escape the synaptic cleft and reach NMDA receptors at neighboring synapses.[162,163] Thus, if glutamate that escaped from a synaptic cleft or was released by astrocytes reached a relatively high concentration in narrow extracellular clefts and diffused from the place of release, it may be able to overcome not only the physical barriers to diffusion[136,137,164] but also the buffering action of the uptake systems present in neurons and astrocytes.[140] It has been suggested that this type of intercellular communication plays a role in LTP and depression as well as during lactation or dehydration, where it can potentiate neurohormonal release,[154,159,165] or in the indirect modulation of the dopaminergic system by excitatory inputs.[166] It should be noted that this type of cell–cell communication is plastic, since the astrocytic isolation of synapses may change over either a short time scale (e.g. during neuronal activity; see Ref. 167) or a long time scale (e.g. during lactation[165,168,169]).

Also, GABA can operate as an extrasynaptic transmitter in several brain regions, and extrasynaptic $GABA_A$ receptors have been shown to have a higher affinity for GABA and slower kinetics of desensitization than the corresponding synaptic $GABA_A$ receptors.[170] This allows them to mediate persistent tonic-inhibitory current. This current is determined by several factors, such as the density of extrasynaptic $GABA_A$ receptors, the proximity of these receptors to the GABA release sources, and the density of GABA transporters near the GABA release sources. In contrast, the $GABA_B$ receptors are mainly located extrasynaptically,[171] suggesting a major role in extrasynaptic GABA VT.

Thus, it is accepted that, via diffusion, the classical neurotransmitters glutamate and GABA can reach receptors at astroglia and at neighboring synapses, affecting the efficacy of transmission.[172] This process is also regulated by the affinity of the glial and neuronal transporters of glutamate and GABA, and also leads to astroglial release of glutamate.[22,173,174]

Summing up, during repetitive stimulation, when the presynaptic terminals of two neighboring synapses are near one another and a paucity of glial membranes is interposed, synaptic spill-over favors their crosstalk. Hence, both synaptic transmission and extrasynaptic VT belong to the fundamental properties of neurons, and both participate in the integrative processes of local circuits.[85,175] In other words, one and the same neuron can release a neurotransmitter that carries out two types of tasks: a highly focused orthodromic signaling that is allowed by the shielding action of neuronal and glial transporters, and a more widespread and diffuse signaling to not only presynaptic but also heterosynaptic structures, detected by high-affinity receptors.[176,177]

A special mode of classical VT that is mainly, but not exclusively, related to the extrasynaptic WT–VT mode is the "metabolic extracellular signal network" (MESN). This mode occurs in ECS, and it has as crucial nodes ecto-enzymes that are capable of producing VT signals from suitable precursors released by cells. These signals can be decoded by high-affinity receptors on the cell membranes. MESNs may be endowed with push and pull signals and with signals capable of triggering and favoring the integration of different responses of the CCNs. A good example of MESNs is the interplay between adenosine triphosphate (ATP) and adenosine (see Figure 8.2), which can be summarized as follows:

1. ATP is secreted mainly by astrocytes, and adenosine is secreted mainly by neurons. ATP released from astrocytes is likely the main source of extracellular ATP[180] and is released by exocytosis.[181] Hence, two of the main components of the CCNs balance the ratio between ATP and adenosine in the ECS.
2. The ATP–adenosine ratio in the ECS and, hence, the adenosine VT communication mode are also under extracellular enzymatic (ecto-5′-nucleotidase) control, since ATP gives rise to adenosine at the level of the ECS. Extracellular concentration of adenosine is maintained by specific nucleoside transporters present in both neurons and astrocytes and by its conversion to inosine.

Hence, astrocytic versus neuronal secretion controls adenosine VT communication mode via the ATP–adenosine ratio in the ECS and the ecto-enzyme activities.

Regarding the ATP–adenosine mediated push–pull mechanisms on blood supply and their modulatory actions on CCNs via their respective high-affinity receptors, it is worth noting the following:

- ATP and adenosine have opposite actions on microvessels, and hence on energy substrate supply.
- ATP acts as a neurotransmitter by binding to several subtypes of purinergic P2 receptors.[182,183] Thus, based on receptor cloning and studying of receptor-induced signal transduction, P2 receptors were divided into P2X ionotropic receptors and P2Y GPCRs.[184] Furthermore, ATP has been demonstrated to act as a cotransmitter with glutamate, noradrenaline, GABA, acetylcholine, and dopamine in the CNS.[185]
- Adenosine inhibits neuronal transmission via A1 receptors; this can result in inhibition of glutamate

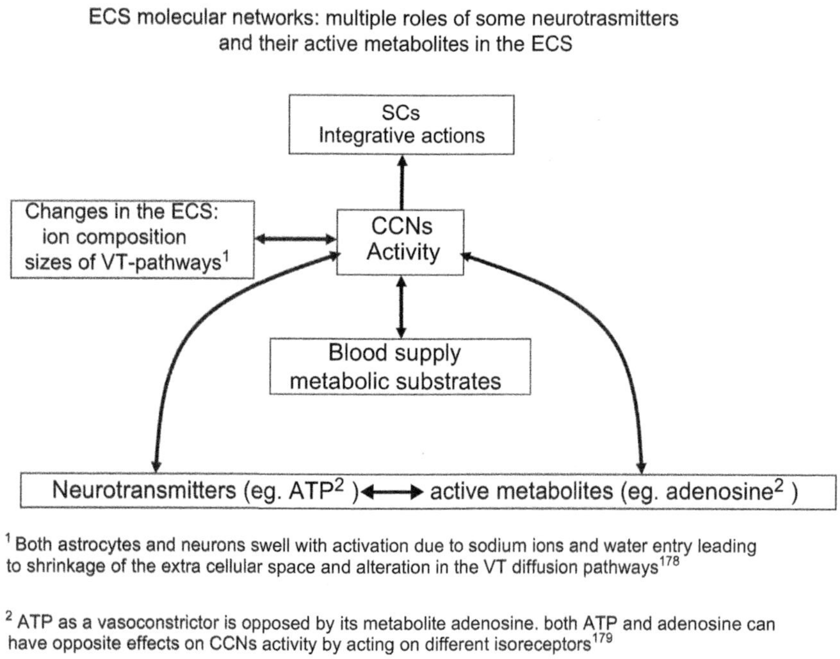
ECS molecular networks: multiple roles of some neurotrasmitters and their active metabolites in the ECS
SCs
Integrative actions
Changes in the ECS:
ion composition
sizes of VT-pathways[1]
CCNs
Activity
Blood supply
metabolic substrates
Neurotransmitters (eg. ATP[2]) active metabolites (eg. adenosine[2])
[1] Both astrocytes and neurons swell with activation due to sodium ions and water entry leading to shrinkage of the extra cellular space and alteration in the VT diffusion pathways[178]
[2] ATP as a vasoconstrictor is opposed by its metabolite adenosine. both ATP and adenosine can have opposite effects on CCNs activity by acting on different isoreceptors[179]

FIGURE 8.2 Schematic representation of the present proposal on the existence of signaling molecular networks based on the synthesis or inactivation of VT signals by the action of ecto-enzymes. In particular, multiple ATP–adenosine interactions are schematically illustrated as an example of the extracellular space (ECS) molecular network concept. For further details, see the text.

release at presynaptic terminals of Schaffer collaterals in the CA1 hippocampus, and in reduction of glutamate release from these fibers.[180,186–188]

- Adenosine can also enhance the release of several neurotransmitters, such as acetylcholine, glutamate, and noradrenaline, via A2 receptors.[189]

Roamer-Type VT

On the basis of new data, there are indications that cells can exchange not only a single message but even a set of messages.[190,191] It has been shown that several messages can be sent via microvesicles (which act as protective containers), dispatched into the ECS, and diffused until the proper targets are reached. This class of intercellular communication belongs, according to our previously stated basic criteria, to the VT mode of communication (no virtually continuous channel). However, note that it often shows the important features of the safety and privacy of the message. Such message safety and privacy can develop only if the proper target cells can recognize the microvesicles through sets of adhesion molecules or receptors. The interaction may be restricted to the plasma membrane, altering the signaling of the cell, or it may lead to their fusion with the plasma membrane or activation of the process of endocytosis, resulting in a decoding of the enclosed signals and in cell–cell communication, as especially demonstrated in the immune system.[191,192]

Different types of microvesicles have been described, and special attention has been paid so far mainly to exosomes and shedding microvesicles, which are the results of specific cellular phenomena (for a review, see Refs 90,192). Even if the field is still far from being described, according to well-accepted criteria for identification of the different classes of microvesicles, the following aspects can be stated:

- Exosomes are microvesicles contained within a special class of endosomes, and they express at their limiting membrane some markers such as Tsg101 and CD9, which also allow their individualization and isolation (for further details, see Ref. 58). Endosomes are membrane-bound organelles that can be classified on the basis of their morphology, their distinct protein and lipid composition, as well as their position within the cell and the cargo that they carry. Thus, they are usually classified as early, late, or recycling endosomes; in particular, late endosomes are a type of multivesicular body (MVB) that contains intraluminal vesicles (ILVs) 30–100 nm in diameter. These ILVs are referred to as exosomes and can be released by fusion of the limiting membrane of the MVB with the plasma membrane. Thus, not only do endosomes transport newly synthesized material from the Golgi complex and endocytosed material from the plasma membrane to various intracellular destinations, but also an alternative fate of MVBs is their exocytic fusion with the plasma membrane,[192] leading to the release of the 30–100 nm ILVs (exosomes) into the extracellular milieu.[193] Exosomes are released both constitutively and in a regulated manner.[192] As far as the signals conveyed to the target cell are concerned, tissue culture studies show that

exosomes can operate as carriers for the intercellular transfer of mtDNA, mRNA, GPCRs, RNAs, and noncoding RNAs.[28,59,192,194]
- Shedding vesicles are microvesicles formed from lipid raft domains of the plasma membrane.[195] The shedding of vesicles is preceded by the budding of small cytoplasmic protrusions, which then detach by fission of their stalk. These vesicles, originating from the plasma membrane, also express specific cell-surface proteins, including integrins and cell adhesion molecules. Therefore, they have the means to bind selectively to, and be taken up by, specific recipient cell types, which express these sets of integrins and cell adhesion molecules. The shedding vesicles may be the vehicle for transferring signalosomes with their receptor mosaics to the target cells. In other words, entire or parts of horizontal molecular networks[196–198] can be transferred by one cell to other cells, creating new transient integrative complex molecular networks in cell populations.

Thus, these data are of substantial interest, in view of the multiple functional roles of the molecules transferred via microvesicles hence via the roamer-type VT.

CONCLUDING REMARKS

Brain integrative actions depend mainly, but not only, on neuronal networks and synaptic transmission. This signaling backbone network is significantly complemented by the other cell types forming the so-called CCNs, including neurons, astrocytes, microglial cells, oligodendroglial cells, ependymal cells, pericytes, and mast cells, in addition to the ECM. Elements of CCNs communicate via two modes of connections, WT and VT, which are not mutually exclusive. Hence, one cell can use both modes. This enlarged view is in agreement with Golgi's proposal that can be paraphrased by stating that different brain cells (neurons and glial cells) present in a certain brain region can operate as a single integrative "province".[81]

Let us discuss some of the main physiological and pathological implications of this new view on CNS organization and intercellular communication modes.

Physiological Implications

It is of the greatest importance to realize that intercellular communication can involve not only transmitters and electrical (ionic) signals, but also genetic information (mtDNA and RNA) and even entire cell organelles, leading to a transient appearance of new proteins in a cell and of new functional properties of a CCN.

Therefore, if fully demonstrated to occur in the brain, these novel forms of WT-TNT and roamer-type VT could represent a new aspect of the extraordinary plasticity of the CNS, offering the possibility of new complex integrative capabilities of brain networks. Although their existence and role in vivo in the CNS are still a matter of investigation and remain to be fully demonstrated, the available experimental data open the possibility that the peculiar features of these intercellular communication modes could be of paramount importance for the integrative actions of the brain CCNs. In this context, it is interesting to cite Smalheiser's proposal that exosomal transfer of proteins and RNAs, especially from the postsynaptic dendrite to the presynaptic terminal, can play a role in synaptic plasticity.[195]

In view of the relevance of GPCRs for brain function and of the evidence that roamer-type VT as well as TNTs could transfer not only mRNA coding for GPCRs but also these receptors as proteins, it has been surmised that, in some instances, VT signals (especially the roamer type) can affect the phenotypic feature of the target cells. This could lead to a new output from the same CCN and, hence, to a polymorphic network.[196,197] The polymorphic network concept[199] suggests the possibility of having a multiform use of the same network following specific changes (e.g. in the intercellular transfer of information). Our data suggest that the Roamer Type of VT can therefore change the operation carried out by some synapses leading to a transient "reuse" by the entire network.

Thus, the concept of reuse of neural circuits[4] can be seen also as a transient reuse of existing neural components, and it may be surmised that this process occurs in the human brain at different time scales:

- Long-term scale: by evolution.
- Intermediate-term scale: by life-long individual experience.
- Short-term scale: from moment to moment, especially as transient reuse responding to external and/or internal inputs impinges on each individual human brain.

In other words, these data and speculations point to the need for careful consideration of several implications of the concept of exaptation and/or redeployment in terms of not simply the brain areas but also the integrative mechanisms at the CCN level, which may be capable of more complex functions.

Pathological Implications

An increasing number of human diseases are known to be caused, either directly or indirectly, by mutations in mtDNA.[200,201] In this context, it should be mentioned that altered mtDNA or mitochondria divorced from their normal endosymbiotic functions within their host cell can become pathogenic entities involved in the initiation and dissemination, via TNTs and/or roamer-type VT, of several pathological conditions.[57]

Exosomal secretion could also have pathological roles in the CNS, especially for conformational protein diseases (CPDs), since a link has been suggested between these vesicles and prion disease pathogenesis.[202] Furthermore, it has been shown that a minute fraction of amyloid-beta (Aβ) peptides can be secreted from the cells in association with exosomes.[203,204] Consistent with this finding, the presence of exosomal proteins has been observed in plaques from AD patient brains,[204] supporting a potential role for exosomes in the pathogenesis of AD.[205]

Actually, increasingly detailed data indicate that prions and the following proteins causing CPDs may diffuse via roamer-type VT[206]:

- Aβ in AD.
- Tau protein in AD, frontotemporal dementia (FTD), and other dementias.
- Superoxide dismutase 1 (SOD1), Tar-DNA binding protein 43 (TDP-43), and fused in sarcoma (FUS) in amyotrophic lateral sclerosis (ALS).
- α-Syn in Parkinson's disease (PD).
- Huntingtin in Huntington's disease (HD).
- Disrupted in schizophrenia 1 (DISC1) in schizophrenia.

GENERAL CONCLUSION

New theoretical models of neuronal networks and new approaches to CNS diseases could be devised by taking into account the complexity of cellular networks that carry out the brain's integrative actions and control the blood supply. In addition, these models must also consider the extreme ductility of the intercellular communication modes as well as the evidence, even if still scarce, of the existence of MESNs that are complex regulatory systems of signals in the ECS, operating mainly via classical VT.

In other words, the CCNs (considered as both trophic and computing devices) and the existence of ECS-based MESNs can open up a new perspective and overcome the dilemma between the vasculo-neural and the neurovascular approaches[27] to CNS disease prevention, treatment, and management.

References

1. Gould SJ, Vrba ES. Exaptation: a missing term in the science of form. *Paleobiology.* 1982;8:4–15.
2. Jacob F. *La logique du vivant. Une histoire de l'hérédité.* Paris: Gallimard Editions; 1970.
3. Xu X, Wang K, Zhang K, et al. A gigantic feathered dinosaur from the lower cretaceous of China. *Nature.* 2012;484:92–95.
4. Anderson ML. Massive redeployment, exaptation, and the functional integration of cognitive operations. *Synthese.* 2007;159: 329–345.
5. Anderson ML. Neural reuse: a fundamental organizational principle of the brain. *Behav Brain Sci.* 2010;33:245–313.
6. Agnati LF, Fuxe K. New concepts on the structure of the neuronal networks: the miniaturization and hierarchical organization of the central nervous system. (Hypothesis). *Biosci Rep.* 1984;4: 93–98.
7. Agnati LF, Guidolin D, Cortelli P, Genedani S, Cela-Conde C, Fuxe K. Neuronal correlates to consciousness. The "Hall of Mirrors" metaphor describing consciousness as an epiphenomenon of multiple dynamic mosaics of cortical functional modules. *Brain Res.* 2012 Jan 11 [Epub ahead of print].
8. Agnati LF, Zoli M, Benfenati F, Pich EM, Grimaldi R, Fuxe K. Aspects of neural plasticity in the central nervous system-II. Numerical classification in neuroanatomy. *Neurochem Int.* 1990;16:419–425.
9. Guidolin D, Albertin G, Guescini M, Fuxe K, Agnati LF. Central nervous system and computation. *Q Rev Biol.* 2011;86:265–285.
10. Agnati LF, Guidolin D, Carone C, Dam M, Genedani S, Fuxe K. Understanding neuronal molecular networks builds on neuronal cellular network architecture. *Brain Res Rev.* 2008;58:379–399.
11. Cajal SR. The structure and connexions of neurons. *Nobel Lecture.* December 12, 1906.
12. Sherrington CS. *The Integrative Action of the Nervous System.* New York: Scribner C. and Sons; 1906.
13. Kandel ER, Schwartz JH, Jessell TM. *Principles of Neural Science.* New York: McGraw-Hill; 2000.
14. Agnati LF, Fuxe K, Zoli M, Ozini I, Toffano G, Ferraguti F. A correlation analysis of the regional distribution of central enkephalin and beta endorphin immunoreactive terminals and of opiate receptors in adult and old male rats. Evidence for the existence of two main types of communication in the central nervous system: the volume transmission and the wiring transmission. *Acta Physiol Scand.* 1986;128:201–207.
15. Agnati LF, Guidolin D, Guescini M, Genedani S, Fuxe K. Understanding wiring and volume transmission. *Brain Res Rev.* 2010;64:137–159.
16. Agnati LF, Leo G, Zanardi A, et al. Volume transmission and wiring transmission from cellular to molecular networks: history and perspectives. *Acta Physiol (Oxf).* 2006;187:329–344.
17. Tanzi E. Sulle modificazione morfologiche funzionali dei dendriti delle cellule nervose. *Rivista di Patologia Nervosa e Mentale.* 1898;3:337–359.
18. Agnati LF, Fuxe K, Nicholson C, Sykova E. Volume transmission revisited. In: *Progress in Brain Research.* Amsterdam: Elsevier; 2000.
19. Agnati LF, Baluska F, Barlow PW, Guidolin D. Mosaic, self-similarity logic, and biological attraction principles: three explanatory instruments in biology. *Commun Integr Biol.* 2009;2:552–563.
20. Agnati LF, Bjelke B, Fuxe K. Volume versus wiring transmission in the brain: a new theoretical frame for neuropsychopharmacology. *Med Res Rev.* 1995;15:33–45.
21. Agnati LF, Guidolin D, Leo G, Carone C, Genedani S, Fuxe K. Receptor–receptor interactions: a novel concept in brain integration. *Prog Neurobiol.* 2010;90:157–175.
22. Fuxe K, Dahlström AB, Jonsson G, et al. The discovery of central monoamine neurons gave volume transmission to the wired brain. *Prog Neurobiol.* 2010;90:82–100.
23. Fuxe K, Marcellino D, Woods AS, et al. Integrated signaling in heterodimers and receptor mosaics of different types of GPCRs of the forebrain: relevance for schizophrenia. *J Neural Transm.* 2009;116:923–939.

24. Agnati LF, Fuxe K. Volume transmission as a key feature of information handling in the central nervous system possible new interpretative value of the Turing's B-type machine. *Prog Brain Res.* 2000;125:3–19.
25. Agnati LF, Cortelli P, Pettersson R, Fuxe K. The concept of trophic units in the central nervous system. *Prog Neurobiol.* 1995;46: 561–574.
26. National Institute of Neurological Disorders and Stroke. Report of the Stroke progress review group. April, 2002; http://www.ninds.nih.gov/find_people/groups/stroke_prg/04_2002_stroke_prg_report.htm. Last accessed: 07.22.2013.
27. Stanimirovic DB, Friedman A. Pathophysiology of the neurovascular unit: disease cause or consequence? *J Cereb Blood Flow Metab.* 2012 Mar 7 [Epub ahead of print].
28. Agnati LF, Guidolin D, Leo G, et al. Possible new targets for GPCR modulation: allosteric interactions, plasma membrane domains, intercellular transfer and epigenetic mechanisms. *J Recept Signal Transduct Res.* 2011;31:315–331.
29. Lorente de Nò R. Architectonics and structure of the cerebral cortex. In: Fulton JF, ed. *Physiology of the Nervous System.* New York: Oxford University Press; 1938:291–330.
30. Mountcastle VB, Davies PW, Berman AL. Response properties of neurons of cat's somatic sensory cortex to peripheral stimuli. *J Neurophysiol.* 1957;20:374–407.
31. Jones EG. Micro-columns in the cerebral cortex. *Proc Natl Acad Sci USA.* 2000;97:5019–5021.
32. Rockland KS, Ichinohe N. Some thoughts on cortical minicolumns. *Exp Brain Res.* 2004;158:265–277.
33. Tanaka K. Columns for complex visual object features in the inferotemporal cortex: clustering of cells with similar but slightly different stimulus selectivities. *Cereb Cortex.* 2003;13:90–99.
34. Rockland KS. Five points on columns. *Front Neuroanat.* 2010;4:22.
35. Faissner A, Pyka M, Geissler M, et al. Contributions of astrocytes to synapse formation and maturation – potential functions of the perisynaptic extracellular matrix. *Brain Res Rev.* 2010;63:26–38.
36. Frischknecht R, Seidenbecher CI. The crosstalk of hyaluronan-based extracellular matrix and synapses. *Neuron Glia Biol.* 2008;4:249–257.
37. Matthews RT, Kelly GM, Zerillo CA, Gray G, Tiemeyer M, Hockfield S. Aggrecan glycoforms contribute to the molecular heterogeneity of perineuronal nets. *J Neurosci.* 2002;22: 7536–7547.
38. Wang D, Fawcett J. The perineuronal net and the control of CNS plasticity. *Cell Tissue Res.* 2012 Mar 23 [Epub ahead of print].
39. Gundelfinger ED, Frischknecht R, Choquet D, Heine M. Converting juvenile into adult plasticity: a role for the brain's extracellular matrix. *Eur J Neurosci.* 2010;31:2156–2165.
40. Rauch U. Extracellular matrix components associated with remodeling processes in brain. *Cell Mol Life Sci.* 2004;61: 2031–2045.
41. Yamaguchi Y. Lecticans: organizers of the brain extracellular matrix. *Cell Mol Life Sci.* 2000;57:276–289.
42. Yong VW, Krekoski CA, Forsyth PA, Bell R, Edwards DR. Matrix metalloproteinases and diseases of the CNS. *Trends Neurosci.* 1998;21:75–80.
43. Dalkara T, Gursoy-Ozdemir Y, Yemisci M. Brain microvascular pericytes in health and disease. *Acta Neuropathol.* 2011;122:1–9.
44. Dore-Duffy P, Cleary K. Morphology and properties of pericytes. *Methods Mol Biol.* 2011;686:49–68.
45. Lee HS, Han J, Bai HJ, Kim KW. Brain angiogenesis in developmental and pathological processes: regulation, molecular and cellular communication at the neurovascular interface. *FEBS J.* 2009;276:4622–4635.
46. Silverman AJ, Sutherland AK, Wilhelm M, Silver R. Mast cells migrate from blood to brain. *J Neurosci.* 2000,20:401–408.
47. Skaper SD, Giusti P, Facci L. Microglia and mast cells: two tracks on the road to neuroinflammation. *FASEB J.* 2012 Apr 19 [Epub ahead of print].
48. Bonkowski D, Katyshev V, Balabanov RD, Borisov A, Dore-Duffy P. The CNS microvascular pericyte: pericyte–astrocyte crosstalk in the regulation of tissue survival. *Fluids Barriers CNS.* 2011;8:8.
49. Balabanov R, Dore-Duffy P. Role of the CNS microvascular pericyte in the blood–brain barrier. *J Neurosci Res.* 1998;53:637–644.
50. Fisher M. Pericyte signaling in the neurovascular unit. *Stroke.* 2009;40:S13–S15.
51. Sims DE. Recent advances in pericyte biology–implications for health and disease. *Can J Cardiol.* 1991;7:431–443.
52. Boyce JA. Mast cells and eicosanoid mediators: a system of reciprocal paracrine and autocrine regulation. *Immunol Rev.* 2007;217:168–185.
53. Wilhelm M, Silver R, Silverman AJ. Central nervous system neurons acquire mast cell products via transgranulation. *Eur J Neurosci.* 2005;22:2238–2248.
54. Nautiyal KM, Ribeiro AC, Pfaff DW, Silver R. Brain mast cells link the immune system to anxiety-like behavior. *Proc Natl Acad Sci USA.* 2008;105:18053–18057.
55. Agnati LF, Zunarelli E, Genedani S, Fuxe K. On the existence of a global molecular network enmeshing the whole central nervous system: physiological and pathological implications. *Curr Protein Pept Sci.* 2006;7:3–15.
56. Apathy S. Das leitende element des nervensystems und sein topographischen beziehungen zu de zellen. *Mittheil Aus der zool Station zu Neapel.* 1897;12:495–748.
57. Agnati LF, Guidolin D, Baluska F, et al. A new hypothesis of pathogenesis based on the divorce between mitochondria and their host cells: possible relevances for the Alzheimer's disease. *Curr Alzheimer Res.* 2010;7:307–322.
58. Guescini M, Genedani S, Stocchi V, Agnati LF. Astrocytes and glioblastoma cells release exosomes carrying mtDNA. *J Neural Transm.* 2010;117:1–4.
59. Guescini M, Leo G, Genedani S, et al. Microvesicle and tunneling nanotube mediated intercellular transfer of g-protein coupled receptors in cell cultures. *Exp Cell Res.* 2012;318:603–613.
60. Holtmaat AJ, Trachtenberg JT, Wilbrecht L, et al. Transient and persistent dendritic spines in the neocortex in vivo. *Neuron.* 2005;45:279–291.
61. Bassett DS, Wymbs NF, Porter MA, Mucha PJ, Carlson JM, Grafton ST. Dynamic reconfiguration of human brain networks during learning. *Proc Natl Acad Sci USA.* 2011;108:7641–7646.
62. da Costa NM, Martin KAC. Whose cortical column would that be? *Front Neuroanat.* 2010;4:16.
63. Meunier D, Lambiotte R, Bullmore ET. Modular and hierarchically modular organization of brain networks. *Front Neurosci.* 2010;4:200.
64. Agnati LF, Ferré S, Leo G, et al. On the molecular basis of the receptor mosaic hypothesis of the engram. *Cell Mol Neurobiol.* 2004;24:501–516.
65. Agnati LF, Guidolin D, Genedani S, et al. How proteins come together in the plasma membrane and function in macromolecular assemblies: focus on receptor mosaics. *J Mol Neurosci.* 2005;26:133–154.
66. Hebb DO. *The Organization of Behavior.* New York: Wiley; 1949.
67. Wang X-J. Synaptic reverberation underlying mnemonic persistent activity. *Trends Neurosci.* 2001;24:455–463.
68. Welzel O, Tischbirek CH, Jung J, et al. Synapse clusters are preferentially formed by synapses with large recycling pool sizes. *PLoS One.* 2010;5:e13514.
69. Harvey CD, Svoboda K. Locally dynamic synaptic learning rules in pyramidal neuron dendrites. *Nature.* 2007;450:1195–1200.

70. Fuxe K, Canals M, Torvinen M, et al. Intramembrane receptor–receptor interactions: a novel principle in molecular medicine. *J Neural Transm.* 2007;114:49–75.
71. Kenakin T, Agnati LF, Caron M, et al. International Workshop at the Nobel Forum, Karolinska Institutet on G protein-coupled receptors: finding the words to describe monomers, oligomers, and their molecular mechanisms and defining their meaning. Can a consensus be reached? *J Recept Signal Transduct Res.* 2010;30:284–286.
72. DeFelipe J, Alonso-Nanclares L, Arellano JI. Microstructure of the neocortex: comparative aspects. *J Neurocytol.* 2002;31:299–316.
73. Benavides-Piccione R, Ballesteros-Yáñez I, DeFelipe J, Yuste R. Cortical area and species differences in dendritic spine morphology. *J Neurocytol.* 2002;31:337–346.
74. Alonso-Nanclares L, Gonzalez-Soriano J, Rodriguez JR, DeFelipe J. Gender differences in human cortical synaptic density. *Proc Natl Acad Sci USA.* 2008;105:14615–14619.
75. Douglas RJ, Koch C, Mahowald M, Martin KA, Suarez HH. Recurrent excitation in neocortical circuits. *Science.* 1995;269: 981–985.
76. Goldman-Rakic PS. Cellular basis of working memory. *Neuron.* 1995;14:477–485.
77. Romo R, Brody CD, Hernández A, Lemus L. Neuronal correlates of parametric working memory in the prefrontal cortex. *Nature.* 1999;399:470–473.
78. Baars BJ. Metaphors of consciousness and attention in the brain. *Trends Neurosci.* 1998;21:58–62.
79. Bach-Y-Rita P. Emerging concepts of brain function. *J Integr Neurosci.* 2005;4:183–205.
80. Descarries L, Seguela P, Watkins KC. Nonjunctional relationship of monoamine axon terminals in the cerebral cortex of adult rat. In: Fuxe K, Agnati LF, eds. *Volume Transmission in the Brain, Novel Mechanisms for Neural Transmission.* New York: Raven Press; 1991:53–62.
81. Golgi C. *La moderna evoluzione delle dottrine e delle conoscenze sulla vita.* XLVII (1). Milano: Rendiconti Regio Istituto Lombardo; 1914.
82. Guillemin R. Peptides in the brain: the new endocrinology of the neuron. *Science.* 1978;202:390–402.
83. Nicholson C. Brain cell microenvironment as a communication channel. In: Schmitt FO, Worden FG, eds. *The Neurosciences: Fourth Study Program.* Cambridge, MA: MIT Press; 1979:457–476.
84. Nieuwenhuys R. Comparative aspects of volume transmission, with sidelight on other forms of intercellular communication. *Prog Brain Res.* 2000;125:49–126.
85. Schmitt FO. Molecular regulators of brain function. A new view. *Neuroscience.* 1984;13:991–1001.
86. Vizi ES, Kiss JP, Lendvai B. Nonsynaptic communication in the central nervous system. *Neurochem Int.* 2004;45:443–451.
87. Vizi ES. *Non-synaptic Interactions between Neurons: Modulation of Neurochemical Transmission.* New York: John Wiley; 1984.
88. Fuxe K, Agnati LF. Two principal modes of electrochemical communication in the brain: volume vs. wiring transmission. In: Fuxe K, Agnati LF, eds. *Volume Transmission in the Brain, Novel Mechanisms for Neural Transmission.* New York: Raven Press; 1991:1–9.
89. Fuxe K, Agnati LF, eds. *Volume Transmission in the Brain, Novel Mechanisms for Neural Transmission.* New York: Raven Press; 1991.
90. Cocucci E, Racchetti G, Meldolesi J. Shedding microvesicles: artefacts no more. *Trends Cell Biol.* 2009;19:43–51.
91. Baluška F, Volkmann D, Barlow PW. Cell–cell channels and their implications for cell theory. In: Baluška F, Volkmann D, Barlow PW, eds. *Cell–Cell Channels.* New York: Landes Bioscience, Georgetown, TX: Springer Science; 2006:1–18.
92. Goncharova LB, Tarakanov AO. Nanotubes at neural and immune synapses. *Curr Med Chem.* 2008;15:210–218.
93. Rustom A, Saffrich R, Markovic I, Walther P, Gerdes H-H. Nanotubular highways for intercellular organelle transport. *Science.* 2004;303:1007–1010.
94. Hopcroft JE, Ullman JD. *Introduction to Automata Theory, Languages and Computation.* Addison-Wesley; 1979.
95. Savtchenko LP, Rusakov DA. The optimal height of the synaptic cleft. *Proc Natl Acad Sci USA.* 2007;104:1823–1828.
96. Bito H. The chemical biology of synapses and neuronal circuits. *Nat Chem Biol.* 2010;6:560–563.
97. Manz BN, Groves JT. Spatial organization and signal transduction at intercellular junctions. *Nat Rev Mol Cell Biol.* 2010;11:342–352.
98. Hervé JC, Bourmeyster N, Sarrouilhe D, Duffy HS. Gap junctional complexes: from partners to functions. *Prog Biophys Mol Biol.* 2007;94:29–65.
99. LeBeau FE, Traub RD, Monyer H, Whittington MA, Buhl EH. The role of electrical signaling via gap junctions in the generation of fast network oscillations. *Brain Res Bull.* 2003;62:3–13.
100. Yeager M, Harris AL. Gap junction channel structure in the early 21st century: facts and fantasies. *Curr Opin Cell Biol.* 2007;19: 521–528.
101. Oviedo-Orta E, Evans WH. Gap junctions and connexin-mediated communication in the immune system. *Biochim Biophys Acta.* 2004;1662:102–112.
102. Theis M, Söhl G, Eiberger J, Willecke K. Emerging complexities in identity and function of glial connexins. *Trends Neurosci.* 2005;28:188–195.
103. Volterra A, Meldolesi J. Astrocytes, from brain glue to communication elements: the revolution continues. *Nat Rev Neurosci.* 2005;6:626–640.
104. Orthmann-Murphy JL, Abrams CK, Scherer SS. Gap junctions couple astrocytes and oligodendrocytes. *J Mol Neurosci.* 2008;35: 101–116.
105. Nagya JI, Dudekb EF, Rashb JE. Update on connexins and gap junctions in neurons and glia in the mammalian nervous system. *Brain Res Rev.* 2004;47:191–215.
106. Oberheim NA, Takano T, Han X, et al. Uniquely hominid features of adult human astrocytes. *Neuroscience.* 2009;29:3276–3287.
107. Pereira A, Furlan FA. Astrocytes and human cognition: modeling information integration and modulation of neuronal activity. *Prog Neurobiol.* 2010;92:405–420.
108. Flores CE, Li X, Bennett MV, Nagy JI, Pereda AE. Interaction between connexin35 and zonula occludens-1 and its potential role in the regulation of electrical synapses. *Proc Natl Acad Sci USA.* 2008;105:12545–12550.
109. Rash JE, Dillman RK, Bilhartz BL, Duffy HS, Whalen LR, Yasumura T. Mixed synapses discovered and mapped throughout mammalian spinal cord. *Proc Natl Acad Sci USA.* 1996;93:4235–4239.
110. Fuxe K, Dahlström A, Höistad M, et al. From the Golgi–Cajal mapping to the transmitter-based characterization of the neuronal networks leading to two modes of brain communication: wiring and volume transmission. *Brain Res Rev.* 2007;55:17–54.
111. Gerdes HH, Carvalho RN. Intercellular transfer mediated by tunneling nanotubes. *Curr Opin Cell Biol.* 2008;20:470–475.
112. Onfelt B, Nedvetzki S, Benninger RK, et al. Structurally distinct membrane nanotubes between human macrophages support long-distance vesicular traffic or surfing of bacteria. *J Immunol.* 2006;177:8476–8483.
113. Sowinski S, Jolly C, Berninghausen O, et al. Membrane nanotubes physically connect T cells over long distances presenting a novel route for HIV-1 transmission. *Nat Cell Biol.* 2008;10:211–219.

114. Gurke S, Barroso JF, Hodneland E, Bukoreshtliev NV, Schlicker O, Gerdes HH. Tunneling nanotube (TNT)-like structures facilitate a constitutive, actomyosin-dependent exchange of endocytic organelles between normal rat kidney cells. *Exp Cell Res.* 2008;314:3669–3683.
115. Belting M, Wittrup A. Nanotubes, exosomes, and nucleic acid-binding peptides provide novel mechanisms of intercellular communication in eukaryotic cells: implications in health and disease. *J Cell Biol.* 2008;183:1187–1191.
116. Koyanagi M, Brandes RP, Haendeler J, Zeiher AM, Dimmeler S. Cell-to-cell connection of endothelial progenitor cells with cardiac myocytes by nanotubes: a novel mechanism for cell fate changes? *Circ Res.* 2005;96:1039–1041.
117. Ambudkar SV, Sauna ZE, Gottesman MM, Szakacs G. A novel way to spread drug resistance in tumor cells: functional intercellular transfer of P-glycoprotein (ABCB1). *Trends Pharmacol Sci.* 2005;26:385–387.
118. Gurke S, Barroso JF, Gerdes HH. The art of cellular communication: tunneling nanotubes bridge the divide. *Histochem Cell Biol.* 2008;129:539–550.
119. Rechavi O, Goldstein I, Kloog Y. Intercellular exchange of proteins: the immune cell habit of sharing. *FEBS Lett.* 2009;583: 1792–1799.
120. Watkins SC, Salter RD. Functional connectivity between immune cells mediated by tunneling nanotubules. *Immunity.* 2005;23: 309–318.
121. Davis DM, Sowinski S. Membrane nanotubes: dynamic long-distance connections between animal cells. *Nat Rev Mol Cell Biol.* 2008;9:431–436.
122. Vidulescu C, Clejan S, O'Connor KC. Vesicle traffic through intercellular bridges in DU 145 human prostate cancer cells. *J Cell Mol Med.* 2004;8:388–396.
123. Aston-Jones G, Segal M, Bloom FE. Brain aminergic axons exhibit marked variability in conduction velocity. *Brain Res.* 1980;195: 215–222.
124. Burbach JP. Neuropeptides and cerebrospinal fluid. *Ann Clin Biochem.* 1982;19:269–277.
125. De Wied D, Jolles J. Neuropeptides derived from pro-opiocortin: behavioral, physiological, and neurochemical effects. *Physiol Rev.* 1982;62:976–1059.
126. Fuxe K, Eneroth P, Gustafsson JA, Löfström A, Skett P. Dopamine in the nucleus accumbens: preferential increase of DA turnover by rat prolactin. *Brain Res.* 1977;122:177–182.
127. Geffen LB, Jessell TM, Cuello AC, Iversen LL. Release of dopamine from dendrites in rat substantia nigra. *Nature.* 1976;260:258–260.
128. Agnati LF, Cortelli P, Biagini G, Bjelke B, Fuxe K. Different classes of volume transmission signals exist in the central nervous system and are affected by metabolic signals, temperature gradients and pressure waves. *Neuroreport.* 1994;6:9–12.
129. Agnati LF, Fuxe K, Baluska F, Guidolin D. Implications of the 'Energide' concept for communication and information handling in the central nervous system. *J Neural Transm.* 2009;116: 1037–1052.
130. Agnati LF, Genedani S, Lenzi PL, et al. Energy gradients for the homeostatic control of brain ECF composition and for VT signal migration: introduction of the tide hypothesis. *J Neural Transm.* 2005;112:45–63.
131. Agnati LF, Zoli M, Strömberg I, Fuxe K. Intercellular communication in the brain: wiring versus volume transmission. *Neuroscience.* 1995;69:711–726.
132. Chen KC, Nicholson C. Changes in brain cell shape create residual extracellular space volume and explain tortuosity behaviour during osmotic challenge. *Proc Natl Acad Sci USA.* 2000;97:8306–8311.
133. Agnati LF, Tarakanov AO, Ferré S, Fuxe K, Guidolin D. Receptor–receptor interactions, receptor mosaics, and basic principles of molecular network organization: possible implications for drug development. *J Mol Neurosci.* 2005;26: 193–208.
134. Hrabětová S, Nicholson C. Chapter 10 Biophysical properties of brain extracellular space explored with ion-selective microelectrodes, integrative optical imaging and related techniques. In: Michael AC, Borland LM, eds. *Electrochemical Methods for Neuroscience.* Boca Raton, FL: CRC Press; 2007.
135. Hrabetová S, Nicholson C. Dextran decreases extracellular tortuosity in thick-slice ischemia model. *J Cereb Blood Flow Metab.* 2000;20:1306–1310.
136. Nicholson C, Sykova E. Extracellular space structure revealed by diffusion analysis. *Trends Neurosci.* 1998;21:207–215.
137. Syková E, Mazel T, Vargová L, Vorísek I, Prokopová-Kubinová S. Extracellular space diffusion and pathological states. *Prog Brain Res.* 2000;125:155–178.
138. Hrabetová S, Hrabe J, Nicholson C. Dead-space microdomains hinder extracellular diffusion in rat neocortex during ischemia. *J Neurosci.* 2003;23:8351–8359.
139. Jansson A. Long distance signalling in volume transmission. Focus on clearance mechanisms. *Prog Brain Res.* 2000;125: 399–413.
140. Rice ME, Cragg SJ. Dopamine spillover after quantal release: rethinking dopamine transmission in the nigrostriatal pathway. *Brain Res Rev.* 2008;58:303–313.
141. Descarries L, Bérubé-Carrière N, Riad M, Bo GD, Mendez JA, Trudeau LE. Glutamate in dopamine neurons: synaptic versus diffuse transmission. *Brain Res Rev.* 2008;58:290–302.
142. Rivera A, Agnati LF, Horvath TL, Valderrama JJ, de La Calle A, Fuxe K. Uncoupling protein 2/3 immunoreactivity and the ascending dopaminergic and noradrenergic neuronal systems. Relevance for volume transmission. *Neuroscience.* 2006;137: 1447–1461.
143. Golgi C. La rete nervosa diffusa degli organi centrali del sistema nervoso. Suo significato fisiologico. Regio Istituto Lombardo di Scienze e Lettere, XXIV. Reprinted in French in: *Archives Italiennes de Biologie.* 1891;15:434–463.
144. Trasatti S. 1799–1999: Alessandro Volta's 'electric pile'. Two hundred years, but it doesn't seem like it. *J Electroanal Chem.* 1999;460:1–4.
145. Yablonskiy DA, Ackerman JJ, Raichle ME. Coupling between changes in human brain temperature and oxidative metabolism during prolonged visual stimulation. *Proc Natl Acad Sci USA.* 2000;97:7603–7608.
146. Agnati LF, Vergoni AV, Leo G, et al. Energy gradients for VT-signal migration in the CNS: studies on melanocortin receptors, mitochondrial uncoupling proteins and food intake. *J Endocrinol Invest.* 2004;27(Suppl 6):23–34.
147. Fuxe K, Rivera A, Jacobsen KX, et al. Dynamics of volume transmission in the brain. Focus on catecholamine and opioid peptide communication and the role of uncoupling protein 2. *J Neural Transm.* 2005;112:65–76.
148. Honorè E. The neuronal background K2P channels: focus on TREK1. *Nat Rev Neurosci.* 2007;8:251–261.
149. Ostrow LW, Sachs F. Mechanosensation and endothelin in astrocytes—hypothetical roles in CNS pathophysiology. *Brain Res Brain Res Rev.* 2005;48:488–508.
150. Puro DG. Stretch-activated channels in human retinal Muller cells. *Glia.* 1991;4:456–460.
151. Paoletti P, Ascher P. Mechanosensitivity of NMDA receptors in cultured mouse central neurons. *Neuron.* 1994;13:645–655.
152. Agnati LF, Genedani S, Leo G, Rivera A, Guidolin D, Fuxe K. One century of progress in neuroscience founded on Golgi and Cajal's

outstanding experimental and theoretical contributions. *Brain Res Rev.* 2007;55:167–189.
153. Celio MR, Spreafico R, De Biasi S, Vitellaro-Zuccarello L. Perineuronal nets: past and present. *Trends Neurosci.* 1998;21:510–515.
154. Oliet SHR, Piet R, Poulain DA. Control of glutamate clearance and synaptic efficacy by glial coverage of neurons. *Science.* 2001;292:923–926.
155. Witcher MR, Park YD, Lee MR, Sharma S, Harris KM, Kirov SA. Three-dimensional relationships between perisynaptic astroglia and human hippocampal synapses. *Glia.* 2010;58:572–587.
156. Cabello N, Gandía J, Bertarelli DC, et al. Metabotropic glutamate type 5, dopamine D_2 and adenosine A_{2a} receptors form higher-order oligomers in living cells. *J Neurochem.* 2009;109:1497–1507.
157. Deitmer JW, Rose CR. Ion changes and signalling in perisynaptic glia. *Brain Res Rev.* 2010;63:113–129.
158. Alle H, Geiger JR. GABAergic spill-over transmission onto hippocampal mossy fiber boutons. *J Neurosci.* 2007;27:942–950.
159. Piet R, Vargova L, Sykova E, Poulain DA, Oliet SHR. Physiological contribution of the astrocytic environment of neurons to intersynaptic crosstalk. *Proc Natl Acad Sci USA.* 2004;101:2151–2155.
160. Gonon F, Burie JB, Jaber M, Benoit-Marand M, Dumartin B, Bloch B. Geometry and kinetics of dopaminergic transmission in the rat striatum and in mice lacking the dopamine transporter. *Prog Brain Res.* 2000;125:291–302.
161. Kullmann DM, Erdemli G, Asztely F. LTP of AMPA and NMDA receptor-mediated signals: evidence for presynaptic expression and extrasynaptic glutamate spill-over. *Neuron.* 1996;17:461–474.
162. Asztely F, Erdemli G, Kullmann DM. Extrasynaptic glutamate spill-over in the hippocampus: dependence on temperature and the role of active glutamate uptake. *Neuron.* 1997;18:281–293.
163. Kullmann DM. Spillover and synaptic cross talk mediated by glutamate and GABA in the mammalian brain. *Prog Brain Res.* 2000;125:339–351.
164. Syková E, Vargová L. Extrasynaptic transmission and the diffusion parameters of the extracellular space. *Neurochem Int.* 2008;52:5–13.
165. Sykova E. Glial diffusion barriers during aging and pathological states. *Prog Brain Res.* 2001;132:339–363.
166. Kiss JP, Zsilla G, Vizi ES. Inhibitory effect of nitric oxide on dopamine transporters: interneuronal communication without receptors. *Neurochem Int.* 2004;45:485–489.
167. Hirrlinger J, Hulsmann S, Kirchhoff F. Astroglial processes show spontaneous motility at active synaptic terminals in situ. *Eur J Neurosci.* 2004;20:2235–2239.
168. Haydon PG. Glia: listening and talking to the synapse. *Nat Rev Neurosci.* 2001;2:185–193.
169. Theodosis DT, Poulain DA. Activity-dependent neuronal–glial and synaptic plasticity in the adult mammalian hypothalamus. *Neuroscience.* 1993;57:501–535.
170. Kullmann DM, Ruiz A, Rusakov DM, Scott R, Semyanov A, Walker MC. Presynaptic, extrasynaptic and axonal $GABA_A$ receptors in the CNS: where and why? *Prog Biophys Mol Biol.* 2005;87:33–46.
171. Charles KJ, Evans ML, Robbins MJ, Calver AR, Leslie RA, Pangalos MN. Comparative immunohistochemical localisation of $GABA_{B1a}$, $GABA_{B1b}$ and $GABA_{B2}$ subunits in rat brain, spinal cord and dorsal root ganglion. *Neuroscience.* 2001;106:447–467.
172. Reichenbach A, Derouiche A, Kirchhoff F. Morphology and dynamics of perisynaptic glia. *Brain Res Rev.* 2010;63:11–25.
173. Fuxe K, Ferré S, Genedani S, Franco R, Agnati LF. Adenosine receptor–dopamine receptor interactions in the basal ganglia and their relevance for brain function. *Physiol Behav.* 2007;92:210–217.
174. Oláh S, Komlósi G, Szabadics J, et al. Output of neurogliaform cells to various neuron types in the human and rat cerebral cortex. *Front Neural Circuits.* 2007;1:4.
175. Agnati LF, Guidolin D, Fuxe K. The brain as a system of nested but partially overlapping networks. Heuristic relevance of the model for brain physiology and pathology. *J Neural Transm.* 2007;114:3–19.
176. Fuxe K, Marcellino D, Rivera A, et al. Receptor–receptor interactions within receptor mosaics. Impact on neuropsychopharmacology. *Brain Res Rev.* 2008;58:415–452.
177. Rusakov DA, Lehreb KP. Perisynaptic asymmetry of glia: new insights into glutamate signalling. *Trends Neurosci.* 2002;25:492–494.
178. Fayuk D, Aitken PG, Somjen GG, Turner DA. Two different mechanisms underlie reversible, intrinsic optical signals in rat hippocampal slices. *J Neurophysiol.* 2002;87:1924–1937.
179. Shetty PK, Galeffi F, Turner DA. Cellular links between neuronal activity and energy homeostasis. *Front Pharmacol.* 2012;3:43.
180. Butt AM. ATP: a ubiquitous gliotransmitter integrating neuron–glial networks. *Semin Cell Dev Biol.* 2011;22:205–213.
181. Pangrsic T, Potokar M, Stenovec M, et al. Exocytotic release of ATP from cultured astrocytes. *J Biol Chem.* 2007;282:28749–28758.
182. Burnstock G. Purinergic cotransmission. *Brain Res Bull.* 1999;50:355–357.
183. Fields RD, Stevens B. ATP: an extracellular signaling molecule between neurons and glia. *Trends Neurosci.* 2000;23:625–633.
184. Majumder P, Trujillo CA, Lopes CG, et al. New insights into purinergic receptor signaling in neuronal differentiation, neuroprotection, and brain disorders. *Purinergic Signal.* 2007;3:317–331.
185. Burnstock G. Purinergic signalling in the CNS. *Open Neurosci J.* 2010;4:24–30.
186. Fowler JC. Escape from inhibition of synaptic transmission during in vitro hypoxia and hypoglycemia in the hippocampus. *Brain Res.* 1992;573:169–673.
187. Lupica CR, Proctor WR, Dunwiddie TV. Presynaptic inhibition of excitatory synaptic transmission by adenosine in rat hippocampus: analysis of unitary EPSP variance measured by whole-cell recording. *J Neurosci.* 1992;12:3753–3764.
188. Zhu PJ, Krnjević K. Adenosine release is a major cause of failure of synaptic transmission during hypoglycaemia in rat hippocampal slices. *Neurosci Lett.* 1993;155:128–131.
189. Sebastião AM, Ribeiro JA. Adenosine A_2 receptor-mediated excitatory actions on the nervous system. *Prog Neurobiol.* 1996;48:167–189.
190. Février B, Raposo G. Exosomes: endosomal-derived vesicles shipping extracellular messages. *Curr Opin Cell Biol.* 2004;16:415–421.
191. Simons M, Raposo G. Exosomes – vesicular carriers for intercellular communication. *Curr Opin Cell Biol.* 2009;21:575–581.
192. Lakkaraju A, Rodriguez-Boulan E. Itinerant exosomes: emerging roles in cell and tissue polarity. *Trends Cell Biol.* 2008;18:199–209.
193. Van Niel G, Porto-Carreiro I, Simoes S, Raposo G. Exosomes: a common pathway for a specialized function. *J Biochem.* 2006;140:13–21.
194. Valadi H, Ekström K, Bossios A, Sjöstrand M, Lee JJ, Lötvall JO. Exosome-mediated transfer of mRNAs and microRNAs is a novel mechanism of genetic exchange between cells. *Nat Cell Biol.* 2007;9:654–659.
195. Smalheiser NR. Exosomal transfer of proteins and RNAs at synapses in the nervous system. *Biol Direct.* 2007;30:2–35.
196. Agnati LF, Ferré S, Lluis C, Franco R, Fuxe K. Molecular mechanisms and therapeutical implications of intramembrane receptor/receptor interactions among heptahelical receptors with examples from the striopallidal GABA neurons. *Pharmacol Rev.* 2003;55:509–550.

197. Agnati LF, Santarossa L, Benfenati F, et al. Molecular basis of learning and memory: modelling based on receptor mosaics. In: Apolloni B, Kurfes F, eds. *From Synapses to Rules*. New York: Kluwer Academic/Plenum Publishers; 2002:165–196.
198. Okamoto T, Schlegel A, Scherer PE, Lisanti MP. Caveolins, a family of scaffolding proteins for organizing "preassembled signaling complexes" at the plasma membrane. *J Biol Chem*. 1998;273:5419–5422.
199. Getting PA, Denkin MS. Tritonia swimming: a model system for integration within rhythmic motor systems. In: Selverston AI, ed. *Model Neural Networks and Behavior*. New York: Plenum Press; 1985.
200. Wallace DC. Mitochondrial diseases in man and mouse. *Science*. 1999;283:1482–1488.
201. Wallace KB, Eells JT, Madeira VM, Cortopassi G, Jones DP. Mitochondria-mediated cell injury. Symposium overview. *Fundam Appl Toxicol*. 1997;38:23–37.
202. Vella LJ, Sharples RA, Nisbet RM, Cappai R, Hill AF. The role of exosomes in the processing of proteins associated with neurodegenerative diseases. *Eur Biophys J*. 2008;37:323–332.
203. Bellingham SA, Guo BB, Coleman BM, Hill AF. Exosomes: vehicles for the transfer of toxic proteins associated with neurodegenerative diseases? *Front Physiol*. 2012;3:124.
204. Rajendran L, Honsho M, Zahn TR, et al. Alzheimer's disease beta-amyloid peptides are released in association with exosomes. *Proc Natl Acad Sci USA*. 2006;103:11172–11177.
205. Ghidoni R, Benussi L, Binetti G. Exosomes: the Trojan horses of neurodegeneration. *Med Hypotheses*. 2008;70:1226–1227.
206. Guest WC, Silverman JM, Pokrishevsky E, O'Neill MA, Grad LI, Cashman NR. Generalization of the prion hypothesis to other neurodegenerative diseases: an imperfect fit. *J Toxicol Environ Health A*. 2011;74:1433–1459.

CHAPTER

9

Electrophysiological Mechanisms of Network Control: Bursting in the Brain—From Cells to Networks

Taufik A. Valiante, Peter L. Carlen

Department of Surgery, Division of Neurosurgery, Toronto, Ontario, Canada; Division of Fundamental Neurobiology, Toronto Western Hospital Research Institute, Toronto Western Hospital, Ontario, Canada; Krembil Neuroscience Center, University Health Network, Toronto, Ontario, Canada

INTRODUCTION

This chapter explores electrophysiological mechanisms of network control: We will focus on burst firing or "bursting", particularly that associated with seizures. We will initially give an overview starting from measurements of large brain circuitry at the level of electroencephalography (EEG), then move to bursting at the cellular level, and end with a discussion of how single-cell activity might be coordinated and influences local and more extended neuronal networks. As noted in Chapter 1, burst firing, along with ephaptic (field effects) and gap junction mechanisms, which are also operative in bursting, are vitally important neurophysiological mechanisms in the control of neuronal networks.

By way of introduction, the term "burst" is rather ill defined; it can be used to describe brain electrical behavior from the level of the scalp EEG to that of a single neuron. The concept of a burst implies a transient increase in activity, with subsequent return to baseline activity levels (Figure 9.1(A)). At the level of a single cell, a burst of spikes is defined as three or more

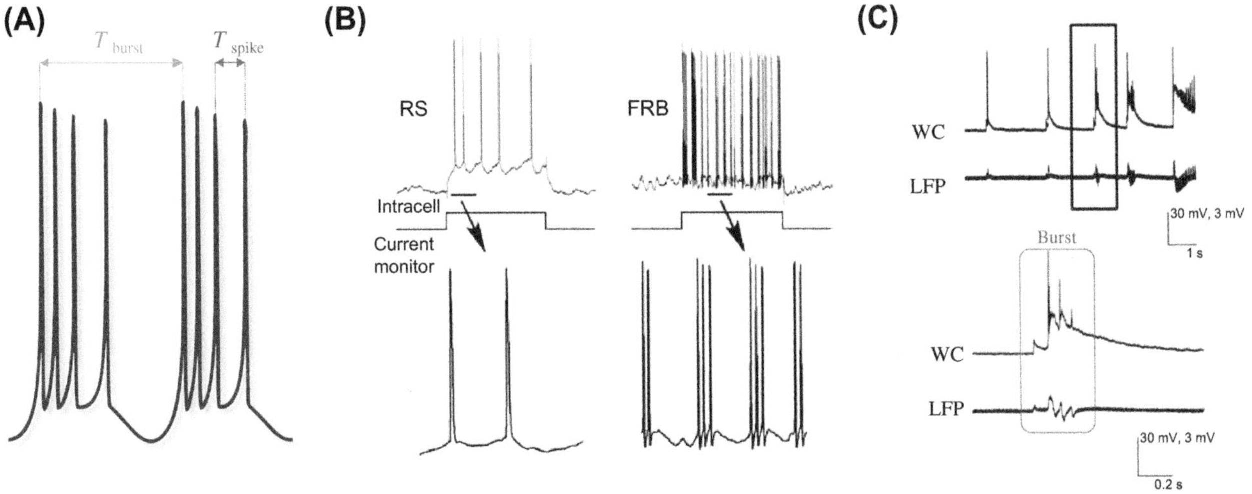

FIGURE 9.1 **Definitions and examples of bursting**. (A) Schematic of a burst, showing the different time scales of measures to characterize such behavior. (B) Different cellular spiking characteristics in response to intracellular current injection. The lower panel depicts expanded regions taken from the upper panel. (*Source: With permission from Ref. 1.*) Regular spiking (RS) and fast-rhythmic bursting (FRB) cells are depicted. (C) Bursting behavior measured at different spatial scales. Note the burst measured in both the whole-cell (WC) recording and the local field potential (LFP). Although both activities appear to be burst-like, they entail different phenomena; nonetheless, they are intimately related. (*Source: With permission from Zhang et al.*[2]) (For color version of this figure, the reader is referred to the online version of this book.)

Neuronal Networks in Brain Function, CNS Disorders, and Therapeutics
http://dx.doi.org/10.1016/B978-0-12-415804-7.00009-5

spikes with interspike intervals (T_{spike}) < 8 ms (see Figure 9.1(A)),[3] usually separated by a relatively silent period. However, a precise definition based on a rigid interspike interval is not really possible.[4] Although both excitatory and inhibitory cells of the brain have the ability to burst,[5,6] it is important to note that a cell's propensity to burst is a state-dependent characteristic.[7] For example, the fast-rhythmic bursting neuron of the thalamus can generate high-frequency tonic firing (at 450 Hz) with strong depolarization; whereas with less vigorous depolarization, it generates bursts of spikes, with the interburst interval (T_{burst}; see Figure 9.1(A)) corresponding to 30–40 Hz[7] (Figure 9.1(B)). When considering brain activity on a larger scale, such as the local field potential (LFP), where activity is averaged over an approximate radius of 250 μm,[8] burst activity can also be observed (see Figure 9.1(C)). In this example, seizure-like events were induced in the whole hippocampus preparation, while simultaneous LFP and whole-cell recordings were performed.[2] It can be seen that a so-called preictal burst in the LFP is associated with intracellular bursting. This observation suggests that activity measured on larger spatial scales can in many ways mimic or reflect what is happening at a smaller scale; in this case, cellular bursting is mimicked by a local network burst. This fractal-like quality of brain activity, where temporal structures appear similar regardless of the scale of observation, suggests but one organizing principle in the brain where activity is structured hierarchically. Such scale-free activity is like that which generates the ubiquitous 1/f spectral signature of brain activity and other complex systems.[9,10] Indeed, many types of oscillatory activities abound in the "awake" and sleeping brain that contribute to the 1/f spectral signature.[11] The organization of such oscillations is not haphazard.[12] Like the "Russian Matryoshka doll" (nesting doll), high-frequency oscillations (HFOs) appear "nested" within lower ones creating a so-called oscillatory hierarchy.[13,14] This nesting or cross-frequency coupling (CFC) is manifested by the control of faster oscillation amplitude by low-frequency phase.[15–18] This temporal waxing and waning of the amplitude of faster oscillations by slower ones engender a burst-like quality to all neural activity. Bursting, in this light, appears to take on a fundamental organizing principle of brain function. We will, however, here review only a small part of this ubiquitous phenomenon.

Scalp EEG

For the electroencephalographer, a burst is defined as "A group of waves which appear and disappear abruptly and are distinguished from background activity by differences in frequency, form and/or amplitude. This term does not imply abnormality and is not a synonym of paroxysm."[19] EEG-measured bursts are usually described in the context of epilepsy, or deep coma. For example, burst suppression is defined as follows: "A pattern characterized by bursts of theta and/or delta waves, at times intermixed with faster waves, and intervening periods of low amplitude (below 20 V). This EEG pattern indicates either severe brain dysfunction or is typical of some anesthetic drugs at certain levels of anesthesia."[19] Epileptiform activity in the form of "interictal spikes" is often found in the scalp EEG of patients with epilepsy, but a major limiting factor is that the scalp EEG can only record synchronous activity emanating from over 6 cm^2 of cortex.[20,21]

Intracranial EEG

A better delineation of brain electrical activity, including bursting, is obtained using intracranial electrodes. Macroelectrode contacts (2–5 mm diameter), which are either surface (subdural electrodes) or depth electrodes implanted within the brain substance itself, are used routinely to localize epileptogenic regions in patients with epilepsy. From these electrodes, spontaneous and evoked (during behavioral tasks) physiological and epileptiform activity can be measured. Such activity represents the summation of many hundreds of thousands of neurons.

Of great recent interest are HFOs. The exact definition of what an HFO represents mechanistically, and whether characterizing a specific range of frequencies as physiological versus pathological is correct, remains unresolved.[22,23] This lack of consensus is currently unavoidable because a mechanistic underpinning for such oscillatory activity is currently lacking. In the human brain, electrocorticographic (ECoG) recordings can detect oscillations between 60 and 200 Hz that are associated with various cognitive tasks.[24] The amplitude of such oscillations appears to be modulated by the phase of low-frequency oscillations, so-called CFC.[15,16] Such HFOs are taken to be physiological, since they are associated with a myriad of brain states, and the strength of CFC depends on the cognitive task.[15] As has been alluded to,[23] HFOs (ripples: 90–200 Hz, and fast ripples: 200–500 Hz; to be discussed in this chapter) come in "packets" and thus represent a high-frequency burst of activity (see Figure 9.2 for an example of a ripple).[26,27] Such an appearance suggests a self-limited process that is likely to be generated by synchronous spiking activity and/or postsynaptic potentials.[23] Such HFOs within the frequency range of 60–200 Hz (which overlaps with ripple frequencies) are also known as "high-gamma activity",[15,28] and such activity accompanies a number of cognitive activities.[29] This high-gamma activity is thought to be generated by asynchronous spiking activity, and thus it has

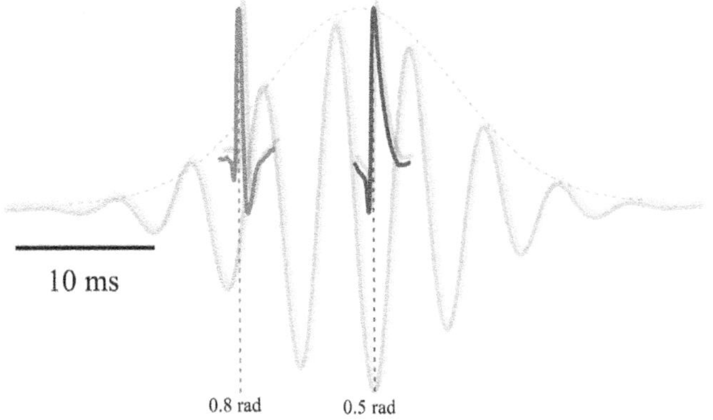

FIGURE 9.2 **Temporal relationship of putative interneurons and pyramidal cells to ripples recorded from the human hippocampus.** This figure summarizes the findings from Ref. 25 that reported the spiking relationship of putative interneurons (red) and pyramidal cells (blue) to ripple oscillations (green). This schematic highlights the burst-like appearance of ripples, which are temporally limited and have a clear peak in amplitude (the gray dotted line represents the amplitude envelope of the ripple). The peak in amplitude corresponds to the time when pyramidal cells are most likely to fire, whereas the interneurons are more like to fire before pyramidal cells earlier in the ripple cycle. In relation to when in the cycle cells will fire, pyramidal cells are more likely to discharge at the trough of the ripple, whereas interneurons discharge approximately 0.5 ms later. The spikes are not on the same time base as the ripple, to demonstrate their waveforms. (The figure is reproduced in color section.)

been suggested that it represents a surrogate measure of population spiking.[30,31] However, quite to the contrary, it has also been argued that such HFOs are generated by synchronous pyramidal cell firing.[16] That HFOs appear to be band-limited events suggests that they are unlikely to be generated by multiunit activity, as power changes are limited to frequencies below 200 Hz.[16] The study by Le Van Quyen et al.[25] highlights the temporal ordering of putative pyramidal cells and interneurons in the generation of ripples in the hippocampi of patients with temporal lobe epilepsy. They showed that interneuronal spiking preceded pyramidal cell spiking. Furthermore, they showed that pyramidal cell spiking was most correlated with the peak amplitude of the ripple event, suggesting a strict ordering of cellular activity in the generation of ripples in the human hippocampus, and that ripples likely represent synchronous pyramidal cell spiking.[25]

Ripple events with frequencies >200 Hz (i.e. fast ripples) are likely pathological, and they may be a sign of abnormal synchronization and a breakdown of inhibitory mechanisms.[23] However, frequency is not everything, as physiological activity has been recorded up to 400 Hz in the sensorimotor cortex of mouse and rat, in response to whisker stimulation.[32] This range of activity falls well within the range of what is usually defined to be the fast-ripple frequency. Thus, whether a specific frequency of activity is pathological likely depends on the structure of the brain from which it is being recorded.[26,27,32,33]

Fast ripples appear to be associated with cellular bursting. This bursting type of behavior has been measured in the hippocampus and cortex, often in epileptogenic tissue, particularly at higher frequencies.[34,35] Using a dense two-dimensional microelectrode array (MEA; $4 \times 4\ mm^2$, 0.4 mm spacing) implanted into the neocortex of epilepsy patients undergoing chronic invasive monitoring, interictal HFOs have been recorded.[36] Most oscillations included fast ripples and were limited to single channels. However, 10% occurred on a larger spatial scale with simultaneous but morphologically distinct detections in multiple channels. These were usually associated with interictal epileptiform discharges, extracellularly measured as spikes or sharp waves. This reflects the multi-scaling quality of bursting activity, occurring mainly in local circuits recorded by one or a few microelectrodes; and when recorded over a larger area, it is measured by a macroelectrode as an interictal spike. Sharp waves in the awake, behaving rat hippocampus are associated with pathological phenomena such as epilepsy and physiological phenomena like slow-wave sleep or behavioral immobility, and they are triggered by population burst of CA3 pyramidal cells.[37]

Bursting activity is also found in other brain regions. Hodaie and colleagues performed single-unit microelectrode recordings in patients who underwent placement of deep-brain stimulation electrodes into the anterior thalamic nucleus for control of intractable epilepsy.[38] Of the 261 neurons recorded, approximately one-half fired in bursts. In 70% of the bursting neurons, the bursts were characterized as low-threshold calcium spike (LTS)-mediated bursts, on the basis of their intraburst firing pattern. In the Parkinsonian globus pallidus internus, Chan and colleagues recorded extracellular single-unit neuronal activity, showing that more than half of the cells were characterized by either aperiodic bursting activity or oscillatory firing, but not both.[39]

There are three questions to consider here: (1) What are the mechanisms underlying the single-unit and local field-measured bursts? (2) How can the bursting in one cell spread to or be coordinated with that of other neurons? And (3) how can cellular bursting influence local and widely spread network activity?

MECHANISMS UNDERLYING THE SINGLE-UNIT AND LOCAL FIELD POTENTIAL–MEASURED BURSTS

Question 1 is addressed by the use of intracellular or whole-cell recordings coupled with local electrical field (extracellular) recordings, which permit study of the underlying ionic and synaptic mechanisms associated with bursting. In many brain areas, there are intrinsically bursting neurons that play physiological roles, and each of these bursting neurons is driven and modulated by specific recurrent mechanisms. Since neuronal bursting is by definition a transient increase in spiking frequency, any mechanism that achieves a transient depolarization causing a burst of a few too many spikes will suffice, including intrinsic ionic conductances and pumps, and/or excitatory postsynaptic potentials (EPSPs) (see Figure 9.3 for a summary of mechanisms). These spikes can be mainly sodium spikes but can also include a strong calcium current component, which is usually manifested by wider spikes.

Bursting behavior is found in cortical pyramidal cells[40,41] and in hippocampal pyramidal cells.[3,42] Much work has been done by the group of Yaari on the intrinsic bursting properties of CA1 hippocampal neurons. Downmodulation of muscarinic-sensitive, subthreshold, and non-inactivating K^+ current (KCNQ/M channels) converts the neuronal firing pattern from simple to complex spiking, whereas upmodulation of these channels exerts the opposite effect.[43] This group also showed that perisomatic persistent Na^+ channels drive spike after-depolarizations and associated bursting in adult CA1 pyramidal cells.[44] Another current of interest that can cause neuronal bursting is spike-triggered calcium influx, which inhibits KV7/M channels, thereby enhancing the spike after-depolarization and neuronal bursting.[45]

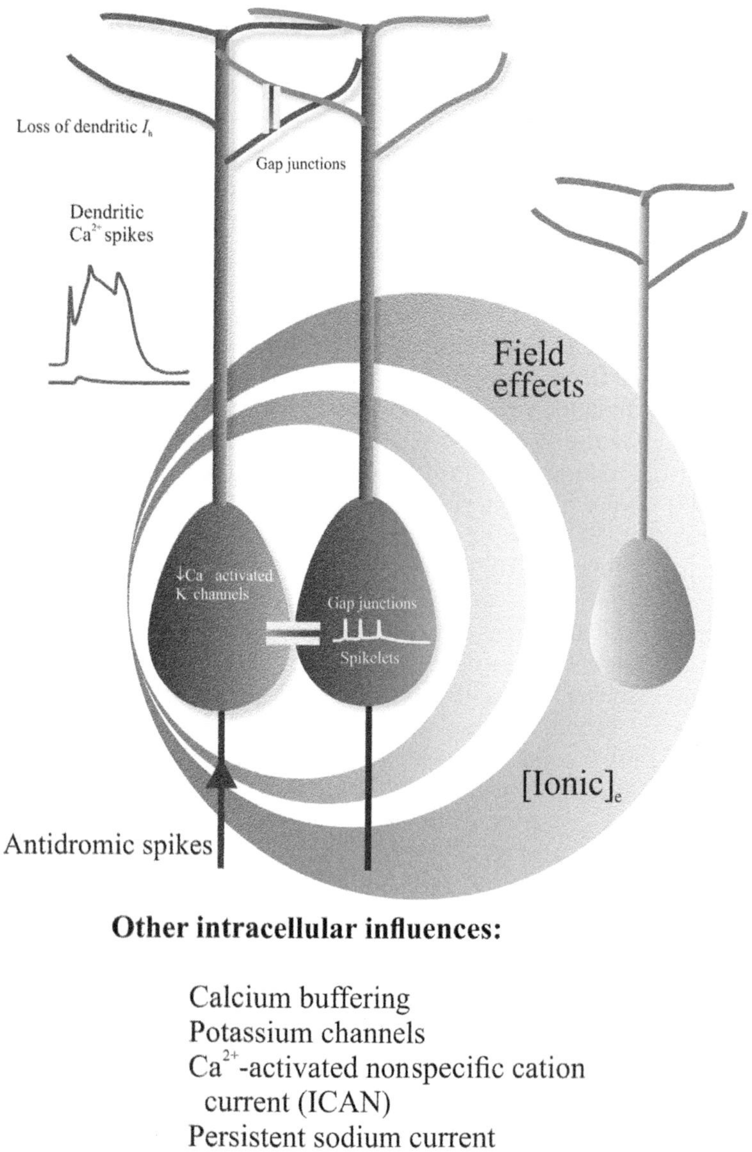

FIGURE 9.3 **Summary of various influences that can generate burst firing evidenced at the cellular level.** Concentration of various extracellular ionic species = [Ionic]$_e$. (For color version of this figure, the reader is referred to the online version of this book.)

Cerebellar Purkinje cells are intrinsically bursting neurons whose spiking and bursting behavior is controlled by the Na^+/K^+ pump.[46] This behavior requires a baseline depolarization and is also strongly modulated by GABAergic input. In the thalamus of several species, thalamocortical neurons show both tonic firing and burst firing. Tonic, Na^+-dependent spiking is initiated when these neurons are depolarized from resting potential levels positive to −55 mV, in both in vivo and in vitro conditions,[47] and this activity persists according to the duration of the membrane depolarization. In contrast, at membrane potential levels negative to −60 mV, such as occurs during slow-wave sleep, de-inactivation of a Ca^{2+} conductance produces, on depolarization, an inward current through T-type Ca^{2+} channels (Cav3.1−3.3), which, if sufficiently large, generates regenerative and Ca^{2+}-dependent spikes, on top of which are activated high-frequency bursts of Na^+ action potentials. In the presence of a Na^+ channel blocker (e.g. tetrodotoxin), the Cav3 conductance is sufficiently large to generate LTSs. When the cells are maintained at a hyperpolarized level, an intrinsic rhythmicity at 2−4 Hz becomes apparent, generated by Ca^{2+} current-based depolarizations and resulting in single or short bursts of spikes, followed by a hyperpolarization and a rapid repolarization before the next burst. This cycle is generated by a combination of Cav3.1−3.3 and I_h cationic currents. This cycle is intimately involved in the mechanisms of sleep.

One of the key components in the respiratory cycle is the pre-Bötzinger complex in the ventrolateral medulla, which, if inactivated, blocks respiratory activity.[48] The autonomous pacemaker activity within respiratory neurons is due to two types of inward currents, the persistent sodium current (I_{NaP}) and the calcium-activated nonspecific cation current (ICAN), which generate intrinsic spiking and bursting activity. These intrinsic membrane currents amplify as well as activate synaptic mechanisms that are critical for the initiation and maintenance of inspiratory activity.

The neuronal bursting mode can play a significant role in information processing. For example, Khosravi-Hashemi and colleagues, recording from and modeling midbrain electrosensory neurons, found that either bursts or isolated spikes could be selectively elicited when the same object moved in opposite directions.[49]

Buzsaki and coworkers discussed the effects of bursting on synaptic plasticity and cell-firing behavior.[50] In in vivo hippocampal recordings, firing rates of individual neurons are relatively constant in an unchanging environment, but they can change in a novel environment. The same group showed a "competition" between single spikes and spike bursts in the in vivo hippocampus and postulated a role for burst discharges in synaptic plasticity. Once a weak input becomes suprathreshold (thereby triggering a spike) by the "teaching" effect of an afferent burst, the consequent reduction of Na^+ channel availability (as a result of the action potential) will reduce the ability of strong inputs to induce a burst. Buzsaki proposed that "the single spike versus burst competition represents a homeostatic regulatory mechanism to maintain synaptic strength and, consequently, firing rate in pyramidal cells."[50]

Afferent bursts can affect their postsynaptic targets as suggested here, or an intrinsic burst in a neuron can provide a feedback signal to the synapses impinging on that neuron. For example, spike bursts cause supralinear summation of EPSPs at pyramidal−pyramidal synapses and pyramidal−interneuron synapses, and they discharge postsynaptic targets more reliably than the same number of single spikes separated by longer intervals.[51] In contrast to individual spikes, bursts can activate postsynaptic *N*-methyl-D-aspartate (NMDA) receptors.[52] Bursts influence synaptic plasticity, but whether this is due to bursting of synaptic afferents to a neuron with postsynaptic modifications, or retrograde effects of a bursting neuron on presynaptic terminals, is still not entirely clear.

Back-propagating action potentials generating neuronal bursting have been proposed to play an important role in neuronal plasticity.[53−55] Sodium-dependent spikes initiated in the axon spread back in a "retrograde" direction into the dendrites, where they become broadened because of an increasing activation of dendritic calcium conductance (thereby creating Ca^{2+} spikes), which increases the local intracellular dendritic calcium concentration.

These Ca^{2+} spikes can then trigger a burst of somatic Na^+-dependent spikes,[56−58] which together with concurrent synaptic depolarization (often in the form of afferent excitatory EPSP bursts) can lead to the induction of long-term potentiation. Action potential−evoked Ca^{2+} spikes demonstrate a cell type−specific profile dependent on that neuronal type's array of voltage-sensitive dendritic Ca^{2+} channels and endogenous buffer capacities, such as those measured in two types of hippocampal inhibitory neurons.[59] In both of these interneuronal types, it was shown that the back-propagating action potential−evoked Ca^{2+} transients summated efficiently during theta-like bursting and were associated with the induction of long-term potentiation at inhibitory synapses onto these neurons.

A subset of CA1 hippocampal neurons can be coupled into transient ensembles by coherent HFOs within sharp-wave ripple complexes (SPW-Rs), which may underlie cognitive functions.[60] These neurons, in contrast to the majority of surrounding silent neurons, fire ectopic action potentials initiated in distal axonal regions and propagate antidromically to the cell body.

This activity is dependent upon $GABA_A$-mediated axonal depolarization and electronic coupling. Facilitation of spontaneous SPW-Rs in hippocampal slices or electrical stimulation of axons reduced synaptic strength, whereas low-level synaptic stimulation delivered after antidromic firing triggered a long-lasting increase in synaptic strength.[61]

Brief afferent synaptic bursting has also been shown to make "unreliable synapses reliable".[52] It is thought that bursts facilitate transmitter release, which in many central mammalian synapses is inconsistently triggered by a single afferent presynaptic action potential. Brief afferent bursts are implicated in synaptic plasticity and information processing. Prolonged bursting, be it presynaptic or postsynaptic in origin, may be a more pathological process that is particularly present in brain hyperexcitability and seizures.

The examples given here, in physiological settings, focus mainly on question 1: What are the mechanisms underlying the single-unit and local field-measured bursts? Many cellular mechanisms for triggering burst behavior in neurons are described, although there are several other mechanisms not mentioned in this chapter because of space constraints.

Burst Propagation and the Network Coordination

We shall now move on to the next level of enquiry, which was embodied in question 2: How can the bursting in one cell spread to or be coordinated with that of other neurons? Here, we will consider synaptic activity, electronic mechanisms (gap junctions), and ephaptic (field effects) and ionic influences as mechanisms that participate in locally measured bursting and oscillatory field activity (summarized in Figure 9.3). This is most commonly studied in the context of seizures, which is the focus of this section.

NEURONAL BURSTING: SEIZURES

On this topic, we are also dealing with a large literature, since neuronal bursting is thought to underlie much of the electrographically measured activity related to both interictal and ictal activity. Mechanisms of seizure-related bursting have been reviewed by Avoli and colleagues.[62] A cross-over between physiological and pathological bursting is the case with SPW-Rs; these are implicated in physiological memory and pathophysiological seizure mechanisms. Behrens and coworkers showed in vitro that in the hippocampal CA3 region, stimuli that induce long-term potentiation,[63] thought by many to be a marker of memory mechanisms, can also generate SPW-Rs, often associated with seizure activity. These SPW-Rs were a manifestation of CA3 burst firing and were dependent upon glutamatergic transmission and gap junctional communication. Our group has demonstrated that low calcium-induced bursting activity is associated with increased gap junctional communication between CA1 pyramidal neurons in vitro.[64] Furthermore, during this calcium-free-induced field burst activity, intracellularly measured coupling potentials in CA1 neurons, called spikelets, were demonstrated.[65] Spikelet amplitudes were unaffected by changes in the neuronal membrane potential. Their pattern of occurrence was indistinguishable from the bursting patterns of action potential firing in these cells under low calcium perfusion, suggesting that they reflected neighboring cell activity.[65] Their presence was eliminated without abolishing spike activity during later perfusion of the hippocampal slice with NH_4Cl, which is associated with intracellular acidification, known to close gap junctional communication.[64] We concluded that these spikelets could have been generated by resistive current flowing through gap junctions, with a superimposed capacitive component. However, later modeling experiments suggested that the in vitro measured spikelets were more likely a manifestation of the simultaneous electric field effects from several local cells whose action potential firing is synchronized.[66] Locally generated ephaptic effects from a locally active and synchronized group or cluster of cells onto interdigitated or adjacent quiescent neurons are certainly important in further synchronizing and also spreading bursting activity.[67,68]

Gap junctional communication is now well recognized as playing a role in the neuronal synchrony associated with bursting activity during seizures.[68,69] More recently, an important role for glial gap junctional communication has also been hypothesized in generating the bursting activity seen with seizures (see reviews by Carlen and Steinhauser and colleagues in Refs 70,71). In several models of epilepsy, enhanced neuronal bursting has been found. Yaari and colleagues showed in rats that after a single episode of status epilepticus, induced by the convulsant pilocarpine, there was upregulation of a Ni^{2+}- and amiloride-sensitive T-type Ca^{2+} current (I(CaT)), which plays a critical role in generating neuronal bursts.[72] It was also shown that the I(CaT) driving bursting is located in the apical dendrites of CA1 neurons. Using the same epilepsy model, they also showed that there was a concomitant increase in the persistent sodium current, which also contributed to intrinsic neuronal bursting.[73] Simeone and coworkers demonstrated that loss of the Kv1.1 potassium channel promoted pathologic sharp waves and HFOs in hippocampal slices in vitro.[74] This corresponds to the findings that some human temporal lobe epilepsies are associated with a functional reduction of the delayed rectifier potassium channel, α-subunit Kv1.1, by either mutation or autoimmune inhibition.

It is important to understand the underlying pathophysiology seen during the transition of a brain region from the interictal state (characterized by isolated EEG spikes) to the ictal state as characterized by repetitive large rhythmic spiking.[26,27] Using human depth recordings, it has been shown that HFOs exhibited increased power during the transition to seizure.[33] These HFOs were localized to the region of primary ictal onset. In vitro, buried in the extracellularly measured recurrent spikes or sharp waves, a statistically significant increasing trend was observed in the subripple (0–100 Hz), ripple (100–200 Hz), and fast-ripple (200–300 Hz) frequency bands during the "preictal" time of transition to seizure from the interictal to the ictal states.[75] Our group[2] has further characterized this transition to seizure, measuring simultaneously the intracellular and extracellular characteristics of interictal, preictal, and ictal bursting (Figure 9.4). In both interneurons and pyramidal CA3 cells, recurrent GABAergic IPSCs predominated interictally and during the early preictal phase, synchronous with extracellularly measured recurrent field potentials (FPs) that under current clamp were associated with postsynaptic bursting behavior. These IPSCs then decreased to zero or reversed polarity by the onset of the higher frequency ictus. However, postsynaptic muscimol-evoked $GABA_A$-mediated currents remained intact. Simultaneously, EPSCs synchronous with the FPs markedly increased to a maximum at the ictal onset. We concluded that the ictal onset was associated with exhaustion of presynaptic release of GABA and unopposed increased glutamatergic responses, as per Figure 9.4. Huberfeld and coworkers also showed that glutamatergic preictal discharges emerged at the transition to seizure in human tissue removed at epilepsy surgery.[77] Figure 9.4 also shows the concomitant rise of extracellular K^+, known to enhance bursting,[78,79] although higher concentrations may terminate an ictus.[80] Just as changes in extracellular K^+ can modify bursting, Boucetta and colleagues showed that fluctuations of extracellular Ca^{2+} during spontaneous network oscillations in vivo changed neuronal firing patterns.[81]

Bursting and Network Activity

We now address Question 3: How can cellular bursting influence local and widely spread network activity? As has been discussed in this chapter, a major determinant of the bursting behavior at the cellular level is intrinsic membrane conductances. However, the brain is highly interconnected,[82,83] follows nonrandom connection patterns,[84–87] and is thus able to generate complex behaviors that "emerge" from this connectedness.[88–90] Such emergent properties are thought to be one of the hallmarks of a complex system, built up from units that, on their own, are unable to generate the activity of the whole[9–11,91] (also see Chapter 30).

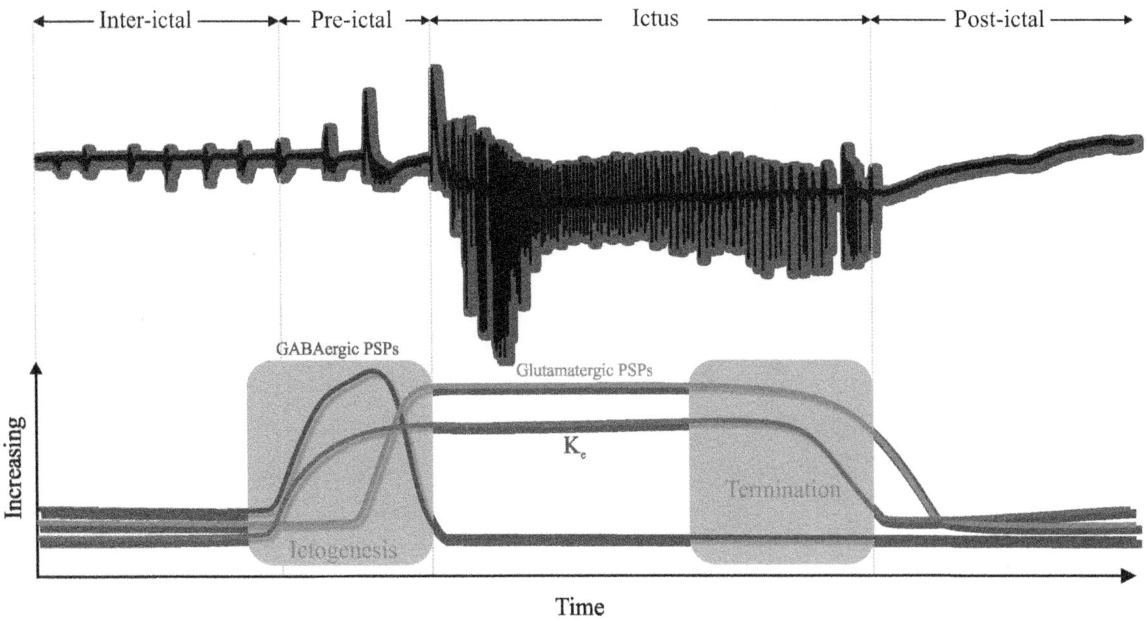

FIGURE 9.4 **Hypothesized time course changes of afferent GABAergic and glutamatergic inputs and extracellular K_e during the interictal, preictal, and ictal states.** Upper traces display a transition to seizure. Bottom traces show the time evolution of the key hypotheses, put onto the longer time base of the uppermost trace. The regions marked "ictogenesis" and "termination" could extend for longer or shorter periods of time. The exact shape and the relative heights of the curves are arbitrary. (For color version of this figure, the reader is referred to the online version of this book.)

One such emergent property is burst generation from a population of cells that themselves are not endowed with bursting abilities. Even at the single-cell level, spiking dynamics can be dissociated from burst generation, suggesting that these are separable phenomena.[92] This dichotomy is supported from modeling studies that have shown that oscillatory burst generation can arise in a model of an avian thalamic nucleus using leaky integrate-and-fire neurons with spike rate adaptation.[93] This model did not include inhibitory activity, suggesting that one could extend this to pathological situations such as epilepsy, which at times has derangements of inhibitory neurotransmission, where bursting could arise in large neuronal populations through feedforward synaptic excitation[93] (Figure 9.5(A)). However, the addition of inhibition to an excitatory system is a critical ingredient in generating the rich repertoire of oscillations[11,96,97] and coherent activity observed within the brain. This coherent activity, often measured as phase coherence,[98] is thought to be the underpinning of distributed processing.[83,98,99] However, inhibition per se does not necessarily engender normal dynamics, as it must exist balanced with excitation at times of physiological activity[100]—too little,[101] too much, and too synchronous[102,103] inhibition can all lead to pathological activity. Specifically in the context of bursting, simulations suggest that even weak inhibition can synchronize networks of bursting neurons that are strongly desynchronized[104] (Figure 9.5(B)). This suggests that, in a system of cells or cells that are prone to bursting or have been rendered prone to bursting by a pathological process, weak inhibition can be strongly synchronizing. In the context of epilepsy, then, intact inhibitory systems with pathological bursting could result in widespread synchronization and epileptiform activity. This is not unlike what is seen in some models of epilepsy[102] (see Chapter 27).

A number of pathological processes are likely involved in the generation of epileptiform activity, not the least of which is exaggerated excitatory synaptic transmission. Such synaptic transmission enhancements (i.e. long-term potentiation and short-term plasticity), when occurring physiologically, are thought to comprise a substrate for permanence in the creation of networks, and as well their dissolution.[105] Bursting activity is thought to strengthen synaptic connections between neurons, either by making synaptic failures less likely[52] or through postsynaptic changes leading to synaptic potentiating[106]; but the role of bursting is different in these two cases. In the first case, it is bursting in the presynaptic neuron that alters release probability, whereas in the second it is postsynaptic bursting that induces short-term plasticity through the release of voltage-dependent blockade of NMDA channels[53,54] and modifications of postsynaptic receptors. In contradistinction to these types of associative synaptic plasticity dependent on ionotropic glutamate receptors, in the hippocampus, theta-burst-patterned activity can induce enhanced bursting in pyramidal cells that is independent of AMPA- or NMDA-type glutamate

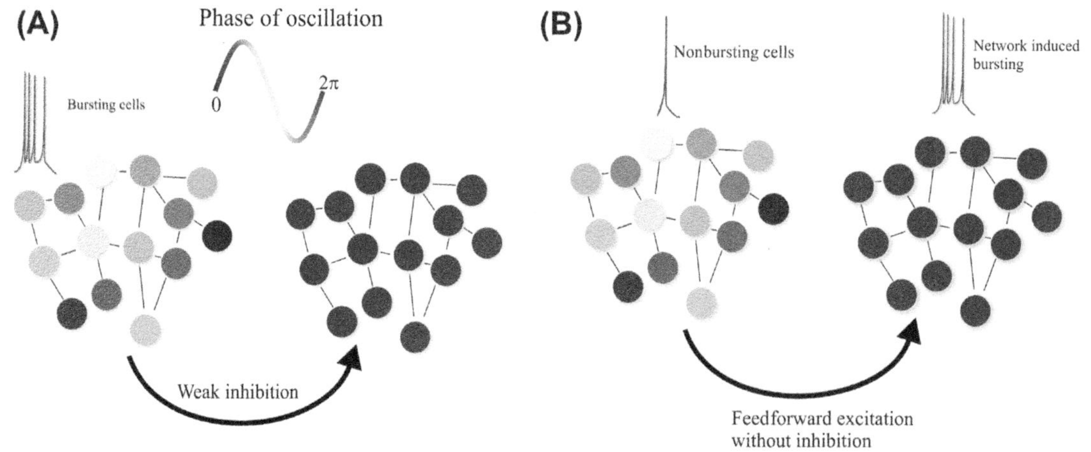

FIGURE 9.5 **Network manifestations of bursting phenomena.**(A) In a population of interconnected but asynchronous cells (the colors depict the phase of the cell's oscillation), a small amount of inhibition can strongly synchronize the population, not unlike that which is seen in the thalamus. The weak inhibition results in de-inactivation of voltage-dependent currents, and thus it provides a synchronizing force to an active population of neurons. From a systems perspective, the fact that the cells are already bursting creates homogeneity in the system, and the inhibition then provides the strong coupling. This can result in a critical state transition[94] from asynchrony to synchrony. Such a mechanism may also underlie how information can be rerouted on a fixed architecture.[95] (B) The organization of a network connection can transform a population of inherently nonbursting cells to bursting through network dynamics. This may be particularly important in the context of epilepsy, where aberrant network interactions could render the population bursting. Invoking the mechanism of (B), preserved inhibition could then strongly synchronize the population if the excitatory interactions are not sufficient to achieve this, resulting in seizures. (The figure is reproduced in color section.)

receptors, but instead requires the activation of metabotropic glutamate receptors and muscarinic acetylcholine receptors.[107] It has also been suggested[107] that such burst-firing plasticity may be involved in state transitions between up and down states of the cortex, which occur coincidently with bursting activity in CA1.[108] In the context of hippocampal function, burst firing from place cells has also been shown to more accurately identify position within a spatial map than single-cell firing taken *in toto*.[109] Thus, bursting may convey more accurate information, albeit in a more compact form. In fact, such a sparse coding scheme, as that arising from bursting within highly correlated firing of neocortical pyramidal cells,[110] may be useful for efficient transmission of information in a noisy environment, and when synaptic failures are frequent.[111]

A prevailing concept, though, to underlie the creation of neuronal assemblies is the communication through coherence (CTC) hypothesis.[112] This hypothesis posits that coherent oscillations between two neuronal populations create windows of excitability that are temporally matched. Communication is enhanced when action potentials arise at peaks of excitation, whereas communication is blocked when action potentials arrive at the nadir of excitability. In this context, the interspike intervals in the presynaptic burst, if matched by postsynaptic membrane potential oscillations, will be more effective at driving a postsynaptic spike. Thus, in this scenario, for ideal communication between two synaptically coupled cells, matching of the precise frequency of spike bursts to postsynaptic subthreshold membrane fluctuations must occur.[113] Such a mechanism has been suggested to be operative up to approximately 100 Hz in a typical cortical pyramidal cell.[113] However, such resonance may be operative at even higher frequencies, with bursting sharpening resonance well up into ripple frequencies (250–450 Hz).[114] Such high-frequency cortical activity has been observed in physiological states in the rat somatosensory cortex in response to vibrissa stimulation,[32] suggesting that such high-frequency resonance may be of physiological import.

Within the CTC framework, one can speak about a number of different frequencies[12] that are thought to create the typical 1/f power spectrum evident in recordings from the awake brain. From a relatively simplistic perspective, specific peaks in the power spectrum or frequency bands likely represent different communication channels. The analogy to a channel may be somewhat strained, since not all frequencies are thought to be involved in long-range communication. For example, it is generally felt that lower frequency oscillations (<30 Hz) are the likely substrate for long-range communication, whereas higher frequencies are more local rhythms.[115,116] Such periodic fluctuations, regardless of frequency, are likely to group cellular spikes at the peaks of excitability. Hence, oscillations per se may be a mechanism for creating burst-like activities in individual cells or groups of neurons (see Figure 9.6). Consider recent evidence from the hippocampus, where theta oscillations were induced optogenetically at theta frequencies.[117] It was shown that such periodic stimulation of the stellate cells of the entorhinal cortex, through a feedforward mechanism, excited interneurons that generated bursts of action potentials at the peaks of excitation (Figure 9.2). It was thus concluded that such CFC where the phase of one oscillation drives the amplitude of another

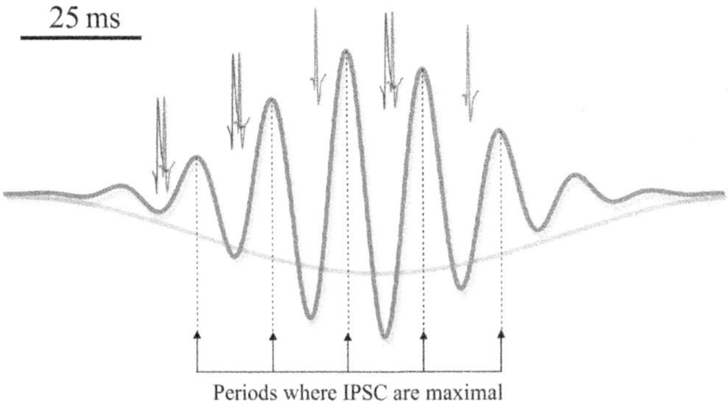

FIGURE 9.6 A feedforward mechanism for bursting and cross-frequency coupling (nesting). A theta oscillation (gray) and associated gamma oscillation (green), with associated spiking of interneurons (red) and excitatory cells (blue). The gamma oscillation is expanded in amplitude to highlight its features relative to the theta oscillation. Within the theta cycle, excitatory cells generate action potentials that excite interneurons. The interneurons feedback onto the excitatory cells, generating inhibitory postsynaptic potentials (IPSPs) in the excitatory cells. These precisely timed IPSPs summate across the population of excitatory cells to generate large sources and hence the strong temporal correlation to the positive-going component of the gamma oscillation. During periods of strong inhibitory cell drive, excitatory cell activity is suppressed. What is not immediately apparent is that each excitatory cell may not discharge on every gamma cycle. However, among a population of excitatory cells, the probability of any one cell discharging is highest at the trough of the theta oscillation, and thus as a population a highly stereotypical envelope of gamma oscillation is generated through this feedback mechanism. The "clock-like" precision of the nested gamma oscillation thus is a population event that is tightly controlled in time by the intrinsic circuitry and temporal organization of cellular discharge. *(Source: This schema has been adapted from Ref. 117.)* Such a "chronocircuit" has been described in the hippocampus as well.[118] This figure also highlights that oscillatory activity; here in this case, the theta oscillation generates periods of increased excitability. Such periods of excitability increase the probability of cells firing at specific times. In the context of the communication through coherence (CTC) hypothesis, such rhythmic gain control is associated with elevated period of neuronal discharge, hence burst generation. Such burst generation, however, need not manifest in individual cells. The burst in fact may be generated by the increased probability of a population of cells increasing their firing rates and/or synchrony during specific time windows, and thus the burst in fact may be a population phenomenon. (The figure is reproduced in color section.)

oscillation, in the context of theta and high-gamma oscillations, is primarily driven by the low-frequency (theta) oscillations. In the context of bursting, then, CFC is an example of how low-frequency oscillations in one population of cells can group action potentials in another population of cells. However, theta to high-gamma CFC is but one example (Figure 9.6). Within the cortex, up and down states that occur at very low frequency are known to regulate HFOs as well.[14] This has been demonstrated in laminar recordings in the human cortex,[119] where, during slow-wave sleep, up states are associated with high-gamma activity that is thought to represent neuronal spiking and postsynaptic potentials.[30,120] In the mouse cortex, using selective optogenetic activation of cortical pyramidal cells, slow oscillations, primarily driven by layer 5 pyramidal cells, induced gamma activity.[121] Such CFC accompanies a number of cognitive activities as well as sleep.[119] Such an oscillatory hierarchy, created by CFC, was initially shown to be operative in the primate brain, where low-frequency oscillations were time locked to the ongoing external stimulus and modulated higher frequency activity.[13] Such CFC is thought to represent some form of neural code, a neural syntax of sorts[122]; the exact meaning of this code, however, remains obscure.

CONCLUSION

In the context of "brain function", what role might bursting play? Is it some type of neural code, or is it just a mechanism for strengthening connections between different cells? An interesting hypothesis has recently been put forward in regard to the layer 5 pyramidal cell,[123] which is able to generate dendritic Ca^{2+} action potentials.[58] The most fascinating aspect of this cell, in addition to its ability to generate dendritic action potentials, is the arrangement of its inputs. It receives nonspecific thalamic inputs as well as feedback and feedforward inputs to its apical tuft and basal dendrites, while specific sensory inputs are received at a more proximal location on the apical dendrite from thalamic inputs terminating in layer 4. It is increasingly accepted that one aspect of brain function involves comparing sensory stimuli to internally generated precepts, in other words, prediction of the sensory stimuli that are received by the brain.[124] Such predictions are thought to be communicated from higher brain regions (feedback), if one describes the brain based on a hierarchical model,[125] to sensory regions, and vice versa (feedforward). A similar feedback and feedforward arrangement can be devised for the thalamus.[125] These brain predictions are then compared to sensory stimuli.[124] Ultimately, such predictive coding has often been thought to require some type of reader or homunculus that compares the prediction and actual sensory stimulus. However, rather interestingly, it has been suggested that the layer 5 pyramidal cell can perform this computation, with the resultant output being burst generation.[123] Burst generation occurs when inputs entering the tuft dendrite arrive at the right time (in relation to the sensory stimulus arriving in layer 4), in the right set of neurons, and of the correct strength. When these criteria are met, a large dendritic calcium action potential is generated, which triggers a burst of Na^{+}-dependent action potentials at the soma—the output to the next processing stage. Thus, in many ways, predictive coding by this schema can be implemented at the level of a single cell, transforming the cerebral cortex into a massively parallel processing unit. The burst of the layer 5 pyramidal cell may thus play a pivotal role in signaling the resultant computations between high-dimensional signals arising from internal predictions and external sensory representations. Thus, bursting may underlie complex behaviors, with mode switching between single spikes to bursting behavior, resulting in significant state changes in the brain and behavioral changes at the level of the entire organism.[20,126,127]

Unanswered Questions

Despite the vast literature on bursting behavior at the single-cell and local-network levels, it is clear that there are many questions left to be explored, some of which are outlined in this section. In fact, we suggest that we have just begun to explore the surface of these complex issues.

1. There continues to be a lack of knowledge regarding the underlying cellular mechanisms of neuronal bursting behavior in many brain regions and the role of various brain pathologies.
2. Drug effects on bursting behavior are poorly understood. For example, the anticonvulsant effects of many clinically used drugs are barely or not at all defined.
3. Linking cellular behavior to locally measured field effects remains problematic. For example, what are the numbers and locations of the cells generating the local fields that reflect bursting behavior? Furthermore, what are the subcellular locations of the current generators of these fields? Do the participating cells change from burst to burst? We suspect that a very dynamic substrate underlies the electrical fields reflecting bursting behavior.
4. At the macro level, how activity in one region spreads and coordinates activity in other regions is still a nascent science. Even more problematic is linking brain rhythms to underlying brain function, which is

surely dependent on more than the measurable electrical activity, and more likely is also tightly linked to underlying biochemical processes. Optogenetics is proving to be a powerful tool in this regard, with the promise of controlling defined cellular targets on a millisecond time scale both in vitro and in vivo.

References

1. Timofeev I, Bazhenov M. Mechanisms and biological role of thalamocortical oscillations. In: Columbus F, ed. *Trends in Chronobiology Research*. Nova Science Publishers; 2005:1–47.
2. Zhang ZJ, Koifman J, Shin DS, Ye H, Zhang L, Valiante TA, Carlen PL. Transition to seizure: ictal discharge is preceded by exhausted presynaptic GABA in the hippocampal CA3 region. *J Neurosci*. 2012;32:2499–2512.
3. Ranck Jr JB. Studies on single neurons in dorsal hippocampal formation and septum in unrestrained rats. I. Behavioral correlates and firing repertoires. *Exp Neurol*. 1973;41(2):461–531.
4. Buzsaki G. How do neurons sense a spike burst? *Neuron*. 2012;73(5):857–859.
5. Steriade M. Impact of network activities on neuronal properties in corticothalamic systems. *J Neurophysiol*. 2001;86(1):1–39.
6. Ascoli GA, Alonso-Nanclares L, Anderson SA, et al. Petilla terminology: nomenclature of features of GABAergic interneurons of the cerebral cortex. *Nat Rev Neurosci*. 2008;9(7): 557–568.
7. Steriade M. Corticothalamic resonance, states of vigilance and mentation. *Neuroscience*. 2000;101(2):243–276.
8. Xing D, Yeh CI, Shapley RM. Spatial spread of the local field potential and its laminar variation in visual cortex. *J Neurosci*. 2009;29(37):11540–11549.
9. Bak P. *How Nature Works: The Science of Self-Organised Criticality*. New York, NY: Copernicus Press; 1996.
10. Prigogine I, Nicolis G. *Self-Organization in Non-equilibrium Systems*. Wiley; 1977.
11. Buzsaki G. *Rhythms of the Brain*. New York: Oxford University Press; 2006.
12. Penttonen M, Buzsaki G. Natural logarithmic relationship between brain oscillators. *Thalamus Relat Syst*. 2003;2:145–152.
13. Lakatos P, Shah AS, Knuth KH, Ulbert I, Karmos G, Schroeder CE. An oscillatory hierarchy controlling neuronal excitability and stimulus processing in the auditory cortex. *J Neurophysiol*. 2005;94(3):1904–1911.
14. Vanhatalo S, Palva JM, Holmes MD, Miller JW, Voipio J, Kaila K. Infraslow oscillations modulate excitability and interictal epileptic activity in the human cortex during sleep. *Proc Natl Acad Sci USA*. 2004;101(14):5053–5057.
15. Canolty RT, Edwards E, Dalal SS, et al. High gamma power is phase-locked to theta oscillations in human neocortex. *Science*. 2006;313(5793):1626–1628.
16. Canolty RT, Knight RT. The functional role of cross-frequency coupling. *Trends Cogn Sci*. 2010;14(11):506–515.
17. Tort AB, Komorowski R, Eichenbaum H, Kopell N. Measuring phase–amplitude coupling between neuronal oscillations of different frequencies. *J Neurophysiol*. 2010;104(2):1195–1210.
18. Tort AB, Kramer MA, Thorn C, et al. Dynamic cross-frequency couplings of local field potential oscillations in rat striatum and hippocampus during performance of a T-maze task. *Proc Natl Acad Sci USA*. 2008;105(51):20517–20522.
19. Deuschl G, Eisen A. Recommendations for the practice of clinical neurophysiology (guidelines of the international federation of clinical neurophysiology). Paper presented at: *Electroencephalogr Clin Neurophysiol Suppl*. 1999.
20. Cooper DC. The significance of action potential bursting in the brain reward circuit. *Neurochem Int*. 2002;41(5):333–340.
21. Tao JX, Baldwin M, Hawes-Ebersole S, Ebersole JS. Cortical substrates of scalp EEG epileptiform discharges. *J Clin Neurophysiol*. 2007;24(2):96–100.
22. Engel Jr J, Bragin A, Staba R, Mody I. High-frequency oscillations: what is normal and what is not? *Epilepsia*. 2009;50(4):598–604.
23. Jefferys JG, Menendez de la Prida L, Wendling F, et al. Mechanisms of physiological and epileptic HFO generation. *Prog Neurobiol*. 2012;98(3):250–264.
24. Uhlhaas PJ, Pipa G, Neuenschwander S, Wibral M, Singer W. A new look at gamma? High- (>60 Hz) gamma-band activity in cortical networks: function, mechanisms and impairment. *Prog Biophys Mol Biol*. 2011;105(1–2):14–28.
25. Le Van Quyen M, Bragin A, Staba R, Crepon B, Wilson CL, Engel Jr J. Cell type-specific firing during ripple oscillations in the hippocampal formation of humans. *J Neurosci*. 2008;28(24): 6104–6110.
26. Bragin A, Engel Jr J, Wilson CL, Fried I, Buzsaki G. High-frequency oscillations in human brain. *Hippocampus*. 1999;9(2): 137–142.
27. Bragin A, Engel Jr J, Wilson CL, Fried I, Mathern GW. Hippocampal and entorhinal cortex high-frequency oscillations (100–500 Hz) in human epileptic brain and in kainic acid–treated rats with chronic seizures. *Epilepsia*. 1999;40(2): 127–137.
28. Crone NE, Miglioretti DL, Gordon B, Lesser RP. Functional mapping of human sensorimotor cortex with electrocorticographic spectral analysis. II. Event-related synchronization in the gamma band. *Brain*. 1998;121(Pt 12):2301–2315.
29. Lachaux JP, Axmacher N, Mormann F, Halgren E, Crone NE. High-frequency neural activity and human cognition: past, present and possible future of intracranial EEG research. *Prog Neurobiol*. 2012;98(3):279–301.
30. Miller KJ. Broadband spectral change: evidence for a macroscale correlate of population firing rate? *J Neurosci*. 2010;30(19): 6477–6479.
31. Manning JR, Jacobs J, Fried I, Kahana MJ. Broadband shifts in local field potential power spectra are correlated with single-neuron spiking in humans. *J Neurosci*. 2009;29(43): 13613–13620.
32. Jones MS, MacDonald KD, Choi B, Dudek FE, Barth DS. Intracellular correlates of fast (>200 Hz) electrical oscillations in rat somatosensory cortex. *J Neurophysiol*. 2000;84(3): 1505–1518.
33. Khosravani H, Mehrotra N, Rigby M, et al. Spatial localization and time-dependant changes of electrographic high frequency oscillations in human temporal lobe epilepsy. *Epilepsia*. 2009;50(4):605–616.
34. Jiruska P, Bragin A. High-frequency activity in experimental and clinical epileptic foci. *Epilepsy Res*. 2011;97(3):300–307.
35. Kohling R, Staley K. Network mechanisms for fast ripple activity in epileptic tissue. *Epilepsy Res*. 2011;97(3):318–323.
36. Schevon CA, Trevelyan AJ, Schroeder CE, Goodman RR, McKhann Jr G, Emerson RG. Spatial characterization of interictal high frequency oscillations in epileptic neocortex. *Brain*. 2009;132(Pt 11):3047–3059.
37. Buzsaki G. Hippocampal sharp waves: their origin and significance. *Brain Res*. 1986;398(2):242–252.
38. Hodaie M, Cordella R, Lozano AM, Wennberg R, Dostrovsky JO. Bursting activity of neurons in the human anterior thalamic nucleus. *Brain Res*. 2006;1115(1):1–8.
39. Chan V, Starr PA, Turner RS. Bursts and oscillations as independent properties of neural activity in the parkinsonian globus pallidus internus. *Neurobiol Dis*. 2011;41(1):2–10.

40. Connors BW, Gutnick MJ. Intrinsic firing patterns of diverse neocortical neurons. *Trends Neurosci.* 1990;13(3):99–104.
41. Gray CM, McCormick DA. Chattering cells: superficial pyramidal neurons contributing to the generation of synchronous oscillations in the visual cortex. *Science.* 1996;274(5284):109–113.
42. Kandel ER, Spencer WA. Electrophysiology of hippocampal neurons. II. After-potentials and repetitive firing. *J Neurophysiol.* 1961;24:243–259.
43. Yue C, Yaari Y. KCNQ/M channels control spike afterdepolarization and burst generation in hippocampal neurons. *J Neurosci.* 2004;24(19):4614–4624.
44. Yue C, Remy S, Su H, Beck H, Yaari Y. Proximal persistent Na^+ channels drive spike afterdepolarizations and associated bursting in adult CA1 pyramidal cells. *J Neurosci.* 2005;25(42):9704–9720.
45. Chen S, Yaari Y. Spike Ca^{2+} influx upmodulates the spike afterdepolarization and bursting via intracellular inhibition of KV7/M channels. *J Physiol.* 2008;586(5):1351–1363.
46. Forrest MD, Wall MJ, Press DA, Feng J. The sodium–potassium pump controls the intrinsic firing of the cerebellar Purkinje neuron. *PLoS One.* 2012;7(12):e51169.
47. Llinas RR, Steriade M. Bursting of thalamic neurons and states of vigilance. *J Neurophysiol.* 2006;95(6):3297–3308.
48. Rekling JC, Feldman JL. PreBotzinger complex and pacemaker neurons: hypothesized site and kernel for respiratory rhythm generation. *Annu Rev Physiol.* 1998;60:385–405.
49. Khosravi-Hashemi N, Chacron MJ. Bursts and isolated spikes code for opposite movement directions in midbrain electrosensory neurons. *PLoS One.* 2012;7(6):e40339.
50. Buzsaki G, Csicsvari J, Dragoi G, Harris K, Henze D, Hirase H. Homeostatic maintenance of neuronal excitability by burst discharges in vivo. *Cereb Cortex.* 2002;12(9):893–899.
51. Thomson AM. Facilitation, augmentation and potentiation at central synapses. *Trends Neurosci.* 2000;23(7):305–312.
52. Lisman JE. Bursts as a unit of neural information: making unreliable synapses reliable. *Trends Neurosci.* 1997;20(1):38–43.
53. Johnston D, Williams S, Jaffe D, Gray R. NMDA-receptor-independent long-term potentiation. *Annu Rev Physiol.* 1992;54:489–505.
54. Spruston N. Pyramidal neurons: dendritic structure and synaptic integration. *Nat Rev Neurosci.* 2008;9(3):206–221.
55. Johnston D, Christie BR, Frick A, et al. Active dendrites, potassium channels and synaptic plasticity. *Philos Trans R Soc Lond B Biol Sci.* 2003;358(1432):667–674.
56. Wong RK, Prince DA, Basbaum AI. Intradendritic recordings from hippocampal neurons. *Proc Natl Acad Sci USA.* 1979; 76(2):986–990.
57. Larkum ME, Nevian T, Sandler M, Polsky A, Schiller J. Synaptic integration in tuft dendrites of layer 5 pyramidal neurons: a new unifying principle. *Science.* 2009;325(5941):756–760.
58. Larkum ME, Zhu JJ, Sakmann B. A new cellular mechanism for coupling inputs arriving at different cortical layers. *Nature.* 1999;398(6725):338–341.
59. Evstratova A, Chamberland S, Topolnik L. Cell type-specific and activity-dependent dynamics of action potential-evoked Ca^{2+} signals in dendrites of hippocampal inhibitory interneurons. *J Physiol.* 2011;589(Pt 8):1957–1977.
60. Bahner F, Weiss EK, Birke G, et al. Cellular correlate of assembly formation in oscillating hippocampal networks in vitro. *Proc Natl Acad Sci USA.* 2011;108(35):E607–E616.
61. Bukalo O, Campanac E, Hoffman DA, Fields RD. Synaptic plasticity by antidromic firing during hippocampal network oscillations. *Proc Natl Acad Sci USA.* 2013;110(13):5175–5180.
62. Avoli M, Louvel J, Pumain R, Kohling R. Cellular and molecular mechanisms of epilepsy in the human brain. *Prog Neurobiol.* 2005;77(3):166–200.
63. Behrens CJ, van den Boom LP, de Hoz L, Friedman A, Heinemann U. Induction of sharp wave-ripple complexes in vitro and reorganization of hippocampal networks. *Nat Neurosci.* 2005;8(11):1560–1567.
64. Perez-Velazquez JL, Valiante TA, Carlen PL. Modulation of gap junctional mechanisms during calcium-free induced field burst activity: a possible role for electronic coupling in epileptogenesis. *J Neurosci.* 1994;14(7):4308–4317.
65. Valiante TA, Perez Velazquez JL, Jahromi SS, Carlen PL. Coupling potentials in CA1 neurons during calcium-free-induced field burst activity. *J Neurosci.* 1995;15(10):6946–6956.
66. Vigmond EJ, Perez Velazquez JL, Valiante TA, Bardakjian BL, Carlen PL. Mechanisms of electrical coupling between pyramidal cells. *J Neurophysiol.* 1997;78(6):3107–3116.
67. Jefferys JG. Nonsynaptic modulation of neuronal activity in the brain: electric currents and extracellular ions. *Physiol Rev.* 1995;75(4):689–723.
68. Perez Velazquez JL, Carlen PL. Gap junctions, synchrony and seizures. *Trends Neurosci.* 2000;23(2):68–74.
69. Carlen PL, Skinner F, Zhang L, Naus C, Kushnir M, Perez Velazquez JL. The role of gap junctions in seizures. *Brain Res Brain Res Rev.* 2000;32(1):235–241.
70. Carlen PL. Curious and contradictory roles of glial connexins and pannexins in epilepsy. *Brain Res.* 2012;1487:54–60.
71. Steinhauser C, Seifert G, Bedner P. Astrocyte dysfunction in temporal lobe epilepsy: K^+ channels and gap junction coupling. *Glia.* 2012;60(8):1192–1202.
72. Yaari Y, Yue C, Su H. Recruitment of apical dendritic T-type Ca^{2+} channels by backpropagating spikes underlies de novo intrinsic bursting in hippocampal epileptogenesis. *J Physiol.* 15, 2007;580(Pt 2):435–450.
73. Chen S, Su H, Yue C, et al. An increase in persistent sodium current contributes to intrinsic neuronal bursting after status epilepticus. *J Neurophysiol.* 2011;105(1):117–129.
74. Simeone TA, Simeone KA, Samson KK, Kim do Y, Rho JM. Loss of the Kv1.1 potassium channel promotes pathologic sharp waves and high frequency oscillations in in vitro hippocampal slices. *Neurobiol Dis.* 2013;54:68–81.
75. Khosravani H, Pinnegar CR, Mitchell JR, Bardakjian BL, Federico P, Carlen PL. Increased high-frequency oscillations precede in vitro low-Mg seizures. *Epilepsia.* 2005;46(8):1188–1197.
76. Zhang ZJ, Valiante TA, Carlen PL. Transition to seizure: from "macro"- to "micro"-mysteries. *Epilepsy Res.* 2011;97(3):290–299.
77. Huberfeld G, Menendez de la Prida L, Pallud J, et al. Glutamatergic pre-ictal discharges emerge at the transition to seizure in human epilepsy. *Nat Neurosci.* 2011;14(5):627–634.
78. Shin DS, Yu W, Fawcett A, Carlen PL. Characterizing the persistent CA3 interneuronal spiking activity in elevated extracellular potassium in the young rat hippocampus. *Brain Res.* 2010;1331:39–50.
79. Traynelis SF, Dingledine R. Potassium-induced spontaneous electrographic seizures in the rat hippocampal slice. *J Neurophysiol.* 1988;59(1):259–276.
80. Bragin A, Penttonen M, Buzsaki G. Termination of epileptic afterdischarge in the hippocampus. *J Neurosci.* 1997;17(7): 2567–2579.
81. Boucetta S, Crochet S, Chauvette S, Seigneur J, Timofeev I. Extracellular Ca^{2+} fluctuations in vivo affect afterhyperpolarization potential and modify firing patterns of neocortical neurons. *Exp Neurol.* 2012.
82. Crick F, Koch C. A framework for consciousness. *Nat Neurosci.* 2003;6(2):119–126.
83. Varela F, Lachaux JP, Rodriguez E, Martinerie J. The brainweb: phase synchronization and large-scale integration. *Nat Rev Neurosci.* 2001;2(4):229–239.

84. Perin R, Berger TK, Markram H. A synaptic organizing principle for cortical neuronal groups. *Proc Natl Acad Sci USA.* 2011;108(13):5419–5424.
85. Perin R, Telefont M, Markram H. Computing the size and number of neuronal clusters in local circuits. *Front Neuroanat.* 2013;7:1.
86. Sporns O. Network attributes for segregation and integration in the human brain. *Curr Opin Neurobiol.* 2013.
87. Song S, Sjostrom PJ, Reigl M, Nelson S, Chklovskii DB. Highly nonrandom features of synaptic connectivity in local cortical circuits. *PLoS Biol.* 2005;3(3):e68.
88. Honey CJ, Kotter R, Breakspear M, Sporns O. Network structure of cerebral cortex shapes functional connectivity on multiple time scales. *Proc Natl Acad Sci USA.* 2007;104(24): 10240–10245.
89. Izhikevich EM. Polychronization: computation with spikes. *Neural Comput.* 2006;18(2):245–282.
90. Eliasmith C, Stewart TC, Choo X, et al. A large-scale model of the functioning brain. *Science.* 2012;338(6111):1202–1205.
91. Hopfield JJ. Neural networks and physical systems with emergent collective computational abilities. *Proc Natl Acad Sci USA.* 1982;79(8):2554–2558.
92. Nowotny T, Rabinovich MI. Dynamical origin of independent spiking and bursting activity in neural microcircuits. *Phys Rev Lett.* 2007;98(12):128106.
93. Shao J, Lai D, Meyer U, Luksch H, Wessel R. Generating oscillatory bursts from a network of regular spiking neurons without inhibition. *J Comput Neurosci.* 2009;27(3):591–606.
94. Scheffer M, Carpenter SR, Lenton TM, et al. Anticipating critical transitions. *Science.* 2012;338(6105):344–348.
95. Battaglia D, Witt A, Wolf F, Geisel T. Dynamic effective connectivity of inter-areal brain circuits. *PLoS Comput Biol.* 2012;8(3): e1002438.
96. Atallah BV, Scanziani M. Instantaneous modulation of gamma oscillation frequency by balancing excitation with inhibition. *Neuron.* 2009;62(4):566–577.
97. Isaacson JS, Scanziani M. How inhibition shapes cortical activity. *Neuron.* 2011;72(2):231–243.
98. Fell J, Axmacher N. The role of phase synchronization in memory processes. *Nat Rev Neurosci.* 2011;12(2):105–118.
99. Siegel M, Donner TH, Engel AK. Spectral fingerprints of large-scale neuronal interactions. *Nat Rev Neurosci.* 2012;13(2): 121–134.
100. Salinas E, Sejnowski TJ. Correlated neuronal activity and the flow of neural information. *Nat Rev Neurosci.* 2001;2(8):539–550.
101. Noebels JL, Avoli M, Rogawski MA. *Jasper's Basic Mechanisms of the Epilepsies [Internet].* 4th ed. Bethesda, MD: National Center for Biotechnology Information (US); 2012.
102. Avoli M, de Curtis M. GABAergic synchronization in the limbic system and its role in the generation of epileptiform activity. *Prog Neurobiol.* 2011;95(2):104–132.
103. Beenhakker MP, Huguenard JR. Neurons that fire together also conspire together: is normal sleep circuitry hijacked to generate epilepsy? *Neuron.* 2009;62(5):612–632.
104. Belykh I, Shilnikov A. When weak inhibition synchronizes strongly desynchronizing networks of bursting neurons. *Phys Rev Lett.* 2008;101(7):078102.
105. Lubenov EV, Siapas AG. Decoupling through synchrony in neuronal circuits with propagation delays. *Neuron.* 2008;58(1):118–131.
106. Markram H, Lubke J, Frotscher M, Sakmann B. Regulation of synaptic efficacy by coincidence of postsynaptic APs and EPSPs. *Science.* 1997;275(5297):213–215.
107. Moore SJ, Cooper DC, Spruston N. Plasticity of burst firing induced by synergistic activation of metabotropic glutamate and acetylcholine receptors. *Neuron.* 2009;61(2):287–300.
108. Battaglia FP, Sutherland GR, McNaughton BL. Hippocampal sharp wave bursts coincide with neocortical "up-state" transitions. *Learn Mem.* 2004;11(6):697–704.
109. Muller RU, Kubie JL, Ranck Jr JB. Spatial firing patterns of hippocampal complex-spike cells in a fixed environment. *J Neurosci.* 1987;7(7):1935–1950.
110. Ohiorhenuan IE, Mechler F, Purpura KP, Schmid AM, Hu Q, Victor JD. Sparse coding and high-order correlations in fine-scale cortical networks. *Nature.* 2010;466(7306):617–621.
111. Stevens CF, Wang Y. Facilitation and depression at single central synapses. *Neuron.* 1995;14(4):795–802.
112. Fries P. A mechanism for cognitive dynamics: neuronal communication through neuronal coherence. *Trends Cogn Sci.* 2005;9(10):474–480.
113. Izhikevich EM, Desai NS, Walcott EC, Hoppensteadt FC. Bursts as a unit of neural information: selective communication via resonance. *Trends Neurosci.* 2003;26(3):161–167.
114. Higgs MH, Spain WJ. Conditional bursting enhances resonant firing in neocortical layer 2–3 pyramidal neurons. *J Neurosci.* 2009;29(5):1285–1299.
115. Kopell N, Ermentrout GB, Whittington MA, Traub RD. Gamma rhythms and beta rhythms have different synchronization properties. *Proc Natl Acad Sci USA.* 2000;97(4): 1867–1872.
116. von Stein A, Chiang C, Konig P. Top-down processing mediated by interareal synchronization. *Proc Natl Acad Sci USA.* 2000;97(26):14748–14753.
117. Pastoll H, Solanka L, van Rossum MC, Nolan MF. Feedback inhibition enables theta-nested gamma oscillations and grid firing fields. *Neuron.* 2013;77(1):141–154.
118. Varga C, Golshani P, Soltesz I. Frequency-invariant temporal ordering of interneuronal discharges during hippocampal oscillations in awake mice. *Proc Natl Acad Sci USA.* 2012;109(40):E2726–E2734.
119. Csercsa R, Dombovari B, Fabo D, et al. Laminar analysis of slow wave activity in humans. *Brain.* 2010;133(9):2814–2829.
120. Ray S, Crone NE, Niebur E, Franaszczuk PJ, Hsiao SS. Neural correlates of high-gamma oscillations (60–200 Hz) in macaque local field potentials and their potential implications in electrocorticography. *J Neurosci.* 2008;28(45):11526–11536.
121. Beltramo R, D'Urso G, Dal Maschio M, et al. Layer-specific excitatory circuits differentially control recurrent network dynamics in the neocortex. *Nat Neurosci.* 2013;16(2):227–234.
122. Buzsaki G. Neural syntax: cell assemblies, synapsembles, and readers. *Neuron.* 2011;68(3):362–385.
123. Larkum M. A cellular mechanism for cortical associations: an organizing principle for the cerebral cortex. *Trends Neurosci.* 2013;36(3):141–151.
124. Bastos AM, Usrey WM, Adams RA, Mangun GR, Fries P, Friston KJ. Canonical microcircuits for predictive coding. *Neuron.* 2012;76(4):695–711.
125. Felleman DJ, Van Essen DC. Distributed hierarchical processing in the primate cerebral cortex. *Cereb Cortex.* 1991;1(1):1–47.
126. Deemyad T, Maler L, Chacron MJ. Inhibition of SK and M channel-mediated currents by 5-HT enables parallel processing by bursts and isolated spikes. *J Neurophysiol.* 2011;105(3):1276–1294.
127. Xu W, Morishita W, Buckmaster PS, Pang ZP, Malenka RC, Sudhof TC. Distinct neuronal coding schemes in memory revealed by selective erasure of fast synchronous synaptic transmission. *Neuron.* 2012;73(5):990–1001.

CHAPTER

10

Network Control Mechanisms—Cellular Milieu

Victor V. Uteshev [1,2], *Alexander G. Gusev* [2,3], *Evgeny A. Sametsky* [2]

[1]Department of Pharmacology and Neuroscience, University of North Texas Health Science Center, Fort Worth, TX, USA, [2]Department of Pharmacology, Southern Illinois University School of Medicine, Springfield, IL, USA, [3]Institute of Neuroscience, University of Oregon, Eugene, OR, USA

INTRODUCTION

Neuronal network function is highly affected by the cellular milieu of neurons in the network, as discussed in Chapter 1. The brain is a highly effective integrator and processor of sensory-motor signaling, which results from the synergistic and coordinated actions of neurons, glial cells, and the external milieu. Brain neurons form functional networks and communicate via chemical and electrical synapses, diffusion transmission (i.e. by releasing neurotransmitters, such as acetylcholine or serotonin, into the extracellular fluid (ECF), where neurotransmitter molecules then progress toward their targets via diffusion[1,2]; see Chapter 8 on volume transmission), and ephaptic transmission (i.e. electrical coupling and potential fields among closely apposed bundles of nerve fibers or neuronal membranes[3]). Therefore, the external milieu supports both neuronal function and interneuronal communication. This chapter discusses the role of the external milieu in the effectiveness of neuronal networks. A variety of biophysical properties of the external milieu contribute to the effectiveness of neuronal network operation, including the presence of specific neuroactive compounds and ions in the ECF, the level of oxygen, the brain temperature, neuronal and glial communication, and the spatiotemporal distribution of inputs.[4,5]

Normal brain function depends on the appropriate interstitial environment, which is separated from the blood by the blood–brain barrier (BBB). Among other functions, the BBB selectively allows hydrophilic compounds into the brain and prevents hydrophobic compounds from entering it, while regulating the transendothelial movement of blood cells, pathogens, and transporting nutrients. For this purpose, endothelial cells exhibit polarized expression of membrane receptors and transporters,[6] whereas an active neurovascular coupling is maintained by tight junctions held by highly specialized endothelial cells, capillary basal lamina, smooth muscle cells, and perivascular astrocytes.[7]

The fluid dynamics in the brain play a vital role in the neuronal network function, with physiologically different compositions of fluid at four levels. At the outermost level, blood is prevented from entering the brain by specialized arrangements at the BBB, as well as at the ventricular ependyma, choroid plexus, and pia mater. This causes permeation of only essential compounds to the cerebrospinal fluid (CSF), and thus ECF, while the entrance of nonessential compounds is blocked. Within the brain parenchyma, the extracellular and intracellular fluids (ICF) contain differential composition of Na^+, K^+, and Ca^{2+} ions vital for nerve conduction.[8] Osmotic homeostasis in the extracellular space (ECS) is facilitated by maintaining a relatively larger volume of the CSF. Ionic composition of the CSF differs from that of plasma, with lower concentrations of Ca^{2+}, K^+, and HCO_3^- and higher concentrations of Mg^{2+} and H^+ in the CSF. Such a difference is maintained by active transport, which is facilitated by a larger number of mitochondria in the endothelial cells of brain capillaries. In the choroid plexus, there is an easy passage of molecules across capillaries, while at the level of the ependyma, nonessential molecules are denied entry. Because of these settings, even excessive changes in the ionic composition of blood plasma have only minor effects on ECF (Figure 10.1); for example, experimental manipulations in the carotid artery (using Ca^{2+}-deficient and Ca^{2+}-rich solutions or hypertonic mannitol solution followed by KCl) did not significantly alter the ionic composition in the ECF of the cortex or hippocampus.[9]

Disintegration of this conditional relationship between blood, CSF, and ECF can be seen in stroke patients, where a clot-caused acute blood flow obstruction produces gross changes in the ECF, triggering depolarization of neurons and astrocytes, neurotransmitter release, and elevation

Neuronal Networks in Brain Function, CNS Disorders, and Therapeutics
http://dx.doi.org/10.1016/B978-0-12-415804-7.00010-1

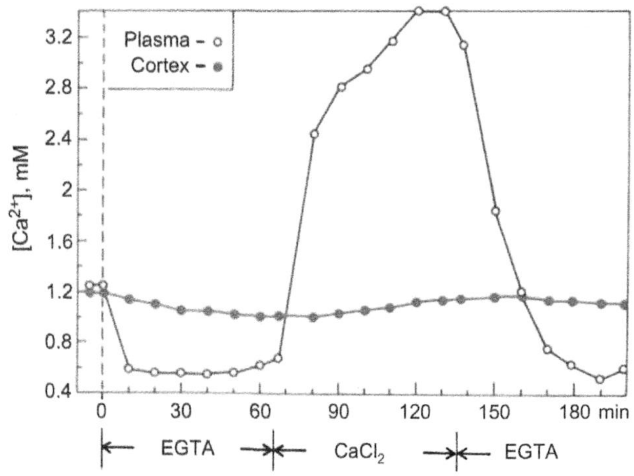

FIGURE 10.1 Effect of acute, severe hypocalcemia and hypercalcemia on the cerebral extracellular Ca^{2+} concentration in a cat.[9] Data from a cat anesthetized with a chloralose–urethane mixture and artificially ventilated. Ca^{2+} in circulating blood was monitored in an extracorporeal arterial loop using an ion-selective electrode in a flow cell. Brain $[Ca^{2+}]_o$ was measured with an ion-selective microelectrode in the neocortex. Blood $[Ca^{2+}]$ was lowered by intravenous infusion of a solution of ethylene glycol tetraacetic acid (EGTA), and it was raised by infusion of $CaCl_2$ solution. *Source: With permission from Refs 9,10.* (For color version of this figure, the reader is referred to the online version of this book.)

in $[K^+]_o$ and $[Ca^{2+}]_i$. The increased permeability of BBB remains one of the major causes of brain damage in a number of neurological conditions such as stroke.[6]

EFFECTS OF THE EXTRACELLULAR IONIC COMPOSITION ON NEURONAL NETWORK ACTIVITY

The ECS represents up to 20% of the total brain volume and provides an essential medium for the transport of nutrients, ions, and oxygen, as the entire vascular system in the brain occupies only about 3% of the brain volume. The ECS is filled with ECF, also called the interstitial fluid, which is in contact with CSF at the ventricles, and both have a similar composition. Diffusion is the predominant means of transporting materials within the ECF.

At sites of high neuronal activity, ECS shrinks by more than 30%. This use-dependent change in the ECS volume could result from the glial response to the focal extracellular K^+ accumulation by a depolarization of the exposed membrane and its propagation along the glial syncytium to sites where the extracellular K^+ concentration has not yet increased, as proposed by Lux.[11] A focal increase in the ECF $[K^+]_o$ increases K^+ influx into glial cells, and as a result, the ECF osmolarity decreases, leading to shrinkage of the ECS volume; whereas at remote sites, K^+ efflux and an increase of the ECS volume are expected.[11]

Ephaptic transmission has been observed in certain central nervous system (CNS) and neuromuscular pathologies such as tinnitus, and is associated with acoustic neuromas,[12] chronically de-enervated muscle,[13] peripheral neuropathy,[14] and cramp.[15] This transmission has also been reported in acutely cut or crushed peripheral nerves,[16] experimental demyelinating disease, and nerve compression, and in the peripheral nervous system of hypocalcemic cats.[3] Moreover, certain geometries of cellular structures (e.g. in the hippocampus) can promote the generation of large extracellular fields that may alter the excitability of neighboring neurons, if they are suitably oriented.[3]

Extracellular ionic composition is sensitive to neuronal activity and plays a vital role in maintaining neuronal network function. The ionic composition of the extracellular milieu contributes to determination of the level of neuronal excitability, ion channel blockade, and synaptic and neuronal activity.[17–21] Under normal physiological conditions, a strong electrochemical gradient exists across the neuronal membrane. In normal ECF, sodium and chloride ion concentrations ($[Na^+]_o$ and $[Cl^-]_o$) are ~140 mM, while the intracellular concentrations of these ions are considerably lower, ~6 mM.[22] The ionic composition of the ECF fluctuates depending on the level of neuronal activity, and the normal equilibrium can be restored but requires energy expenditure. Therefore, a delicate balance in the ionic composition of the external milieu is required for the generation and propagation of action potentials and the regulation of osmotic balance, pH, and neuronal volume.[23,24]

Potassium Ions

Potassium is a major player in the generation of an electrochemical gradient across the neuronal membrane. The concentration of K^+ ions is high ($[K^+]_i$ ~ 140 mM) in the ICF and low ($[K^+]_o$ ~ 3 mM) in the ECF.[22] An increase in $[K^+]_o$ causes depolarization and, thus, increases the excitability of neurons and neurotransmitter release. $[K^+]_o$ is regulated by active transport (i.e. Na^+–K^+ ATPase, K^+–Cl^- cotransporters, and Na^+–K^+–Cl^- transporters) in both neurons and astrocytes; however, astrocytes can take up K^+ ions by diffusion using inward-rectifying K^+ channels.[25]

In the brain, normal $[K^+]_o$ ranges between 2.7 and 3.5 mM, which is lower than in the rest of the body. This has protective significance as substantial increases in $[K^+]_o$ can produce adverse effects.[26] An increase in $[K^+]_o$ may occur during normal or excessive physiological neural activity. For example, visual stimuli can make transient 0.5 mM increments in $[K^+]_o$, and skin tactile stimuli, depending on the severity, can raise $[K^+]_o$ by 0.4–3.0 mM in the spinal cord.[9,27]

Calcium Ions

The $[Ca^{2+}]_o$ is near 1.5 mM, while $[Ca^{2+}]_i$ is >10,000-fold lower.[28] During perinatal development, $[Ca^{2+}]_o$ is 20–30% higher than in adults.[29] Neurons spend ~15% of energy for clearing Ca^{2+}, which can be toxic. The Ca^{2+} ion efflux takes place through high-affinity but low-capacity Ca^{2+}-ATPase pumps as well as low-affinity but high-capacity Na^+-Ca^{2+} exchangers.[30,31] Ca^{2+} ions are required for synaptic neurotransmission because release of synaptic vesicles from presynaptic active zones is Ca^{2+} dependent.[32,33] Ca^{2+} ions also act as intracellular second messengers, initiating cellular apoptosis, cytoprotection, protein phosphorylation, and gene expression. Many normal physiological functions are Ca^{2+} dependent, but an excess of intracellular Ca^{2+} or a lack of the optimal balance between Ca^{2+} entry and clearance may destroy neuronal integrity and cause neuronal death.[34]

There is now good evidence to support the notion that Ca^{2+} ions can act as primary messengers as well. An increased $[Ca^{2+}]_o$ stimulates spontaneous release of glutamate in the neurons.[35] Thus, in hippocampal slices, neurotransmitter release increases when $[Ca^{2+}]_o$ is raised from 1.2 to 1.8 mM and decreases when $[Ca^{2+}]_o$ is lowered to 0.8 mM.[26,36] External cations, particularly divalent ones, attracted by negative membrane surface potential, form a thin, diffuse double ionic layer near the membrane surface that acts as an electric screen reducing the originating surface potential[37] and decrease the Ca^{2+} permeability of ligand-gated ion channels (e.g. *N*-methyl-D-aspartate receptors (NMDARs)).[38] However, at chemical synapses, an increase in $[Ca^{2+}]_o$ facilitates, but an increase in $[Mg^{2+}]$ inhibits, neurotransmitter release.[39]

Magnesium Ions

Intracellular $[Mg^{2+}]$ is typically approximately fourfold higher than $[Mg^{2+}]_o$. This ratio is maintained by ion pumps and intracellular binding sites. Physiological concentrations of Mg^{2+} ions in the ECF (~1 mM) play an important role in the regulation of neurotransmitter release, neuronal excitability, and electrolyte kinetics.[26,40] Mg^{2+} ions block Ca^{2+}-permeable ion channels, and reduce neurotransmitter release and NMDAR activation.[21,41,42] Mg^{2+} ions have been hypothesized to produce antidepressant effects by facilitating serotonergic, adrenergic, and dopaminergic receptor activation.[43] Moreover, Mg^{2+} deficiency may cause apathy, anxiety, and psychosis, as significantly depressed levels of Mg^{2+} are detected in the CSF of individuals with depression and schizophrenia.[44,45]

Chloride Ions

Extracellular $[Cl^-]_o$ is regulated by changes in neuronal permeability to Cl^- ions and active transport, such as $Na^+-K^+-Cl^-$ transporters, K^+-Cl^- cotransporters, and $Cl^--HCO_3^-$ exchangers that maintain electrochemical gradient and, therefore, require consumption of energy.[46] In the normal CSF, $[Cl^-]_o$ is ~130 mM.[47,48] The intracellular concentrations of Cl^- vary among neuronal subtypes depending on the levels of expression of K^+-Cl^- and $Na^+-K^+-2Cl^-$ cotransporters.[49] For example, during embryonic and postnatal development, Cl^--permeable GABA receptor-mediated ion channels excite neurons.[50] These channels become inhibitory upon CNS maturation. However, in the absence or deficiency of these Cl^- transporters, regulation of intracellular Cl^- concentration and conductance becomes impaired.[49]

EFFECTS OF OXYGEN ON NEURONAL ACTIVITY

Oxygen is essential for ATP synthesis and energy metabolism. In the absence of sufficient supplies of oxygen (and glucose), the energy demand of active neurons can no longer be met, and failure of the Na^+/K^+-ATPase pump causes a rapid loss of the neuronal transmembrane electrochemical gradient. As a result, the brain tissues undergo transient spreading (SD) or terminal anoxic (AnD) depolarizations and loss of electrical activity. Although the exact mechanisms responsible for SD and AnD in specific populations of central neurons are not known, increased extracellular levels of glutamate and K^+ ions as well as activation of various voltage-gated (e.g. Na^+, K^+, and Ca^{2+}) and ligand-gated (e.g. NMDAR/mediated) ion channels have been detected and hypothesized to make critical contributions to oxygen and glucose deprivation-induced neuronal injury in ex vivo models of ischemia.[51–55] By contrast, the activation of highly Ca^{2+}-permeable $\alpha 7$ nicotinic acetylcholine receptor (nAChR)-mediated ion channels can be neuroprotective, and these effects may be neuronal-type specific.[56] The exact mechanism of $\alpha 7$ nAChR-mediated neuroprotection is not known but may involve the activation of JAK2/AKT/Bcl2-dependent pathways.[57–59] By contrast, excessive levels of oxygen can be neurotoxic due to increased production of reactive oxygen species.[60] Ex vivo and in vitro studies routinely employ high levels (e.g. 95%) of oxygen and thus may cause oxygen neurotoxicity, excessive neuronal activity, and damage,[60,61] confounding data interpretation. Accordingly, reduced levels of oxygen (e.g. 20–40%) in ex vivo and in vitro preparations have been suggested.[62]

EFFECTS OF OSMOLARITY ON NEURONAL ACTIVITY

Under physiological conditions, ECF osmolarity remains constant on both sides of the BBB. However, pathophysiological changes in osmolarity create an osmotic gradient on either side of the BBB that then permits water movement, leading to either cerebral inflation (osmotic edema) or cerebral dehydration. In the case of cerebral edema, the brain tends to modify the ECF molecular composition to accommodate volume changes. In hypotonic plasma conditions, the brain expels osmotic molecules, such as amino acids, polyols, trimethylamines, and electrolytes, to prevent or reduce edematous conditions, and a reverse situation takes place in hypertonic conditions. Severe osmotic edema in the brain can result from water intoxication, acute hyponatremia, or rapidly changing hyperosmolarity. However, even mild changes, such as moderate hyponatremia, can impair normal brain osmoregulation.[63]

During edematic conditions in the brain, water moves into the ECF, causing brain swelling and elevation of intracranial pressure. The decreased osmolarity of the ECF has been shown to enhance synaptic transmission in vitro[9] and promotes seizures.[64] Hypo-osmolarity has been shown to increase K^+ currents in hippocampal neurons in a selective and neuron-specific manner.[65] Hypo-osmolarity has also been reported to activate (via neuronal swelling) stretch-sensitive or inactivate stretch-inactivated ion channels.[66] Furthermore, NMDAR-mediated Ca^{2+} channels and voltage-activated Ca^{2+} channels in cultured neurons also appear to be sensitive to osmolarity of the ECF.[67] Furosemide (an agent that reduces neuronal swelling) exhibits antiepileptiform activity in vitro and in vivo by nonsynaptic modulation of hippocampal interneuron excitability under the conditions of cell swelling and reduced ECS.[68] By contrast, an elevated osmolarity of the ECF decreases synaptic transmission as well as voltage-gated Na^+, K^+, and Ca^{2+} currents, leading to coma.

EFFECTS OF pH ON NEURONAL ACTIVITY

Neurotransmission and ion channel conductance are affected by extracellular pH. ATP hydrolysis causes acidification of the ECF[69] and promotes activation of pH-sensitive neurons. Over 90% of CNS neurons respond to pH 7 with an inward current, while mild elevations in the ECF pH (pH 7.1–7.2) can excite neurons and increase their spontaneous firing. While alkalosis leads to hyperexcitability, acidosis reduces neuronal excitability. In the brain, a pH drop of ~0.2 could be achieved by the activity-mediated acidification of the ECF.[70] Greater levels of acidification (~0.5) have also been reported in the retina of rabbits under physiological conditions.[71] Among the ligand-gated ion channels, protons inhibit glutamate currents but stimulate GABA currents.[72]

To detect changes in the ECF pH, neurons express specialized acid-sensing channels, which are the proton-gated Na^+ channels capable of detecting $[H^+]_o$ and generating depolarizing currents when extracellular pH drops to 6.9–5.0.[73] These sensors belong to the family of voltage-insensitive, amiloride-sensitive epithelial Na^+ channel–degenerin (ENaC–DEG).[74,75] The intracellular pH in central neurons is slightly more acidic than in the ECF. The ECF in turn is slightly more acidic (pH 7.3, 50 nM $[H^+]$) compared to blood (pH 7.4, 40 nM $[H^+]$).[70,76] CO_2 can freely pass through the BBB, and thus the respiratory alkalosis and acidosis can alter the neuronal activity in both the CNS and the peripheral nervous system (PNS).

EFFECTS OF TEMPERATURE ON NEURONAL ACTIVITY

Neuronal and synaptic properties, such as the resting membrane potential and neuronal input resistance, the frequency of spontaneous firing, the properties of action potential, and the efficacy of synaptic neurotransmission, are sensitive to the brain's temperature. Lowering the brain's temperature produces a larger Ca^{2+} influx in a single action potential of neocortical cells and increases spillover of neurotransmitters in the hippocampus.[77,78] Hypothermia reduces the brain's metabolism, energy, and oxygen utilization; inhibits glutamate while increasing brain-derived neurotrophic factors; and suppresses mitochondrial function. These changes lead to a decline in the production of free radicals and oxidative stress and the inhibition of apoptosis. Swelling and pro-inflammatory mechanisms also are inhibited.[79]

Lowering temperature increases Ca^{2+} influx, reduces Mg^{2+} block of NMDAR channels, and reduces the threshold for synaptic plasticity because a subthreshold tetanus stimulation becomes suprathreshold at lower temperatures, causing neuroplasticity.[80] A slight reduction in the brain temperature (2–3 °C) in ischemic rats resulted in a pronounced neuroprotection, as under these conditions ~60% of the hippocampus completely recovered from ischemia.[81] Hypothermia (~32 °C) has been shown to prevent ischemia-induced cellular mortality in gerbils, and these effects were also linked to the inhibition of Ca^{2+}- and calmodulin-dependent protein kinase-II.[82] Brain cooling has a favorable effect on traumatic brain injury, excitotoxicity, cerebral blood flow and metabolism, nitric oxide production, and apoptosis. In near-term sheep fetuses, brain cooling is effective in reducing the extent of brain injury even when it is initiated up to 5.5 h after brain ischemia.[83] In a randomized controlled trial, Shankaran et al.[83] evaluated the whole-body cooling effect in term infants (first 6–72 h of life) with moderate or severe hypoxic-ischemic encephalopathy. They reported that whole-body hypothermia reduced the risk of death or disability in the subjects.[83] In infants with hypoxic-ischemic encephalopathy, moderate hypothermia is associated with a consistent reduction in death and neurological impairment at 18 months.[84] However, an excessive drop in the ECF temperature (>10 °C) may cause a complete neuronal inactivation.[85] It should be noted that ex vivo and in vitro studies routinely use subphysiological (e.g. room) temperatures; thus, certain corrections for temperature dependence of the observed effects may need to be made for data interpretation.

EFFECTS OF GLIAL CELLS ON NEURONAL ACTIVITY

Glial cells, especially astrocytes, play an essential role in maintaining the ionic composition of the ECF (see Chapter 12 on glia). Astrocytes remove unused neurotransmitter molecules and contribute to setting the ECF pH and focal $[K^+]$.[86–89] Glial cells can provide a temporary storage of K^+ ions.[90] Moreover, a number of transporters for H^+ and HCO_3^- are found on the astrocyte membrane, suggesting that H^+ and HCO_3^- ions can also be stored by astrocytes in a fashion similar to that for K^+ ions. Elevated $[K^+]_i$ depolarizes glial cells and stimulates glial $NaHCO_3$ uptake, resulting in the glial cytoplasmic alkalinization and acidification of ECF.[9] This mechanism allows astrocytes to modulate the ECF pH, and a developmental role of glial cells in generation of the activity-dependent acidic shift has been discussed: the ECF becomes more acidic as the animal matures.[88] Abnormalities in the function of astrocytes are associated with certain neurological disorders such as neuropathic pain, epilepsy, Alzheimer's disease, schizophrenia, and depression.[91]

EXTRACELLULAR IONS AND EX VIVO MODELS OF SEIZURE

There is a strong correlation between the brain's susceptibility to seizures and the ionic composition of the ECF. Seizures lead to marked changes in the ECF's ionic contents, while inadequate (i.e. excessive or deficient) ionic composition of the ECF may cause seizures. Specifically, elevated $[K^+]_o$ is a characteristic feature of epileptic seizures. Active neurons, glial cells, and a damaged BBB may contribute to the elevated $[K^+]_o$ associated with seizures,[92] while elevated $[K^+]_o$ (~10–12 mM) can produce seizure-like activity in the brain tissue ex vivo.[93] In addition to seizure-like activity, elevations in $[K^+]_o$ can also lead to spreading depression.[94] Moreover, 4-aminopyridine (4-AP), a K^+ channel blocker, induces recurrent interictal events and causes epileptiform synchronization and increased transmitter release from inhibitory and excitatory synaptic terminals.[94] Similarly, seizures and spreading depression are associated with a substantial (~0.5 mM) reduction in $[Ca^{2+}]_o$ during interictal epileptiform discharges, up to 1.2 mM during epileptic seizures, and it can decline to 0.08 mM in spreading depression.[95]

In ex vivo and in vitro settings, lowering $[Mg^{2+}]_o$ in artificial ECF generates epileptic-like seizure discharges in hippocampal slices due to a reduced Mg^{2+} block of pre- and postsynaptic voltage- and ligand-gated Ca^{2+} ion channels and decreased membrane surface charge.[21] This low-Mg^{2+} model of seizures is commonly used in experiments testing the effects of antiepileptic drugs[96] in acute hippocampal slices and intact whole hippocampi.[97–100] In individuals with epilepsy, the ECF concentration of Mg^{2+} is lower than in people without epilepsy, and intravenous administration of Mg^{2+} ions leads to seizure suppression.[21] The seizure-like activity induced by low Mg^{2+} in brain slices significantly increases with increased $[K^+]_o$ (3.5–5 mM) because of a depolarizing shift in the resting membrane potential,[21] but the strength of seizures induced by an Mg^{2+}-free ECF can be reversed by $GABA_A$ receptor agonists.[101]

Brain Cooling and Seizures

Lowering temperature suppresses seizures in the chemically induced animal model of epilepsy.[102,103] Hypothermia can also be effective for postanoxic encephalopathy and intracranial pressure reduction. However, it is clinically ineffective in status epilepticus[79] despite promising results obtained in animals.[104]

Spreading Depression and Ionic Homeostasis

Spreading depression is a transient propagation of electrochemical disturbance in the cortex characterized by substantial shifts in the extracellular ionic concentrations of K^+ (elevation), Na^+, Ca^{2+}, and Cl^- (drop) ions[105]; loss of neural activity; and changes in the ionic distribution.[106] Although realistic models of spreading depression have been developed,[107] effective preventive strategies have yet to be found.

Ischemia and Extracellular Milieu

Most central neurons are highly sensitive to hypoxic stress, which may lead to disruption of ionic homeostasis via enhanced K^+ efflux and Na^+, Ca^{2+}, and Cl^- influx,[108] leading to neuronal injury and death. During hypoxia, $[Na^+]_o$ drops sharply from ~140 mM to about ~60 mM in the hippocampus[52,106] and ~40 mM in hypoglossal neurons[109]; while $[Ca^{2+}]_o$ decreases from ~1.5 mM to ~0.5 mM and $[Ca^{2+}]_i$ increases from <100 nM to micromolar levels in hippocampal, cortical, and thalamic neurons.[110] By contrast, $[K^+]_o$ increases slowly in the initial stages of hypoxia and reaches its equilibrium within several minutes. This slow increase is followed by the second fast and large increase in $[K^+]_o$, reaching peak values of 25–100 mM depending on the animal's age, the brain region, and the severity of hypoxic insult. During the recovery phase, $[K^+]_o$ declines rapidly to the pretreatment level with a brief overshoot. These changes

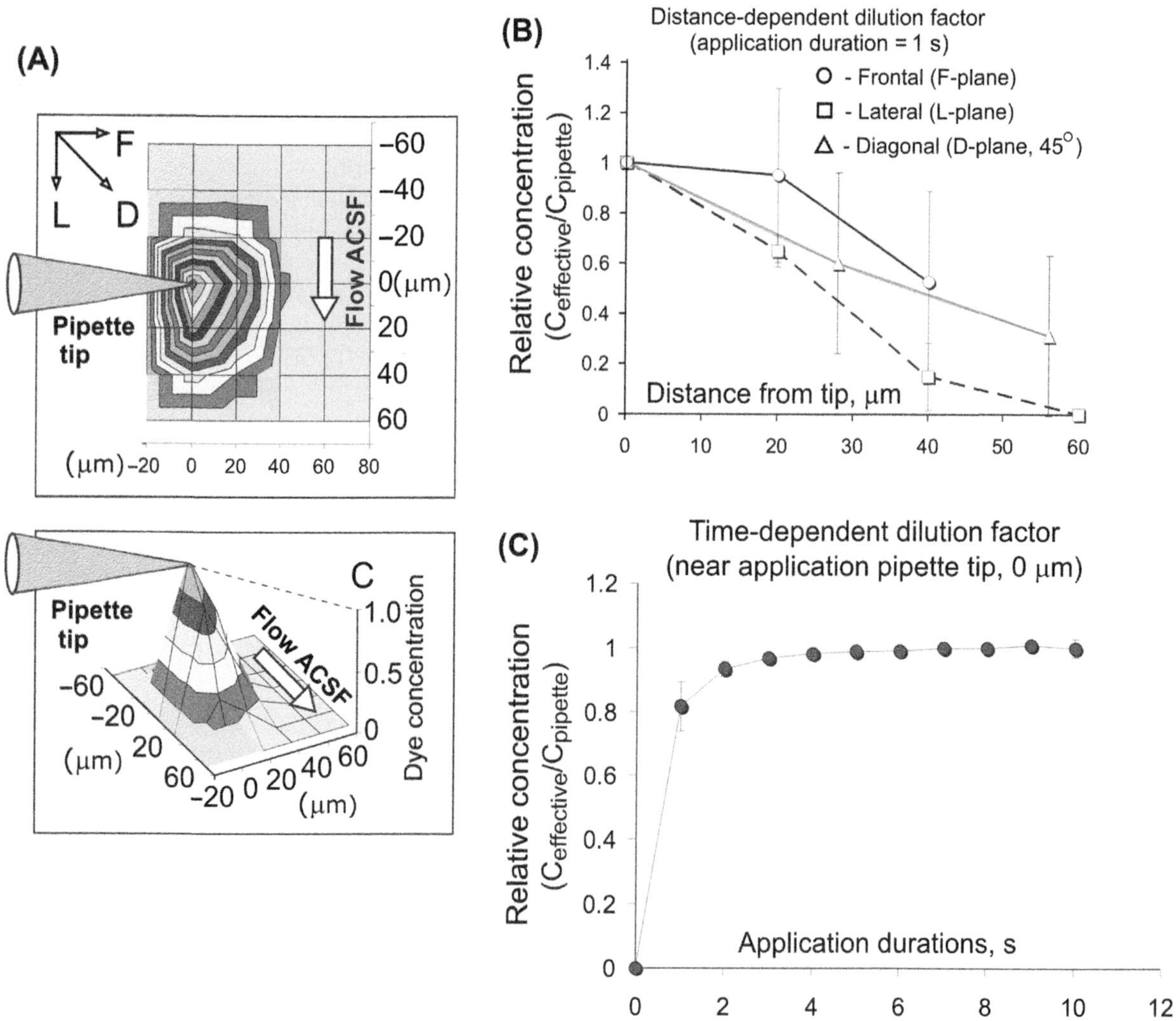

FIGURE 10.2 **Distance and time dependence of drug diffusion in the ECS in acute hypothalamic brain slices.** To model the diffusion of drugs in the ECS of acute brain slices, the distance and time distributions of a fluorescent tracer pressure, applied within the tuberomammillary nucleus of the hypothalamus in acute hypothalamic slices, were investigated. The concentration of the tracer in the vicinity of the application pipette is expected to be somewhat lower than the original concentration of tracer in the application pipette due to diffusion. (A) To evaluate the drug concentration profile during pressure puffs (application pressure: 10 psi), application pipettes (application tip diameter: 0.2 μm) were filled with 50 μM Ca-Green-1 fluorescent dye, and fluorescent intensities were measured in the frontal (F), lateral (L), and diagonal (D) directions at different distances (0, 20, 40, and 60 μm) from the tip of application pipette. The slight asymmetry in the dye concentration profile along the lateral axis is due to the presence of a constant flow of oxygenated artificial cerebrospinal fluid (ACSF) (1 ml/min) within the experimental chamber to keep the brain tissue alive during the experiment. The flow direction is indicated by an open arrow. (B) Evaluation of the dye concentration profiles in the F-, L-, and D- planes. Ratios ($C_{effective}/C_{pipette}$) of fluorescent intensities were detected at various distances from the application tip ($C_{effective}$) and compared to the fluorescent intensity ($C_{pipette}$) detected near the tip during a 1 s puff. Concentrations of dye inside and outside the application pipette were postulated to be proportionate to the detected fluorescent intensities. Distance increments of 20 μm were employed along the F- and L- axes. An increment of $20\sqrt{2}$ μm was employed for the D-axis. (C) The fluorescent intensity corresponding to different puff durations (i.e. 0–10 s) of dye application was recorded near the tip of the application pipette (i.e. 0 μm) and then normalized to the intensity obtained at prolonged application durations (e.g. 8 s). The saturating concentration of dye near the tip during a prolonged application (>8 s) was postulated to be equal to the original concentration of dye in the application pipette. (For color version of this figure, the reader is referred to the online version of this book.)

are more profound in the intact brain compared to in ex vivo settings.[110]

EVALUATION OF DISTANCE AND TIME DEPENDENCE OF DRUG DIFFUSION IN THE EXTRACELLULAR SPACE

Due to diffusion, the effective concentrations of focally applied drugs near the recorded neurons are expected to be somewhat lower than the original drug concentration in the application pipette. Differences in the applied and original concentrations of drugs can be evaluated using fluorescent tracers. Two factors determine the error in the applied concentration: the distance between the application pipette tip and the neuron (distance factor; Figure 10.2(A) and (B)) and the application duration (time factor; Figure 10.2(C)). To evaluate the drug concentration profile and thus the effective concentrations applied to neurons, application pipettes (tip diameter: ~0.2 μm) were filled with 50 μM Ca-Green-1 fluorescent dye (Life Technologies, Grand Island, NY), and fluorescent intensities were measured upon a single puff (application pressure: 10 psi) in frontal (F), lateral (L), and diagonal (D) directions at different distances (0, 20, 40, 60 μm) from the tip of the application pipette (Figure 10.2(A) and (B)) during various application durations (Figure 10.2(C)). In these experiments, the tuberomammillary nucleus of the posterior hypothalamus in acute hypothalamic slices was used.

The fluorescent intensities corresponding to different durations (0–10 s) of dye applications were recorded at the tip of the application pipette (0 μm) and then normalized to the intensity obtained at prolonged application durations (e.g. 8 s; Figure 10.2(C)). The concentration of dye at the tip (0 μm) during saturating, prolonged applications (>8 s) was postulated to be equal to the original dye concentration in the application pipette (i.e. 50 μM). The dye concentrations were then assumed to be proportionate to relative intensities of corresponding fluorescent responses. The results of these experiments demonstrate that drugs dissipate very rapidly (>50% within 40 μm) as a function of distance from the point of application within the ECS (Figure 10.2). This approach provides a reliable method of evaluation of drug diffusion and structural anisotropy within specific brain regions ex vivo and in vitro. Therefore, a focal (<100 μm) drug administration within the ECS is practically achievable.

CONCLUSION

A balanced ionic composition of the internal and external milieus is essential for neuronal survival and normal function of neuronal networks. Deviations from the ionic homeostasis are observed during periods of excessive neuronal activity that are characterized by excessive neuronal depolarization and complete or partial loss of the plasma and/or mitochondrial transmembrane electrochemical gradients as detected in epileptic seizures, cerebral ischemia, and anoxic and spreading depression. Although the types of intracellular and extracellular ions that allow neuronal activity are known, the list of plasma membrane and mitochondrial ion channels and pores permeable to those ions and activated by specific pathological conditions remains incomplete. Determining the mechanisms and links among these ions, proteins, and specific pathologies is a formidable challenge waiting to be resolved.

References

1. Agnati LF, Zoli M, Stromberg I, Fuxe K. Intercellular communication in the brain: wiring versus volume transmission. *Neuroscience.* 1995;69(3):711–726.
2. Faingold CL. Emergent properties of CNS neuronal networks as targets for pharmacology: application to anticonvulsant drug action. *Prog Neurobiol.* 2004;72(1):55–85.
3. Jefferys JG. Nonsynaptic modulation of neuronal activity in the brain: electric currents and extracellular ions. *Physiol Rev.* 1995;75(4):689–723.
4. Klausberger T, Magill PJ, Marton LF, et al. Brain-state- and cell-type-specific firing of hippocampal interneurons in vivo. *Nature.* 2003;421(6925):844–848.
5. Parker D. Neuronal network analyses: premises, promises and uncertainties. *Philos Trans R Soc Lond B Biol Sci.* 2010;365(1551):2315–2328.
6. Weiss N, Miller F, Cazaubon S, Couraud PO. The blood–brain barrier in brain homeostasis and neurological diseases. *Biochim Biophys Acta.* 2009;1788(4):842–857.
7. Kovacs R, Papageorgiou I, Heinemann U. Slice cultures as a model to study neurovascular coupling and blood brain barrier in vitro. *Cardiovasc Psychiatry Neurol.* 2011;2011:646958.
8. Go KG. The normal and pathological physiology of brain water. *Adv Tech Stand Neurosurg.* 1997;23:47–142.
9. Somjen GG. Ion regulation in the brain: implications for pathophysiology. *Neuroscientist.* 2002;8(3):254–267.
10. Somjen GG, Allen BW, Balestrino M, Aitken PG. Pathophysiology of pH and Ca^{2+} in bloodstream and brain. *Can J Physiol Pharmacol.* 1987;65(5):1078–1085.
11. Lux HD, Heinemann U, Dietzel I. Ionic changes and alterations in the size of the extracellular space during epileptic activity. *Adv Neurol.* 1986;44:619–639.
12. Eggermont JJ. On the pathophysiology of tinnitus; a review and a peripheral model. *Hear Res.* 1990;48(1–2):111–123.
13. Roth G. Myo-axonal ephaptic responses and their F waves in case of chronic denervation. *Electroencephalogr Clin Neurophysiol.* 1993;89(4):252–260.
14. Serra G, Aiello I, De Grandis D, Tugnoli V, Carreras M. Muscle-nerve ephaptic excitation in some repetitive after-discharges. *Electroencephalogr Clin Neurophysiol.* 1984;57(5):416–422.
15. Jansen PH, Joosten EM, Vingerhoets HM. Muscle cramp: main theories as to aetiology. *Eur Arch Psychiatry Neurol Sci.* 1990;239(5):337–342.

16. Feasby TE, Bostock H, Sears TA. Conduction in regenerating dorsal root fibres. *J Neurol Sci*. 1981;49(3):439–454.
17. Armstrong CM, Cota G. Calcium ion as a cofactor in Na channel gating. *Proc Natl Acad Sci USA*. 1991;88(15):6528–6531.
18. Bennett E, Urcan MS, Tinkle SS, Koszowski AG, Levinson SR. Contribution of sialic acid to the voltage dependence of sodium channel gating. A possible electrostatic mechanism. *J Gen Physiol*. 1997;109(3):327–343.
19. Feng Z, Durand DM. Low-calcium epileptiform activity in the hippocampus in vivo. *J Neurophysiol*. 2003;90(4):2253–2260.
20. Hanck DA, Sheets MF. Extracellular divalent and trivalent cation effects on sodium current kinetics in single canine cardiac Purkinje cells. *J Physiol*. 1992;454:267–298.
21. Isaev D, Ivanchick G, Khmyz V, et al. Surface charge impact in low-magnesium model of seizure in rat hippocampus. *J Neurophysiol*. 2012;107(1):417–423.
22. Hansen AJ. Effect of anoxia on ion distribution in the brain. *Physiol Rev*. 1985;65(1):101–148.
23. Cui J, Yang H, Lee US. Molecular mechanisms of BK channel activation. *Cell Mol Life Sci*. 2009;66(5):852–875.
24. Hu S, Sheng WS, Lokensgard JR, Peterson PK. Morphine induces apoptosis of human microglia and neurons. *Neuropharmacology*. 2002;42(6):829–836.
25. Frohlich F, Bazhenov M, Iragui-Madoz V, Sejnowski TJ. Potassium dynamics in the epileptic cortex: new insights on an old topic. *Neuroscientist*. 2008;14(5):422–433.
26. Rausche G, Igelmund P, Heinemann U. Effects of changes in extracellular potassium, magnesium and calcium concentration on synaptic transmission in area CA1 and the dentate gyrus of rat hippocampal slices. *Pflugers Arch*. 1990;415(5):588–593.
27. Heinemann U, Schaible HG, Schmidt RF. Changes in extracellular potassium concentration in cat spinal cord in response to innocuous and noxious stimulation of legs with healthy and inflamed knee joints. *Exp Brain Res*. 1990;79(2):283–292.
28. Uteshev VV, Knot HJ. Somatic Ca^{2+} dynamics in response to choline-mediated excitation in histaminergic tuberomammillary neurons. *Neuroscience*. 2005;134(1):133–143.
29. Jones HC, Keep RF. Brain fluid calcium concentration and response to acute hypercalcaemia during development in the rat. *J Physiol*. 1988;402:579–593.
30. Brown EM. Physiology and pathophysiology of the extracellular calcium-sensing receptor. *Am J Med*. 1999;106(2):238–253.
31. Guerini D, Coletto L, Carafoli E. Exporting calcium from cells. *Cell Calcium*. 2005;38(3–4):281–289.
32. Ikeda K, Yanagawa Y, Bekkers JM. Distinctive quantal properties of neurotransmission at excitatory and inhibitory autapses revealed using variance-mean analysis. *J Neurosci*. 2008;28(50):13563–13573.
33. Rozov A, Burnashev N, Sakmann B, Neher E. Transmitter release modulation by intracellular Ca^{2+} buffers in facilitating and depressing nerve terminals of pyramidal cells in layer 2/3 of the rat neocortex indicates a target cell-specific difference in presynaptic calcium dynamics. *J Physiol*. 2001;531(Pt 3):807–826.
34. Uteshev VV. α7 nicotinic ACh receptors as a ligand-gated source of Ca^{2+} ions: the search for a Ca^{2+} optimum. *Adv Exp Med Biol*. 2012;740:603–638.
35. Vyleta NP, Smith SM. Spontaneous glutamate release is independent of calcium influx and tonically activated by the calcium-sensing receptor. *J Neurosci*. 2011;31(12):4593–4606.
36. Balestrino M, Aitken PG, Somjen GG. The effects of moderate changes of extracellular K^+ and Ca^{2+} on synaptic and neural function in the CA1 region of the hippocampal slice. *Brain Res*. 1986;377(2):229–239.
37. Grahame DC. The electrical double layer and the theory of electrocapillarity. *Chem Rev*. 1947;41:441–501.
38. Uteshev VV. Evaluation of Ca^{2+} permeability of nicotinic acetylcholine receptors in hypothalamic histaminergic neurons. *Acta Biochim Biophys Sin (Shanghai)*. 2010;42(1):8–20.
39. Hille B. *Ion Channels of Excitable Membranes*. 3rd ed. Sunderland, MA: Sinauer Associates, Inc.; 2001.
40. McLeod Jr JR, Shen M, Kim DJ, Thayer SA. Neurotoxicity mediated by aberrant patterns of synaptic activity between rat hippocampal neurons in culture. *J Neurophysiol*. 1998;80(5):2688–2698.
41. Billard JM. Ageing, hippocampal synaptic activity and magnesium. *Magnes Res*. 2006;19(3):199–215.
42. Nowak L, Bregestovski P, Ascher P, Herbet A, Prochiantz A. Magnesium gates glutamate-activated channels in mouse central neurons. *Nature*. 1984;307:462–465.
43. Eby 3rd GA, Eby KL. Magnesium for treatment-resistant depression: a review and hypothesis. *Med Hypotheses*. 2010;74(4):649–660.
44. Levine J, Stein D, Rapoport A, Kurtzman L. High serum and cerebrospinal fluid Ca/Mg ratio in recently hospitalized acutely depressed patients. *Neuropsychobiology*. 1999;39(2):63–70.
45. Pliszka SR, Rogeness GA. Calcium and magnesium in children with schizophrenia and major depression. *Biol Psychiatry*. 1984;19(6):871–876.
46. Vilas GL, Johnson DE, Freund P, Casey JR. Characterization of an epilepsy-associated variant of the human Cl^-/HCO_3^- exchanger AE3. *Am J Physiol Cell Physiol*. 2009;297(3):C526–C536.
47. Donato T, Shapira Y, Artru A, Powers K. Effect of mannitol on cerebrospinal fluid dynamics and brain tissue edema. *Anesth Analg*. 1994;78(1):58–66.
48. Ramkissoon A, Coovadia HM. Chloride levels in meningitis. *S Afr Med J*. 1988;73(9):522–523.
49. Zhu L, Lovinger D, Delpire E. Cortical neurons lacking KCC2 expression show impaired regulation of intracellular chloride. *J Neurophysiol*. 2005;93(3):1557–1568.
50. Owens DF, Kriegstein AR. Developmental neurotransmitters? *Neuron*. 2002;36(6):989–991.
51. Ben-Ari Y. Galanin and glibenclamide modulate the anoxic release of glutamate in rat CA3 hippocampal neurons. *Eur J Neurosci*. 1990;2(1):62–68.
52. Muller M, Somjen GG. Na^+ dependence and the role of glutamate receptors and Na^+ channels in ion fluxes during hypoxia of rat hippocampal slices. *J Neurophysiol*. 2000;84(4):1869–1880.
53. Rader RK, Lanthorn TH. Experimental ischemia induces a persistent depolarization blocked by decreased calcium and NMDA antagonists. *Neurosci Lett*. 1989;99(1–2):125–130.
54. Rossi DJ, Oshima T, Attwell D. Glutamate release in severe brain ischaemia is mainly by reversed uptake. *Nature*. Jan 20, 2000;403(6767):316–321.
55. Tanaka E, Yamamoto S, Kudo Y, Mihara S, Higashi H. Mechanisms underlying the rapid depolarization produced by deprivation of oxygen and glucose in rat hippocampal CA1 neurons in vitro. *J Neurophysiol*. 1997;78(2):891–902.
56. Kalappa BI, Sun F, Johnson SR, Jin K, Uteshev VV. A positive allosteric modulator of α7 nAChRs augments neuroprotective effects of endogenous nicotinic agonists in cerebral ischemia. Br J Pharmacol. 2013; in press.
57. Akaike A, Takada-Takatori Y, Kume T, Izumi Y. Mechanisms of neuroprotective effects of nicotine and acetylcholinesterase inhibitors: role of alpha4 and alpha7 receptors in neuroprotection. *J Mol Neurosci*. 2010;40(1–2):211–216.
58. Del Barrio L, Martin-de-Saavedra MD, Romero A, et al. Neurotoxicity induced by okadaic acid in the human neuroblastoma SH-SY5Y line can be differentially prevented by alpha7 and beta2* nicotinic stimulation. *Toxicol Sci*. 2011;123(1):193–205.
59. Shimohama S. Nicotinic receptor-mediated neuroprotection in neurodegenerative disease models. *Biol Pharm Bull*. 2009;32(3):332–336.

60. Mulkey DK, Henderson 3rd RA, Olson JE, Putnam RW, Dean JB. Oxygen measurements in brain stem slices exposed to normobaric hyperoxia and hyperbaric oxygen. *J Appl Physiol.* 2001;90(5):1887–1899.
61. Dean JB, Mulkey DK, Henderson 3rd RA, Potter SJ, Putnam RW. Hyperoxia, reactive oxygen species, and hyperventilation: oxygen sensitivity of brain stem neurons. *J Appl Physiol.* 2004;96(2):784–791.
62. D'Agostino DP, Putnam RW, Dean JB. Superoxide ($^{*}O_2^-$) production in CA1 neurons of rat hippocampal slices exposed to graded levels of oxygen. *J Neurophysiol.* 2007;98(2):1030–1041.
63. Boulard G, Marguinaud E, Sesay M. Osmotic cerebral oedema: the role of plasma osmolarity and blood brain barrier. *Ann Fr Anesth Reanim.* 2003;22(3):215–219.
64. Ballyk BA, Quackenbush SJ, Andrew RD. Osmotic effects on the CA1 neuronal population in hippocampal slices with special reference to glucose. *J Neurophysiol.* 1991;65(5):1055–1066.
65. Baraban SC, Bellingham MC, Berger AJ, Schwartzkroin PA. Osmolarity modulates K^+ channel function on rat hippocampal interneurons but not CA1 pyramidal neurons. *J Physiol.* 1997;498(Pt 3):679–689.
66. Oliet SH, Bourque CW. Gadolinium uncouples mechanical detection and osmoreceptor potential in supraoptic neurons. *Neuron.* 1996;16(1):175–181.
67. Paoletti P, Ascher P. Mechanosensitivity of NMDA receptors in cultured mouse central neurons. *Neuron.* 1994;13(3):645–655.
68. Hochman DW, Baraban SC, Owens JW, Schwartzkroin PA. Dissociation of synchronization and excitability in furosemide blockade of epileptiform activity. *Science.* 1995;270(5233):99–102.
69. Dmitriev AV, Mangel SC. Retinal pH reflects retinal energy metabolism in the day and night. *J Neurophysiol.* 2004;91(6):2404–2412.
70. Chesler M. Regulation and modulation of pH in the brain. *Physiol Rev.* 2003;83(4):1183–1221.
71. Dmitriev AV, Mangel SC. Circadian clock regulation of pH in the rabbit retina. *J Neurosci.* 2001;21(8):2897–2902.
72. Traynelis SF, Cull-Candy SG. Proton inhibition of *N*-methyl-D-aspartate receptors in cerebellar neurons. *Nature.* May 24, 1990;345(6273):347–350.
73. Duan B, Wang YZ, Yang T, et al. Extracellular spermine exacerbates ischemic neuronal injury through sensitization of ASIC1a channels to extracellular acidosis. *J Neurosci.* Feb 9, 2011; 31(6):2101–2112.
74. Meltzer RH, Kapoor N, Qadri YJ, Anderson SJ, Fuller CM, Benos DJ. Heteromeric assembly of acid-sensitive ion channel and epithelial sodium channel subunits. *J Biol Chem.* 2007;282(35):25548–25559.
75. Petroff EY, Price MP, Snitsarev V, et al. Acid-sensing ion channels interact with and inhibit BK K^+ channels. *Proc Natl Acad Sci USA.* 2008;105(8):3140–3144.
76. Tombaugh GC. Intracellular pH buffering shapes activity-dependent Ca^{2+} dynamics in dendrites of CA1 interneurons. *J Neurophysiol.* 1998;80(4):1702–1712.
77. Borst JG, Sakmann B. Calcium current during a single action potential in a large presynaptic terminal of the rat brainstem. *J Physiol.* 1998;506(Pt 1):143–157.
78. Kullmann DM, Asztely F. Extrasynaptic glutamate spillover in the hippocampus: evidence and implications. *Trends Neurosci.* 1998;21(1):8–14.
79. Rossetti AO. What is the value of hypothermia in acute neurologic diseases and status epilepticus? *Epilepsia.* 2011;52(Suppl. 8):64–66.
80. McNaughton BL, Shen J, Rao G, Foster TC, Barnes CA. Persistent increase of hippocampal presynaptic axon excitability after repetitive electrical stimulation: dependence on *N*-methyl-D-aspartate receptor activity, nitric-oxide synthase, and temperature. *Proc Natl Acad Sci USA.* 1994;91(11):4830–4834.
81. Busto R, Dietrich WD, Globus MY, Valdes I, Scheinberg P, Ginsberg MD. Small differences in intraischemic brain temperature critically determine the extent of ischemic neuronal injury. *J Cereb Blood Flow Metab.* 1987;7(6):729–738.
82. Churn SB, Taft WC, Billingsley MS, Blair RE, DeLorenzo RJ. Temperature modulation of ischemic neuronal death and inhibition of calcium/calmodulin-dependent protein kinase II in gerbils. *Stroke.* 1990;21(12):1715–1721.
83. Shankaran S, Laptook AR, Ehrenkranz RA, et al. Whole-body hypothermia for neonates with hypoxic-ischemic encephalopathy. *N Engl J Med.* 2005;353(15):1574–1584.
84. Edwards AD, Brocklehurst P, Gunn AJ, et al. Neurological outcomes at 18 months of age after moderate hypothermia for perinatal hypoxic ischaemic encephalopathy: synthesis and meta-analysis of trial data. *BMJ.* 2010;340:c363.
85. Michalski A, Wimborne BM, Henry GH. The effect of reversible cooling of cat's primary visual cortex on the responses of area 21a neurons. *J Physiol.* 1993;466:133–156.
86. Araque A, Navarrete M. Glial cells in neuronal network function. *Philos Trans R Soc Lond B Biol Sci.* 2010;365(1551):2375–2381.
87. Bordey A, Sontheimer H. Postnatal development of ionic currents in rat hippocampal astrocytes in situ. *J Neurophysiol.* 1997;78(1):461–477.
88. Erlichman JS, Leiter JC. Glia modulation of the extracellular milieu as a factor in central CO_2 chemosensitivity and respiratory control. *J Appl Physiol.* 2010;108(6):1803–1811.
89. Sykova E, Chvatal A. Glial cells and volume transmission in the CNS. *Neurochem Int.* 2000;36(4–5):397–409.
90. Ballanyi K, Grafe P, ten Bruggencate G. Ion activities and potassium uptake mechanisms of glial cells in guinea-pig olfactory cortex slices. *J Physiol.* 1987;382:159–174.
91. Casanova MF, Stevens JR, Brown R, Royston C, Bruton C. Disentangling the pathology of schizophrenia and paraphrenia. *Acta Neuropathol.* 2002;103(4):313–320.
92. Durand DM, Park EH, Jensen AL. Potassium diffusive coupling in neural networks. *Philos Trans R Soc Lond B Biol Sci.* 2010;365(1551):2347–2362.
93. Gabriel S, Njunting M, Pomper JK, et al. Stimulus and potassium-induced epileptiform activity in the human dentate gyrus from patients with and without hippocampal sclerosis. *J Neurosci.* 2004;24(46):10416–10430.
94. Kohling R, Avoli M. Methodological approaches to exploring epileptic disorders in the human brain in vitro. *J Neurosci Methods.* 2006;155(1):1–19.
95. Hablitz JJ, Heinemann U, Lux HD. Step reductions in extracellular Ca^{2+} activate a transient inward current in chick dorsal root ganglion cells. *Biophys J.* 1986;50(4):753–757.
96. Albus K, Wahab A, Heinemann U. Standard antiepileptic drugs fail to block epileptiform activity in rat organotypic hippocampal slice cultures. *Br J Pharmacol.* 2008;154(3):709–724.
97. Derchansky M, Shahar E, Wennberg RA, et al. Model of frequent, recurrent, and spontaneous seizures in the intact mouse hippocampus. *Hippocampus.* 2004;14(8):935–947.
98. Khalilov I, Dzhala V, Medina I, et al. Maturation of kainate-induced epileptiform activities in interconnected intact neonatal limbic structures in vitro. *Eur J Neurosci.* 1999;11(10):3468–3480.
99. Quilichini PP, Diabira D, Chiron C, Ben-Ari Y, Gozlan H. Persistent epileptiform activity induced by low Mg^{2+} in intact immature brain structures. *Eur J Neurosci.* 2002;16(5):850–860.
100. Wu C, Shen H, Luk WP, Zhang L. A fundamental oscillatory state of isolated rodent hippocampus. *J Physiol.* 2002;540(Pt 2):509–527.

101. Jones RS. Ictal epileptiform events induced by removal of extracellular magnesium in slices of entorhinal cortex are blocked by baclofen. *Exp Neurol*. 1989;104(2):155–161.
102. Fujii M, Inoue T, Nomura S, et al. Cooling of the epileptic focus suppresses seizures with minimal influence on neurologic functions. *Epilepsia*. 2012;53(3):485–493.
103. Rothman S, Yang XF. Local cooling: a therapy for intractable neocortical epilepsy. *Epilepsy Curr*. 2003;3(5):153–156.
104. Schmitt FC, Buchheim K, Meierkord H, Holtkamp M. Anticonvulsant properties of hypothermia in experimental status epilepticus. *Neurobiol Dis*. 2006;23(3):689–696.
105. Tong CK, Chesler M. Modulation of spreading depression by changes in extracellular pH. *J Neurophysiol*. 2000;84(5):2449–2457.
106. Muller M, Somjen GG. Na^+ and K^+ concentrations, extra- and intracellular voltages, and the effect of TTX in hypoxic rat hippocampal slices. *J Neurophysiol*. 2000;83(2):735–745.
107. Kager H, Wadman WJ, Somjen GG. Simulated seizures and spreading depression in a neuron model incorporating interstitial space and ion concentrations. *J Neurophysiol*. 2000;84(1):495–512.
108. Chao D, Xia Y. Ionic storm in hypoxic/ischemic stress: can opioid receptors subside it? *Prog Neurobiol*. 2010;90(4):439–470.
109. Jiang C, Xia Y, Haddad GG. Role of ATP-sensitive K^+ channels during anoxia: major differences between rat (newborn and adult) and turtle neurons. *J Physiol*. 1992;448:599–612.
110. Silver IA, Erecinska M. Intracellular and extracellular changes of $[Ca^{2+}]$ in hypoxia and ischemia in rat brain in vivo. *J Gen Physiol*. 1990;95(5):837–866.

CHAPTER

11

Neuronal Network Mechanisms—Sex and Development

Aristea S. Galanopoulou[1], *Solomon L. Moshé*[1,2]

[1]Saul R. Korey Department of Neurology, Dominick P. Purpura Department of Neuroscience and Comprehensive Einstein/Montefiore Epilepsy Center, Albert Einstein College of Medicine, Bronx, NY, USA, [2]Department of Pediatrics, Albert Einstein College of Medicine, Bronx, NY, USA

INTRODUCTION

The brain is organized into neuronal networks, many of which coordinate specific functions and/or behaviors. These can be fundamental physiologic functions, such as learning (e.g. Chapter 13) and motor activity (Chapter 17). However, if disrupted, abnormal network activity may give rise to pathological demonstrations of a disease process, such as dementia, movement disorders (Chapter 25), or epileptic motor seizures (e.g. Chapter 26). The plasticity of neuronal networks is evident from the ongoing transformation of their function during brain development or their adaptive changes occurring under the influence of environmental (Chapter 28) or endocrine interactions during the sexual differentiation of the brain.

Gamma-aminobutyric acid (GABA) signaling has been of particular interest in understanding neuronal network plasticity, both because it is one of the major neurotransmitter systems and also because it regulates brain development. The main subtypes of GABA receptors are ligand-gated Cl^- channels, such as $GABA_A$ receptors, and metabotropic receptors ($GABA_B$ receptors). $GABA_A$ receptors normally cause neuronal hyperpolarization in mature neurons, via influx of Cl^-, and inhibition of neuronal activity. They are pentameric channels composed of a variety of subunits, but they typically have two α and two β subunits, whereas the fifth subunit may vary: it is usually a γ in most receptors or a δ subunit in extrasynaptic $GABA_A$ receptors.[1,2] Early in the development in most neurons, however, $GABA_A$ receptor activation has depolarizing effects, due to the predominance of cation chloride cotransporters that maintain high intracellular Cl^- concentrations (Na^+–K^+–Cl^- cotransporter NKCC1) over cotransporters that extrude Cl^- (K^+–Cl^- cotransporter KCC2).[1–5] The early depolarizing effects of $GABA_A$ receptor activation, seen in immature neurons, have been shown to be necessary for normal brain development.[6–8] On the other hand, $GABA_B$ receptors hyperpolarize neurons by increasing K^+ conductance postsynaptically, or they reduce presynaptic Ca^{++} content and neurotransmitter release.

Here, we will highlight some of the developmental processes that transform the network output, as a function of development and sex, in selected neuronal networks involved in seizure control: the basal ganglia, limbic structures such as the hippocampus, and a corticothalamic network. We will describe an overview of the structure and function of these networks and some of the molecular and electrophysiological mechanisms altering their physiology and function in an age- and sex-dependent manner, focusing on GABA receptors. Finally, we will discuss the potential implications for their role in the pathogenesis of neurological diseases, such as epilepsy.

BASAL GANGLIA

The basal ganglia consist of the striatum (caudate and putamen), globus pallidus externa (GPe) and interna (GPi; also called the entopeduncular nucleus), subthalamic nucleus (STN), and substantia nigra (SN). The SN is

Neuronal Networks in Brain Function, CNS Disorders, and Therapeutics
http://dx.doi.org/10.1016/B978-0-12-415804-7.00011-3

traditionally divided into two major parts: the pars compacta (SNC) and pars reticulata (SNR).[9] The SNC contains almost exclusively dopaminergic neurons, the loss of which is implicated in Parkinson's disease. In contrast, the SNR contains predominantly GABAergic neurons, and only a minority of dopaminergic neurons is located in its posterior region (Figure 11.1). There is evidence that the adult SNR contains topographically distinct regions[10]; we have also identified that the anterior (SNRant) and posterior SNR (SNRpost) may have different functional roles in seizure propagation and control, regulation of rotatory behavior, and histochemical features.[11–14]

The prevailing hypothesis suggests that cortical glutamatergic projections activate striatal neurons, which in turn may either activate or inhibit thalamocortical

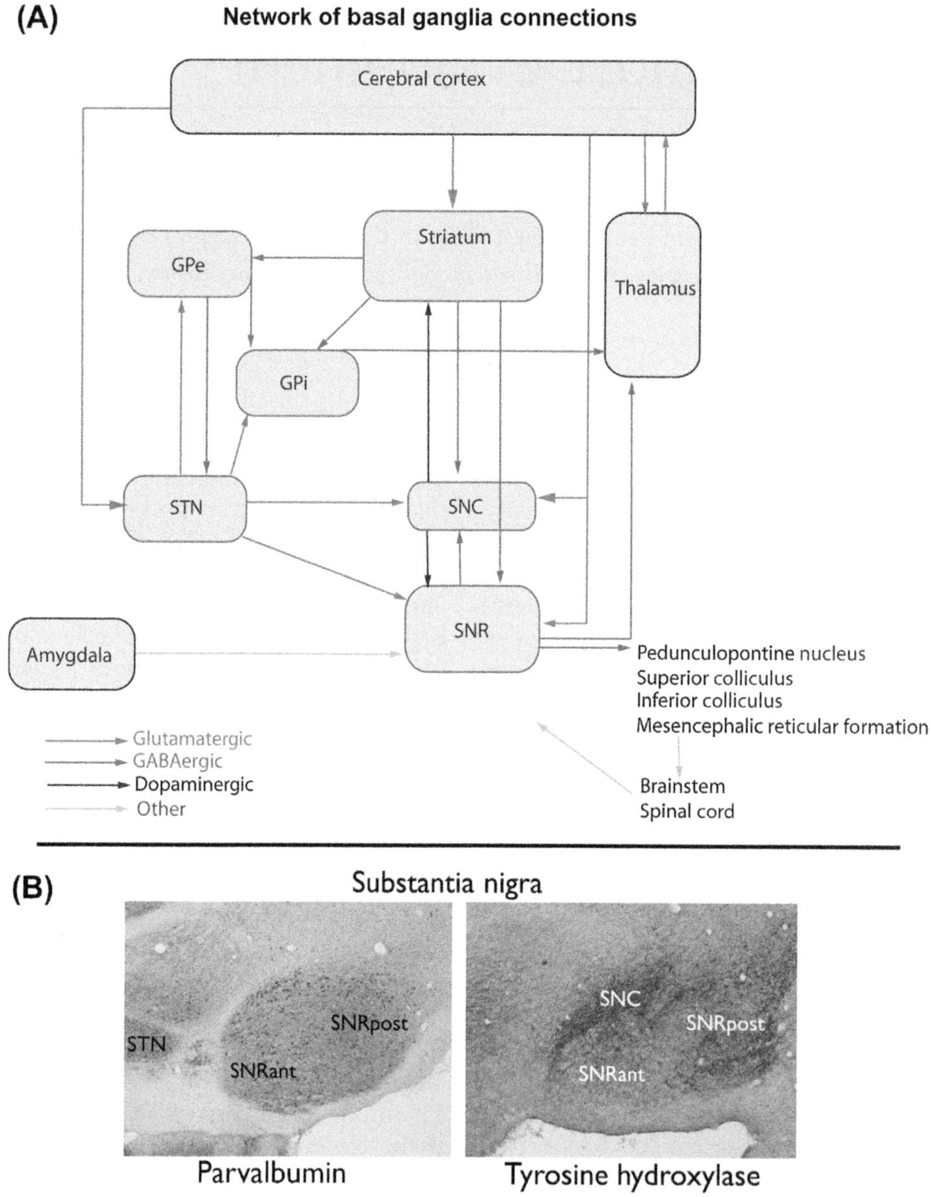

FIGURE 11.1 **The circuitry of connections within and beyond the basal ganglia and substantia nigra regional organization.** (A) The basal ganglia nuclei are shown here with the yellow boxes. The direct pathway involves striatal projections to the GPi–SNR and subsequently to the thalamus. The indirect pathway traverses through the striatum toward the GPe and STN, which then activates the SNR. (B) The SN consists of two distinct regions with different functions in seizure control. Sagittal sections of a PN30 rat SN are shown here, stained either with anti-parvalbumin antibody (left panel) to indicate the majority of GABAergic neurons or with antityrosine hydroxylase antibody to label dopaminergic neurons in the SNC or SNRpost. The SNRant consists of almost exclusively GABAergic neurons (parvalbumin-positive). Regional differences in the connectivity of the two regions have been reported, but these have not yet been fully described.[10,15] GPe: globus pallidum externa; GPi: globus pallidum interna; STN: subthalamic nucleus; SNR: substantia nigra pars reticulata; SNC: substantia nigra pars compacta. (The figure is reproduced in color section.)

projection neurons depending upon whether they engage the direct or indirect basal ganglia pathway. Activation of the direct pathway involves activation of the striatum and inhibition of the GPi and SNR, and subsequently relieves their inhibitory effect upon the thalamus, resulting in further activation of the thalamocortical input (Figure 11.1). In contrast, striatal projections toward the indirect pathway inhibit GPe GABAergic neurons, relieving their inhibition from STN, which via activation of the SNR GABAergic neurons inhibit the thalamocortical projections (Figure 11.1). The basal ganglia also receive input from limbic structures as well as send efferents to the pedunculopontine nucleus and superior colliculus, which project to other brainstem sites and to the spinal cord. As a result, they play a central role in motor control, eye gaze, sleep, and cognitive processes, acting as gatekeepers for the information processing. A computational model of gating information processing and memory formation was proposed recently[16]; according to this, activation of the indirect ("NoGo") pathway is equivalent to closing the SNR gate and inactivating the thalamocortical path, and as a result the frontal cortex maintains the acquired information. In contrast, activation of the direct ("Go") pathway suppresses the SNR output, opening the gate and allowing the update of working memory in the cortex. The effects may be even more complicated when one takes into account the regional differences in the functions of SNRant and SNRpost.

The basic functions served by the basal ganglia—movement control, cognition, and behavior—are normal fundamental differentiating features of the two sexes but also change as a function of age and development. Under pathological conditions, basal ganglia may play a key role in the control of seizure expression or propagation, acting as a gate to limbic, corticothalamic, or corticoreticular networks.[13,17–29] Furthermore, pathological processes affecting the basal ganglia may lead to movement disorders, such as Parkinson's disease, tic disorders, and stereotypies. Many of these disorders exhibit age- and sex-specific features and different natural histories in male versus female patients. Seizures at younger ages tend to be more common in boys, epileptic syndromes may follow age- and sex-specific patterns of susceptibility,[30,31] and sex differences in the patterns of interictal hypometabolism in temporal lobe epilepsy patients are reported to exist.[32,33] Parkinson's disease may be more frequent in men than in women,[34] but women may have more severe nonmotor symptoms than men.[35] Tourette syndrome is three times more prevalent in boys than in girls. As a result, age and sex differences in the biology and function of basal ganglia, under both physiological and pathological conditions, might be expected. Here, we will summarize some of the progress done on age- and sex-specific influences in basal ganglia function, using as a paradigm the SNR and its role in seizure control.

Age- and sex-specific development of SNR function in seizure control. In vitro and in vivo studies in rodents demonstrate that the SNR undergoes functional changes through development that mature in a sex- and region-specific manner. In vivo, these have been extensively studied using the flurothyl seizure model, whereby exposure of rodents to flurothyl ether, a chemoconvulsant, provokes clonic and tonic-clonic generalized seizures with easily quantifiable latencies. Intranigral bilateral infusions of a GABAergic agonist, muscimol, elicit proconvulsant effects in PN15 male rats by accelerating the latency to clonic seizure.[13,17,26,36] At postnatal day 30 (PN30), a muscimol-sensitive anticonvulsant region emerges from the SNRant, whereas the SNRpost retains its muscimol-sensitive proconvulsant function through adulthood.[13] The same antero-posterior regional differentiation of the SNR in older ages is also seen with other $GABA_A$ receptor agonists, although some qualitative differences in output are seen (Table 11.1).[13,26,36–42] In females, however, muscimol infusions in the SNR do not produce proconvulsant effects at any of the studied ages (PN15–PN30), whereas the anticonvulsant effects of nigral muscimol infusions first appear at a younger age (PN25).[13] Furthermore, intranigral activation of $GABA_A$ receptors accelerates the appearance of flurothyl-induced tonic-clonic seizures in PN15–PN30 male rats, but not in adult male rats or in age-matched females.[43]

The anticonvulsant action of nigral infusions of $GABA_A$ receptor agonists on the clonic seizure threshold may be due to downstream inhibition of the pedunculopontine tegmental nucleus and subsequently of downstream brainstem and spinal cord networks.[27–29,44] However, the developmental and regional specifications of the SNR role in seizure control extend to other methods of altering SNR activity, which are not necessarily directly related to GABA neurotransmission. These treatments include intranigral infusions of inhibitors of *N*-methyl-D-aspartate (NMDA) receptors or electrical stimulation of the SNR[9,45] (Table 11.1).

Regarding the molecular, electrophysiological, and structural factors underlying the age- and sex-specific function of the SNR, the sex-specific developmental differences in the function of the GABA-sensitive seizure-controlling SNR neurons may be due both to local factors that relate to GABA receptor structure and function (Table 11.2) and to distant effects that relate to the different output of the SNR neurons to downstream structures. The local GABA-related differences are summarized in Table 11.2. Overall, these findings support a gradual developmental acquisition of faster kinetics in the $GABA_A$ receptor inhibitory postsynaptic currents (IPSCs), which is attributed to a replacement of the $\alpha3$ by the $\alpha1$ subunit.[47] Such changes may render the

TABLE 11.1 Effects of SNR Infusions or Electrical Stimulation on Flurothyl Seizure Threshold for Clonic Seizures in Male Rats

Drug	Pharmacologic effect	PN15–16	Adult	References
Muscimol	$GABA_A$ receptor agonist	Proconvulsant	Anticonvulsant (SNRant); proconvulsant (SNRpost)	13,26,36,37
Phenobarbital	$GABA_A$ receptor agonist	Anticonvulsant	Anticonvulsant	38
Zolpidem	α1-preferring $GABA_A$ receptor agonist	Anticonvulsant	Anticonvulsant (SNRant); no effect (SNRpost)	39
GVG	GABA aminotransferase inhibitor	No effect	Anticonvulsant (SNRant); proconvulsant (SNRpost)	38,40,41
ZAPA	Low-affinity $GABA_A$ receptor site agonist	Anticonvulsant (low dose); proconvulsant (high dose)	Anticonvulsant (SNRant); proconvulsant (SNRpost)	41
THIP	$GABA_A$ receptor agonist (high affinity for $\alpha4/\delta$ receptors)	Proconvulsant	Anticonvulsant (low doses); proconvulsant (high doses)	42
Bicuculline	$GABA_A$ receptor antagonist	Proconvulsant	Proconvulsant (SNRant); no effect (SNRpost)	36,37,41
Baclofen	$GABA_B$ receptor agonist	Anticonvulsant	No effect	13,25,38
CGP 35348	$GABA_B$ receptor antagonist	Proconvulsant	No effect	38
CGP 36742	$GABA_B$ receptor antagonist	Proconvulsant	No effect	38
AP7	NMDA receptor inhibitor	No effect	Anticonvulsant (SNRant); proconvulsant (SNRpost)	9
Electrical stimulation		Anticonvulsant	Anticonvulsant (SNRant); no effect (SNRpost)	

Effect of infusions in anterior SNR; AP7: (DL-2-amino-7-phosphonoheptanoic acid); GVG: Gamma-vinyl GABA; THIP: 4,5,6,7-tetrahydroisoxazolo[5,4-c]pyridin-3-ol; ZAPA: (Z)-3-[(aminoiminomethyl)thio]prop-2-enoic acid.

TABLE 11.2 Developmental and Sex-Specific Differences in Components of GABAergic System of the Rat SNRant

Factor	Age	Male versus female (M vs F)	References
$GABA_A$ receptor α1 mRNA		PN15, PN30: M < F	12
$GABA_A$ receptor α1-ir (somatic)	M, F: PN5, PN15 < PN30	PN5: M < F; PN15, PN30: M = F	47
$GABA_A$ receptor α3-ir (somatic)	M: PN5 > PN30 F: PN5 > PN15 > PN30	PN5: M < F; PN15, PN30: M = F	47
$GABA_A$ receptor IPSC frequencies	M, F: increases between PN15 to PN30	PN5–9: M > F; PN12–32: M = F	47
$GABA_A$ receptor IPSC amplitudes	M, F: increases between PN15 to PN30	PN5–9, PN28–32: M > F; PN12–15: M = F	47
$GABA_A$ receptor IPSC decay and rise times	M, F: decrease between PN5 to PN30	PN28–32: M < F; PN5–15: M = F	47
KCC2 mRNA	M: PN15 < PN30, adult; F: PN15 < PN30	PN5, PN30: M < F	11
Egaba	Egaba becomes hyperpolarizing: M: at PN16.6 F: at PN9.8		11,48
Number of GABA-ir neurons		PN15, PN30: M < F	12
Muscimol effects (systemic administration)		PN15 M: increase in KCC2 mRNA and pCREB-ir; PN15 F: no effect	49
Muscimol binding		Adult wood mice: M < F	50

Egaba: reversal potential for $GABA_A$ receptor responses; F: female; IPSC: inhibitory postsynaptic current; ir: immunoreactivity; M: male.

SNR capable of synchronizing its responses to faster frequency inputs in older subjects.

In addition, the SNR GABAergic neurons in younger rodents, males in particular, tend to have less effective $GABA_A$ receptor inhibition due to either lower receptor expression or the presence of depolarizing $GABA_A$ receptor signaling.[11,47,48] In the rodent SNR, the maturation of $GABA_A$ receptor signaling from depolarizing to hyperpolarizing is delayed in males compared to females, based on KCC2 mRNA expression, synaptic GABA receptor responses using a gramicidin-perforated patch clamp, and muscimol-induced calcium rises using fura-2 AM (fura-2 acetoxymethyl ester) imaging.[11,48] The mechanisms behind the sex differences and developmental shift in $GABA_A$ receptor signaling are currently unknown, although several factors have been proposed, including sex hormones,[51] neuronal activity, GABA signaling, and other gene regulatory factors.[1,52] A possible scenario proposed to lead to the earlier appearance of hyperpolarizing $GABA_A$ receptor responses in female rat SNR is the perinatal surge of testosterone in newborn males, which, through conversion to estradiol, locally keeps suppressed the expression of KCC2, delaying the developmental increase in its expression.[51]

Beyond rendering $GABA_A$ receptor inhibition less effective at this early postnatal age, $GABA_A$ receptor–mediated depolarizations are also necessary for normal neuronal development.[3,11,52] In vivo knockout or pharmacologic inhibition of NKCC1, or overexpression of KCC2 during the embryonic and/or early postnatal period when cortical neurons are expected to have depolarizing $GABA_A$ receptor responses, results in the abnormal development of excitatory synapses and, to a lesser extent, of GABAergic synapses as well as abnormalities in neurodevelopment.[6–8] It is therefore hypothesized that the longer presence of depolarizing $GABA_A$ receptor responses in the early postnatal male SNR, compared to that of the female, may be important for the sexual differentiation of its function.[52] In regard to the development of the proconvulsant muscimol-sensitive SNR function in PN15 male rats, this was shown to be induced by the early perinatal testosterone surge that normally occurs in newborn male pups, with a critical period between PN0 and PN2.[53]

Another contributing factor to the regional diversity in the functional output of the SNR could be their projections to different downstream targets. It has been reported recently that rostral and caudal SNR target different thalamic nuclei.[15] However, further studies are needed to outline when these connections are formed in males and females and to determine if they are pertinent to the observed differences in seizure control.

Clinical relevance: The possible clinical scenarios that relate to the experiments discussed in this section may relate to the efficiency of GABA-acting drugs to engage the SNR into inhibiting the expression or propagation of a seizure in the setting of a proconvulsant insult. $GABA_A$ receptor agonists would appear, therefore, to be less potent in engaging the SNR-related pathways that control seizure onset and propagation in younger ages, particularly in males. This may be one of the mechanisms underlying, possibly, the less potent antiseizure effects of benzodiazepines and other GABA-acting drugs early in life.[54–56] In fact, the age- and sex-related differences in $GABA_A$ receptor composition in the SNR pinpoint the possibility that, perhaps, individualized treatments using $GABA_A$ receptor agonists with higher specificity for the receptors expressed at the studied age and sex group may be more useful and effective than the existing treatment protocols, which are based on efficacy derived from population studies.

Enhanced GABAergic input to the SNR may also occur once a seizure starts, due to the abundant GABAergic afferents to the SNR (Figure 11.1). In this setting, activation of $GABA_A$ receptors in the SNR may alter SNR activity and its output and, therefore, affect the spread and generalization of seizure activity. GABA-mediated inhibition of SNRant neurons would therefore be expected to inhibit their activity and reduce their GABAergic output to downstream targets. In this case, however, the presence, degree, and type of inhibition (phasic versus tonic) of the SNR would depend upon the type of predominantly expressed $GABA_A$ receptors in the SNR as well as the presence of $GABA_A$ receptor–mediated hyperpolarization or depolarization in vivo. For instance, the presence of in vivo depolarizing $GABA_A$ receptor responses may weaken the GABA-mediated inhibition, which will then depend upon shunting inhibition only,[57] whereas it might generate paradoxical excitatory (i.e. proconvulsant) effects at seizure onset that would increase SNR efferent output. Also, the balance between tonic and phasic $GABA_A$ receptor–mediated responses would also influence the pattern of downstream effects (rhythmic or oscillatory versus tonic) and potentially the clinical manifestations cumulating into rhythmic or clonic electroclinical seizure patterns or tonic seizures. Of equal importance is the impact of such changes upon memory update and maintenance in the cortex, which may become important when considering not only the age- and sex-specific cognitive processes but also the cognitive comorbidities of seizures, epilepsies, and basal ganglia disorders.[16]

Temporal Lobe Network

The medial temporal lobe structures include the dentate gyrus (DG), hippocampus, subiculum, presubiculum, parasubiculum, and entorhinal, perirhinal, and parahippocampal cortices. These are important in long-term memory formation but are also one of the most commonly affected networks in seizures and epilepsies. The basic "trisynaptic" pathway entails afferents from layer II of the entorhinal cortex to the DG (the *perforant pathway*), projections from the granule neurons of the dentate to the CA3 pyramidal neurons (the *mossy fiber pathway*), and projections from the CA3 pyramidal neurons to CA1 (*Schaffer collaterals*) (Figure 11.2). Finally, CA1 efferents are sent to the subiculum, and subicular efferents to the cortical areas. The finer control of this circuit is more complex due to the influence of local interneurons, interactions with the contralateral hippocampus, antidromic connections (i.e. CA3 to the hilus or DG), or those between the CA1–CA3 neurons and the cortex. Under pathologic conditions, such as temporal lobe epilepsy, abnormal reorganization of the network can be done due to the concurrent cellular loss, neo-neurogenesis, and aberrant redirection of mossy fiber projections back to the DG (i.e. *mossy fiber sprouting*).[58]

The numerous connections between the temporal lobe and other brain regions may underlie the significant variability in symptoms of epileptic seizures in patients with temporal lobe epilepsy. These may include fear or olfactory auras (originating from the amygdala, hippocampus, and parahippocampal areas), experiential auras (or somatic motor symptoms without automatisms) (originating from the temporal neocortex), visceral sensations or automatisms (originating from the amygdala and hippocampus), impaired consciousness, sleep–wake influences or generalization of seizures (originating from the brainstem and the thalamocortical network), and reproductive disorders (originating from the hypothalamus).[59–62]

A study comparing the age-related semiological features of seizures from young patients with temporal lobe epilepsy reported that early in life there was a higher prevalence of motor symptoms, which gradually subsided or became less overt at older ages.[63,64] However, other semiological features, like emotional signs, vegetative signs, or auras, had similar frequencies across ages.[64] These findings tend to indicate the asynchronous pattern of brain development and cross-regional connectivity, which emphasizes the importance of considering neuronal network function within the appropriate maturational context of an individual.

The structure, function, and connectivity of the temporal lobe network undergo significant changes during development, as exemplified in Figure 11.3 for the male hippocampus. These include the progressive maturation of excitatory and inhibitory synaptic connections, the migration and differentiation of neurons, a balance between tonic and phasic or depolarizing versus hyperpolarizing $GABA_A$ receptor inhibition, and the type of glutamatergic receptor responses. Numerous studies have described that, early in development, hippocampal neurons are depolarized by $GABA_A$ receptors, and, gradually, over the course of the first 2–3 postnatal weeks hyperpolarizing $GABA_A$ receptor responses appear.[2–4,65–67] In addition, acquisition of hyperpolarizing $GABA_A$ receptor responses occurs earlier in females than in males due to sex differences in the expression of cation chloride cotransporters, like KCC2 and NKCC1.[67] Again, these age- and sex-specific differences in GABA signaling, therefore, not

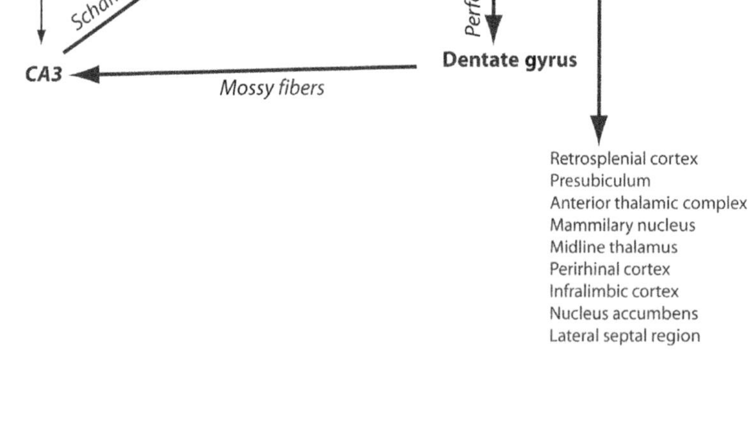

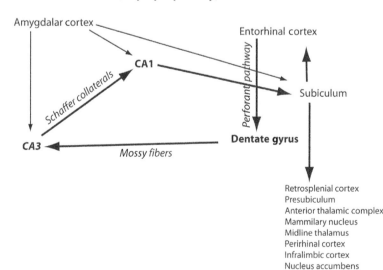

FIGURE 11.2 **The basic hippocampal circuit (trisynaptic pathway).** The perforant pathway introduces cortical input to the dentate gyrus. The mossy fiber pathway projects from the dentate granule cells to the CA3 pyramidal neurons. The Schaffer collaterals project from the CA3 to the CA1 pyramidal neurons. CA1 projections to the subiculum and subsequent efferents back to the cortex as well as other brain regions facilitate the spread of the activity.

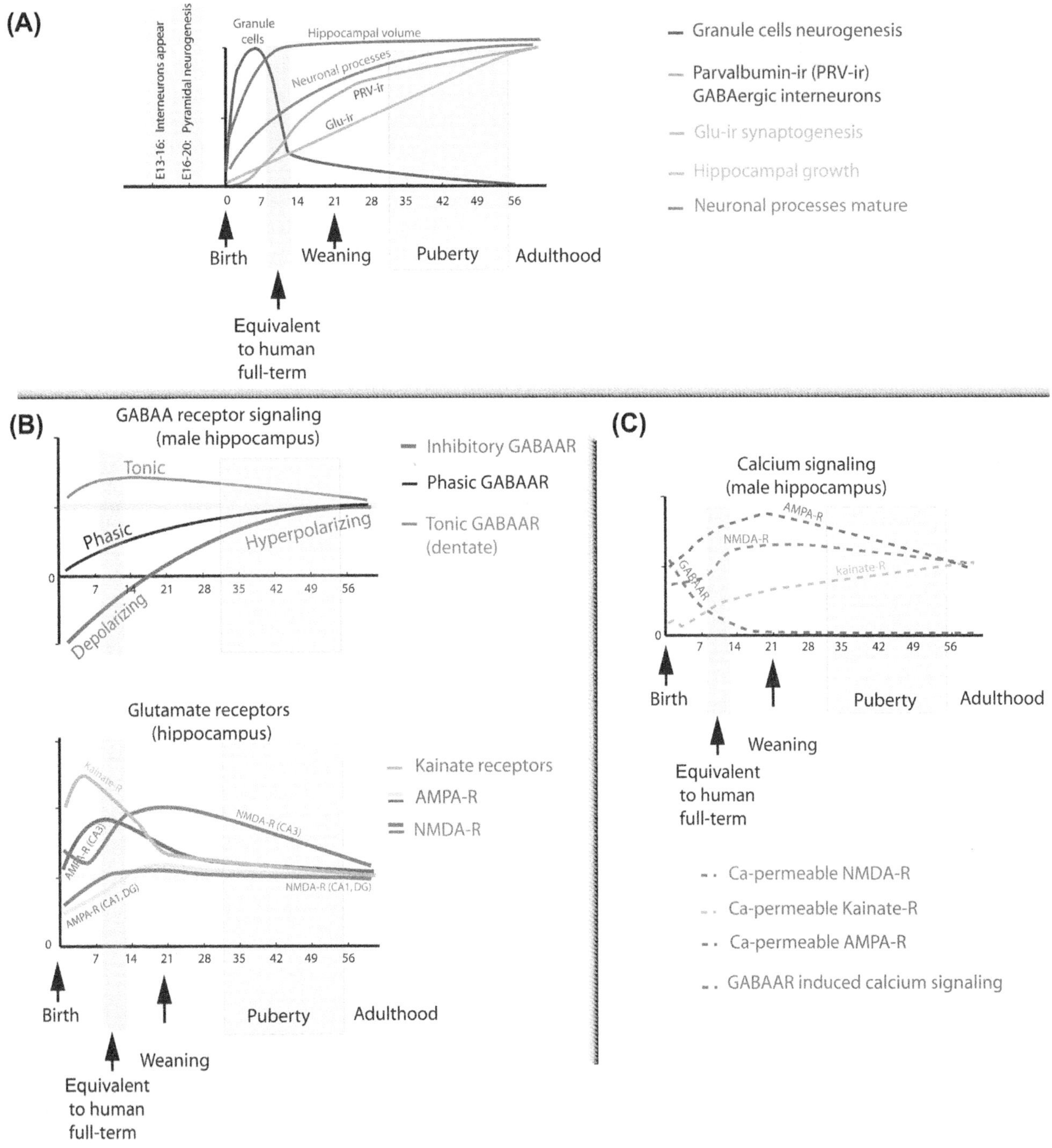

FIGURE 11.3 Developmental changes in the hippocampus of male rodents. (A) Developmental changes in neurogenesis, excitatory (glutamatergic: Glu-ir) and GABAergic synaptogenesis, and hippocampal growth in rodents.[69] *(Source: Modified from Ref. 69 with permission from John Wiley and Sons.)* (B) Developmental changes in tonic, phasic, and depolarizing versus hyperpolarizing $GABA_A$ receptor responses[65,67,70,71] (upper panel) and of kainic acid,[72] NMDA, and AMPA receptor expression in the rat male hippocampus[71,73] (lower panel). Region, sex, and cell type differences are also reported. (C) Developmental changes in $GABA_A$ or glutamate receptor–induced increases in intracellular calcium in the male rat hippocampus, based on E-gaba studies, and the relative expression of calcium-permeable glutamatergic receptors.[67,72,74,75] (The figure is reproduced in color section.)

only are likely to impact the network communication protocols through direct electrophysiological effects but also may result in long-term developmental changes driven by calcium signaling cascades activated in GABAergic neurons only when GABA is inducing depolarization. Indeed, sex differences in the phosphorylation of the transcriptional factor *cAMP responsive element binding protein* (pCREB) by systemic injection of muscimol have been shown preferentially in male but not in female hippocampal neurons.[80]

The widespread connectivity and significant plasticity of the temporal lobe make it particularly vulnerable to exogenous influences that leave their imprint upon its structural and functional features. These may include stressful factors or pathological conditions, such as prior seizures, or drugs. For instance, prior seizures and stress may alter the reversal potential of $GABA_A$ receptor postsynaptic responses (E-gaba) and $GABA_A$ receptor function, and $GABA_A$ receptor expression in manners that depend upon age and sex.[67,76,77] As a result, the protocol of communication within the temporal lobe structures may change, often in a pathologic manner that predisposes and facilitates epileptic seizures or abnormal behaviors. For instance, in vitro electrophysiological and histopathological evidence from postsurgical human epileptic temporal lobes suggests that the epileptic state is associated with an aberrant reversal of E-gaba to the depolarizing state.[78–82]

Although significant debate has arisen recently about the technical issues that may contribute to the appearance of in vitro depolarizing $GABA_A$ receptor responses,[83] the evidence favoring the developmental and sex-specific differences in $GABA_A$ receptor signaling comes from a number of in vivo and in vitro studies that support the presence of depolarizing in vivo responses.[1,52] These studies correlate the in vitro electrophysiological GABA responses with the expression of the cation chloride cotransporters in the intact brain; in vitro fluorescent imaging techniques; in vivo, in vitro, and in culture experiments using a cation chloride cotransporter knockout; as well as the age- and sex-specific differences in the effects of in vivo–administered drugs that concur with the in vitro observations.

CORTICOTHALAMIC NETWORK

The thalamus is important in trafficking sensory information in the brain from and toward the cortex, changing its gating pattern as a function of the sensory state (sleep or awake). The principal sensory relay thalamic neurons have reciprocal glutamatergic connections with the cerebral cortex. The nucleus thalami reticularis, on the other hand, consisting mainly of GABAergic neurons, receives both cortical and thalamic afferents but also controls the activity of thalamocortical relay neurons via GABAergic projections. In addition, midline thalamic nuclei project to the cerebral cortex and striatum but also receive afferents from the brainstem, basal forebrain, and hypothalamus.[84,85]

Corticothalamic networks may drive the generation of rhythmic oscillatory activities, such as sleep spindles, but under pathological conditions, these may be transformed into characteristic epileptic discharges, such as spike-and-slow-wave discharges (SWDs), or may allow the spread of epileptic activities and secondary generalization of seizures. $GABA_A$ and $GABA_B$ receptors again play important roles in modulating the activity and expression of epileptic SWDs, as they are pacing the bursting activity of thalamic relay neurons.[84–87] The exact mechanisms underlying the age- and sex-specific features of absence epilepsies are still unknown, although a hypothesis for a possible role of developmental changes in the expression or function of $GABA_A$ receptors has been proposed.[88]

An interesting hypothesis implicating the thalamocortical network into the occasionally observed electroclinical uncoupling of neonatal seizures was proposed by Glykys et al.[89] Thalamic neurons exhibit hyperpolarizing $GABA_A$ receptor signaling very early in life, at ages when cortical neurons are still depolarized by GABA.[89] As a result, treatment of neonatal seizures with $GABA_A$ receptor agonists, like phenobarbital, can suppress epileptic activity in thalamic neurons but not in cortical neurons, resulting in a clinical suppression of seizure activity but a persistence of electrographic cortically generated seizure activity. However, the appearance of hyperpolarizing $GABA_A$ receptor responses across the whole seizure-controlling network is more complex as more caudal structures, like the SNR, do not manifest hyperpolarizing $GABA_A$ receptor responses until the second or third week of postnatal life, depending on the sex. The exact sequence of effects of these GABA-acting antiseizure drugs, through the whole seizure-controlling network, needs better clarification.

CONCLUSIONS

The regional specification of the brain into networks and their extensive interactions has allowed for the focused utilization of resources to optimally perform a task. The interconnectivity between neuronal networks allows for the coordination of different tasks and behaviors (see Chapter 29). The complex array of inputs and outputs to other systems, as well as biological or environmental cues, permits the adaptation of cognitive and behavioral processes to the circumstances existing each moment according to an age- and sex-specific manner. As a result, the normal basic protocols of network operation, as we have come to recognize them using simple and reproducible experimental setups, may drastically change in real life in manners that can be highly individualized (also see Chapter 28). In addition, the concept of abnormal expression and function is very relevant and context limited, as the example of depolarizing $GABA_A$ receptor activity indicates: it can be normal in very young ages but pathologic in later stages of development. It is therefore important to develop methods to achieve live, individualized monitoring of targets with sufficient temporal and spatial resolution, which will help establish correlations between target and network activity. This will be invaluable for not only providing proof-of-concept evidence for the roles of specific target mechanisms in the pathogenesis of a disease but also facilitating the implementation of individualized therapies.

Acknowledgments

Studies at Albert Einstein College of Medicine were supported by grants from NINDS/NICHD NS62947 and NS45243, NIH/NINDS NS 20253 and NS078333, CURE, PACE Foundation, Autism Speaks, the Heffer Family Medical Foundation, the Siegel Family Charitable Foundation, and the Eunice Kennedy Shriver National Institute of Child Health & Human Development of the National Institutes of Health (NIH) under Award Number P30HD071593.

References

1. Galanopoulou AS. GABA(A) receptors in normal development and seizures: friends or foes? *Curr Neuropharmacol.* 2008;6:1–20.
2. Farrant M, Kaila K. The cellular, molecular and ionic basis of GABA(A) receptor signalling. *Prog Brain Res.* 2007;160:59–87.
3. Ben-Ari Y. Excitatory actions of gaba during development: the nature of the nurture. *Nat. Rev. Neurosci.* 2002;3:728–739.
4. Rivera C, Voipio J, Payne JA, et al. The K+/Cl- co-transporter KCC2 renders GABA hyperpolarizing during neuronal maturation. *Nature.* 1999;397:251–255.
5. Plotkin MD, Snyder EY, Hebert SC, et al. Expression of the Na-K-2Cl cotransporter is developmentally regulated in postnatal rat brains: a possible mechanism underlying GABA's excitatory role in immature brain. *J. Neurobiol.* 1997;33:781–795.
6. Wang DD, Kriegstein AR. Blocking early GABA depolarization with bumetanide results in permanent alterations in cortical circuits and sensorimotor gating deficits. *Cereb. Cortex.* 2011;21:574–587.
7. Wang DD, Kriegstein AR. GABA regulates excitatory synapse formation in the neocortex via NMDA receptor activation. *J. Neurosci.* 2008;28:5547–5558.
8. Cancedda L, Fiumelli H, Chen K, et al. Excitatory GABA action is essential for morphological maturation of cortical neurons in vivo. *J. Neurosci.* 2007;27:5224–5235.
9. Veliskova J, Liptakova S, Hussain S. The effects of N-methyl-D-aspartate antagonist 2-amino-7-phosphonoheptanoic acid microinfusions into the adult male rat substantia nigra pars reticulata are site-specific. *Neurosci Lett.* 2001;316:108–110.
10. Deniau JM, Chevalier G. The lamellar organization of the rat substantia nigra pars reticulata: distribution of projection neurons. *Neuroscience.* 1992;46:361–377.
11. Galanopoulou AS, Kyrozis A, Claudio OI, et al. Sex-specific KCC2 expression and GABA(A) receptor function in rat substantia nigra. *Exp. Neurol.* 2003;183:628–637.
12. Ravizza T, Friedman LK, Moshe SL, et al. Sex differences in GABA(A)ergic system in rat substantia nigra pars reticulata. *Int. J. Dev. Neurosci.* 2003;21:245–254.
13. Veliskova J, Moshe SL. Sexual dimorphism and developmental regulation of substantia nigra function. *Ann. Neurol.* 2001;50:596–601.
14. Velisek L, Veliskova J, Ravizza T, et al. Circling behavior and [14C]2-deoxyglucose mapping in rats: possible implications for autistic repetitive behaviors. *Neurobiol Dis.* 2005; 18:346–355.
15. Gulcebi MI, Ketenci S, Linke R, et al. Topographical connections of the substantia nigra pars reticulata to higher-order thalamic nuclei in the rat. *Brain Res. Bull.* 2012;87:312–318.
16. O'Reilly RC. Biologically based computational models of high-level cognition. *Science.* 2006;314:91–94.
17. Sperber EF, Veliskova J, Germano IM, et al. Age-dependent vulnerability to seizures. *Adv. Neurol.* 1999;79:161–169.
18. Sabatino M, Ferraro G, Vella N, et al. Nigral influence on focal epilepsy. *Neurophysiol Clin.* 1990;20:189–201.
19. Depaulis A, Snead 3rd OC, Marescaux C, et al. Suppressive effects of intranigral injection of muscimol in three models of generalized non-convulsive epilepsy induced by chemical agents. *Brain Res.* 1989;498:64–72.
20. Garant DS, Gale K. Infusion of opiates into substantia nigra protects against maximal electroshock seizures in rats. *J. Pharmacol. Exp. Ther.* 1985;234:45–48.
21. De Sarro G, Meldrum BS, Reavill C. Anticonvulsant action of 2-amino-7-phosphonoheptanoic acid in the substantia nigra. *Eur J. Pharmacol.* 1984;106:175–179.
22. Iadarola MJ, Gale K. Substantia nigra: site of anticonvulsant activity mediated by gamma-aminobutyric acid. *Science.* 1982;218:1237–1240.
23. Veliskova J, Velsek L, Moshe SL. Subthalamic nucleus: a new anticonvulsant site in the brain. *Neuroreport.* 1996;7:1786–1788.
24. Veliskova J, Moshe SL. Update on the role of substantia nigra pars reticulata in the regulation of seizures. *Epilepsy Curr.* 2006;6:83–87.
25. Sperber EF, Wurpel JN, Moshe SL. Evidence for the involvement of nigral GABAB receptors in seizures of rat pups. *Brain Res. Dev. Brain Res.* 1989;47:143–146.
26. Moshe SL, Albala BJ. Nigral muscimol infusions facilitate the development of seizures in immature rats. *Brain Res.* 1984;315:305–308.
27. Kreindler A, Zuckermann E, Steriade M, et al. Electro-clinical features of convulsions induced by stimulation of brain stem. *J. Neurophysiol.* 1958;21:430–436.
28. Browning RA. Role of the brain-stem reticular formation in tonic-clonic seizures: lesion and pharmacological studies. *Fed. Proc.* 1985;44:2425–2431.
29. Browning RA, Nelson DK, Mogharreban N, et al. Effect of midbrain and pontine tegmental lesions on audiogenic seizures in genetically epilepsy-prone rats. *Epilepsia.* 1985;26:175–183.
30. Benn EK, Hauser WA, Shih T, et al. Estimating the incidence of first unprovoked seizure and newly diagnosed epilepsy in the low-income urban community of Northern Manhattans, New York City. Epilepsia. 2008;49:1431–9.
31. Annegers JF, Hauser WA, Lee JR, et al. Incidence of acute symptomatic seizures in Rochester, Minnesota, 1935-1984. *Epilepsia.* 1995;36:327–333.
32. Savic I, Engel Jr J. Sex differences in patients with mesial temporal lobe epilepsy. *J. Neurol Neurosurg Psychiatry.* 1998;65:910–912.
33. Nickel J, Jokeit H, Wunderlich G, et al. Gender-specific differences of hypometabolism in mTLE: implication for cognitive impairments. *Epilepsia.* 2003;44:1551–1561.
34. Gordon PH, Mehal JM, Holman RC, et al. Parkinson's disease among American Indians and Alaska natives: A nationwide prevalence study. *Mov. Disord.* 2012.

35. Martinez-Martin P, Falup Pecurariu C, Odin P, et al. Gender-related differences in the burden of non-motor symptoms in Parkinson's disease. *J. Neurol.* 2012;259:1639–1647.
36. Sperber EF, Wong BY, Wurpel JN, et al. Nigral infusions of muscimol or bicuculline facilitate seizures in developing rats. *Brain Res.* 1987;465:243–250.
37. Sperber EF, Wurpel JN, Zhao DY, et al. Evidence for the involvement of nigral GABAA receptors in seizures of adult rats. *Brain Res.* 1989;480:378–382.
38. Velisek L, Veliskova J, Ptachewich Y, et al. Age-dependent effects of gamma-aminobutyric acid agents on flurothyl seizures. *Epilepsia.* 1995;36:636–643.
39. Veliskova J, Loscher W, Moshe SL. Regional and age specific effects of zolpidem microinfusions in the substantia nigra on seizures. *Epilepsy Res.* 1998;30:107–114.
40. Xu SG, Garant DS, Sperber EF, et al. Effects of substantia nigra gamma-vinyl-GABA infusions on flurothyl seizures in adult rats. *Brain Res.* 1991;566:108–114.
41. Veliskova J, Velisek L, Nunes ML, et al. Developmental regulation of regional functionality of substantial nigra GABAA receptors involved in seizures. *Eur. J. Pharmacol.* 1996;309:167–173.
42. Xu SG, Garant DS, Sperber EF, et al. The proconvulsant effect of nigral infusions of THIP on flurothyl-induced seizures in rat pups. *Brain Res. Dev. Brain Res.* 1992;68:275–277.
43. Velisek L, Veliskova J, Giorgi FS, et al. Sex-specific control of flurothyl-induced tonic-clonic seizures by the substantia nigra pars reticulata during development. *Exp. Neurol.* 2006;201:203–211.
44. Okada R, Negishi N, Nagaya H. The role of the nigrotegmental GABAergic pathway in the propagation of pentylenetetrazol-induced seizures. *Brain Res.* 1989;480:383–387.
45. Wurpel JN, Sperber EF, Moshe SL. Age-dependent differences in the anticonvulsant effects of 2-amino-7-phosphono-heptanoic acid or ketamine infusions into the substantia nigra of rats. *Epilepsia.* 1992;33:439–443.
46. Velisek L, Veliskova J, Moshe SL. Electrical stimulation of substantia nigra pars reticulata is anticonvulsant in adult and young male rats. *Exp. Neurol.* 2002;173:145–152.
47. Chudomel O, Herman H, Nair K, et al. Age- and gender-related differences in GABAA receptor-mediated postsynaptic currents in GABAergic neurons of the substantia nigra reticulata in the rat. *Neuroscience.* 2009;163:155–167.
48. Kyrozis A, Chudomel O, Moshe SL, et al. Sex-dependent maturation of GABAA receptor-mediated synaptic events in rat substantia nigra reticulata. *Neurosci. Lett.* 2006;398:1–5.
49. Galanopoulou AS. Sex- and cell-type-specific patterns of GABAA receptor and estradiol-mediated signaling in the immature rat substantia nigra. *Eur. J. Neurosci.* 2006;23:2423–2430.
50. Canonaco M, Tavolaro R, Facciolo RM, et al. Sexual dimorphism of GABAA receptor levels in subcortical brain regions of a woodland rodent (Apodemus sylvaticus). *Brain Res. Bull.* 1996;40:187–194.
51. Galanopoulou AS, Alm EM, Veliskova J. Estradiol reduces seizure-induced hippocampal injury in ovariectomized female but not in male rats. *Neurosci Lett.* 2003;342:201–205.
52. Galanopoulou AS. Sexually dimorphic expression of KCC2 and GABA function. *Epilepsy Res.* 2008;80:99–113.
53. Giorgi FS, Veliskova J, Chudomel O, et al. The role of substantia nigra pars reticulata in modulating clonic seizures is determined by testosterone levels during the immediate postnatal period. *Neurobiol Dis.* 2007;25:73–79.
54. Hasson H, Kim M, Moshe SL. Effective treatments of prolonged status epilepticus in developing rats. *Epilepsy Behav.* 2008;13:62–69.
55. Dzhala VI, Brumback AC, Staley KJ. Bumetanide enhances phenobarbital efficacy in a neonatal seizure model. *Ann. Neurol.* 2008;63:222–235.
56. Sankar R, Painter MJ. Neonatal seizures: after all these years we still love what doesn't work. *Neurology.* 2005;64:776–777.
57. Staley KJ, Mody I. Shunting of excitatory input to dentate gyrus granule cells by a depolarizing GABAA receptor-mediated postsynaptic conductance. *J. Neurophysiol.* 1992;68:197–212.
58. Galanopoulou AS, Vidaurre J, Moshe SL. Under what circumstances can seizures produce hippocampal injury: evidence for age-specific effects. *Dev. Neurosci.* 2002;24:355–363.
59. Gil-Nagel A, Risinger MW. Ictal semiology in hippocampal versus extrahippocampal temporal lobe epilepsy. *Brain.* 1997;120(Pt 1):183–192.
60. Blumenfeld H. Consciousness and epilepsy: why are patients with absence seizures absent? *Prog Brain Res.* 2005;150:271–286.
61. Herzog AG, Coleman AE, Jacobs AR, et al. Interictal EEG discharges, reproductive hormones, and menstrual disorders in epilepsy. *Ann. Neurol.* 2003;54:625–637.
62. Herzog AG, Coleman AE, Jacobs AR, et al. Relationship of sexual dysfunction to epilepsy laterality and reproductive hormone levels in women. *Epilepsy Behav.* 2003;4:407–413.
63. Fogarasi A, Jokeit H, Faveret E, et al. The effect of age on seizure semiology in childhood temporal lobe epilepsy. *Epilepsia.* 2002;43:638–643.
64. Fogarasi A, Tuxhorn I, Janszky J, et al. Age-dependent seizure semiology in temporal lobe epilepsy. *Epilepsia.* 2007;48:1697–1702.
65. Khazipov R, Khalilov I, Tyzio R, et al. Developmental changes in GABAergic actions and seizure susceptibility in the rat hippocampus. *Eur. J. Neurosci.* 2004;19:590–600.
66. Tyzio R, Minlebaev M, Rheims S, et al. Postnatal changes in somatic gamma-aminobutyric acid signalling in the rat hippocampus. *Eur. J. Neurosci.* 2008;27:2515–2528.
67. Galanopoulou AS. Dissociated gender-specific effects of recurrent seizures on GABA signaling in CA1 pyramidal neurons: role of GABA(A) receptors. *J. Neurosci.* 2008;28:1557–1567.
68. Auger AP, Hexter DP, McCarthy MM. Sex difference in the phosphorylation of cAMP response element binding protein (CREB) in neonatal rat brain. *Brain Res.* 2001;890:110–117.
69. Danglot L, Triller A, Marty S. The development of hippocampal interneurons in rodents. *Hippocampus.* 2006;16:1032–1060.
70. Holter NI, Zylla MM, Zuber N, et al. Tonic GABAergic control of mouse dentate granule cells during postnatal development. *Eur. J. Neurosci.* 2010;32:1300–1309.
71. Galanopoulou AS, Moshe SL. In search of epilepsy biomarkers in the immature brain: goals, challenges and strategies. *Biomark Med.* 2011;5:615–628.
72. Ritter LM, Vazquez DM, Meador-Woodruff JH. Ontogeny of ionotropic glutamate receptor subunit expression in the rat hippocampus. *Brain Res. Dev. Brain Res.* 2002;139:227–236.
73. Insel TR, Miller LP, Gelhard RE. The ontogeny of excitatory amino acid receptors in rat forebrain—I. N-methyl-D-aspartate and quisqualate receptors. *Neuroscience.* 1990;35:31–43.
74. Pellegrini-Giampietro DE, Zukin RS, Bennett MV, et al. Switch in glutamate receptor subunit gene expression in CA1 subfield of hippocampus following global ischemia in rats. *Proc. Natl. Acad. Sci. U S A.* 1992;89:10499–10503.
75. Rakhade SN, Jensen FE. Epileptogenesis in the immature brain: emerging mechanisms. *Nat. Rev. Neurol.* 2009;5:380–391.
76. Brooks-Kayal AR, Raol YH, Russek SJ. Alteration of epileptogenesis genes. *Neurotherapeutics.* 2009;6:312–318.
77. Brooks-Kayal AR. Rearranging receptors. *Epilepsia.* 2005;46(suppl 7):29–38.

78. Huberfeld G, Wittner L, Clemenceau S, et al. Perturbed chloride homeostasis and GABAergic signaling in human temporal lobe epilepsy. *J. Neurosci.* 2007;27:9866–9873.
79. Miles R, Blaesse P, Huberfeld G, et al. Chloride homeostasis and GABA signaling in temporal lobe epilepsy. In: Noebels JL, Avoli M, Rogawski MA, et al. (Eds) Jasper's Basic Mechanisms of the Epilepsies. 4th ed. Bethesda (MD) 2012.
80. Cohen I, Navarro V, Clemenceau S, et al. On the origin of interictal activity in human temporal lobe epilepsy in vitro. *Science.* 2002;298:1418–1421.
81. Munoz A, Mendez P, DeFelipe J, et al. Cation-chloride cotransporters and GABA-ergic innervation in the human epileptic hippocampus. *Epilepsia.* 2007;48:663–673.
82. Palma E, Amici M, Sobrero F, et al. Anomalous levels of Cl- transporters in the hippocampal subiculum from temporal lobe epilepsy patients make GABA excitatory. *Proc. Natl. Acad Sci. U S A.* 2006;103:8465–8468.
83. Bregestovski P, Bernard C, Excitatory GABA. How a Correct Observation May Turn Out to be an Experimental Artifact. *Front Pharmacol.* 2012;3:65.
84. Coulter DA. *Thalamocortical Anatomy and Physiology Philadelphia.* Lippincott-Raven Publishers; 1997.
85. Blumenfeld H, McCormick DA. Corticothalamic inputs control the pattern of activity generated in thalamocortical networks. *J. Neurosci.* 2000;20:5153–5162.
86. Walker MC, Kullmann DM. Tonic GABAA Receptor-Mediated Signaling in Epilepsy. In: Noebels JL, Avoli M, Rogawski MA, et al. (Eds) Jasper's Basic Mechanisms of the Epilepsies. 4th ed. Bethesda (MD)2012.
87. Han HA, Cortez MA, Snead OC. GABAB Receptor and Absence Epilepsy. In: Noebels JL, Avoli M, Rogawski MA, et al. (Eds) Jasper's Basic Mechanisms of the Epilepsies. 4th ed. Bethesda (MD)2012.
88. Li H, Huguenard JR, Fisher RS. Gender and age differences in expression of GABAA receptor subunits in rat somatosensory thalamus and cortex in an absence epilepsy model. *Neurobiol Dis.* 2007;25:623–630.
89. Glykys J, Dzhala VI, Kuchibhotla KV, et al. Differences in cortical versus subcortical GABAergic signaling: a candidate mechanism of electroclinical uncoupling of neonatal seizures. *Neuron.* 2009;63:657–672.

CHAPTER

12

Astrocytic Regulation of Synapses, Neuronal Networks, and Behavior

Michael M. Halassa[1], *Marcello D'Ascenzo*[2], *Anna Boccaccio*[3], *Tommaso Fellin*[3]

[1]Department of Psychiatry, Massachusetts General Hospital, Boston, MA, USA, [2]Institute of Human Physiology, Medical School, Università Cattolica, Rome, Italy, [3]Department of Neuroscience and Brain Technologies, Istituto Italiano di Tecnologia, Genova, Italy

INTRODUCTION

In the mammalian central nervous system, astrocytes are intimately associated with neurons. This structural association forms the basis for the physiological communication between these two cell types. Astrocytes enwrap neuronal processes[1,2] and are essential for a number of supportive functions, such as synaptic glutamate uptake, glutamate recycling, K^+ buffering, and lactate secretion.[3,4] In addition, astrocytes are capable of releasing chemical transmitters in a process termed gliotransmission.[5–8] We will review recent experimental evidence showing that gliotransmission modulates fundamental aspects of brain function from synaptic transmission to neuronal excitability, cortical oscillations, and behavior.

ASTROCYTIC-NEURONAL STRUCTURAL ASSOCIATION

In contrast to the star-shaped structure revealed by metal impregnation methods and glial fibrillary acidic protein (GFAP) staining, astrocytes are now appreciated to exhibit a much more complex morphology. In fact, a study in which astrocytes were electroporated with lipophilic dyes in situ showed that GFAP staining reveals only 15% of the astrocytic volume.[9] The rest of the astrocyte, which includes secondary, tertiary, and fine processes, remains invisible to classical staining methods (Figure 12.1).

Lipophilic dye filling[9] and molecular genetic labeling of astrocytes with the green fluorescent protein (GFP)[11] have shown that these cells occupy nonoverlapping

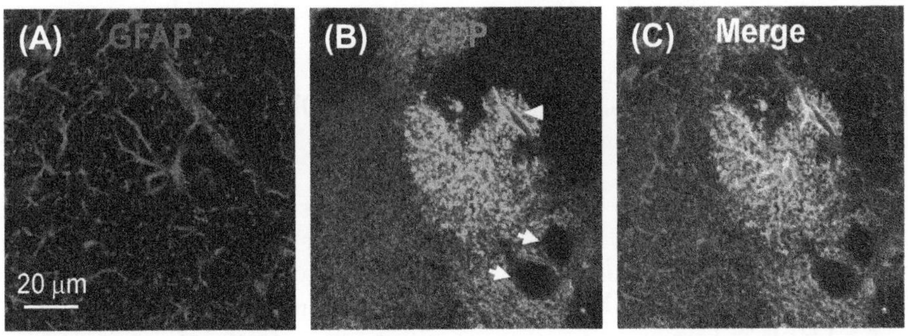

FIGURE 12.1 **Astrocytic morphology and structural relationship with neurons**. (A) Immunostaining against the glial-specific protein GFAP reveals only a limited portion of the astrocytic structure, composed mainly of primary processes. (B) When the fluorescent marker GFP is specifically expressed in a subpopulation of astrocytes, fine higher order processes become visible, revealing the complexity of the astrocytic morphology. Astrocytes contact neuronal cell bodies (arrows in B) and blood vessels (arrowhead in B). Images in A–B are merged in (C). (*Source: Reproduced with permission from Ref. 10.*) (The figure is reproduced in color section.)

Neuronal Networks in Brain Function, CNS Disorders, and Therapeutics
http://dx.doi.org/10.1016/B978-0-12-415804-7.00012-5

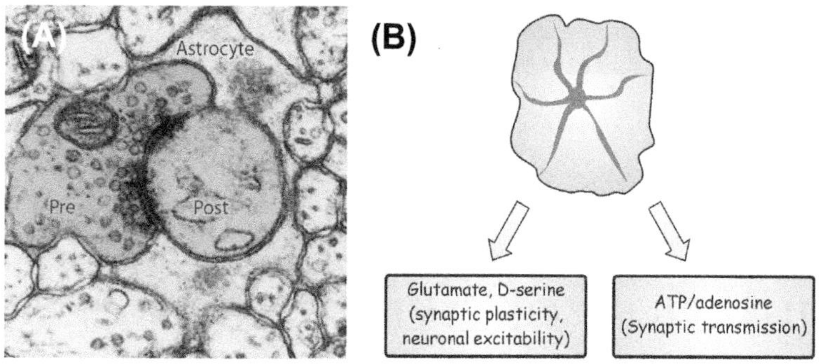

FIGURE 12.2 **Astrocytes modulate neuronal function by releasing different chemical transmitters.** (A) The structural basis of the concept of the tripartite synapse is shown in this electron microscopy image. The astrocytic process (green) enwraps both the presynaptic (red) and postsynaptic (orange) terminals. (*Source: Reproduced with permission from Ref. 12.*) (B) Astrocytes release glutamate and D-serine that, by activating NMDA receptors, modulate synaptic plasticity, neuronal excitability, and synchrony. Astrocytes also release ATP, which is degraded to adenosine and strongly suppresses synaptic transmission by activating adenosine A1 receptors. (*Source: Modified from Ref. 13.*) (The figure is reproduced in color section.)

territories both in the hippocampus and in the cortex. Furthermore, a single cortical astrocyte enwraps, on average, four neuronal cell bodies and hundreds of dendrites.[11] On an ultrastructural level, the astrocytic process is opposed to the pre- and postsynaptic neuronal terminals of most synapses (Figure 12.2(A)), and it has been estimated that an astrocyte contacts ~100,000 synapses.[2] The highly organized structure of astrocytes and their close association with neurons suggest that astrocytes could play a role in the regulation of neuronal function. Indeed, following seminal studies performed in the early 1990s,[14,15] the term "tripartite synapse" was coined by Haydon and colleagues,[5] highlighting the partnership of astrocytes and neurons and its importance in synaptic physiology (see the "Gliotransmission" section).

Time lapse confocal microscopy in slice cultures has demonstrated that astrocytic processes dynamically contact dendritic spines,[16,17] and electron micrography of the supraoptic nucleus has shown that the astrocytic coverage of synapses of that region is highly dependent on the hormonal state of the animal[18]; virgin rats show high astrocytic coverage of synapses, while in lactating animals astrocytic processes withdraw from synapses, dramatically impacting synaptic physiology.[19] Thus, rather than being static components of the tripartite synapse, astrocytic processes are highly dynamic structures whose coverage of the pre- and postsynaptic terminals can impact neuronal excitability and synaptic plasticity.

GLIOTRANSMISSION: THE RELEASE OF CHEMICAL TRANSMITTERS BY ASTROCYTES

Gliotransmission is an umbrella term that describes the release of chemical transmitters from astrocytes through different cellular mechanisms. For example, astrocytes release the transmitter glutamate via exocytosis, anion channels, and hemichannels.[20] The list of molecules released by astrocytes is long and includes, among others, adenosine-5′-triphosphate (ATP), D-serine, glutamate, brain-derived neurotropic factor (BDNF), neuropeptide Y (NPY), tumor necrosis factor alpha (TNF-α), and atrial natriuretic peptide (ANP) (for reviews, see Refs 6,8,13,21).

Out of the several potential pathways of gliotransmission, vesicular release is arguably best understood from a cellular and physiological point of view. Experimental evidence suggests that astrocytes express a number of vesicular proteins, including synaptobrevin II, cellubrevin, SNAP23, Munc18, and complexin.[22] This allows astrocytes to release chemicals in a soluble *N*-ethylamide attachment protein receptor (SNARE)-dependent manner. Furthermore, astrocytes express synaptotagmin IV, a key regulator of SNARE-dependent release in these cells.[22]

Astrocytes release ATP, D-serine, glutamate, BDNF, and NPY in a vesicular manner.[23–27] Whether these gliotransmitters are packaged in overlapping vesicle pools remains an open question. However, recent evidence suggests that ATP and glutamate are packaged in distinct vesicles in cultured astrocytes.[23]

COMPLEXITY OF ASTROCYTE-TO-NEURON COMMUNICATION

Several studies have investigated the role of chemical transmitter release from astrocytes in different aspects of neuronal function. For example, Oliet and colleagues demonstrated that D-serine released by astrocytes acts as a co-agonist of synaptic *N*-methyl-D-aspartate (NMDA) receptors to boost NMDA-mediated currents.[19] The availability of D-serine at synapses has a profound impact on synaptic metaplasticity (the plasticity of synaptic plasticity). Decreasing the synaptic availability of this gliotransmitter either by enzymatic degradation or by withdrawal of the astrocytic process results in favoring the induction of long-term depression (LTD) over long-term potentiation (LTP) following a high-frequency stimulus.[19] Thus, by regulating the activity of neuronal NMDA receptors, astrocytic D-serine controls synaptic metaplasticity.

In addition to D-serine, astrocytes release glutamate that acts on both presynaptic metabotropic glutamate (mGluRs)[28] and postsynaptic NMDA receptors.[29,30] Activation of presynaptic mGluRs by astrocytic glutamate leads to a transient increase in the release probability of these terminals. Enhanced release probability becomes long lasting when astrocytic glutamate release coincides with postsynaptic neuronal depolarization.[28] Activation of postsynaptic NMDA receptors by astrocytic glutamate generates slow inward currents (SICs).[29–33] These events occur with a high degree of synchrony in closely spaced (<100 μm) neurons.[30,34,35] When recorded in current clamp, neuronal depolarization induced by glutamate release from astrocytes leads to firing of single as well as multiple action potentials,[36] demonstrating that gliotransmission can impact neuronal excitability.

In addition to providing an excitatory drive for synaptic transmission and neuronal excitability, astrocytes can exert suppressive actions on neurons. For example (as discussed in this chapter), astrocytes release ATP, which, upon rapid degradation to adenosine, acts on A1 receptors to inhibit synaptic transmission.[37,38] Astrocytic release of ATP can be both spontaneous and activity dependent, providing both a tonic and a phasic suppression of synaptic transmission.[38]

In summary, astrocytes release a variety of neuroactive molecules that deeply impact fundamental brain functions such as synaptic plasticity, neuronal excitability, and synchrony (Figure 12.2). As described here, it is important to emphasize that different gliotransmitters can have different, even opposing, effects on synapses.[12] For example, by targeting NMDA receptors, D-serine and glutamate provide excitatory drive to neuronal networks, while adenosine inhibits synaptic release of neurotransmitters by activating A1 receptors. Whether the same astrocyte is able to release different gliotransmitters under different conditions is not known. In addition, how a neuronal network is able to integrate the synergistic and opposing actions of different gliotransmitters is an exciting area of future investigations.

The generation of genetically engineered mice to inhibit vesicular gliotransmission revealed that ATP is a primary gliotransmitter in vivo.[38] Inhibiting this pathway revealed a role for astrocytic purines in the coordination of synaptic networks, in the control of spontaneous cortical rhythms[10] and in the modulation of sleep-related behaviors.[39] Therefore, for the rest of this chapter, we mainly focus on experimental results that were obtained with the use of transgenic mice and that point to a central role of astrocytic release of ATP in brain physiology and behavior.

VESICULAR ATP RELEASE FROM ASTROCYTES AND ITS FUNCTIONAL CONSEQUENCES ON NEURONAL FUNCTION

Although considered organs of degradation, lysosomes are known to be secretion competent in a number of cell types, including melanocytes and hematopoietic cells.[40] Incubating cultured astrocytes with styryl dyes results in labeling a pool of recycling vesicles, which includes lysosomes.[23,41] In one study,[23] the stimulation of astrocytes by ATP or glutamate resulted in partial destaining of *N*-(3-triethylammoniumpropyl)-4-(4-(diethylamino)styryl)pyridinium dibromide (FM2-10), a fluorescent dye for labeling lysosomes, suggesting a "kiss-and-run" mode of fusion of these organelles. Incubating cultured astrocytes with BAPTA-AM resulted in the inhibition of lysosomal exocytosis, suggesting that this process is Ca^{2+} dependent. Subcellular fractionation experiments and confocal imaging of Mant-ATP, a fluorescent ATP analog, show that lysosomes contain high levels of ATP, suggesting that lysosomes may be the organelles' mediating vesicular purinergic gliotransmission.[23] The fact that astrocytes are enriched with genes involved in lysosomal biogenesis[42] is consistent with this notion.

In addition to lysosomes, astrocytic dense core vesicles have been shown to contain high levels of ATP that are able to release this purine in a tetanus-toxin and Ca^{2+}-sensitive manner.[43] Whether lysosomal or dense core vesicle-dependent release of ATP represents the primary source of purinergic gliotransmission in vivo remains an open question.

Astrocytic ATP can directly excite neurons by activating purinergic receptors, or it can be degraded to adenosine and act on neuronal adenosine receptors. For example, by activating $P2X_7$ receptors on magnocellular neurons (MCN), hypothalamic astrocytes cause an increase in AMPA receptor surface expression on these neurons and thus an increase in neuronal excitability.[44] Astrocytes can be activated by neuromodulators such as norepinephrine, which cause ATP release from these glia and the resulting consequences on neuronal excitability. Interestingly, when astrocytic function is inhibited, the excitatory action of norepinephrine on MCN neurons is abolished, suggesting that astrocytes in certain situations can be the primary transducers of neuromodulatory inputs. Given that astrocytes have recently been shown to impact sleep[39,45] (discussed in this chapter), a process that is highly dependent on neuromodulation, the role of astrocytes in transducing neuromodulatory input may have far-reaching implications in understanding neuronal network function and sleep physiology.

Molecular genetics, including the generation of astrocyte-specific transgenic animals, has allowed for a cleaner approach to investigating the role of astrocytes in synaptic physiology, neuronal network function, and behavior. One such model, developed by Haydon and colleagues, introduced a dominant negative SNARE (dnSNARE) into astrocytes in a conditional manner.[38] Using the well-established Tet-Off system, this model allows for doxycycline-mediated control of gliotransmission. The generation of the "dnSNARE mouse" allowed for establishing a role of astrocytic purines in coordinating synaptic networks. That is, in a paper by Pascual et al., the authors showed that astrocytes release ATP that, after rapid degradation to adenosine, exerts a tonic suppression of excitatory synaptic transmission in the hippocampus. Brain slices derived from dnSNARE mice showed an enhancement of basal CA3–CA1 synaptic transmission, a phenotype that was rescued by perfusing these slices with ATP. The effect of ATP depended on the activity of 5′ectonucleotidases, the enzyme that converts ATP to adenosine, demonstrating that adenosine, and not ATP, is the molecule mediating the rescue of the dnSNARE phenotype. Furthermore, this important study showed that astrocytic purinergic signaling is dynamically recruited by high-frequency stimulation of certain synapses, to suppress nearby inactive synapses in a process termed heterosynaptic suppression.

GLIOTRANSMISSION MODULATES NETWORK ACTIVITY AND CORTICAL RHYTHMS IN VIVO

All the experimental evidence described so far has been obtained in brain slice preparation, but whether gliotransmission influences neuronal activity in vivo is not known. A recent study[10] addresses this issue and demonstrates that astrocytes modulate slow oscillations, a cortical rhythm that characterizes non-rapid-eye-movement (NREM) sleep.[46,47]

Urethane-anesthetized mice are a good model for the study of slow oscillations because, under this type of anesthesia, slow oscillations represent the main spontaneous rhythm in the cortex. This cortical oscillation consists of spontaneous bursts of synchronous activity (also called upstates) intermingled with silent periods (named downstates) at a frequency of <1 Hz. By using local field potential recordings in vivo and comparing slow oscillations in wild-type (WT) and in transgenic mice with impaired gliotransmission (dnSNARE), the authors found significantly reduced power of the slow oscillations in transgenic compared to control mice.[10] Importantly, these results were confirmed with patch-clamp recordings in vivo from pyramidal neurons of the superficial layers of the somatosensory cortex (Figure 12.3). Neurons in dnSNARE mice have a lower probability of being in the upstate compared to the same neurons in a WT animal. The reduced upstate probability is due to the shorter duration of the upstates and prolonged duration of the downstates (Figure 12.3).

These results demonstrate that the impairment of gliotransmission results in altered network activity and

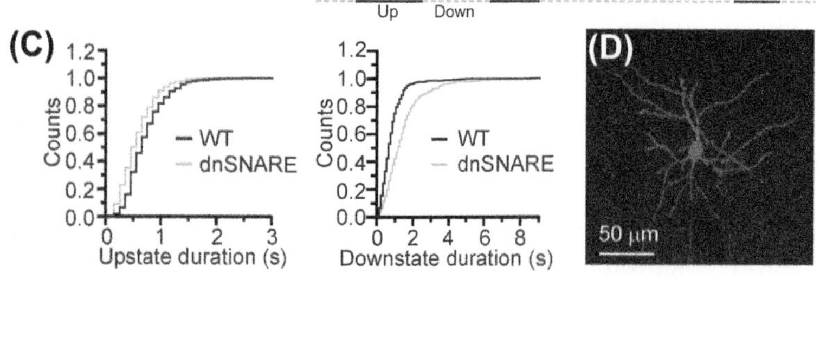

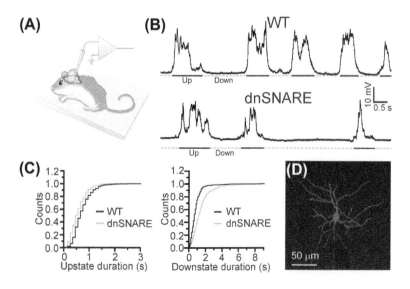

FIGURE 12.3 **Inhibition of gliotransmission results in altered neuronal activity in vivo.** (A–B) In vivo patch-clamp recordings from cortical neurons demonstrate that inhibition of gliotransmission (dnSNARE mouse) results in altered slow oscillations in the cortex (B). (C) Shorter upstate (left) and prolonged downstate (right) durations are observed in dnSNARE compared to WT animals. The morphological reconstruction of a recorded cell is shown in (D). (*Source: Reproduced with permission from Ref. 10.*) (For color version of this figure, the reader is referred to the online version of this book.)

show that the communication between astrocytes and neurons plays an active role in the modulation of neuronal function and rhythmogenesis in vivo.

To understand the mechanisms by which the inhibition of gliotransmission results in altered network activity, the authors investigated the effect of dnSNARE expression into astrocytes on cortical synapses, which are known to be of fundamental importance in the generation of slow oscillations.[48–50] Two main effects were observed: first, dnSNARE expression in astrocytes leads to a hypofunction of NMDA receptors at cortical synapses. Second, block of gliotransmission results in a decrease of the tonic level of extracellular adenosine and, as a consequence, in the loss of the tonic A1 receptor-mediated suppression of cortical synapses. Thus, on the one side, astrocytes boost NMDA receptor function, while, on the other, they tonically suppress synaptic activity by activating presynaptic A1 receptors. The integration of these two opposing effects on cortical synapses is likely to be responsible for the altered slow-oscillation activity that is observed in transgenic dnSNARE mice. Indeed, co-application of NMDA and A1 receptor antagonists in WT animals, to partially mimic the effect of dnSNARE expression on cortical synapses, results in a reduction of slow oscillations similar to that observed in the dnSNARE mouse.[10]

Given that slow oscillations are a brain rhythm characterizing NREM sleep, the authors also tested whether slow oscillations were affected in dnSNARE mice in freely behaving animals during natural sleep. A fundamental property of sleep is that its intensity is a function of prior wakefulness, that is, sleep is homeostatically regulated: the more a subject is awake, the higher the intensity of subsequent sleep is. Slow oscillations correlate with sleep intensity (otherwise called sleep pressure). Specifically, slow oscillations are increased when sleep pressure is high, and they are decreased when sleep pressure is low. Using chronic electroencephalogram (EEG) recordings in WT and dnSNARE mice, the authors found that, under conditions of high homeostatic sleep-pressure when slow oscillations are boosted, the power of slow oscillations was significantly reduced in dnSNARE animals compared to controls. In contrast, when sleep pressure is low and slow oscillations are decreased, no difference could be observed between WT and dnSNARE animals.[10]

ASTROCYTES REGULATE SLEEP-RELATED BEHAVIORS

In addition to regulating sleep-related rhythms, we have recently shown that astrocytes directly regulate sleep behavior[39] (see Chapter 21). Sleep is an ancient behavior that is regulated by a circadian clock (see Chapter 14), which controls the timing and entrainment of sleep to environmental stimuli such as the light–dark cycle and food availability, and by a homeostatic process that regulates sleep intensity as a function of prior wakefulness. Recent studies[51] have shown that understanding why lost sleep has to be compensated may be key to understanding why one needs to sleep at all. Slow-wave activity (SWA) in the NREM sleep EEG has been shown to correlate with sleep intensity.[52] Given that the EEG is thought to sample cortical subthreshold synaptic potentials, Tononi and colleagues hypothesized that an enhancement in cortical synaptic transmission underlies the increase in SWA when sleep pressure is high. An elegant paper by Tononi's group[53] has shown that wakefulness is accompanied by an enhancement of cortical synaptic transmission, while sleep is accompanied by a reduction in cortical synaptic transmission. This was paralleled by biochemical evidence showing that NMDA receptor function is enhanced during wakefulness to promote LTP-like processes, while the opposite occurs during sleep. Thus, one leading hypothesis of sleep function states that cortical synapses are strengthened by wake-dependent sensory experience and that sleep is required for synaptic scaling to reduce energy and space demand. This hypothesis is supported by the fact that sleep is dominated by slow oscillations, which are in the right frequency range for inducing LTD-like processes that may underlie synaptic scaling.[54]

Adenosine is known to be an important homeostatic sleep factor. Adenosine levels in the brain correlate with the amount of prior wakefulness, the introduction of adenosine into the brain promotes sleep, and blocking adenosine action can attenuate sleep (and sleep drive).[55,56] Given that astrocytes control adenosine levels in the brain, we used the dnSNARE mouse (which is known to have a deficiency in astrocytic adenosine accumulation) to test whether astrocytes are involved in this fundamental process.

Our studies[39] showed that dnSNARE mice exhibit an attenuated SWA phenotype under baseline conditions and following a 6 h period of sleep deprivation (Figure 12.4(A) and (B)). This is accompanied by resilience to the effect of sleep deprivation on learning and memory. This means that when WT animals are sleep deprived following a novel object recognition task, their memory consolidation is impaired, and when tested 18 h later, they exhibit deficits in memory expression. dnSNARE mice, on the other hand, are completely immune to the effect of sleep deprivation on recognition memory (Figure 12.4(C) and (D)). Furthermore, both the sleep and memory phenotypes are mimicked in WT animals when adenosine A1 receptors are antagonized by delivering 8-cyclopentyltheophylline (CPT), an A1 receptor antagonist, into brain ventricles using osmotic minipumps.[39] Thus, astrocytic adenosine

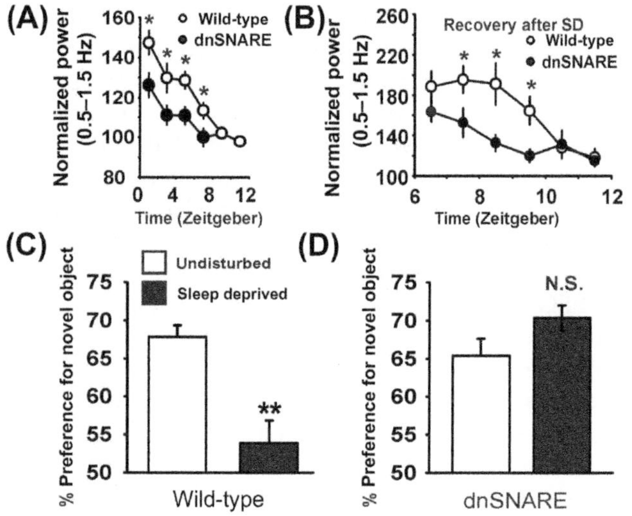

FIGURE 12.4 **Gliotransmission modulates sleep homeostasis and sleep-related behaviors.** (A–B) During the light phase (A) or following a period of sleep deprivation (SD) (B), low-frequency slow-wave activity (SWA) is reduced in the dnSNARE when compared to WT animals. (C–D) Sleep deprivation impairs novel object recognition in WT (C) but not in dnSNARE (D) animals. (*Source: Reproduced with permission from Ref. 39.*)

regulates mammalian sleep homeostasis and cognitive consequences of sleep loss. Given Tononi's hypothesis of sleep function and centrality of homeostatic regulation of this behavior to its role in brain function, understanding the details of astrocytic regulation of sleep homeostasis, including their potential role in transducing wake/sleep-promoting neuromodulatory input into different brain regions, may be vital to ultimately understand why we sleep.

ASTROCYTIC NEUROMODULATION CONTRIBUTES TO FEEDBACK CONTROL OF BREATHING

Astrocytes, besides contacting hundreds of neuronal processes, multiple cell bodies, and thousands of synapses, are also intimately associated with microvasculature, onto which they extend several end-feet.[57] Astrocytes therefore are in the right position to quickly relay blood-borne stimuli to the activities of neuronal networks. A remarkable example of how astrocytes serve as a vascular-neuronal interface is provided by a recent study[58] that focused on the central nervous mechanisms underlying the chemosensory control of breathing.

Breathing in vertebrates is a fundamental behavior present from birth until death. Homeostatic control of breathing is achieved by feedback loops involving chemical receptors in the peripheral circulation and in the central nervous system. Central respiratory chemoreception refers specifically to the mechanism by which an increase in brain PCO_2 (hypercapñia) stimulates breathing in order to maintain the arterial PCO_2 value within a few mmHg of the steady-state level (~40 mmHg).[59] The dominant theory of central respiratory chemoreception is that CO_2 works indirectly through its effect on pH, which stimulates different neuronal populations located near the ventral surface (VS) of the medulla oblongata of the brainstem, in particular on the overlapping retrotrapezoid nucleus–parafacial respiratory group.[60] Despite this general scheme, which includes the notion that neurons are the unique cells able to sense brain CO_2 (or pH), Gourine and colleagues have recently proposed that astrocytes fulfill an equivalent role.[58] In elegant experiments, they show that in anesthetized and artificially ventilated rats, a modest acidification (0.2 pH) of the solution covering the surgically exposed brainstem VS causes an immediate increase in intracellular Ca^{2+} in VS astrocytes expressing the genetically encoded Ca^{2+} sensor Case12.[58] Ca^{2+} excitation of VS astrocytes in response to acidification has been observed also in in vitro preparations such as acute brainstem slices of adult rats, organotypic brainstem slice cultures, and dissociated VS astrocytes. Hypercapnia-evoked $[Ca^{2+}]$ increase in VS astrocytes also leads to release of ATP, which promotes a Ca^{2+} influx into neighboring astrocytes through ionotropic purinergic P2X receptors and, consequently, local propagation of astrocytic Ca^{2+} excitation.

Calcium imaging and patch-clamp recordings from neurons within the retrotrapezoid nucleus (RTN) revealed that reversible membrane depolarization of these neurons induced by changes in pH is largely mediated by prior release of ATP through the activation of metabotropic P2Y receptors.[58] This finding prompted the authors to test whether released ATP from astrocytes was responsible for the increased activity of RTN neurons. In order to mimic pH-evoked Ca^{2+} excitation in astrocytes, they used an adenoviral vector in which the mutated version of the light-sensitive channelrhodopsin-2 is fused to a far-red-shifted fluorescent protein, Katushka 1.3, and expressed in brainstem astrocytes using enhanced GFAP promoter. Selective optogenetic stimulation of VS astrocytes in organotypic brainstem slices triggered immediate ATP release and evoked long-lasting depolarization of RTN neurons via an ATP-dependent mechanism. Importantly, an illumination-evoked Ca^{2+} increase in VS astrocytes triggered robust activation of the respiratory network in vivo. In particular, Gourine et al. reported that in anesthetized and artificially ventilated rats, unilateral illumination of astrocytes in the brainstem VS triggered robust respiratory activity, and this response was blocked by ATP receptor antagonist MRS2179. Moreover, the same effect was observed in animals breathing normally.[58]

The results of this study have been recently strengthened by new evidence demonstrating that brainstem-cultured astrocytes are functionally specialized to sense changes in pH and respond to acidification with enhanced vesicular release of ATP.[61] In particular, by using total internal reflection fluorescence (TIRF) microscopy, Kasymov and colleagues found that 35% of cultured brainstem astrocytes respond to acidification with an increased rate of exocytosis of ATP-containing vesicular compartments. Interestingly, this effect, which required intracellular Ca^{2+} signaling and was independent of autocrine ATP action, was completely absent in cortical cultured astrocytes. Moreover, they found a higher level of expression of genes encoding proteins associated with ATP vesicular transport and fusion in brainstem astrocytes compared to cortical astrocytes. Although this study did not reveal the mechanism(s) underlying the high sensitivity of brainstem astrocytes to changes in pH, it demonstrates that brainstem astrocytes, in contrast to cortical astrocytes, possess specific signaling properties that link changes in extracellular pH to exocytosis of ATP-containing vesicles.

Taken together, all these multifaceted studies led the authors to propose a mechanism by which VS astrocytes regulate breathing in vivo. Specifically, the acidification-evoked $[Ca^{2+}]$ increase in VS astrocytes leads to release into the extracellular space of ATP that stimulates metabotropic P2Y receptors and thus depolarizes neurons in the adjacent and overlapping RTN. Consequently, the increased rate of action potential firing of the RTN neurons propagates to the pre-Bötzinger neurons that ultimately induce stimulation of inspiratory muscle activities. These studies thereby not only indicate that astrocytes are capable of sensing the pH$-PCO_2$ level of the arterial blood entering the brainstem but also provide a remarkable example of glial participation in complex behavior.

CONCLUDING REMARKS

In this chapter, we summarized some of the most recent evidence highlighting the importance of astrocytes in brain function. Based on these results, a new view of astrocytes is emerging in which, besides providing structural and metabolic support to neurons, astrocytes also have signaling capabilities. Indeed, in different experimental systems from cultured cells to slice and in vivo preparations, astrocytes have been shown to release chemical transmitters. These transmitters can modulate several aspects of neuronal function from the activity of single synapses to that of neuronal networks. For example, D-serine and ATP released by astrocytes control synaptic transmission and plasticity. Moreover, inhibition of transmitter release from these cells results in altered rhythmogenesis in the cortex in vivo and in the alteration of sleep-related behaviors. These results open a new horizon in the study of astrocytic function and suggest that the understanding of brain properties under physiological and pathological conditions,[7,13,62,63] in particular in the context of neuromodulation, will necessarily go through a better understanding of astrocytic complex biology.

Acknowledgments

This work was supported by Telethon-Italy (GGP10138), San Paolo "Programma in Neuroscienze", and FIRB (RBAP11X42L) to T.F.

References

1. Peters A, Palay SL, Webster HD. *The Fine Structure of the Nervous System*. 3rd ed. Oxford, New York: Oxford University Press; 1991.
2. Ventura R, Harris KM. Three-dimensional relationships between hippocampal synapses and astrocytes. *J Neurosci.* 1999;19:6897–6906.
3. Volterra A, Magistretti PJ, Haydon PG. *The Tripartite Synapse: Glia in Synaptic Transmission*. Oxford, UK: Oxford University Press; 2002.
4. Kettenmann H, Ransom BR. *Neuroglia*. 1st ed. New York, Oxford: Oxford University Press; 1995.
5. Araque A, Parpura V, Sanzgiri RP, Haydon PG. Tripartite synapses: glia, the unacknowledged partner. *Trends Neurosci.* 1999;22:208–215.
6. Haydon PG. GLIA: listening and talking to the synapse. *Nat Rev Neurosci.* 2001;2:185–193.
7. Volterra A, Meldolesi J. Astrocytes, from brain glue to communication elements: the revolution continues. *Nat Rev Neurosci.* 2005;6:626–640.
8. Halassa MM, Fellin T, Haydon PG. The tripartite synapse: roles for gliotransmission in health and disease. *Trends Mol Med.* 2007;13:54–63.
9. Bushong EA, Martone ME, Jones YZ, Ellisman MH. Protoplasmic astrocytes in CA1 stratum radiatum occupy separate anatomical domains. *J Neurosci.* 2002;22:183–192.
10. Fellin T, Halassa MM, Terunuma M, et al. Endogenous nonneuronal modulators of synaptic transmission control cortical slow oscillations in vivo. *Proc Natl Acad Sci USA.* 2009;106: 15037–15042.
11. Halassa MM, Fellin T, Takase H, Dong JH, Haydon PG. Synaptic islands defined by the territory of a single astrocyte. *J Neurosci.* 2007;27:6473–6477.
12. Fellin T, Pascual O, Haydon PG. Astrocytes coordinate synaptic networks: balanced excitation and inhibition. *Physiology.* 2006;21:208–215.
13. Fellin T. Communication between neurons and astrocytes: relevance to the modulation of synaptic and network activity. *J Neurochem.* 2009;108:533–544.
14. Cornell-Bell AH, Finkbeiner SM, Cooper MS, Smith SJ. Glutamate induces calcium waves in cultured astrocytes: long-range glial signaling. *Science.* 1990;247:470–473.

15. Parpura V, Basarsky TA, Liu F, Jeftinija K, Jeftinija S, Haydon PG. Glutamate-mediated astrocyte-neuron signalling. *Nature*. 1994;369:744–747.
16. Hirrlinger J, Hulsmann S, Kirchhoff F. Astroglial processes show spontaneous motility at active synaptic terminals in situ. *Eur J Neurosci*. 2004;20:2235–2239.
17. Haber M, Zhou L, Murai KK. Cooperative astrocyte and dendritic spine dynamics at hippocampal excitatory synapses. *J Neurosci*. 2006;26:8881–8891.
18. Theodosis DT, Poulain DA, Oliet SH. Activity-dependent structural and functional plasticity of astrocyte–neuron interactions. *Physiol Rev*. 2008;88:983–1008.
19. Panatier A, Theodosis DT, Mothet JP, et al. Glia-derived D-serine controls NMDA receptor activity and synaptic memory. *Cell*. 2006;125:775–784.
20. Fellin T, Carmignoto G. Neurone-to-astrocyte signalling in the brain represents a distinct multifunctional unit. *J Physiol*. 2004;559:3–15.
21. Auld DS, Robitaille R. Glial cells and neurotransmission: an inclusive view of synaptic function. *Neuron*. 2003;40: 389–400.
22. Zhang Q, Fukuda M, Van Bockstaele E, Pascual O, Haydon PG. Synaptotagmin IV regulates glial glutamate release. *Proc Natl Acad Sci USA*. 2004;101:9441–9446.
23. Zhang Z, Chen G, Zhou W, et al. Regulated ATP release from astrocytes through lysosome exocytosis. *Nat Cell Biol*. 2007;9:945–953.
24. Pangrsic T, Potokar M, Stenovec M, et al. Exocytotic release of ATP from cultured astrocytes. *J Biol Chem*. 2007;282: 28749–28758.
25. Mothet JP, Pollegioni L, Ouanounou G, Martineau M, Fossier P, Baux G. Glutamate receptor activation triggers a calcium-dependent and SNARE protein-dependent release of the gliotransmitter D-serine. *Proc Natl Acad Sci USA*. 2005;102: 5606–5611.
26. Bergami M, Santi S, Formaggio E, et al. Uptake and recycling of pro-BDNF for transmitter-induced secretion by cortical astrocytes. *J Cell Biol*. 2008;183:213–221.
27. Krzan M, Stenovec M, Kreft M, et al. Calcium-dependent exocytosis of atrial natriuretic peptide from astrocytes. *J Neurosci*. 2003;23:1580–1583.
28. Perea G, Araque A. Astrocytes potentiate transmitter release at single hippocampal synapses. *Science*. 2007;317:1083–1086.
29. Parri HR, Gould TM, Crunelli V. Spontaneous astrocytic Ca^{2+} oscillations in situ drive NMDAR-mediated neuronal excitation. *Nat Neurosci*. 2001;4:803–812.
30. Fellin T, Pascual O, Gobbo S, Pozzan T, Haydon PG, Carmignoto G. Neuronal synchrony mediated by astrocytic glutamate through activation of extrasynaptic NMDA receptors. *Neuron*. 2004;43:729–743.
31. Nestor MW, Mok LP, Tulapurkar ME, Thompson SM. Plasticity of neuron–glial interactions mediated by astrocytic EphARs. *J Neurosci*. 2007;27:12817–12828.
32. Navarrete M, Araque A. Endocannabinoids mediate neuron–astrocyte communication. *Neuron*. 2008;57:883–893.
33. Shigetomi E, Bowser DN, Sofroniew MV, Khakh BS. Two forms of astrocyte calcium excitability have distinct effects on NMDA receptor-mediated slow inward currents in pyramidal neurons. *J Neurosci*. 2008;28:6659–6663.
34. Angulo MC, Kozlov AS, Charpak S, Audinat E. Glutamate released from glial cells synchronizes neuronal activity in the hippocampus. *J Neurosci*. 2004;24:6920–6927.
35. Kozlov AS, Angulo MC, Audinat E, Charpak S. Target cell-specific modulation of neuronal activity by astrocytes. *Proc Natl Acad Sci USA*. 2006;103:10058–10063.
36. Fellin T, Gomez-Gonzalo M, Gobbo S, Carmignoto G, Haydon PG. Astrocytic glutamate is not necessary for the generation of epileptiform neuronal activity in hippocampal slices. *J Neurosci*. 2006;26:9312–9322.
37. Zhang JM, Wang HK, Ye CQ, et al. ATP released by astrocytes mediates glutamatergic activity-dependent heterosynaptic suppression. *Neuron*. 2003;40:971–982.
38. Pascual O, Casper KB, Kubera C, et al. Astrocytic purinergic signaling coordinates synaptic networks. *Science*. 2005;310: 113–116.
39. Halassa MM, Florian C, Fellin T, et al. Astrocytic modulation of sleep homeostasis and cognitive consequences of sleep loss. *Neuron*. 2009;61:213–219.
40. Blott EJ, Griffiths GM. Secretory lysosomes. *Nat Rev Mol Cell Biol*. 2002;3:122–131.
41. Li D, Ropert N, Koulakoff A, Giaume C, Oheim M. Lysosomes are the major vesicular compartment undergoing Ca^{2+}-regulated exocytosis from cortical astrocytes. *J Neurosci*. 2008;28:7648–7658.
42. Cahoy JD, Emery B, Kaushal A, et al. A transcriptome database for astrocytes, neurons, and oligodendrocytes: a new resource for understanding brain development and function. *J Neurosci*. 2008;28:264–278.
43. Coco S, Calegari F, Pravettoni E, et al. Storage and release of ATP from astrocytes in culture. *J Biol Chem*. 2003;278: 1354–1362.
44. Gordon GR, Baimoukhametova DV, Hewitt SA, Rajapaksha WR, Fisher TE, Bains JS. Norepinephrine triggers release of glial ATP to increase postsynaptic efficacy. *Nat Neurosci*. 2005;8:1078–1086.
45. Halassa MM, Fellin T, Haydon PG. Tripartite synapses: roles for astrocytic purines in the control of synaptic physiology and behavior. *Neuropharmacology*. 2009;57:343–346.
46. Steriade M, Nunez A, Amzica F. A novel slow (<1 Hz) oscillation of neocortical neurons in vivo – depolarizing and hyperpolarizing components. *J Neurosci*. 1993;13: 3252–3265.
47. Steriade M. Grouping of brain rhythms in corticothalamic systems. *Neuroscience*. 2006;137:1087–1106.
48. Sanchez-Vives MV, McCormick DA. Cellular and network mechanisms of rhythmic recurrent activity in neocortex. *Nat Neurosci*. 2000;3:1027–1034.
49. Shu YS, Hasenstaub A, McCormick DA. Turning on and off recurrent balanced cortical activity. *Nature*. 2003;423: 288–293.
50. Timofeev I, Grenier F, Bazhenov M, Sejnowski TJ, Steriade M. Origin of slow cortical oscillations in deafferented cortical slabs. *Cereb Cortex*. 2000;10:1185–1199.
51. Cirelli C, Tononi G. Is sleep essential? *PLoS Biol*. 2008;6:e216.
52. Franken P, Chollet D, Tafti M. The homeostatic regulation of sleep need is under genetic control. *J Neurosci*. 2001;21:2610–2621.
53. Vyazovskiy VV, Cirelli C, Pfister-Genskow M, Faraguna U, Tononi G. Molecular and electrophysiological evidence for net synaptic potentiation in wake and depression in sleep. *Nat Neurosci*. 2008;11:200–208.
54. Esser SK, Hill SL, Tononi G. Sleep homeostasis and cortical synchronization: I. Modeling the effects of synaptic strength on sleep slow waves. *Sleep*. 2007;30:1617–1630.
55. Basheer R, Strecker RE, Thakkar MM, McCarley RW. Adenosine and sleep–wake regulation. *Prog Neurobiol*. 2004; 73:379–396.
56. Porkka-Heiskanen T, Kalinchuk A, Alanko L, Urrila A, Stenberg D. Adenosine, energy metabolism, and sleep. *Scientific World Journal*. 2003;3:790–798.

57. Simard M, Arcuino G, Takano T, Liu QS, Nedergaard M. Signaling at the gliovascular interface. *J Neurosci*. 2003;23:9254–9262.
58. Gourine AV, Kasymov V, Marina N, et al. Astrocytes control breathing through pH-dependent release of ATP. *Science*. 2010;329:571–575.
59. Guyenet PG, Stornetta RL, Bayliss DA. Central respiratory chemoreception. *J Comp Neurol*. 2010;518:3883–3906.
60. Mulkey DK, Stornetta RL, Weston MC, et al. Respiratory control by ventral surface chemoreceptor neurons in rats. *Nat Neurosci*. 2004;7:1360–1369.
61. Kasymov V, Larina O, Castaldo C, et al. Differential sensitivity of brainstem versus cortical astrocytes to changes in pH reveals functional regional specialization of astroglia. *J Neurosci*. 2013;33:435–441.
62. Haydon PG, Carmignoto G. Astrocyte control of synaptic transmission and neurovascular coupling. *Physiol Rev*. 2006; 86:1009–1031.
63. Witcher MR, Ellis TL. Astroglial networks and implications for therapeutic neuromodulation of epilepsy. *Front Comput Neurosci*. 2012;6:61.

CHAPTER

13

The Fear Memory Network

Glenn E. Schafe

Department of Psychology and Center for Study of Gene Structure and Function, Hunter College, The City University of New York, New York, NY, USA

Pavlovian fear conditioning has become the paradigm of choice to study the mechanisms of mammalian associative memory and those of anxiety disorders that are characterized by persistent, unwanted fear memories. In this chapter, I first review what is known about the neuronal network underlying simple forms of Pavlovian fear conditioning, including an in-depth look at the mechanisms underlying synaptic plasticity and memory formation in the amygdala and throughout the wider fear network. Next, I review more complex aspects of fear learning, including a discussion of the neuronal network and mechanisms underlying contextual fear conditioning and fear extinction. Finally, I briefly summarize what is known about the fear-learning system of the human brain and its relevance for understanding and treating anxiety disorders that are characterized by acquired fears.

AN OVERVIEW OF PAVLOVIAN FEAR CONDITIONING

Classical or Pavlovian fear conditioning has long been a tool of behavioral psychology to study simple forms of associative learning in the mammal. In this paradigm, an animal (or human) learns to fear an initially emotionally neutral stimulus (the conditioned stimulus (CS)) that acquires aversive properties after being paired with a noxious stimulus (the unconditioned stimulus (US)). First used by J.B. Watson and his colleague Rosalie Rayner in the now-infamous studies on "Little Albert",[1] fear conditioning is now most widely studied in rodents, where a discrete cue (such as a tone, light, or odor; i.e. a CS) is paired with a brief electric shock to the feet (a US). Before conditioning, the CS does not elicit fearful behavior. After as little as one CS–US pairing, however, the animal begins to exhibit a range of conditioned responses (CRs), both to the tone CS and to the context in which conditioning occurs (e.g. the conditioning chamber). In rats, these CRs include "freezing" or immobility (the rat's species-typical behavioral response to a threatening stimulus), autonomic and endocrine alterations (such as changes in heart rate and blood pressure, defecation, and increased levels of circulating stress hormones), and the potentiation of reflexes like the acoustic startle response.[2–6] The study of the neurobiological mechanisms underlying Pavlovian fear conditioning has accelerated considerably in recent years, not only because it represents an ideal model for the study of associative memory formation from a neural and molecular perspective[7,8] but also because of its potential clinical relevance to psychiatric disorders such as posttraumatic stress disorder (PTSD) that are characterized by unusually strong and persistent traumatic memories.[9,10]

THE AMYGDALA AND FEAR CONDITIONING

The neuroanatomical pathways underlying the acquisition and expression of Pavlovian fear conditioning have been extensively well defined over the last several decades. This is particularly true for the "auditory fear conditioning" paradigm, where an animal learns to fear a tone (CS) that is paired with an aversive presentation of a foot shock (US), although similar mechanisms have been proposed for fear conditioning to a visual CS.[3,11] Auditory fear conditioning involves transmission of auditory CS and somatosensory US information to the lateral nucleus of the amygdala (LA), a region that lesion and functional inactivation studies have consistently shown to be critical for fear learning.[12–16] Cytologically, the LA contains populations of glutamatergic pyramidal and inhibitory neurons whose morphological characteristics are similar to those found in the cortex, with the

Neuronal Networks in Brain Function, CNS Disorders, and Therapeutics
http://dx.doi.org/10.1016/B978-0-12-415804-7.00013-7

exception that the LA is not a layered structure.[17,18] The LA itself can be further subdivided into dorsal (LAd) and ventral regions (LAv).[18] Anatomical tract tracing studies have shown that neurons in the LAd, and to a lesser extent the LAv, receive direct glutamatergic projections from areas of the auditory thalamus and cortex, specifically from the medial division of the medial geniculate body and the posterior intralaminar nucleus (MGm–PIN) and cortical area TE3.[19–24] Neurophysiological recording studies have indicated that inputs from each of these auditory areas synapse onto single neurons in the LAd,[25] where they converge with inputs from the somatosensory US.[26] The US input pathways to the LA have been studied in less detail, but they are generally thought to involve transmission along both subcortical and cortical routes. Previous studies have suggested that lesions of both the thalamic PIN and the insular cortex may be critical for transmitting US information to the LA.[27] Furthermore, direct stimulation of the PIN has been shown to be an effective US in an auditory fear-conditioning paradigm.[28,29]

Thalamic and cortical inputs to the LA, although both capable of mediating fear learning,[30] are widely believed to carry different types of CS information to the LA. The thalamic route (often called the "low road") is believed to be critical for rapidly transmitting crude aspects of the CS to the LA, while the cortical route (known as the "high road") is believed to carry highly refined information to the amygdala.[7] In support of this hypothesis, lesions of MGm–PIN have been shown to impair simple forms of auditory fear conditioning that involve presentation of a pure (e.g. 1–10 kHz) tone CS,[31,32] while lesions of the auditory cortex have no effect on this type of conditioning[32,33] (but see Ref. 34). Thus, the thalamic pathway between the MGm–PIN and the LA appears to be sufficient to support certain forms of auditory fear conditioning. However, when conditioning depends on the ability of the animal to make fine discriminations between different auditory CSs or when the CS is a complex auditory cue such as an ultrasonic vocalization, cortical regions appear to play a critical role in processing and transmitting CS information to the LA.[35–37] Thus, both pathways likely contribute to fear learning depending on the nature and complexity of the CS.

During the retrieval or expression of a fear memory, the LA engages the central nucleus of the amygdala (CE), which traditionally has been thought of as the principal output nucleus of the fear-learning system.[7] The CE itself is a heterogeneous structure containing several subnuclei, including the lateral central amygdala (CEl), the medial central amygdala (CEm), and the capsular division of the central amygdala (CEc).[18] Interestingly, each of these subnuclei appears to be largely composed of GABAergic neurons that resemble those found in the striatum.[38] The LA projects to the CE by

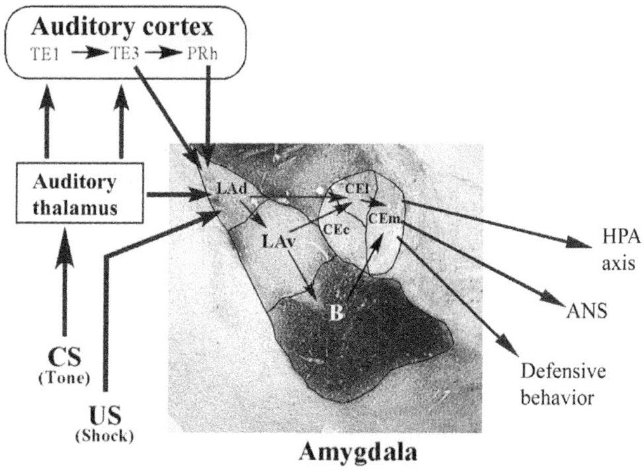

FIGURE 13.1 **Information flow within the fear system.** Auditory fear conditioning involves the transmission of CS sensory information from areas of the auditory thalamus and cortex to the dorsal division of the lateral amygdala (LA), where it can converge with incoming somatosensory information from the foot shock US. It is in the LA that alterations in synaptic transmission are thought to encode key aspects of the learning. During fear expression, the LA engages the central nucleus of the amygdala (CE) both directly and by way of projections from the adjacent basal amygdala (B). The medial division of the CE (CEm) projects widely to many areas of the forebrain and brainstem that control the expression of fear CRs, including freezing, hypothalamic–pituitary–adrenal (HPA) axis activation, and alterations in cardiovascular activity. LAd: dorsolateral amygdala; LAv: ventrolateral amygdala; B: basal nucleus of the amygdala; CEc: capsular division of the CE; CEl: lateral central nucleus; CEm: medial division of the central nucleus.

one of two routes: both directly and by way of the adjacent basal nucleus of the amygdala (see Figure 13.1). The direct route involves monosynaptic excitatory projections to the CEl, which in turn sends an inhibitory projection to neurons of the CEm. The indirect route involves direct projections to the basal amygdala (B), which projects to the CEm directly and by way of nearby GABAergic intercalated cell masses (ICMs) that lie between the LA–B and the CE.[39–41] The net result of transmission through either pathway is that CEm projection neurons are disinhibited.[42] The CEm, in turn, is known to project widely to areas of the forebrain, hypothalamus, and brainstem that control behavioral, endocrine, and autonomic CRs associated with fear learning.[2–6] Projections from the CEm to the midbrain periaqueductal gray, for example, have been shown to be particularly important for mediating behavioral and endocrine responses such as freezing and hypoalgesia[43–45] (see Chapter 32), while projections to the lateral hypothalamus have been implicated in the control of conditioned cardiovascular responses.[46] Importantly, while lesions of these individual areas can selectively impair expression of individual CRs, damage to the CE interferes with the expression of all fear CRs.[7] Thus, the CE acts to coordinate the collection of hardwired, and typically species-specific, responses that underlie fear behavior.

SYNAPTIC PLASTICITY IN THE AMYGDALA AND FEAR CONDITIONING

The LA not only is the recipient of sensory information about the CS and US but also is thought to be a critical site of synaptic plasticity underlying fear learning.[7,47,48] In support of this view, studies have shown that individual cells in LAd alter their neurophysiological response properties when CS and US are paired during fear conditioning. For example, LAd neurons that are initially weakly responsive to an auditory cue respond vigorously to that same cue after fear conditioning.[49–54] This change in the responsiveness of LAd cells that occurs as the result of CS–US pairing has contributed to the view that neural plasticity in the LA encodes key aspects of fear learning and memory storage.[47,48,55,56] Importantly, these training-related changes in LA unit activity are not a simple reflection of the fact that the animal is expressing fear behavior. Repa and colleagues, for example, have shown that conditional changes in spike firing of single LA neurons occur either on or before the first trial in which fear responding is observed.[53] Furthermore, Goosens and colleagues observed that CS-elicited spike firing of LA neurons can be dissociated altogether from the expression of fear.[57] Using a differential fear-conditioning paradigm in which one CS was paired with shock (CS+) and another not (CS−), they showed that only the CS+ elicited conditional changes in spike firing of LA neurons; if the CS− was presented in an environment where the rat was expressing high levels of contextual fear memory, there was no observable change in CS-elicited unit activity.[57] Furthermore, the CS+ was observed to elicit robust changes in unit activity even when the CE was inactivated using a local anesthetic, lidocaine, and the rat was rendered incapable of expressing fear.[57] Collectively, these findings suggest that training-related changes in LA unit activity are determined by the associative history of the CS and are not influenced by the motivational or behavioral state of the animal.

Long-Term Potentiation as a Mechanism of Fear Learning

The training-related change in the responsiveness of LA neurons to a tone CS during and after fear conditioning suggests that alterations in excitatory synaptic transmission in the LA might be critical for fear conditioning. Accordingly, it has been proposed that a mechanism akin to long-term potentiation (LTP), an experimentally induced form of synaptic plasticity that was initially discovered in the hippocampus,[58] may underlie fear learning in the LA. At its core, LTP involves a change in the weight of an initially weak input after that input has been paired with a strong input,[59,60] a process that is widely believed to be accompanied at the cellular level by the growth of new synaptic connections. As such, LTP and associative fear memory formation, in which an initially ineffective CS becomes effective after pairing with an aversive US, share a number of core conceptual features. Experimentally, LTP has been demonstrated, both in vivo and in vitro, in each of the major sensory input pathways to the LA, including the thalamic and cortical auditory pathways.[61–67] Furthermore, fear conditioning itself has been shown to lead to neurophysiological changes in the LA in a manner that is very similar to those observed following artificial LTP induction, and these changes persist over days.[54,68] Finally, fear conditioning has been shown to share a common biochemical and molecular substrate with that of LTP, including the involvement of *N*-methyl-D-aspartate (NMDA) receptor (NMDAR)-driven activation of protein kinase signaling cascades[69,70] (see Chapter 27), the activation of transcription factors,[71] the de novo synthesis of mRNA and protein,[72,73] the regulation of immediate early genes,[74–76] and structural changes at LA synapses.[77,78]

DISTRIBUTED VERSUS LOCAL PLASTICITY IN THE AMYGDALA

While numerous studies have suggested that the LA is a critical locus of synaptic plasticity underlying fear memory acquisition and storage, it has become clear that LA synapses are not the only critical synapses in the amygdala that undergo changes that are associated with fear memory formation. Several recent studies, for example, have suggested that a distributed, rather than localized, network of plasticity in the wider amygdala underlies fear learning.[79,80]

Distributed Plasticity within the LA

The distributed view of plasticity underlying fear learning begins in the LA itself, where plasticity at two sets of synapses has been linked to fear learning, and in unique ways. While most studies that have documented training-induced alterations in synaptic plasticity have focused on a single population of cells in the LAd,[49–52,54] Repa and colleagues have documented plastic changes in two populations of cells in the LA.[53] The first is the traditionally studied dorsal population in the LAd that shows enhanced firing to the CS in the initial stages of training and testing. These so-called transiently plastic cells exhibit short-latency changes (within 10–15 ms after tone onset) that are consistent with the involvement of rapid, monosynaptic thalamic input, and are sensitive to extinction if the CS is not continuously reinforced. The second population of cells occupies a more ventral position in the LAd and in the dorsal regions of the LAv. In contrast to the transiently plastic cells, these more ventral cells exhibit enhanced firing to the CS throughout training and testing, and they do not appear to be sensitive to extinction; that is, they continue to fire to the CS even after the behavioral response is extinguished. Furthermore, these "long-term plastic cells" exhibit longer latencies (within 30–40 ms after tone onset), indicative of a polysynaptic pathway. Thus, it has been hypothesized that a network of neurons within the LA is responsible for triggering and storing fear memories, respectively.[53,79]

Distributed Plasticity within Amygdala Nuclei

In recent years, interest has also grown in the idea that distributed plasticity between amygdala nuclei may also be critical for fear learning. This idea first gained traction following a report from LeDoux and colleagues showing that the CE, traditionally thought of solely as an "output" structure, may also be an important locus of fear memory acquisition and storage.[81] In that study, functional inactivation restricted to either the LA or CE impaired acquisition of auditory fear conditioning. Furthermore, infusion of the protein synthesis inhibitor anisomycin into the CE impaired fear memory consolidation, that is, rats had intact short-term memory but impaired long-term memory.[81] These findings suggest that the CE plays an important role not only in fear expression, but also in the acquisition and consolidation of fear learning.

How might the CE participate in fear memory acquisition and consolidation? Since the CE, and particularly the CEm, also appears to be a recipient of auditory[82–85] and somatosensory[86,87] information, one possibility is that the CE encodes in parallel the same type of association that is encoded in the LA. In support of this idea, Paré and colleagues have shown that high-frequency stimulation of the auditory thalamus induces an NMDAR-dependent form of LTP in CEm neurons.[88] Furthermore, under certain circumstances, the CE has been shown to be capable of mediating fear learning if the LA is compromised.[89] A second possibility is that plasticity in the LA and CE proceeds in a serial manner, such that plasticity and memory formation in the CE depend on prior plasticity in the LA. This view has been advocated in a model by Paré and colleagues that proposes that plasticity in the LA enables CEm neurons to encode plasticity that is essential for fear conditioning, resulting in distributed plasticity and memory formation throughout the amygdala.[80] The mechanism by which this distributed plasticity between the LA and CE occurs is at present unknown, but it likely involves projections from the LA to CEm neurons via the nearby ICMs, which lie between the LA and CE.[41,90] Additional experiments employing single-unit recording techniques in both the LA and CEm will be required to determine how these two regions influence one another during fear conditioning.

PLASTICITY BEYOND THE AMYGDALA

While the evidence outlined in this chapter has supported the notion that fear memories are acquired and stored in the LA via an associative LTP-like process, other evidence suggests that regions of the wider fear network outside of the LA may also participate in fear memory formation. It has long been recognized, for example, that auditory fear conditioning induces associative alterations in the activity of neurons not only in the LA but also in the auditory cortex[91,92] and the auditory thalamus.[93,94] Cells within the MGm–PIN and auditory cortical area TE3, like those in LA, rapidly develop increased firing to the CS during and after auditory fear conditioning.[91–93,95–97] Furthermore, receptive field analysis of the MGm–PIN and TE3 during auditory fear conditioning shows the development and maintenance of highly specific plasticity, including shifts of tuning to the frequency of the CS.[94,98,99] These findings suggest that plastic changes in afferent regions of the wider fear network may also be critical for some aspects of fear memory formation and/or storage. Interestingly, a number of studies have indicated that training-induced plasticity in thalamic and cortical regions is driven by the LA,[100–102] suggesting the intriguing possibility that training-induced plasticity in the LA may act to promote plastic changes throughout the wider fear network during the process of fear memory acquisition and storage. However, studies have also suggested that plastic changes in regions afferent to the LA may not be critical for fear memory formation. Poremba and Gabriel, for example, showed that, under certain circumstances, fear memories can be acquired without accompanying thalamic plasticity,[102] a finding consistent with that of Maren and colleagues.[101] Together, these findings suggest that training-induced neurophysiological changes in the MGm–PIN are not essential for the acquisition of fear conditioning per se. However, it remains possible that these distributed neurophysiological changes reflect alterations in sensory or perceptual processing associated with emotional memory formation.

CONTEXTUAL FEAR CONDITIONING

In a typical auditory fear-conditioning experiment, the animal learns to fear not only the tone CS that is paired with the aversive US but also the context in which conditioning occurs. This so-called contextual fear conditioning may also be induced by the presentation of an aversive US alone within a novel environment. In the laboratory, fear to the context is measured by returning the rat to the conditioning chamber on the test day and measuring freezing behavior.[2,103]

In comparison to auditory fear conditioning, much less is known about the neuronal network underlying contextual fear. Much of the work examining the neuroanatomical substrates of contextual fear has relied on lesion and functional inactivation methods, and, as in auditory fear conditioning, the amygdala appears to play an essential role. For example, lesions of the amygdala, including the LA and basal nucleus, have been shown to disrupt both acquisition and expression of contextual fear conditioning,[104–106] as has reversible functional inactivation targeted to the LA.[15] Furthermore, like auditory fear conditioning, contextual fear conditioning is similarly characterized by the involvement of NMDARs and protein kinase signaling cascades,[69,107–110] de novo mRNA synthesis,[72] and the regulation of immediate early genes[111] in the amygdala. Collectively, these findings suggest that essential aspects of contextual fear memory are encoded and stored in the amygdala via alterations in some of the same intracellular signaling mechanisms that underlie acquisition and consolidation of auditory fear conditioning. Very little data, however, exist that allow us to distinguish between the types of involvement of different amygdala subnuclei in contextual fear, although lesion evidence suggests that the LA and anterior basal nuclei are critical.[112] The CE is, of course, essential for the expression of contextual fear learning, as it is for auditory fear conditioning.[112] It remains unknown, however, whether the CE is also required for the acquisition and/or consolidation of contextual fear, or whether distributed plasticity within the LA underlies contextual fear learning.

The hippocampus also plays a critical role in contextual fear conditioning, presumably by forming a contextual representation of the training environment and transmitting that information as a "contextual CS" to the amygdala during fear conditioning.[113,114] Early studies showed that electrolytic and neurotoxic lesions of the dorsal hippocampus disrupt contextual, but not auditory, fear conditioning.[104,106,115,116] Posttraining lesions appear to be the most effective; pretraining lesions of the hippocampus have occasionally been shown to be without effect.[116] This is presumably because the animal uses a nonhippocampal (or so-called elemental) strategy to acquire fear to the contextual cues of the environment in the absence of an intact hippocampus. Posttraining lesions of the hippocampus, however, are effective at impairing contextual fear only if given shortly after training. If rats are given dorsal hippocampal lesions 28 days after training, there is no memory impairment.[115] This "retrograde gradient" of recall suggests that hippocampal-dependent memories are gradually stabilized over time in other regions of the brain for permanent storage, an idea that is consistent with the findings of hippocampal-dependent declarative memory research in humans.[117] The exact mechanism whereby these "remote" contextual fear memories are consolidated remains unknown, but it is thought to involve LTP-like changes in signaling between the hippocampus and regions of the cortex that make up the individual elements of the contextual representation.[118]

TURNING FEAR OFF: FEAR EXTINCTION

Fear extinction is a process whereby repeated presentations of the CS in the absence of the aversive US lead to a weakening of the expression of fear CRs. At the behavioral level, it has long been appreciated that extinction does not "erase" the original fear memory but instead creates a new inhibitory memory that competes with the expression of the original CS–US memory. Extinguished memories, for example, are well known to be subject to "spontaneous recovery", in which the original CR may reappear after time has passed.[119] Furthermore, reexposure to an aversive US is often sufficient to "reinstate" a well-extinguished fear memory.[120] Finally, extinguished fear memories are expressed in a context-specific manner; the original fear CR will "renew" when the CS is presented outside of the extinction context.[121,122] Each of these observations argues strongly that the original CS–US association remains intact after extinction learning, and that the extinction memory itself acts to regulate or gate the expression of fear CRs.[8,123] While fear extinction has been well characterized at the behavioral level, until recently comparatively little was known about its neurobiological substrates. Within the last decade, however, work in a number of laboratories has implicated several structures that make up the "extinction network", including the prefrontal cortex, amygdala, and hippocampus.

The medial prefrontal cortex (mPFC) and in particular the ventral mPFC (also known as the infralimbic cortex, or IL) appear to play important roles in fear extinction. Early studies, for example, showed that selective lesions of the ventral mPFC retard the extinction of fear to an auditory CS while having no effect on initial fear acquisition.[124,125] Furthermore, neurons in the mPFC alter their response properties as the result of extinction.[126,127] Interestingly, studies by Quirk and colleagues suggest that the mPFC may not be necessary for fear extinction per se, but rather for the consolidation of extinction memory. For example, rats with IL lesions are able to extinguish normally within a session (e.g. show evidence of extinction memory in the short term), but show impaired extinction memory between sessions that are separated by at least a day.[128] Furthermore, neurons in the IL show no evidence of firing to a tone CS within an extinction session, but fire strongly after the extinction memory has been consolidated.[129] Furthermore, artificial stimulation of the IL that resembles responding in an extinguished rat is sufficient to inhibit behavioral expression of fear in nonextinguished rats.[129] Thus, it appears that the mPFC plays an essential role in long-term retention and/or expression of fear extinction. The question of whether the mPFC is a "site of storage" of extinction or rather simply a region that is necessary for the long-term expression of extinguished memories has only begun to be explored. Findings have indicated, however, that extinction training regulates the intrinsic excitability of IL neurons[130] and the expression of the immediate early gene cFos in regions of the mPFC.[131] Furthermore, intra-mPFC infusion of inhibitors of protein kinase signaling pathways and de novo protein synthesis impair long-term recall of fear extinction,[131,132] and direct infusions of brain-derived neurotrophic factor (BDNF) into the IL can mimic the effects of extinction training.[133] These findings collectively suggest that essential aspects of the plasticity underlying extinction memory are localized in the mPFC.

Pharmacological and neurophysiological evidence has suggested that the amygdala may also be a critical site of plasticity underlying fear extinction. Infusions of NMDAR antagonists or inhibitors of protein kinase signaling cascades into the LA have been shown to impair fear extinction.[134–137] Conversely, both systemic and intra-LA infusions of D-cycloserine, a partial agonist of the NMDAR, facilitate fear extinction.[138] More recently, Ressler and colleagues showed that signaling via BDNF in the amygdala is critical to the consolidation of fear extinction.[139] These experiments collectively suggest that some type of activity-dependent synaptic plasticity must take place in the amygdala during fear extinction learning, as it does during initial learning. Interestingly, Lüthi and colleagues have recently shown that distinct populations of neurons within the basal nucleus of the amygdala encode fear and extinction learning.[140,141] In that study, "fear" neurons showed increased firing during and after fear conditioning that diminished with extinction, while "extinction" neurons showed increased firing throughout fear extinction.[140] Interestingly, fear neurons within the basal nucleus have been shown to be reciprocally connected with the mPFC.[140,141] Furthermore, the mPFC projects to GABAergic ICMs that are situated between the lateral and basal amygdala and the CE,[142] which may be important for regulating fear responses.[41,80,123,143] In agreement with this hypothesis, Quirk and colleagues have shown that stimulation of the mPFC neurons blunts the activity of CE neurons that are critical for the expression of fear responses.[143] Furthermore, chemical stimulation of the IL with the $GABA_A$ antagonist picrotoxin leads to an increase in cFos expression within the ICMs,[144] and selective lesions of the ICMs impair the expression of fear extinction.[145]

One of the more interesting facts about memories that have undergone extinction is that they are context specific. That is, an extinguished fear memory remains extinguished only in the context in which extinction has taken place, but it can return or "renew" in a different context.[121,122] Not surprisingly, recent studies have indicated that the hippocampus plays an important role in the contextual modulation of fear extinction. Maren and colleagues, for example, have shown that training-induced neurophysiological responses in the LA readily extinguish within a fear extinction session, but this neural representation of extinction, like the behavior itself, is specific to the context in which extinction has taken place.[146] Furthermore, functional inactivation of the dorsal or ventral regions of the hippocampus using the $GABA_A$ agonist muscimol can impair the context-specific expression of fear extinction,[147–149] and renewal of an extinguished fear memory has been shown to be associated with cFos expression in the ventral hippocampus.[150] Lüthi and colleagues have further demonstrated that activity in "fear" neurons within the basal amygdala rapidly reemerges after extinction if the animal is tested in a different context.[140] The mechanisms by which the hippocampus mediates context-specific expression of fear extinction remain unclear, but it has been proposed that projections from the hippocampus to both the mPFC and the amygdala may be critical.[146,151]

FEAR LEARNING IN HUMANS AND ITS RELEVANCE TO ANXIETY DISORDERS

In recent years, considerable progress has been made in understanding how the human fear-learning system is organized, and what features it shares with the fear-learning system of lower vertebrates. In this section, I will briefly summarize these findings and provide a brief overview of their relevance for understanding and treating anxiety disorders such as PTSD. For a more comprehensive look at this topic, see Refs 152,153.

The Human Fear-Learning System: Lesion and fMRI Studies

Consistent with studies in rodents, lesions of the amygdala in humans have been observed to impair fear conditioning.[154,155] Fear conditioning in human subjects is typically accomplished by pairing a visual cue (e.g. a blue square; i.e. the CS) with either mild electric shock to the skin or an aversive high-amplitude (i.e. 100 dB or more) noise (US). Conditioned fear is then measured by changes in skin conductance upon presentation of the CS. Interestingly, damage to the amygdala in humans produces deficits in conditioned emotional responding to a CS, even though the declarative knowledge of the CS–US contingency remains intact.[154] That is, a patient with amygdala damage will not respond fearfully to the CS after it has been paired with an aversive US, but he or she is capable of stating that the CS was previously presented and followed by the US. Interestingly, patients with selective hippocampal damage exhibit the converse effect; they will respond fearfully to the CS but cannot tell you why.[154]

Studies using fMRI have found that fear conditioning leads to increases in BOLD response in the human amygdala.[156,157] These changes largely mirror what has been observed in neurophysiological studies of amygdala activity in rodents, namely, increases in CS-elicited amygdala activity during and after fear conditioning, and a corresponding attenuation of CS-elicited amygdala activity with extinction of the behavioral response.[157,158] Furthermore, as suggested by the animal work, the human fear-learning system appears preferentially suited to use subcortical low-road information during fear learning. Whalen and colleagues observed increased amygdala activation to "masked" presentation of fearful faces. Here, the emotional faces were presented too quickly to be consciously perceived by the subjects.[159,160] Similarly, Morris and colleagues observed CS-elicited increases in amygdala activity to masked "unseen" faces.[161] Furthermore, when the activity of the amygdala during fear conditioning was cross-correlated with the activity in other regions of the brain, the strongest correlations were seen with subcortical (thalamic and collicular) rather than cortical areas, further emphasizing the importance of the direct thalamo-amygdala pathway in the human brain.[161]

More recent studies have examined fear extinction in the human brain. Consistent with studies using rodents, extinction of fear in human subjects is associated with an increase in BOLD response in the mPFC,[158,162] and the thickness of the mPFC has been observed to be correlated with extinction memory.[163]

Relevance to Anxiety Disorders

The rapid progress made in identifying the fear network in both rodent models and, more recently, the human brain has provided an opportunity for researchers to examine how this network might be altered in psychological disorders such as PTSD. An early study observed that amygdala activity is enhanced in Vietnam veterans with PTSD during the presentation of combat-relevant sounds,[164] as well as in combat veterans viewing either masked[165] or overtly[166] fearful faces that are presented to them. At the cortical level, decreased mPFC volumes have been observed in patients with PTSD,[167] and patients with PTSD exhibit impairments in fear extinction recall as well as retrieval-related mPFC activity during recall of extinction memory.[168]

The observed impairments in mPFC cortical volumes and activity in PTSD suggest that patients with this disorder may not fully benefit from exposure-based therapies that rely upon fear extinction procedures.[152] Accordingly, recent work has begun to explore pharmacological means by which to augment fear extinction in PTSD patients. Inspired by the findings from rodent studies showing facilitation of fear extinction following both systemic and intra-LA infusions of the partial NMDAR agonist D-cycloserine,[138] one recent study found preliminary support for the use of D-cycloserine in augmenting exposure-based therapy in patients with PTSD.[169] While preliminary, these findings suggest that pharmacological treatments derived from the study of fear extinction in rodent models may hold promise for the treatment of anxiety disorders, including PTSD, in which acquired fears play a prominent role.[170]

CONCLUSIONS

Within the last several decades, it is clear that a considerable amount has been learned about the neural pathways and key synaptic events underlying fear learning in the amygdala and throughout the wider fear network of the brain. These findings provide a foundation for the continued study of the neuronal basis of emotional learning and memory at the cellular level. Importantly, they also provide us with a set of tools to continue our analysis of more complex and clinically relevant aspects of fear learning, including contextual control of learned fear and fear extinction, that may be relevant for understanding and treating psychological disorders such as PTSD.

Acknowledgments

This work was supported in part by the National Institutes of Health (grant no. MH 073949) and by Yale University.

References

1. Watson JB, Rayner R. Conditioned emotional reactions. 1920. *Am Psychol.* 2000;55(3):313–317.
2. Blanchard RJ, Blanchard DC. Crouching as an index of fear. *J Comp Physiol Psychol.* 1969;67(3):370–375.
3. Davis M. Neurobiology of fear responses: the role of the amygdala. *J Neuropsychiatry Clin Neurosci.* 1997;9(3):382–402.
4. Kapp BS, Frysinger RC, Gallagher M, Haselton JR. Amygdala central nucleus lesions: effect on heart rate conditioning in the rabbit. *Physiol Behav.* 1979;23(6):1109–1117.

5. LeDoux JE, Iwata J, Cicchetti P, Reis DJ. Different projections of the central amygdaloid nucleus mediate autonomic and behavioral correlates of conditioned fear. *J Neurosci*. 1988;8(7):2517–2529.
6. Roozendaal B, Koolhaas JM, Bohus B. Attenuated cardiovascular, neuroendocrine, and behavioral responses after a single footshock in central amygdaloid lesioned male rats. *Physiol Behav*. 1991;50(4):771–775.
7. LeDoux JE. Emotion circuits in the brain. *Annu Rev Neurosci*. 2000; 23:155–184.
8. Maren S, Quirk GJ. Neuronal signalling of fear memory. *Nat Rev Neurosci*. 2004;5(11):844–852.
9. Pitman RK, Shalev AY, Orr SP. Posttraumatic stress disorder: emotion, conditioning, & memory. In: Gazzaniga MS, ed. *The New Cognitive Neurosciences*. Cambridge: MIT Press; 2000.
10. Tronson NC, Taylor JR. Molecular mechanisms of memory reconsolidation. *Nat Rev Neurosci*. 2007;8(4):262–275.
11. Davis M. The role of the amygdala in fear-potentiated startle: implications for animal models of anxiety. *Trends Pharmacol Sci*. 1992;13(1):35–41.
12. Campeau S, Davis M. Involvement of the central nucleus and basolateral complex of the amygdala in fear conditioning measured with fear-potentiated startle in rats trained concurrently with auditory and visual conditioned stimuli. *J Neurosci*. 1995;15(3 Pt 2):2301–2311.
13. Helmstetter FJ, Bellgowan PS. Effects of muscimol applied to the basolateral amygdala on acquisition and expression of contextual fear conditioning in rats. *Behav Neurosci*. 1994;108(5):1005–1009.
14. LeDoux JE, Cicchetti P, Xagoraris A, Romanski LM. The lateral amygdaloid nucleus: sensory interface of the amygdala in fear conditioning. *J Neurosci*. 1990;10(4):1062–1069.
15. Muller J, Corodimas KP, Fridel Z, LeDoux JE. Functional inactivation of the lateral and basal nuclei of the amygdala by muscimol infusion prevents fear conditioning to an explicit conditioned stimulus and to contextual stimuli. *Behav Neurosci*. 1997;111(4):683–691.
16. Wilensky AE, Schafe GE, LeDoux JE. The amygdala modulates memory consolidation of fear-motivated inhibitory avoidance learning but not classical fear conditioning. *J Neurosci*. 2000; 20(18):7059–7066.
17. McDonald AJ. Cytoarchitecture of the central amygdaloid nucleus of the rat. *J Comp Neurol*. 1982;208(4):401–418.
18. Pitkanen A, Savander V, LeDoux JE. Organization of intra-amygdaloid circuitries in the rat: an emerging framework for understanding functions of the amygdala [published erratum appears in *Trends Neurosci*. Feb 1998;21(2):52] [see comments]. *Trends Neurosci*. 1997;20(11):517–523.
19. Bordi F, LeDoux J. Sensory tuning beyond the sensory system: an initial analysis of auditory response properties of neurons in the lateral amygdaloid nucleus and overlying areas of the striatum. *J Neurosci*. 1992;12(7):2493–2503.
20. Doron NN, Ledoux JE. Organization of projections to the lateral amygdala from auditory and visual areas of the thalamus in the rat [published erratum appears in *J Comp Neurol*. Feb 14, 2000; 417(3):385–386]. *J Comp Neurol*. 1999;412(3):383–409.
21. LeDoux JE, Farb CR. Neurons of the acoustic thalamus that project to the amygdala contain glutamate. *Neurosci Lett*. 1991; 134(1):145–149.
22. LeDoux JE, Ruggiero DA, Reis DJ. Projections to the subcortical forebrain from anatomically defined regions of the medial geniculate body in the rat. *J Comp Neurol*. 1985;242(2):182–213.
23. McDonald AJ. Cortical pathways to the mammalian amygdala. *Prog Neurobiol*. 1998;55(3):257–332.
24. Romanski LM, LeDoux JE. Information cascade from primary auditory cortex to the amygdala: corticocortical and corticoamygdaloid projections of temporal cortex in the rat. *Cereb Cortex*. 1993;3(6):515–532.
25. Li XF, Stutzmann GE, LeDoux JE. Convergent but temporally separated inputs to lateral amygdala neurons from the auditory thalamus and auditory cortex use different postsynaptic receptors: in vivo intracellular and extracellular recordings in fear conditioning pathways. *Learn Mem*. 1996;3(2–3):229–242.
26. Romanski LM, Clugnet MC, Bordi F, LeDoux JE. Somatosensory and auditory convergence in the lateral nucleus of the amygdala. *Behav Neurosci*. 1993;107(3):444–450.
27. Shi C, Davis M. Pain pathways involved in fear conditioning measured with fear- potentiated startle: lesion studies. *J Neurosci*. 1999;19(1):420–430.
28. Cruikshank SJ, Edeline JM, Weinberger NM. Stimulation at a site of auditory-somatosensory convergence in the medial geniculate nucleus is an effective unconditioned stimulus for fear conditioning. *Behav Neurosci*. 1992;106(3):471–483.
29. Kwon JT, Choi JS. Cornering the fear engram: long-term synaptic changes in the lateral nucleus of the amygdala after fear conditioning. *J Neurosci*. 2009;29(31):9700–9703.
30. Romanski LM, LeDoux JE. Equipotentiality of thalamo-amygdala and thalamo-cortico-amygdala circuits in auditory fear conditioning. *J Neurosci*. 1992;12(11):4501–4509.
31. LeDoux JE, Sakaguchi A, Iwata J, Reis DJ. Interruption of projections from the medial geniculate body to an archi-neostriatal field disrupts the classical conditioning of emotional responses to acoustic stimuli. *Neuroscience*. 1986;17(3):615–627.
32. LeDoux JE, Sakaguchi A, Reis DJ. Subcortical efferent projections of the medial geniculate nucleus mediate emotional responses conditioned to acoustic stimuli. *J Neurosci*. 1984;4(3):683–698.
33. Romanski LM, LeDoux JE. Bilateral destruction of neocortical and perirhinal projection targets of the acoustic thalamus does not disrupt auditory fear conditioning. *Neurosci Lett*. 1992;142(2): 228–232.
34. Boatman JA, Kim JJ. A thalamo-cortico-amygdala pathway mediates auditory fear conditioning in the intact brain. *Eur J Neurosci*. 2006;24(3):894–900.
35. Bang SJ, Brown TH. Perirhinal cortex supports acquired fear of auditory objects. *Neurobiol Learn Mem*. 2009;92(1):53–62.
36. Jarrell TW, Gentile CG, Romanski LM, McCabe PM, Schneiderman N. Involvement of cortical and thalamic auditory regions in retention of differential bradycardiac conditioning to acoustic conditioned stimuli in rabbits. *Brain Res*. 1987;412(2):285–294.
37. Lindquist DH, Jarrard LE, Brown TH. Perirhinal cortex supports delay fear conditioning to rat ultrasonic social signals. *J Neurosci*. 2004;24(14):3610–3617.
38. McDonald AJ. Neurons of the lateral and basolateral amygdaloid nuclei: a Golgi study in the rat. *J Comp Neurol*. 1982;212(3):293–312.
39. Pape HC, Pare D. Plastic synaptic networks of the amygdala for the acquisition, expression, and extinction of conditioned fear. *Physiol Rev*. 2010;90(2):419–463.
40. Pare D, Smith Y. Intrinsic circuitry of the amygdaloid complex: common principles of organization in rats and cats. *Trends Neurosci*. 1998;21(6):240–241.
41. Paré D, Smith Y. The intercalated cell masses project to the central and medial nuclei of the amygdala in cats. *Neuroscience*. 1993; 57(4):1077–1090.
42. Ehrlich I, Humeau Y, Grenier F, Ciocchi S, Herry C, Luthi A. Amygdala inhibitory circuits and the control of fear memory. *Neuron*. 2009;62(6):757–771.
43. De Oca BM, DeCola JP, Maren S, Fanselow MS. Distinct regions of the periaqueductal gray are involved in the acquisition and expression of defensive responses. *J Neurosci*. 1998;18(9): 3426–3432.
44. Helmstetter FJ, Landeira-Fernandez J. Conditional hypoalgesia is attenuated by naltrexone applied to the periaqueductal gray. *Brain Res*. 1990;537(1–2):88–92.

45. Helmstetter FJ, Tershner SA. Lesions of the periaqueductal gray and rostral ventromedial medulla disrupt antinociceptive but not cardiovascular aversive conditional responses. *J Neurosci*. 1994; 14(11 Pt 2):7099–7108.
46. Iwata J, LeDoux JE, Reis DJ. Destruction of intrinsic neurons in the lateral hypothalamus disrupts the classical conditioning of autonomic but not behavioral emotional responses in the rat. *Brain Res*. 1986;368(1):161–166.
47. Blair HT, Schafe GE, Bauer EP, Rodrigues SM, LeDoux JE. Synaptic plasticity in the lateral amygdala: a cellular hypothesis of fear conditioning. *Learn Mem*. 2001;8(5):229–242.
48. Maren S. Neurobiology of Pavlovian fear conditioning. *Annu Rev Neurosci*. 2001;24:897–931.
49. Blair HT, Tinkelman A, Moita MA, LeDoux JE. Associative plasticity in neurons of the lateral amygdala during auditory fear conditioning. *Ann N Y Acad Sci*. 2003;985:485–487.
50. Maren S. Auditory fear conditioning increases CS-elicited spike firing in lateral amygdala neurons even after extensive overtraining. *Eur J Neurosci*. 2000;12(11):4047–4054.
51. Quirk GJ, Armony JL, LeDoux JE. Fear conditioning enhances different temporal components of tone-evoked spike trains in auditory cortex and lateral amygdala. *Neuron*. 1997;19(3): 613–624.
52. Quirk GJ, Repa C, LeDoux JE. Fear conditioning enhances short-latency auditory responses of lateral amygdala neurons: parallel recordings in the freely behaving rat. *Neuron*. 1995;15(5): 1029–1039.
53. Repa JC, Muller J, Apergis J, Desrochers TM, Zhou Y, LeDoux JE. Two different lateral amygdala cell populations contribute to the initiation and storage of memory. *Nat Neurosci*. 2001;4(7):724–731.
54. Rogan MT, Staubli UV, LeDoux JE. Fear conditioning induces associative long-term potentiation in the amygdala. *Nature*. 1997; 390(6660):604–607.
55. Fanselow MS, LeDoux JE. Why we think plasticity underlying Pavlovian fear conditioning occurs in the basolateral amygdala. *Neuron*. 1999;23(2):229–232.
56. Schafe GE, Nader K, Blair HT, LeDoux JE. Memory consolidation of Pavlovian fear conditioning: a cellular and molecular perspective. *Trends Neurosci*. 2001;24(9):540–546.
57. Goosens KA, Hobin JA, Maren S. Auditory-evoked spike firing in the lateral amygdala and Pavlovian fear conditioning: mnemonic code or fear bias? *Neuron*. 2003;40(5):1013–1022.
58. Bliss TV, Lømo T. Long-lasting potentiation of synaptic transmission in the dentate area of the anaesthetized rabbit following stimulation of the perforant path. *J Physiol (Lond)*. 1973;232(2): 331–356.
59. Barrionuevo G, Brown TH. Associative long-term potentiation in hippocampal slices. *Proc Natl Acad Sci USA*. 1983;80(23): 7347–7351.
60. Brown TH, Chapman PF, Kairiss EW, Keenan CL. Long-term synaptic potentiation. *Science*. 1988;242(4879):724–728.
61. Chapman PF, Kairiss EW, Keenan CL, Brown TH. Long-term synaptic potentiation in the amygdala. *Synapse*. 1990;6(3):271–278.
62. Clugnet MC, LeDoux JE. Synaptic plasticity in fear conditioning circuits: induction of LTP in the lateral nucleus of the amygdala by stimulation of the medial geniculate body. *J Neurosci*. 1990; 10(8):2818–2824.
63. Doyère V, Schafe GE, Sigurdsson T, LeDoux JE. Long-term potentiation in freely moving rats reveals asymmetries in thalamic and cortical inputs to the lateral amygdala. *Eur J Neurosci*. 2003;17(12):2703–2715.
64. Huang YY, Kandel ER. Postsynaptic induction and PKA-dependent expression of LTP in the lateral amygdala. *Neuron*. 1998;21(1): 169–178.
65. Maren S, Fanselow MS. Synaptic plasticity in the basolateral amygdala induced by hippocampal formation stimulation in vivo. *J Neurosci*. 1995;15(11):7548–7564.
66. Rogan MT, LeDoux JE. LTP is accompanied by commensurate enhancement of auditory-evoked responses in a fear conditioning circuit. *Neuron*. 1995;15(1):127–136.
67. Weisskopf MG, Bauer EP, LeDoux JE. L-type voltage-gated calcium channels mediate NMDA-independent associative long-term potentiation at thalamic input synapses to the amygdala. *J Neurosci*. 1999;19(23):10512–10519.
68. McKernan MG, Shinnick-Gallagher P. Fear conditioning induces a lasting potentiation of synaptic currents in vitro. *Nature*. 1997; 390(6660):607–611.
69. Rodrigues SM, Schafe GE, LeDoux JE. Intraamygdala blockade of the NR2B subunit of the NMDA receptor disrupts the acquisition but not the expression of fear conditioning. *J Neurosci*. 2001; 21(17):6889–6896.
70. Schafe GE, Atkins CM, Swank MW, Bauer EP, Sweatt JD, LeDoux JE. Activation of ERK/MAP kinase in the amygdala is required for memory consolidation of pavlovian fear conditioning. *J Neurosci*. 2000;20(21):8177–8187.
71. Josselyn SA, Shi C, Carlezon Jr WA, Neve RL, Nestler EJ, Davis M. Long-term memory is facilitated by cAMP response element-binding protein overexpression in the amygdala. *J Neurosci*. 2001;21(7):2404–2412.
72. Bailey DJ, Kim JJ, Sun W, Thompson RF, Helmstetter FJ. Acquisition of fear conditioning in rats requires the synthesis of mRNA in the amygdala. *Behav Neurosci*. 1999;113(2):276–282.
73. Schafe GE, LeDoux JE. Memory consolidation of auditory pavlovian fear conditioning requires protein synthesis and protein kinase A in the amygdala. *J Neurosci*. 2000;20(18):RC96.
74. Maddox SA, Monsey MS, Schafe GE. Early growth response gene 1 (Egr-1) is required for new and reactivated fear memories in the lateral amygdala. *Learn Mem*. 2011;18(1):24–38.
75. Maddox SA, Schafe GE. The activity-regulated cytoskeletal-associated protein (Arc/Arg3.1) is required for reconsolidation of a Pavlovian fear memory. *J Neurosci*. 2011;31(19):7073–7082.
76. Ploski JE, Pierre VJ, Smucny J, et al. The activity-regulated cytoskeletal-associated protein (Arc/Arg3.1) is required for memory consolidation of pavlovian fear conditioning in the lateral amygdala. *J Neurosci*. 2008;28(47):12383–12395.
77. Ostroff LE, Cain CK, Bedont J, Monfils MH, Ledoux JE. Fear and safety learning differentially affect synapse size and dendritic translation in the lateral amygdala. *Proc Natl Acad Sci USA*. 2010; 107(20):9418–9423.
78. Ostroff LE, Cain CK, Jindal N, Dar N, Ledoux JE. Stability of presynaptic vesicle pools and changes in synapse morphology in the amygdala following fear learning in adult rats. *J Comp Neurol*. 2012;520(2):295–314.
79. Medina JF, Christopher Repa J, Mauk MD, LeDoux JE. Parallels between cerebellum- and amygdala-dependent conditioning. *Nat Rev Neurosci*. 2002;3(2):122–131.
80. Paré D, Quirk GJ, Ledoux JE. New vistas on amygdala networks in conditioned fear. *J Neurophysiol*. 2004;92(1):1–9.
81. Wilensky AE, Schafe GE, Kristensen MP, LeDoux JE. Rethinking the fear circuit: the central nucleus of the amygdala is required for the acquisition, consolidation, and expression of pavlovian fear conditioning. *J Neurosci*. 2006;26(48):12387–12396.
82. Frankland PW, Cestari V, Filipkowski RK, McDonald RJ, Silva AJ. The dorsal hippocampus is essential for context discrimination but not for contextual conditioning. *Behav Neurosci*. 1998;112(4): 863–874.
83. LeDoux JE, Ruggiero DA, Forest R, Stornetta R, Reis DJ. Topographic organization of convergent projections to the thalamus

from the inferior colliculus and spinal cord in the rat. *J Comp Neurol.* 1987;264(1):123–146.
84. Linke R, Braune G, Schwegler H. Differential projection of the posterior paralaminar thalamic nuclei to the amygdaloid complex in the rat. *Exp Brain Res.* 2000;134(4):520–532.
85. Turner BH, Herkenham M. Thalamoamygdaloid projections in the rat: a test of the amygdala's role in sensory processing. *J Comp Neurol.* 1991;313(2):295–325.
86. Bernard JF, Besson JM. The spino(trigemino)pontoamygdaloid pathway: electrophysiological evidence for an involvement in pain processes. *J Neurophysiol.* 1990;63(3):473–490.
87. Jasmin L, Burkey AR, Card JP, Basbaum AI. Transneuronal labeling of a nociceptive pathway, the spino-(trigemino-) parabrachio-amygdaloid, in the rat. *J Neurosci.* 1997;17(10): 3751–3765.
88. Samson RD, Pare D. Activity-dependent synaptic plasticity in the central nucleus of the amygdala. *J Neurosci.* 2005;25(7): 1847–1855.
89. Zimmerman JM, Rabinak CA, McLachlan IG, Maren S. The central nucleus of the amygdala is essential for acquiring and expressing conditional fear after overtraining. *Learn Mem.* 2007; 14(9):634–644.
90. Royer S, Martina M, Pare D. An inhibitory interface gates impulse traffic between the input and output stations of the amygdala. *J Neurosci.* 1999;19(23):10575–10583.
91. Bakin JS, Weinberger NM. Classical conditioning induces CS-specific receptive field plasticity in the auditory cortex of the guinea pig. *Brain Res.* 1990;536(1–2):271–286.
92. Edeline JM, Weinberger NM. Receptive field plasticity in the auditory cortex during frequency discrimination training: selective retuning independent of task difficulty. *Behav Neurosci.* 1993; 107(1):82–103.
93. Gabriel M, Saltwick SE, Miller JD. Conditioning and reversal of short-latency multiple-unit responses in the rabbit medial geniculate nucleus. *Science.* 1975;189(4208):1108–1109.
94. Weinberger NM. Learning-induced changes of auditory receptive fields. *Curr Opin Neurobiol.* 1993;3(4):570–577.
95. Birt D, Olds M. Associative response changes in lateral midbrain tegmentum and medial geniculate during differential appetitive conditioning. *J Neurophysiol.* 1981;46(5):1039–1055.
96. Hennevin E, Maho C, Hars B. Neuronal plasticity induced by fear conditioning is expressed during paradoxical sleep: evidence from simultaneous recordings in the lateral amygdala and the medial geniculate in rats. *Behav Neurosci.* 1998;112(4):839–862.
97. Weinberger N. Sensory plasticity and learning: the magnocellular medial geniculate nucleus of the auditory system. In: Woody CD, ed. *Conditioning: Representation of Involved Neural Function.* New York: Plenum; 1982:697–710.
98. Edeline JM, Weinberger NM. Associative retuning in the thalamic source of input to the amygdala and auditory cortex: receptive field plasticity in the medial division of the medial geniculate body. *Behav Neurosci.* 1992;106(1):81–105.
99. Lennartz RC, Weinberger NM. Frequency-specific receptive field plasticity in the medial geniculate body induced by pavlovian fear conditioning is expressed in the anesthetized brain. *Behav Neurosci.* 1992;106(3):484–497.
100. Armony JL, Quirk GJ, LeDoux JE. Differential effects of amygdala lesions on early and late plastic components of auditory cortex spike trains during fear conditioning. *J Neurosci.* 1998;18(7): 2592–2601.
101. Maren S, Yap SA, Goosens KA. The amygdala is essential for the development of neuronal plasticity in the medial geniculate nucleus during auditory fear conditioning in rats. *J Neurosci.* 2001;21(6):RC135.
102. Poremba A, Gabriel M. Amygdalar efferents initiate auditory thalamic discriminative training-induced neuronal activity. *J Neurosci.* 2001;21(1):270–278.
103. Fanselow MS. Conditioned and unconditional components of post-shock freezing. *Pavlov J Biol Sci.* 1980;15(4):177–182.
104. Kim JJ, Rison RA, Fanselow MS. Effects of amygdala, hippocampus, and periaqueductal gray lesions on short- and long-term contextual fear. *Behav Neurosci.* 1993;107(6):1093–1098.
105. Maren S. Overtraining does not mitigate contextual fear conditioning deficits produced by neurotoxic lesions of the basolateral amygdala. *J Neurosci.* 1998;18(8):3088–3097.
106. Phillips RG, LeDoux JE. Differential contribution of amygdala and hippocampus to cued and contextual fear conditioning. *Behav Neurosci.* 1992;106(2):274–285.
107. Goosens KA, Holt W, Maren S. A role for amygdaloid PKA and PKC in the acquisition of long-term conditional fear memories in rats. *Behav Brain Res.* 2000;114(1–2):145–152.
108. Kim JJ, DeCola JP, Landeira-Fernandez J, Fanselow MS. *N*-methyl-D-aspartate receptor antagonist APV blocks acquisition but not expression of fear conditioning. *Behav Neurosci.* 1991; 105(1):126–133.
109. Rodrigues SM, Bauer EP, Farb CR, Schafe GE, LeDoux JE. The group I metabotropic glutamate receptor mGluR5 is required for fear memory formation and long-term potentiation in the lateral amygdala. *J Neurosci.* 2002;22(12):5219–5229.
110. Rodrigues SM, Farb CR, Bauer EP, LeDoux JE, Schafe GE. Pavlovian fear conditioning regulates Thr^{286} autophosphorylation of Ca^{2+}/calmodulin-dependent protein kinase II at lateral amygdala synapses. *J Neurosci.* 2004;24(13):3281–3288.
111. Malkani S, Wallace KJ, Donley MP, Rosen JB. An egr-1 (zif268) antisense oligodeoxynucleotide infused into the amygdala disrupts fear conditioning. *Learn Mem.* 2004;11(5):617–624.
112. Goosens KA, Maren S. Contextual and auditory fear conditioning are mediated by the lateral, basal, and central amygdaloid nuclei in rats. *Learn Mem.* 2001;8(3):148–155.
113. Barrientos RM, O'Reilly RC, Rudy JW. Memory for context is impaired by injecting anisomycin into dorsal hippocampus following context exploration. *Behav Brain Res.* 2002;134(1–2): 299–306.
114. Fanselow MS, Poulos AM. The neuroscience of mammalian associative learning. *Annu Rev Psychol.* 2005;56:207–234.
115. Kim JJ, Fanselow MS. Modality-specific retrograde amnesia of fear. *Science.* 1992;256(5057):675–677.
116. Maren S, Aharonov G, Fanselow MS. Neurotoxic lesions of the dorsal hippocampus and Pavlovian fear conditioning in rats. *Behav Brain Res.* 1997;88(2):261–274.
117. Milner B, Squire LR, Kandel ER. Cognitive neuroscience and the study of memory. *Neuron.* 1998;20(3):445–468.
118. Frankland PW, O'Brien C, Ohno M, Kirkwood A, Silva AJ. Alpha-CaMKII-dependent plasticity in the cortex is required for permanent memory. *Nature.* 2001;411(6835):309–313.
119. Pavlov IP. *Conditioned Reflexes.* London: Oxford University Press; 1927.
120. Rescorla RA, Heth CD. Reinstatement of fear to an extinguished conditioned stimulus. *J Exp Psychol Anim Behav Process.* 1975;1(1): 88–96.
121. Bouton ME, Bolles RC. Contextual control of the extinction of conditioned fear. *Learn Motiv.* 1979;10:445–466.
122. Bouton ME, Ricker ST. Renewal of extinguished responding in a second context. *Anim Learn Behav.* 1994;22:317–324.
123. Quirk GJ, Gehlert DR. Inhibition of the amygdala: key to pathological states? *Ann N Y Acad Sci.* 2003;985:263–272.
124. Morgan MA, LeDoux JE. Differential contribution of dorsal and ventral medial prefrontal cortex to the acquisition and

extinction of conditioned fear in rats. *Behav Neurosci.* 1995; 109(4):681–688.
125. Morgan MA, Romanski LM, LeDoux JE. Extinction of emotional learning: contribution of medial prefrontal cortex. *Neurosci Lett.* 1993;163(1):109–113.
126. Garcia R, Vouimba RM, Baudry M, Thompson RF. The amygdala modulates prefrontal cortex activity relative to conditioned fear. *Nature.* 1999;402(6759):294–296.
127. Herry C, Vouimba RM, Garcia R. Plasticity in the mediodorsal thalamo-prefrontal cortical transmission in behaving mice. *J Neurophysiol.* 1999;82(5):2827–2832.
128. Quirk GJ, Russo GK, Barron JL, Lebron K. The role of ventromedial prefrontal cortex in the recovery of extinguished fear. *J Neurosci.* 2000;20(16):6225–6231.
129. Milad MR, Quirk GJ. Neurons in medial prefrontal cortex signal memory for fear extinction. *Nature.* 2002;420(6911):70–74.
130. Santini E, Quirk GJ, Porter JT. Fear conditioning and extinction differentially modify the intrinsic excitability of infralimbic neurons. *J Neurosci.* 2008;28(15):4028–4036.
131. Santini E, Ge H, Ren K, Pena de Ortiz S, Quirk GJ. Consolidation of fear extinction requires protein synthesis in the medial prefrontal cortex. *J Neurosci.* 2004;24(25):5704–5710.
132. Hugues S, Chessel A, Lena I, Marsault R, Garcia R. Prefrontal infusion of PD098059 immediately after fear extinction training blocks extinction-associated prefrontal synaptic plasticity and decreases prefrontal ERK2 phosphorylation. *Synapse.* 2006;60(4):280–287.
133. Peters J, Dieppa-Perea LM, Melendez LM, Quirk GJ. Induction of fear extinction with hippocampal-infralimbic BDNF. *Science.* 2010;328(5983):1288–1290.
134. Davis M. Role of NMDA receptors and MAP kinase in the amygdala in extinction of fear: clinical implications for exposure therapy. *Eur J Neurosci.* 2002;16(3):395–398.
135. Falls WA, Miserendino MJ, Davis M. Extinction of fear-potentiated startle: blockade by infusion of an NMDA antagonist into the amygdala. *J Neurosci.* 1992;12(3):854–863.
136. Herry C, Trifilieff P, Micheau J, Luthi A, Mons N. Extinction of auditory fear conditioning requires MAPK/ERK activation in the basolateral amygdala. *Eur J Neurosci.* 2006;24(1):261–269.
137. Lu KT, Walker DL, Davis M. Mitogen-activated protein kinase cascade in the basolateral nucleus of amygdala is involved in extinction of fear-potentiated startle. *J Neurosci.* 2001;21(16):RC162.
138. Walker DL, Ressler KJ, Lu KT, Davis M. Facilitation of conditioned fear extinction by systemic administration or intra-amygdala infusions of D-cycloserine as assessed with fear-potentiated startle in rats. *J Neurosci.* 2002;22(6):2343–2351.
139. Chhatwal JP, Stanek-Rattiner L, Davis M, Ressler KJ. Amygdala BDNF signaling is required for consolidation but not encoding of extinction. *Nat Neurosci.* 2006;9(7):870–872.
140. Herry C, Ciocchi S, Senn V, Demmou L, Muller C, Luthi A. Switching on and off fear by distinct neuronal circuits. *Nature.* 2008;454(7204):600–606.
141. Herry C, Ferraguti F, Singewald N, Letzkus JJ, Ehrlich I, Luthi A. Neuronal circuits of fear extinction. *Eur J Neurosci.* 2010;31(4): 599–612.
142. McDonald AJ, Mascagni F, Guo L. Projections of the medial and lateral prefrontal cortices to the amygdala: a *Phaseolus vulgaris* leucoagglutinin study in the rat. *Neuroscience.* 1996; 71(1):55–75.
143. Quirk GJ, Likhtik E, Pelletier JG, Pare D. Stimulation of medial prefrontal cortex decreases the responsiveness of central amygdala output neurons. *J Neurosci.* 2003;23(25):8800–8807.
144. Berretta S, Pantazopoulos H, Caldera M, Pantazopoulos P, Pare D. Infralimbic cortex activation increases c-Fos expression in intercalated neurons of the amygdala. *Neuroscience.* 2005;132(4): 943–953.
145. Likhtik E, Popa D, Apergis-Schoute J, Fidacaro GA, Pare D. Amygdala intercalated neurons are required for expression of fear extinction. *Nature.* 2008;454(7204):642–645.
146. Hobin JA, Goosens KA, Maren S. Context-dependent neuronal activity in the lateral amygdala represents fear memories after extinction. *J Neurosci.* 2003;23(23):8410–8416.
147. Corcoran KA, Desmond TJ, Frey KA, Maren S. Hippocampal inactivation disrupts the acquisition and contextual encoding of fear extinction. *J Neurosci.* 2005;25(39):8978–8987.
148. Corcoran KA, Maren S. Hippocampal inactivation disrupts contextual retrieval of fear memory after extinction. *J Neurosci.* 2001;21(5):1720–1726.
149. Hobin JA, Ji J, Maren S. Ventral hippocampal muscimol disrupts context-specific fear memory retrieval after extinction in rats. *Hippocampus.* 2006;16(2):174–182.
150. Knapska E, Maren S. Reciprocal patterns of c-Fos expression in the medial prefrontal cortex and amygdala after extinction and renewal of conditioned fear. *Learn Mem.* 2009;16(8):486–493.
151. Orsini CA, Kim JH, Knapska E, Maren S. Hippocampal and prefrontal projections to the basal amygdala mediate contextual regulation of fear after extinction. *J Neurosci.* 2011;31(47): 17269–17277.
152. Milad MR, Rauch SL, Pitman RK, Quirk GJ. Fear extinction in rats: implications for human brain imaging and anxiety disorders. *Biol Psychol.* 2006;73(1):61–71.
153. Phelps EA, LeDoux JE. Contributions of the amygdala to emotion processing: from animal models to human behavior. *Neuron.* 2005;48(2):175–187.
154. Bechara A, Tranel D, Damasio H, Adolphs R, Rockland C, Damasio AR. Double dissociation of conditioning and declarative knowledge relative to the amygdala and hippocampus in humans. *Science.* 1995;269(5227):1115–1118.
155. LaBar KS, LeDoux JE, Spencer DD, Phelps EA. Impaired fear conditioning following unilateral temporal lobectomy in humans. *J Neurosci.* 1995;15(10):6846–6855.
156. Buchel C, Morris J, Dolan RJ, Friston KJ. Brain systems mediating aversive conditioning: an event-related fMRI study. *Neuron.* 1998; 20(5):947–957.
157. LaBar KS, Gatenby JC, Gore JC, LeDoux JE, Phelps EA. Human amygdala activation during conditioned fear acquisition and extinction: a mixed-trial fMRI study. *Neuron.* 1998;20(5): 937–945.
158. Phelps EA, Delgado MR, Nearing KI, LeDoux JE. Extinction learning in humans: role of the amygdala and vmPFC. *Neuron.* 2004;43(6):897–905.
159. Whalen PJ, Kagan J, Cook RG, et al. Human amygdala responsivity to masked fearful eye whites. *Science.* 2004;306(5704):2061.
160. Whalen PJ, Rauch SL, Etcoff NL, McInerney SC, Lee MB, Jenike MA. Masked presentations of emotional facial expressions modulate amygdala activity without explicit knowledge. *J Neurosci.* 1998;18(1):411–418.
161. Morris JS, Ohman A, Dolan RJ. A subcortical pathway to the right amygdala mediating "unseen" fear. *Proc Natl Acad Sci USA.* 1999; 96(4):1680–1685.
162. Milad MR, Wright CI, Orr SP, Pitman RK, Quirk GJ, Rauch SL. Recall of fear extinction in humans activates the ventromedial prefrontal cortex and hippocampus in concert. *Biol Psychiatry.* 2007;62(5):446–454.
163. Milad MR, Quinn BT, Pitman RK, Orr SP, Fischl B, Rauch SL. Thickness of ventromedial prefrontal cortex in humans is correlated with extinction memory. *Proc Natl Acad Sci USA.* 2005; 102(30):10706–10711.
164. Liberzon I, Taylor SF, Amdur R, et al. Brain activation in PTSD in response to trauma-related stimuli. *Biol Psychiatry.* 1999;45(7): 817–826.

165. Rauch SL, Whalen PJ, Shin LM, et al. Exaggerated amygdala response to masked facial stimuli in posttraumatic stress disorder: a functional MRI study. *Biol Psychiatry.* 2000;47(9):769–776.
166. Shin LM, Wright CI, Cannistraro PA, et al. A functional magnetic resonance imaging study of amygdala and medial prefrontal cortex responses to overtly presented fearful faces in posttraumatic stress disorder. *Arch Gen Psychiatry.* 2005;62(3):273–281.
167. Rauch SL, Shin LM, Segal E, et al. Selectively reduced regional cortical volumes in post-traumatic stress disorder. *Neuroreport.* 2003;14(7):913–916.
168. Milad MR, Pitman RK, Ellis CB, et al. Neurobiological basis of failure to recall extinction memory in posttraumatic stress disorder. *Biol Psychiatry.* 2009;66(12):1075–1082.
169. de Kleine RA, Hendriks GJ, Kusters WJ, Broekman TG, van Minnen A. A randomized placebo-controlled trial of D-cycloserine to enhance exposure therapy for posttraumatic stress disorder. *Biol Psychiatry.* 2012;71(11):962–968.
170. Krystal JH. Enhancing prolonged exposure therapy for posttraumatic stress disorder with D-cycloserine: further support for treatments that promote experience-dependent neuroplasticity. *Biol Psychiatry.* 2012;71(11):932–934.

CHAPTER

14

Orchestration of the Circadian Clock Network by the Suprachiasmatic Nucleus

Shelley A. Tischkau[1], *Stacey L. Krager*[2]

[1]Department of Pharmacology, Southern Illinois University School of Medicine, Springfield, IL, USA,
[2]Department of Internal Medicine, Southern Illinois University School of Medicine, Springfield, IL, USA

INTRODUCTION

A compelling argument can be proffered that the most ubiquitous and persistent environmental factor present throughout the evolution of modern species is the revolution of the Earth about its own axis, creating a solar day that consists of a 24 h window of light and darkness. This recurrent pattern endows a sense of time to organisms that live on this planet. The significance of the ability to discern time is accentuated by the presence of an internal mechanism for keeping time on a 24 h (circadian) scale, inherent in the genetic framework of living organisms ranging from cyanobacteria to human mammals. The internal, molecular program drives circadian oscillations within the organism that manifest at the molecular, biochemical, physiological, and behavioral levels. Importantly, these oscillations allow anticipatory responses to changes in the environment and promote survival.[1,2]

Circadian patterns are characterized by events that recur during the subjective day or the light portion of the 24 h period and the subjective night or the dark part of the 24 h period.[3,4] Thus, organisms maintain physiological synchrony with the light–dark environment. The two defining characteristics of the circadian timing system are perseverance of oscillation under constant environmental conditions, which define these rhythms as self-sustained and endogenously generated, and the ability to adapt to environmental change, particularly to changes in the environmental light–dark cycle. Rhythms have been studied in whole animals, individual tissues, organs, and cell culture models. Perhaps the most obvious of all circadian rhythms is the behavioral rest–activity cycle, which has been the subject of intense study, providing a behavioral standard for investigation of rhythmicity. Circadian cycles are also expressed in physiology and gene expression. Some examples of rhythms include *Neurospora crassa* asexual spore production, leaf movements in plants, photosynthesis and nitrogen fixation in cyanobacteria,[5,6] the firing rate of the suprachiasmatic nucleus (SCN) in mammals, clock gene expression levels, and metabolic glucose uptake.[3]

Coherent circadian rhythms in mammals may be viewed as an organismic network, with a central node located in the SCN of the ventral hypothalamus, the so-called master clock. Although individual neurons within the SCN are independent oscillators,[7,8] rhythm generation for the organism is considered an emergent property (see Chapter 30) of these paired nuclei.[9] The location of the SCN, nestled in the optic chiasm, with its connection to the external environment through a direct, monosynaptic connection from the retina via specialized retinal ganglion cells,[10–14] allows the nucleus to monitor environmental levels of illumination, which can then be integrated, and information based upon these data are transmitted to the rest of the organism through a variety of neuroendocrine mechanisms. Thus, circadian rhythmicity is accomplished by the intricate coordination of a neuroendocrine network. In its most simple form, the network is composed of three components: (1) the oscillator, (2) input to the oscillator, and (3) output from the oscillator. This chapter describes the nature of rhythmicity by examining the molecular and cellular basis for building an oscillator, evidence that justifies the SCN as the master oscillator, the array of afferent information that accesses the oscillator, and, finally, the neuroendocrine mechanisms that allow the SCN to transmit timing information throughout the body.

Neuronal Networks in Brain Function, CNS Disorders, and Therapeutics
http://dx.doi.org/10.1016/B978-0-12-415804-7.00014-9

THE CELLULAR BASIS OF CIRCADIAN RHYTHMICITY

"Clock genes" within cells are a driving force underlying the generation of self-sustained circadian rhythmicity at the cellular level. In the 40+ years since the discovery of the first reported clock gene in *Drosophila*, Period,[15] a variety of approaches involving spontaneous and inducible mutations in organisms ranging from fruit flies to humans have produced an emerging picture of a highly conserved general mechanism for generating circadian rhythmicity. Some of these genes, known as clock genes, are Period (Per), Frequency (Frq), Clock (Clk), Cryptochrome (Cry), and Brain muscle ARNT-like1 (Bmal1). Although the genes and corresponding proteins that form core clock components vary across phyla, the mechanistic basis behind the generation of a circadian cycle remains highly conserved. The molecular basis for circadian rhythmicity is encoded in interlocking transcriptional and translational feedback loops.[16] The generation of the cycle is started by gene transcription, with translation of the transcript into a protein leading to a negative feedback loop. The protein or downstream target then inhibits additional transcription. The original protein product must then be removed for the loop to maintain functionality. Within the SCN, molecular generation of circadian rhythms is dependent upon the function of a core negative feedback loop.[2,17] In mammals, the constitutively expressed CLOCK (circadian locomotor output cycles kaput, or CLK) protein forms a heteromeric transcription factor with the oscillating BMAL1 protein through interacting PAS (Period–ARNT–SIM) domains; this complex binds to promoters of Cry (Cryptochrome) and Per (Period) and drives their transcription. In turn, CRY and PER proteins heterodimerize, and, in a typical negative feedback manner, move into the nucleus and inhibit their own transcription by acting as transcriptional repressors at CLK–BMAL1 directed sites.[17,18] This feedback is marked by a 6 h delay in the Per–Cry component, likely due to extensive posttranslational modifications of the various clock components (Figure 14.1).[19,20] Progressive phosphorylation of PER and CRY proteins by casein kinase 1ε/δ and AMPK (AMP kinase), respectively, leads to polyubiquitination by complexes of E3 ligases and, ultimately, to their degradation at the 26S proteosome.[21–25] This degradation toward the end of the circadian cycle releases transcriptional repression and allows CLK–BMAL1 transcription to begin anew, thus triggering a new biological day. This core cycle takes approximately 24 h to complete.

Regulation of the CLK–BMAL1 complex by ancillary feedback loops provides stability to the molecular oscillator. E-box elements in the promoters of nuclear receptors Rev-erbα and RORα also provide a mechanism for the regulation of transcription of these genes by CLK–BMAL1. In turn, the rhythmic expression of

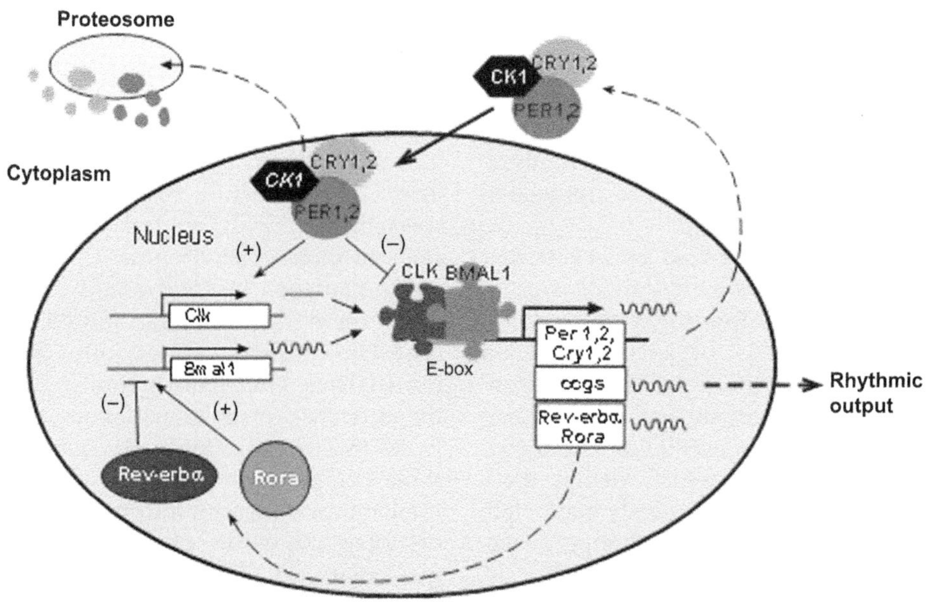

FIGURE 14.1 The core molecular clock. CLK–BMAL1 drives the expression of genes containing E-box promoter elements. In the core loop, CLK–BMAL1 drives transcription of Pers and Crys, dependent upon the availability of BMAL1. Per–Cry heterodimers feedback to inhibit CLK–BMAL1 activity. Per–Cry is phosphorylated and subsequently degraded by the proteosome. An accessory loop regulates BMAL1. CLK–BMAL1 also drives production of Rev-erbα and Rora, which have opposing effects on production of BMAL1. Finally, CLK–BMAL1 drives production of clock control genes (ccgs). (For color version of this figure, the reader is referred to the online version of this book.)

Bmal1 is determined by the opposing actions of these two genes, which compete for binding to ROR elements in the Bmal1 promoter. RORα drives transcription of Bmal1, whereas REV-ERBα inhibits Bmal1 expression.[26,27] Posttranslational modifications and epigenetic mechanisms are also important for regulation of the CLK–BMAL1 complex.[28] CLK appears to incur several posttranslational effects on its dimerization partner, BMAL1, including SUMOylation and acetylation.[29,30] SUMOylation and ubiquitination of BMAL1 are important for its circadian expression and its activity.[29,31] Recruitment of CLK–BMAL1 is mediated by a histone methyltransferase; CLK has intrinsic histone acetyltransferase activity, which promotes the unwinding of the DNA and enhances transcriptional activation of CLK's target genes.[32] Transcriptional activity of the CLK–BMAL1 complex is inhibited by SIRT1, which is expressed in a circadian fashion in antiphase with CLK–BMAL1 activity and acts as a histone deacetylase to directly oppose the histone acetyltransferase activity of CLK.[33,34]

The intracellular workings of the circadian clock are not restricted to a series of transcriptional or translational events with associated enzymatic posttranslational modifications of the transcriptional machinery. In fact, transcriptional regulation may not even be required to build a cellular clock, as elegantly indicated in studies of the cyanobacterial clock, where rhythmicity has been demonstrated in a cell-free system, making use of three bacterial proteins (kaiA, kaiB, and kaiC) together with adenosine triphosphate (ATP).[35] Clearly, other cellular events are essential for regulating the transcriptional clockwork. Membrane potential, intracellular calcium levels, and cyclic adenosine monophosphate (cAMP) are important and likely interrelated with respect to their regulation of intrinsic rhythmicity of neurons comprising the master clock in the SCN.[36–41] Firing rate rhythms of SCN neurons are calcium dependent.[42] The calcium-dependent potassium channel, BK, regulates rhythmic SCN neuronal firing; loss of the BK channel significantly elevates the neuronal firing rate at night, suppressing the robustness of rhythmicity.[43,44] Rhythmic oscillations in intracellular cAMP are also required to maintain the firing-rate rhythms of individual neurons.[39] Similarly, membrane depolarization,[45] intracellular calcium flux,[36,37] and cAMP are all coupled to the rhythmic expression of clock genes within the SCN.[38,39,42] Cre-elements are located in the promoters of the Per1 and Per2 genes[46]; activation of Cre-containing genes, as well as oscillations in Per1 and Per2 expression, is required for rhythmic firing of SCN neurons.[9,47–49] Collectively, the available data paint a complex picture suggestive of a complex intracellular network whose interrelationships ultimately coalesce into expression of a circadian rhythm within individual neurons of the SCN.

SCN AS THE MASTER CLOCK

The fact that circadian rhythms persist when animals are placed in constant environmental conditions establishes the notion that rhythmicity is produced endogenously rather than being a product of exposure to the alternating cycles of light and dark that comprise our environment. This inspired an anatomical search for the location of the "master" clock. As a follow-up to electron microscopic studies that demonstrated direct synaptic connectivity from the retina,[50] lesion studies revealed a loss of rhythmicity upon selective destruction of the SCN of the basal hypothalamus.[51,52] Transplantation of SCN or SCN2.2 cells (an immortalized cell line derived from the rat SCN) into arrhythmic animals restores many aspects of circadian rhythmicity, even if the transplant does not establish synaptic connections.[53–58] More importantly, transplantation studies using the tau mutant hamster, which has an endogenous period that is approximately 2 h shorter than that of a normal hamster, demonstrate that when rhythms are restored, the expressed period is determined by the transplanted SCN.[59] SCN transplants will even impose rhythmicity when placed into a genetically arrhythmic host.[60] SCN slices retain a circadian rhythm in electrical activity, even after 3 weeks in culture[61–65]; biochemical analyses reveal that slices also display 24 h rhythms in glucose utilization and production of certain peptides.[66–68] Collectively, these studies solidify the conclusion that the SCN is the master pacemaker.

The SCN is a bilateral nucleus nestled in the optic chiasm in the ventral portion of the anterior hypothalamus; each SCN contains approximately 10,000 neurons in mice and 45,000 in humans. SCN neurons are small in diameter (~10 μm), are tightly packed, and have simple dendritic structure with relatively few connections.[69] Electrical activity recordings of dissociated and dispersed SCN neurons suggest that all SCN neurons are independently rhythmic,[8] and thus each SCN neuron has pacemaker properties. However, not all SCN neurons are functionally equivalent.[70] The SCN is, in fact, a heterogeneous network of neurons, which have largely been defined according to their neuropeptide content.[71,72] The SCN is anatomically divided into two major regions defined by neuropeptide content, afferent and efferent connections, although this model likely minimizes the inherent complexity of the structure (Figure 14.2) (reviewed in Ref. 69). Whereas significant species variability exists, the consensus is that vasoactive intestinal peptide (VIP) and gastrin-releasing peptide (GRP) define the "core", while

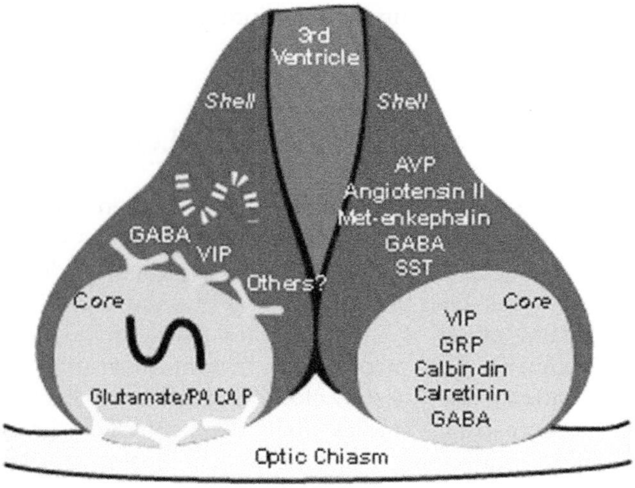

FIGURE 14.2 **General structure of the heterogeneous SCN.** SCN is divided into core and shell regions. The core contains the primary oscillator, which drives oscillations in the shell. VIP, GABA, and others are projected as neurotransmitters that provide coupling between core and shell. The core also receives the primary input, especially from the RHT, via glutamate and PACAP release. Core neurons express VIP and GRP, as well as calbindin, calretinin, and GABA. Shell neurons express AVP, angiotensin II, met-enkephalin, GABA, and somatostatin (SST). (For color version of this figure, the reader is referred to the online version of this book.)

arginine vasopressin (AVP) is the most abundant neuropeptide expressed in the neurons of the "shell".[73] Located in the ventrolateral region of the nucleus and directly adjacent to the optic chiasm, neurons in the core are synaptically connected to the retinohypothalamic tract (RHT), thus defining the site for input to the SCN from the optic nerve. Core neurons also express calbindin, calretinin, and neurotensin, as well as gamma aminobutyric acid (GABA), the amino acid neurotransmitter.[73] Cholecystokinin, glutamate, somatostatin, and substance P are also found in the SCN.[73] Core neurons project extensively into the shell. Shell neurons are located in the dorsomedial region of the nucleus, partially envelope the core, and express AVP, angiotensin II, met-enkephalin, and GABA. There is little reciprocal innervation from the shell to the core.[74] Efferent pathways emanate from both core and shell primarily into adjacent hypothalamic nuclei, with limited projections to the thalamus, forebrain, and periaqueductal gray.[73,74]

The neuronal circuitry of the SCN produces rhythmicity through intricate coupling of individual oscillators. Studies of dispersed cultures of SCN neurons reveal that each individual neuron is an independent oscillator. In culture, however, the period of individual SCN neuronal oscillations ranges from 20 to 28 h, suggesting variability in their oscillatory nature.[8] More recent studies confirm that SCN neurons vary widely in their expression of neuropeptides, pacemaking ability, and responsiveness to stimuli and in the rhythms that they control.[70,75] Thus, despite significant heterogeneity, individual oscillators must synchronize to form a coherent circuit in order to generate a rhythm whose oscillatory period is remarkably stable. The SCN in vivo displays exceptional synchrony. Communication among neurons in the nucleus produces an oscillatory network where individual components demonstrate unity in period, although phasing and amplitude of the oscillation remain distinctly different in the core compared to the shell. Neurons of the shell are distinctly rhythmic in vivo, as measured by gene expression, neuropeptide production, and electrical activity.[69,70,75] The amplitude of the rhythm in core neurons is less robust; these neurons, however, are acutely responsive to stimulation by light information processed through the RHT.[69]

Close examination reveals that the oscillation follows a highly ordered progression of activation that spreads across the SCN. The PER2–luciferase reporter demonstrates that activation occurs first in the dorsomedial shell region, which is dominated by AVP-expressing neurons, and spreads ventrally and laterally toward and into the VIP-rich core.[69,76] This oscillatory behavior is consistent with measures of rhythmic VIP and AVP release from the SCN; VIP release peaks earlier in the day than does AVP.[77,78] Functional coupling exists throughout the nucleus. When the core and shell are separated in vitro, coherent rhythmicity is lost in the shell but not in the core.[76] When the core is selectively lesioned in vivo, sparing the shell, circadian rhythms in locomotion, body temperature, heart rate, and hormone secretion are lost.[79,80] Thus, it is the core that maintains an essential synchrony and drives the circadian output necessary to achieve physiological and behavioral rhythmicity.

The mechanisms for functional coupling between core and shell remain elusive. Application of tetrodotoxin, which inhibits sodium channels and, therefore, synaptic activity, abolishes synchronized rhythms throughout the nucleus, suggesting that neurotransmission is required for coupling and synchrony.[76] A number of candidate molecules have been investigated for a role in coupling within the SCN network. Application of GABA can synchronize the firing rate in cultures of dispersed SCN neurons and can reset the phase of SCN slices.[81] In contrast, the $GABA_A$ receptor antagonist bicuculline can alter the activity of SCN slices in a manner reminiscent of separating core and shell, suggesting that GABA release from the core affects synchrony with the shell.[82] A circadian rhythm in GABA release and in the frequency of inhibitory postsynaptic currents has been demonstrated.[83] There is consensus that SCN neurons are nearly ubiquitously GABAergic, as is the expression of both $GABA_A$ and $GABA_B$ receptors.[70]

Evidence that VIP acts as a synchronizing factor is rapidly accumulating. VIP is released in a circadian manner from SCN slices in vitro. Application of VIP can alter the circadian phase both in vitro and in vivo. VIP is extensively expressed in core neurons; approximately 15% of the total SCN neurons are VIPergic.[73] The VIP receptor $VPAC_2$ is found throughout the SCN. Importantly, most if not all AVP-expressing shell neurons contain the $VPAC_2$ receptor.[78] Mice with a genetic deletion of VIP and the $VPAC_2$ receptor display distinct deficits in rhythms that suggest significantly diminished coupling.[84,85] A majority of mice of either phenotype have the unique characteristic of expressing multiple free-running circadian periods simultaneously.[86] The SCN of these mice displays reduced amplitudes in the rhythms of clock genes and neuronal activity. SCN synchrony is severely diminished in the SCN of these animals. Synchrony and rhythmicity are restored by treating VIP-deficient neuronal cultures with a $VPAC_2$ receptor agonist.[70]

Using the criteria that a synchronizing agent should be expressed in the SCN, particularly in core neurons, with cognate receptors located in the shell; should be released in a circadian manner; and should have effects on the SCN phase when applied exogenously, it is apparent that several other neurotransmitters warrant investigation. Primary among these are GRP, neurotensin, and prokineticin 2. Exogenous GRP can cause phase shifting in wild-type neurons and restore coupling in the $VPAC_2$ receptor-deficient mice.[70] Furthermore, gap junctions may play a role in intra-SCN coupling. Connexins are expressed in the SCN, and dye coupling can be demonstrated where a dye will appear in an adjacent neuron following injection into a neighboring cell. Electrical coupling is evident and more prevalent during subjective day.[87] Animals lacking connexin-36 lose electrical coupling and display reduced-amplitude circadian rhythms.[88] The preponderance of available evidence suggests that gap junctions couple cells within the core to each other and cells within the shell to each other, but that gap junctions do not connect core neurons to shell neurons. Thus, it seems that gap junctions provide strength in coupling within neurons of the same general type.

INPUT TO THE SCN

The SCN generates stable, endogenous rhythms. The period of this rhythmicity, albeit species specific, is usually either slightly shorter or longer than 24 h. Thus, daily minor adjustments of the clock are necessary to maintain alignment of physiological rhythms with the 24 h cycle imposed by the rotation of the Earth about its axis. This process is termed "entrainment". Also, physiological rhythms must adjust to larger changes in environmental light, such as occurs after transcontinental travel. This type of clock resetting is termed a phase shift. Zeitgebers are environmental signals that serve as adjustment cues to the circadian cycle that allow for both entrainment and phase shifting. Among a multitude of zeitgebers, prominent examples include light, food availability, predator presence, and temperature. Zeitgebers must gain access to the SCN clock in order to induce changes. Typically, afferent pathways are categorized into those arriving at the SCN from photic and nonphotic sources. Neuroanatomical information bombards the SCN, with stimuli arising from the RHT and the geniculohypothalamic tract (GHT), through the thalamic intergeniculate leaflet (IGL) and clusters of nuclei in the base of the brainstem that control sleep and are known as the median raphe nuclei (Figure 14.3)[89] (also see Chapter 21). Afferent signals from each of these sources impinge primarily, although not exclusively, on neurons associated with the SCN core.[89] Afferent information to the shell region arises primarily from other hypothalamic nuclei and, as detailed in this chapter, from the core.

Light is the most prominent and most extensively studied zeitgeber that affects the SCN network. Nocturnal light is perceived as an error signal by the SCN, which responds by resetting the circadian phase in a characteristic manner defined as a phase response curve (PRC). Light in the early night is perceived as a lengthening of the day; the clock responds by adjusting its phase such that the oscillation occurs later on subsequent days, which is designated a phase delay. Light in the late night is perceived as an early onset of the subsequent day. The clock responds by jumping ahead, termed a "phase advance".[4,69] Photic cues transmit light signals directly to the SCN from the retina via the RHT, a monosynaptic connection involving a specialized group of retinal ganglion cells that express the photopigment melanopsin. Classic lesion studies that underscored the importance of the RHT to circadian entrainment were critical to defining the "circadian visual system", and ultimately to the discovery of the SCN as the master clock.[90] Electrical stimulation of the RHT mimics the effects of light, causing phase delays in early night and phase advance in late night. Glutamate, an excitatory amino acid, is the primary neurotransmitter that conveys the light signal to the SCN. RHT stimulation causes release of glutamate; application of glutamate to the SCN mimics the effects of light (reviewed in Ref. 91). Pituitary adenylate cyclase-activating peptide (PACAP), and to a lesser extent aspartate and substance P, are coreleased with glutamate and have modulatory effects on phase resetting.[91] Although both *N*-methyl-D-aspartate

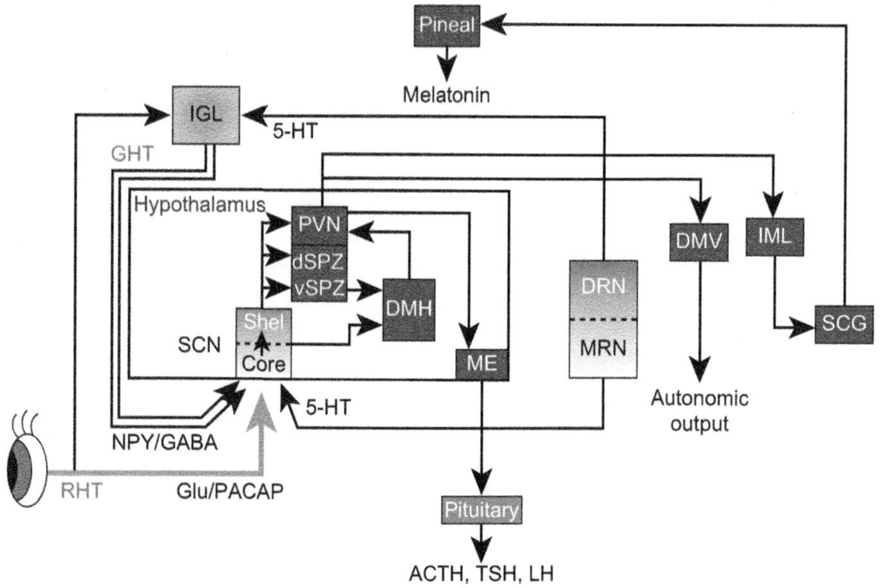

FIGURE 14.3 Afferent and efferent pathways associated with the SCN. A simplified version of the afferent and efferent connections of the SCN is shown. Photic input (orange) arises from the RHT (glutamate and PACAP) directly and from the GHT (GABA and NPY) indirectly. Nonphotic input (red) arrives from the DRN, indirectly from the IGL (GABA and NPY) and directly from the MRN (serotonin an 5-HT). Output pathways are shown in blue. Primary outputs are to the hypothalamus, via the subparaventricular zone (dSPV, mSPV), PVN, and DMH. Autonomic output arises from the PVN connection in the dorsal motor nucleus of the vagus (DMV). The hypothalamic–pituitary axis is controlled primarily via output from the PVN to the median eminence (ME). Melatonin is controlled via a multisynaptic pathway from the PVN to the IML, SCG, and then the pineal. (For color version of this figure, the reader is referred to the online version of this book.)

(NMDA) and non-NMDA glutamate receptors are involved in transmitting the light signal, NMDA receptors are necessary and sufficient to achieve phase resetting. NMDA administration mimics the effects of light, and inhibition of NMDA receptors blocks light- and glutamate-induced phase resetting.[91]

Activation of NMDA receptors initiates a series of intracellular events within core SCN neurons, ultimately allowing them to adjust their phase. The ensuing rise in intracellular calcium prompts activation of voltage-sensitive calcium channels. Calcium activates nitric oxide synthase (NOS) to produce nitric oxide (NO).[92] Signaling downstream of NO is more complex and dependent on the time of day. Early-night phase delays proceed following NO-dependent activation of ryanodine receptors (RYR).[93] In the late night, activation of NOS by light induces phase resetting through a process that depends on activation of protein kinase G (PKG).[93–95] Protein kinase A (PKA), calcium- and calmodulin-dependent protein kinase II (CaMKII), and two members of the mitogen-activated protein kinase (MAPK) family, ERK and JNK, are also activated by light[91] (also see Chapter 7).

Ultimately, light-induced phase resetting requires engagement of the molecular clockworks. The mechanism for the required elevation in Per1 and Per2 is phosphorylation and activation of the transcription factor, Ca^{2+}/cAMP responsive binding protein (CREB).[46,48,49] The rise in intracellular calcium in response to glutamatergic signaling induced by light leads to activation of a number of protein kinases, including CaMKII and MAPK throughout the night, and, in turn, to phosphorylation of CREB and activation of CRE-mediated gene expression.[48,96] Inhibition of CREB phosphorylation and CREB-mediated transcription blocks both light-induced Per1 elevation and phase shifts. Both Per1 and Per2 contain CRE elements in their promoters that are activated after light stimulation at night in the SCN.[46] Light and/or glutamate increase levels of Per1 and Per2 transcripts in the SCN. Inhibition of Per1 and Per2, using antisense oligonucleotides, blocks the phase-shifting effects of light in the SCN.[47,49]

The projection of the RHT directly onto the SCN is clearly important for the circadian network. An additional projection of the RHT, the IGL, is also involved. The SCN receives indirect input from the RHT through this connection with the IGL and, subsequently, the GHT.[97,98] Photic information arriving in the SCN from the GHT likely is associated with the ability of the SCN to adjust circadian timing in the face of changes in the seasonal photoperiod. Neuropeptide Y and GABA are the primary neurotransmitters associated with GHT afferents to the SCN.[99,100] NPY-deficient mice have altered abilities to adapt to changes in photoperiod. Information processed by the IGL is not, however, restricted to photic events. Nonphotic information arrives in the IGL via a connection with the brainstem dorsal raphe nucleus.[101] Thus, the GHT provides the SCN with information that likely endows its ability to integrate photic information with nonphotic cues.[102]

Finally, a direct afferent projection arrives in the SCN via the median raphe nucleus.[72,89] This pathway is a major nonphotic input to the SCN and is primarily serotonergic in content. Application of serotonin to the SCN causes phase resetting throughout the day through activation of cAMP/PKA-dependent signal transduction. Serotonergic terminals synapse most commonly on only the VIP neurons of the core SCN, although some connectivity with VP-containing neurons of the shell is also observed. Information from the median raphe enters the SCN at the same access point as the retinal input from the RHT.[89] Thus, it is not surprising that application of serotonin can modulate the light-signaling pathway. The common access point for RHT, GHT, and median raphe fibers reveals a neuroanatomical basis for integration of photic and nonphotic information within the SCN. The information gathered by the SCN via the RHT, GHT, and raphe nucleus is then processed and transmitted to the peripheral regions of the brain and body and utilized for pacemaker function.

GATING OF THE SCN

The SCN circadian clock is a self-timekeeper that monitors temporal progress over any proximate 24 h period. Inherent in the clock mechanism is a plasticity that allows for altering the timing of events when the environment signals that change is necessary. The SCN itself temporally gates the access of afferent signals, thereby restricting the window of access of information entering the clock.[3,4] For example, light gains access to the resetting mechanism of the clockworks only during the night. When the clock is exposed to light during "subjective" day (the time that would be day in under-constant-darkness conditions), there is no effect on the timing of subsequent rhythms. Specific chemical stimuli, such as serotonin, melatonin, acetylcholine, and a host of other neurotransmitters, will also affect clock timing only during those specific times or domains of the cycle when they are viewed as a sort of error message.

The access of afferent information to the resetting mechanism of the SCN may be divided into a series of four specific time domains, termed day, night, dusk, and dawn.[3] These domains are characterized by available access to signal transduction pathways that can be activated only by specific afferent signals. The daytime period is generally altered by the stimuli that couple to cAMP/PKA-dependent signaling pathways.[3,4] Elevation of cAMP using membrane-permeable cAMP analogs, or agonists that couple to cAMP signaling pathways, such as serotonin and PACAP, alter the phase of the SCN circadian rhythm only when applied during the day. The nighttime period adjusts through cGMP and cGMP-dependent protein kinase activation via a cholinergic stimulus.[3,4] Environmental light cues also play a role in the nighttime period. In this case, calcium and NO are introduced through glutamate transmission. The dusk and dawn periods are sensitive to phase resetting by the hormone melatonin, most likely through activation of signal transduction cascades associated with protein kinase C.[3,4]

SCN OUTPUT

Possibly the most important function of the SCN is to act as a relay, transmitting time-of-day information from the external environment to the rest of the body and thereby providing a mechanism for physiological synchronization among all organ systems. SCN output can be neuroanatomic, via the autonomic nervous system, or neuroendocrine.[17] Changes in SCN firing rate and consequent neurotransmitter release provide the prominent mechanism for production of rhythmic output by the SCN, although humoral signals may also make a significant contribution. Evidence for humoral regulation of SCN output derives from studies using encapsulated fetal SCN transplants that cannot make synaptic contact; these transplants restore rhythmicity in locomotor activity in animals with prior SCN lesion[58] presumably by volume transmission (Chapter 8). The nature of humoral regulation of circadian locomotor activity remains largely unknown; however, factors that may be secreted by the SCN that have effects on behavior include prokineticin-2, transforming growth factor α (TGFα), and cardiotrophin-like cytokine (CLC).[103] Interestingly, not all rhythms can be rescued with encapsulated transplants, suggesting that certain rhythms, especially those associated with the endocrine system (e.g. melatonin and corticosterone), require neuronal hardwiring and synaptic transmission.[55,104]

Four major efferent pathways emanate from the SCN (Figure 14.3); the targets have been defined as endocrine neurons in the hypothalamus, autonomic neurons of the paraventricular nucleus (PVN) of the hypothalamus, hypothalamic neurons that then relay information to other brain regions, and a smaller subset of neurons outside the hypothalamus.[105–107] Thus, the most extensive connections are found locally within the hypothalamus, with particularly extensive connections to the hypothalamic subparaventricular zone (sPVZ). The arcuate nucleus (ARC), bed nucleus of the stria terminalis (BNST), dorsomedial hypothalamus (DMH), lateral septum (LS), and preoptic area (POA) are all local brain regions that receive SCN efferents. The thalamic habenula (HB), PVN, and IGL are other known SCN efferent pathways.[103] Notably, SCN projection neurons exhibit topographic organization, as determined by anterograde and retrograde labeling.[108] Projections to the medial preoptic area (MPOA), dorsomedial and paraventricular hypothalamic nuclei, bed nucleus of stria terminalis, paraventricular thalamic nucleus, zona incerta, and medial sPVZ arise primarily from neurons of the SCN shell, although a few core neurons may innervate these areas.[108] The lateral sPVZ, peri-suprachiasmatic region, and LS receive input primarily from the SCN core, with some sparse input from the shell.

SCN efferents synapse with three specific neuronal types, defined as endocrine neurons, preautonomic neurons, and intermediate neurons.[107] The SCN-associated neurons of the DMH, the MPOA, and the sPVZ have been identified as intermediate neurons.[109] These neurons are thought to be the integrative messengers of circadian information with other hypothalamic inputs. Information carried on these pathways is relayed to the autonomic and endocrine neurons. The neuronal group characterized as the endocrine neurons is located in the PVN, POA, and ARC and is defined by its release of corticotropin-releasing hormone (CRH) and gonadotropin-releasing hormone (GnRH). These neurons have long been recognized as a reliable target for regulation by the biological clock, and their direct connection to the SCN has been demonstrated through anatomical tracing experiments.[110,111] The preautonomic neurons of the brainstem and spinal cord have also been targeted as an SCN output pathway.[112]

A prevalent concept regarding SCN output held that the nucleus functioned as a whole, generating timing information and sending it out as a single, homogeneous signal. Recent evidence now reveals this to be an oversimplification of the mechanism by which the SCN generates output signals. Circadian rhythmicity is prevalent in myriad aspects of physiology, with the peaks and troughs of various parameters occurring at different times over the course of a day. For example, in humans peak levels of the hormone melatonin occur at night, peak activity occurs during the day, cortisol secretion peaks in the morning, and blood pressure peaks in the afternoon. Each of these is controlled by output from the SCN. SCN anatomy demonstrates that the SCN is not a homogeneous population of neurons, as previously thought, but rather contains heterogeneous populations of neurons that can be phenotypically categorized according to neurotransmitter content, acrophase (time of the peak firing rate), and targets.[107] Electrophysiological analysis of single neurons indicates that subpopulations of neurons with different peaks in firing rate exist within the SCN. Summation of electrical activity yields the familiar activity rhythm of the SCN with its acrophase that occurs near midday.[113,114] Furthermore, real-time analysis of Per1 expression tracked with a short-lived green fluorescent protein reveals four subpopulations of SCN neurons. The largest group (~60%) shows peak Per1 expression at midday, which correlates with the ensemble electrical activity rhythm. The other smaller groups peak 3–4 h earlier, 3–4 h later, and during the night.[115,116]

A wealth of transmitter combinations is associated with SCN efferent neurons that include the classical neurotransmitters, glutamate and GABA, as well as several neuropeptides, especially VIP and AVP.[117–119] Of the ~10,000 neurons comprising the individual SCN in mice, up to 30% contain GABA colocalized with a neuropeptide transmitter.[120–122] Vasopressin is linked to target areas of the MPOA, the periventricular and subparaventricular nucleus, the DMH, and the PVN of the hypothalamus.[108,123–125] Approximately one-third of SCN neurons contain GABA[118]; GABAergic neurotransmission conveys timing information and inhibits melatonin production during the day. Glutamate neurotransmission from SCN efferent neurons targets hypothalamic sites, particularly the PVN. The coexpression and cooperation among these neurotransmitters allow the SCN to project distinct signals to different regions of the brain.[126] These chemical signals are used to coordinate daily activities of the whole organism, through their interactions with both parasympathetic and sympathetic branches of the autonomic nervous system, and with neuroendocrine output pathways. Output pathways control a vast array of physiological and behavioral events, only a few of which are outlined throughout the rest of this section.

SCN CONTROL OF LOCOMOTOR ACTIVITY

Locomotor activity (see Chapter 17) has long been the most utilized behavioral model for assessing circadian rhythmicity. In comparison with knowledge regarding input to the SCN, intra-SCN structure, and coupling, the mechanisms that underlie the transmission of efferent circadian information from the SCN to control the activity involved in sleep and wakefulness remain relatively unknown. Recent studies have identified prokineticin 2 (PK2), TGFα, and CLC as SCN-derived molecules that function in circadian regulation of locomotor activity.[103] PK2 is expressed in the SCN in a rhythmic manner with a peak during the day, and it is directly regulated by CLK:BMAL1.[127] Its cognate receptor is located in brain regions that receive direct input from the SCN. PK2 has inhibitory effects on locomotor activity in mice.[127] Intracerebroventricular administration of PK2 during the night inhibits activity in nocturnal mice. Reduced SCN levels of PK2 in a transgenic mouse that expresses a mutant form of the Huntington's gene are associated with an increase in daytime activity. The effect of PK2 from the SCN may occur via its direct connection with the PVN; PK2 has an excitatory effect on PVN neurons (reviewed in Ref. 128). TGFα is also rhythmically expressed in the SCN, and its infusion into the third ventricle disrupts circadian sleep–wake cycles by inhibiting locomotor activity. Epidermal growth factor (EGF) receptors are located in the sPVZ, a major site for SCN output.[129] Mutations in EGF receptors cause increased locomotor activity. Similarly, CLC has inhibitory effects on locomotor activity when infused into the third ventricle at a time when its expression by a subset of vasopressin-expressing SCN neurons is lowest. Its receptors are located along the third ventricle in a region known to be populated by SCN efferents. The effects of all three molecules, TGFα, PK2, and CLC, are independent of the core molecular clockworks, in a manner consistent with each of these acting as an output of the clock.

SCN CONTROL OF THE ADRENAL GLAND

Strong evidence links circadian expression of glucocorticoids to entrainment of peripheral clocks.[105] Dexamethasone can shift the phase of oscillators in peripheral tissues and restore oscillations in gene expression in the liver of SCN-lesioned mice.[17] Promoters of the core clock elements, Bmal1, Cry1, Per1, and Per2, contain glucocorticoid response elements, providing a mechanism for glucocorticoid regulation of the core clockworks. The stress hormone cortisol, or corticosterone in rodents, displays strong diurnal rhythmicity, with peak expression occurring just prior to awakening. In rodents, the corticosterone peak occurs, therefore, in the late part of the day.[130] The corticosterone rhythm is likely mediated by two distinct pathways emanating from the SCN. SCN-derived AVP neurons project to the PVN, where they can be found in proximity with CRH-releasing neurons. However, AVP inhibits the release of corticosterone. In fact, the AVP rhythm precedes that of corticosterone in the rodent. AVP peaks early in the day and begins to decline as corticosterone rises. Typically, AVP has a stimulatory effect on the postsynaptic cell. Thus, the inhibitory effect on corticosterone release is likely mediated by a GABA-containing interneuron. Moreover, the corticosterone rhythm is not heavily dependent upon a rhythm in adrenocorticotrophic hormone (ACTH) secretion. Rather, there is a distinct rhythm in adrenal gland sensitivity to ACTH, which is likely mediated through a multisynaptic relay from the SCN, through the PVN, the spinal cord, and, ultimately, the adrenal cortex.[130]

SCN CONTROL OF THE FEMALE REPRODUCTIVE CYCLE

The hypothalamic–pituitary–gonadal axis provides another example of the circadian control of endocrine physiology.[131] In spontaneously ovulating animals, the ovulation-triggering luteinizing hormone (LH) surge occurs on the day of proestrus, typically just prior to the onset of activity. The LH surge proceeds only when a precisely timed signal from the SCN occurs in the presence of the high levels of estrogen produced as ovarian follicles approach maturity (reviewed in Ref. 131). Circadian regulation of the female reproductive cycle is mediated through SCN innervation of a complex hypothalamic network. GnRH neurons contain a molecular clock, the phase of which is altered by signals that reset the SCN circadian clock.[132] The SCN projects directly onto a subset of GnRH neurons,[133] as well as indirectly onto estrogen-responsive kisspeptin-containing neurons in the anteroventral periventricular nucleus (AVPV) and gonadotropin inhibitory hormone–containing neurons in the dorsomedial nucleus of the hypothamalus.[131] VIPergic neurons arising in the core of the SCN synapse with $VPAC_2$ receptor-containing GnRH neurons. The production of VIP by the SCN is important for triggering the activity of the GnRH neurons on the day of proestrus.[131] Estrogen receptor α, the receptor subtype that mediates the positive feedback effect of estrogen in the hypothalamus, is notably absent in the SCN-receptive GnRH neuronal population.[131,134] Thus, the integration of the circadian signal with the hormonal milieu must occur at an intermediate site. The AVPV is likely a key regulatory site (reviewed in Ref. 131). The AVPV receives afferent information from AVP-expressing neurons that arise in the SCN core. AVPV neurons express estrogen receptor α, project directly onto GnRH neurons, and are active at the time of the LH surge. Clock mutant mice display reduced levels of AVP in the SCN and do not produce an endogenous LH surge.[135] AVP production by the SCN occurs consequent to GnRH secretion, and injection of AVP into the MPOA can produce an LH surge in SCN-lesioned animals. The AVPV neurons use the RFamide peptide kisspeptin to integrate the circadian and estrogen signals (reviewed in Ref. 136). Kisspeptin is upregulated by estrogen in the AVPV, and kisspeptin neurons are activated at the time of the LH surge. Finally, the SCN projects onto a population of neurons in the dorsomedial nucleus of the hypothalamus that express gonadotropin inhibitory hormone; production of this peptide suppresses the LH surge.[137,138] The projections of the gonadotropin inhibitory hormone–containing neurons, in turn, lie in close apposition to those of GnRH neurons. It appears, then, that activation of the SCN in the proper hormonal environment stimulates GnRH neurons through a direct VIP-mediated signal and an indirect AVP-mediated signal with the kisspeptin-containing neurons of the AVPV and through inhibition of the gonadotropin inhibitory hormone–containing neurons of the DMH.

SCN CONTROL OF THE PINEAL GLAND

Perhaps the most widely recognized endocrine system under the control of the SCN is the pineal gland and the production of its primary output, melatonin (reviewed in Ref. 139). Melatonin is well known as the hormone of night. The duration of melatonin production parallels the length of the night. Thus, by providing an internal definition of night length, melatonin provides a physiological measure of seasonality. Melatonin production is regulated by the SCN and, in turn, feeds back to modulate circadian clock function. SCN ablation abolishes the melatonin rhythm. SCN regulation of pineal melatonin secretion is mediated through an indirect, multisynaptic pathway involving complex regulation and numerous neurotransmitters.[140] GABAergic SCN efferents project to the PVN. Autonomic neurons of the PVN project onto the intermediolateral nucleus of the spinal cord, which projects to the superior cervical ganglion. Melatonin production is stimulated by the release of norepinephrine from the SCG terminals onto the pineal gland.[141,142] During the day, spontaneous activity of SCN neurons releases GABA onto the PVN, which suppresses glutamatergic output of this pathway, and inhibits synthesis and secretion of melatonin. A glutamatergic signal from the SCN to the PVN, present at night, can stimulate the production of melatonin.[143,144]

Melatonin is implicated in the regulation of a vast array of processes important in the maintenance of health. Melatonin regulates reproduction in seasonally active species. The antioxidant properties of melatonin have led to investigation of it as an anticancer agent. More recently, the discovery of melatonin receptors on β-cells in the pancreas, and reports of increased insulin secretion in melatonin receptor–deficient mice, have implicated melatonin in control of blood glucose. More established, however, is the role of melatonin in the regulation of sleep and circadian rhythmicity. Ramelteon is a relatively selective melatonin receptor agonist approved by the US Food and Drug Administration (FDA) for treatment of insomnia. Although an output of the clock, melatonin feeds back to modulate clock function and synchronize rhythms through actions on Rev-erbα.[139] Melatonin application at dawn and dusk can reset the rhythm of the SCN clock.[3]

SCN CONTROL OF METABOLISM

The central nervous system places a high demand on the body for glucose, which it can neither synthesize nor store. The liver and pancreas are key organs in maintaining the optimal blood glucose levels required for brain function. Given the diurnal variation in activity, as well as time-of-day dependent variations in food intake, it is therefore not surprising that the SCN regulates levels of metabolic hormones, including insulin, glucagon, gastrin, and leptin, as well as blood glucose through actions on glucose production by the liver and insulin production by the pancreas (reviewed in Ref. 145). Rhythms in key aspects of these metabolic parameters exist and are not dependent upon the temporal information provided by feeding behavior. Projections of the SCN synapse on autonomic neurons in the PVN. Anatomical evidence suggests that these AVP-expressing SCN efferents can influence both sympathetic and parasympathetic outflow from the hypothalamus, depending upon whether GABA or glutamate is co-expressed with AVP.[145] In the case of metabolism, these clock-derived outputs contribute to the sympathetic input to the liver that controls hepatic production of glucose. Similarly, a balance of sympathetic and parasympathetic input to adipose tissue that regulates lipogenesis and lipolysis is tied to the SCN.[145]

CIRCADIAN RHYTHMS IN HEALTH AND DISEASE

Circadian rhythmicity is a ubiquitous phenomenon that allows adaptive synchronization of physiological processes to an external environment where light and darkness vary with 24 h periodicity. Rhythmicity is apparent at every level of organization, ranging from gene expression to behavior, and it controls a vast array of processes, including many behaviors, hormone levels, blood pressure, body temperature, liver function, and many others. Although the incidence of rhythmicity has long been described, the role of the clock in disease remains underinvestigated. Moreover, considerations of clock function with respect to clinical therapeutic value are largely ignored. Increasingly, however, evidence is accumulating to demonstrate that clock disruption can cause disease (reviewed in Ref. 146). The "jet lag" associated with rapid changes in time zones can produce insomnia and impaired cognitive function.[147] Shift workers experience increased incidences of certain types of cancer; metabolic disorders, including type 2 diabetes; cardiovascular disease; and psychiatric impairments.[146] Recent evidence suggests that uncoupling of the central clock in the SCN from peripheral clocks, such as the liver, can be detrimental to health and may induce metabolic syndrome.[148] In mice, genetic disruption of the circadian clock has revealed numerous functional impairments. CLK mutant mice, as well as Bmal1- and Rev-erbα-deficient mice, display impaired glucose and lipid metabolism. Per-mutant mice are cancer-prone, whereas Cry-deficient mice are cancer-resistant. Cry,

ROR, and PAR bZIP knockouts display problems with xenobiotic metabolism and regulation of detoxification in the liver (reviewed in Ref. 146). Moreover, circadian rhythmicity undoubtedly affects the therapeutic efficacy of drugs by influencing pharmacokinetics and pharmacodynamics. Thus, the circadian clock network represents a vastly untapped resource for the development of new therapeutics. Clearly, a better understanding of the hierarchical circadian clock network will reveal its important contributions to health and disease.

CONCLUSIONS

In today's 24/7 society, exposure to light at night from the television or computer, and work demands and lifestyle choices that increase nighttime activity and daytime sleep, place increasing demands on our circadian system. Disruption of this clock network, through chronic jet lag and shift work, leads to illness, underscoring the importance of the circadian system in maintenance of health. The circadian clock network was once the object of scientific study simply because it provided a clean example of a simple behavior (activity rhythms) controlled directly by the function of a discrete number of genes. However, the importance of the circadian clock network in health and disease has only begun to be realized. In mammals, the SCN remains the central driving force in managing this network and maintaining functional synchrony with the environment. The development of transgenic mice, as well as the discovery of human polymorphisms in core clock genes, has revealed that a dysfunctional clock contributes to a wide array of disease states ranging from sleep disorders and psychiatric illnesses to cancer and metabolic disease. Understanding of the complex neuroendocrine events that sustain a healthy circadian system is paramount to the development of novel "chrono"-therapies that target the circadian system in a variety of disease states.

References

1. Menaker M, Takahashi JS, Eskin A. The physiology of circadian pacemakers. *Annu Rev Physiol*. 1978;40:501–526.
2. Takahashi JS, Hong HK, Ko CH, McDearmon EL. The genetics of mammalian circadian order and disorder: implications for physiology and disease. *Nat Rev Genet*. 2008;9:764–775.
3. Gillette MU, Mitchell JW. Signaling in the suprachiasmatic nucleus: selectively responsive and integrative. *Cell Tissue Res*. 2002;309:99–107.
4. Gillette MU, Tischkau SA. Suprachiasmatic nucleus: the brain's circadian clock. *Recent Prog Horm Res*. 1999;54:33–58 discussion 58–39.
5. Kramer C. Rhythmic conidiation in *Neurospora crassa*. *Methods Mol Biol*. 2007;362:49–65.
6. Young MW, Kay SA. Time zones: a comparative genetics of circadian clocks. *Nat Rev Genet*. 2001;2:702–715.
7. Honma S, Shirakawa T, Katsuno Y, Namihira M, Honma K. Circadian periods of single suprachiasmatic neurons in rats. *Neurosci Lett*. 1998;250:157–160.
8. Welsh DK, Logothetis DE, Meister M, Reppert SM. Individual neurons dissociated from rat suprachiasmatic nucleus express independently phased circadian firing rhythms. *Neuron*. 1995;14:697–706.
9. Tischkau SA, Gillette MU. Oligodeoxynucleotide methods for analyzing the circadian clock in the suprachiasmatic nucleus. *Methods Enzymol*. 2005;393:593–610.
10. Do MT, Yau KW. Intrinsically photosensitive retinal ganglion cells. *Physiol Rev*. 2010;90:1547–1581.
11. Hannibal J. Neurotransmitters of the retino-hypothalamic tract. *Cell Tissue Res*. 2002;309:73–88.
12. Hannibal J, Fahrenkrug J. Melanopsin: a novel photopigment involved in the photoentrainment of the brain's biological clock? *Ann Med*. 2002;34:401–407.
13. Moore RY. Retinohypothalamic projection in mammals: a comparative study. *Brain Res*. 1973;49:403–409.
14. Moore RY, Lenn NJ. A retinohypothalamic projection in the rat. *J Comp Neurol*. 1972;146:1–14.
15. Konopka RJ, Benzer S. Clock mutants of *Drosophila melanogaster*. *Proc Natl Acad Sci USA*. 1971;68:2112–2116.
16. Reppert SM, Weaver DR. Coordination of circadian timing in mammals. *Nature*. 2002;418:935–941.
17. Mohawk JA, Green CB, Takahashi JS. Central and peripheral circadian clocks in mammals. *Annu Rev Neurosci*. 2012;35:445–462.
18. Kwon I, Choe HK, Son GH, Kim K. Mammalian molecular clocks. *Exp Neurobiol*. 2011;20:18–28.
19. Gallego M, Virshup DM. Post-translational modifications regulate the ticking of the circadian clock. *Nat Rev Mol Cell Biol*. 2007;8:139–148.
20. Virshup DM, Eide EJ, Forger DB, Gallego M, Harnish EV. Reversible protein phosphorylation regulates circadian rhythms. *Cold Spring Harb Symp Quant Biol*. 2007;72:413–420.
21. Akashi M, Tsuchiya Y, Yoshino T, Nishida E. Control of intracellular dynamics of mammalian period proteins by casein kinase I epsilon (CKIepsilon) and CKIdelta in cultured cells. *Mol Cell Biol*. 2002;22:1693–1703.
22. Busino L, Bassermann F, Maiolica A, et al. SCFFbxl3 controls the oscillation of the circadian clock by directing the degradation of cryptochrome proteins. *Science*. 2007;316:900–904.
23. Eide EJ, Woolf MF, Kang H, et al. Control of mammalian circadian rhythm by CKIepsilon-regulated proteasome-mediated PER2 degradation. *Mol Cell Biol*. 2005;25:2795–2807.
24. Lamia KA, Sachdeva UM, DiTacchio L, et al. AMPK regulates the circadian clock by cryptochrome phosphorylation and degradation. *Science*. 2009;326:437–440.
25. Shirogane T, Jin J, Ang XL, Harper JW. SCFbeta-TRCP controls clock-dependent transcription via casein kinase 1-dependent degradation of the mammalian period-1 (Per1) protein. *J Biol Chem*. 2005;280:26863–26872.
26. Jetten AM. Retinoid-related orphan receptors (RORs): critical roles in development, immunity, circadian rhythm, and cellular metabolism. *Nucl Recept Signal*. 2009;7:e003.
27. Preitner N, Damiola F, Lopez-Molina L, et al. The orphan nuclear receptor REV-ERBα controls circadian transcription within the positive limb of the mammalian circadian oscillator. *Cell*. 2002;110:251–260.
28. Masri S, Zocchi L, Katada S, Mora E, Sassone-Corsi P. The circadian clock transcriptional complex: metabolic feedback intersects with epigenetic control. *Ann N Y Acad Sci*. 1264:103–109.
29. Cardone L, Hirayama J, Giordano F, Tamaru T, Palvimo JJ, Sassone-Corsi P. Circadian clock control by SUMOylation of BMAL1. *Science*. 2005;309:1390–1394.

30. Hirayama J, Sahar S, Grimaldi B, et al. CLOCK-mediated acetylation of BMAL1 controls circadian function. *Nature*. 2007;450:1086–1090.
31. Lee J, Lee Y, Lee MJ, et al. Dual modification of BMAL1 by SUMO2/3 and ubiquitin promotes circadian activation of the CLOCK/BMAL1 complex. *Mol Cell Biol*. 2008;28:6056–6065.
32. Grimaldi B, Nakahata Y, Sahar S, et al. Chromatin remodeling and circadian control: master regulator CLOCK is an enzyme. *Cold Spring Harb Symp Quant Biol*. 2007;72:105–112.
33. Grimaldi B, Nakahata Y, Kaluzova M, Masubuchi S, Sassone-Corsi P. Chromatin remodeling, metabolism and circadian clocks: the interplay of CLOCK and SIRT1. *Int J Biochem Cell Biol*. 2009;41:81–86.
34. Nakahata Y, Kaluzova M, Grimaldi B, et al. The NAD^+-dependent deacetylase SIRT1 modulates CLOCK-mediated chromatin remodeling and circadian control. *Cell*. 2008;134:329–340.
35. Nakajima M, Imai K, Ito H, et al. Reconstitution of circadian oscillation of cyanobacterial KaiC phosphorylation in vitro. *Science*. 2005;308:414–415.
36. Ikeda M, Sugiyama T, Wallace CS, et al. Circadian dynamics of cytosolic and nuclear Ca^{2+} in single suprachiasmatic nucleus neurons. *Neuron*. 2003;38:253–263.
37. Ikeda M, Yoshioka T, Allen CN. Developmental and circadian changes in Ca^{2+} mobilization mediated by $GABA_A$ and NMDA receptors in the suprachiasmatic nucleus. *Eur J Neurosci*. 2003;17:58–70.
38. Nahm SS, Farnell YZ, Griffith W, Earnest DJ. Circadian regulation and function of voltage-dependent calcium channels in the suprachiasmatic nucleus. *J Neurosci*. 2005;25:9304–9308.
39. O'Neill JS, Maywood ES, Chesham JE, Takahashi JS, Hastings MH. cAMP-dependent signaling as a core component of the mammalian circadian pacemaker. *Science*. 2008;320:949–953.
40. Shibata S, Moore RY. Development of neuronal activity in the rat suprachiasmatic nucleus. *Brain Res*. 1987;431:311–315.
41. Shibata S, Newman GC, Moore RY. Effects of calcium ions on glucose utilization in the rat suprachiasmatic nucleus in vitro. *Brain Res*. 1987;426:332–338.
42. Lundkvist GB, Kwak Y, Davis EK, Tei H, Block GD. A calcium flux is required for circadian rhythm generation in mammalian pacemaker neurons. *J Neurosci*. 2005;25:7682–7686.
43. Kent J, Meredith AL. BK channels regulate spontaneous action potential rhythmicity in the suprachiasmatic nucleus. *PLoS One*. 2008;3:e3884.
44. Meredith AL, Wiler SW, Miller BH, et al. BK calcium-activated potassium channels regulate circadian behavioral rhythms and pacemaker output. *Nat Neurosci*. 2006;9:1041–1049.
45. de Jeu M, Hermes M, Pennartz C. Circadian modulation of membrane properties in slices of rat suprachiasmatic nucleus. *Neuroreport*. 1998;9:3725–3729.
46. Travnickova-Bendova Z, Cermakian N, Reppert SM, Sassone-Corsi P. Bimodal regulation of mPeriod promoters by CREB-dependent signaling and CLOCK/BMAL1 activity. *Proc Natl Acad Sci USA*. 2002;99:7728–7733.
47. Akiyama M, Kouzu Y, Takahashi S, et al. Inhibition of light- or glutamate-induced mPer1 expression represses the phase shifts into the mouse circadian locomotor and suprachiasmatic firing rhythms. *J Neurosci*. 1999;19:1115–1121.
48. Obrietan K, Impey S, Smith D, Athos J, Storm DR. Circadian regulation of cAMP response element-mediated gene expression in the suprachiasmatic nuclei. *J Biol Chem*. 1999;274:17748–17756.
49. Tischkau SA, Mitchell JW, Tyan SH, Buchanan GF, Gillette MU. Ca^{2+}/cAMP response element-binding protein (CREB)-dependent activation of Per1 is required for light-induced signaling in the suprachiasmatic nucleus circadian clock. *J Biol Chem*. 2003;278:718–723.
50. Hendrickson AE, Wagoner N, Cowan WM. An autoradiographic and electron microscopic study of retino-hypothalamic connections. *Z Zellforsch Mikrosk Anat*. 1972;135:1–26.
51. Moore RY, Eichler VB. Loss of a circadian adrenal corticosterone rhythm following suprachiasmatic lesions in the rat. *Brain Res*. 1972;42:201–206.
52. Stephan FK, Zucker I. Circadian rhythms in drinking behavior and locomotor activity of rats are eliminated by hypothalamic lesions. *Proc Natl Acad Sci USA*. 1972;69:1583–1586.
53. Earnest DJ, Liang FQ, Ratcliff M, Cassone VM. Immortal time: circadian clock properties of rat suprachiasmatic cell lines. *Science*. 1999;283:693–695.
54. Hakim H, DeBernardo AP, Silver R. Circadian locomotor rhythms, but not photoperiodic responses, survive surgical isolation of the SCN in hamsters. *J Biol Rhythms*. 1991;6:97–113.
55. Lehman MN, Silver R, Gladstone WR, Kahn RM, Gibson M, Bittman EL. Circadian rhythmicity restored by neural transplant. Immunocytochemical characterization of the graft and its integration with the host brain. *J Neurosci*. 1987;7:1626–1638.
56. LeSauter J, Lehman MN, Silver R. Restoration of circadian rhythmicity by transplants of SCN "micropunches". *J Biol Rhythms*. 1996;11:163–171.
57. Ralph MR, Foster RG, Davis FC, Menaker M. Transplanted suprachiasmatic nucleus determines circadian period. *Science*. 1990;247:975–978.
58. Silver R, LeSauter J, Tresco PA, Lehman MN. A diffusible coupling signal from the transplanted suprachiasmatic nucleus controlling circadian locomotor rhythms. *Nature*. 1996;382:810–813.
59. Guo H, Brewer JM, Lehman MN, Bittman EL. Suprachiasmatic regulation of circadian rhythms of gene expression in hamster peripheral organs: effects of transplanting the pacemaker. *J Neurosci*. 2006;26:6406–6412.
60. Sujino M, Masumoto KH, Yamaguchi S, van der Horst GT, Okamura H, Inouye ST. Suprachiasmatic nucleus grafts restore circadian behavioral rhythms of genetically arrhythmic mice. *Curr Biol*. 2003;13:664–668.
61. Bos NP, Mirmiran M. Circadian rhythms in spontaneous neuronal discharges of the cultured suprachiasmatic nucleus. *Brain Res*. 1990;511:158–162.
62. Green DJ, Gillette R. Circadian rhythm of firing rate recorded from single cells in the rat suprachiasmatic brain slice. *Brain Res*. 1982;245:198–200.
63. Groos G, Hendriks J. Circadian rhythms in electrical discharge of rat suprachiasmatic neurones recorded in vitro. *Neurosci Lett*. 1982;34:283–288.
64. Inouye ST, Kawamura H. Persistence of circadian rhythmicity in a mammalian hypothalamic "island" containing the suprachiasmatic nucleus. *Proc Natl Acad Sci USA*. 1979;76:5962–5966.
65. Shibata S, Oomura Y, Kita H, Hattori K. Circadian rhythmic changes of neuronal activity in the suprachiasmatic nucleus of the rat hypothalamic slice. *Brain Res*. 1982;247:154–158.
66. Flood DG, Gibbs FP. Species difference in circadian [^{14}C] 2-deoxyglucose uptake by suprachiasmatic nuclei. *Brain Res*. 1982;232:200–205.
67. Gillette MU, Reppert SM. The hypothalamic suprachiasmatic nuclei: circadian patterns of vasopressin secretion and neuronal activity in vitro. *Brain Res Bull*. 1987;19:135–139.
68. Schwartz WJ, Gainer H. Suprachiasmatic nucleus: use of ^{14}C-labeled deoxyglucose uptake as a functional marker. *Science*. 1977;197:1089–1091.
69. Yan L, Karatsoreos I, Lesauter J, et al. Exploring spatiotemporal organization of SCN circuits. *Cold Spring Harb Symp Quant Biol*. 2007;72:527–541.

70. Aton SJ, Herzog ED. Come together, right...now: synchronization of rhythms in a mammalian circadian clock. *Neuron.* 2005;48: 531–534.
71. Cassone VM, Speh JC, Card JP, Moore RY. Comparative anatomy of the mammalian hypothalamic suprachiasmatic nucleus. *J Biol Rhythms.* 1988;3:71–91.
72. Morin LP, Allen CN. The circadian visual system, 2005. *Brain Res Rev.* 2006;51:1–60.
73. Abrahamson EE, Moore RY. Suprachiasmatic nucleus in the mouse: retinal innervation, intrinsic organization and efferent projections. *Brain Res.* 2001;916:172–191.
74. Leak RK, Card JP, Moore RY. Suprachiasmatic pacemaker organization analyzed by viral transynaptic transport. *Brain Res.* 1999;819:23–32.
75. Antle MC, Silver R. Orchestrating time: arrangements of the brain circadian clock. *Trends Neurosci.* 2005;28:145–151.
76. Yamaguchi S, Isejima H, Matsuo T, et al. Synchronization of cellular clocks in the suprachiasmatic nucleus. *Science.* 2003;302:1408–1412.
77. Nakamura W, Honma S, Shirakawa T, Honma K. Regional pacemakers composed of multiple oscillator neurons in the rat suprachiasmatic nucleus. *Eur J Neurosci.* 2001;14:666–674.
78. Shinohara K, Honma S, Katsuno Y, Abe H, Honma K. Two distinct oscillators in the rat suprachiasmatic nucleus in vitro. *Proc Natl Acad Sci USA.* 1995;92:7396–7400.
79. Honma S, Shirakawa T, Nakamura W, Honma K. Synaptic communication of cellular oscillations in the rat suprachiasmatic neurons. *Neurosci Lett.* 2000;294:113–116.
80. Shirakawa T, Honma S, Katsuno Y, Oguchi H, Honma KI. Synchronization of circadian firing rhythms in cultured rat suprachiasmatic neurons. *Eur J Neurosci.* 2000;12:2833–2838.
81. Liu C, Reppert SM. GABA synchronizes clock cells within the suprachiasmatic circadian clock. *Neuron.* 2000;25:123–128.
82. Albus H, Vansteensel MJ, Michel S, Block GD, Meijer JH. A GABAergic mechanism is necessary for coupling dissociable ventral and dorsal regional oscillators within the circadian clock. *Curr Biol.* 2005;15:886–893.
83. Itri J, Colwell CS. Regulation of inhibitory synaptic transmission by vasoactive intestinal peptide (VIP) in the mouse suprachiasmatic nucleus. *J Neurophysiol.* 2003;90:1589–1597.
84. Colwell CS, Michel S, Itri J, et al. Disrupted circadian rhythms in VIP- and PHI-deficient mice. *Am J Physiol Regul Integr Comp Physiol.* 2003;285:R939–R949.
85. Harmar AJ, Marston HM, Shen S, et al. The $VPAC_2$ receptor is essential for circadian function in the mouse suprachiasmatic nuclei. *Cell.* 2002;109:497–508.
86. Aton SJ, Colwell CS, Harmar AJ, Waschek J, Herzog ED. Vasoactive intestinal polypeptide mediates circadian rhythmicity and synchrony in mammalian clock neurons. *Nat Neurosci.* 2005;8: 476–483.
87. Colwell CS. Rhythmic coupling among cells in the suprachiasmatic nucleus. *J Neurobiol.* 2000;43:379–388.
88. Long MA, Jutras MJ, Connors BW, Burwell RD. Electrical synapses coordinate activity in the suprachiasmatic nucleus. *Nat Neurosci.* 2005;8:61–66.
89. Morin LP. Neuroanatomy of the extended circadian rhythm system. *Exp Neurol.* 2012.
90. Johnson RF, Moore RY, Morin LP. Loss of entrainment and anatomical plasticity after lesions of the hamster retinohypothalamic tract. *Brain Res.* 1988;460:297–313.
91. Golombek DA, Rosenstein RE. Physiology of circadian entrainment. *Physiol Rev.* 2010;90:1063–1102.
92. Ding JM, Chen D, Weber ET, Faiman LE, Rea MA, Gillette MU. Resetting the biological clock: mediation of nocturnal circadian shifts by glutamate and NO. *Science.* 1994;266:1713–1717.
93. Ding JM, Buchanan GF, Tischkau SA, et al. A neuronal ryanodine receptor mediates light-induced phase delays of the circadian clock. *Nature.* 1998;394:381–384.
94. Mathur A, Golombek DA, Ralph MR. cGMP-dependent protein kinase inhibitors block light-induced phase advances of circadian rhythms in vivo. *Am J Physiol.* 1996;270:R1031–R1036.
95. Weber ET, Gannon RL, Rea MA. cGMP-dependent protein kinase inhibitor blocks light-induced phase advances of circadian rhythms in vivo. *Neurosci Lett.* 1995;197:227–230.
96. Obrietan K, Impey S, Storm DR. Light and circadian rhythmicity regulate MAP kinase activation in the suprachiasmatic nuclei. *Nat Neurosci.* 1998;1:693–700.
97. Harrington ME. The ventral lateral geniculate nucleus and the intergeniculate leaflet: interrelated structures in the visual and circadian systems. *Neurosci Biobehav Rev.* 1997;21:705–727.
98. Morin LP, Blanchard JH. Forebrain connections of the hamster intergeniculate leaflet: comparison with those of ventral lateral geniculate nucleus and retina. *Vis Neurosci.* 1999;16:1037–1054.
99. Harrington ME, Nance DM, Rusak B. Neuropeptide Y immunoreactivity in the hamster geniculo-suprachiasmatic tract. *Brain Res Bull.* 1985;15:465–472.
100. Moore RY, Card JP. Intergeniculate leaflet: an anatomically and functionally distinct subdivision of the lateral geniculate complex. *J Comp Neurol.* 1994;344:403–430.
101. Glass JD, Grossman GH, Farnbauch L, DiNardo L. Midbrain raphe modulation of nonphotic circadian clock resetting and 5-HT release in the mammalian suprachiasmatic nucleus. *J Neurosci.* 2003;23:7451–7460.
102. Meyer-Bernstein EL, Morin LP. Differential serotonergic innervation of the suprachiasmatic nucleus and the intergeniculate leaflet and its role in circadian rhythm modulation. *J Neurosci.* 1996;16:2097–2111.
103. Dibner C, Schibler U, Albrecht U. The mammalian circadian timing system: organization and coordination of central and peripheral clocks. *Annu Rev Physiol.* 2010;72:517–549.
104. Meyer-Bernstein EL, Jetton AE, Matsumoto SI, Markuns JF, Lehman MN, Bittman EL. Effects of suprachiasmatic transplants on circadian rhythms of neuroendocrine function in golden hamsters. *Endocrinology.* 1999;140:207–218.
105. Buijs RM, Kalsbeek A. Hypothalamic integration of central and peripheral clocks. *Nat Rev Neurosci.* 2001;2:521–526.
106. Kalsbeek A, Palm IF, La Fleur SE, et al. SCN outputs and the hypothalamic balance of life. *J Biol Rhythms.* 2006;21:458–469.
107. Kalsbeek A, Perreau-Lenz S, Buijs RM. A network of (autonomic) clock outputs. *Chronobiol Int.* 2006;23:201–215.
108. Leak RK, Moore RY. Topographic organization of suprachiasmatic nucleus projection neurons. *J Comp Neurol.* 2001;433: 312–334.
109. Saper CB, Lu J, Chou TC, Gooley J. The hypothalamic integrator for circadian rhythms. *Trends Neurosci.* 2005;28:152–157.
110. Buijs RM, Markman M, Nunes-Cardoso B, Hou YX, Shinn S. Projections of the suprachiasmatic nucleus to stress-related areas in the rat hypothalamus: a light and electron microscopic study. *J Comp Neurol.* 1993;335:42–54.
111. Vrang N, Larsen PJ, Mikkelsen JD. Direct projection from the suprachiasmatic nucleus to hypophysiotrophic corticotropin-releasing factor immunoreactive cells in the paraventricular nucleus of the hypothalamus demonstrated by means of *Phaseolus vulgaris*-leucoagglutinin tract tracing. *Brain Res.* 1995;684:61–69.
112. Teclemariam-Mesbah R, Kalsbeek A, Pevet P, Buijs RM. Direct vasoactive intestinal polypeptide-containing projection from the suprachiasmatic nucleus to spinal projecting hypothalamic paraventricular neurons. *Brain Res.* 1997;748:71–76.
113. Schaap J, Albus H, VanderLeest HT, Eilers PH, Detari L, Meijer JH. Heterogeneity of rhythmic suprachiasmatic nucleus

neurons: implications for circadian waveform and photoperiodic encoding. *Proc Natl Acad Sci USA*. 2003;100:15994–15999.
114. Schaap J, Pennartz CM, Meijer JH. Electrophysiology of the circadian pacemaker in mammals. *Chronobiol Int*. 2003;20:171–188.
115. LeSauter J, Yan L, Vishnubhotla B, et al. A short half-life GFP mouse model for analysis of suprachiasmatic nucleus organization. *Brain Res*. 2003;964:279–287.
116. Quintero JE, Kuhlman SJ, McMahon DG. The biological clock nucleus: a multiphasic oscillator network regulated by light. *J Neurosci*. 2003;23:8070–8076.
117. Buijs RM, Wortel J, Hou YX. Colocalization of gamma-aminobutyric acid with vasopressin, vasoactive intestinal peptide, and somatostatin in the rat suprachiasmatic nucleus. *J Comp Neurol*. 1995;358:343–352.
118. Castel M, Morris JF. Morphological heterogeneity of the GABAergic network in the suprachiasmatic nucleus, the brain's circadian pacemaker. *J Anat*. 2000;196(Pt 1):1–13.
119. Hermes ML, Coderre EM, Buijs RM, Renaud LP. GABA and glutamate mediate rapid neurotransmission from suprachiasmatic nucleus to hypothalamic paraventricular nucleus in rat. *J Physiol*. 1996;496(Pt 3):749–757.
120. Madeira MD, Andrade JP, Lieberman AR, Sousa N, Almeida OF, Paula-Barbosa MM. Chronic alcohol consumption and withdrawal do not induce cell death in the suprachiasmatic nucleus, but lead to irreversible depression of peptide immunoreactivity and mRNA levels. *J Neurosci*. 1997;17:1302–1319.
121. Moore RY, Speh JC. GABA is the principal neurotransmitter of the circadian system. *Neurosci Lett*. 1993;150:112–116.
122. Sofroniew MV, Weindl A. Identification of parvocellular vasopressin and neurophysin neurons in the suprachiasmatic nucleus of a variety of mammals including primates. *J Comp Neurol*. 1980;193:659–675.
123. Kalsbeek A, Teclemariam-Mesbah R, Pevet P. Efferent projections of the suprachiasmatic nucleus in the golden hamster (*Mesocricetus auratus*). *J Comp Neurol*. 1993;332:293–314.
124. Watts AG, Swanson LW. Efferent projections of the suprachiasmatic nucleus: II. Studies using retrograde transport of fluorescent dyes and simultaneous peptide immunohistochemistry in the rat. *J Comp Neurol*. 1987;258:230–252.
125. Watts AG, Swanson LW, Sanchez-Watts G. Efferent projections of the suprachiasmatic nucleus: I. Studies using anterograde transport of *Phaseolus vulgaris* leucoagglutinin in the rat. *J Comp Neurol*. 1987;258:204–229.
126. Jagota A, de la Iglesia HO, Schwartz WJ. Morning and evening circadian oscillations in the suprachiasmatic nucleus in vitro. *Nat Neurosci*. 2000;3:372–376.
127. Cheng MY, Bullock CM, Li C, et al. Prokineticin 2 transmits the behavioural circadian rhythm of the suprachiasmatic nucleus. *Nature*. 2002;417:405–410.
128. Zhou QY, Cheng MY. Prokineticin 2 and circadian clock output. *FEBS J*. 2005;272:5703–5709.
129. Kramer A, Yang FC, Snodgrass P, et al. Regulation of daily locomotor activity and sleep by hypothalamic EGF receptor signaling. *Science*. 2001;294:2511–2515.
130. Kalsbeek A, Buijs RM. Output pathways of the mammalian suprachiasmatic nucleus: coding circadian time by transmitter selection and specific targeting. *Cell Tissue Res*. 2002;309:109–118.
131. Williams 3rd WP, Kriegsfeld LJ. Circadian control of neuroendocrine circuits regulating female reproductive function. *Front Endocrinol (Lausanne)*. 2012;3:60.
132. Hickok JR, Tischkau SA. In vivo circadian rhythms in gonadotropin-releasing hormone neurons. *Neuroendocrinology*. 2010;91:110–120.
133. Van der Beek EM, Horvath TL, Wiegant VM, Van den Hurk R, Buijs RM. Evidence for a direct neuronal pathway from the suprachiasmatic nucleus to the gonadotropin-releasing hormone system: combined tracing and light and electron microscopic immunocytochemical studies. *J Comp Neurol*. 1997;384:569–579.
134. Herbison AE, Theodosis DT. Localization of oestrogen receptors in preoptic neurons containing neurotensin but not tyrosine hydroxylase, cholecystokinin or luteinizing hormone-releasing hormone in the male and female rat. *Neuroscience*. 1992;50:283–298.
135. Miller BH, Olson SL, Turek FW, Levine JE, Horton TH, Takahashi JS. Circadian clock mutation disrupts estrous cyclicity and maintenance of pregnancy. *Curr Biol*. 2004;14:1367–1373.
136. Khan AR, Kauffman AS. The role of kisspeptin and RFamide-related peptide-3 neurones in the circadian-timed preovulatory luteinising hormone surge. *J Neuroendocrinol*. 2011;24:131–143.
137. Kriegsfeld LJ. Driving reproduction: RFamide peptides behind the wheel. *Horm Behav*. 2006;50:655–666.
138. Kriegsfeld LJ, Mei DF, Bentley GE, et al. Identification and characterization of a gonadotropin-inhibitory system in the brains of mammals. *Proc Natl Acad Sci USA*. 2006;103:2410–2415.
139. Borjigin J, Zhang LS, Calinescu AA. Circadian regulation of pineal gland rhythmicity. *Mol Cell Endocrinol*. 2012;349:13–19.
140. Kalsbeek A, Garidou ML, Palm IF, et al. Melatonin sees the light: blocking GABA-ergic transmission in the paraventricular nucleus induces daytime secretion of melatonin. *Eur J Neurosci*. 2000;12:3146–3154.
141. Drijfhout WJ, van der Linde AG, de Vries JB, Grol CJ, Westerink BH. Microdialysis reveals dynamics of coupling between noradrenaline release and melatonin secretion in conscious rats. *Neurosci Lett*. 1996;202:185–188.
142. Drijfhout WJ, van der Linde AG, Kooi SE, Grol CJ, Westerink BH. Norepinephrine release in the rat pineal gland: the input from the biological clock measured by in vivo microdialysis. *J Neurochem*. 1996;66:748–755.
143. Buijs RM, van Eden CG, Goncharuk VD, Kalsbeek A. The biological clock tunes the organs of the body: timing by hormones and the autonomic nervous system. *J Endocrinol*. 2003;177:17–26.
144. Perreau-Lenz S, Kalsbeek A, Garidou ML, et al. Suprachiasmatic control of melatonin synthesis in rats: inhibitory and stimulatory mechanisms. *Eur J Neurosci*. 2003;17:221–228.
145. Kalsbeek A, Scheer FA, Perreau-Lenz S, et al. Circadian disruption and SCN control of energy metabolism. *FEBS Lett*. 2011;585:1412–1426.
146. Sukumaran S, Almon RR, DuBois DC, Jusko WJ. Circadian rhythms in gene expression: relationship to physiology, disease, drug disposition and drug action. *Adv Drug Deliv Rev*. 62:904–917.
147. Waterhouse J, Reilly T, Atkinson G, Edwards B. Jet lag: trends and coping strategies. *Lancet*. 2007;369:1117–1129.
148. Wang C, Xu CX, Krager SL, Bottum KM, Liao DF, Tischkau SA. Aryl hydrocarbon receptor deficiency enhances insulin sensitivity and reduces PPAR-α pathway activity in mice. *Environ Health Perspect*. 2011;119:1739–1744.

CHAPTER

15

mTOR Signaling in Cortical Network Development

Tiffany V. Lin, Angelique Bordey

Departments of Neurosurgery and Cellular and Molecular Physiology, Yale University School of Medicine, New Haven, CT, USA

INTRODUCTION

The development of functional cortical networks is a complex process that begins with corticogenesis in utero, further develops with axonal growth and dendritic arborization, and continues throughout life with pruning and tuning of synaptic connections. Aberrations in any of these processes, from neurogenesis to synaptic plasticity, have the potential to disrupt normal network functionality. Often, the results of such disruptions include epilepsy and cognitive dysfunction, which can significantly impact quality of life. One major player throughout cortical network development is the mammalian target of rapamycin (mTOR). This is evidenced by the association of hyperactive mTOR with malformations of cortical development (MCDs),[1] which can arise from disruptions to any stage of cortical development. Additionally, there is strong evidence that mTOR signaling is necessary for neuronal polarity, axon guidance, dendrite outgrowth, and synaptic plasticity.[2] With such widespread effects on cortical development, it makes sense that mTOR is directly involved in several genetic disorders with neurological sequelae (e.g. tuberous sclerosis and neurofibromatosis) and is also implicated in a long list of neuropsychiatric syndromes and disorders (including fragile X syndrome, autism, schizophrenia, and Alzheimer's and Parkinson's diseases).[2,3] Therefore, there is enormous potential for the medical benefit in developing better models of mTOR-associated disorders and clarifying mTOR's basic functions in cortical development. In this chapter, we provide a concise overview of what is known about mTOR's role in several stages of cortical network development and outline strategies that we are pursuing to better understand the in vivo effects of aberrant mTOR signaling during corticogenesis.

BACKGROUND

Corticogenesis and Cortical Network Development

In mammals, the cortex is a six-layered structure that develops in an inside-out manner, with newly born neurons migrating past earlier-born neurons to form successively more superficial layers.[4,5] Neural progenitors lining the ventricle give rise to pyramidal projection neurons that will eventually form local cortical and long-range subcortical and cortico-cortical circuits. In mice, neurogenesis of cortical projection neurons begins around embryonic day 11.5 (E11.5) with asymmetric division of radial glia in the ventricular zone (VZ).[6–8] The radial glia also produce a population of intermediate progenitor cells that contribute to cortical pyramidal neuron production.[8] The newly born neurons migrate radially to the cortical plate along the scaffolding provided by the basal processes of the radial glia, which extend from the VZ, where the glial cell body is located, to the pial surface.[9,10] By E17.5, nearly all of the cortical projection neurons have been born, although migration of the most recently born neurons to their residing layer is ongoing through the early postnatal period.

For normal cortical network formation to occur, not only do neurons need to migrate to the appropriate layer, but also local and long-range connections must be properly established. This requires projection neuron subtype specification as well as functional synaptic connectivity through axon and dendrite outgrowth. Although it appears that much subtype specification is tied to laminar position and is determined by birth date, postmitotic neurons are also influenced by subsequent molecular signals. While the complexity of

Neuronal Networks in Brain Function, CNS Disorders, and Therapeutics
http://dx.doi.org/10.1016/B978-0-12-415804-7.00015-0

these signals is beyond the scope of this chapter (for a review, see Ref. 11), some subtype and laminar-specific transcription factors that are critical for specification include Sox5 for layer 6, Ctip2 and Fezf2 for layer 5 subcortical projection neurons, and Satb2 for upper layer callosal projection neurons.

Contemporaneous with and following migration and subtype specification, appropriate connectivity and synapse formation must be established for effective communication and network function. During migration, the polarization of neurons occurs to specify axons from dendrites, and axon extension begins. Then, only after reaching their final position in the cortex do neurons begin to elaborate their dendritic arbors, providing the substrate for synaptic connections. Both axon and dendrite morphogenesis are dictated by neuronal activity as well as environmental and intrinsic signals, many of which are shared by both types of processes.[12,13] With the foundations laid, the final step is to connect neurons into a functional network through synapse formation. These connections will be established, optimized, and pruned in an activity-dependent manner through the remainder of the organism's life.

mTOR Signaling

The protein mTOR is a serine–threonine kinase that acts as the primary catalytic domain in two distinct protein complexes: mTOR complex 1 (mTORC1) and mTORC2. The core components of mTORC1 are mLST8[14] and Raptor[15,16] in addition to mTOR, whereas mTORC2 contains mammalian lethal with SEC13 protein 8 (mLST8),[17] Rictor,[18,19] and Sin1.[18] The downstream effects of the complexes differ greatly, and this chapter focuses on the role of mTORC1. mTORC1 is regulated in response to a number of inputs that are important to central nervous system (CNS) signaling. These include glutamate at *N*-methyl-D-aspartate (NMDA) receptors and metabotropic glutamate receptors (mGluR),[20,21] reelin,[22] and growth factors like insulin[23] and brain-derived neurotrophic factor.[24,25] These inputs alter mTOR activity through signaling pathways such as Ras–ERK and PI3K–Akt, which typically converge on the immediate upstream regulators of mTOR: TSC1/2 (a complex composed of hamartin (TSC1) and tuberin (TSC2)) and Ras-homolog enriched in brain (Rheb). Rheb, a small GTPase, activates mTORC1 signaling when bound to guanosine triphosphate (GTP), although the mechanism by which it does this is still uncertain.[26] Whereas Rheb is a positive regulator of mTORC1 activity, TSC1/2 negatively regulates mTORC1 activity. It does this through TSC2's GTPase activating protein (GAP) activity toward Rheb,[27–30] which drives Rheb toward its inactive guanosine diphosphate (GDP)-bound state. Specific pharmacological inhibition of mTORC1 activity has typically been accomplished using rapamycin, although there are major pitfalls to its use, as will be discussed in this chapter.

The primary downstream function of mTOR signaling is protein translation regulation. Canonically, this is achieved through phosphorylation of downstream targets, including p70 S6 kinases (S6Ks, including S6K1 and also the related S6K2) and eukaryotic initiation factor 4E (eIF4E) binding proteins (4E-BPs).[31] Phosphorylation of S6K1 leads to phosphorylation of the ribosomal protein S6, among other targets; phosphorylation of 4E-BP causes it to unbind from eIF4E, leaving it free to bind and recruit mRNAs to the translational complex.[32] These changes are traditionally thought to promote the translation of mRNAs containing 5′ terminal oligopyrimidine (TOP) motifs, allowing for increased translation of specific but large subsets of mRNAs. Indeed, this is borne out by a recent screen of mTOR-regulated mRNAs.[33] While S6Ks and 4E-BPs are the best studied targets of mTORC1, there are many more that are not discussed here (for comprehensive mTOR signaling pathways, see Ref. 34). A simplified schematic of mTORC1 signaling is shown in Figure 15.1.

Role of mTORC1 in Cortical Development and Integration

Corticogenesis

Despite mTOR's involvement in MCDs, surprisingly little research has explored the function of mTOR on corticogenesis. In some nonneuronal cell types, mTOR signaling is necessary for cytoskeletal remodeling and migration.[35] However, studies performed on neuronal migration have not demonstrated a necessity for mTOR signaling. For example, while Ras–ERK and PI3K–Akt signaling are necessary for hepatocyte growth factor–triggered neuronal migration, loss of mTOR signaling using rapamycin does not affect this type of migration in culture.[36] In vivo, brain-specific Rheb knockout animals with strongly impaired mTOR signaling show mostly normal cortical structure with intact lamination.[37] Cortical thickness was decreased by 35%, but total neuronal nuclear antigen-positive ($NeuN^+$) cell counts remained the same, suggesting that the loss of thickness was driven by nonneuronal cells, neuropil, or myelination. Indeed, the major change observed was decreased postnatal myelination as indicated by a strong decrease in levels of myelin proteins; this was accompanied by fewer mature oligodendrocytes despite equal numbers of oligodendrocyte progenitors. Although there is not yet any convincing evidence for a requirement of mTOR signaling in corticogenesis, the amount of research in this area is limited, and a thorough understanding of its role in neurogenesis,

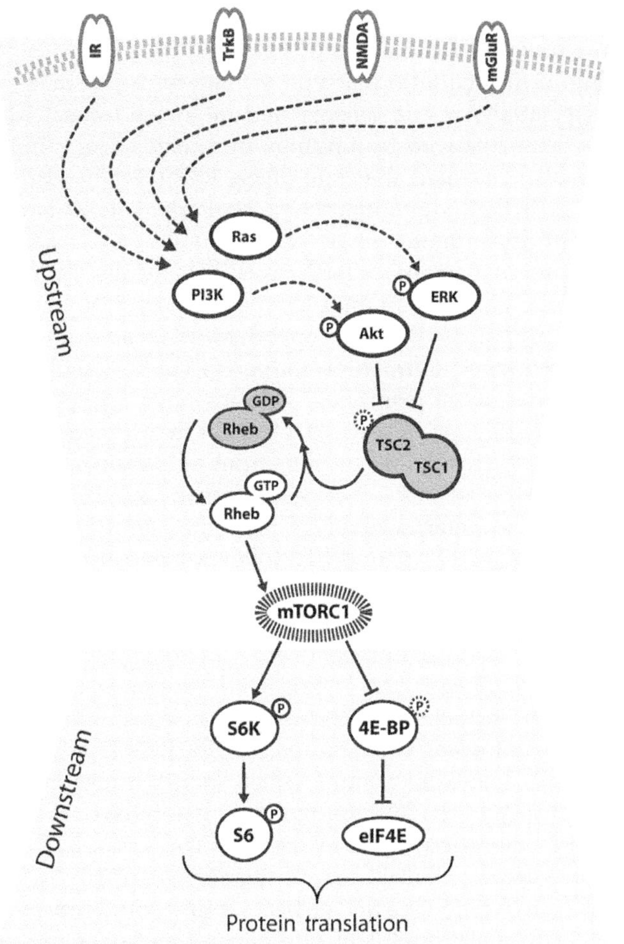

FIGURE 15.1 A simplified map of mTORC1 signaling. *Upstream*: Several signals important for CNS signaling can activate mTORC1 signaling through major signaling pathways such as PI3K–Akt and Ras–ERK. These subsequently converge upon the upstream regulator of mTOR: the TSC1–TSC2 complex (TSC1/2). TSC1/2 negatively regulates mTOR by acting as a GTPase activating protein toward the small GTPase, Rheb. GTP-bound Rheb activates mTORC1 signaling. *Downstream*: mTORC1 phosphorylates S6Ks and 4E-BPs. This allows S6K to phosphorylate its downstream targets, including the ribosomal protein S6, and it causes 4E-BP to unbind from eIF4E. Both of these events have the functional effect of increasing mRNA translation and protein expression. Lines with arrows indicate activation, and T-capped lines indicate inhibition. A "P" encircled by a solid line indicates activating phosphorylation; a dashed circle indicates inhibitory phosphorylation. Dashed lines indicate that multiple steps between the connected molecules have been condensed.

migration, and specification of cortical projection neurons has yet to be elucidated.

Although mTOR's endogenous function during corticogenesis is unclear, we do know that mTOR signaling is capable of affecting cortical development. Indeed, hyperactive mTOR is associated with at least one subtype of MCDs known as focal cortical dysplasias (FCDs). This association suggests that mTOR gain-of-function can exert a strong influence on corticogenesis (for a review, see Ref. 1). FCDs are cytoarchitectural aberrations of the cortex that are characterized by dyslamination and the presence of misoriented and dysmorphic cells. Tuberous sclerosis is a classic focal cortical dysplasia syndrome with a known genetic origin: mutations to either of the genes that comprise the tuberous sclerosis complex (i.e. *TSC1* or *TSC2*), the upstream negative regulator of mTOR.[38,39] The majority of these patients develop tubers, focal cortical malformations after which the disorder is named. Outside of tuberous sclerosis, type IIb focal cortical dysplasias are typically characterized by increased mTORC1 signaling as measured by phosphorylated S6K1 and S6 immunoreactivity.[40] Hemimegalencephaly is another subtype of MCD that can result in overgrowth and cytoarchitectural aberrations in whole or large parts of entire cerebral hemispheres. Recently, it was found that almost one-third of hemimegencephaly patients in a sample had somatic mutations in genes coding for PI3K, Akt3, or mTOR in tissue resected from the affected hemisphere that was not seen in peripheral blood samples taken from the patients.[41]

Neuronal Morphology

Axons, dendrites, and spines are the structural basis of neuronal communication, with axons providing the output and dendrites and spines receiving and integrating incoming information. Developmentally, axon outgrowth is the earliest of these processes to occur in the growth of a neuron. Inhibition of mTOR impairs axon specification[42,43] and also alters the growth cone response to guidance cues. Work in *Xenopus* retinal growth cones showed that not only are components of the mTOR signaling pathway present in growth cones,[44] but also rapamycin impairs growth cone response to the repellent signals Sempahorin-3A and Slit2 and the chemoattractant Netrin-1.[44,45] In rodents, it appears that repulsive signaling by EphrinAs (EphAs) also requires proper mTOR signaling.[46] In cultured wild-type neurons, EphA1 exposure downregulates mTOR signaling. However, upregulation of mTOR signaling in cultured retinal ganglion cells through expression of constitutively active or wild-type Rheb, as well as by knockout of one *Tsc2* allele, results in impaired growth cone collapse in response to EphA1. Accordingly, the same study found that a *Tsc2* heterozygous ($Tsc2^{+/-}$) mouse model of tuberous sclerosis exhibits abnormalities in retinal projections to the lateral geniculate nucleus that mirror those of EphA-deficient animals.

Regulation of dendritic arborization by mTOR signaling has been consistently demonstrated in vitro. Inhibition of mTOR by rapamycin in hippocampal slice culture and primary hippocampal neuron culture results in less complex dendritic trees.[47–49] This is also true following short hairpin RNA (shRNA) knockdown of Raptor.[49] Driving PI3K–Akt pathways using constitutively active PI3K and Akt had the opposite effect, making dendrites hypertrophic.[47–49] This overgrowth is mTOR dependent, as evidenced by rescue with rapamycin or shRaptor. While the in vitro studies are in agreement, few studies have looked at mTOR's role in dendritic arborization in vivo. One group used a mouse model with floxed *Tsc1* alleles (*Tsc1*$^{fl/fl}$). These animals were allowed to develop with two functional copies of *Tsc1*, but viral vectors expressing Cre were injected into the hippocampus at postnatal day 14 (P14). Ten to fourteen days after viral transfection, the researchers observed no visible alterations in the dendritic morphology of transfected CA1 pyramidal neurons, although quantification was not presented.[50] However, it is possible that either 10 or 14 days would not be enough time for a distinct change in dendritic outgrowth to occur and/or that increasing mTOR signaling 2 weeks into postnatal development is too late to induce changes. Other in vivo data pointing to a role for mTOR in dendrite growth come from the fact that other regulators of neuronal morphology, like reelin, require mTOR activity to effect their changes.[22]

Finally, like dendrite morphology, mTOR's effects on spine morphology and density have been explored both in vitro and in vivo, but with mixed conclusions. In vitro, chronic rapamycin decreases both spine and filopodia densities in dissociated hippocampal neurons.[48] Furthermore, the same study showed that hyperactivation of PI3K and Akt increased filopodia density in an mTOR-dependent manner. Cre-treated organotypic slice cultures from floxed *Tsc1* animals (as well as slice cultures transfected with shRNAs against *Tsc2*) have decreased spine density, but increased spine length and spine head width.[51] However, it was found that these changes were not mTOR dependent. The aforementioned in vivo study employing virally mediated Cre expression in P14 *Tsc1*$^{fl/fl}$ mice also found no changes in spine density or length.[50]

Plasticity

While network wiring during development is important for laying the framework for network communication, changes in synaptic strength as well as synapse formation and loss are dynamic processes that occur throughout life. These changes in connectivity are commonly thought to be the cellular processes underlying learning. Synaptic plasticity, namely, long-term potentiation (LTP) and long-term depression (LTD), describes the phenomenon by which the strength of synaptic connections between two neurons can be altered by virtue of the strength and pattern of signaling between them. mTOR's role in maintaining the protein synthesis-dependent, late phase of plasticity is one of its most studied effects in the CNS. In the late 1990s, it was initially demonstrated that rapamycin could block long-term facilitation, a type of long-term plasticity, in dissociated Aplysia sensory and motor neurons.[52] This has been followed by findings in rodent hippocampus that also revealed that late-phase LTP (L-LTP) also requires mTOR signaling.[20,53,54] Similarly, L-LTD is also mTOR dependent.[21]

Upregulation of mTOR signaling results in more complex changes in plasticity. For LTD, TSC models show impaired mGluR-dependent LTD and possibly low-frequency stimulation-induced LTD.[55,56] Acute hippocampal slices from *Tsc2*$^{+/-}$ mice have an enhanced LTP phenotype.[57] That is, a protocol that typically only produces early LTP in sections from wild-type mice produces L-LTP in *Tsc2*$^{+/-}$ mice. However, a rat TSC model that is also heterozygous for *Tsc2* (also known as Eker rats) displayed impaired LTP following an L-LTP induction protocol.[55] While these results appear to be in opposition to one another, neither study directly contradicts the other. That is, Ehninger et al.[57] did not explore the differences between *Tsc2*$^{+/-}$ and wild-type mice following an L-LTP induction protocol, and von der Brelie et al.[55] did not look at early LTP protocols in the Eker rats. Indeed, a 4E-BP2 knockout animal, which should mimic at least some aspects of mTOR upregulation, exhibited both types of LTP alterations seen in the two TSC models.[58] One could speculate that strong stimulation with L-LTP induction on a hyperactive mTOR background could result in a lack of translational control that may be detrimental to maintaining lasting plasticity. However, that same mTOR hyperactivity could enhance LTP following a weaker, subthreshold, early LTP induction stimulus.

Taken together, there is a large amount of evidence for the influence of mTOR across nearly all stages of cortical network development, including structural organization, wiring, and maintenance. These cellular- and network-level changes also translate to functional and behavioral consequences. MCDs are commonly associated with epilepsy, with reports of 70–75% of patients presenting with seizures.[59] Similarly, seizures occur in >80% of tuberous sclerosis patients.[60] Additionally, disorders with hyperactive mTOR signaling are often characterized by cognitive dysfunction,[61,62] which cannot be fully explained by seizures and cortical malformations.[63] This is reflected in animal research as well: both hyperactive mTOR in TSC disease models without seizures (i.e. *Tsc2*$^{+/-}$ and *Tsc1*$^{+/-}$) and inhibition of mTOR signaling with rapamycin result in learning and memory impairments.[57,64–72] However, the molecular mechanisms by which aberrant mTOR leads to these neurological manifestations are still poorly understood. In order to be able to precisely dissect these mechanisms, we must have better access to and genetic control of mTOR activity during development than has previously

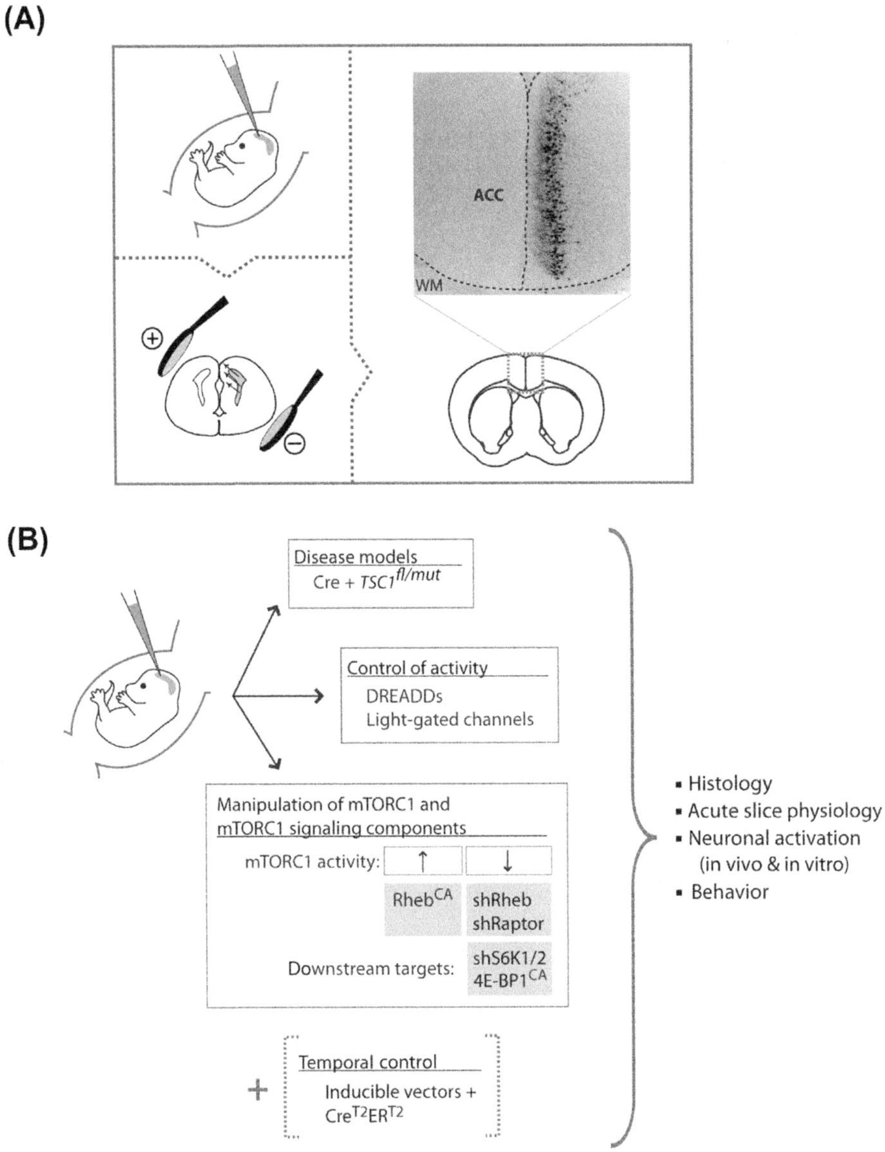

FIGURE 15.2 In utero electroporation. (A) Illustration of in utero electroporation procedures beginning with the injection of DNA constructs in the embryo; current injection across the head of the animal to drive constructs toward the region of interest; and an example of an E15 electroporated cortex (and contralateral, nonelectroporated cortex) at postnatal day 7 (P7). ACC: anterior cingulate cortex; WM: white matter. (B) Potential uses for IUE for the study of mTOR signaling and related disorders.

been achieved with pharmacological or transgenic tools alone.

METHODS: IN UTERO ELECTROPORATION

Our laboratory is interested in mTOR across multiple levels, including basic understanding of mTOR function as well as disorders of mTOR signaling. The primary method we employ to investigate how mTOR signaling affects developmental processes and network formation in the cortex is in utero electroporation (IUE). IUE allows us to manipulate cortical development in a focal manner by selectively introducing DNA-expressing constructs in the neural progenitors of targeted cortical regions in utero. The focal nature of our technique is advantageous for investigating both the basic science and disease sides of our interests. It enables us to understand the basic functions of mTOR by disrupting a subset of cells in an otherwise normally developing animal. While transgenic animals are good models of disease, disruption of function throughout the whole organism or the system of interest can make it difficult to separate the direct contributions of mTOR function from secondary effects resulting from other sequelae. For disease models, cortical dysplasias often occur following somatic mutations on either a normal background or one already altered by germline mutations. By creating focal disruptions and combining IUE with transgenic models, we can more closely recreate the molecular underpinnings of these lesions.

IUE involves a laparotomy of a pregnant mouse to gain access to the uterine horns, injection of DNA constructs into the lateral ventricles of the embryos, and using pulses of current through electrode paddles to introduce the constructs into the neural progenitors lining the ventricles (Figure 15.2(A)).[73,74] The uterine horns are then placed back into the abdominal cavity, and the embryos allowed to develop as usual. The placement of the electrodes during electroporation determines the regional targeting of specific cortical regions. Furthermore, the embryonic stage at the time of electroporation allows us to target specific cortical layers. For

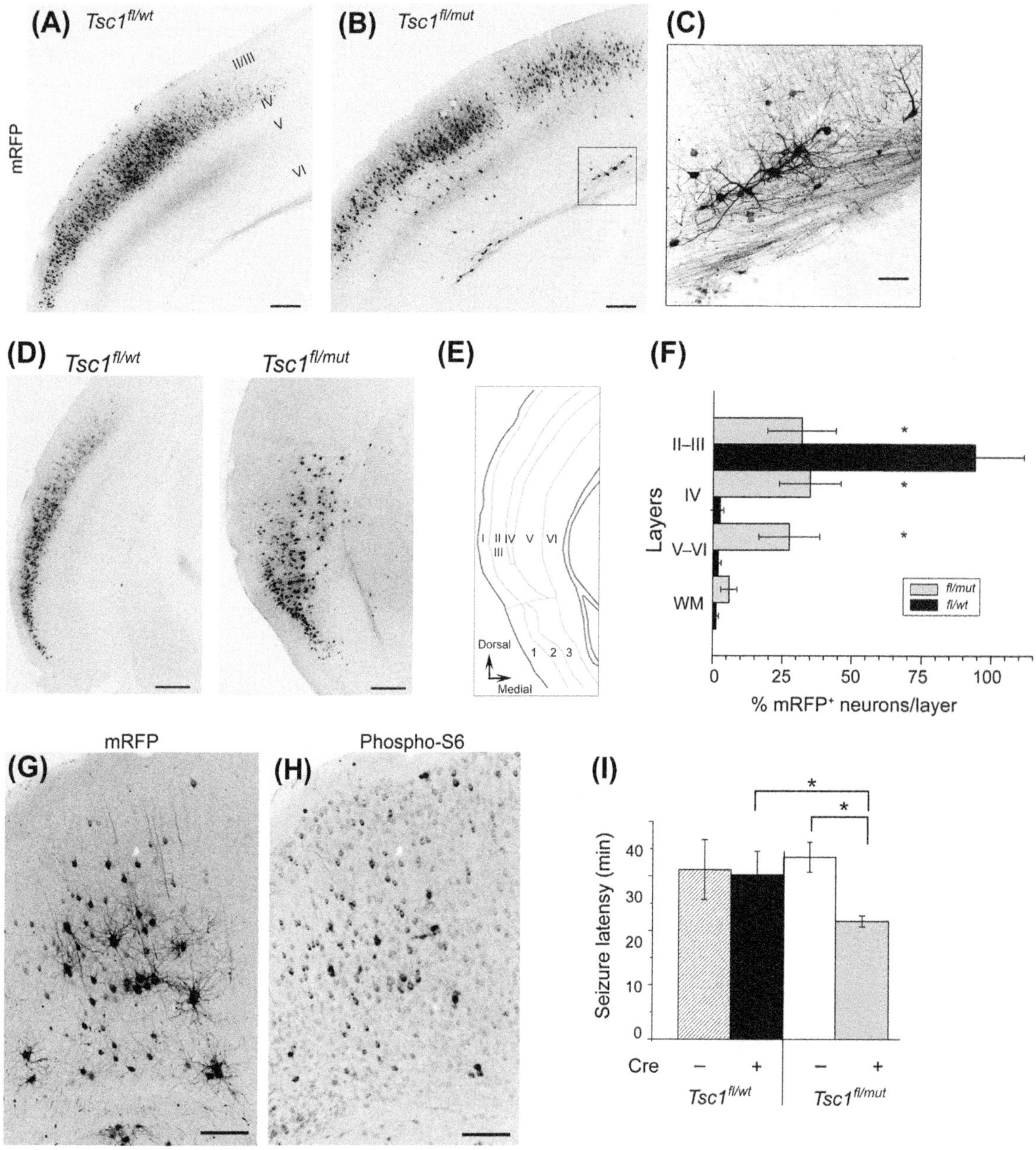

FIGURE 15.3 ***Tsc1* deletion in utero recapitulates aspects of cortical malformations seen in tuberous sclerosis patients.** (A and B) Micrographs of electroporated cells from coronal sections of P28 $Tsc1^{fl/wt}$ (A) and $Tsc1^{fl/mut}$ (B) mice electroporated at E16 with monomeric red fluorescent protein (mRFP) and Cre-expressing plasmids. Scale bar: 140 μm. (C) Enlarged view of white-matter heterotopia from the boxed area in (B). Scale bar: 70 μm. (D) Micrographs of electroporated cells in coronal sections from P28 $Tsc1^{fl/wt}$ controls and $Tsc1^{fl/mut}$ mice electroporated with mRFP and Cre at E15. (E) Diagram of a coronal section detailing the structure of the cortex in the areas shown in (D). (F) Bar graph illustrating the percent distribution of electroporated cells through the cortex and white matter (WM). (G and H) Micrographs depicting the immunoreactivity for phosphorylated S6 (H) in $mRFP^+$ electroporated cells (G) from $Tsc1^{fl/mut}$ mice. Scale bar: 70 μm. (I) Latency to pentylenetetrazole-induced seizures in $Tsc1^{fl/wt}$ and $Tsc1^{fl/mut}$ mice, with and without Cre electroporation. *: $p < 0.05$ (unpaired student t-test). (*Source: All images reprinted from Ref. 79 with permission.*)

example, electroporation at E15 means that constructs are expressed only in upper layer neurons that are born at and soon after that embryonic age. Accordingly, targeting at earlier dates, such as E11–E12, results in electroporation of deep-layer neurons. Dilution of the electroporated plasmids over time leads to a limited number of cells that will express the introduced constructs. We find that electroporation at E15 results in positive expression of electroporated constructs in pyramidal neurons of cortical layers 2/3, but it does not result in expression in astrocytes that are generated by radial glia following neurogenesis.

By providing access to the developing cortex, IUE allows us to apply the wide range of molecular tools normally used postnatally. This means gene or shRNA expression for gain-of-function or loss-of-function manipulations, respectively; the use of inducible and conditional constructs for increased temporal and anatomical specificity; a combination with floxed transgenic animals for genomic deletion; and the use of synthetic ligand receptors and optogenetics to manipulate neuronal activity (Figure 15.2(B)).

CURRENT RESEARCH

Disease Models

Despite being able to model the background genotype of tuberous sclerosis patients, it has been difficult to recapitulate many of the neuropathological aspects of the disease in rodent models. In particular, the hallmark structural feature, tubers, has been difficult to recreate, with a tuber being reported in a single Eker rat.[75] However, there is evidence that these malformations form following a "second hit" mutation that occurs somatically during development, resulting in a loss of function of the remaining functional *TSC1* or *TSC2* allele (i.e. loss of heterozygosity).[76,77] Therefore, it could be that the rarity of these second mutations in animal models is responsible for the rarity of tubers in *Tsc1* or *Tsc2* heterozygous rodent models. Indeed, tuber formation was induced by irradiation of Eker rats.[78] However, the general mutagenic nature of irradiation means that it could also be causing mutations in unrelated genes.

Our laboratory therefore set out to mimic this loss of heterozygosity in select cortical progenitor populations by combining transgenic animals with IUE.[79] Mice that were heterozygous for *Tsc1* ($Tsc1^{wt/mut}$) were bred with mice in which both Tsc1 alleles were floxed ($Tsc1^{fl/fl}$), yielding animals that had one floxed allele and one null allele ($Tsc1^{fl/mut}$). This recapitulates the background genotype of human patients, who are heterozygous for either *TSC1* or *TSC2*. On this background, we used IUE to electroporate a Cre-expressing construct and therefore knocked out the remaining functional allele in a discrete area of the cortex. This allowed us to model the somatic loss-of-heterozygosity that is believed to underlie the formation of tubers in tuberous sclerosis patients. Use of this strategy creates a disease model that closely follows the genetic profile of TSC patients and the focal two-hit nature of tubers. As a control, Cre-electroporated $Tsc1^{fl/wt}$ littermates were used.

Using this model, we were able to generate both white-matter heterotopias and tuber-like lesions (Figure 15.3).[79] Following electroporation at a later embryonic stage (E16), heterotopias were observed in the white matter (Figure 15.3(A)–(C)). Electroporation at E15 to target the birth date of layer 2/3 neurons resulted in tuber-like formations (Figure 15.3(D)). Whereas almost all electroporated cells in control animals migrated and integrated into the appropriate layer, only 32% of the Cre-electroporated $Tsc1^{null}$ cells did (Figure 15.3(F)). Instead, the majority of cells integrated into deeper lamina and within the white matter. In agreement with the total loss of Tsc1 expression and elevated mTOR signaling, these displaced neurons had significantly higher levels of phosphorylated S6, as measured by immunoreactivity (Figure 15.3(G) and (H)). The electroporated cells also had enlarged cell bodies and were occasionally multinucleated, both features of cells in cortical tubers. However, unlike clinical tubers, we did not observe the mixed neuroglial markers seen in a subset of cytomegalic cells (i.e. giant cells). Behaviorally, the mice also showed decreased pentylenetetrazol-induced seizure latency (Figure 15.3(I)).

Although our and others' inability to recapitulate all aspects of the cortical lesions seen in patients could be a function of the technical approach, it is also possibly due to the inherent differences between rodent models and humans. This is illustrated by the fact that even between rodent models (i.e. between mice and rats), the same technical manipulations do not always yield the same outcomes.[80] With these caveats in mind, however, rodent models still are the most efficient option for laying the groundwork for understanding a disease state and normal function in complex systems. Going forward, we hope that our model will be useful for examining potential molecular targets for rescue of these heterotopias and tuber-like lesions. Furthermore, since MCDs are strongly associated with epilepsy, this model provides the opportunity to better understand the connectivity of these lesions to the surrounding cortex and identify sites of hyperexcitability.

Control of Neuronal Activity

One way of addressing the question of connectivity is through co-electroporation of constructs that allow for specific stimulation of tubers and displaced neurons.

Using conventional electrophysiological methods would allow for specific stimulation of electroporated cells, but only on a single-cell level. Attempts to stimulate larger numbers of neurons using stimulation electrodes would result in the stimulation of normal tissue as well. To circumvent these limitations, we plan to use electroporation of both synthetic ligand-gated receptors (designer receptors exclusively activated by designer drugs, or DREADDs) as well as light-gated channels (e.g. channelrhodopsin). Since only cells electroporated with these exogenous constructs will be excited by the external stimulus (either a synthetic ligand or light), it is possible to achieve activation of displaced neurons in a specific manner.

DREADDs, as their name suggests, are engineered G-protein coupled receptors (GPCRs) that are activated only by a synthetic ligand. Since these peptides are not present endogenously, injection of the ligand in vivo or application to slices in vitro allows for specific activation of those cells expressing the designer GPCR. One such receptor is the human muscarinic M_3 designer receptor hM3Dq, which is activated exclusively by clozapine-N-oxide (CNO).[81] Inhibitory DREADDs have also been developed.[81] The benefit of this system is that, unlike channel rhodopsins, there is no need for invasive access to the brain for in vivo activation. However, unlike the light-gated channels, the temporal control is imprecise both in vivo and in vitro. When given in vivo, activity begins to spike 5–10 min following CNO injection and will last longer than 50 min, even with low doses.[82] In vitro, bath application of CNO results in strong burst firing within 5 min after application and continues for up to 15 min after the start of the washout.[82]

Light-gated channels have been used extensively since their initial development as a tool for control of neuronal activity in 2005.[83] Expression of channelrhodopsin-2, an algal light-gated nonspecific cation channel, allows for precise temporal activation of neurons with membrane depolarization occurring within ~2 ms of exposure to 470 nm light and deactivation times of ~10 ms after removal of light stimulus.[83,84] Since 2005, many other light-gated channels have been discovered or developed for experimental use, including the bacterial light-gated chloride pump halorhodopsin, which produces light-stimulated inhibition.[85] In addition to the more precise temporal control provided by optogenetics over ligand-gated channels, there is greater spatial control as well. That is, introduction of CNO either in bath or through peripheral injection will result in stimulation of all DREADD-expressing cells in the slice or in the organism, respectively. With the right equipment, photostimulation can be used to excite single cells in acute slices[86] or narrow areas of tissue in vivo.[87]

Manipulation of mTORC1 Signaling during Cortical Development

While the *Tsc1$^{fl/mut}$* mouse allows us to model one of the few identified genetic causes of MCDs, most MCDs do not occur in people with known genetic disorders. However, with a large percentage of MCD resections pointing to hyperactive mTOR signaling, it is important to explore the question of how mTORC1 signaling specifically affects corticogenesis. Since the TSC1/2 complex has known non-mTORC1 effects, it is therefore necessary to more directly target mTOR. In so doing, we hope to answer questions about what the specific effects of mTOR signaling are and to investigate the developmental questions that have been posed in vitro, but have yet to be resolved in vivo. Does upregulation of mTOR in vivo throughout development alter the dendritic growth of pyramidal neurons? Is mTOR upregulation alone sufficient to induce MCDs?

However, the question of how to more directly target mTOR is a complex one. As mentioned in this chapter, mTOR can act in multiple complexes with distinct functions. Thus, whereas one would typically directly target a gene of interest to dissect its function, overexpressing or knocking down mTOR has the potential to affect both mTORC1 and mTORC2 signaling. Since we are most interested in the function of mTORC1, we must paradoxically turn to indirect targets in order to gain specificity. Thus, to increase mTORC1 signaling, we plan to use a mutant form of its immediate upstream regulator, Rheb. This mutant, RhebS16H or Rheb^{CA}, preferentially binds GTP even in the presence of TSC1/2 GAP activity,[88] making it constitutively active.

Downregulation of mTORC1 activity can be achieved either with shRNA knockdown of Rheb or the mTORC1 component Raptor. Since we cannot rule out non-mTORC1 effects of Rheb, shRaptor can also be used to rescue any phenotypes seen with Rheb manipulation to ensure that the changes seen are mTOR dependent. Further molecular dissection can be done using constructs that counter the effects of mTOR on downstream targets. Expression of a constitutively active 4E-BP1 (F113A, or 4E-BP^{CA}) results in decreased association with the mTORC1 complex, resistance to phosphorylation by mTORC1, and increased binding to eIF4E following insulin-induced stimulation of mTOR activity.[89] Eliminating the function of S6Ks requires knockdown of both S6K1 and S6K2 in order to avoid compensation. A single shRNA can be used to target both S6Ks,[90] or a cocktail of multiple shRNAs can be used.

The aforementioned constructs can be used in either a constitutive or inducible manner. That is, they can be expressed from the point of electroporation onward, or temporal control can be added using the Cre–Lox system. This can be accomplished by adding a floxed stop sequence in front of the shRNA or gene sequence in the construct and co-electroporation of an inducible Cre vector (e.g. $Cre^{T2}ER^{T2}$). With an inducible strategy, it is possible to isolate the effects of mTOR activity changes at different stages of development, and we can also ask whether rescue can be achieved in adulthood or must be resolved during development.

UNANSWERED QUESTIONS AND FUTURE RESEARCH

Loss of mTORC1 Signaling

Although mTOR signaling has been studied extensively in the disease context, the basic function of mTOR signaling in CNS development is still poorly understood, especially in vivo. Previous work has approached this question by using pharmacological inhibition by rapamycin. However, there are several disadvantages to using rapamycin. First, the systemic nature of pharmacological treatments means a lack of anatomical specificity in targeting. Additionally, although it is commonly touted as an mTORC1-specific inhibitor, rapamycin has been shown in culture and in vivo to affect mTORC2 signaling with chronic use.[91–93] Finally, not only is rapamycin nonspecific, but also it does not inhibit all aspects of mTORC1 signaling,[94–96] providing a more complete blockade of S6K1 phosphorylation than that of 4E-BP1. Taken together, the nature of rapamycin limits its usefulness for understanding both the comprehensive and specific effects of mTORC1.

Few have explored the effects of losing mTOR function using genetic deletion; however, this is likely due in part to the lack of viable approaches. Knockouts of mTORC1 components are often embryonic lethal,[97] and only recently have CNS- or forebrain-specific conditional knockouts been employed. One study used a combined approach with heterozygous mTOR knockout combined with a low concentration of rapamycin that appeared to affect mTORC1 signaling in the $mTOR^{+/-}$, but not wild-type, animals.[54] Interesting purely genetic models that have been generated include the brain-specific Rheb knockout mentioned in this chapter,[37] as well as a floxed Raptor mouse[98] that was recently used for a CamKII-specific knockout.[99] In addition to their use to study the effects of mTOR loss throughout the brain, these floxed models would be especially useful in conjunction with electroporation of Cre to better understand cell autonomous developmental effects of mTOR signaling.

Downstream Targets

Up until now, much of the research concerning mTOR has focused primarily on mTOR itself, its upstream regulators, and immediate downstream targets. However, as a regulator of translation, mTOR's potential range of influence is enormous. Understanding what specific agents are responsible for carrying out particular effects of mTOR signaling can shed light on the basic mechanisms of network development and maintenance, and it can also provide potential candidates for therapeutic targets. Although rapamycin is a pharmacological mTOR inhibitor that is already available for clinical use, its aforementioned disadvantages (i.e. lack of specificity and incomplete inhibition) mean that it may be unable to ameliorate all the effects that arise from hyperactivation and will certainly have additional peripheral side effects.

To this end, several microarray and RNA-sequencing screens of mTOR-regulated translation have been conducted to generate a database of downstream targets.[24,33,100] However, many of these have employed rapamycin to determine mTOR dependence, which would mean the results might both be missing targets and include false positives. A recent study looked at polyribosome-associated mRNAs altered by the general mTOR inhibitor Torin, which provides a more complete inhibition of signaling (albeit for both mTORC1 and mTORC2).[33] The data from this screen are an important resource for mTOR researchers; however, the utility for those investigating the CNS is diminished by the authors' use of cultured mouse embryonic fibroblasts. This means that many neuron-relevant, and certainly neuron-specific, transcripts could be missing. To date, the only published screen done in neurons was a more narrow study using cultured cortical and hippocampal neurons to look at rapamycin-dependent brain-derived neurotropic factor (BDNF)-induced translation.[24] While this yielded a concise and interesting set of regulated mRNAs, including many coding for synapse-associated proteins, it is limited by its use of rapamycin and the narrow focus of the manipulation. Furthermore, dissociated cultured neurons cannot speak to how mTOR acts in the in vivo developmental system.

The ability to look at in vivo translational regulation in specific cell populations has been made possible in the past 5 years with the engineering of conditionally expressed tagged ribosomal proteins. The first of these, translating ribosome affinity purification (TRAP), uses expression of an enhanced green fluorescent protein (EGFP)-tagged L10a ribosomal protein driven by cell-specific promoters to achieve exclusive expression of the tagged protein in tissues or cell populations of interest.[101,102] A similar tool, the RiboTag system, was developed independently[103]; this technology uses Cre-driven conditional expression of a hemagglutinin tagged ribosomal protein L22 driven by its endogenous promoter. In both cases, the tagged nature of the ribosomal proteins allows for pulldown of polyribosomes from specific cell populations out of tissues and isolation of their associated mRNAs (i.e. actively translated mRNAs). These can then be used for sequencing or microarray analysis. Using these engineered ribosomal proteins, one could perform transcriptomic analysis of mTOR-regulated mRNA translation in vivo with regional specificity (i.e. targeting certain areas of the brain and/or in specific neuronal subtypes) and temporal specificity (i.e. by taking lysates at different developmental time points).

Collectively, the body of mTOR research in the CNS has revealed the range and depth of mTOR's influence on the formation and maintenance of cortical networks in both normal and disease states. Up until this point, research has focused on signals upstream and immediately downstream of mTOR. However, recent methodological and technological advances enable researchers to explore the downstream mechanisms by which mTOR exerts its effects with greater precision and depth. We believe that IUE provides one of the best methods to explore both disease-related and basic mechanistic questions since it opens up a wide range of molecular tools to be employed in vivo during corticogenesis. The knowledge that comes from these new avenues of research has the potential to provide candidate targets for future therapeutic use as well as contribute to the understanding of normal and pathological corticogenesis.

CONCLUSION

Our understanding of corticogenesis has improved exponentially over the past decades. In parallel, advances in molecular genetics have revealed that genetic mutations during embryonic development can result in defects in corticogenesis and generate cortical malformations. Mutations in components of the mTOR signaling pathway can contribute to these malformations, but our understanding of the molecular etiology of cortical malformations lags behind the wealth of knowledge on corticogenesis. We and others hope to close this gap by manipulating mTOR activity and downstream effectors and examine the impact on corticogenesis and circuit formation. Approaches such as IUE combined with novel tools to manipulate both single-cell and circuit activity and to screen proteomic or transcriptomic changes allow us to pursue these questions.

References

1. Crino PB. mTOR: a pathogenic signaling pathway in developmental brain malformations. *Trends Mol Med.* 2011;17(12):734–742.
2. Swiech L, Perycz M, Malik A, Jaworski J. Role of mTOR in physiology and pathology of the nervous system. *Biochim Biophys Acta.* 2008;1784(1):116–132.
3. Hoeffer CA, Klann E. mTOR signaling: at the crossroads of plasticity, memory and disease. *Trends Neurosci.* 2010;33(2): 67–75.
4. Angevine Jr JB, Sidman RL. Autoradiographic study of cell migration during histogenesis of cerebral cortex in the mouse. *Nature.* 1961;192:766–768.
5. Rakic P. Neurons in rhesus monkey visual cortex: systematic relation between time of origin and eventual disposition. *Science.* 1974;183(4123):425–427.
6. Chenn A, McConnell SK. Cleavage orientation and the asymmetric inheritance of Notch1 immunoreactivity in mammalian neurogenesis. *Cell.* 1995;82(4):631–641.
7. Malatesta P, Hartfuss E, Götz M. Isolation of radial glial cells by fluorescent-activated cell sorting reveals a neuronal lineage. *Development.* 2000;127(24):5253–5263.
8. Noctor SC, Martínez-Cerdeño V, Ivic L, Kriegstein AR. Cortical neurons arise in symmetric and asymmetric division zones and migrate through specific phases. *Nat Neurosci.* 2004;7(2):136–144.
9. Rakic P. Mode of cell migration to the superficial layers of fetal monkey neocortex. *J Comp Neurol.* 1972;145(1):61–83.
10. Noctor SC, Flint AC, Weissman TA, Dammerman RS, Kriegstein AR. Neurons derived from radial glial cells establish radial units in neocortex. *Nature.* 2001;409(6821):714–720.
11. Kwan KY, Šestan N, Anton ES. Transcriptional co-regulation of neuronal migration and laminar identity in the neocortex. *Development.* 2012;139(9):1535–1546.
12. McAllister AK. Cellular and molecular mechanisms of dendrite growth. *Cereb Cortex.* 2000;10(10):963–973.
13. Jan Y-N, Jan LY. The control of dendrite development. *Neuron.* 2003;40(2):229–242.
14. Kim D-H, Sarbassov DD, Ali SM, et al. GβL, a positive regulator of the rapamycin-sensitive pathway required for the nutrient-sensitive interaction between raptor and mTOR. *Mol Cell.* 2003;11(4):895–904.
15. Hara K, Maruki Y, Long X, et al. Raptor, a binding partner of target of rapamycin (TOR), mediates TOR action. *Cell.* 2002;110(2):177–189.
16. Kim D-H, Sarbassov DD, Ali SM, et al. mTOR interacts with raptor to form a nutrient-sensitive complex that signals to the cell growth machinery. *Cell.* 2002;110(2):163–175.
17. Jacinto E, Loewith R, Schmidt A, et al. Mammalian TOR complex 2 controls the actin cytoskeleton and is rapamycin insensitive. *Nat Cell Biol.* 2004;6(11):1122–1128.
18. Jacinto E, Facchinetti V, Liu D, et al. SIN1/MIP1 maintains rictor-mTOR complex integrity and regulates Akt phosphorylation and substrate specificity. *Cell.* 2006;127(1):125–137.
19. Sarbassov DD, Ali SM, Kim D-H, et al. Rictor, a novel binding partner of mTOR, defines a rapamycin-insensitive and raptor-independent pathway that regulates the cytoskeleton. *Curr Biol.* 2004;14(14):1296–1302.
20. Cammalleri M, Lütjens R, Berton F, et al. Time-restricted role for dendritic activation of the mTOR-p70S6K pathway in the induction of late-phase long-term potentiation in the CA1. *Proc Natl Acad Sci USA.* 2003;100(24):14368–14373.
21. Hou L, Klann E. Activation of the phosphoinositide 3-kinase-Akt-mammalian target of rapamycin signaling pathway is required for metabotropic glutamate receptor-dependent long-term depression. *J Neurosci.* 2004;24(28):6352–6361.
22. Jossin Y, Goffinet AM. Reelin signals through phosphatidylinositol 3-kinase and Akt to control cortical development and through mTor to regulate dendritic growth. *Mol Cell Biol.* 2007;27(20):7113–7124.
23. Chung J, Grammer TC, Lemon KP, Kazlauskas A, Blenis J. PDGF- and insulin-dependent pp70S6k activation mediated by phosphatidylinositol-3-OH kinase. *Nature.* 1994;370(6484):71–75.

24. Schratt GM, Nigh EA, Chen WG, Hu L, Greenberg ME. BDNF regulates the translation of a select group of mRNAs by a mammalian target of rapamycin-phosphatidylinositol 3-kinase-dependent pathway during neuronal development. *J Neurosci.* 2004;24(33):7366–7377.
25. Slipczuk L, Bekinschtein P, Katche C, Cammarota M, Izquierdo I, Medina JH. BDNF activates mTOR to regulate GluR1 expression required for memory formation. *PLoS One.* 2009;4(6):e6007.
26. Avruch J, Long X, Lin Y, et al. Activation of mTORC1 in two steps: Rheb-GTP activation of catalytic function and increased binding of substrates to raptor1. *Biochem Soc Trans.* 2009;37(1):223.
27. Garami A, Zwartkruis FJT, Nobukuni T, et al. Insulin activation of Rheb, a mediator of mTOR/S6K/4E-BP signaling, is inhibited by TSC1 and 2. *Mol Cell.* 2003;11(6):1457–1466.
28. Inoki K, Li Y, Xu T, Guan K-L. Rheb GTPase is a direct target of TSC2 GAP activity and regulates mTOR signaling. *Genes Dev.* 2003;17(15):1829–1834.
29. Tee AR, Manning BD, Roux PP, Cantley LC, Blenis J. Tuberous sclerosis complex gene products, Tuberin and Hamartin, control mTOR signaling by acting as a GTPase-activating protein complex toward Rheb. *Curr Biol.* 2003;13(15):1259–1268.
30. Zhang Y, Gao X, Saucedo LJ, Ru B, Edgar BA, Pan D. Rheb is a direct target of the tuberous sclerosis tumour suppressor proteins. *Nat Cell Biol.* 2003;5(6):578–581.
31. Burnett PE, Barrow RK, Cohen NA, Snyder SH, Sabatini DM. RAFT1 phosphorylation of the translational regulators p70 S6 kinase and 4E-BP1. *Proc Natl Acad Sci USA.* 1998;95(4):1432–1437.
32. Ma XM, Blenis J. Molecular mechanisms of mTOR-mediated translational control. *Nat Rev Mol Cell Biol.* 2009;10(5):307–318.
33. Thoreen CC, Chantranupong L, Keys HR, Wang T, Gray NS, Sabatini DM. A unifying model for mTORC1-mediated regulation of mRNA translation. *Nature.* 2012;485(7396):109–113.
34. Caron E, Ghosh S, Matsuoka Y, et al. A comprehensive map of the mTOR signaling network. *Mol Syst Biol.* 2010;6:453.
35. Qian Y, Corum L, Meng Q, et al. PI3K induced actin filament remodeling through Akt and p70S6K1: implication of essential role in cell migration. *Am J Physiol Cell Physiol.* 2004;286(1): C153–C163.
36. Segarra J, Balenci L, Drenth T, Maina F, Lamballe F. Combined signaling through ERK, PI3K/AKT, and RAC1/p38 is required for met-triggered cortical neuron migration. *J Biol Chem.* 2006; 281(8):4771–4778.
37. Zou J, Zhou L, Du X-X, et al. Rheb1 is required for mTORC1 and myelination in postnatal brain development. *Dev Cell.* 2011;20(1): 97–108.
38. European Chromosome 16 Tuberous Sclerosis Consortium. Identification and characterization of the tuberous sclerosis gene on chromosome 16. *Cell.* 1993;75(7):1305–1315.
39. van Slegtenhorst M, de Hoogt R, Hermans C, et al. Identification of the tuberous sclerosis gene TSC1 on chromosome 9q34. *Science.* 1997;277(5327):805–808.
40. Orlova KA, Tsai V, Baybis M, et al. Early progenitor cell marker expression distinguishes type II from type I focal cortical dysplasias. *J Neuropathol Exp Neurol.* 2010;69(8):850–863.
41. Lee JH, Huynh M, Silhavy JL, et al. De novo somatic mutations in components of the PI3K–AKT3–mTOR pathway cause hemimegalencephaly. *Nat Genet.* 2012.
42. Li Y-H, Werner H, Püschel AW. Rheb and mTOR regulate neuronal polarity through Rap1B. *J Biol Chem.* 2008;283(48): 33784–33792.
43. Morita T, Sobue K. Specification of neuronal polarity regulated by local translation of CRMP2 and Tau via the mTOR-p70S6K pathway. *J Biol Chem.* 2009;284(40):27734–27745.
44. Campbell DS, Holt CE. Chemotropic responses of retinal growth cones mediated by rapid local protein synthesis and degradation. *Neuron.* 2001;32(6):1013–1026.
45. Piper M, Anderson R, Dwivedy A, et al. Signaling mechanisms underlying Slit2-induced collapse of *Xenopus* retinal growth cones. *Neuron.* 2006;49(2):215–228.
46. Nie D, Di Nardo A, Han JM, et al. Tsc2-Rheb signaling regulates EphA-mediated axon guidance. *Nat Neurosci.* 2010;13(2):163–172.
47. Jaworski J, Spangler S, Seeburg DP, Hoogenraad CC, Sheng M. Control of dendritic arborization by the phosphoinositide-3′-kinase-Akt-mammalian target of rapamycin pathway. *J Neurosci.* 2005;25(49):11300–11312.
48. Kumar V, Zhang M-X, Swank MW, Kunz J, Wu G-Y. Regulation of dendritic morphogenesis by Ras–PI3K–Akt–mTOR and Ras–MAPK signaling pathways. *J Neurosci.* 2005;25(49): 11288–11299.
49. Urbanska M, Gozdz A, Swiech LJ, Jaworski J. Mammalian target of rapamycin complex 1 (mTORC1) and 2 (mTORC2) control the dendritic arbor morphology of hippocampal neurons. *J Biol Chem.* 2012.
50. Bateup HS, Takasaki KT, Saulnier JL, Denefrio CL, Sabatini BL. Loss of Tsc1 in vivo impairs hippocampal mGluR-LTD and increases excitatory synaptic function. *J Neurosci.* 2011;31(24): 8862–8869.
51. Tavazoie SF, Alvarez VA, Ridenour DA, Kwiatkowski DJ, Sabatini BL. Regulation of neuronal morphology and function by the tumor suppressors Tsc1 and Tsc2. *Nat Neurosci.* 2005;8(12): 1727–1734.
52. Casadio A, Martin KC, Giustetto M, et al. A transient, neuron-wide form of CREB-mediated long-term facilitation can be stabilized at specific synapses by local protein synthesis. *Cell.* 1999;99(2):221–237.
53. Tang SJ, Reis G, Kang H, Gingras A-C, Sonenberg N, Schuman EM. A rapamycin-sensitive signaling pathway contributes to long-term synaptic plasticity in the hippocampus. *Proc Natl Acad Sci USA.* 2002;99(1):467–472.
54. Stoica L, Zhu PJ, Huang W, Zhou H, Kozma SC, Costa-Mattioli M. Selective pharmacogenetic inhibition of mammalian target of Rapamycin complex I (mTORC1) blocks long-term synaptic plasticity and memory storage. *Proc Natl Acad Sci USA.* 2011;108(9):3791–3796.
55. von der Brelie C, Waltereit R, Zhang L, Beck H, Kirschstein T. Impaired synaptic plasticity in a rat model of tuberous sclerosis. *Eur J Neurosci.* 2006;23(3):686–692.
56. Auerbach BD, Osterweil EK, Bear MF. Mutations causing syndromic autism define an axis of synaptic pathophysiology. *Nature.* 2011;480(7375):63–68.
57. Ehninger D, Han S, Shilyansky C, et al. Reversal of learning deficits in a $Tsc2^{+/-}$ mouse model of tuberous sclerosis. *Nat Med.* 2008;14(8):843–848.
58. Banko JL, Poulin F, Hou L, DeMaria CT, Sonenberg N, Klann E. The translation repressor 4E-BP2 is critical for eIF4F complex formation, synaptic plasticity, and memory in the hippocampus. *J Neurosci.* 2005;25(42):9581–9590.
59. Leventer RJ, Phelan EM, Coleman LT, Kean MJ, Jackson GD, Harvey AS. Clinical and imaging features of cortical malformations in childhood. *Neurology.* 1999;53(4):715–722.
60. Chu-Shore CJ, Major P, Camposano S, Muzykewicz D, Thiele EA. The natural history of epilepsy in tuberous sclerosis complex. *Epilepsia.* 2010;51(7):1236–1241.
61. Krab LC, Goorden SMI, Elgersma Y. Oncogenes on my mind: ERK and MTOR signaling in cognitive diseases. *Trends Genet.* 2008;24(10):498–510.

62. Ehninger D, de Vries PJ, Silva AJ. From mTOR to cognition: molecular and cellular mechanisms of cognitive impairments in tuberous sclerosis. *J Intellect Disabil Res*. 2009;53(10):838–851.
63. O'Callaghan FJK, Harris T, Joinson C, et al. The relation of infantile spasms, tubers, and intelligence in tuberous sclerosis complex. *Arch Dis Child*. 2004;89(6):530–533.
64. Goorden SMI, van Woerden GM, van der Weerd L, Cheadle JP, Elgersma Y. Cognitive deficits in $Tsc1^{+/-}$ mice in the absence of cerebral lesions and seizures. *Ann Neurol*. 2007;62(6):648–655.
65. Dash PK, Orsi SA, Moore AN. Spatial memory formation and memory-enhancing effect of glucose involves activation of the tuberous sclerosis complex-mammalian target of rapamycin pathway. *J Neurosci*. 2006;26(31):8048–8056.
66. Parsons RG, Gafford GM, Helmstetter FJ. Translational control via the mammalian target of rapamycin pathway is critical for the formation and stability of long-term fear memory in amygdala neurons. *J Neurosci*. 2006;26(50):12977–12983.
67. Bekinschtein P, Katche C, Slipczuk LN, et al. mTOR signaling in the hippocampus is necessary for memory formation. *Neurobiol Learn Mem*. 2007;87(2):303–307.
68. Sui L, Wang J, Li B-M. Role of the phosphoinositide 3-kinase-Akt-mammalian target of the rapamycin signaling pathway in long-term potentiation and trace fear conditioning memory in rat medial prefrontal cortex. *Learn Mem*. 2008;15(10):762–776.
69. Myskiw JC, Rossato JI, Bevilaqua LRM, Medina JH, Izquierdo I, Cammarota M. On the participation of mTOR in recognition memory. *Neurobiol Learn Mem*. 2008;89(3):338–351.
70. Glover EM, Ressler KJ, Davis M. Differing effects of systemically administered rapamycin on consolidation and reconsolidation of context vs. cued fear memories. *Learn Mem*. 2010;17(11):577–581.
71. Gafford GM, Parsons RG, Helmstetter FJ. Consolidation and reconsolidation of contextual fear memory requires mammalian target of rapamycin-dependent translation in the dorsal hippocampus. *Neuroscience*. 2011;182:98–104.
72. Deli A, Schipany K, Rosner M, et al. Blocking mTORC1 activity by rapamycin leads to impairment of spatial memory retrieval but not acquisition in C57BL/6J mice. *Behav Brain Res*. 2012;229(2):320–324.
73. Saito T, Nakatsuji N. Efficient gene transfer into the embryonic mouse brain using in vivo electroporation. *Dev Biol*. 2001;240(1): 237–246.
74. Saito T. In vivo electroporation in the embryonic mouse central nervous system. *Nat Protoc*. 2006;1(3):1552–1558.
75. Mizuguchi M, Takashima S, Yamanouchi H, Nakazato Y, Mitani H, Hino O. Novel cerebral lesions in the Eker rat model of tuberous sclerosis: cortical tuber and anaplastic ganglioglioma. *J Neuropathol Exp Neurol*. 2000;59(3):188–196.
76. Crino PB, Aronica E, Baltuch G, Nathanson KL. Biallelic TSC gene inactivation in tuberous sclerosis complex. *Neurology*. 2010;74(21):1716–1723.
77. van Eeghen AM, Black ME, Pulsifer MB, Kwiatkowski DJ, Thiele EA. Genotype and cognitive phenotype of patients with tuberous sclerosis complex. *Eur J Hum Genet*. 2012;20(5):510–515.
78. Wenzel HJ, Patel LS, Robbins CA, Emmi A, Yeung RS, Schwartzkroin PA. Morphology of cerebral lesions in the Eker rat model of tuberous sclerosis. *Acta Neuropathol*. 2004;108(2):97–108.
79. Feliciano DM, Su T, Lopez J, Platel J-C, Bordey A. Single-cell Tsc1 knockout during corticogenesis generates tuber-like lesions and reduces seizure threshold in mice. *J Clin Invest*. 2011;121(4): 1596–1607.
80. Ramos RL, Bai J, LoTurco JJ. Heterotopia formation in rat but not mouse neocortex after RNA interference knockdown of DCX. *Cereb Cortex*. 2006;16(9):1323–1331.
81. Armbruster BN, Li X, Pausch MH, Herlitze S, Roth BL. Evolving the lock to fit the key to create a family of G protein-coupled receptors potently activated by an inert ligand. *Proc Natl Acad Sci USA*. 2007;104(12):5163–5168.
82. Alexander GM, Rogan SC, Abbas AI, et al. Remote control of neuronal activity in transgenic mice expressing evolved G protein-coupled receptors. *Neuron*. 2009;63(1):27–39.
83. Boyden ES, Zhang F, Bamberg E, Nagel G, Deisseroth K. Millisecond-timescale, genetically targeted optical control of neural activity. *Nat Neurosci*. 2005;8(9):1263–1268.
84. Ishizuka T, Kakuda M, Araki R, Yawo H. Kinetic evaluation of photosensitivity in genetically engineered neurons expressing green algae light-gated channels. *Neurosci Res*. 2006;54(2): 85–94.
85. Zhang F, Wang L-P, Brauner M, et al. Multimodal fast optical interrogation of neural circuitry. *Nature*. 2007;446(7136):633–639.
86. Papagiakoumou E, Anselmi F, Bègue A, et al. Scanless two-photon excitation of channelrhodopsin-2. *Nat Methods*. 2010; 7(10):848–854.
87. Aravanis AM, Wang L-P, Zhang F, et al. An optical neural interface: in vivo control of rodent motor cortex with integrated fiberoptic and optogenetic technology. *J Neural Eng*. 2007;4(3): S143–S156.
88. Yan L, Findlay GM, Jones R, Procter J, Cao Y, Lamb RF. Hyper-activation of mammalian target of rapamycin (mTOR) signaling by a gain-of-function mutant of the Rheb GTPase. *J Biol Chem*. 2006;281(29):19793–19797.
89. Wang L, Rhodes CJ, Lawrence Jr JC. Activation of mammalian target of rapamycin (mTOR) by insulin is associated with stimulation of 4EBP1 binding to dimeric mTOR complex 1. *J Biol Chem*. 2006;281(34):24293–24303.
90. Bae EJ, Xu J, Oh DY, et al. Liver-specific p70 S6 kinase depletion protects against hepatic steatosis and systemic insulin resistance. *J Biol Chem*. 2012;287(22):18769–18780.
91. Sun S-Y, Rosenberg LM, Wang X, et al. Activation of Akt and eIF4E survival pathways by rapamycin-mediated mammalian target of rapamycin inhibition. *Cancer Res*. 2005;65(16):7052–7058.
92. Sarbassov DD, Ali SM, Sengupta S, et al. Prolonged rapamycin treatment inhibits mTORC2 assembly and Akt/PKB. *Mol Cell*. 2006;22(2):159–168.
93. Lamming DW, Ye L, Katajisto P, et al. Rapamycin-induced insulin resistance is mediated by mTORC2 loss and uncoupled from longevity. *Science*. 2012;335(6076):1638–1643.
94. Fingar DC, Richardson CJ, Tee AR, Cheatham L, Tsou C, Blenis J. mTOR controls cell cycle progression through its cell growth effectors S6K1 and 4E-BP1/eukaryotic translation initiation factor 4E. *Mol Cell Biol*. 2004;24(1):200–216.
95. Thoreen CC, Kang SA, Chang JW, et al. An ATP-competitive mammalian target of rapamycin inhibitor reveals rapamycin-resistant functions of mTORC1. *J Biol Chem*. 2009;284(12): 8023–8032.
96. Wang X, Beugnet A, Murakami M, Yamanaka S, Proud CG. Distinct signaling events downstream of mTOR cooperate to mediate the effects of amino acids and insulin on initiation factor 4E-binding proteins. *Mol Cell Biol*. 2005;25(7):2558–2572.
97. Guertin DA, Stevens DM, Thoreen CC, et al. Ablation in mice of the mTORC components raptor, rictor, or mLST8 reveals that mTORC2 is required for signaling to Akt-FOXO and PKCα, but not S6K1. *Dev Cell*. 2006;11(6):859–871.
98. Bentzinger CF, Romanino K, Cloëtta D, et al. Skeletal muscle-specific ablation of raptor, but not of rictor, causes metabolic changes and results in muscle dystrophy. *Cell Metab*. 2008;8(5):411–424.
99. Lustenberger RM, Wolfer DP, Vogt KE, Rüegg MA. The role of mTOR complex 1 in synapse function and plasticity. *Poster Presented at: Society for Neuroscience Annual Meeting*. Washington, DC; November 2011.

100. Grolleau A, Bowman J, Pradet-Balade B, et al. Global and specific translational control by rapamycin in T cells uncovered by microarrays and proteomics. *J Biol Chem.* 2002;277(25):22175–22184.
101. Heiman M, Schaefer A, Gong S, et al. A translational profiling approach for the molecular characterization of CNS cell types. *Cell.* 2008;135(4):738–748.
102. Doyle JP, Dougherty JD, Heiman M, et al. Application of a translational profiling approach for the comparative analysis of CNS cell types. *Cell.* 2008;135(4):749–762.
103. Sanz E, Yang L, Su T, Morris DR, McKnight GS, Amieux PS. Cell-type-specific isolation of ribosome-associated mRNA from complex tissues. *Proc Natl Acad Sci USA.* 2009;106(33):13939–13944.

CHAPTER

16

Network Control Mechanisms—Synaptogenesis and Epilepsy Development

Kevin Staley [1], *Jonas Dyhrfjeld-Johnsen* [2], *Waldemar Swiercz* [1], *F. Edward Dudek* [3]

[1]Department of Neurology, Massachusetts General Hospital, Harvard Medical School, Boston, MA, USA, [2]Sensorion, Montpellier, France, [3]Department of Neurosurgery, University of Utah, Salt Lake City, UT, USA

Synaptogenesis can occur as a result of various types of brain injury, including that which can lead to the development of central nervous system disorders.

After brain injury, some patients develop epilepsy. The fraction of brain-injured patients who develop epilepsy can be as low as 2–3% for a closed head injury without major sequelae[1] to more than 70% for the most severely injured patients.[2] The epilepsy develops over time intervals that vary from months to many years, suggesting that the changes subserving epilepsy occur slowly. A widely held hypothesis is that the interval between injury and epilepsy, commonly referred to as the latent period, represents the time needed for the formation of new circuitry in the region of brain injury.[3] Experimental evidence of axon sprouting after brain injury[4–6] supports this idea. But sprouting was originally described as a self-repair mechanism,[7] and in the majority of brain-injured patients, sprouting is thought to subserve a reparative role that makes possible the reconstitution of essential brain functions such as ambulation, communication, and skilled hand use after injury.[8] Here, we consider the question: what goes wrong in the circuit repair process in the patients who develop epilepsy after brain injury?

One possibility is that these patients are predisposed to epilepsy as a consequence of various subclinical channelopathies[9] that are phenotypically unmasked after injury (the so-called second hit hypothesis). This implies that brain injury lowers the seizure threshold and that patients with a lower seizure threshold before the brain injury may experience a reduction in seizure threshold that is sufficient to engender spontaneous seizures (i.e. the development of epilepsy). While this is likely to explain some cases of epilepsy after brain injury, it does not explain why only a fraction of genetically homogeneous rodents develop epilepsy after brain injury (e.g. Ref. 10). Another possibility arises from the observation that clinical brain injury is most often traumatic or ischemic, and these injuries result in heterogeneous deficits—the circuit damage varies greatly from patient to patient in terms of lost neurons, inputs, and outputs. As mentioned here, as the injury becomes more severe, the incidence of epilepsy increases. This suggests that an important determinant of whether a patient develops epilepsy after brain injury is the nature of the damage to the circuit. A corollary to this idea is that epilepsy depends on the details of the consequent repair. If we knew the rules governing this repair, we might be able to better predict who is at risk for epilepsy after injury, the length of the latent period between injury and the development of epilepsy, and perhaps the best time points and methods for intervention.

To understand circuit repair, we need to understand circuit formation. A wealth of technologies are now available to address this basic but difficult problem, including activity-dependent imaging of neural networks, high-density multielectrode recordings, photo uncaging of caged neurotransmitter agonists, and a variety of molecular methods for labeling neurons[11] and synaptic connections.[12] Unfortunately, the overwhelming complexity of brain development has perforce left many relevant questions unaddressed to date.[13] Some of these questions are surprisingly, almost embarrassingly, basic. For example: what strategies do neurons use to choose postsynaptic partners? In other words, how do neurons go about the task of wiring the brain? We don't have good answers

Neuronal Networks in Brain Function, CNS Disorders, and Therapeutics
http://dx.doi.org/10.1016/B978-0-12-415804-7.00016-2

for this basic question because, although the connectivity of regions and types of cells is beginning to be understood,[14] the connectivity of individual neurons is extraordinarily difficult to determine.

Consider the problem of feedback inhibition, in which the firing of action potentials by a principal neuron results in activation of a local interneuron and release of the inhibitory neurotransmitter gamma-aminobutyric acid (GABA) at an inhibitory synapse on the principal neuron. Feedback inhibition is presumed to be the major means of control of the level of network activity in the brain and, thus, an important endogenous anti-epileptic mechanism. There is abundant evidence that interneurons receive glutamatergic input and make inhibitory connections on principal cells. But what drives the interneuron to fire? Does a single pyramidal cell firing cause the interneuron to fire? Release of GABA at an inhibitory synapse is very effective at preventing action potentials in the postsynaptic neuron.[15] Thus, when an interneuron fires, if it releases GABA at all of its thousands of outputs,[16] then all of those thousands of postsynaptic principal neurons will be temporarily silenced. Because of the large impact of the firing of a single interneuron, the rules governing the excitation of interneurons are very important for understanding neural network function.

What are the rules for interneuron excitation? We know from paired recordings of principal cells and interneurons, as well as combined intra- and extracellular recordings, that interneurons fire after the activation of a solitary excitatory input synapse about one-third of the time.[17] Thus, the firing of an interneuron most often requires coordinated activation of its excitatory inputs. This brings us to a closely related question: what are the excitatory inputs to an interneuron? What principal neurons comprise the "input field" of the interneuron? Do neighboring principal neurons activate common interneurons? In other words, are interneuron input fields composed of clumps of neighboring principal cells, or are the input fields more widely distributed? Is there a strategy by which principal neurons decide whether to synapse on a particular inhibitory interneuron? *Without knowledge of these questions, we can't really create realistic artificial neural networks to study brain function.* And while these are therefore important questions, more fundamental questions for control of network excitability may be: what is the relationship between an interneuron's inputs and its outputs? Are the input cells the same as output cells? Interneuron inputs and outputs are beginning to be studied with genetic anatomical approaches,[18] but reciprocal connections and the relationships between inputs and outputs are very hard to determine with anatomical techniques. Paired recordings of principal cells and basket cells suggest that there is not a 1:1 correspondence between an interneuron's input field and its output field.[19] In other words, just because a pyramidal cell has an excitatory postsynaptic connection to an interneuron, this does not mean that the interneuron has a reciprocal inhibitory postsynaptic connection to the principal cell. However, we do not know this for certain because paired recordings between principal cells and interneurons are performed in brain slices, where an enormous fraction of the connectivity has been lost in the process of slicing[20] (Chapter 1).

To address the problem of circuit repair after brain injury while avoiding the massive de-afferentation and de-efferentation of acute slices, we studied organotypic slice cultures. These cultures are composed of 400 μm thick hippocampal slices that are placed in an incubator and kept at an interface between culture media and 5% CO_2 in room air. Using standard culture techniques,[21,22] we found that these cultures become "epileptic" (i.e. they exhibit neuronal firing that mimics that seen in epilepsy) over the course of the first 7–10 days in vitro, displaying recurrent epileptiform discharges resembling both interictal and ictal activity recorded from patients.[23–25]

The brain slice cultures comprise a wonderful model of epilepsy after brain injury, because the process of slicing mimics the diffuse axonal injury that occurs during trauma. The natural increase in connectivity that occurs over the first weeks in culture[26] appears to drive the epileptogenesis, because inhibiting this connectivity prevents the epilepsy.[24] Others had previously demonstrated that organotypic slices become epileptic,[27,28] but this point remains somewhat controversial. Investigators who do not think organotypic slice cultures are epileptic tend to use the cultures within the first week after slicing, i.e. before the onset of most of the epileptic activity,[23,25] and record in the presence of high concentrations of divalent cations, which suppress epileptiform activity.

When considering epileptogenic circuit alterations that occur after brain injury, the first question might be: are the synaptic properties changed as a consequence of injury, repair, interictal spiking, or seizures? We found the synaptic changes to be modest (Figure 16.1), supporting the idea that circuit changes rather than changes in cellular or synaptic properties are likely to underlie the development of epilepsy in this model of posttraumatic epileptogenesis. Interestingly, seizures tended to depress synaptic strength, whereas interictal activities tended to increase synaptic strength. However, both activities are present in chronic epilepsy, and thus it was not surprising to find that the net changes in synaptic strength were fairly modest, in line with what would be predicted from theories of synaptic homeostasis, and in line with what other investigators have reported in organotypic slices.[29,30] In our modeling studies,[31] these changes were not sufficient to engender epilepsy.

If the observed changes in synaptic weighting are not sufficient to engender epilepsy, what is? Pharmacological

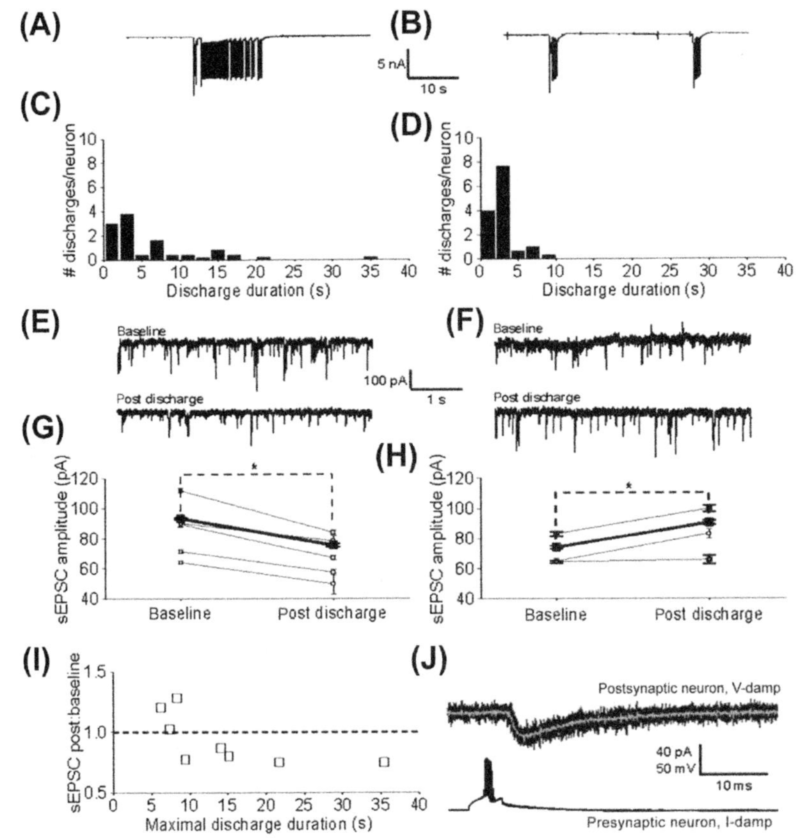

FIGURE 16.1 Synaptic plasticities induced by ictal versus interictal activity. Whole-cell recordings from CA3 pyramidal cells in organotypic slices. **Ictal recordings are on the left** (A, C, E, G), and **interictal recordings are on the right** (B, D, F, H). In these preliminary experiments, epileptiform activity was recorded in the presence of $GABA_A$ and $GABA_B$ blockers in standard artificial cerebrospinal fluid (3.5 mM $K^+{}_o$, 2 mM $Mg^{2+}{}_o$, and $Ca^{2+}{}_o$) at 14DIV. Top row: Ictal (A) and interictal (B) discharges. Second row: Epileptiform discharge duration histograms for slices exhibiting a combination of ictal and interictal (C) versus only interictal (D) discharges (interictal < 10 s). Most slices demonstrate both activities at 21DIV. Third row: Whole-cell recordings of spontaneous excitatory postsynaptic currents before and after ictal (E) and interictal (F) discharges. Fourth row: Neurons recorded in slices with both interictal and ictal discharges demonstrate depotentiation (G), whereas neurons from slices exhibiting only interictal discharge exhibit primarily long-term potentiation (H). (I) Direction of synaptic plasticity versus the maximum duration of epileptiform activity recorded supports. (J) Demonstration of the feasibility of paired, synaptically connected recordings of CA3 pyramidal cells in organotypic slices. (For color version of this figure, the reader is referred to the online version of this book.)

disinhibition leads robustly to burst behavior in vitro[32] rather than occasional seizures admixed with interictal activity, as is seen in epileptic patients and experimental subjects. This indicates that epilepsy cannot be explained by a simple lack of inhibition. Along these lines, most epileptic patients function quite well for the vast majority of the time during which they are not seizing, indicating that the alterations that cause epilepsy must be relatively subtle—more subtle, for example, than a pharmacological blockade of inhibition. These considerations bring us back to the circuit: if neurons are connected in a particular fashion, can the pattern of connectivity engender epilepsy?

We used a simplified 10,000-neuron model[31] to begin to address this question. A 100×100 matrix of integrate-and-fire glutamatergic neurons was inhibited by a 15×15 matrix of feedback interneurons. In this model, a low rate of spontaneous glutamate release from presynaptic terminals would occasionally sum to generate action potentials in the postsynaptic neurons. This activity could build locally, but it was quenched before activating the entire network by two strong inhibitory features of the network: GABAergic interneurons and activity-dependent depression at the excitatory glutamatergic synapses.[33] Thus, excessive local activity would lead to activity-dependent depression of the presynaptic terminals of the spiking neurons. Activity-dependent depression recovers with a sufficiently slow time constant (about 8 s) so that activity could not be sustained and local action potential rates dropped back to baseline. Depending on the local wiring strategy for interneurons, GABAergic inhibition could also quench local bursts of activity. This brings into focus the importance of the wiring strategy for interneuron inputs and outputs; for these models, we used distance-dependent stochastic connectivity for pyramidal cell—pyramidal cell connections, pyramidal cell—interneuron connections, and interneuron—pyramidal cell connections.

At baseline, no epileptiform activity was present. Reduction in inhibition caused bursting behavior that was reminiscent of interictal activity, but no seizures. However, several patterns of injury and reparative connectivity engendered interictal spikes as well as occasional seizures. A schematic of one of these patterns of injury is illustrated in Figure 16.2.

When the network geometry was made inhomogeneous, seizure activity could be generated when activity propagated through the network sufficiently slowly and sparsely that synapses recovered from activity-dependent depression before the activity

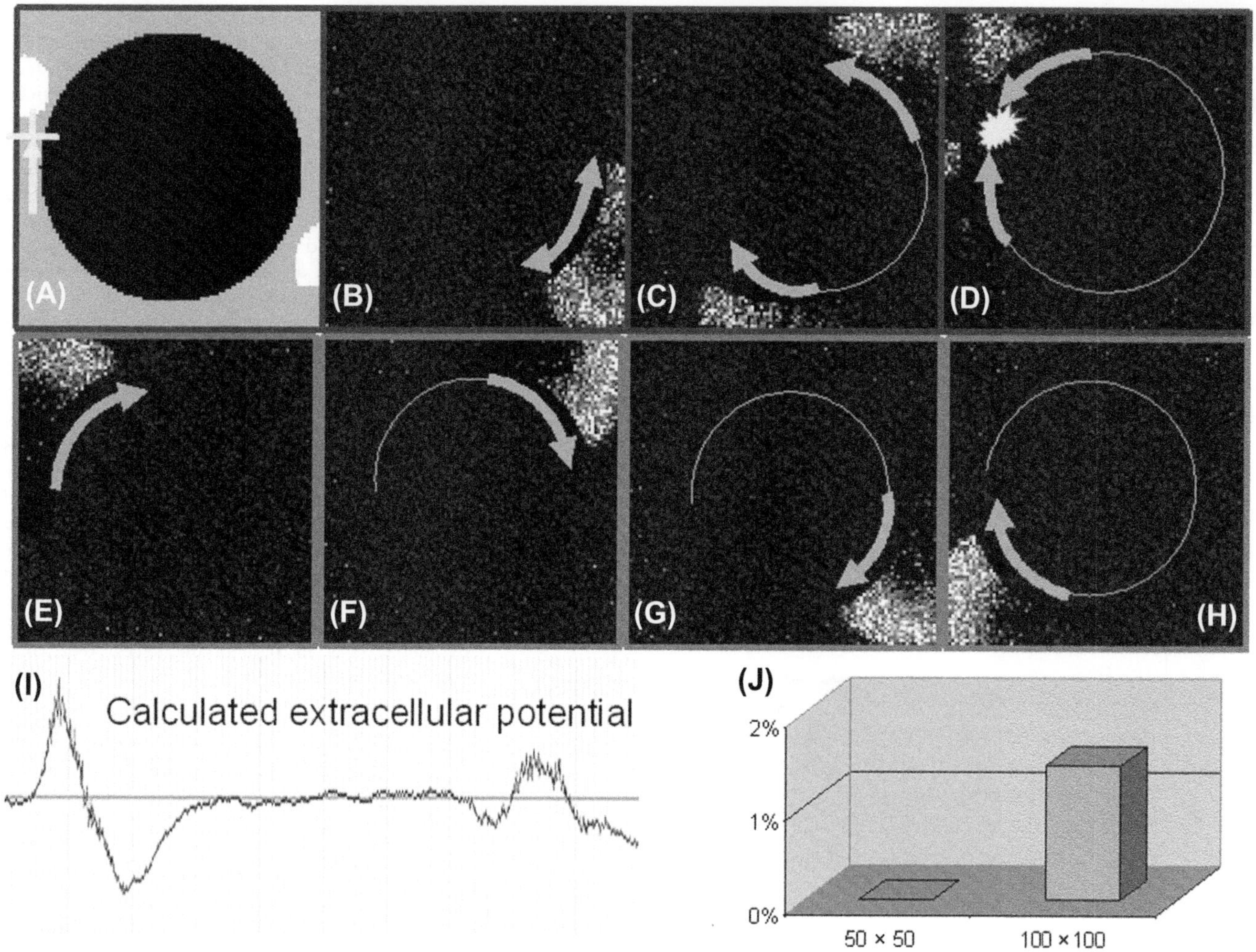

FIGURE 16.2 **Epileptogenic effects of circuit changes.** (A) Features of neuronal circuitry that can be painted onto a template using standard drawing tools. The 100 × 100 pyramidal cell network has been modified by a central area of complete cell loss (solid black circle), areas of partial cell loss (gray areas), and areas of preserved cell density (white areas). The higher cell density and connectivity cause most bursts to arise from these two areas. The upper-left white area also has feedback inhibition (a yellow diode symbol) from preserved interneurons. This reduces the probability of counterclockwise propagation of excitation. (B–D) A spontaneous network ignition from the lower right island of preserved cell density. The waves of excitation meet in the upper-left corner and annihilate each other. (E–H) A burst ignited in the island of preserved cell density in the upper-left corner successfully propagates through multiple cycles. (I) The extracellular potential calculated over two cycles for the activity shown in (E–H) demonstrates local rhythmic activity, in this case sharp waves in the delta band, as has been seen at the onset of some focal seizures in human epilepsy. (J) The proportion of spontaneously generated waves of excitation that is reentrant. A smaller network (50 × 50 neurons) cannot generate reentrant waves because the time required to traverse the longest path in the network is shorter than the refractory period of the synapses at the start of the path. The 100 × 100 neuron network illustrated here generated sustained reentry about 1% of the time (the other trials generated spikes) due to the high probability that a wave of excitation would die as a consequence of running into a refractory area caused by spontaneous activity arising elsewhere in the network. This provides a mechanism for the clinically important but unexplained high ratio of interictal-to-ictal activity. (For interpretation of the references to color in this figure legend, the reader is referred to the online version of this book.)

returned to their area of the network. Thus, seizure activity appeared as a propagating wave, which has also been observed in experimental seizures in vivo.[34] The sparser the activity, the fewer glutamatergic synapses were depressed, and the more rapidly an area recovered after the traveling wave of excitability passed through. The rapidity with which an area recovered was an important determinant as to whether the activity could be sustained, or whether a subsequent traveling wave of activity would encounter a section of the network that was still refractory due to activity-dependent depression of glutamatergic synapses; in the latter case, the traveling wave would break up, and synchronous activity would stop. If the activity was too sparse, it would also die out. Thus, we found that interneurons were important for maintaining the level of local activity, where specific, intermediate intensities of activity were more likely to engender sustained traveling waves of reentrant seizure activity. The importance of inhibition in this model brings up the interesting finding that recovery of inhibition is also an important feature of in vivo epileptogenesis.[35] That is, by the time that seizures begin, injury-induced disinhibition has been repaired. This may not be a coincidence if a particular level of inhibition is needed to sustain seizure activity.

Figure 16.2 illustrates a "donut" circuit morphology in which traveling waves developed in the surviving tissue that surrounded a large area of injury in the network. While this was an easy topology to create and recreate, there are many other circuit inhomogeneities that could engender seizure activity. To summarize our preliminary findings:

1. Some network topologies engender seizure activity. These tend to be inhomogeneous networks where the spread of activity is limited in a way that favors reentry of the activity (e.g. traveling waves of activity).
2. Sustained seizure activity was observed as traveling waves of local activation of principal cells and interneurons.
3. For seizure activity to be sustained, a local section of the network needed to recover from activity-dependent depression of glutamatergic synapses before activity reentered that portion of the network.
4. Sparse local activity was much more readily sustained than intense local activity, because sparse activity did not cause as much activity-dependent synaptic depression. This is why blocking all inhibition did not cause seizures—the entire network rapidly and intensely activated, resulting in widespread synaptic depression that quenched all synchronous activity.[36] This type of intense, disinhibited activity causes periodic bursting of the entire network, with the time between bursts largely determined by the rate of recovery from synaptic depression.[33,37]

These modeling studies demonstrate the importance of the nature of the brain injury. Some patterns of injury to the neural network are much more likely to engender reentrant activity than others.

What of the recovery of the network by sprouting? As discussed earlier in the chapter, very little is known about the strategies that neurons use to connect to each other during normal brain development,[13,14] and essentially nothing is known about the strategies that neurons use to reconnect to each other after injury. For example, how important a determinant is the principle of synaptic homeostasis? This is the idea that neurons require a certain amount of inputs or outputs per unit time. Inputs are generally considered to be synaptic activity, and outputs are generally measured as action potentials or calcium transients. In the absence of these inputs and outputs, for example after brain injury and de-afferentation, neurons alter their properties and perhaps connectivity to reestablish their preferred quantity of inputs or outputs. There is compelling experimental evidence to support the idea of neuronal homeostasis,[38] which may drive key elements of epileptogenesis.[39] What are the details of the implementation of this principle?

This important question awaits detailed studies of the evolution of an epileptic focus. With the advent of in vivo two-photon microscopy and transgenic fluorophores, this question is nearly within reach. The outlines can be discerned. For example, clinical studies have already confirmed one prediction of the homeostatic model: several standard anticonvulsants do not prevent the development of epilepsy after head injury.[40] In the organotypic slice culture model of posttraumatic epilepsy, anticonvulsants suppress seizures transiently, but epilepsy develops consistently despite the continued presence of a commonly used anticonvulsant (phenytoin).[23] The in vitro data exclude the commonly posited problems with compliance that may have contributed to the lack of efficacy of anticonvulsants in the human trials.

In vitro experiments can extend the findings to include blocking of interictal spiking, and even blocking most synaptic activity with agents such as tetrodotoxin and broad-spectrum glutamate receptor antagonists, which are not feasible in vivo. These agents prevented seizures but did not prevent epileptogenesis—when they were washed off, robust epilepsy was evident. This is consistent with the predictions of the homeostatic model, in which neurons strive for a particular number of inputs and outputs and a particular activity level. Such striving in the setting of limited input and output options could create the levels of positive feedback necessary to engender seizures.

Blocking the creation of these inputs and outputs, for example by preventing a sufficiently anabolic neuronal state through blockade of the mammalian target of rapamycin (mTOR) pathway (see Chapter 15), has been demonstrated to prevent the development of epilepsy in vivo[41] and in vitro,[24] although there are likely important caveats to these findings that continue to be elucidated.[42] Our in vitro data suggest that all sprouting is inhibited by mTOR antagonists. Thus, after brain injury, both beneficial and harmful circuit repairs are likely to be inhibited by mTOR antagonists.

In the coming years, we look forward to the elucidation of the connectivity rules governing circuit formation and repair. Knowledge of these rules is fundamental both to our understanding of the genesis of epilepsy and to successful interventions that inhibit epileptogenic circuit alterations but do not compromise the rebuilding of circuits that subserve normal brain function.

References

1. Annegers JF, Hauser A, Coan SP, Rocca WA. A population-based study of seizures after traumatic brain injuries. *N Engl J Med.* 1998;338(1):20–24.
2. Jennet B. *Epilepsy after Non-missile Head Injuries.* Chicago: Year Book Medical; 1973.
3. Dudek FE, Staley KJ. The time course and circuit mechanisms of acquired epileptogenesis. In: Noebels JL, Avoli M, Rogawski MA, Olsen RW, Delgado-Escueta AV, eds. *Jasper's Basic Mechanisms of the Epilepsies [Internet].* 4th ed. Bethesda, MD: National Center for Biotechnology Information (US); 2012.
4. Sutula T, He XX, Cavazos J, Scott G. Synaptic reorganization in the hippocampus induced by abnormal functional activity. *Science.* 1988;239(4844):1147–1150.
5. Tauck DL, Nadler JV. Evidence of functional mossy fiber sprouting in hippocampal formation of kainic acid-treated rats. *J Neurosci.* 1985;5(4):1016–1022.
6. Wuarin JP, Dudek FE. Electrographic seizures and new recurrent excitatory circuits in the dentate gyrus of hippocampal slices from kainate-treated epileptic rats. *J Neurosci.* 1996;16(14): 4438–4448.
7. Steward O, Vinsant SL. Identification of the cells of origin of a central pathway which sprouts following lesions in mature rats. *Brain Res.* 1978;147(2):223–243.
8. Cramer SC, Sur M, Dobkin BH, et al. Harnessing neuroplasticity for clinical applications. *Brain.* 2011;134(Pt 6): 1591–1609.
9. Klassen T, Davis C, Goldman A, et al. Exome sequencing of ion channel genes reveals complex profiles confounding personal risk assessment in epilepsy. *Cell.* 2011;145(7):1036–1048.
10. Bolkvadze T, Pitkänen A. Development of post-traumatic epilepsy after controlled cortical impact and lateral fluid-percussion-induced brain injury in the mouse. *J Neurotrauma.* 2012;29(5):789–812.
11. Weissman TA, Sanes JR, Lichtman JW, Livet J. Generating and imaging multicolor Brainbow mice. *Cold Spring Harb Protoc.* 2011;2011(7):763–769.
12. Fino E, Packer AM, Yuste R. The logic of inhibitory connectivity in the neocortex. *Neuroscientist.* 2012 [Epub ahead of print] PMID: 22922685.
13. Alivisatos AP, Chun M, Church GM, et al. Neuroscience. The brain activity map. *Science.* 2013;339(6125):1284–1285.
14. Thomson AM, Lamy C. Functional maps of neocortical local circuitry. *Front Neurosci.* 2007;1(1):19–42.
15. Miles R, Tóth K, Gulyás AI, Hájos N, Freund TF. Differences between somatic and dendritic inhibition in the hippocampus. *Neuron.* 1996;16(4):815–823.
16. Lasztóczi B, Tukker JJ, Somogyi P, Klausberger T. Terminal field and firing selectivity of cholecystokinin-expressing interneurons in the hippocampal CA3 area. *J Neurosci.* 2011;31(49): 18073–18093.
17. Bazelot M, Dinocourt C, Cohen I, Miles R. Unitary inhibitory field potentials in the CA3 region of rat hippocampus. *J Physiol.* 2010;588(Pt 12):2077–2090.
18. Inan M, Blázquez-Llorca L, Merchán-Pérez A, Anderson SA, DeFelipe J, Yuste R. Dense and overlapping innervation of pyramidal neurons by chandelier cells. *J Neurosci.* 2013;33(5): 1907–1914.
19. Zhang W, Buckmaster PS. Dysfunction of the dentate basket cell circuit in a rat model of temporal lobe epilepsy. *J Neurosci.* 2009; 29(24):7846–7856.
20. Dzhala V, Valeeva G, Glykys J, Khazipov R, Staley K. Traumatic alterations in GABA signaling disrupt hippocampal network activity in the developing brain. *J Neurosci.* 2012;32(12): 4017–4031.
21. Gähwiler BH, Thompson SM, Muller D. Preparation and maintenance of organotypic slice cultures of CNS tissue. *Curr Protoc Neurosci.* 2001 Chapter 6:Unit 6.
22. Stoppini L, Buchs PA, Muller D. A simple method for organotypic cultures of nervous tissue. *J Neurosci Methods.* 1991;37(2): 173–182.
23. Berdichevsky Y, Dzhala V, Mail M, Staley KJ. Interictal spikes, seizures and ictal cell death are not necessary for post-traumatic epileptogenesis in vitro. *Neurobiol Dis.* 2012; 45(2):774–785.
24. Berdichevsky Y, Dryer AM, Saponjian Y, Mahoney MM, Pimentel CA, Lucini CA, Usenovic M, Staley KJ. PI3K-Akt signaling activates mTOR-mediated epileptogenesis in organotypic hippocampal culture model of post-traumatic epilepsy. J Neurosci. May 2013; 33(21):9056-9067.
25. Dyhrfjeld-Johnsen J, Berdichevsky Y, Swiercz W, Sabolek H, Staley KJ. Interictal spikes precede ictal discharges in an organotypic hippocampal slice culture model of epileptogenesis. *J Clin Neurophysiol.* 2010;27(6):418–424.
26. De Simoni A, Griesinger CB, Edwards FA. Development of rat CA1 neurones in acute versus organotypic slices: role of experience in synaptic morphology and activity. *J Physiol.* 2003; 550(Pt 1):135–147.
27. Bausch SB, McNamara JO. Contributions of mossy fiber and CA1 pyramidal cell sprouting to dentate granule cell hyperexcitability in kainic acid-treated hippocampal slice cultures. *J Neurophysiol.* 2004;92(6):3582–3595.
28. McBain CJ, Boden P, Hill RG. Rat hippocampal slices 'in vitro' display spontaneous epileptiform activity following long-term organotypic culture. *J Neurosci Methods.* 1989;27(1):35–49.
29. Muller D, Buchs PA, Stoppini L. Time course of synaptic development in hippocampal organotypic cultures. *Brain Res Dev Brain Res.* 1993;71(1):93–100.
30. Pavlidis P, Madison DV. Synaptic transmission in pair recordings from CA3 pyramidal cells in organotypic culture. *J Neurophysiol.* 1999;81(6):2787–2797.
31. Swiercz W, Cios K, Hellier J, Yee A, Staley K. Effects of synaptic depression and recovery on synchronous network activity. *J Clin Neurophysiol.* 2007;24(2):165–174.
32. Miles R, Wong RKS, Traub RD. Synchronized afterdischarges in the hippocampus: contribution of local synaptic interactions. *Neuroscience* 1984;(12):1179–1189.
33. Jones J, Stubblefield EA, Benke TA, Staley KJ. Desynchronization of glutamate release prolongs synchronous CA3 network activity. *J Neurophysiol.* 2007;97(5):3812–3818.
34. Viventi J, Kim DH, Vigeland L, et al. Flexible, foldable, actively multiplexed, high-density electrode array for mapping brain activity in vivo. *Nat Neurosci.* 2011;14(12):1599–1605.
35. Thind KK, Yamawaki R, Phanwar I, Zhang G, Wen X, Buckmaster PS. Initial loss but later excess of GABAergic synapses with dentate granule cells in a rat model of temporal lobe epilepsy. *J Comp Neurol.* 2010;518(5):647–667.
36. Sabolek HR, Swiercz WB, Lillis KP, et al. A candidate mechanism underlying the variance of interictal spike propagation. *J Neurosci.* 2012;32(9):3009–3021.
37. Staley KJ, Bains JS, Yee A, Hellier J, Longacher JM. Statistical model relating CA3 burst probability to recovery from

burst-induced depression at recurrent collateral synapses. *J Neurophysiol*. 2001;86(6):2736–2747.

38. Turrigiano G. Homeostatic synaptic plasticity: local and global mechanisms for stabilizing neuronal function. *Cold Spring Harb Perspect Biol*. 2012;4(1):a005736.
39. Houweling AR, Bazhenov M, Timofeev I, Steriade M, Sejnowski TJ. Homeostatic synaptic plasticity can explain post-traumatic epileptogenesis in chronically isolated neocortex. *Cereb Cortex*. 2005;15(6):834–845.
40. Temkin NR. Preventing and treating posttraumatic seizures: the human experience. *Epilepsia*. 2009;50(Suppl. 2):10–13.
41. Zeng LH, Rensing NR, Wong M. The mammalian target of rapamycin signaling pathway mediates epileptogenesis in a model of temporal lobe epilepsy. *J Neurosci*. 2009;29(21): 6964–6972.
42. Buckmaster PS, Lew FH. Rapamycin suppresses mossy fiber sprouting but not seizure frequency in a mouse model of temporal lobe epilepsy. *J Neurosci*. 2011;31(6):2337–2347.

CHAPTER

17

The Brain and Spinal Cord Networks Controlling Locomotion

Larry M. Jordan [1], *Urszula Sławińska* [2]

[1]Department of Physiology, Spinal Cord Research Centre, University of Manitoba, Winnipeg, MB, Canada,
[2]Department of Neurophysiology, Nencki Institute of Experimental Biology PAS, Warsaw, Poland

The neural networks that control locomotion, a basic motor act that occurs in all vertebrates, are remarkably well preserved in all species. The most basic of the locomotor networks is located in the spinal cord, and it provides the necessary muscle synergies responsible for the swimming movements, undulatory movements, and limb movements that underlie the capacity for progression.[1–4] This spinal network, known as the central pattern generator (CPG) for locomotion, is activated and controlled by specific supraspinal structures.[1,2,5–11] Figure 17.1 summarizes the major connections of the brain regions that are responsible for the control of locomotion. The final pathway from the brain to the spinal cord that activates the CPG consists of several different descending reticulospinal (RS) systems. The RS neurons are activated by specific structures in the brainstem that constitute the mesencephalic locomotor region (MLR), which includes the cuneiform nucleus (CN), the pedunculopontine nucleus (PPN), and surrounding structures, and which receives input and control from forebrain, diencephalic, limbic, and basal ganglia structures that engage the midbrain locomotor areas for the full range of locomotor tasks available to the animals. There is considerable sensory feedback from the limb that contributes to the locomotor capability of the spinal CPG. Forebrain and brainstem locomotor centers that initiate and control locomotion are now known to be important for controlling locomotion in all vertebrate species (for reviews, see Refs 5,6,11–16). Structures including the cerebral cortex, the diencephalon, the limbic system, and the basal ganglia and its output nuclei contribute to the activation of the spinal CPG. In decerebrate animals, where the basal ganglia, diencephalic, limbic, and other forebrain structures are absent, locomotion can occur spontaneously or can be evoked from the midbrain locomotor areas, indicating that locomotion can occur with only brainstem structures intact. Output from the cerebellum is able to elicit activity in the locomotor CPG as well, but like many of the other structures that are sufficient for activation of locomotion, it is not required. It appears that there are many redundancies in the brain systems that are capable of eliciting locomotion under different circumstances.

DESCENDING CONTROL OF LOCOMOTION

The medial brainstem area containing locomotor RS cells has been proposed as a brainstem substrate for action selection.[17] Corticoreticular–RS interneuronal connections appear to operate as a flexible control system for the control of movements, including those that combine goal-directed locomotion with other motor actions.[18] The cortical production of locomotion occurs at the RS level, based upon pyramidal tract stimulation, with the pyramidal tract interrupted below the stimulus site, producing locomotion through a brainstem relay.[19] Microstimulation studies[20,21] show that the medial reticular formation (MRF) produces movement responses, and electrical or chemical stimulation of the MRF produces locomotion and activates spinal excitatory and inhibitory interneurons of the CPG that project to motoneurons.[22] Others have also found

http://dx.doi.org/10.1016/B978-0-12-415804-7.00017-4

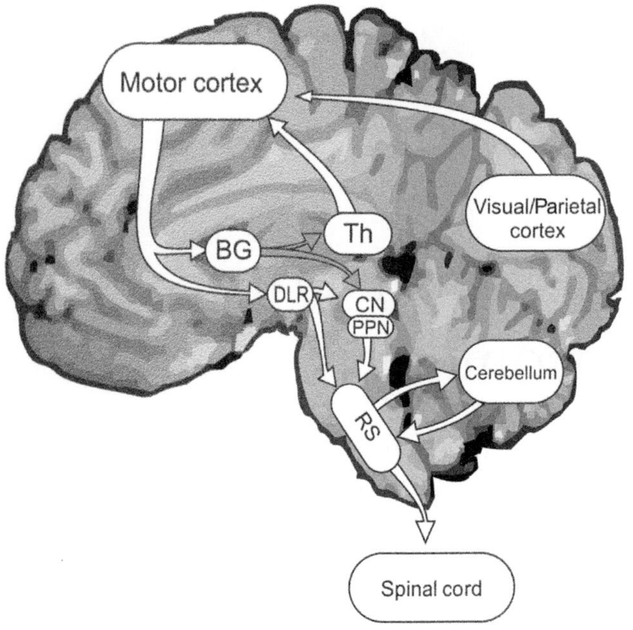

FIGURE 17.1 The main contributors to the network in the brain for control of locomotion are superimposed on a sagittal view of the human brain. The white arrows represent excitatory projections, while shaded arrows represent inhibitory connections. The motor cortex can select a locomotor task by activating the basal ganglia (BG), where the striatum provided inhibition to the BG output neurons of the globus pallidus. The globus pallidus and homologous basal ganglia output neurons tonically inhibit the major components of the MLR, the cuneiform nucleus (CN) and the pedunculopontine nucleus (PPN), so that BG activation leads to disinhibition of the MLR nuclei, resulting in the initiation of locomotion through a relay in reticulospinal (RS) neurons. The BG output is monitored and fed back to the cortex via the thalamus (Th). Another route for activation of the midbrain locomotor neurons is by excitation of the widespread neuronal systems included in the diencephalic locomotor region (DLR), which can elicit locomotion either via activating CN and/or PPN or by projections to the RS locomotor areas. The various DLR and MLR areas can be recruited to produce locomotion due to activation from the cortex, limbic structures, and other parts of the brain in a variety of conditions (e.g. arousal, exploration, and escape) where locomotion is an appropriate output. Multiple RS neuron groups are able to activate the spinal CPG for locomotion.

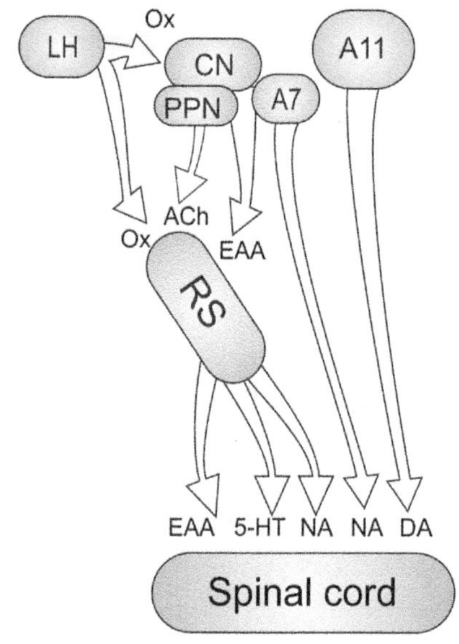

FIGURE 17.2 Diagram showing the main components of the reticulospinal (RS) projections to the spinal cord to activate the locomotor CPG. The RS systems that are effective for eliciting locomotion are distinguishable based upon their transmitter content. Pathways containing excitatory amino acids (EAA) such as glutamate project from magnocellular and gigantocellular parts of the RS system to the spinal cord. Other RS pathways arise in the 5-hydroxytryptamine (5-HT) and noradrenergic (NA) regions of the medulla. The RS systems are known to be activated from the lateral hypothalamus (LH), which includes an orexinergic (Ox) pathway, and from the components of the MLR, including the cuneiform nucleus (CN) and the pedunculopontine nucleus (PPN). CN and PPN provide glutamatergic (excitatory amino acid, or EAA) input to RS neurons, and PPN also produces RS activation due to a cholinergic (acetylcholine, or ACh) projection. There is a newly described orexinergic input to neurons of the CN for initiation of locomotion. Another putative component of the MLR is the A7 noradrenergic group of neurons found at the junction of the midbrain and the pons, in a site where electrical stimulation elicits locomotion. These cells project directly to the spinal cord. A dopaminergic (DA) pathway, thought to arise from the All group of dopamine-containing neurons of the hypothalamus, may also be an important descending pathway for the initiation of locomotion in some species.

that stimulation of RS neurons in the medulla elicits locomotion.[23–25]

Many neurotransmitters in descending pathways originating in the brain activate the spinal locomotor CPG (Figure 17.2), including noradrenaline (NA), dopamine (DA), 5-hydroxytryptamine (5-HT), excitatory amino acids (EAA) such as glutamate, and acetylcholine (reviewed in Refs 26–28). The inhibitory neurotransmitters glycine and gamma-aminobutyric acid (GABA) also contribute to the control of CPG neurons. The first descending system that was implicated in the control of locomotion was the noradrenergic system, based upon the finding that L-DOPA administration could produce a pattern of reflex responses suggesting a locomotor organization.[29,30] Stimulation of flexor reflex afferents (FRAs) produced late long-lasting discharges in ipsilateral flexor nerves (Figure 17.3(A)), while contralateral FRAs produced similar responses in extensor motoneurons (reviewed in Ref. 32). Stimulation of brainstem neurons that are the source of a noradrenergic pathway to the spinal cord (A7) can elicit locomotion.[33] This region is known to provide the noradrenergic innervation of the ventral horn.[34] However, specific lesions of the noradrenergic fibers in the spinal cord did not abolish spontaneous or MLR-evoked locomotion.[35] This is due to the significant redundancy in descending pathways capable of eliciting locomotion.[36–38] In chronic spinal cat preparations, intrathecal injections of the noradrenergic $alpha_2$ receptor agonist clonidine elicited locomotion, while

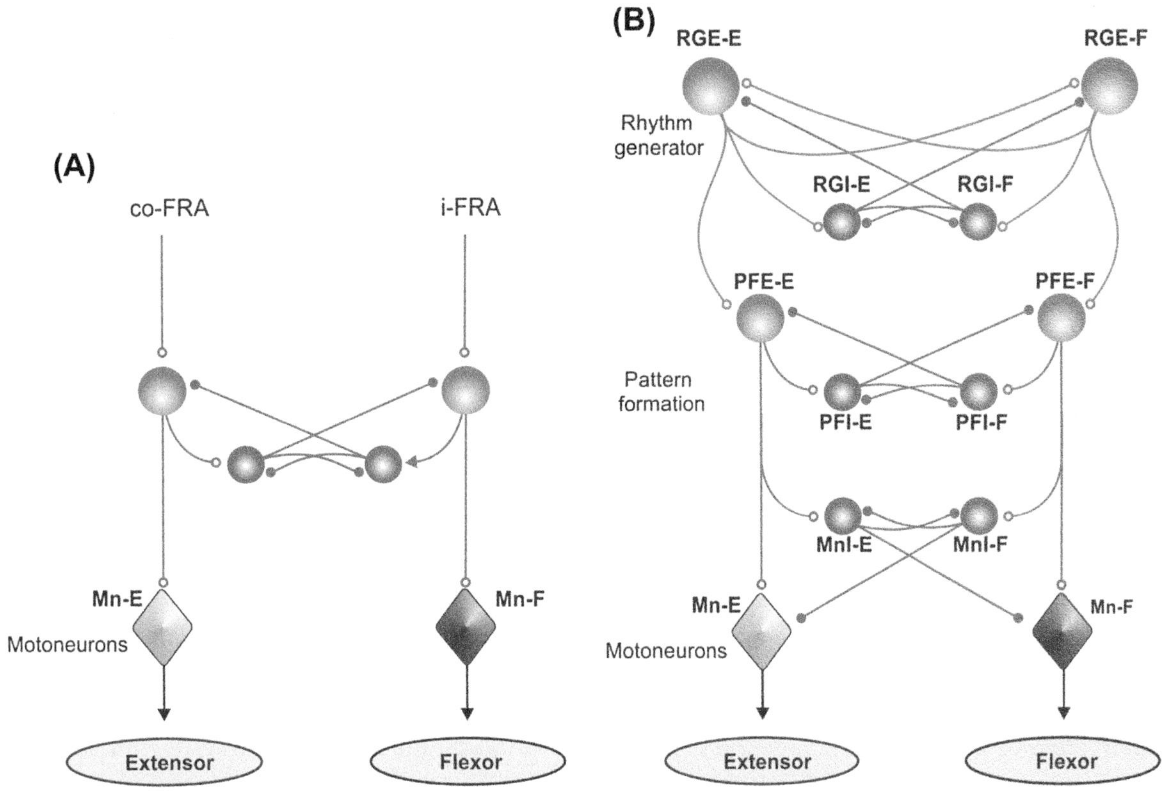

FIGURE 17.3 Models of the CPG. (A) The half-center model of Graham-Brown, as modified by Lundberg to explain the findings in L-DOPA-treated spinal cats. Stimulation of ipsilateral flexor-reflex afferents (iFRAs) produced late-long lasting excitation of flexor motoneurons, while stimulation of contralateral flexor reflex afferents (co-FRAs) produced similar excitation of extensor motoneurons. The L-DOPA treatment produced locomotion in the spinal cat preparation, and the half-center model was proposed as a plausible organization to explain these findings. (B) A computational model of spinal locomotor circuitry with a two-level CPG.[31] Rhythm generator (RG) and pattern formation (PF) networks represent the two levels of the CPG. The excitatory RGE-E (rhythm generator—extensor) and RGE-F (rhythm generator—flexor) populations reciprocally inhibit each other via the inhibitory RG populations RGI. The PF excitatory populations (PFE) reciprocally inhibit each other through the PF inhibitory populations (PFI). The RGE-E and RGE-F populations have recurrent excitatory connections. Locomotion is initiated by a tonic excitatory drive (from MLR and/or MRF) to both the RG and PF populations. The locomotor rhythm and the durations of the flexor and extensor phases are determined by the RG network that controls the activity of the PF network by direct excitation of PFE neurons (and inhibition to PFE neurons mediated by the RGI populations—not shown). PFE population activity produces a phase-specific activation of the corresponding group of synergist motoneuron (Mn-E and Mn-F) pools. Phase-dependent inhibition of motoneurons is produced by the MnI-E and MnI-F populations whose activity is regulated by excitation from the PF network and inhibition from MnI neurons. IaINs are included in the MnI population, and inhibition from Renshaw cells (not shown) as well as mutual inhibitory connections between the MnI populations can also control MnI rhythmicity. (For color version of this figure, the reader is referred to the online version of this book.)

intrathecal yohimbine, an $alpha_2$ receptor antagonist, impaired locomotion in intact cats.[39] Intraspinal injections of clonidine were effective in a restricted area of the midlumbar spinal cord in cats.[40,41] In freely moving rats, intrathecal administration of yohimbine produced transient paralysis,[42] consistent with a role for the descending noradrenergic pathway in the production of locomotion.

In rodents, 5-HT is the most potent neurotransmitter that elicits locomotion in the isolated neonatal spinal cord.[43] Precursors or agonists of 5-HT can elicit locomotion in spinal rats, mice, and rabbits, but not in spinal cats (reviewed in Ref. 28). Stimulation of a specific area in the medulla containing 5-HT neurons, the parapyramidal region (PPR), gives rise to locomotion in the isolated brainstem–spinal cord preparation of neonatal rats.[44] 5-HT_{2A} and 5-HT_7 receptors are both able to activate the CPG, and the 5-HT_{2A} receptor increases the excitability of motoneurons. A combination of 5-HT_{2A} and 5-HT_7 receptor agonists is more effective than either alone in eliciting locomotion in rats with complete spinal transections.[45] A prominent action of 5-HT acting at these receptors is to control intra- and interlimb coordination.[27,46] Partial restoration of coordinated locomotion in spinal rats occurs after intraspinal grafting of 5-HT neurons, which is blocked by a 5-HT antagonist.[47] Efforts to restore locomotion after spinal cord injury have targeted regeneration or regrowth in the 5-HT pathway.

A putative dopaminergic system descending from the A11 group of dopaminergic neurons of the hypothalamus (reviewed in Refs 27,28) is implicated in locomotor control. DA agonists are necessary for eliciting locomotor activity in the isolated in vitro functionally mature mouse spinal cord[48] and are sufficient for activating the locomotor CPG in neonatal preparations.[49–51] The dopaminergic activation of the CPG is mediated by D1 receptors in the mouse spinal cord.[52] DA is less effective than other neurotransmitters for eliciting locomotion in spinal animals, but it appears to be required for 5-HT-induced locomotion.[53] The dopaminergic pathway originates in the A11 group of dopaminergic neurons, which is located in the posterior hypothalamus.

Locomotion is elicited by application of several transmitters and neuromodulators into the MRF (Figure 17.2). Cholinergic activation via muscarinic receptors is effective in cats[23] and rats,[24] consistent with a cholinergic input from the PPN. In a transgenic mouse line in which Cre-recombinase is selectively expressed in 5-HT neurons (ePet–Cre mice), a conditional pseudorabies virus that replicates only in Cre-expressing neurons was injected into the serotonergic area of the caudal medulla.[54] Retrograde labeling was observed in PPN, showing that medullary 5-HT neurons receive input from PPN. Stimulation of PPN in brainstem slices produced prolonged responses in RS neurons located immediately anterior to the inferior olive, in a region including the magnocellular reticular formation (pars alpha), the ventral reticular nucleus (pars alpha), and the PPR, referred to as the medioventral medulla (MED) by Garcia-Rill and coworkers[55] and the MRF by Jordan's group.[56] A cholinergic agonist excited the MED or MRF cells, an effect blocked by a muscarinic antagonist.

EAA are also effective when injected into the MRF,[24,56] as would be expected from glutamatergic input from the CN.[57] A recent study[57] using vesicular glutamate transporter 2–channelrhodopsin2–yellow fluorescent protein (Vglut2–ChR2–YFP) mouse demonstrated that ChR2–YFP expressed in Vglut2-positive cells could be activated by photo-stimulation to initiate locomotor-like activity in vitro. This effect was blocked by spinal application of kynurenic acid, which acts, in part, to block glutamate receptors and is consistent with a descending glutamatergic system from RS neurons of the MRF.[58] Intrathecal application of other glutamate antagonists blocks MLR-induced locomotion in decerebrate cats, and agonists of glutamate elicit locomotion when applied directly to the spinal cord.[59] In spinal cats, intrathecal *N*-methyl-D-aspartate (NMDA) application enhanced locomotor performance.[60] Intrathecal applications of the NMDA antagonist D(–)-2-amino-5-phosphonopentanoic acid (AP5) in intact cats only slightly perturbed locomotion, but in chronic spinal cats it blocked locomotion completely. In isolated spinal cords from neonatal rats and functionally mature mice, NMDA facilitates locomotor activity.[48,61]

Orexin-A injections into the MRF (gigantocellular reticular nucleus, dorsal to the pyramidal tract) elicit locomotion.[25] This same area produces locomotion when stimulated electrically, and it overlaps with the RS locomotor area (Figure 17.2).

THE LOCOMOTOR AREAS OF THE BRAIN FOR SELECTION OF LOCOMOTION

Mesencephalon

The MLR was originally defined in the decerebrate cat preparation as an area beneath the inferior colliculus, using an electrode placement defined by the external features of the brain. Electrodes were placed in an area identified as CN.[62,63] The anatomical definition of the MLR in the cat has been confirmed many times over in several different laboratories.[64–69] MLR stimulation (CN) in the intact cat produced arousal, sometimes accompanied by a startle response, then locomotor activity proceeding to fast walking, running, and jumping, similar to escape behavior.[70]

The identity of the neurons comprising the MLR remains controversial, however. Garcia-Rill and coworkers[64,71,72] focused on a site in a more medial area of the midbrain 2–3 mm lateral to the midline. They used anterograde and retrograde labeling to define projections from the more medial MLR sites to a lateral area corresponding to Probst's tract.[72] They suggested that Probst's tract, a major output pathway for the PPN, and the pontomedullary locomotor strip (PLS) are coextensive. Electrical stimulation of the PLS produces locomotion,[73,74] and it has been defined not as a fiber pathway but as a series of local neurons that are synaptically connected. Previous workers[66] described the PLS as a column of cells extending from the MLR through the brainstem to the upper cervical levels. Neurons within the PLS project to cells of the medial and lateral reticular formation.[75] Cooling to block PLS and MRF synaptic transmission showed that the MRF and not the PLS is likely to be the pathway for normal production of locomotion.[76] The PLS was shown to correspond closely to the spinal nucleus and tract of the trigeminal nerve, and drug applications into this area facilitated locomotion that could then be evoked by exteroceptive stimulation in the peripheral receptive fields of the trigeminal nerve. This suggests that the PLS stimulus activates sensory input from the face, and gives rise to locomotion in much the same way as sensory input does at the spinal level. The medial MLR region appears to activate the cells of the spinal nucleus of the trigeminal nerve, and not a system of neurons dedicated to the control of locomotion. The medial MLR sites may activate portions of the mesencephalic nucleus of the trigeminal nerve, the sensory neurons providing proprioceptive information from the muscles of mastication. Thus, the medial MLR–PLS locomotor system is likely the vestige of a primitive system described in lamprey, whereby input from the head leads to escape swimming.[77] Subsequent work in mammalian models has focused on the projections from the lateral MLR region originally described by Shik and coworkers[73,74] and its relay through the MRF.

In contrast to the results in cat decerebrate preparations, similar experiments in rats revealed effective sites in both the CN and PPN.[78,79] The PPN contains both cholinergic and glutamatergic neurons, and Garcia-Rill has continued to maintain that the MLR corresponds almost exclusively to the PPN cholinergic neurons.[80] Other workers, however, found effective sites in the CN of rat brainstem, with no overlap with cholinergic regions of the midbrain.[81] They described the PPN as "distinctly ventral to our MLR". In anaesthetized intact rats, stimulation in the mesencephalon in the CN, the deep layers of the superior colliculus, and the more rostral mesencephalic reticular nucleus was shown to be effective.[82] Well-coordinated quadrupedal stepping was elicited in anaesthetized rats by stimulation of the periaqueductal gray, the CN, and lateral aspects of the PPN.[83] More recently, Takakusaki[84] has clearly shown that stimulation of the CN produces locomotion in the decerebrate cat, while PPN stimulation gives rise to decreased muscle tone. A possible explanation for the differences between cat and rat preparations is that the cholinergic neurons of the rat PPN are more important for locomotion than in the cat. In a study using the activity-dependent marker c-fos as a probe for active cells, cholinergic cells of the rat PPN were shown to be relatively inactive during a locomotor task, while numerous CN neurons were labeled.[6]

Midbrain stimulation in decerebrate macaque monkeys also elicits locomotion.[85] The effective stimulus sites were described as the CN and the superior cerebellar peduncle. Midbrain stimulation was also effective for eliciting locomotor activity in decerebrated marmoset monkeys (*Callithrix jacchus*), but the neurons activated were not identified.[86] A lesion occupying a large portion of the midbrain containing the MLR region in humans resulted in gait failure.[87] It is clear that patients with freezing of gait (FOG) have gray matter atrophy in the MLR.[88] In human subjects with Parkinson's disease where MLR stimulation has been attempted to restore locomotion in cases of FOG, the PPN was the initial target.[89] This approach has been disappointing, however, and more recent studies have described the CN and subcuneiform nuclei (sCN) as more effective sites for improving gait than the PPN.[90,91] Functional imaging of imagined gait has shown activity in the MLR, with the CN and the periaqueductal gray most active,[88] and recordings during mimicked steps in human subjects' sCN neurons increased their firing.[92] Some role for the PPN is possible, however, because lesioning of cholinergic mesencephalic neurons produced postural and gait defects in monkeys.[93] Functional imaging of imagined gait showed increased activity in CN as well as PPN.[93]

In lamprey, the MLR and the PPN may be separate structures. In this species, the MLR appears to be a nucleus containing cholinergic neurons that is located dorsal to the PPN and projects to RS locomotor command neurons.[94] Forebrain and brainstem areas for control of locomotion that are homologous with mammalian structures serving the same purpose are found in lamprey. The MLR of this species sends glutamatergic and cholinergic messages to RS neurons to activate swimming.[95]

Diencephalon

There is a broad area in the diencephalon (Figure 17.1) that can be stimulated to produce locomotion, and it has several names, including the subthalamic locomotor region (SLR) or the diencephalic locomotor region (DLR).[16,96] In mammals, the effective sites for evoking locomotion include the fields of Forel and the zona incerta and surrounding areas.[10,97–101] SLR lesions eliminated voluntary locomotion for a restricted period of time, but after 12 days voluntary locomotion began to return.[97] During the initial reduced locomotion period, MLR stimulation restored locomotion. SLR stimulation in intact cats produced exploratory-like behavior.[70] In intact rats, lateral hypothalamus stimulation caused the animals to walk with head movements indicative of exploration. The locomotion started after a period of sniffing, which is typical of exploratory behavior.[102] These authors also stimulated the posterior hypothalamus, where the response was escape-like vigorous locomotion and running.

The diencephalon contains a projection from the hippocampus and amygdala to the nucleus accumbens and onward to the subpallidal region and the MLR,[103] and there are inputs from the lateral hypothalamic area to the MLR as well as the RS locomotor command neurons.[104] Under some behavioral circumstances, the MLR is a necessary relay for the production of locomotion from limbic structures.[105]

Orexin (Ox) neurons (Figure 17.2) are located in the perifornical lateral hypothalamus and project to the mesopontine tegmentum, including the MLR. The lateral hypothalamic sites containing Ox neurons[106] overlap extensively with the sites in the lateral and posterior hypothalamus that effectively elicit locomotion in intact rats.[102,107] This area may also overlap with the effective sites for evoking locomotion within the nearby fields of Forel and the zona incerta.[10,98] Ox neurons in the lateral hypothalamus express c-fos after an exploratory locomotor task in cats[108] or after locomotion on an activity wheel,[109] and are implicated in the control of exploratory locomotion. Orexin injected into the CN in cats produces locomotion, and when applied to the PPN, it suppressed PPN-induced muscle atonia.[84] Locomotion is impaired in $Ox^{-/-}$ mice, and intraventricular application of an Ox receptor antagonist impaired locomotion in wild-type mice.[109] Locomotion induced by stimulation of the lateral hypothalamic area occurs despite lesions in the MLR,[97] and lateral hypothalamus neurons terminate on RS neurons in the medulla.[110] Orexin-containing fibers contact 5-HT neurons in the medulla, including the raphe pallidus, the raphe obscurus, and the PPR.[111] As described in this chapter, the PPR[44] is one of the descending command structures of the MRF able to elicit locomotion. Figure 17.2 shows a diagram illustrating the possible role of lateral hypothalamic orexinergic neurons in the control of locomotion.

Basal Ganglia

The basal ganglia (Figure 17.1) are thought to form a mechanism for action selection, with output through the globus pallidus interna (GPi) and the substantia nigra pars reticulate (SNr).[15,16] Both receive input from the substantia nigra *pars compacta* (SNc) and the PPN, and they both project directly to brainstem locomotor centers.[94,112] Their output neurons are GABAergic inhibitory neurons,[113] and they have a high level of resting activity, keeping MLR neurons under tonic inhibition. Subpopulations of basal ganglia output neurons project to different brainstem motor centers, thereby preventing them from being activated unless the inhibitory control is blocked through basal ganglia input. The striatum contains neurons that are difficult to activate, but once recruited they provide a powerful inhibition of the GPi and SNr, so that the MLR neurons are disinhibited and thus become active enough to elicit locomotion.[114] Optogenetic stimulation of the striatal neurons of the pathway to the globus pallidus in mice facilitated ambulatory behavior.[115] Pallidal projections to the MLR were described by Garcia-Rill and coworkers.[69] In the cat, the entopeduncular nucleus (EN), homologous to the globus pallidus in higher mammals and a major output route for the basal ganglia, was retrogradely labeled and antidromically activated from the CN within the MLR.

Cerebral Cortex

The motor cortex contributes to precision walking that requires an exact foot placement, such as on an uneven terrain.[116–119] The role of the motor cortex is considered to be facultative rather than essential because cortical lesions have so little effect on the ability of most animals to walk.[119,120] For example,[121] it was shown that cats with a bilateral pyramidotomy exhibit major locomotor deficits only when challenged to walk either from rung to rung on a horizontal ladder or along the surface of a curved pipe. Thus, the major contribution of the motor cortex during locomotion occurs when the animal modifies its basic locomotor rhythm to accommodate an uneven locomotor terrain. During gait modifications, subpopulations of motor cortical neurones modify the magnitude and phase of the electromyograpic (EMG) activity of all muscles involved in the movement. Different limb trajectories can be produced by differentially modifying cortical activity.[122] The motor cortex plays a small role in the planning of gait modifications for visual control of walking, however. Instead, the posterior parietal cortex appears to contribute to this function. Lesions to the parietal cortex lead to errors in forelimb placement in relation to an advancing obstacle. They also result in deficits in forelimb–hindlimb coordination.[119]

Spinal Cord

The spinal cord contains the basic organization (CPG) needed to provide coordinated locomotor movements.[1–4,123] This is demonstrated by the fact that animals with a complete spinal cord transection can engage in locomotion with appropriate sequencing of muscle activity of the hindlimbs, coordination of the left and right hindlimbs, and alternating activity in flexor and extensor muscles around a joint. It was demonstrated over a century ago that the spinal cord contains the entire neural network necessary to produce "spinal stepping"[124–126] without input from the brain or from sensory afferents to the spinal cord. Activation of noradrenergic $alpha_2$ receptors in the spinal cord was shown to produce locomotion in spinal cats,[29,30,127,128] and this finding led to the development of the notion of a CPG for locomotion in mammals. It also sparked a modern revival of interest in the control of locomotion in vertebrates. Subsequent work demonstrated that locomotor output recorded in peripheral muscle nerves can be elicited in a variety of preparations with blockage of neuromuscular transmission (fictive locomotion), which is further evidence supporting the CPG concept.

The development of in vitro fictive locomotion preparations using isolated neonatal rat or mouse spinal cord (reviewed in Ref. 129) has accelerated our understanding of the organization of the CPG. It is now clear that the locomotor CPG is distributed along the spinal cord, and it can be activated at different levels by inputs or neurotransmitters that activate the neurons in a specific area of the spinal cord. In spinal cats, noradrenergic activation of the CPG requires neurons in the L3–L4 segments,[130] while more rostral segments are particularly important in rodents. When neurons in L1–L2 of the intact adult rat were destroyed by kainate injection, voluntary locomotion was greatly impaired, in contrast to the results of injections of kainate elsewhere in the spinal cord.[131]

Models of the CPG

Graham-Brown[132] proposed a spinal CPG that could produce the rhythmic alternating activity of flexor and extensor motoneurons during locomotion, and it was termed the "half-center" model (Figure 17.3(A)). This idea was later tested by Lundberg and colleagues in experiments on spinal interneurons involved in flexion reflexes, in an effort to determine if such reflexes could serve as the basic building blocks of the circuitry responsible for mammalian locomotion.[29,30,133] This half-center CPG organization contains two groups of excitatory neurons that directly control the activity of flexor and extensor muscles. Mutual inhibitory interconnections between the flexor- and extensor-related excitatory neurons are the basis for the rhythmic activity, assuring that the antagonist neuron groups cannot be active simultaneously. A process described as "fatigue" was proposed as the means to reduce excitation in the active excitatory neurons, and this resulted in release of the inhibitory input to the antagonist neurons and hence switching from flexion to extension and from extension to flexion. This "fatigue" process could be explained by the presence of a spike-frequency adaptation in the CPG neurons. Various iterations of this model have appeared in the intervening years, culminating in the model illustrated in Figure 17.3(B). This model, proposed by McCrea and Rybak,[31] consists of a two-level CPG with a common rhythm generator (RG) that controls the operation of the pattern formation (PF) circuitry responsible for motoneuron activation. This two-level CPG organization has been investigated with a computational model that includes populations of spinal interneurons and motoneurons modeled in the Hodgkin–Huxley style, with persistent sodium currents (I_{NaP}) as key elements of their cellular properties. Their simulations demonstrate that a two-level CPG can reproduce experimental results, such as spontaneous deletions of motoneuron activity and a variety of effects of afferent stimulation. The two-level concept is based largely on the observation that deletions of motoneuron activity during an ongoing rhythm, such as extensor motoneuron silencing for one or more steps while the flexor rhythm continues, can occur without changing the timing of the next step. This has been termed a "nonresetting deletion", in contrast to deletions that are associated with a change in the timing of subsequent steps.[9,134] This organization accounts for the independent control of motoneuron activity and the locomotor rhythm, so that the rhythm can be altered without changes in the level of motoneuron activity,[135] and motoneuron activity can be changed without altering the locomotor cycle.[136–138] A further element of this organization is the presence of a "reciprocity module",[9] where one set of excitatory interneurons (PFE neurons) drives both its agonist motoneurons and the inhibitory interneurons (PFI neurons) to the antagonist motoneurons.[139]

An important role for persistent sodium currents (I_{NaP}) in the production of locomotion has been suggested by the actions of drugs that influence I_{NaP} on fictive locomotion in rat,[140] mouse,[141] and salamander[142] spinal cord, and on interneurons in the ventral horn, including cells implicated in the control of locomotion.[141,143–146] In the McCrea–Rybak model, I_{NaP} is used as the basis for interneuron firing. It seems likely that some CPG neurons will be characterized by the presence of I_{NaP}.

The final common pathway for production of movement is through spinal motoneurons, and their properties are altered during locomotion, so that they become more excitable and more easily recruited (reviewed in Ref. 147). Box 17.1 provides a simplified summary of the changes in motoneurons that occur in going from the resting condition to the locomotor state. These changes are an integral part of the processes that are activated when locomotion is initiated, but the details of the mechanisms giving rise to these changes are just beginning to be examined.

CPG INTERNEURONS

A number of identified spinal cord interneurons are known to be active during locomotion, based largely on studies using fictive locomotion. Intracellular recordings from motoneurons revealed the presence of rhythmic membrane potential oscillations termed locomotor drive potentials (LDPs).[148,149] These oscillations were shown to consist of excitatory synaptic input alternating with inhibitory synaptic input.[150–152] The interneurons responsible for the LDP have not been identified, but some of the physiologically identified interneuron types are candidates for these roles, and for the various roles in the CPG defined in the McCrea and Rybak model described in this chapter.

Ia Inhibitory Interneurons (IaINs)

Reciprocal inhibition of motoneurons is provided by IaINs, and they are active during locomotion in phase with motoneurons to the homonymous muscle from which the Ia afferents that excite them arise.[151,153,154] They project to motoneurons of antagonists muscles to

BOX 17.1

SUMMARY OF THE CHANGES IN MOTONEURONS THAT OCCUR IN GOING FROM THE RESTING CONDITION TO THE LOCOMOTOR STATE

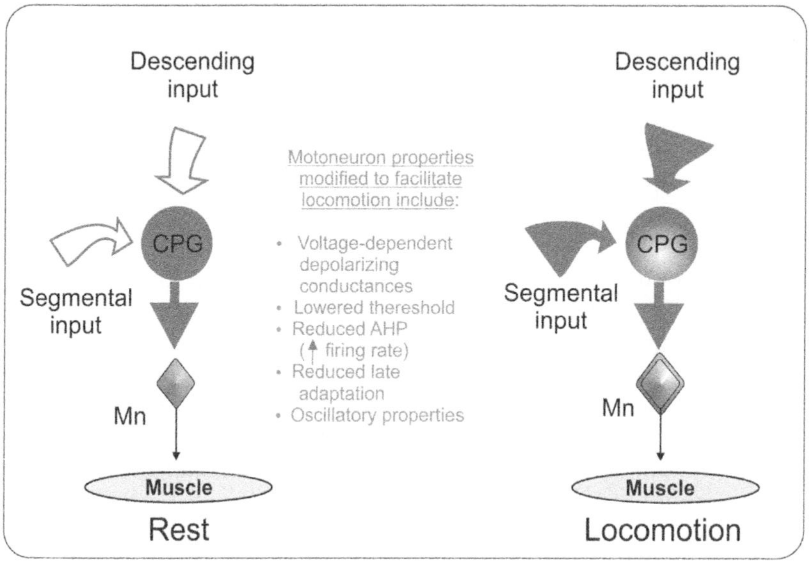

inhibit them. They provide part, but not all, of the inhibitory phase of the motoneuron LDP. If they are physiologically inactivated due to stimulation of the Renshaw cells (RCs) that inhibit them, the inhibitory phase of the LDP is not abolished. In the McCrea-Rybak model (Figure 17.3(B)), they form part of the MnI population.

Renshaw Cells

RCs were the first spinal cord interneuron class to be physiologically identified. They are responsible for recurrent inhibition of motoneurons and IaINs, and they are rhythmically active concurrently with the population of IaINs that they are known to inhibit during locomotion.[154,155] Pharmacological inactivation of RCs during locomotion by blocking their synaptic drive from motoneuron recurrent collaterals does not perturb the rhythm, but it increases the firing of both IaINs and motoneurons.[156]

Cholinergic Propriospinal Neurons

Cholinergic propriospinal neurons of the spinal cord are active during locomotion based upon c-fos labeling and electrophysiological recording, and among these is a population of commissural cholinergic neurons that are vigorously active during ipsilateral extension.[157] There is also a small cluster of spinal cholinergic interneurons in lamina VIII (V0c; see the "V0 Interneurons" section) that represents the sole source of C bouton inputs to motoneurons and controls motoneuron excitability by reducing the amplitude of the afterhyperpolarization (AHP).

INTERNEURONS IDENTIFIED ON THE BASIS OF PROGENITOR DOMAIN

Recent developments in developmental neurobiology have led to the identification of a number of spinal interneurons that may play diverse roles in the control of locomotion.[158] The identity of these various populations is based upon their expression of specific transcription factors that are important for specifying each phenotype during development. It is possible to achieve permanent labeling of spinal subpopulations in the mouse using Cre expression that is driven from a promoter transiently expressed in a defined progenitor domain. The

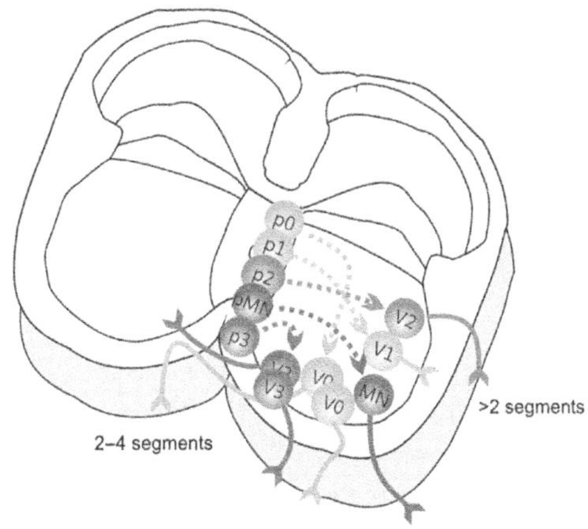

	Progenitors	Postmitotic		Transmitter	Axonal projection	
V0	Dbx1/2	?	V0d	GABA/Glycine 70%	Commissural	MN ?
		Evx1/2	V0v	Glutamate 25%	Commissural	MN ?
		Pitx2	V0c	Acetylcholine 5%	Ipsilateral/Bilateral	MN IaIN ?
V1	Dbx2	En1	RC	GABA/Glycine	Ipsilateral	MN IaIN
			IaIN			MN IaIN
			75% ?			?
V2	Lhx3/4	Lhx3, Chx10 (EphA4)	V2a	Glutamate	Ipsilateral	MN V0
		GATA2/3	V2b	GABA/Glycine		?
pMN	Nkx6-1	Hb9	MN	Acetylcholine	Perhipheral	Muscles
V3	Nkx2-2, Nkx6-1	Sim1	V3s	Glutamate	Commissural 85%	MN RC IaIN V2
			V3r		Ipsilateral 15%	
?	?	Hb9	?	Glutamate	Ipsilateral	MN ?

FIGURE 17.4 Diagram representing the progenitor domains (p0–p3) that give rise to ventral spinal interneuron groups (V0–V3). The transcription factors that characterize the progenitor domains and the postmitotic interneuron subgroups are illustrated. Where possible the transmitter phenotypes of the interneuron subgroups are given, along with their known sites of termination. Motoneuron progenitors and their associated transcription factors are also illustrated. Interneurons that express Hb9 (similar to motoneurons) are also illustrated, although the cardinal progenitor group that produces them is not known. V0d: dorsal V0 interneurons; V0v: ventral V0 interneurons; V0c: cholinergic V0 interneurons; RCs: Renshaw cells; IaIN: Ia inhibitory interneurons; V2a: excitatory V2 interneurons; V2b: inhibitory V2 interneurons; MN: motoneurons; V3s: V3 interneurons producing synchrony; V3r: V3 interneurons with connections expected of rhythm-generating layer neurons. (The figure is reproduced in color section.)

cross between such Cre mice and a ubiquitous reporter mouse strain leads to the expression of a reporter protein such as green fluorescent protein (GFP) upon Cre recombination. This strategy permanently labels postmitotic neurons as they differentiate. Figure 17.4 summarizes the interneurons that have been characterized using such a strategy. The neurons identified in this manner that are located in the ventral horn have been the targets for investigation into their possible roles during locomotion, and their properties and putative roles in locomotion have been extensively reviewed.[159–164]

The canonical progenitor domains p0–p3 give rise to postmitotic classes of interneurons that are further defined by the expression of specific transcription factors. As shown in Figure 17.4, they give rise to four classes of ventral postmitotic interneuron subclasses (V0–V3) defined by the expression of specific transcription factors. Details about the anatomy and physiology of the interneuron subclasses are now emerging, along with experiments in which these neurons are selectively silenced, that allow suggestions about their roles in the control of locomotion to be made.

V0 Interneurons

P0 progenitors are defined by expression of the homeobox gene Dbx1, and they give rise to three interneuron subclasses: V0d, V0v, and V0c. Evx1/2 expression defines postmitotic V0d (dorsal and inhibitory) commissural neurons. V0v (ventral and excitatory) commissural neurons have not yet been associated with any postmitotic transcription factor. A type of ipsilateral (and possibly bilateral) V0c (ipsilateral and bilateral cholinergic) neuron expresses the postmitotic transcription factor Pitx1. V0 neurons are rhythmically active during locomotion,[165] and ablation of Dbx1 neurons impairs left–right coordination in neonatal spinal cord preparations.[166] Although commissural cells have been extensively studied during fictive locomotion (reviewed in Refs 129,167,168), and they must be responsible for left–right alternation, commissural cells within a segment of the spinal cord are not essential for locomotion, because locomotion can proceed unperturbed after midsagittal sections of the spinal cord for several segments (reviewed in Ref. 169). Thus, a small contingent of commissural interneurons crossing at some distance from the affected motoneuron groups is sufficient for maintaining left–right alternation.

The V0c ipsilateral subclass, expressing the transcription factor Pitx2, has been identified as a new class of physiologically and anatomically defined interneuron group. They are lamina VIII cholinergic cells that project to ipsilateral motoneurons and form cholinergic C-terminals.[170,171] They act via M2 muscarinic receptors to reduce the AHP of motoneurons, thus controlling their excitability. The AHP is reduced during fictive locomotion,[172] and silencing the V0c neurons limits motoneuron output during a locomotor task.[171] V0c interneurons also project to IaINs, so they not only control the activity of motoneurons but also influence the interneurons that are responsible for inhibition of antagonist motoneurons.[173] They are also known to receive 5-HT terminals, making them likely targets for the brainstem 5-HT locomotor system.

V1 Interneurons

V1 interneurons are all ipsilateral inhibitory interneurons, and they include all RCs and some IaINs. Most V1 interneurons have not been physiologically identified, but this class does not appear to include the inhibitory interneurons responsible for much of the hyperpolarized phase of the motoneuron LDP. Ablation or acute silencing of these neurons reduces locomotor speed,[174] but it does not reduce the hyperpolarized phase of the LDP. It is clear that another progenitor domain likely is responsible for other inhibitory interneuron development, because IaINs persist after V1 ablation.[175]

In swimming vertebrates such as zebrafish and tadpoles, there is a simpler relationship between embryonic progenitor domains and mature categories of spinal interneurons. For example, embryonic V1 interneurons generate one type of interneuron in zebrafish and tadpoles[176,177] but several subtypes in mammals,[178,179] including RCs and some Ia inhibitory interneurons (IaINs). Approximately 75% of V1 interneurons are neither RCs nor IaINs, and their physiological identification has not been established.

V2 Interneurons

The p2 domain gives rise to excitatory **V2a-INs** and inhibitory **V2b-INs** in mammals, but V2a-INs in zebrafish differentiate into one type of IN, excitatory circumferential ipsilateral descending (CiD) IN, with functional differences based on the time of neurogenesis. Early-born V2a-CiD-INs are dorsally located and are active during escape or fast swimming, while later born neurons are ventrally located and active during sustained swimming.[180,181] In zebrafish, these last-order excitatory interneurons terminating on motoneurons are essential components of the CPG. In limbed vertebrates such as mice, however, **V2a-INs** maintain contacts with motoneurons, but ablation only disrupts left–right coordination.[182,183] They may make up a part of the PFE population in the McCrea–Rybak model (Figure 17.3) that is important for control of the contralateral CPGs, but they clearly do not provide a major portion of the rhythmic excitatory input to motoneurons during locomotion. They are excited by 5-HT, but they do not appear to have conditional bursting properties.[184]

V2b-INs are inhibitory neurons that project to motoneurons. They may form part of the MnI group, but their action during locomotion is unknown. They may also be candidates for the other inhibitory populations in the McCrea–Rybak model, including RGI and PFI.

V3 Interneurons

V3-INs (glutamatergic) are mostly commissural, although some 15% are ipsilateral. Ablation of V3-INs reduces the "robustness" of the locomotor rhythm, interfering with coordination.[185] The commissural ones (V3s) appear to be responsible for synchrony[186] when inhibitory influences are removed. Because they project to V2-INs, V3r interneurons are candidate RGE neurons in the McCrea–Rybak model. They are not pacemaker cells, however, and they do not respond to 5-HT, so they may not form a major component of the RG layer.

Hb9 Interneurons

Defined by postnatal expression of the transcription factor Hb9,[187,188] these neurons have received considerable attention as potential rhythm-generating cells (RGE in the McCrea–Rybak model). Their potential role in locomotion has been extensively reviewed.[129,189,190] They are rhythmically active during fictive locomotion, they receive input from 5-HT fibers, and they are activated by primary afferent fibers. They display postinhibitory rebound, a characteristic of RGE in other species, and they have conditional bursting properties that appear in the presence of substances that elicit locomotion in the isolated mouse spinal cord. They are not derived from any of the known cardinal progenitors, and ablation of these neurons has not been accomplished. Their pattern of activity during fictive locomotion has indicated that they may not be essential for rhythm generation, because they commence firing after the ventral root of the same segment.[191] Nevertheless, without a clear demonstration that the recorded motoneurons are driven by the recorded Hb9 cells, such a conclusion is tentative, and definition of the role played by Hb9 neurons in locomotion must await future experiments.

It is clear from the foregoing that none of the genetically identified interneuron subgroups have clearly defined functional roles in locomotion. Further refinement of the transcription factor code can be expected to improve this situation. It is also clear that the physiological identification of none of the groups of neurons proposed in the McCrea–Rybak model has been accomplished. Current knowledge from both perspectives suggests many hypotheses that can be subjected to rigorous testing, and it can be hoped that such approaches will be fruitful.

SENSORY CONTROL OF LOCOMOTION

Despite the fact that sensory input is not necessary for the basic pattern of locomotion to occur, the CPG is under very potent control from descending pathways and from sensory afferents. These effects have been reviewed extensively.[2,192,193] Sensory input to the CPG serves several vital functions, including inducing or permitting locomotion, preventing or stopping locomotion, and correcting ongoing steps depending on the task or the phase of locomotion (e.g. the ability to step over obstacles). Locomotor activity can alter afferent control, such as changing a reflex from inhibitory to excitatory, sometimes in a phase-dependent manner. Afferent input is also controlled by presynaptic inhibition, which varies extensively depending upon the step cycle.

Cutaneous Afferents

Paramount among the effects of afferent input is the ability of sensory stimulation to activate the locomotor CPG. The CPG can be activated by activity in a variety of peripheral afferents. In rodents, tail stimulation[194] produces a stepping response in rats with a complete spinal transection (spinal rat). A similar approach has been used in cats, where perineal and/or tail stimuli are used to elicit locomotion in chronic spinal cats.[126,195] Tail stimulation and electrical stimulation of the cauda equine are effective means of eliciting fictive locomotion in isolated rodent spinal cord preparations.[51,196–201] Dorsal root stimulation can also produce locomotor activity.[128,202] The ability of peripheral afferent activation to activate the locomotor CPG probably underlies the effectiveness of epidural stimulation and intraspinal microstimulation to restore locomotion.[203,204]

Cutaneous receptors on the plantar surface of the paw[205–207] can facilitate locomotion or initiate stepping.[208] Denervation of the hindpaw eliminates the recovery of locomotion after spinal cord injury that could not be overcome by extensive training.[207] Local anesthetic applied to the paw in spinal rats[45] showed that inputs from the plantar surface of the foot are essential for facilitation of stepping by loading of the limb. Cutaneous receptors on the back are able to stop ongoing locomotor activity.[209,210]

Cutaneous input has the ability to modify locomotor output, as demonstrated by the stumbling corrective response.[211,212] This is a response to cutaneous stimulation of the dorsal surface of the paw during the swing phase of locomotion. This results in flexion of the limb, followed by stepping over the obstacle and placing the foot in front of it. This occurs in spinal animals as well as in fictive locomotion.[213] When the same stimulus is applied during the stance phase of locomotion, the response is reversed, so that flexion does not occur, but there is increased extension.[214]

Proprioceptive Afferents

Proprioceptors responding to hip extension were considered by Sherrington[126] to be responsible for the initiation of the swing phase of locomotion. Hip extension beyond a particular point is necessary for the initiation of the swing phase of locomotion,[215] and hip movements can reset and entrain the locomotor rhythm,[135,216,217] with hip extension leading to flexor bursts. Hip joint capsule denervation was without effect, and low-threshold stretch-sensitive muscle afferents appear to be responsible for the influence of hip movement to prolong extension and initiate flexion.[135] Movements about the hip joint were shown to have a potent effect on the locomotor rhythm, with increased hip extension resulting in increased frequency of fictive locomotion.

Loading, based on current knowledge of the central actions of proprioceptors, has been reviewed in detail.[31,193] Load receptors in muscles of the rat[218] and cat[137,219–221] can facilitate locomotion. The strategy of loading of extensor muscles in human subjects with spinal cord injury[222,223] and in spinal animals[218,224,225] has been used to facilitate recovery of locomotion.

Muscle stretch or vibration of the hip flexor muscles during the stance phase of locomotion leads to early onset of the swing phase,[226] implicating muscle spindle afferents in flexor muscles as a possible source of afferent input that could account for the restoration of plantar stepping. Muscle spindle afferents are also effective for controlling the timing of the phases of the locomotor cycle.[136,137] Activation of Golgi tendon organs is sufficient[219–221] for positive force feedback effects to prolong the stance phase of locomotion.

CLINICAL APPLICATIONS

A Locomotor CPG in Primates and Humans

Early work on the presence of a CPG in macaque monkeys (*Macaca fascicularis*) did not support this concept,[85] despite the use of agents that were known to induce spinal locomotion in lower animals. Some years later, however, administration of a variety of pharmacological agents to acutely spinalized marmoset monkeys (*C. jacchus*) in the absence of phasic afferent input to the spinal cord elicited fictive locomotion, showing clearly that primates possess a CPG for locomotion similar to that observed in lower animals.[86]

Bussel and coworkers[227] examined a patient with a complete spinal cord section who exhibited rhythmical contractions (0.5 Hz frequency) of the trunk and lower limb extensor muscles, and they interpreted these observations as support for the presence of a CPG in humans. In 1994, Calancie et al.[228] described the "first well-defined example of a central RG for stepping in the adult human." A 37-year-old male with an injury to the cervical spinal cord regained some movement of the arms and fingers and limited movement in the lower limbs. When lying supine and extending his hips, the subject's lower limbs engaged in stepping movements. "The movements (1) involved alternating flexion and extension of his hips, knees, and ankles; (2) were smooth and rhythmic; (3) were forceful enough that the subject soon became uncomfortable due to excessive muscle 'tightness' and an elevated body temperature; and (4) could not be stopped by voluntary effort."[228] Calancie and his colleagues concluded that "these data represent the clearest evidence to date that such a [CPG] network does exist in man." Other clear evidence comes from the use of epidural stimulation in humans, in an effort to activate the spinal CPG directly with electrical stimulation.[229] In these studies, human subjects with complete paralysis of the legs were induced to perform coordinated stepping movements when the spinal cord was stimulated. Nadeau et al.[230] described a patient with a complete spinal cord transection at T5 who spontaneously developed frequent continuous rhythmic activity of the lower trunk and legs. They concluded, "The rhythmic activity observed in the patient appeared related to the activation of a spinal pattern generator akin to what has been described in most animal species after complete spinal lesions."

Activation of the Spinal CPG in Spinal Cord Injury

Efforts to restore locomotion in patients with spinal cord injuries and other disease states associated with loss of walking movements include locomotor training, epidural stimulation of the spinal cord or deep brain stimulation (DBS), and pharmacological activation of the CPG. It has been possible to restore coordinated, weight-supported, upright bipedal treadmill locomotion in rodents with a total spinal cord transection using a combination of pharmacological and electrical means of activating the CPG, together with locomotor training.[231] A substantial contribution to this recovery is likely activation of the CPG from cutaneous afferents arising in the hindpaw.[45] Epidural stimulation has been shown to have benefit in a human subject with spinal cord injury.[232] It enabled full weight-bearing standing for up to 25 min with assistance provided only for balance. Locomotor-like patterns could be produced when stimulation parameters were optimized for stepping. Several months after implantation of the epidural electrodes, the patient recovered voluntary control of some leg movements, but only during epidural stimulation. DBS with electrodes placed in brain locomotor regions has been suggested as a means of restoring locomotion in cases of partial spinal cord injury, but this has not yet been systematically tested.

DBS in Parkinson's Disease

Oscillatory rhythms in different frequency ranges are thought to coherently bind cooperating neuronal assemblies. Selection of locomotor output by the basal ganglia is proposed to be associated with gamma oscillations (20–100 Hz), particularly in the PPN,[233] and this has been emphasized as a criterion for DBS site selection to restore locomotion in cases of Parkinsonism with freezing gait.[234] The limbic output that selects locomotor activity, however, is associated instead with theta rhythm, which is first described in the hippocampus of the rat as oscillations (6–11 Hz) that appeared at locomotion onset. Theta rhythms (4–12 Hz) occur in several cortical and subcortical regions, including the striatum. Phase coupling in goal-directed behavior involving the hippocampus and the striatum is governed by theta oscillations and not by gamma oscillations.[235] Consistent with this, observations in PPN slices show that although there is gamma activity in PPN neurons excited by depolarizing current injection, cholinergic and glutamatergic excitation was associated with a marked increase in theta rhythm.[233] Theta rhythm recorded in human PPN is correlated with the speed of gait,[236] but gamma peaks were not observed during gait or at rest. Just prior to the onset of an episode of freezing gait, there was a significant drop in theta rhythm.

Other locomotor areas in the rat have been shown to express theta rhythm during locomotion, and these include the SLR and the posterior hypothalamus.[102,237] In these studies, the sites for recording that displayed the theta rhythm were determined to be effective for eliciting locomotion, and then extracellular field potentials were recorded during spontaneous and induced locomotion. Posterior hypothalamus stimulation with GABA antagonists also elicits locomotor movements,[238] and lesions of the posterior hypothalamus reduce both voluntary movement and theta frequency during movement.[239] Theta and alpha (8–12 Hz) rhythm in the globus pallidus internum, which is a target for DBS in dystonia and involved in the selection of locomotor behavior, increases during treadmill locomotion in human subjects.[240]

Taken together, these studies suggest that an oscillatory rhythm that coherently binds cooperating neuronal assemblies involved in locomotion is more likely to be the theta rhythm and not the gamma rhythm. This may have important clinical implications, because currently neurosurgeons are using gamma band activity as a search criterion for the selection of sites suitable for DBS to restore normal gait.[241] Structures displaying a theta rhythm may be better targets for DBS to restore locomotion.[236] These authors found that the best outcome in freezing gait patients was achieved when the DBS stimulus was applied at the site of maximal theta activity (termed "alpha" in this chapter and defined as 7–12 Hz).

CONCLUDING REMARKS

This review of the networks of neurons controlling locomotion has focused on the recent knowledge extending that available in numerous reviews of the subject over the past decade. We have emphasized the aspects of locomotor control that have been adopted for clinical application. We discussed the importance of MLR structures in the use of DBS to provide improved gait in freezing gait experienced by patients with Parkinson's disease. The controversy about the relative roles of the PPN and CN in the initiation of locomotion, and their importance in various species, has re-emerged in this context. The opportunities for using optogenetics and other newly developed techniques to specifically test hypotheses about the role of these nuclei are evident. A new interpretation of data showing theta rhythm activity in the various locomotor-controlling structures of the brain gives new impetus to the investigation and clinical use of rhythmic activity in populations of locomotor neurons. The intriguing possibility that extracellular rhythms in brain areas such as limbic structures, diencephalon, and the basal ganglia can be significant in binding together different structures to produce locomotion has emerged. It seems likely that emphasis should be shifted from gamma to theta rhythms for the identification of suitable targets for DBS to correct gait abnormalities. A specific pathway from the medullary 5-HT neurons to the spinal cord that originates in the PPR, a lateral component of these nuclei outside of the midline areas previously presumed to be responsible for this effect, has been defined. The importance of the descending 5-HT system for the production is now well recognized, and it is the target of many efforts to restore locomotion after spinal cord injury. New interpretations of the effects of DLR stimulation have emerged recently. For example, the orexinergic pathway from hypothalamic neurons projecting to both the MLR and MRF may explain the efficacy of lateral hypothalamus stimulation for the production of locomotion. The importance of a dopaminergic pathway from the hypothalamus in the production of locomotion in mice has prompted new interest in the dopaminergic pathways involved in the initiation of locomotion. Specific noradrenergic nuclei that should be investigated in greater detail to reveal their role in the production of locomotion are also identified. The role of sensory feedback from the plantar surface of the foot has now received recognition as an important contributing factor to the potentiation of stepping that occurs with loading of the limb, adding to the interest in proprioceptors that has dominated this field. New genetic tools for the identification of CPG interneurons have produced a surge in the discovery of new subclasses of interneurons. Methods to selectively delete selected neurons from the system have suggested important roles for newly identified interneuron subclasses in the spinal cord CPG. All of this portends that a new understanding of the brain and spinal cord systems for controlling locomotion is on the horizon.

References

1. Rossignol S. Neural control of stereotypic limb movements. In: Rowell LB, Shepherd JT, eds. *Handbook of Physiology, Section 12, Exercise: Regulation and Integration of Multiple Systems*. New York: Oxford University Press; 1996:173–216.
2. Rossignol S, Dubuc R, Gossard JP. Dynamic sensorimotor interactions in locomotion. *Physiol Rev.* 2006;86(1):89–154.
3. Grillner S. *Control of Locomotion in Bipeds, Tetrapods, and Fish*. Vol. 2. Baltimore, MD: Waverly Press; 1981.
4. Grillner S. Neurobiological bases of rhythmic motor acts in vertebrates. *Science*. 1985;228(4696):143–149.
5. Armstrong DM. Supraspinal contributions to the initiation and control of locomotion in the cat. *Prog Neurobiol*. 1986;26(4):273–361.
6. Jordan LM. Initiation of locomotion in mammals. *Ann N Y Acad Sci*. 1998;860:83–93.
7. Shik ML, Orlovsky GN. Neurophysiology of locomotor automatism. *Physiol Rev.* 1976;56(3):465–501.

8. Whelan PJ. Control of locomotion in the decerebrate cat. *Prog Neurobiol.* 1996;49(5):481–515.
9. Jordan LM. Brainstem and spinal cord mechanisms for the initiation of locomotion. In: Shimamura M, Grillner S, Edgerton VR, eds. *Neurobiological Basis of Human Locomotion.* Tokyo: Japan Scientific Societies Press; 1991:3–21.
10. Orlovsky GN. Spontaneous and induced locomotion of the thalamic cat. *Biophysics.* 1969;14:1154–1162.
11. Orlovsky GN, Deliagina TG, Grillner S. *Neuronal Control of Locomotion from Mollusc to Man.* New York: Oxford University Press; 1999.
12. Dubuc R, Brocard F, Antri M, et al. Initiation of locomotion in lampreys. *Brain Res Rev.* 2008;57(1):172–182.
13. Grillner S, Dubuc R. Control of locomotion in vertebrates: spinal and supraspinal mechanisms. *Adv Neurol.* 1988;47:425–453.
14. Jordan LM. Initiation of locomotion from the mammalian brainstem. In: Grillner S, Stein PSG, Stuart DG, Forssberg H, Herman RM, eds. *Neurobiology of Vertebrate Locomotion.* London: Macmillan Press; 1986:21–37.
15. Grillner S, Georgopoulos AP, Jordan LM. Selection and initiation of motor behavior. In: Stein PSG, Grillner S, Selverston AI, Stuart DG, eds. *Neurons, Networks, and Motor Behavior.* Cambridge, MA: MIT Press; 1997:3–19.
16. Grillner S, Wallen P, Saitoh K, Kozlov A, Robertson B. Neural bases of goal-directed locomotion in vertebrates—an overview. *Brain Res Rev.* 2008;57(1):2–12.
17. Humphries MD, Gurney K, Prescott TJ. Is there a brainstem substrate for action selection? *Philos Trans R Soc Lond B Biol Sci.* 2007;362(1485):1627–1639.
18. Matsuyama K, Mori F, Nakajima K, Drew T, Aoki M, Mori S. Locomotor role of the corticoreticular-reticulospinal-spinal interneuronal system. *Prog Brain Res.* 2004;143:239–249.
19. Shik ML, Orlovskii GN, Severin FV. Locomotion of the mesencephalic cat evoked by pyramidal stimulation. *Biofizika.* 1968;13(1):127–135.
20. Drew T, Rossignol S. Functional organization within the medullary reticular formation of intact unanesthetized cat. I. Movements evoked by microstimulation. *J Neurophysiol.* 1990;64(3): 767–781.
21. Drew T, Rossignol S. Functional organization within the medullary reticular formation of intact unanesthetized cat. II. Electromyographic activity evoked by microstimulation. *J Neurophysiol.* 1990;64(3):782–795.
22. Noga BR, Kriellaars DJ, Brownstone RM, Jordan LM. Mechanism for activation of locomotor centers in the spinal cord by stimulation of the mesencephalic locomotor region. *J Neurophysiol.* 2003;90(3):1464–1478.
23. Garcia-Rill E, Skinner RD. The mesencephalic locomotor region. I. Activation of a medullary projection site. *Brain Res.* 1987;411(1): 1–12.
24. Kinjo N, Atsuta Y, Webber M, Kyle R, Skinner RD, Garcia-Rill E. Medioventral medulla-induced locomotion. *Brain Res Bull.* 1990;24(3):509–516.
25. Mileykovskiy BY, Kiyashchenko LI, Siegel JM. Muscle tone facilitation and inhibition after orexin-a (hypocretin-1) microinjections into the medial medulla. *J Neurophysiol.* 2002;87(5): 2480–2489.
26. Alford S, Schwartz E, Viana di Prisco G. The pharmacology of vertebrate spinal central pattern generators. *Neuroscientist.* 2003; 9(3):217–228.
27. Jordan LM, Liu J, Hedlund PB, Akay T, Pearson KG. Descending command systems for the initiation of locomotion in mammals. *Brain Res Rev.* 2008;57(1):183–191.
28. Miles GB, Sillar KT. Neuromodulation of vertebrate locomotor control networks. *Physiology (Bethesda).* 2011;26(6):393–411.
29. Jankowska E, Jukes MG, Lund S, Lundberg A. The effect of DOPA on the spinal cord. 6. Half-centre organization of interneurones transmitting effects from the flexor reflex afferents. *Acta Physiol Scand.* 1967;70(3):389–402.
30. Jankowska E, Jukes MG, Lund S, Lundberg A. The effect of DOPA on the spinal cord. 5. Reciprocal organization of pathways transmitting excitatory action to alpha motoneurones of flexors and extensors. *Acta Physiol Scand.* 1967;70(3):369–388.
31. McCrea DA, Rybak IA. Organization of mammalian locomotor rhythm and pattern generation. *Brain Res Rev.* 2008;57(1): 134–146.
32. Hultborn H, Nielsen JB. Spinal control of locomotion—from cat to man. *Acta Physiol (Oxf).* 2007;189(2):111–121.
33. Steeves JD, Jordan LM, Lake N. The close proximity of catecholamine-containing cells to the 'mesencephalic locomotor region' (MLR). *Brain Res.* 1975;100(3):663–670.
34. Bruinstroop E, Cano G, Vanderhorst VG, et al. Spinal projections of the A5, A6 (locus coeruleus), and A7 noradrenergic cell groups in rats. *J Comp Neurol.* 2012;520(9):1985–2001.
35. Steeves JD, Schmidt BJ, Skovgaard BJ, Jordan LM. Effect of noradrenaline and 5-hydroxytryptamine depletion on locomotion in the cat. *Brain Res.* 1980;185(2):349–362.
36. Górska T, Bem T, Majczyński H, Zmysłowski W. Unrestrained walking in cats with partial spinal lesions. *Brain Res Bull.* 1993;32(3):241–249.
37. Rossignol S, Barriere G, Alluin O, Frigon A. Re-expression of locomotor function after partial spinal cord injury. *Physiology (Bethesda).* 2009;24:127–139.
38. Loy DN, Magnuson DS, Zhang YP, et al. Functional redundancy of ventral spinal locomotor pathways. *J Neurosci.* 2002;22(1):315–323.
39. Giroux N, Reader TA, Rossignol S. Comparison of the effect of intrathecal administration of clonidine and yohimbine on the locomotion of intact and spinal cats. *J Neurophysiol.* 2001;85(6): 2516–2536.
40. Delivet-Mongrain H, Leblond H, Rossignol S. Effects of localized intraspinal injections of a noradrenergic blocker on locomotion of high decerebrate cats. *J Neurophysiol.* 2008;100(2):907–921.
41. Marcoux J, Rossignol S. Initiating or blocking locomotion in spinal cats by applying noradrenergic drugs to restricted lumbar spinal segments. *J Neurosci.* 2000;20(22):8577–8585.
42. Majczyński H, Cabaj A, Sławińska U, Górska T. Intrathecal administration of yohimbine impairs locomotion in intact rats. *Behav Brain Res.* 2006;175(2):315–322.
43. Schmidt BJ, Jordan LM. The role of serotonin in reflex modulation and locomotor rhythm production in the mammalian spinal cord. *Brain Res Bull.* 2000;53(5):689–710.
44. Liu J, Jordan LM. Stimulation of the parapyramidal region of the neonatal rat brain stem produces locomotor-like activity involving spinal 5-HT_7 and 5-HT_{2A} receptors. *J Neurophysiol.* 2005;94(2):1392–1404.
45. Sławińska U, Majczyński H, Dai Y, Jordan LM. The upright posture improves plantar stepping and alters responses to serotonergic drugs in spinal rats. *J Physiol (Lond).* 2012;590(Pt 7):1721–1736.
46. Liu J, Akay T, Hedlund PB, Pearson KG, Jordan LM. Spinal 5-HT_7 receptors are critical for alternating activity during locomotion: in vitro neonatal and in vivo adult studies using 5-HT_7 receptor knockout mice. *J Neurophysiol.* 2009;102(1):337–348.
47. Majczyński H, Maleszak K, Cabaj A, Sławińska U. Serotonin-related enhancement of recovery of hind limb motor functions in spinal rats after grafting of embryonic raphe nuclei. *J Neurotrauma.* 2005;22(5):590–604.
48. Jiang Z, Carlin KP, Brownstone RM. An in vitro functionally mature mouse spinal cord preparation for the study of spinal motor networks. *Brain Res.* 1999;816(2):493–499.

49. Kiehn O, Kjaerulff O. Spatiotemporal characteristics of 5-HT and dopamine-induced rhythmic hindlimb activity in the in vitro neonatal rat. *J Neurophysiol.* 1996;75(4):1472–1482.
50. Barriere G, Mellen N, Cazalets JR. Neuromodulation of the locomotor network by dopamine in the isolated spinal cord of newborn rat. *Eur J Neurosci.* 2004;19(5):1325–1335.
51. Whelan P, Bonnot A, O'Donovan MJ. Properties of rhythmic activity generated by the isolated spinal cord of the neonatal mouse. *J Neurophysiol.* 2000;84(6):2821–2833.
52. Lapointe NP, Rouleau P, Ung RV, Guertin PA. Specific role of dopamine D_1 receptors in spinal network activation and rhythmic movement induction in vertebrates. *J Physiol (Lond).* 2009; 587(Pt 7):1499–1511.
53. Madriaga MA, McPhee LC, Chersa T, Christie KJ, Whelan PJ. Modulation of locomotor activity by multiple 5-HT and dopaminergic receptor subtypes in the neonatal mouse spinal cord. *J Neurophysiol.* 2004;92(3):1566–1576.
54. Braz JM, Enquist LW, Basbaum AI. Inputs to serotonergic neurons revealed by conditional viral transneuronal tracing. *J Comp Neurol.* 2009;514(2):145–160.
55. Mamiya K, Bay K, Skinner RD, Garcia-Rill E. Induction of long-lasting depolarization in medioventral medulla neurons by cholinergic input from the pedunculopontine nucleus. *J Appl Physiol.* 2005;99(3):1127–1137.
56. Noga BR, Kettler J, Jordan LM. Locomotion produced in mesencephalic cats by injections of putative transmitter substances and antagonists into the medial reticular formation and the pontomedullary locomotor strip. *J Neurosci.* 1988;8(6):2074–2086.
57. Hägglund M, Borgius L, Dougherty KJ, Kiehn O. Activation of groups of excitatory neurons in the mammalian spinal cord or hindbrain evokes locomotion. *Nat Neurosci.* 2010;13(2):246–252.
58. Reed WR, Shum-Siu A, Magnuson DS. Reticulospinal pathways in the ventrolateral funiculus with terminations in the cervical and lumbar enlargements of the adult rat spinal cord. *Neuroscience.* 2008;151(2):505–517.
59. Douglas JR, Noga BR, Dai X, Jordan LM. The effects of intrathecal administration of excitatory amino acid agonists and antagonists on the initiation of locomotion in the adult cat. *J Neurosci.* 1993;13(3):990–1000.
60. Chau C, Giroux N, Barbeau H, Jordan L, Rossignol S. Effects of intrathecal glutamatergic drugs on locomotion I. NMDA in short-term spinal cats. *J Neurophysiol.* 2002;88(6):3032–3045.
61. Cowley KC, Schmidt BJ. A comparison of motor patterns induced by *N*-methyl-D-aspartate, acetylcholine and serotonin in the in vitro neonatal rat spinal cord. *Neurosci Lett.* 1994;171(1–2):147–150.
62. Shik ML, Severin FV, Orlovskii GN. Control of walking and running by means of electric stimulation of the midbrain. *Biofizika.* 1966;11(4):659–666.
63. Shik ML, Severin FV, Orlovskii GN. Structures of the brain stem responsible for evoked locomotion. *Fiziol Zh SSSR Im I M Sechenova.* 1967;53(9):1125–1132.
64. Garcia-Rill E, Skinner RD, Jackson MB, Smith MM. Connections of the mesencephalic locomotor region (MLR) I. Substantia nigra afferents. *Brain Res Bull.* 1983;10(1):57–62.
65. Garcia-Rill E, Skinner RD, Fitzgerald JA. Chemical activation of the mesencephalic locomotor region. *Brain Res.* 1985;330(1):43–54.
66. Mori S, Shik ML, Yagodnitsyn AS. Role of pontine tegmentum for locomotor control in mesencephalic cat. *J Neurophysiol.* 1977;40(2): 284–295.
67. Steeves JD, Jordan LM. Autoradiographic demonstration of the projections from the mesencephalic locomotor region. *Brain Res.* 1984;307(1–2):263–276.
68. Jell RM, Elliott C, Jordan LM. Initiation of locomotion from the mesencephalic locomotor region: effects of selective brainstem lesions. *Brain Res.* 1985;328(1):121–128.
69. Garcia-Rill E, Skinner RD, Gilmore SA. Pallidal projections to the mesencephalic locomotor region (MLR) in the cat. *Am J Anat.* 1981;161(3):311–321.
70. Mori S, Sakamoto T, Ohta Y, Takakusaki K, Matsuyama K. Site-specific postural and locomotor changes evoked in awake, freely moving intact cats by stimulating the brainstem. *Brain Res.* 1989;505(1):66–74.
71. Garcia-Rill E. Connections of the mesencephalic locomotor region (MLR) III. Intracellular recordings. *Brain Res Bull.* 1983;10(1): 73–81.
72. Garcia-Rill E, Skinner RD, Gilmore SA, Owings R. Connections of the mesencephalic locomotor region (MLR) II. Afferents and efferents. *Brain Res Bull.* 1983;10(1):63–71.
73. Shik ML, Iagodnitsyn AS. Reactions of cat hindbrain "locomotor strip" neurons to microstimulation. *Neirofiziologiia.* 1978;10(5): 510–518.
74. Shik ML, Iagodnitsyn AS. Pontobulbar "locomotor strip". *Neirofiziologiia.* 1977;9(1):95–97.
75. Budakova NN, Shik ML. Walking does not require continuity of the medullar "locomotion strip". *Biull Eksp Biol Med.* 1980;89(1): 3–6.
76. Shefchyk SJ, Jell RM, Jordan LM. Reversible cooling of the brainstem reveals areas required for mesencephalic locomotor region evoked treadmill locomotion. *Exp Brain Res.* 1984;56(2): 257–262.
77. Viana Di Prisco GV, Pearlstein E, Robitaille R, Dubuc R. Role of sensory-evoked NMDA plateau potentials in the initiation of locomotion. *Science.* 1997;278(5340):1122–1125.
78. Skinner RD, Garcia-Rill E. The mesencephalic locomotor region (MLR) in the rat. *Brain Res.* 1984;323(2):385–389.
79. Johnels B, Steg G. A mechanographic method for measurement of locomotor activity in rats. Effects of dopaminergic drugs and electric stimulation of the brainstem. *J Neurosci Methods.* 1982; 6(1–2):17–27.
80. Garcia-Rill E, Homma Y, Skinner RD. Arousal mechanisms related to posture and locomotion: 1. Descending modulation. *Prog Brain Res.* 2004;143:283–290.
81. Coles SK, Iles JF, Nicolopoulos-Stournaras S. The mesencephalic centre controlling locomotion in the rat. *Neuroscience.* 1989;28(1): 149–157.
82. Mel'nikova ZL. Locomotion of rats induced by stimulation of the mesencephalon. *Vestn Moskov Univ Biol.* 1975;2:45–51.
83. Ross GS, Sinnamon HM. Forelimb and hindlimb stepping by the anesthetized rat elicited by electrical stimulation of the pons and medulla. *Physiol Behav.* 1984;33(2):201–208.
84. Takakusaki K. Forebrain control of locomotor behaviors. *Brain Res Rev.* 2008;57(1):192–198.
85. Eidelberg E, Walden JG, Nguyen LH. Locomotor control in macaque monkeys. *Brain.* 1981;104(Pt 4):647–663.
86. Fedirchuk B, Nielsen J, Petersen N, Hultborn H. Pharmacologically evoked fictive motor patterns in the acutely spinalized marmoset monkey (*Callithrix jacchus*). *Exp Brain Res.* 1998;122(3): 351–361.
87. Masdeu JC, Alampur U, Cavaliere R, Tavoulareas G. Astasia and gait failure with damage of the pontomesencephalic locomotor region. *Ann Neurol.* 1994;35(5):619–621.
88. Snijders AH, Leunissen I, Bakker M, et al. Gait-related cerebral alterations in patients with Parkinson's disease with freezing of gait. *Brain.* 2011;134(Pt 1):59–72.
89. Mazzone P, Lozano A, Stanzione P, et al. Implantation of human pedunculopontine nucleus: a safe and clinically relevant target in Parkinson's disease. *Neuroreport.* 2005;16(17):1877–1881.
90. Ferraye MU, Debu B, Fraix V, et al. Effects of pedunculopontine nucleus area stimulation on gait disorders in Parkinson's disease. *Brain.* 2010;133(Pt 1):205–214.

91. Alam M, Schwabe K, Krauss JK. The pedunculopontine nucleus area: critical evaluation of interspecies differences relevant for its use as a target for deep brain stimulation. *Brain.* 2011;134(Pt 1):11–23.
92. Piallat B, Chabardes S, Torres N, et al. Gait is associated with an increase in tonic firing of the sub-cuneiform nucleus neurons. *Neuroscience.* 2009;158(4):1201–1205.
93. Karachi C, Grabli D, Bernard FA, et al. Cholinergic mesencephalic neurons are involved in gait and postural disorders in Parkinson disease. *J Clin Invest.* 2010;120(8):2745–2754.
94. Stephenson-Jones M, Ericsson J, Robertson B, Grillner S. Evolution of the basal ganglia; dual output pathways conserved throughout vertebrate phylogeny. *J Comp Neurol.* 2012. http://dx.doi.org/10.1002/cne.23087 [Epub ahead of print].
95. Le Ray D, Juvin L, Ryczko D, Dubuc R. Chapter 4—Supraspinal control of locomotion: the mesencephalic locomotor region. *Prog Brain Res.* 2011;188:51–70.
96. El Manira A, Pombal MA, Grillner S. Diencephalic projection to reticulospinal neurons involved in the initiation of locomotion in adult lampreys *Lampetra fluviatilis. J Comp Neurol.* 1997;389(4): 603–616.
97. Sirota MG, Shik ML. Locomotion of the cat on stimulation of the mesencephalon. *Fiziol Zh SSSR Im I M Sechenova.* 1973;59(9): 1314–1321.
98. Waller WH. Progression movements elicited by subthalamic stimulation. *J Neurophysiol.* 1940;3:300–3007.
99. Parker SM, Sinnamon HM. Forward locomotion elicited by electrical stimulation in the diencephalon and mesencephalon of the awake rat. *Physiol Behav.* 1983;31(5):581–587.
100. Milner KL, Mogenson GJ. Electrical and chemical activation of the mesencephalic and subthalamic locomotor regions in freely moving rats. *Brain Res.* 1988;452(1–2):273–285.
101. Kasicki S, Korczyński R, Romaniuk JR, Sławińska U. Two locomotor strips in the diencephalon of thalamic cats. *Acta Neurobiol Exp (Wars).* 1991;51(5–6):137–143.
102. Sławińska U, Kasicki S. Theta-like rhythm in depth EEG activity of hypothalamic areas during spontaneous or electrically induced locomotion in the rat. *Brain Res.* 1995;678(1–2):117–126.
103. Mogenson GJ, Ciriello J, Garland J, Wu M. Ventral pallidum projections to mediodorsal nucleus of the thalamus: an anatomical and electrophysiological investigation in the rat. *Brain Res.* 1987;404(1–2):221–230.
104. Sinnamon HM. Preoptic and hypothalamic neurons and the initiation of locomotion in the anesthetized rat. *Prog Neurobiol.* 1993;41(3):323–344.
105. Brudzynski SM, Mogenson GJ. Association of the mesencephalic locomotor region with locomotor activity induced by injections of amphetamine into the nucleus accumbens. *Brain Res.* 1985;334(1): 77–84.
106. Nambu T, Sakurai T, Mizukami K, Hosoya Y, Yanagisawa M, Goto K. Distribution of orexin neurons in the adult rat brain. *Brain Res.* 1999;827(1–2):243–260.
107. Marciello M, Sinnamon HM. Locomotor stepping initiated by glutamate injections into the hypothalamus of the anesthetized rat. *Behav Neurosci.* 1990;104(6):980–990.
108. Torterolo P, Yamuy J, Sampogna S, Morales FR, Chase MH. Hypocretinergic neurons are primarily involved in activation of the somatomotor system. *Sleep.* 2003;26(1):25–28.
109. Anaclet C, Parmentier R, Ouk K, et al. Orexin/hypocretin and histamine: distinct roles in the control of wakefulness demonstrated using knock-out mouse models. *J Neurosci.* 2009;29(46): 14423–14438.
110. Orlovsky GN. Work of reticulospinal neurones during locomotion. *Biofizika.* 1970;15:728–737.
111. Berthoud HR, Patterson LM, Sutton GM, Morrison C, Zheng H. Orexin inputs to caudal raphe neurons involved in thermal, cardiovascular, and gastrointestinal regulation. *Histochem Cell Biol.* 2005;123(2):147–156.
112. Stephenson-Jones M, Samuelsson E, Ericsson J, Robertson B, Grillner S. Evolutionary conservation of the basal ganglia as a common vertebrate mechanism for action selection. *Curr Biol.* 2011;21(13):1081–1091.
113. Grillner S, Hellgren J, Menard A, Saitoh K, Wikstrom MA. Mechanisms for selection of basic motor programs—roles for the striatum and pallidum. *Trends Neurosci.* 2005;28(7):364–370.
114. Garcia-Rill E. The basal ganglia and the locomotor regions. *Brain Res.* 1986;396(1):47–63.
115. Kravitz AV, Freeze BS, Parker PR, et al. Regulation of parkinsonian motor behaviours by optogenetic control of basal ganglia circuitry. *Nature.* 2010;466(7306):622–626.
116. Beloozerova IN, Sirota MG. The role of the motor cortex in the control of vigour of locomotor movements in the cat. *J Physiol (Lond).* 1993;461:27–46.
117. Beloozerova IN, Sirota MG. The role of the motor cortex in the control of accuracy of locomotor movements in the cat. *J Physiol (Lond).* 1993;461:1–25.
118. Bretzner F, Drew T. Motor cortical modulation of cutaneous reflex responses in the hindlimb of the intact cat. *J Neurophysiol.* 2005;94(1):673–687.
119. Drew T, Andujar JE, Lajoie K, Yakovenko S. Cortical mechanisms involved in visuomotor coordination during precision walking. *Brain Res Rev.* 2008;57(1):199–211.
120. Armstrong DM. The supraspinal control of mammalian locomotion. *J Physiol (Lond).* 1988;405:1–37.
121. Liddell EG, Phillips CG. Striatal and pyramidal lesions in the cat. *Brain.* 1946;69(4):264–279.
122. Drew T, Kalaska J, Krouchev N. Muscle synergies during locomotion in the cat: a model for motor cortex control. *J Physiol.* 2008;586(5):1239–1245.
123. Majczyński H, Sławińska U. Locomotor recovery after thoracic spinal cord lesions in cats, rats and humans. *Acta Neurobiol Exp (Wars).* 2007;67(3):235–257.
124. Graham-Brown T. The intrinsic factors in the act of progression in the mammal. *Proc R Soc B.* 1911;84:308–319.
125. Graham-Brown T. *Rhythmic Movements: A Contribution to the Study of the Central Nervous System.* Edinburgh: University of Edinburgh; 1912.
126. Sherrington CS. Flexion-reflex of the limb, crossed extension reflex, and reflex stepping and standing. *J Physiol (Lond).* 1910;40: 28–121.
127. Forssberg H, Grillner S. The locomotion of the acute spinal cat injected with clonidine i.v. *Brain Res.* 1973;50(1):184–186.
128. Grillner S, Zangger P. On the central generation of locomotion in the low spinal cat. *Exp Brain Res.* 1979;34(2):241–261.
129. Kiehn O. Locomotor circuits in the mammalian spinal cord. *Annu Rev Neurosci.* 2006;29:279–306.
130. Langlet C, Leblond H, Rossignol S. Mid-lumbar segments are needed for the expression of locomotion in chronic spinal cats. *J Neurophysiol.* 2005;93(5):2474–2488.
131. Magnuson DS, Lovett R, Coffee C, et al. Functional consequences of lumbar spinal cord contusion injuries in the adult rat. *J Neurotrauma.* 2005;22(5):529–543.
132. Graham-Brown T. On the nature of the fundamental activity of the nervous centres; together with an analysis of the conditioning of rhythmic activity in progression, and a theory of the evolution of function in the nervous system. *J Physiol (Lond).* 1914;48(1):18–46.
133. Lundberg A. Half-centres revisited. *Adv Physiol Sci.* 1981;1: 155–167.

134. Lafreniere-Roula M, McCrea DA. Deletions of rhythmic motoneuron activity during fictive locomotion and scratch provide clues to the organization of the mammalian central pattern generator. *J Neurophysiol*. 2005;94(2):1120–1132.
135. Kriellaars DJ, Brownstone RM, Noga BR, Jordan LM. Mechanical entrainment of fictive locomotion in the decerebrate cat. *J Neurophysiol*. 1994;71(6):2074–2086.
136. Perreault M-C, Angel MJ, Guertin P, McCrea DA. Effects of stimulation of hindlimb flexor group II muscle afferents during fictive locomotion. *J Physiol (Lond)*. 1995;487:211–220.
137. Guertin P, Angel M, Perreault M-C, McCrea DA. Ankle extensor group I afferents excite extensors throughout the hindlimb during MLR-evoked fictive locomotion in the cat. *J Physiol (Lond)*. 1995;487(1):197–209.
138. Stecina K, Quevedo J, McCrea DA. Parallel reflex pathways from flexor muscle afferents evoking resetting and flexion enhancement during fictive locomotion and scratch in the cat. *J Physiol (Lond)*. 2005;569(Pt 1):275–290.
139. Hamm TM, Trank TV, Turkin VV. Correlations between neurograms and locomotor drive potentials in motoneurons during fictive locomotion: implications for the organization of locomotor commands. *Prog Brain Res*. 1999;123:331–339.
140. Tazerart S, Viemari JC, Darbon P, Vinay L, Brocard F. Contribution of persistent sodium current to locomotor pattern generation in neonatal rats. *J Neurophysiol*. 2007;98(2):613–628.
141. Zhong G, Masino MA, Harris-Warrick RM. Persistent sodium currents participate in fictive locomotion generation in neonatal mouse spinal cord. *J Neurosci*. 2007;27(17):4507–4518.
142. Ryczko D, Charrier V, Ijspeert A, Cabelguen JM. Segmental oscillators in axial motor circuits of the salamander: distribution and bursting mechanisms. *J Neurophysiol*. 2010;104(5):2677–2692.
143. Dai Y, Jordan LM. Multiple patterns and components of persistent inward current with serotonergic modulation in locomotor activity-related neurons in Cfos-EGFP mice. *J Neurophysiol*. 2010;103(4):1712–1727.
144. Tazerart S, Vinay L, Brocard F. The persistent sodium current generates pacemaker activities in the central pattern generator for locomotion and regulates the locomotor rhythm. *J Neurosci*. 2008; 28(34):8577–8589.
145. Theiss RD, Kuo JJ, Heckman CJ. Persistent inward currents in rat ventral horn neurones. *J Physiol (Lond)*. 2007;580(Pt 2):507–522.
146. Ziskind-Conhaim L, Wu L, Wiesner EP. Persistent sodium current contributes to induced voltage oscillations in locomotor-related hb9 interneurons in the mouse spinal cord. *J Neurophysiol*. 2008; 100(4):2254–2264.
147. Brownstone RM. Beginning at the end: repetitive firing properties in the final common pathway. *Prog Neurobiol*. 2006;78(3–5): 156–172.
148. Shefchyk SJ, Jordan LM. Motoneuron input-resistance changes during fictive locomotion produced by stimulation of the mesencephalic locomotor region. *J Neurophysiol*. 1985;54(5):1101–1108.
149. Jordan LM. Factors determining motoneuron rhythmicity during fictive locomotion. In: Roberts A, Roberts B, eds. *Neural Origin of Rhythmic Movements*. Great Britain: Society for Experimental Biology; 1983:423–444.
150. Shefchyk SJ, Jordan LM. Excitatory and inhibitory postsynaptic potentials in alpha-motoneurons produced during fictive locomotion by stimulation of the mesencephalic locomotor region. *J Neurophysiol*. 1985;53(6):1345–1355.
151. Pratt CA, Jordan LM. Ia inhibitory interneurons and Renshaw cells as contributors to the spinal mechanisms of fictive locomotion. *J Neurophysiol*. 1987;57(1):56–71.
152. Orsal D, Perret C, Cabelguen JM. Evidence of rhythmic inhibitory synaptic influences in hindlimb motoneurons during fictive locomotion in the thalamic cat. *Exp Brain Res*. 1986;64(1):217–224.
153. Feldman AG, Orlovsky GN. Activity of interneurons mediating reciprocal 1a inhibition during locomotion. *Brain Res*. 1975;84(2): 181–194.
154. McCrea DA, Pratt CA, Jordan LM. Renshaw cell activity and recurrent effects on motoneurons during fictive locomotion. *J Neurophysiol*. 1980;44(3):475–488.
155. Pratt CA, Jordan LM. Recurrent inhibition of motoneurons in decerebrate cats during controlled treadmill locomotion. *J Neurophysiol*. 1980;44(3):489–500.
156. Noga BR, Shefchyk SJ, Jamal J, Jordan LM. The role of Renshaw cells in locomotion: antagonism of their excitation from motor axon collaterals with intravenous mecamylamine. *Exp Brain Res*. 1987;66(1):99–105.
157. Huang A, Noga BR, Carr PA, Fedirchuk B, Jordan LM. Spinal cholinergic neurons activated during locomotion: localization and electrophysiological characterization. *J Neurophysiol*. 2000;83(6):3537–3547.
158. Jessell TM. Neuronal specification in the spinal cord: inductive signals and transcriptional codes. *Nat Rev Genet*. 2000;1(1):20–29.
159. Grossmann KS, Giraudin A, Britz O, Zhang J, Goulding M. Genetic dissection of rhythmic motor networks in mice. *Prog Brain Res*. 2010;187:19–37.
160. Brownstone RM, Bui TV. Spinal interneurons providing input to the final common path during locomotion. *Prog Brain Res*. 2010;187:81–95.
161. Goulding M. Circuits controlling vertebrate locomotion: moving in a new direction. *Nat Rev Neurosci*. 2009;10(7):507–518.
162. Kiehn O, Dougherty KJ, Hagglund M, Borgius L, Talpalar A, Restrepo CE. Probing spinal circuits controlling walking in mammals. *Biochem Biophys Res Commun*. 2010;396(1):11–18.
163. Kiehn O. Development and functional organization of spinal locomotor circuits. *Curr Opin Neurobiol*. 2011;21(1):100–109.
164. Arber S. Motor circuits in action: specification, connectivity, and function. *Neuron*. 2012;74(6):975–989.
165. Dyck J, Gosgnach S. Whole cell recordings from visualized neurons in the inner laminae of the functionally intact spinal cord. *J Neurophysiol*. 2009;102(1):590–597.
166. Lanuza GM, Gosgnach S, Pierani A, Jessell TM, Goulding M. Genetic identification of spinal interneurons that coordinate left-right locomotor activity necessary for walking movements. *Neuron*. 2004;42(3):375–386.
167. Kiehn O, Quinlan KA, Restrepo CE, et al. Excitatory components of the mammalian locomotor CPG. *Brain Res Rev*. 2008;57(1):56–63.
168. Jankowska E. Spinal interneuronal networks in the cat: elementary components. *Brain Res Rev*. 2008;57(1):46–55.
169. Cowley KC, Zaporozhets E, Schmidt BJ. Propriospinal transmission of the locomotor command signal in the neonatal rat. *Ann N Y Acad Sci*. 2010;1198:42–53.
170. Miles GB, Hartley R, Todd AJ, Brownstone RM. Spinal cholinergic interneurons regulate the excitability of motoneurons during locomotion. *Proc Natl Acad Sci USA*. 2007;104(7):2448–2453.
171. Zagoraiou L, Akay T, Martin JF, Brownstone RM, Jessell TM, Miles GB. A cluster of cholinergic premotor interneurons modulates mouse locomotor activity. *Neuron*. 2009;64(5):645–662.
172. Brownstone RM, Jordan LM, Kriellaars DJ, Noga BR, Shefchyk SJ. On the regulation of repetitive firing in lumbar motoneurones during fictive locomotion in the cat. *Exp Brain Res*. 1992;90(3): 441–455.
173. Siembab VC, Smith CA, Zagoraiou L, Berrocal MC, Mentis GZ, Alvarez FJ. Target selection of proprioceptive and motor axon synapses on neonatal V1-derived Ia inhibitory interneurons and Renshaw cells. *J Comp Neurol*. 2010;518(23):4675–4701.
174. Gosgnach S, Lanuza GM, Butt SJ, et al. V1 spinal neurons regulate the speed of vertebrate locomotor outputs. *Nature*. 2006; 440(7081):215–219.

175. Wang Z, Li L, Goulding M, Frank E. Early postnatal development of reciprocal Ia inhibition in the murine spinal cord. *J Neurophysiol.* 2008;100(1):185–196.
176. Higashijima S, Masino MA, Mandel G, Fetcho JR. Engrailed-1 expression marks a primitive class of inhibitory spinal interneuron. *J Neurosci.* 2004;24(25):5827–5839.
177. Li WC, Higashijima S, Parry DM, Roberts A, Soffe SR. Primitive roles for inhibitory interneurons in developing frog spinal cord. *J Neurosci.* 2004;24(25):5840–5848.
178. Sapir T, Geiman EJ, Wang Z, et al. Pax6 and engrailed 1 regulate two distinct aspects of Renshaw cell development. *J Neurosci.* 2004;24(5):1255–1264.
179. Alvarez FJ, Jonas PC, Sapir T, et al. Postnatal phenotype and localization of spinal cord V1 derived interneurons. *J Comp Neurol.* 2005;493(2):177–192.
180. Kimura Y, Okamura Y, Higashijima S. alx, a zebrafish homolog of Chx10, marks ipsilateral descending excitatory interneurons that participate in the regulation of spinal locomotor circuits. *J Neurosci.* 2006;26(21):5684–5697.
181. McLean DL, Fetcho JR. Spinal interneurons differentiate sequentially from those driving the fastest swimming movements in larval zebrafish to those driving the slowest ones. *J Neurosci.* 2009;29(43):13566–13577.
182. Crone SA, Quinlan KA, Zagoraiou L, et al. Genetic ablation of V2a ipsilateral interneurons disrupts left-right locomotor coordination in mammalian spinal cord. *Neuron.* 2008;60(1):70–83.
183. Crone SA, Zhong G, Harris-Warrick R, Sharma K. In mice lacking V2a interneurons, gait depends on speed of locomotion. *J Neurosci.* 2009;29(21):7098–7109.
184. Zhong G, Droho S, Crone SA, et al. Electrophysiological characterization of V2a interneurons and their locomotor-related activity in the neonatal mouse spinal cord. *J Neurosci.* 2010;30(1):170–182.
185. Zhang Y, Narayan S, Geiman E, et al. V3 spinal neurons establish a robust and balanced locomotor rhythm during walking. *Neuron.* 2008;60(1):84–96.
186. Rabe N, Gezelius H, Vallstedt A, Memic F, Kullander K. Netrin-1-dependent spinal interneuron subtypes are required for the formation of left-right alternating locomotor circuitry. *J Neurosci.* 2009;29(50):15642–15649.
187. Wilson JM, Hartley R, Maxwell DJ, et al. Conditional rhythmicity of ventral spinal interneurons defined by expression of the Hb9 homeodomain protein. *J Neurosci.* 2005;25(24):5710–5719.
188. Hinckley CA, Hartley R, Wu L, Todd A, Ziskind-Conhaim L. Locomotor-like rhythms in a genetically distinct cluster of interneurons in the mammalian spinal cord. *J Neurophysiol.* 2005; 93(3):1439–1449.
189. Brownstone RM, Wilson JM. Strategies for delineating spinal locomotor rhythm-generating networks and the possible role of Hb9 interneurones in rhythmogenesis. *Brain Res Rev.* 2008;57(1): 64–76.
190. Gosgnach S. The role of genetically-defined interneurons in generating the mammalian locomotor rhythm. *Integr Comp Biol.* 2011;51(6):903–912.
191. Kwan AC, Dietz SB, Webb WW, Harris-Warrick RM. Activity of Hb9 interneurons during fictive locomotion in mouse spinal cord. *J Neurosci.* 2009;29(37):11601–11613.
192. Pearson KG. Generating the walking gait: role of sensory feedback. *Prog Brain Res.* 2004;143:123–129.
193. Pearson KG. Role of sensory feedback in the control of stance duration in walking cats. *Brain Res Rev.* 2008;57(1):222–227.
194. Meisel RL, Rakerd B. Induction of hindlimb stepping movements in rats spinally transected as adults or as neonates. *Brain Res.* 1982;240(2):353–356.
195. Afelt Z. Reflex activity in chronic spinal cats. *Acta Neurobiol Exp (Wars).* 1970;30(2):129–144.
196. Lev-Tov A, Delvolve I, Kremer E. Sacrocaudal afferents induce rhythmic efferent bursting in isolated spinal cords of neonatal rats. *J Neurophysiol.* 2000;83(2):888–894.
197. Delvolve I, Gabbay H, Lev-Tov A. The motor output and behavior produced by rhythmogenic sacrocaudal networks in spinal cords of neonatal rats. *J Neurophysiol.* 2001;85(5):2100–2110.
198. Gordon IT, Whelan PJ. Monoaminergic control of cauda-equina-evoked locomotion in the neonatal mouse spinal cord. *J Neurophysiol.* 2006;96(6):3122–3129.
199. Berry JA, Biedlingmaier JF, Whelan PJ. In vitro resistance to bacterial biofilm formation on coated fluoroplastic tympanostomy tubes. *Otolaryngol Head Neck Surg.* 2000;123(3):246–251.
200. Norreel JC, Pflieger JF, Pearlstein E, Simeoni-Alias J, Clarac F, Vinay L. Reversible disorganization of the locomotor pattern after neonatal spinal cord transection in the rat. *J Neurosci.* 2003;23(5): 1924–1932.
201. Smith JC, Feldman JL, Schmidt BJ. Neural mechanisms generating locomotion studied in mammalian brain stem-spinal cord in vitro. *FASEB J.* 1988;2(7):2283–2288.
202. Marchetti C, Beato M, Nistri A. Alternating rhythmic activity induced by dorsal root stimulation in the neonatal rat spinal cord in vitro. *J Physiol (Lond).* 2001;530(Pt 1):105–112.
203. Gaunt RA, Prochazka A, Mushahwar VK, Guevremont L, Ellaway PH. Intraspinal microstimulation excites multisegmental sensory afferents at lower stimulus levels than local alpha-motoneuron responses. *J Neurophysiol.* 2006;96(6):2995–3005.
204. Barthelemy D, Leblond H, Rossignol S. Characteristics and mechanisms of locomotion induced by intraspinal microstimulation and dorsal root stimulation in spinal cats. *J Neurophysiol.* 2007;97(3):1986–2000.
205. Duysens J, Pearson KG. The role of cutaneous afferents from the distal hindlimb in the regulation of the step cycle of thalamic cats. *Exp Brain Res.* 1976;24:245–255.
206. Bouyer LJ, Rossignol S. Contribution of cutaneous inputs from the hindpaw to the control of locomotion. I. Intact cats. *J Neurophysiol.* 2003;90(6):3625–3639.
207. Bouyer LJ, Rossignol S. Contribution of cutaneous inputs from the hindpaw to the control of locomotion. II. Spinal cats. *J Neurophysiol.* 2003;90(6):3640–3653.
208. Giszter SF, Davies MR, Graziani V. Motor strategies used by rats spinalized at birth to maintain stance in response to imposed perturbations. *J Neurophysiol.* 2007;97(4):2663–2675.
209. Viala G, Buser P. Inhibition of spinal locomotor activity by a special method of somatic stimulation in rabbits. *Exp Brain Res.* 1974;21(3):275–284.
210. Viala G, Orsal D, Buser P. Cutaneous fiber groups involved in the inhibition of fictive locomotion in the rabbit. *Exp Brain Res.* 1978;33(2):257–267.
211. Forssberg H, Grillner S, Rossignol S. Phasic gain control of reflexes from the dorsum of the paw during spinal locomotion. *Brain Res.* 1977;132(1):121–139.
212. Forssberg H. Stumbling corrective reaction: a phase-dependent compensatory reaction during locomotion. *J Neurophysiol.* 1979; 42(4):936–953.
213. Quevedo J, Stecina K, Gosgnach S, McCrea DA. Stumbling corrective reaction during fictive locomotion in the cat. *J Neurophysiol.* 2005;94(3):2045–2052.
214. Forssberg H, Grillner S, Rossignol S. Phase dependent reflex reversal during walking in chronic spinal cats. *Brain Res.* 1975; 85(1):103–107.
215. Grillner S, Rossignol S. On the initiation of the swing phase of locomotion in chronic spinal cats. *Brain Res.* 1978;146:269–277.
216. Andersson O, Grillner S. Peripheral control of the cat's step cycle. II. Entrainment of the central pattern generators for locomotion

by sinusoidal hip movements during 'fictive locomotion'. *Acta Physiol Scand.* 1983;118:229–239.

217. Andersson O, Grillner S. Peripheral control of the cat's step cycle. I. Phase dependent effects of ramp-movements of the hip during 'fictive locomotion'. *Acta Physiol Scand.* 1981;113:89–101.
218. Timoszyk WK, Nessler JA, Acosta C, et al. Hindlimb loading determines stepping quantity and quality following spinal cord transection. *Brain Res.* 2005;1050(1–2):180–189.
219. Conway BA, Hultborn H, Kiehn O. Proprioceptive input resets central locomotor rhythm in the spinal cat. *Exp Brain Res.* 1987;68:643–656.
220. Duysens J, Pearson KG. Inhibition of flexor burst generation by loading ankle extensor muscles in walking cats. *Brain Res.* 1980;187(2):321–332.
221. Pearson KG, Ramirez JM, Jiang W. Entrainment of the locomotor rhythm by group Ib afferents from ankle extensor muscles in spinal cats. *Exp Brain Res.* 1992;90:557–566.
222. Dietz V. Evidence for a load receptor contribution to the control of posture and locomotion. *Neurosci Biobehav Rev.* 1998;22(4):495–499.
223. Harkema SJ, Hurley SL, Patel UK, Requejo PS, Dobkin BH, Edgerton VR. Human lumbosacral spinal cord interprets loading during stepping. *J Neurophysiol.* 1997;77:797–811.
224. Timoszyk WK, De Leon RD, London N, Roy RR, Edgerton VR, Reinkensmeyer DJ. The rat lumbosacral spinal cord adapts to robotic loading applied during stance. *J Neurophysiol.* 2002;88(6): 3108–3117.
225. de Leon RD, Kubasak MD, Phelps PE, et al. Using robotics to teach the spinal cord to walk. *Brain Res Brain Res Rev.* 2002; 40(1–3):267–273.
226. Hiebert GW, Whelan PJ, Prochazka A, Pearson KG. Contribution of hind limb flexor muscle afferents to the timing of phase transitions in the cat step cycle. *J Neurophysiol.* 1996;75(3):1126–1137.
227. Bussel B, Roby-Brami A, Azouvi P, Biraben A, Yakovleff A, Held JP. Myoclonus in a patient with spinal cord transection. Possible involvement of the spinal stepping generator. *Brain.* 1988;111(Pt 5):1235–1245.
228. Calancie B, Needham-Shropshire B, Jacobs P, Willer K, Zych G, Green BA. Involuntary stepping after chronic spinal cord injury. Evidence for a central rhythm generator for locomotion in man. *Brain.* 1994;117(Pt 5):1143–1159.
229. Dimitrijevic MR, Gerasimenko Y, Pinter MM. Evidence for a spinal central pattern generator in humans. *Ann N Y Acad Sci.* 1998;860:360–376.
230. Nadeau S, Jacquemin G, Fournier C, Lamarre Y, Rossignol S. Spontaneous motor rhythms of the back and legs in a patient with a complete spinal cord transection. *Neurorehabil Neural Repair.* 2010;24(4):377–383.
231. Courtine G, Gerasimenko Y, van den Brand R, et al. Transformation of nonfunctional spinal circuits into functional states after the loss of brain input. *Nat Neurosci.* 2009;12(10):1333–1342.
232. Harkema S, Gerasimenko Y, Hodes J, et al. Effect of epidural stimulation of the lumbosacral spinal cord on voluntary movement, standing, and assisted stepping after motor complete paraplegia: a case study. *Lancet.* 2011;377(9781):1938–1947.
233. Simon C, Kezunovic N, Ye M, et al. Gamma band unit activity and population responses in the pedunculopontine nucleus. *J Neurophysiol.* 2010;104(1):463–474.
234. Garcia-Rill E, Simon C, Smith K, Kezunovic N, Hyde J. The pedunculopontine tegmental nucleus: from basic neuroscience to neurosurgical applications: arousal from slices to humans: implications for DBS. *J Neural Transm.* 2011;118(10):1397–1407.
235. Tort AB, Kramer MA, Thorn C, et al. Dynamic cross-frequency couplings of local field potential oscillations in rat striatum and hippocampus during performance of a T-maze task. *Proc Natl Acad Sci USA.* 2008;105(51):20517–20522.
236. Thevathasan W, Pogosyan A, Hyam JA, et al. Alpha oscillations in the pedunculopontine nucleus correlate with gait performance in Parkinsonism. *Brain.* 2012;135(Pt 1):148–160.
237. Sławińska U, Kasicki S. The frequency of rat's hippocampal theta rhythm is related to the speed of locomotion. *Brain Res.* 1998;796(1–2):327–331.
238. Waldrop TG, Bauer RM, Iwamoto GA. Microinjection of GABA antagonists into the posterior hypothalamus elicits locomotor activity and a cardiorespiratory activation. *Brain Res.* 1988;444(1): 84–94.
239. Robinson TE, Whishaw IQ. Effects of posterior hypothalamic lesions on voluntary behavior and hippocampal electroencephalograms in the rat. *J Comp Physiol Psychol.* 1974;86(5):768–786.
240. Singh A, Kammermeier S, Plate A, Mehrkens JH, Ilmberger J, Botzel K. Pattern of local field potential activity in the globus pallidus internum of dystonic patients during walking on a treadmill. *Exp Neurol.* 2011;232(2):162–167.
241. Shimamoto SA, Larson PS, Ostrem JL, Glass GA, Turner RS, Starr PA. Physiological identification of the human pedunculopontine nucleus. *J Neurol Neurosurg Psychiatry.* 2010;81(1): 80–86.

CHAPTER

18

The Brainstem Respiratory Network

Tara G. Bautista[1], *Teresa E. Pitts*[2], *Paul M. Pilowsky*[3], *Kendall F. Morris*[4]

[1]The Florey Institute of Neuroscience and Mental Health, Melbourne, VIC, Australia, [2]Department of Physiological Sciences, University of Florida, Gainesville, FL, USA, [3]The Heart Research Institute, Sydney, NSW, Australia, [4]Department of Molecular Pharmacology and Physiology, University of South Florida College of Medicine, Tampa, FL, USA

FUNCTIONS OF THE BRAINSTEM RESPIRATORY NETWORK

The respiratory system works with the cardiovascular system to subserve the most basic of life-sustaining functions, that is, to supply tissues with oxygen (O_2), remove carbon dioxide (CO_2), and maintain a normal acid–base balance. The most studied activity of this system is "eupnea", or quiet, awake breathing, and research has focused primarily on defining the brainstem respiratory network—that is, the respiratory central pattern generator (CPG). However, it should be emphasized that beyond this basic function, the networks that control respiration are also vitally important in a host of other behaviors. Homeostasis, often even survival, demands that these behaviors, including swallow, cough, emesis, expiration reflex, micturition, defecation, parturition, suckling, locomotion, vocalization, and sleep, be exquisitely coordinated with breathing. It has therefore been suggested that the respiratory brainstem CPG (discussed in this chapter) be extended to reflect not only the networks generating eupnea but also the concept of "behavioral control assemblies". It has therefore been suggested that previous terminology such as brainstem "centers" and CPGs, discussed here, be extended to the concept of behavioral control assemblies composed of neurons that operate cooperatively in circuits and are transiently configured to process and store information related to the regulation of a given behavior.[1–3]

ANATOMY OF THE RESPIRATORY SYSTEM

The central control of respiratory rhythm and pattern is performed by a network of neurons within the brainstem that operates under drives from chemoreceptors (that sense O_2 and CO_2 concentrations and pH) and sleep–wake centers. Eupnea is often divided into three phases: inspiration, postinspiration, and expiration.[4–6] During inspiration, airflow into the lungs is principally due to the contraction of the diaphragm, which is innervated by the phrenic nerve. Phrenic motoneurons are located within the ventral horn of the cervical spinal cord. Structures in the upper airway (including muscles of the tongue, pharynx, and larynx) provide airflow resistance.[7–19] This resistance is provided by paired intrinsic laryngeal muscles that manipulate vocal cord length, tension, and position, thus affecting the glottic aperture. Motoneurons that supply laryngeal muscles are located in the caudal brainstem, in the vicinity of the nucleus retroambiguus.[20] The laryngeal abductor (posterior cricoarytenoid) muscle dilates the vocal cords during inspiration, and laryngeal adductor muscles (thyroarytenoid, lateral cricoarytenoid, and interarytenoids) partially narrow the vocal folds during the postinspiratory phase.[21] As with other upper airway muscles, laryngeal muscles exhibit a decline in tone during sleep.[22] Importantly, laryngeal abduction and adduction play important roles in upper airway reflexes such as swallow,[23] expiration reflex,[24] and cough, which protect the lower airways from the aspiration of irritants that can result in morbidity and mortality.[25–29] During eupneic expiration, the continued outflow of air from the lungs is usually due to passive lung recoil, with minimal activity in respiratory-related motor outputs. In contrast, "forced breathing" during exercise or lung disease involves the recruitment of expiratory muscles such as the abdominal and internal intercostal muscles, which can generate a more forceful expiratory airflow.

The brainstem contains several types of neurons that are active preferentially during the specific phases of the respiratory cycle. They are often referred to by their

Neuronal Networks in Brain Function, CNS Disorders, and Therapeutics
http://dx.doi.org/10.1016/B978-0-12-415804-7.00018-6

active phase (i.e. inspiratory, postinspiratory, or expiratory). Some neurons are phase spanning (i.e. are active to varying extents across respiratory phases). It is important to note that neurons that may not have overt respiratory modulation may be still considered "respiratory" neurons; that is, they significantly contribute to the control of breathing (e.g. tonically active chemosensitive neurons[30]). The opposite is also true; neurons that have respiratory-modulated activity may not be essential in the control of respiration, including cardiac vagal preganglionic neurons[31–35] and presympathetic neurons.[36–40]

Historically, the neuronal network that generates the three phases of eupnea has been divided into three groups that are bilaterally distributed along the neuraxis (Figure 18.1).[4,6] These are (1) a subnucleus of the nucleus tractus solitarius (NTS)—the dorsal respiratory group (DRG) in the caudal, dorsomedial medulla; (2) the ventral respiratory group (VRG) in the ventrolateral medulla; and (3) the pontine respiratory group (PRG) in the dorsolateral pons. Recently, it has become accepted that neurons in other regions of the brainstem, most notably the raphé, and the chemosensory retrotrapezoidal nucleus (which overlaps with the parafacial respiratory group; together, they are known as the retrotrapezoid and parafacial nuclei, or RTN/PF), can have profound modulatory influences on the generation of the breathing pattern.[41–45]

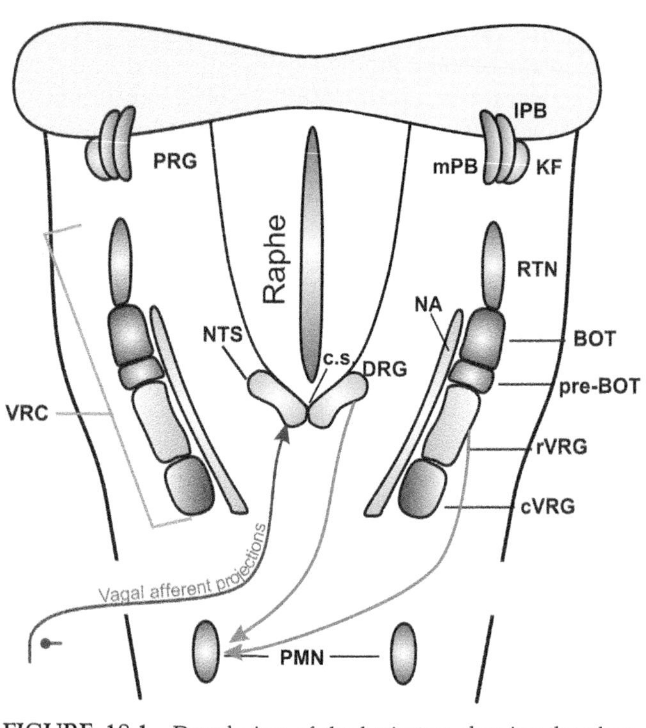

FIGURE 18.1 Dorsal view of the brainstem showing the placement of the three bilateral cell groups and the midline raphé that produce and modulate the respiratory rhythm. These include the pontine respiratory group (PRG), ventral respiratory column (VRC), and dorsal respiratory group (DRG). Vagal afferent neurons carrying information from pulmonary stretch receptors terminate in the caudal ventrolateral subnucleus of the nucleus of the solitary tract (NTS), in the vicinity of the DRG. Sources of premotor input to phrenic motoneurons (PMN) in the spinal cord include the neurons in the DRG and the rostral ventral respiratory group (rVRG). Sources of premotor input to phrenic motoneurons (PMN) in the spinal cord include the neurons in the DRG and the rostral ventral respiratory group (rVRG). Also shown is the midline raphé complex. lPB: lateral parabrachial nucleus; mPB: medial parabrachial nucleus; KF: Kölliker–Fuse nucleus; RTN: retrotrapezoid nucleus; BOT: Bötzinger complex; pre-BOT: pre-Bötzinger complex; cVRG: caudal ventral respiratory group; NA: nucleus ambiguus; c.s.: central canal. (For color version of this figure, the reader is referred to the online version of this book.)

DORSAL RESPIRATORY GROUP

The DRG is a subnucleus of the NTS, which contains a classically defined cluster of respiratory-modulated, mostly inspiratory neurons. A subset of these neurons is bulbospinal and premotor to predominantly contralateral phrenic motoneurons.[46–48] "Pump cells" are another important group of neurons in this region; they receive monosynaptic excitatory inputs from slowly adapting lung stretch receptors, which signal the volume of the lungs.[46] Pump cells project to the different compartments of the VRG,[49] including the commissural NTS,[49] the PRG,[49] and the RTN/PF.[50] Pump cell function is instrumental in the Hering–Breuer reflex, in which further lung inflation, above a certain lung volume, is prevented by the termination of inspiration.[51]

VENTRAL RESPIRATORY COLUMN

The ventral respiratory column (VRC) is a contiguous column in the medulla that extends in the caudal direction from the caudal pole of the facial motor nucleus (VIIn) to the spino-medullary junction.[52–54] The VRC lies ventrolateral to the nucleus ambiguus (NA), which comprises several premotoneurons and motoneurons that are related to respiration (e.g. laryngeal motoneurons), digestion (e.g. esophageal motoneurons), and control of the heart (e.g. cardiac vagal motoneurons). The VRC is also dorsal and medial to neurons critical for the tonic and reflex sympathetic control of blood pressure.[55–59] The VRC is subdivided rostrocaudally into at least three compartments,[54,60] which are discussed throughout the rest of this section.

Bötzinger Complex

A subset of neurons within the Bötzinger complex are expiratory modulated and provide widespread inhibition of other respiratory-modulated neurons of the VRC, the DRG, the PRG, and other respiratory-related areas, including the medullary raphé.[61,62] Bötzinger augmenting-expiratory neurons are bulbospinal and monosynaptically inhibit phrenic motoneurons.[63–65] Decrementing-expiratory neurons are mainly propriobulbar (i.e. without projections to phrenic motoneurons).[64,66]

The Bötzinger complex plays a critical role in determining the length of postinspiration and expiration during eupnea.[67] The Bötzinger complex also integrates reflexes that elicit a temporary arrest of breathing ("apnea") by initiating, and/or prolonging the duration of, these phases (e.g. the Hering–Breuer reflex and superior laryngeal nerve stimulation).[11,68–70] Activation of the Bötzinger complex with excitatory amino acids results in the cessation of respiratory rhythm at the expiratory phase.[52,54] Coronal transection immediately caudal to this nucleus completely abolishes all expiratory motor output.[67,71]

Current research suggests that the mechanism underlying the termination of inspiration during eupnea, or the "inspiratory off switch", exists within the rostral half of the VRC (i.e. the Bötzinger and pre-Bötzinger complexes).[72–75] Inspiratory termination is initiated by late inspiratory neurons (the "reversible inspiratory off switch"), which are active just prior to the transition from inspiration to postinspiration–expiration. This transition is completed with the recruitment of postinspiratory- and decrementing-expiratory neurons (the "irreversible inspiratory off switch"). The current theory is largely based on the observations (1) that the peak firing of late-inspiratory and decrementing-expiratory neurons is coincident with the cessation of firing of augmenting-inspiratory neurons that are presumably phrenic premotoneurons, and (2) of known monosynaptic inhibitory inputs from the former to latter types of neurons.[76,77]

Bötzinger neurons are further involved in the regulation of upper airway muscle activity, demonstrating drastic changes in activity during swallow, cough, and sneeze.[78–81]

Pre-Bötzinger

The pre-Bötzinger complex is a cluster of neurons contiguous with the caudal end of the Bötzinger region.[60] It is composed of small, propriobulbar, preinspiratory modulated neurons containing vesicular glutamatergic transporter 2 (VGLUT2) that also express the neurokinin 1 receptor.[82,83] Stimulation of the pre-Bötzinger complex with excitatory amino acids elicits destabilization of the respiratory rhythm and tachypnea, with or without increases in tonic phrenic activity.[52,54,84]

The pre-Bötzinger complex is thought to be crucial in the generation of eupneic respiratory rhythm. In isolation (i.e. coronal slice preparations), the pre-Bötzinger complex produces a rhythm in the adjacent hypoglossal motor neurons, which can be recorded on the attached hypoglossal nerve.[85,86] Destruction of neurokinin 1 receptor positive structures in the pre-Bötzinger complex in rodents severely disrupts inspiration and abolishes rhythmic activity in phrenic and vagus nerves in vivo and in situ.[67,87] In goats, acute ablation of the pre-Bötzinger complex results in irreversible apnea[88]; however, with gradual destruction (e.g. over 30 days), respiratory rhythm initially exhibits state-dependent perturbation, but plasticity within respiratory networks enables ongoing respiratory rhythm so that arterial blood gases remain normal during wakefulness and sleep.[89,90] Neumueller et al.[90] suggests that anatomical changes within the hypoglossal and medial parabrachialis nucleus contribute to network plasticity.

A subset of pre-Bötzinger neurons possess "pacemaker"-like properties by demonstrating intrinsic bursting when synaptically isolated using low-Ca^{2+} and high-Mg^{2+} solutions and/or cocktails of drugs that inhibit fast synaptic transmission.[91–93] This intrinsic property was previously proposed to "drive" the respiratory rhythm. Specific blockers of pacemaker currents in the pre-Bötzinger complex, in vitro and in vivo, prevent hypoxic-induced gasping but do not perturb eupneic respiratory rhythm.[94–96]

The Ventral Respiratory Group

Although some researchers refer to the entire VRC as the VRG, others have referred to only the portions of the VRC caudal to the pre-Bötzinger as the VRG.

1. The *rostral VRG* contains the bulk of phrenic premotoneurons, which are the augmenting-inspiratory neurons that are bulbospinal and monosynaptically excite phrenic motoneurons using glutamate as a neurotransmitter.[82] Excitation of the more caudal portion of the rostral VRG, where the phrenic premotoneurons are most concentrated, reportedly has no effect on respiratory rhythm.[54,97] In contrast, stimulating the rostral and dorsal portions of the rostral VRG can cause changes in respiratory rhythm as presumably respiratory interneurons are affected.[98]
2. The *caudal VRG* contains expiratory-modulated neurons that activate motoneurons in the thoracic and lumbar spinal cord innervating the accessory muscles of expiration (i.e. the abdominal and internal intercostal muscles) during forced breathing.[99,100] The caudal VRG also contains pharyngeal and laryngeal premotoneurons.[101,102] Expiratory modulation of caudal VRG neurons may originate from excitatory inputs from the RTN/PF,[71] perhaps the Bötzinger complex.[103] Bradypnea or apnea

elicited during microinjection of excitatory amino acids into the caudal VRG has been attributed to activation of rostrally projecting interneurons.[52,54] The general consensus, however, is that caudal VRG neurons are not critically involved in respiratory rhythmogenesis during eupnea.[4] Disfacilitation of the caudal VRG by antagonism of glutamatergic receptors fails to affect inspiratory and expiratory duration and, ultimately, respiratory frequency.[104]

The caudal VRG is involved in behaviors that require modulation of the expiratory phase. Like the Bötzinger complex, the caudal VRG is implicated in upper airway reflex behaviors involving expiratory prolongation, including cough[105] and emesis.[106] Caudal VRG neurons that receive descending inputs from the periaqueductal gray in the midbrain represent the last common relay in the coordination of respiration and vocalization, the latter being initiated preferentially during postinspiration and expiration.[101]

Pontine Respiratory Group

The PRG encompasses the parabrachial and Kölliker–Fuse nuclei within the dorsolateral pons. The PRG contains several types of respiratory-modulated neurons, especially phase spanning (i.e. peak activity is during the transitions between inspiration and expiration).[107,108] Anatomical and cross-correlation studies suggest a dense reciprocal innervation between PRG neurons with VRC.[74,109,110] PRG neurons are also known to directly project onto phrenic motoneurons[82] and are laryngeal adductor premotoneurons.[108]

The PRG is strongly implicated in engaging the medullary inspiratory off switch in the absence of vagally mediated lung stretch receptor information (the Hering–-Breuer reflex) to terminate inspiration. Stimulation of the PRG results in an abrupt cessation of the inspiratory phase of breathing, and it alters the expression of the postinspiratory phase.[67,73,75] In vagotomized animals, pontine inactivation by either transection or local blockade of excitatory neurotransmission results in loss of the postinspiratory phase and apneusis.[111] A similar apneustic response can be obtained by injection of somatostatin (acting on SST2a receptors) into the Bötzinger complex.[112]

The PRG has an important role in the coordination and adaptation of the medullary respiratory rhythm to sensory information (e.g. from pulmonary stretch receptors, peripheral chemoreceptors, and laryngeal irritant receptors) by modulating the medullary respiratory circuitry.[113–115] The PRG receives considerable efferent projections from the NTS, the major termination site for several sensory afferent neurons.[116,117] It also receives central chemoreceptor information from the RTN/PF[44] and from nasal trigeminal afferents.[118] In particular, the PRG is implicated in phase resetting of the respiratory rhythm in response to sensory afferent information. Unilateral and partial PRG lesions abolish the expiratory prolongation and subsequent respiratory phase resetting following swallows evoked by superior laryngeal nerve stimulation.[114,119] Lateral PRG lesions abolish the tachypnea elicited during hypoxia and hypercapnia,[120,121] and reversible blockade eliminates entrainment of breathing by somatic afferent neurons.[115]

Retrotrapezoid and Parafacial Nuclei

The RTN/PF is located superficially between the ventral medullary surface and the facial motor nucleus,[109] has reciprocal VRG connections,[109,110] and projects to the PRG.[44] The RTN is a vital brainstem center that processes chemosensory information and coordinates respiratory adjustments to such information. The RTN receives input regarding the partial pressure of O_2 and CO_2 in blood from peripheral chemoreceptors via the commissural NTS.[50] It also directly detects increased CO_2 partial pressure.[44,50] RTN CO_2-sensitive neurons are glutamatergic, nonaminergic, and noncholinergic; contain the homeobox transcription factor Phox2b; and express the neurokinin 1 receptor.[43,122,123] A large subset of RTN neurons also express preprogalanin mRNA.[41–43] RTN neurons fire tonically, but become respiratory modulated at high CO_2 partial pressure in the blood.[103,124] Focal acidification of the RTN[125] or specific photostimulation of Phox2B-expressing CO_2-sensitive RTN neurons[44] causes vigorous and long-lasting increases in phrenic nerve activity.

The RTN overlaps with the PF, a region described in *en bloc* brainstem and spinal cord preparation of neonatal rat containing neurons that are intrinsically sensitive to hypercapnia and possess a biphasic preinspiratory and postinspiratory firing pattern.[126,127] A subset of PF neurons expresses neurochemical markers similar to those of RTN neurons.[128] Various lines of research suggest that the PF could be a dominant respiratory oscillator that paces pre-Bötzinger neurons, at least in neonates,[127] or alternatively an expiratory oscillator that couples with the pre-Bötzinger inspiratory oscillator during forced breathing to activate accessory muscles of expiration.[129]

Raphé

Neurons in the medullary raphé complex (the obscurus, magnus, and pallidus) are the primary source of serotonin in the brainstem and spinal cord.[130–132] In rat, electrical stimulation of the different raphé compartments by excitatory amino acids can cause either a bradypnea leading to apnea (magnus and obscurus) or tachypnea (pallidus), with or without tonic activity in the diaphragm.[133] In the cat, electrical stimulation of the raphé obscurus results in long-term increases in respiratory frequency and tidal volume.[134]

The medullary raphé complex is another key site in processing chemosensory information. Multiarray cell recordings during peripheral chemoreceptor activation demonstrate increases (25%) or decreases (15%) in caudal raphé nuclei neuron activity; however, the serotonergic phenotype of the neurons was not verified.[135,136] Interestingly, changes in respiration due to focal acidification of the medullary raphé differ across the sleep–wake cycle.[137] Raphé neurons, many of which are serotenergic, may also alter the ventilatory response to hypoxia by modulating the NTS processing of peripheral chemoreceptor inputs. Retrograde tracing from the NTS labels serotonergic neurons in all compartments of the medullary raphé, in particular the raphé magnus.[138] Electrical and glutamatergic activation of the raphé magnus significantly blunts the increased activation of chemosensitive NTS neurons following intravenous cyanide injection.[139] The raphé may also affect the hypoxic response by modulating the excitability of phrenic motoneurons.[55]

INTERACTIONS WITH OTHER NETWORKS AND RECONFIGURATION FOR AIRWAY PROTECTION

Swallow and cough are the two most critical behaviors that interact with breathing to protect the airway.

Swallow

Swallow is a motor act including oral, pharyngeal, and esophageal phases.[140,141] Of significant interest is the pharyngeal phase of swallow, due to its anatomical and functional interaction with the respiratory system.[140,142–144] The pharyngeal phase is a reflex, stereotypical motor act involving muscles of the oral cavity, pharynx, larynx, and upper esophagus, as well as those of inspiration. The tongue propels the bolus from the oral cavity, and it is diverted around the larynx (which is elevated under the chin) and propelled through the upper esophageal sphincter.[145–147] Functional apnea during swallowing is achieved by adduction of the vocal folds and ventricular folds (false vocal folds), and inversion of the epiglottis over the laryngeal vestibule.[145–147] The majority of swallows are triggered by saliva or mucus in the oral and/or pharyngeal cavity to maintain a clear upper airway.[148]

The swallow CPG is located within the brainstem, involving two principal clusters of neurons in the regions of the DRG and the VRC.[140,149,150] A significant omission in the current model of the swallowing pattern generator is the changes in respiratory motor output that occur concurrent with swallow. Moreover, the current model of the swallowing pattern generator does not account for the participation of respiratory-modulated neurons in the generation of the swallow motor pattern; for example, previous investigations demonstrate that DRG and VRC neurons exhibit swallow-related burst activity, as well as responses to single-pulse superior laryngeal nerve stimulation.[11,61,151,152]

DRG neurons that show swallow-related activity are probably the first point of interaction between the swallow and respiratory pattern generators. Using intracellular recording in decerebrate cat, Gestreau et al.[151] reported that a majority of bulbospinal inspiratory-modulated neurons in the NTS are depolarized and exhibit a burst of action potentials during swallow. Propriobulbar inspiratory-modulated neurons in the NTS are also activated in parallel with swallow.[151] This inspiratory neuronal activity is hypothesized to be responsible for the "schluckatmung" production (i.e. the phrenic burst that accompanies swallow, otherwise termed "swallow breath").[153,154] Phrenic activity during swallowing has been reported in cats,[151] rats,[155] goats,[114] and humans (adult and infant).[156,157] The role of this inspiratory activity in the coordination of breathing and swallowing and the biomechanics of bolus movement has not been fully established, but it is a promising line of research into swallow–breathing interactions.

Cough

The function of cough is to remove fluids, mucus, and/or foreign bodies from the respiratory tract by the generation of high-velocity expiratory airflows. These airflows during cough are generated by a complex and sequential motor pattern involving three phases: inspiration, compression, and expulsion.[25,158–165] The inspiratory phase of cough is generated by a large burst of activity in inspiratory muscles, such as the diaphragm and inspiratory intercostal muscles.[25,158–165] The compressive phase of cough involves rapidly increasing expiratory thoracic and abdominal muscle activity produced by laryngeal closure by contraction of laryngeal adductor muscles.[25,158–165] The large increase in intrapleural pressure generated during the compression phase produces very high airflows (up to 12 l/s in humans) when the larynx opens and the expulsive phase begins. The expulsive phase is characterized by extremely large bursts of activity in expiratory thoracic and abdominal muscles.[25,158–165]

Similar to the discussion given here on the role of sensory afferents in the modulation of breathing, cough is also elicited and/or modulated by these afferents. In the lower airways, pulmonary stretch receptors, rapidly adapting "irritant" receptors, and pulmonary C-fibers can all influence the production of cough.[166–172] Stimulation of rapidly adapting receptors (RARs) will reliably elicit cough.[173] Pulmonary stretch receptors have a permissive role in the production of cough induced by stimulation of the trachea and bronchi and a facilitatory role in cough in response to laryngeal stimulation.[174,175] The exact role of pulmonary C-fibers in the production of cough is more controversial, with some groups supporting an excitatory role[176] and others supporting an inhibitory role.[177] Recently, a subset of dedicated "cough receptors" has been identified in the guinea pig.[166,167,178]

Sensory information from the aforementioned pulmonary afferents is processed in the brainstem, where the basic central elements responsible for the production of cough as well as breathing are located. Pulmonary vagal afferent information is processed by second-order interneurons located near and in various subnuclei of the NTS.[178,179] These interneurons include pump cells, second-order RAR relay neurons,[25,164,165] laryngeal second-order relay neurons,[179] and relay neurons mediating pulmonary C-fiber reflexes.[178,179] Presumably, all of these groups of interneurons could contribute to the production of cough under different conditions.

Neurons that participate in the regulation of motor drive to chest wall, abdominal, and upper airway muscles are located in separate medullary regions, the DRG, PRG, and VRC.[25,80,164,165,180–182] Previous work has shown that most DRG and VRC neurons, including those responsible for production of the respiratory drive, have discharge patterns that are appropriate for contribution to the cough motor pattern.[25,80,164,165,180–182]

SUMMARY

The current hypotheses explaining the neurogenesis of swallow, cough, and breathing suggest that overlapping networks of neurons mediate their coordination and production. Clearly, swallow, cough, and breathing are different behaviors. However, networks can participate in such different behaviors by dynamic alteration of the excitability of key elements, presynaptic modulation of afferent sensory signals, and/or recruitment of previously silent elements, to name a few. These processes represent *reconfiguration*. It has been suggested that this reconfiguration represents a decision process that evaluates incoming sensory information and decides whether to continue the respiratory rhythm and pattern as is, or produce an airway protective behavior that temporarily modulates respiration—both with the ultimate goal of ensuring long-term ventilation.

References

1. Pitts T, Morris K, Lindsey B, Davenport P, Poliacek I, Bolser D. Co-ordination of cough and swallow in vivo and in silico. *Exp Physiol*. 2012;97(4):469–473.
2. O'Connor R, Segers LS, Morris KF, et al. A joint computational respiratory neural network-biomechanical model for breathing and airway defensive behaviors. *Front Physiol*. 2012;3.
3. Bolser DC, Pitts TE, Morris KF. The use of multiscale systems biology approaches to facilitate understanding of complex control systems for airway protection. *Curr Opin Pharmacol*. 2011.
4. Bianchi AL, Denavit-Saubie M, Champagnat J. Central control of breathing in mammals: neuronal circuitry, membrane properties, and neurotransmitters. *Physiol Rev*. 1995;75(1):1–45.
5. Ezure K. Information processing at the nucleus tractus solitarii and respiratory rhythm generation. *Respir Res*. 2001;2(Suppl. 1): 2.3.
6. Richter DW, Spyer KM. Studying rhythmogenesis of breathing: comparison of in vivo and in vitro models. *Trends Neurosci*. 2001;24(8):464–472.
7. Bautista TG, Burke PG, Sun QJ, Berkowitz RG, Pilowsky PM. The generation of post-inspiratory activity in laryngeal motoneurons: a review. *Adv Exp Med Biol*. 2010;669:143–149.
8. Bautista TG, Xing T, Fong AY, Pilowsky PM. Recurrent laryngeal nerve activity exhibits a 5-HT-mediated long-term facilitation and enhanced response to hypoxia following acute intermittent hypoxia in rat. *J Appl Physiol*. 2012;112(7):1144–1156.
9. Bautista TG, Sun QJ, Pilowsky PM. Expiratory-modulated laryngeal motoneurons exhibit a hyperpolarization preceding depolarization during superior laryngeal nerve stimulation in the in vivo adult rat. *Brain Res*. 2012;1445:52–61.
10. Sun QJ, Chum JM, Bautista TG, Pilowsky PM, Berkowitz RG. Neuronal mechanisms underlying the laryngeal adductor reflex. *Ann Otol Rhinol Laryngol*. 2011;120(11):755–760.
11. Sun QJ, Bautista TG, Berkowitz RG, Zhao WJ, Pilowsky PM. The temporal relationship between non-respiratory burst activity of expiratory laryngeal motoneurons and phrenic apnoea during stimulation of the superior laryngeal nerve in rat. *J Physiol*. 2011;589(Pt 7):1819–1830.
12. Bautista TG, Sun QJ, Zhao WJ, Pilowsky PM. Cholinergic inputs to laryngeal motoneurons functionally identified in vivo in rat: a combined electrophysiological and microscopic study. *J Comp Neurol*. 2010;518(24):4903–4916.
13. Pilowsky PM, Sun QJ, Berkowitz RG, Goodchild AK. Serotonin inputs to inspiratory laryngeal motoneurons in the rat. *J Comp Neurol*. 2002;451(1):91–98.
14. Pilowsky PM, Sun QJ, Berkowitz RG, Goodchild AK. Substance P inputs to laryngeal motoneurons in the rat. *Respir Physiol Neurobiol*. 2003;137(1):11–18.
15. Berkowitz RG, Chalmers J, Sun QJ, Pilowsky P. Intracellular recording from posterior cricoarytenoid motoneurons in the rat. *Ann Otol Rhinol Laryngol*. 1999;108(12):1120–1125.
16. Berkowitz RG, Sun QJ, Pilowsky PM. Congenital bilateral vocal cord paralysis and the role of glycine. *Ann Otol Rhinol Laryngol*. 2005;114(6):494–498.
17. Sun QJ, Berkowitz RG, Pilowsky PM. $GABA_A$ mediated inhibition and post-inspiratory pattern of laryngeal constrictor motoneurons in rat. *Respir Physiol Neurobiol*. 2008;162(1):41–47.
18. Sun QJ, Pilowsky P, Minson J, Arnolda L, Chalmers J, Llewellyn-Smith IJ. Close appositions between tyrosine hydroxylase immunoreactive boutons and respiratory neurons in the rat ventrolateral medulla. *J Comp Neurol*. 1994;340(1):1–10.
19. Sun QJ, Berkowitz RG, Pilowsky PM. Response of laryngeal motoneurons to hyperventilation induced apnea in the rat. *Respir Physiol Neurobiol*. 2005;146(2–3):155–163.

20. Bieger D, Hopkins DA. Viscerotopic representation of the upper alimentary tract in the medulla oblongata in the rat: the nucleus ambiguus. *J Comp Neurol.* 1987;262(4):546–562.
21. Kuna ST, Bedi DG, Ryckman C. Effect of nasal airway positive pressure on upper airway size and configuration. *Am Rev Respir Dis.* 1988;138(4):969–975.
22. Sherrey JH, Pollard MJ, Megirian D. Respiratory functions of the inferior pharyngeal constrictor and sternohyoid muscles during sleep. *Exp Neurol.* 1986;92(1):267–277.
23. Doty R, Bosma J. An electromyographic analysis of reflex deglutition. *J Neurophysiol.* 1956;19:44–60.
24. Poliacek I, Rose MJ, Corrie LWC, et al. Short reflex expirations (expiration reflexes) induced by mechanical stimulation of the trachea in anesthetized cats. *Cough.* 2008;4(1):1.
25. Shannon R, Baekey D, Morris K, Lindsey B. Brainstem respiratory networks and cough. *Pulm Pharmacol.* 1996;9(5–6):343–347.
26. Thach BT. Maturation of cough and other reflexes that protect the fetal and neonatal airway. *Pulm Pharmacol Ther.* 2007;20(4):365–370.
27. Widdicombe J. Neurophysiology of the cough reflex. *Eur Respir J.* 1995;8(7):1193–1202.
28. Widdicombe J, Chung KF. Cough. *Pulm Pharmacol Ther.* 2007;20(4):305–306.
29. Widdicombe J, Fontana G. Cough: what's in a name? *Eur Respir J.* 2006;28(1):10–15.
30. Guyenet PG, Stornetta RL, Abbott SBG, Depuy SD, Fortuna MG, Kanbar R. Central CO_2 chemoreception and integrated neural mechanisms of cardiovascular and respiratory control. *J Appl Physiol.* 2010;108(4):995–1002.
31. Dergacheva O, Griffioen KJ, Neff RA, Mendelowitz D. Respiratory modulation of premotor cardiac vagal neurons in the brainstem. *Respir Physiol Neurobiol.* 2010;174(1–2):102–110.
32. Dergacheva O, Kamendi H, Wang X, et al. 5-HT_2 receptors modulate excitatory neurotransmission to cardiac vagal neurons within the nucleus ambiguus evoked during and after hypoxia. *Neuroscience.* 2009;164(3):1191–1198.
33. Dergacheva O, Kamendi H, Wang X, et al. The role of 5-HT_3 and other excitatory receptors in central cardiorespiratory responses to hypoxia: implications for sudden infant death syndrome. *Pediatr Res.* 2009;65(6):625–630.
34. Dergacheva O, Griffioen KJ, Wang X, Kamendi H, Gorini C, Mendelowitz D. 5-HT_2 receptor subtypes mediate different long-term changes in GABAergic activity to parasympathetic cardiac vagal neurons in the nucleus ambiguus. *Neuroscience.* 2007;149(3):696–705.
35. Griffioen KJ, Gorini C, Jameson H, Mendelowitz D. Purinergic P2X receptors mediate excitatory transmission to cardiac vagal neurons in the nucleus ambiguus after hypoxia. *Hypertension.* 2007;50(1):75–81.
36. Boychuk CR, Woerman AL, Mendelowitz D. Modulation of bulbospinal rostral ventral lateral medulla neurons by hypoxia/hypercapnia but not medullary respiratory activity. *Hypertension.* 2012;60(6):1491–1497.
37. Miyawaki T, Goodchild AK, Pilowsky PM. Evidence for a tonic GABA-ergic inhibition of excitatory respiratory-related afferents to presympathetic neurons in the rostral ventrolateral medulla. *Brain Res.* 2002;924(1):56–62.
38. Miyawaki T, Minson JB, Arnolda LF, Chalmers JP, Llewellyn-Smith IJ, Pilowsky PM. Role of excitatory amino acid receptors in cardiorespiratory coupling in the ventrolateral medulla. *Am J Physiol.* 1996;271:R1221–R1230.
39. Miyawaki T, Pilowsky P, Sun QJ, et al. Central inspiration increases barosensitivity of neurons in rat rostral ventrolateral medulla. *Am J Physiol.* 1995;268(4 Pt 2):R909–R918.
40. Pilowsky P. Good vibrations? Respiratory rhythms in the central control of blood pressure. *Clin Exp Pharmacol Physiol.* 1995;22(9):594–604.
41. Spirovski D, Li Q, Pilowsky PM. Brainstem galanin-synthesizing neurons are differentially activated by chemoreceptor stimuli and represent a subpopulation of respiratory neurons. *J Comp Neurol.* 2012;520(1):154–173.
42. Pilowsky PM, Lung MSY, Spirovski D, McMullan S. Differential regulation of the central neural cardiorespiratory system by metabotropic neurotransmitters. *Philos Trans R Soc Lond B Biol Sci.* 2009;364:2537–2552.
43. Stornetta RL, Spirovski D, Moreira TS, et al. Galanin is a selective marker of the retrotrapezoid nucleus in rats. *J Comp Neurol.* 2009;512(3):373–383.
44. Abbott SBG, Stornetta RL, Socolovsky CS, West GH, Guyenet PG. Photostimulation of channelrhodopsin-2 expressing ventrolateral medullary neurons increases sympathetic nerve activity and blood pressure in rats. *J Physiol.* 2009;587(23):5613–5631.
45. Abbott SB, Stornetta RL, Coates MB, Guyenet PG. Phox2b-expressing neurons of the parafacial region regulate breathing rate, inspiration, and expiration in conscious rats. *J Neurosci.* 2011;31(45):16410–16422.
46. Berger AJ. Dorsal respiratory group neurons in the medulla of cat: spinal projections, responses to lung inflation and superior laryngeal nerve stimulation. *Brain Res.* 1977;135(2):231–254.
47. Fedorko L, Merrill EG, Lipski J. Two descending medullary inspiratory pathways to phrenic motoneurones. *Neurosci Lett.* 1983;43(2–3):285–291.
48. Averill DB, Cameron WE, Berger AJ. Neural elements subserving pulmonary stretch receptor-mediated facilitation of phrenic motoneurons. *Brain Res.* 1985;346(2):378–382.
49. Ezure K, Tanaka I, Saito Y, Otake K. Axonal projections of pulmonary slowly adapting receptor relay neurons in the rat. *J Comp Neurol.* 2002;446(1):81–94.
50. Takakura AC, Moreira TS, Colombari E, West GH, Stornetta RL, Guyenet PG. Peripheral chemoreceptor inputs to retrotrapezoid nucleus (RTN) CO_2-sensitive neurons in rats. *J Physiol.* 2006;572(Pt 2):503–523.
51. McCrimmon DR, Monnier A, Hayashi F, Zuperku EJ. Pattern formation and rhythm generation in the ventral respiratory group. *Clin Exp Pharmacol Physiol.* 2000;27(1–2):126–131.
52. Chitravanshi VC, Sapru HN. Phrenic nerve responses to chemical stimulation of the subregions of ventral medullary respiratory neuronal group in the rat. *Brain Res.* 1999;821(2):443–460.
53. Ott MM, Nuding SC, Segers LS, Lindsey BG, Morris KF. Ventrolateral medullary functional connectivity and the respiratory and central chemoreceptor-evoked modulation of retrotrapezoid-parafacial neurons. *J Neurophysiol.* 2011;105(6):2960–2975.
54. Monnier A, Alheid GF, McCrimmon DR. Defining ventral medullary respiratory compartments with a glutamate receptor agonist in the rat. *J Physiol.* 2003;548(Pt 3):859–874.
55. Pilowsky PM, Jiang C, Lipski J. An intracellular study of respiratory neurons in the rostral ventrolateral medulla of the rat and their relationship to catecholamine-containing neurons. *J Comp Neurol.* 1990;301(4):604–617.
56. Pilowsky PM, Lipski J, Prestidge R, Jiang C. Dual fluorescence combined with a two-color immunoperoxidase technique: a new way of visualizing diverse neuronal elements. *J Neurosci Methods.* 1991;36(2–3):185–193.
57. Pilowsky P, Llewellyn-Smith IJ, Arnolda L, Lipski J, Minson J, Chalmers J. Are the ventrally projecting dendrites of respiratory neurons a neuroanatomical basis for the chemosensitivity of the ventral medulla oblongata? *Sleep.* 1993;16(Suppl. 8):S53–S55.

58. Pilowsky P, Llewellyn-Smith IJ, Lipski J, Minson J, Arnolda L, Chalmers J. Projections from inspiratory neurons of the ventral respiratory group to the subretrofacial nucleus of the cat. *Brain Res.* 1994;633(1–2):63–71.
59. Sun QJ, Minson J, Llewellyn-Smith IJ, Arnolda L, Chalmers J, Pilowsky P. Botzinger neurons project towards bulbospinal neurons in the rostral ventrolateral medulla of the rat. *J Comp Neurol.* 1997;388(1):23–31.
60. Sun QJ, Goodchild AK, Chalmers JP, Pilowsky PM. The pre-Botzinger complex and phase-spanning neurons in the adult rat. *Brain Res.* 1998;809(2):204–213.
61. Jiang C, Lipski J. Extensive monosynaptic inhibition of ventral respiratory group neurons by augmenting neurons in the Botzinger complex in the cat. *Exp Brain Res.* 1990;81(3): 639–648.
62. Nunez-Abades PA, Morillo AM, Pasaro R. Brainstem connections of the rat ventral respiratory subgroups: afferent projections. *J Auton Nerv Syst.* 1993;42(2):99–118.
63. Fedorko L, Merrill EG. Axonal projections from the rostral expiratory neurones of the Botzinger complex to medulla and spinal cord in the cat. *J Physiol.* 1984;350:487–496.
64. Tian GF, Peever JH, Duffin J. Botzinger-complex expiratory neurons monosynaptically inhibit phrenic motoneurons in the decerebrate rat. *Exp Brain Res.* 1998;122(2):149–156.
65. Ellenberger HH, Feldman JL. Monosynaptic transmission of respiratory drive to phrenic motoneurons from brainstem bulbospinal neurons in rats. *J Comp Neurol.* 1988;269(1):47–57.
66. Ezure K, Manabe M. Decrementing expiratory neurons of the Botzinger complex. II. Direct inhibitory synaptic linkage with ventral respiratory group neurons. *Exp Brain Res.* 1988;72(1): 159–166.
67. Smith JC, Abdala AP, Koizumi H, Rybak IA, Paton JF. Spatial and functional architecture of the mammalian brain stem respiratory network: a hierarchy of three oscillatory mechanisms. *J Neurophysiol.* 2007;98(6):3370–3387.
68. Feldman JL, Cohen MI. Relation between expiratory duration and rostral medullary expiratory neuronal discharge. *Brain Res.* 1978;141(1):172–178.
69. Hayashi F, Coles SK, McCrimmon DR. Respiratory neurons mediating the Breuer–Hering reflex prolongation of expiration in rat. *J Neurosci.* 1996;16(20):6526–6536.
70. Bongianni F, Mutolo D, Carfi M, Fontana GA, Pantaleo T. Respiratory neuronal activity during apnea and poststimulatory effects of laryngeal origin in the cat. *J Appl Physiol.* 2000;89(3): 917–925.
71. Abdala AP, Rybak IA, Smith JC, Paton JF. Abdominal expiratory activity in the rat brainstem-spinal cord in situ: patterns, origins and implications for respiratory rhythm generation. *J Physiol.* 2009;587(Pt 14):3539–3559.
72. Haji A, Okazaki M, Yamazaki H, Takeda R. Physiological properties of late inspiratory neurons and their possible involvement in inspiratory off-switching in cats. *J Neurophysiol.* 2002;87(2): 1057–1067.
73. Okazaki M, Takeda R, Yamazaki H, Haji A. Synaptic mechanisms of inspiratory off-switching evoked by pontine pneumotaxic stimulation in cats. *Neurosci Res.* 2002;44(1):101–110.
74. Segers LS, Nuding SC, Dick TE, et al. Functional connectivity in the pontomedullary respiratory network. *J Neurophysiol.* 2008;100(4):1749–1769.
75. Morschel M, Dutschmann M. Pontine respiratory activity involved in inspiratory/expiratory phase transition. *Philos Trans R Soc Lond B Biol Sci.* 2009;364(1529):2517–2526.
76. Richter DW. Generation and maintenance of the respiratory rhythm. *J Exp Biol.* 1982;100:93–107.
77. Pierrefiche O, Champagnat J, Richter DW. Calcium-dependent conductances control neurones involved in termination of inspiration in cats. *Neurosci Lett.* 1995;184(2):101–104.
78. Oku Y, Tanaka I, Ezure K. Activity of bulbar respiratory neurons during fictive coughing and swallowing in the decerebrate cat. *J Physiol.* 1994;480(Pt 2):309–324.
79. Davenport PW, Bolser DC, Morris KF. Swallow remodeling of respiratory neural networks. *Head Neck.* 2011;33(Suppl. 1): S8–S13.
80. Baekey DM, Morris KF, Gestreau C, Li Z, Lindsey BG, Shannon R. Medullary respiratory neurones and control of laryngeal motoneurones during fictive eupnoea and cough in the cat. *J Physiol.* 2001;534(Pt 2):565–581.
81. Shiba K, Nakazawa K, Ono K, Umezaki T. Multifunctional laryngeal premotor neurons: their activities during breathing, coughing, sneezing, and swallowing. *J Neurosci.* 2007;27(19): 5156–5162.
82. Dobbins EG, Feldman JL. Brainstem network controlling descending drive to phrenic motoneurons in rat. *J Comp Neurol.* 1994;347(1):64–86.
83. Makeham JM, Goodchild AK, Pilowsky PM. NK1 receptor and the ventral medulla of the rat: bulbospinal and catecholaminergic neurons. *Neuroreport.* 2001;12(17):3663–3667.
84. Solomon IC, Edelman NH, Neubauer JA. Patterns of phrenic motor output evoked by chemical stimulation of neurons located in the pre-Botzinger complex in vivo. *J Neurophysiol.* 1999;81(3): 1150–1161.
85. Smith JC, Ellenberger HH, Ballanyi K, Richter DW, Feldman JL. Pre-Botzinger complex: a brainstem region that may generate respiratory rhythm in mammals. *Science.* 1991;254(5032): 726–729.
86. Carroll MS, Viemari JC, Ramirez JM. Patterns of inspiratory phase-dependent activity in the in vitro respiratory network. *J Neurophysiol.* 2013;109(2):285–295.
87. Gray PA, Janczewski WA, Mellen N, McCrimmon DR, Feldman JL. Normal breathing requires preBotzinger complex neurokinin-1 receptor-expressing neurons. *Nat Neurosci.* 2001;4(9):927–930.
88. Wenninger JM, Pan LG, Klum L, et al. Large lesions in the pre-Botzinger complex area eliminate eupneic respiratory rhythm in awake goats. *J Appl Physiol.* 2004;97(5):1629–1636.
89. Krause KL, Forster HV, Kiner T, et al. Normal breathing pattern and arterial blood gases in awake and sleeping goats after near total destruction of the presumed pre-Botzinger complex and the surrounding region. *J Appl Physiol.* 2009;106(2):605–619.
90. Neumueller S, Hodges MR, Krause K, et al. Anatomic changes in multiple brainstem nuclei after incremental, near-complete neurotoxic destruction of the pre-Botzinger Complex in adult goats. *Respir Physiol Neurobiol.* 2011;175(1):1–11.
91. Koshiya N, Smith JC. Neuronal pacemaker for breathing visualized in vitro. *Nature.* 1999;400(6742):360–363.
92. Johnson SM, Smith JC, Funk GD, Feldman JL. Pacemaker behavior of respiratory neurons in medullary slices from neonatal rat. *J Neurophysiol.* 1994;72(6):2598–2608.
93. Pena F, Ramirez JM. Endogenous activation of serotonin-2A receptors is required for respiratory rhythm generation in vitro. *J Neurosci.* 2002;22(24):11055–11064.
94. Pace RW, Mackay DD, Feldman JL, Del Negro CA. Role of persistent sodium current in mouse preBotzinger Complex neurons and respiratory rhythm generation. *J Physiol.* 2007;580(Pt 2): 485–496.
95. Paton JF, Abdala AP, Koizumi H, Smith JC, St-John WM. Respiratory rhythm generation during gasping depends on persistent sodium current. *Nat Neurosci.* 2006;9(3):311–313.

96. Del Negro CA, Morgado-Valle C, Feldman JL. Respiratory rhythm: an emergent network property? *Neuron*. 2002;34(5): 821–830.
97. Feldman JL, McCrimmon DR, Speck DF. Effect of synchronous activation of medullary inspiratory bulbo-spinal neurones on phrenic nerve discharge in cat. *J Physiol*. 1984;347: 241–254.
98. Alheid GF, Gray PA, Jiang MC, Feldman JL, McCrimmon DR. Parvalbumin in respiratory neurons of the ventrolateral medulla of the adult rat. *J Neurocytol*. 2002;31(8–9):693–717.
99. Miller AD, Ezure K, Suzuki I. Control of abdominal muscles by brain stem respiratory neurons in the cat. *J Neurophysiol*. 1985;54(1):155–167.
100. Saji M, Miura M. Thoracic expiratory motor neurons of the rat: localization and sites of origin of their premotor neurons. *Brain Res*. 1990;507(2):247–253.
101. Holstege G. Anatomical study of the final common pathway for vocalization in the cat. *J Comp Neurol*. 1989;284(2):242–252.
102. Boers J, Klop EM, Hulshoff AC, de Weerd H, Holstege G. Direct projections from the nucleus retroambiguus to cricothyroid motoneurons in the cat. *Neurosci Lett*. 2002;319(1):5–8.
103. Fortuna MG, West GH, Stornetta RL, Guyenet PG. Botzinger expiratory-augmenting neurons and the parafacial respiratory group. *J Neurosci*. 2008;28(10):2506–2515.
104. Bongianni F, Mutolo D, Nardone F, Pantaleo T. Ionotropic glutamate receptors mediate excitatory drive to caudal medullary expiratory neurons in the rabbit. *Brain Res*. 2005;1056(2): 145–157.
105. Poliacek I, Corrie LWC, Wang C, Rose MJ, Bolser DC. Microinjection of DLH into the region of the caudal ventral respiratory column in the cat: evidence for an endogenous cough-suppressant mechanism. *J Appl Physiol*. 2007;102(3): 1014–1021.
106. Umezaki T, Zheng Y, Shiba K, Miller AD. Role of nucleus retroambigualis in respiratory reflexes evoked by superior laryngeal and vestibular nerve afferents and in emesis. *Brain Res*. 1997;769(2):347–356.
107. Dick TE, Bellingham MC, Richter DW. Pontine respiratory neurons in anesthetized cats. *Brain Res*. 1994;636(2):259–269.
108. Dutschmann M, Herbert H. The Kolliker-Fuse nucleus gates the postinspiratory phase of the respiratory cycle to control inspiratory off-switch and upper airway resistance in rat. *Eur J Neurosci*. 2006;24(4):1071–1084.
109. Smith JC, Morrison DE, Ellenberger HH, Otto MR, Feldman JL. Brainstem projections to the major respiratory neuron populations in the medulla of the cat. *J Comp Neurol*. 1989;281(1): 69–96.
110. Ellenberger HH, Feldman JL. Brainstem connections of the rostral ventral respiratory group of the rat. *Brain Res*. 1990;513(1):35–42.
111. Fung ML, Wang W, St John WM. Involvement of pontile NMDA receptors in inspiratory termination in rat. *Respir Physiol*. 1994;96(2–3):177–188.
112. Burke PG, Abbott SB, McMullan S, Goodchild AK, Pilowsky PM. Somatostatin selectively ablates post-inspiratory activity after injection into the Botzinger complex. *Neuroscience*. 2010;167(2): 528–539.
113. Dick TE, Shannon R, Lindsey BG, et al. Pontine respiratory-modulated activity before and after vagotomy in decerebrate cats. *J Physiol*. 2008;586(Pt 17):4265–4282.
114. Bonis J, Neumueller S, Marshall B, et al. The effects of lesions in the dorsolateral pons on the coordination of swallowing and breathing in awake goats. *Respir Physiol Neurobiol*. 2011;175(2): 272–282.
115. Potts JT, Rybak IA, Paton JF. Respiratory rhythm entrainment by somatic afferent stimulation. *J Neurosci*. 2005;25(8): 1965–1978.
116. Loewy AD, Burton H. Nuclei of the solitary tract: efferent projections to the lower brain stem and spinal cord of the cat. *J Comp Neurol*. 1978;181(2):421–449.
117. Ricardo JA, Koh ET. Anatomical evidence of direct projections from the nucleus of the solitary tract to the hypothalamus, amygdala, and other forebrain structures in the rat. *Brain Res*. 1978;153(1):1–26.
118. Dutschmann M, Herbert H. The Kolliker-Fuse nucleus mediates the trigeminally induced apnoea in the rat. *Neuroreport*. 1996;7(8): 1432–1436.
119. Oku Y, Dick TE. Phase resetting of the respiratory cycle before and after unilateral pontine lesion in cat. *J Appl Physiol*. 1992;72(2):721–730.
120. Song G, Poon CS. Lateral parabrachial nucleus mediates shortening of expiration and increase of inspiratory drive during hypercapnia. *Respir Physiol Neurobiol*. 2009;165(1):9–12.
121. Song G, Poon CS. Lateral parabrachial nucleus mediates shortening of expiration during hypoxia. *Respir Physiol Neurobiol*. 2009;165(1):1–8.
122. Connelly CA, Ellenberger HH, Feldman JL. Are there serotonergic projections from raphe and retrotrapezoid nuclei to the ventral respiratory group in the rat? *Neurosci Lett*. 1989;105(1–2): 34–40.
123. Lazarenko RM, Milner TA, Depuy SD, et al. Acid sensitivity and ultrastructure of the retrotrapezoid nucleus in Phox2b-EGFP transgenic mice. *J Comp Neurol*. 2009;517(1):69–86.
124. Guyenet PG, Mulkey DK, Stornetta RL, Bayliss DA. Regulation of ventral surface chemoreceptors by the central respiratory pattern generator. *J Neurosci*. 2005;25(39):8938–8947.
125. Li A, Nattie EE. Focal central chemoreceptor sensitivity in the RTN studied with a CO_2 diffusion pipette in vivo. *J Appl Physiol*. 1997;83(2):420–428.
126. Onimaru H, Homma I. Respiratory rhythm generator neurons in medulla of brainstem–spinal cord preparation from newborn rat. *Brain Res*. 1987;403(2):380–384.
127. Onimaru H, Ikeda K, Kawakami K. Phox2b, RTN/pFRG neurons and respiratory rhythmogenesis. *Respir Physiol Neurobiol*. 2009;168(1–2):13–18.
128. Onimaru H, Ikeda K, Kawakami K. CO_2-sensitive preinspiratory neurons of the parafacial respiratory group express Phox2b in the neonatal rat. *J Neurosci*. 2008;28(48):12845–12850.
129. Janczewski WA, Feldman JL. Distinct rhythm generators for inspiration and expiration in the juvenile rat. *J Physiol*. 2006;570(Pt 2):407–420.
130. Arita H, Ichikawa K, Sakamoto M. Serotonergic cells in nucleus raphe pallidus provide tonic drive to posterior cricoarytenoid motoneurons via 5-hydroxytryptamine$_2$ receptors in cats. *Neurosci Lett*. 1995;197(2):113–116.
131. Bonham AC. Neurotransmitters in the CNS control of breathing. *Respir Physiol*. 1995;101(3):219–230.
132. Lindsay AD, Feldman JL. Modulation of respiratory activity of neonatal rat phrenic motoneurones by serotonin. *J Physiol*. 1993;461:213–233.
133. Verner TA, Goodchild AK, Pilowsky PM. A mapping study of cardiorespiratory responses to chemical stimulation of the midline medulla oblongata in ventilated and freely breathing rats. *Am J Physiol Regul Integr Comp Physiol*. 2004;287(2): R411–R421.
134. Millhorn DE. Stimulation of raphe (obscurus) nucleus causes long-term potentiation of phrenic nerve activity in cat. *J Physiol*. 1986;381:169–179.

135. Morris KF, Arata A, Shannon R, Lindsey BG. Long-term facilitation of phrenic nerve activity in cats: responses and short time scale correlations of medullary neurones. *J Physiol.* 1996;490(Pt 2): 463–480.
136. Morris KF, Shannon R, Lindsey BG. Changes in cat medullary neurone firing rates and synchrony following induction of respiratory long-term facilitation. *J Physiol.* 2001;532(Pt 2): 483–497.
137. Nattie EE, Li A. CO_2 dialysis in the medullary raphe of the rat increases ventilation in sleep. *J Appl Physiol.* 2001;90(4): 1247–1257.
138. Thor KB, Helke CJ. Serotonin- and substance P-containing projections to the nucleus tractus solitarii of the rat. *J Comp Neurol.* 1987;265(2):275–293.
139. Perez H, Ruiz S. Medullary responses to chemoreceptor activation are inhibited by locus coeruleus and nucleus raphe magnus. *Neuroreport.* 1995;6(10):1373–1376.
140. Jean A. Brain stem control of swallowing: neuronal network and cellular mechanisms. *Physiol Rev.* 2001;81(2):929–969.
141. Miller A. The neurobiology of swallowing and dysphagia. *Dev Disabil Res Rev.* 2008;14:77–86.
142. Dick T, Oku Y, Romaniuk J, Cherniack N. Interaction between central pattern generators for breathing and swallowing in the cat. *J Physiol.* 1993;465(1):715.
143. Feroah TR, Forster H, Fuentes CG, et al. Effects of spontaneous swallows on breathing in awake goats. *J Appl Physiol.* 2002;92(5): 1923–1935.
144. Feroah TR, Forster H, Fuentes CG, et al. Contributions from rostral medullary nuclei to coordination of swallowing and breathing in awake goats. *J Appl Physiol.* 2002;93(2):581–591.
145. Schultz JL, Perlman AL, VanDaele DJ. Laryngeal movement, oropharyngeal pressure, and submental muscle contraction during swallowing. *Arch Phys Med Rehabil.* 1994;75(2): 183–188.
146. Thexton AJ, Crompton AW, German RZ. Electromyographic activity during the reflex pharyngeal swallow in the pig: Doty and Bosma (1956) revisited. *J Appl Physiol.* 2007;102(2):587–600.
147. Thexton AJ, Crompton AW, Owerkowicz T, German RZ. Impact of rhythmic oral activity on the timing of muscle activation in the swallow of the decerebrate pig. *J Neurophysiol.* 2009;101(3): 1386–1393.
148. Pommerenke WT. A study of the sensory areas eliciting the swallow reflex. *Am J Physiol.* 1928;84:36–41.
149. Ootani S, Umezaki T, Shin T, Murata Y. Convergence of afferents from the SLN and GPN in cat medullary swallowing neurons. *Brain Res Bull.* 1995;37(4):397–404.
150. Yamamura K, Kitagawa J, Kurose M, et al. Neural mechanisms of swallowing and effects of taste and other stimuli on swallow initiation. *Biol Pharm Bull.* 2010;33(11):1786–1790.
151. Gestreau C, Milano S, Bianchi AL, Grelot L. Activity of dorsal respiratory group inspiratory neurons during laryngeal-induced fictive coughing and swallowing in decerebrate cats. *Exp Brain Res.* 1996;108(2):247–256.
152. Saito Y, Ezure K, Tanaka I, Osawa M. Activity of neurons in ventrolateral respiratory groups during swallowing in decerebrate rats. *Brain Dev.* 2003;25(5):338–345.
153. Ingelfinger FJ. Esophageal motility. *Physiol Rev.* 1958;38(4): 533–584.
154. Hukuhara T, Okada H. Effects of deglutition upon the spike discharges of neurones in the respiratory center. *Jpn J Physiol.* 1956;6(2):162–166.
155. Saito Y, Ezure K, Tanaka I. Swallowing-related activities of respiratory and non-respiratory neurons in the nucleus of solitary tract in the rat. *J Physiol.* 2002;540(Pt 3):1047–1060.
156. Hårdemark Cedborg AI, Sundman E, Bodén K, et al. Co-ordination of spontaneous swallowing with respiratory airflow and diaphragmatic and abdominal muscle activity in healthy adult humans. *Exp Physiol.* 2009;94(4):459–468.
157. Wilson S, Thach B, Brouillette R, Abu-Osba Y. Coordination of breathing and swallowing in human infants. *J Appl Physiol.* 1981;50(4):851.
158. Bolser DC. Fictive cough in the cat. *J Appl Physiol.* 1991;71(6): 2325–2331.
159. Dicpinigaitis PV. Experimentally induced cough. *Pulm Pharmacol Ther.* 2007;20(4):319–324.
160. Fontana GA, Lavorini F. Cough motor mechanisms. *Respir Physiol Neurobiol.* 2006;152(3):266–281.
161. Pitts T, Bolser D, Rosenbek J, Troche M, Sapienza C. Voluntary cough production and swallow dysfunction in Parkinson's disease. *Dysphagia.* 2008;23(3):297–301.
162. Pitts T, Troche MS, Carnaby-Mann G, Rosenbek JC, Okun MS, Sapienza CM. Utilizing voluntary cough to detect penetration and aspiration during oropharyngeal swallowing in Parkinson's disease. *Chest.* 2010.
163. Ross BB, Gramiak R, Rahn H. Physical dynamics of the cough mechanism. *J Appl Physiol.* 1955;8(3):264–268.
164. Shannon R, Baekey D, Morris K, Nuding S, Segers L, Lindsey B. Production of reflex cough by brainstem respiratory networks. *Pulm Pharmacol Ther.* 2004;17(6):369–376.
165. Shannon R, Baekey DM, Morris KF, Lindsey BG. Ventrolateral medullary respiratory network and a model of cough motor pattern generation. *J Appl Physiol.* 1998;84(6):2020.
166. Canning BJ. Anatomy and neurophysiology of the cough reflex. *Chest.* 2006;129(Suppl. 1):33S.
167. Canning BJ. The cough reflex in animals: relevance to human cough research. *Lung.* 2008;186(Suppl. 1):S23–S28.
168. Canning BJ, Mazzone SB, Meeker SN, Mori N, Reynolds SM, Undem BJ. Identification of the tracheal and laryngeal afferent neurones mediating cough in anaesthetized guinea pigs. *J Physiol.* 2004;557(2):543–558.
169. Lieu T, Undem BJ. Neuroplasticity in vagal afferent neurons involved in cough. *Pulm Pharmacol Ther.* 2011;24(3):276–279.
170. Moore KA, Undem BJ, Weinreich D. Antigen inhalation unmasks NK-2 tachykinin receptor-mediated responses in vagal afferents. *Am J Respir Crit Care Med.* 2000;161(1):232.
171. Muroi Y, Undem BJ. Targeting peripheral afferent nerve terminals for cough and dyspnea. *Curr Opin Pharmacol.* 2011;11(3):254–264.
172. Myers AC, Kajekar R, Undem BJ. Allergic inflammation-induced neuropeptide production in rapidly adapting afferent nerves in guinea pig airways. *Am J Physiol-Lung Cell Mol Physiol.* 2002;282(4):L775.
173. Ezure K, Otake K, Lipski J, Wong She RB. Efferent projections of pulmonary rapidly adapting receptor relay neurons in the cat. *Brain Res.* 1991;564(2):268–278.
174. Hanacek J, Davies A, Widdicombe JG. Influence of lung stretch receptors on the cough reflex in rabbits. *Respiration.* 1984;45(3): 161–168.
175. Sant'Ambrogio G, Sant'Ambrogio FB, Davies A. Airway receptors in cough. *Bull Eur Physiopathol Respir.* 1984;20(1):43–47.
176. Forsberg K, Karlsson JA. Cough induced by stimulation of capsaicin-sensitive sensory neurons in conscious guinea-pigs. *Acta Physiol Scand.* 1986;128(2):319–320.
177. Tatar M, Webber SE, Widdicombe JG. Lung C-fibre receptor activation and defensive reflexes in anaesthetized cats. *J Physiol.* 1988;402:411–420.
178. Canning BJ. Encoding of the cough reflex. *Pulm Pharmacol Ther.* 2007;20(4):396–401.

179. Haji A, Ohi Y, Kimura S. Cough-related neurons in the nucleus tractus solitarius of decerebrate cats. *Neuroscience*. 2012;218: 100–109.
180. Baekey DM, Morris KF, Nuding SC, Segers LS, Lindsey BG, Shannon R. Medullary raphe neuron activity is altered during fictive cough in the decerebrate cat. *J Appl Physiol*. 2003;94(1): 93–100.
181. Baekey DM, Morris KF, Nuding SC, Segers LS, Lindsey BG, Shannon R. Ventrolateral medullary respiratory network participation in the expiration reflex in the cat. *J Appl Physiol*. 2004;96(6): 2057–2072.
182. Segers LS, Nuding SC, Vovk A, et al. Discharge identity of medullary inspiratory neurons is altered during repetitive fictive cough. *Front Physiol*. 2012;3:223.

CHAPTER

19

Visual Network

Moran Furman

Department of Neurology, Yale University School of Medicine, New Haven, CT, USA

INTRODUCTION

In the 1830s, the Swiss crystallographer Louis A. Necker discovered that cubic crystals appeared, when observed under a microscope, to flip back and forth in three dimensions (3D), as if magically inverting their internal structure. In his attempts to solve this mystery, he realized that a similar perceptual phenomenon is experienced when looking at a simple two-dimensional (2D) drawing of a cube (Figure 19.1). Thus, it was not the actual structure of the crystals under Necker's microscope that was changing over time, but the interpretation of the visual system when presented with an ambiguous stimulus.[1]

The Necker-cube illusion illustrates how the visual system is actively and dynamically engaged in interpreting the visual scene captured by the eyes. The visual system decomposes the scene using local feature detectors that are sensitive to specific visual features—color, texture, motion, and so on. These local features are then assembled into a meaningful, coherent percept, based on rules, expectations, and prior experiences acquired during development and over the course of evolution. These remarkable computations are implemented in a network of cortical and subcortical brain areas. Proper functioning of these central nervous system (CNS) structures underlies normal visual functions. Damage to these structures due to injury or neurological disease impairs vision, sometimes in intriguing, almost bizarre manners, emphasizing the complexity underlying the seemingly effortless act of seeing.[2–4] Due to the importance of vision to human behavior, visual impairments can have a profound and debilitating impact on patients' quality of life. Emerging neurostimulation and other neuroengineering techniques are paving the way for novel therapeutic approaches for treating blindness and impaired vision.[5–9]

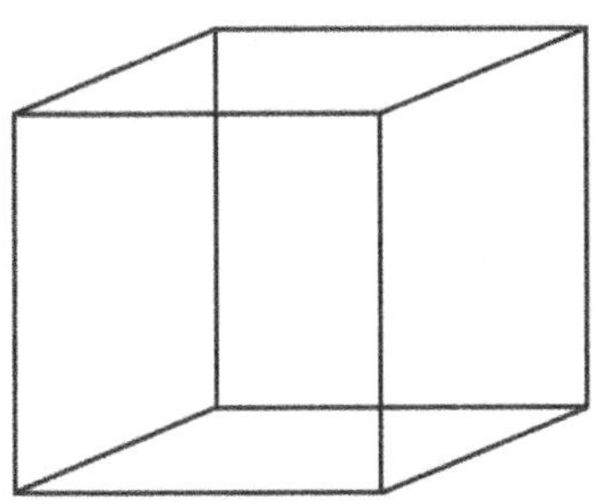

FIGURE 19.1 The Necker cube illusion. A two-dimensional drawing of a cube is normally perceived as a 3D structure appearing in one of two possible configurations. When observed continuously over tens of seconds, perception will typically alternate back and forth between the two 3D shapes.

Visual systems vary considerably among mammalian species, and these differences need to be taken into account while interpreting experiments from animal models. Yet, many principles as well as details of the organization and function of the visual system have been well preserved over the course of mammalian evolution. In recent years, there has been a growing use of mice and rats for the study of vision, partly due to rapid advances in molecular, optogenetic, imaging, and behavioral techniques applicable mainly to rodents.[10–15] Generally, this chapter examines the visual system from the human–primate perspective, with reference to other species, including rodents, where indicated. The first part of the chapter provides an overview of brain networks subserving visual processing, and the second part discusses how neural activity in these brain regions correlates with conscious visual experience.

RETINAL CIRCUITS FOR INITIAL VISUAL PROCESSING

Light enters the eye through the lens and forms a 2D image of the visual field on the retina, which lines the

Neuronal Networks in Brain Function, CNS Disorders, and Therapeutics
http://dx.doi.org/10.1016/B978-0-12-415804-7.00019-8

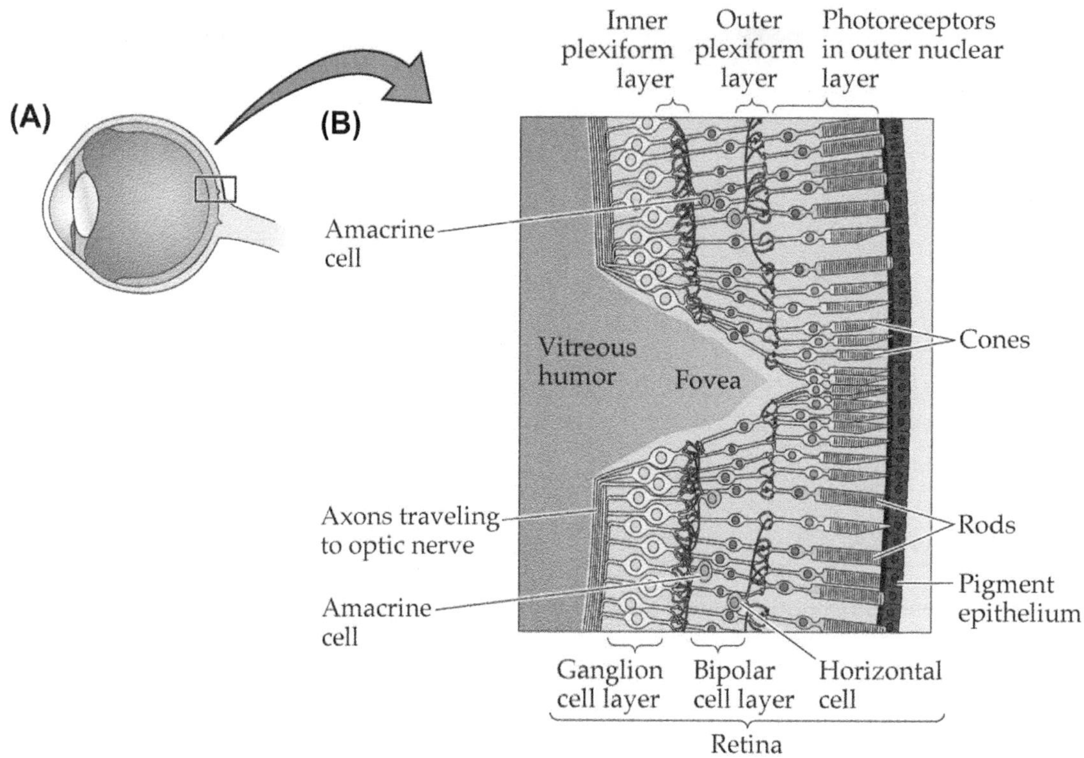

FIGURE 19.2 **The retina.** (A) Light enters the eye through the lens and forms an image on the retina, which lines the inner surface of the eye. (B) Magnified view of the retina in the region around the fovea. The fovea corresponds to the central fixation point, where visual acuity is maximal. The retina is a layered structure composed of neurons and glial cells. Rod and cone photoreceptors are located in the outermost layer of the retina, farthest from the lens. Therefore, light traverses the entire thickness of the retina to reach them, except in the fovea, where light reaches photoreceptors with minimal distortion. Bipolar, horizontal, and amacrine cells mediate signals from photoreceptors to retinal ganglion cells (RGCs). RGCs project their axons to the optic nerve and to the brain. (*Source: Reproduced, with permission, from Blumenfeld H. Neuroanatomy through Clinical Cases. 2nd ed. Sinauer Associates, Inc.; 2010.*) (For color version of this figure, the reader is referred to the online version of this book.)

inner surface of the eye (Figure 19.2). The retina is a layered network of neurons and glial cells, described anatomically in detail by Ramon y Cajal over a century ago.[16] During embryonic development, the retina originates as an outgrowth of the brain. Thus, despite its peripheral location, the retina is in fact considered part of the CNS.

Light is captured in the retina by three classes of photoreceptor cells: rods, cones, and the more recently discovered melanopsin-expressing intrinsically photosensitive retinal ganglion cells (ipRGCs). In humans, rods outnumber cones by about 20:1. Rods have relatively poor spatial and temporal resolution, are not color sensitive, and support vision in low-level light conditions. In contrast, cones have relatively high spatial and temporal resolution, are color sensitive, and are active during daylight. As mentioned here, cones are fewer in number than rods, but they are much more densely represented in the fovea, where visual acuity is highest. The third class of photosensitive retinal neurons, ipRGCs, and their downstream pathways are involved in the regulation of circadian rhythms, pupillary light reflex, and other "nonvisual" responses to light that rely on light levels but are not directly involved in the analysis of visual images.[17]

Rods and cones send signals to bipolar cells, which in turn synapse onto retinal ganglion cells (RGCs) that send their axons into the optic nerve. In addition to this feedforward, "vertical" pathway, two classes of retinal interneurons form lateral connections with nearby bipolar and ganglion cells: horizontal cells and amacrine cells. All of these classes of retinal neurons can be further divided into multiple subclasses based on morphological, physiological, and molecular signatures.[18] Retinal networks, through their vertical-lateral architecture, implement intricate image-processing computations, which achieve at least two major goals. The first is information compression: there are roughly 125 million photoreceptors in the retina but only about 1.3 million RGCs that send their axons to the brain. The second goal of retinal processing is calculation of invariances. Invariant recognition, which continues in higher visual centers in the brain, allows detection of objects' properties such as color, shape, and size

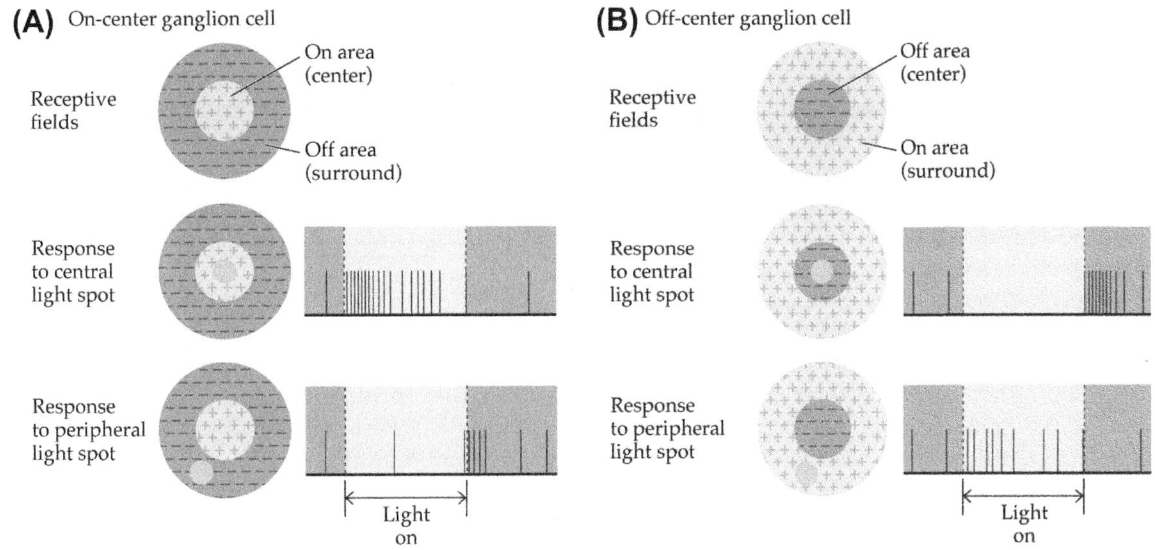

FIGURE 19.3 **Center-surround receptive fields of retinal ganglion cells (RGCs).** Schematic receptive field and response pattern of an on-center (A) and off-center (B) RGC. An on-center RGC responds with a train of action potentials to the presence of a light spot in the center of the receptive field, and it is inhibited by light in the surround. Conversely, off-center RGCs are excited by light in the surround but inhibited by light in the center of the receptive field. (*Source: Reproduced, with permission, from Blumenfeld H. Neuroanatomy through Clinical Cases. 2nd ed. Sinauer Associates, Inc.; 2010.*) (For color version of this figure, the reader is referred to the online version of this book.)

independently from variations in the visual stimulus resulting from changes in illumination, distance, viewing angle, and more.

RGCs have center-surround receptive fields (see Figure 19.3 for further details). That is, these neurons respond best to intensity differences between a central region and a surrounding region of the visual field. Similar receptive fields are also encountered in subcortical visual regions. However, most *cortical* neurons in the visual system have more sophisticated response properties, reflecting a higher level of visual analysis.

Curiously, the retinas of mammals, including humans, not only project to the brain but also receive input from the brainstem, via axons originating from serotonergic and histaminergic neurons in the dorsal raphe and hypothalamus, respectively. These neurons are part of the ascending arousal system (see Chapter 22), suggesting that these "retinopetal" projections may modulate visual processing with correlation to arousal levels.[19] Although the number of retinopetal axons is small, they branch extensively in the retina.

Remarkably, neural networks in the retina, at least in lower vertebrates, possess not only spatial image-processing capabilities at any moment in time but also sophisticated and adaptive temporal pattern recognition mechanisms, which signal novelty or omissions in repetitive trains of stimuli.[20]

Thus, neural circuits in the retina, the earliest stage of visual processing, display many of the hallmarks characteristics of visual systems in general, including parallel, interacting streams of information processing; top-down modulation; invariant pattern recognition; and experience-based expectations and predictions.[21]

SUBCORTICAL VISUAL PATHWAYS

The retina projects to several subcortical nuclei. The two projections that mediate vision, in contrast to light-dependent nonvisual functions, are those to the lateral geniculate nucleus (LGN) of the thalamus and the superior colliculus (SC) in the midbrain (Figure 19.5). In both regions, as in many areas of the visual cortex, retinal inputs are retinotopically organized, meaning that nearby locations in the retina project to neighboring locations in the target, thus forming a "map" of the visual field. The LGN projects to the primary visual cortex, which is discussed later in this chapter.

The LGN has six layers. The two ventral layers are the magnocellular layers. The magnocellular layers relay information from M cells of the retina, which have large receptive fields and respond best to gross features and movement, and are not color sensitive or only slightly so. The four remaining layers of the LGN are the parvocellular layers, which relay information from retinal P cells, which have small receptive fields, and are sensitive to fine visual details and color. Intralaminar LGN neurons also relay color information.[22] Like in the retina, neurons in the LGN have small center-surround concentric receptive fields. Axons from ipsilateral and contralateral retinas synapse onto different layers of the LGN. Thus, the overall architecture of parallel processing streams, carrying information about particular aspects of sensory inputs, is preserved from the retina to the LGN.

Traditionally, the LGN has been viewed as a relatively passive relay station of visual information from the retina to the cortex, partly because of the similarity of receptive field properties of RGCs and LGN neurons. Also, early studies found little modulation of LGN activity in response to selective attention and other cognitive influences, although later findings revised this account.[23,24] Anatomically, the LGN is ideally positioned for early regulatory modulation of information transmission. In fact, retinal afferents form only a minority of the input to the LGN. About 90% of the input to the LGN comes from three other sources (with roughly equal contributions): (1) GABAergic inhibitory inputs from the thalamic reticular nucleus (TRN), (2) cholinergic inputs from the pedunculopontine tegmental (PPT) nucleus and the parabigeminal nucleus (PBN) of the brainstem, and (3) glutamatergic cortico-thalamic feedback projections from V1.[25] Physiologically, regulation of LGN transmission may involve various mechanisms, including transitions between burst and tonic firing modes[26,27] and modulating synchrony and correlation among LGN neurons[28] (see Chapter 9).

The SC like the LGN, receives direct input from the retina. The SC is a midbrain region involved in eye movements and spatial attention. Retinal inputs form a retinotopic map in the upper layers of the SC. The SC also receives sensory input from other modalities, including auditory and somatosensory inputs, and the maps of these multisensory inputs are spatially aligned.[29] The SC projects to the association cortex via relays in the pulvinar and lateral posterior nucleus of the thalamus (see "The colliculo-pulvinar-cortical pathway").

The nonmammalian homolog of the SC, the optic tectum, embodies the whole visual system in many vertebrates. In mammals, and particularly higher mammals, the dominance of the SC as a visual center is reduced, whereas the geniculo-cortical pathway plays a more central role in visual processing. In mice, for instance, at least 70% of RGCs project to the SC.[30] In cats, the number is down to about 50%,[31] and in monkeys 10%.[32] Nevertheless, the visual pathway initiating in the retino-collicular projection plays important functions in directing visual attention and in rapid visual processing, particularly of motion.

The SC forms dense reciprocal connections with the PBN, which is sometimes referred to as a satellite of the SC. The projection from the SC to the PBN is excitatory and utilizes the neuropeptide substance P, whereas the back projection is cholinergic. The PBN also projects to other brain structures such as the thalamus and the amygdala. The SC—PBN loop is involved in spatial attention and possibly also supports the subconscious processing of emotional content of visual stimuli as revealed following damage to the primary visual cortex.[33,34]

THE COLLICULO-PULVINAR-CORTICAL PATHWAY

The pulvinar is the largest nucleus in the primate thalamus, but it has been studied much less than the LGN. The superficial layers of the SC relay to the dorsal visual cortex (middle-temporal (MT), V3) via the inferior pulvinar.[35–37] Fast transmission along this pathway may mediate rapid motion detection and saliency processing. The colliculo-pulvinar pathway to the cortex is also involved in perceptual stability during rapid saccadic eye movements.[38,39] The pulvinar, like the LGN, receives GABAergic input from the TRN and cholinergic input from brainstem regions.[40]

The importance of the pulvinar for attention and visual processing is emphasized by lesion studies. Patients with pulvinar lesions show deficits in (1) attending to the contralesional field, (2) filtering out distracter information, and (3) binding visual features based on spatial information.[41–43] Reversible silencing of the pulvinar in monkeys causes visuo-spatial hemineglect and impairment in visually guided behavior such as reaching and grasping.[44,45] Together, these findings suggest critical involvement of the pulvinar in several aspects of spatial cognition.

THE PRIMARY VISUAL CORTEX

The LGN projects to the primary visual cortex (also referred to as V1, striate cortex, or area 17) via the optic radiations, in which axons from the ipsi- and contralateral retinal layers of the LGN are intermingled. V1, like many parts of the visual pathways, is retinotopically organized.[46] In primates, it spans over 10% of the neocortex.[47] Since the pioneering work of Hubel and Wiesel,[48,49] decades of research on V1 have revealed phenomenal sophistication in its organization and function.[50–55] To a certain extent, different stimulus attributes such as form, color, and movement are processed by separate groups of neurons in V1, and this segregation into processing streams is reflected also in the output projections of V1 and the organization of its downstream target areas (Figure 19.4). For instance, cytochrome oxidase staining of V1 reveals patches of stains known as blobs; color-sensitive neurons without orientation selectivity are concentrated in these blobs, whereas cells between the blobs have little color selectivity but are orientation selective.[52] A fraction of V1

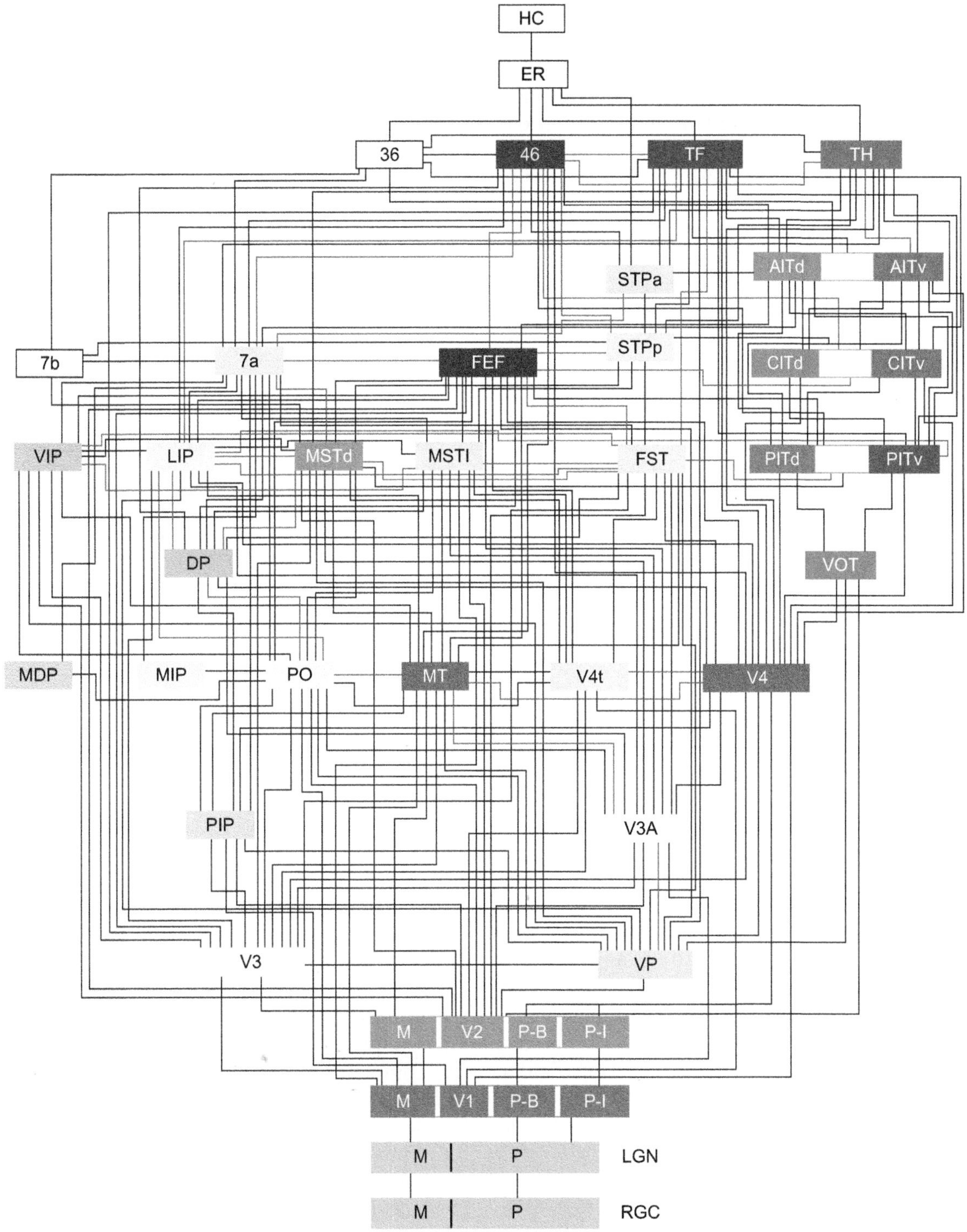

FIGURE 19.4 **Distributed hierarchical processing in the visual cortex of the macaque monkey.** The visual system is organized in a parallel, interacting processing stream, organized in a semihierarchical structure. Area V1 (the primary visual cortex) projects directly and indirectly to a large network of extrastriate visual areas that specialize in processing specific aspects of the visual scene (see the text for details). RGCs: retinal ganglion cells; LGN: lateral geniculate nucleus; M: magnocellular pathway; P: parvocellular pathway. (*Source: Reproduced, with permission, from Felleman DJ, Van Essen DC. Distributed hierarchical processing in the primate cerebral cortex. Cereb Cortex. 1991;1:1–47.*) (For color version of this figure, the reader is referred to the online version of this book.)

neurons can be classified as simple cells, which respond selectively to an oriented line that is either brighter or darker than the background, whereas the majority of V1 cells are complex cells and respond to orientation independently of contrast. Receptive fields of V1 neurons are relatively small, particularly in the fovea, and thus provide a detailed feature-based representation of the visual field at a high spatial resolution.

Inputs originating from each eye are kept largely separate in layer IV, the input layer of the cortex, but converge onto binocular cells in layers II, III, V, and VI. As a consequence of this binocular convergence, some cells in V1 are sensitive to disparity (the difference in location of a stimulus on the two retinas), a key component in binocular depth perception.[56,57]

VENTRAL AND DORSAL CORTICAL PATHWAYS FOR VISUAL PROCESSING

V1 projects to several cortical visual areas. The impressive network of visually related areas downstream of V1 consists of over 30 regions, which together span more than 50% of the primate neocortex (Figure 19.4). The visual cortex is organized in a generally hierarchical structure, blurred to some extent by massive feedback connectivity as well as reciprocal connections among many of the visual areas. Additionally, cortical visual areas have extensive connections with a variety of subcortical structures, including nuclei in the forebrain (amygdala, claustrum, and caudate nucleus), thalamus (pulvinar and reticular nucleus), midbrain (SC), brainstem (pons), hypothalamus, and more.[47]

Anatomically, the plethora of extrastriate visual areas can be roughly organized into two processing streams: one courses ventrally, terminating in the inferior temporal lobe; and the other runs dorsally through the MT and middle-superior-temporal (MST) areas, culminating in association areas of the parietal lobe such as the lateral-intraparietal (LIP) area (Figure 19.5). Ungerleider and Mishkin[58] coined the idea of a ventral "what" pathway, involved in visual recognition of objects, versus a dorsal "where" pathway concerned with spatial relationships among objects and visual guidance toward them. A related but alternative view, proposed by Goodale and Milner,[59] focuses on a "perception vs action" dichotomy. In this interpretation, the ventral pathway ("perception") contains visual representations that can be used for cognitive operations such as object recognition and memory, whereas the dorsal pathway ("action") provides real-time visual guidance for motor actions such as eye movements and manual grasping. Increasing evidence suggests that a number of visual properties, such as shape recognition, are processed in both pathways.[60] Interestingly, a two-stream organization

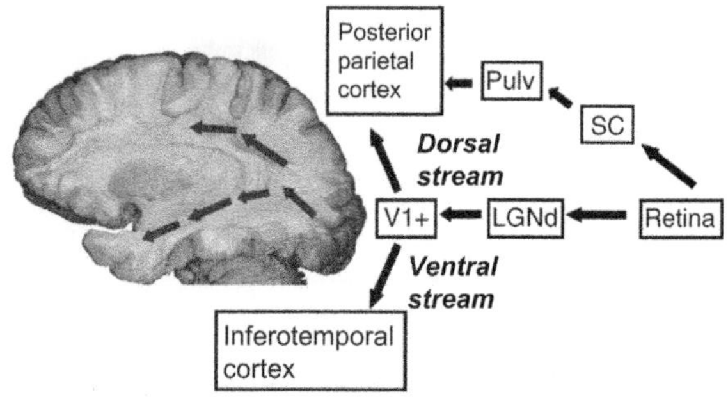

FIGURE 19.5 **Ventral and dorsal cortical pathways.** Overall organization of the ventral and dorsal cortical streams and their input pathways. Cortical areas downstream of V1 can be roughly organized into two processing streams. The ventral stream culminates in areas of the inferior temporal lobe, and it is involved primarily in object recognition and related perceptual functions. The dorsal stream culminates in association areas of the parietal lobe, and it is involved in spatial relationships among objects and visual guidance for motor actions. V1 receives visual input via the retino-geniculate pathway. A second visual pathway initiating in the retina conveys visual information to the parietal cortex via the superior-colliculus and thalamic pulvinar. In higher mammals, this colliculo-pulvinar-cortical pathway is less dominant than the retino-geniculate pathway, but it plays important roles in eye movements, spatial attention, and rapid motion processing. (*Source: Reproduced, with permission, from Wandell BA, et al. Visual field maps in human cortex. Neuron. 2007;56:366–383.*) (For color version of this figure, the reader is referred to the online version of this book.)

analogous to the ventral-dorsal organization in primates was recently revealed in the mouse visual cortex.[61] This suggests that certain layout principles of visual network organization are well conserved across mammalian species.

Generally, as one proceeds from V1 to higher regions in the visual hierarchy, neurons encode more complex stimulus properties, and their receptive fields become progressively larger.[60,62] For instance, most neurons in MT and MST are motion sensitive and are selective to target motion in a particular direction or specific optic flow patterns.[60,63] Most neurons in the infero-temporal (IT) complex specialize in shape processing, and they include neurons selective to faces,[64] 3D shapes,[65] contour features,[66] and more. Interestingly, visual areas in the "intermediate" level of the visual hierarchy are some of the hardest to characterize. Area V4, for instance, is central for color and shape processing,[67–69] but it also plays important roles in target selection, attention, depth perception, figure–ground segregation, and even motion processing.[70–72]

THE NEURAL BASIS OF CONSCIOUS VISUAL EXPERIENCE

"Conscious experience" is an inherently subjective phenomenon. Accordingly, the term has generated vigorous debates over its meaning and whether it can be approached at all using standard scientific methods. In this chapter, "conscious visual experience" refers to the specific contents of vision in situations where this content can be clearly and consistently reported by experimental subjects. As an example, one may consider a motion picture. At 24 frames per second, the sequence of images in a movie elicits an unambiguous percept of continuous motion; this differs fundamentally from the "frozen movement" percept elicited by the same images presented, say, at one frame per second. The contents of the visual experience when watching the movie at its normal speed (i.e. continuous motion) are consistently reported by subjects, and the neural basis of this percept can be then examined experimentally.

How does neural activity across the visual system relate to conscious visual experience? This question has been addressed using several approaches, including (1) lesion studies in human patients and animal models, and (2) electrophysiology, imaging, and other techniques combined with psychophysical paradigms designed to detect neural correlates of conscious visual experience.

LOSS OF VISUAL AWARENESS FOLLOWING LOCALIZED LESIONS IN THE VISION NETWORK

Focal lesions to V1 cause loss of visual awareness in corresponding locations of the contralateral visual field (scotomas). In fact, historically, the retinotopic organization of V1 was first established based on scotomas in soldiers with occipital bullet wounds from the Russo-Japanese War and World War I.[73,74] Interestingly, in certain cases patients are not aware of their focal loss of vision due to the "filling-in" phenomenon.[75,76] Global unilateral lesions of V1 cause a loss, or a dramatic reduction of awareness to visual stimuli in the whole contralateral visual field. Notably, patients with V1 lesions often retain residual visual abilities in their "blind" visual field (a phenomenon called "blindsight"). In forced-choice psychophysical tasks, these patients can discriminate the presence, location, orientation, color, and movement of stimuli significantly above chance, despite reporting no awareness to the stimuli.[77–80] Whereas some researchers argued for complete loss of visual awareness in blindsight, other studies indicated that some patients do retain residual awareness in their blind field, particularly of moving objects.[80–83] It is possible that these visual impressions are so degraded or different from normal vision that, unless carefully examined, patients tend to report them as lack of visual awareness. Some blindsight patients have described their visual impressions in the "blind" field as "black moving on black", or flashes of light seen behind a screen.

The residual visual abilities in blindsight involve subcortical pathways to the extrastriate cortex that bypass V1. Originally, the colliculo-pulvinar-cortical pathway was proposed as the main route for the visual abilities in blindsight,[77,84] but more recent evidence suggests that the LGN and its projections to areas other than V1 critically contribute to the residual visual capabilities in blindsight.[85]

Why does damage to V1 so profoundly disrupt conscious experience if visual information is transmitted to the extrastriate cortex via alternative routes? One possibility is that damage to V1 deprives extrastriate areas of much of their input, so that residual activity in these areas is insufficient to elicit a conscious percept. In other words, according to this model, awareness does not necessarily have "access" to V1, but V1 is necessary to activate other regions that are crucial for awareness. Another possibility is that neural activity in V1 itself is somehow crucial for visual awareness, despite the fact that we are not aware of the neural activity in V1, or at least much of it, as discussed in the "Neural Correlates of Perceived Stimulus Properties" section. According to this model, it is not just the reduced "drive" to extrastriate areas after V1 lesions that impairs visual awareness but also the absence of V1 activity by itself.

Interestingly, focal lesions of most extrastriate areas do not impair visual awareness, despite the fact that neural activity in many of these areas is tightly correlated with conscious experience (discussed in this chapter). Such lesions transiently or permanently damage processing of specific visual attributes, sometimes with profoundly debilitating impact on patients' lives.[2,4,86,87] Lesions to V2, for instance, impair perceptual grouping but do not affect acuity or contrast sensitivity[88]; lesions to MT and MST impair motion perception[89–91]; lesions to V4 and putatively V8 impair color perception[92,93]; and inferior temporal lobe lesions can cause deficits in the recognition of faces and objects, as well as other shape-related perceptual impairments.[2,3,94,95]

Extrastriate lesions that do impair visual awareness are those of the superior temporal gyrus and, to a lesser degree, posterior parietal lobe. These lesions may cause profound deficits in attention. Patients with unilateral lesions often show contralateral spatial neglect,[96,97] and bilateral lesions can lead to a more profound deficit called Balint's syndrome in which patients have deficits in shifting attention and in visual guided movements.[98]

NEURAL CORRELATES OF PERCEIVED STIMULUS PROPERTIES

How does neural activity across the visual system relate to conscious visual perception? Does "awareness" have "access" to the information encoded in the activity of neurons in V1, for instance, or perhaps only to activity in higher cortical areas?

When two colors of the same brightness alternate at a certain frequency, subjects perceive either an alternating pattern ("flicker") or, if the frequency is high enough, a merged single and unchanging color. Humans and monkeys are aware of the flicker at frequencies up to about 10 Hz. The question arises: Do neurons in V1 respond to the alternating colors at frequencies above 10 Hz? Interestingly, the answer is yes. Recordings in alert monkeys show that the majority of color-opponent neurons in V1, like those in the retina and LGN, respond robustly at frequencies of 30 Hz and beyond, and their activity follows the temporal pattern of the stimulus.[99] This provides clear evidence of a visual signal that is encoded in V1 but not perceived.

How can one explain this dissociation between V1 activity and perception? Crick and Koch argued that awareness has access to neural activity in high-level extrastriate areas that project directly to the frontal cortex, but not to V1.[100] An alternate, perhaps more plausible assumption is that the relationship between V1 and awareness is dynamic, flexible, and situation dependent, rather than hard wired.[101] For instance, during isoluminant flicker, the activity of V1 color-opponent neurons may not be perceived, potentially due to the lack of co-activation of color-insensitive neurons.[99] Generally, the response properties of V1 neurons are ideally suited for providing the neural basis of awareness to fine details, such as minute facial expressions. Thus, face perception under normal conditions is likely to require both neural activity in object-selective regions such as the IT complex, where faces can be categorized and recognized, and activity in V1 that encodes small, local features.

Eye movements are another domain where the relationship between perception and neural activity can be examined in detail. I will focus on two types of eye movements: saccades and smooth pursuit. Saccades are rapid eye movements aimed at redirecting the fovea, where acuity is maximal, to an object of interest. During a saccade, the image on the retina quickly shifts from one point to another. If spatial perception was directly linked to the image on the retina, we would perceive a jump of the visual space during each saccade. However, we normally perceive the visual environment as stable. Von Helmholz postulated over 150 years ago that spatial stability during eye movements is achieved by integrating two signals: visual information arriving from the eyes, and an internal extraretinal signal, likely a copy of the motor signal sent to the eyes.[102] In recent decades, extensive research on the visual system during saccades has confirmed Von Helmholz's hypothesis (Figure 19.6). In V1, receptive fields have fixed retinal coordinates. Thus, during saccades, the receptive fields of V1 neurons shift from one point in space to another. Information encoded in these neurons is therefore dissociated from perception. However, in many extrastriate visual areas, as well as in the frontal eye field (FEF) in the frontal cortex and SC, neurons exhibit "shifting receptive fields", meaning that during saccade preparation, a neuron's sensitivity shifts from one retinal location to another in a manner that preserves sensitivity to a fixed location in the external space. Shifting receptive fields in areas such as the FEF necessarily imply the presence of not only a retinal input but also an extraretinal signal related to the eye movement itself, as originally hypothesized by Von Helmholz. The copy of the motor signal to the perceptual system is often referred to as corollary discharge,[38] and it is likely to involve signals conveyed via the SC to the pulvinar and from there to parietal and frontal cortical areas.[39]

As with saccades, spatial stability during pursuit eye movements involves integration of retinal and motor-related signals in extrastriate cortical areas. In contrast to saccades, pursuit eye movements are smooth and relatively slow rotations of the eyeball, aimed at tracking moving objects. The retinal image of the pursued object is nearly stable, but we perceive the target as moving (although, interestingly, perceptual estimates of target velocity err systematically[103]). V1 neurons, and also most MT neurons, encode motion in retinal coordinates. Thus, neural activity in these regions is not well correlated with perceived motion. However, neurons in area MST integrate retinal and nonretinal signals to generate representation of motion in external coordinates, a process called pursuit compensation. In a way, pursuit compensation reflects the ability to distinguish between self-generated and externally generated visual motion. Interestingly, pursuit compensation is impaired in schizophrenia, and the degree of the impairment correlates well with the degree of delusions of influence, in which patients attribute external sources to their thoughts or action.[104] Apart from schizophrenia, deficits in pursuit compensation can result from extrastriate lesions. In one intriguing case report, a patient perceived during pursuit the stationary world as moving in a direction opposite to his eye movement; that is, he perceived the retinal image movement per se, uncorrected for eye movements. This seemingly subtle impairment resulted in nausea, vertigo, and severe limitations in everyday-life activities.[87]

Multistable stimuli offer another set of tools for studying the relationship between neural activity and visual perception. Multistable perception emerges when sensory information is ambiguous, and it can be interpreted in two or more mutually exclusive ways. The Necker cube, presented in the "Introduction" to this chapter, is an example of an ambiguous image that results in bistable perception. Another example is

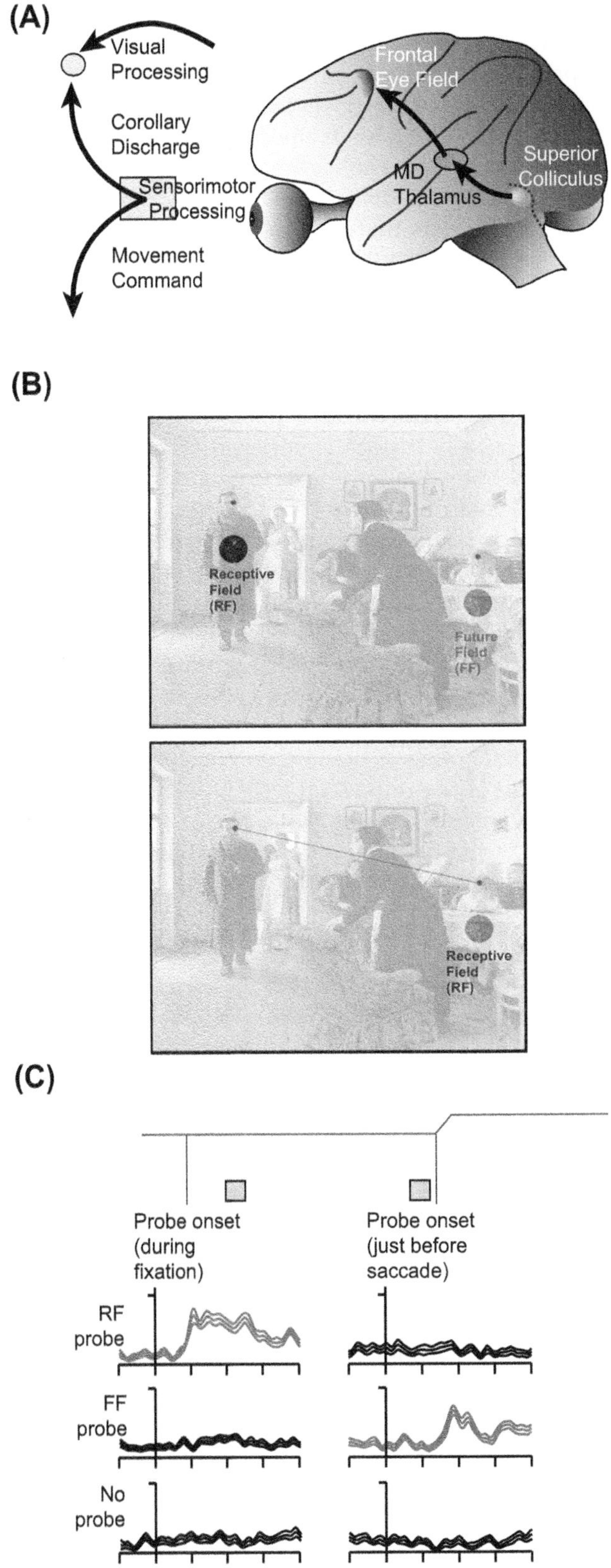

binocular rivalry, in which two different images are presented to the two eyes. In binocular rivalry, subjects perceive at any moment only one of the two images, with spontaneous alterations between the two images. Binocular rivalry allows dissociating between neural activity related to the unchanging stimulus and neural activity related to the alternating percept.[105,106] Early physiological studies concluded that neural activity in the LGN and V1 had little influence on the resolution of binocular rivalry. Subsequently, functional magnetic resonance imaging (fMRI) studies demonstrated clear effects of binocular rivalry on blood oxygenation level dependent (BOLD) signals in V1.[107,108] The discrepancy between electrophysiological and fMRI studies may relate to the fact that low-frequency power of the local field potential (LFP) in early cortical areas is more closely related to the perceptual awareness than spiking activity, and LFP in turn more strongly correlates with fMRI BOLD signals than with spiking activity.[109,110] Whereas the role of V1 in multistable perception is strongly debated, the involvement of extrastriate visual areas is more firmly established. In many extrastriate areas, both electrophysiological and fMRI experiments show clear correlations between subjective perception and neural activity.[105,111] Importantly, some brain regions also show a response to the suppressed stimuli during binocular rivalry. For instance, activity in the amygdala and superior temporal sulcus is associated with the emotional content of suppressed stimuli.[112,113]

FIGURE 19.6 **Spatial stability during eye movements is achieved through integration of visual and motor signals.** During eye movements, the visual system "compensates" for shifts in the location of the retinal image, to generate visual representations in externally based coordinates ("spatial stability"). Whereas early visual areas, such as V1, encode information in purely retinal coordinates, higher association areas of the cortex, such as the LIP in the parietal lobe and the FEF in the frontal lobe, adjust their responses during eye movements to compensate for the shift in the retinal image. Perception correlates with neural representations in higher association areas but does not correlate with retinal representations in the early visual areas. Eye movement compensation is achieved by integrating visual signals, and a motor signal that is a copy ("corollary discharge") of the movement command is sent to the eyes (A, left). The superior colliculus, for instance, sends motor commands to generate eye movements, and at the same time it projects through the medial dorsal nucleus of the thalamus (MD) to the FEF (A, right). During saccadic eye movements, neurons in the FEF exhibit "shifting receptive fields" (B, C). To probe the responses properties of these neurons, visual stimuli are presented before and after an eye movement in their receptive field (RF), as well as in their "future field" (FF), which corresponds to the RF after the eye movement (B). Notably, shortly prior to the eye movement, these neurons become nonresponsive to stimuli in the RF but respond robustly to stimuli in the FF (C). (*Source: Reproduced, with permission, from Wurtz RH. Neuronal mechanisms of visual stability. Vision Res. 2008;48:2070–2089.*) (The figure is reproduced in color section.)

CONCEPTUAL MODEL: BRAIN NETWORKS FOR VISUAL AWARENESS

This last section proposes a conceptual framework regarding the relationship between neural activity across the visual system and visual awareness. The proposed framework draws upon the more general theory of Plum and Posner concerning brain networks underlying states of consciousness.[114] Plum and Posner distinguished between two brain systems: those that regulate the *level of consciousness*, and those that provide the *content of consciousness*.

The systems regulating the *level of consciousness* consist of cortico-subcortical networks spanning high-order cortical areas such as the frontal and temporal-parietal association areas, as well as subcortical areas, including the basal forebrain, hypothalamus, thalamus, and upper brainstem activating systems. Blumenfeld proposed to refer to this collection of brain networks as the "consciousness system", in analogy to the sensory, motor, and other cortical-subcortical systems in the brain.

Brain systems that provide the *content of consciousness* include those underlying sensory and motor processing, memory, and emotions/drives. As distinct from the level of consciousness, the content of consciousness can be view as the substrate—it is what we are conscious of.

Along similar lines, and within the context of vision, one could again distinguish between two visual subsystems: one that regulates the *level or presence* of visual awareness, and one that provides the *contents* of the visual conscious experience.

The subsystem regulating the level or presence of visual awareness coincides in part with the more general system controlling the level of consciousness as a whole: being conscious is necessary, but not sufficient, for experiencing vision. Anatomically, many subcortical components of the "consciousness system" (which regulates the overall level of consciousness) project directly to critical visual centers. For instance, the TRN and cholinergic brainstem regions project to the LGN and pulvinar, and serotonergic and histaminergic neurons in the brainstem project to the retina. Optogenetic techniques, which permit selective stimulation or inhibition of specific cell types in the brain, are paving the way for examining the roles of these individual pathways during visual processing. In addition to the aforementioned structures, the subsystem regulating the level or presence of visual awareness also contains components that are specific to vision. When these vision-specific components are damaged or silenced, conscious vision is impaired without necessarily impairing consciousness in general. Key brain regions that specifically regulate the level of visual awareness include V1, the LGN, the pulvinar, and the superior-temporal gyrus. As discussed in this chapter, damage to any of these regions results in loss or dramatic reduction of visual awareness in the corresponding part of the visual field.

The second visual subsystem, the one that provides the contents of visual experience, includes many regions in the elaborate network of extrastriate visual areas, such as V2, V4, MT and MST, the IT complex, and also the SC, and the connections of all these areas to subcortical regions such as the amygdala. These areas specialize in processing specific aspects of the visual experience, such as color, texture, motion, shape, spatial relationships, emotional contents, and more. Damage to these areas robs visual experience of specific visual attributes, but it does not cause loss of visual awareness. The two visual subsystems, which regulate the level or presence of visual awareness versus the contents of visual experience, partially overlap and are strongly interconnected.

The immense complexity and richness of the human visual system (more than 50% of the cortex is involved in visual processing) humble any attempt to summarize its function and organization. Our current knowledge and understanding of the visual system are likely to be just the tip of the proverbial iceberg. Nevertheless, decades of intense research have led to unprecedented progress in the fascinating quest of understanding the neural basis of visual cognition.

References

1. Necker LA. Observations on some remarkable optical phenomena seen in Switzerland; and on an optical phenomenon which occurs on viewing a figure of a crystal or geometrical solid. *Lond Edinb Philos Mag J Sci*. 1832;1(5):329–337.
2. Blumenfeld H. *Neuroanatomy through Clinical Cases*. Sinauer; 2002.
3. Sacks OW. *The Man Who Mistook His Wife for a Hat and Other Clinical Tales*. Touchstone; 1998.
4. Ramachandran VS, Blakeslee S. *Phantoms in the Brain: Probing the Mysteries of the Human Mind*. Harper Perennial; 1999.
5. Pearson R, Barber A, Rizzi M, et al. Restoration of vision after transplantation of photoreceptors. *Nature*. 2012.
6. Theogarajan L. Strategies for restoring vision to the blind: current and emerging technologies. *Neurosci Lett*. 2012.
7. Busskamp V, Roska B. Optogenetic approaches to restoring visual function in retinitis pigmentosa. *Curr Opin Neurobiol*. 2011.
8. Golan L, Reutsky I, Farah N, Shoham S. Design and characteristics of holographic neural photo-stimulation systems. *J Neural Eng*. 2009;6:066004.
9. Cepko CL. Emerging gene therapies for retinal degenerations. *J Neurosci*. 2012;32(19):6415–6420.
10. Harvey CD, Coen P, Tank DW. Choice-specific sequences in parietal cortex during a virtual-navigation decision task. *Nature*. 2012;484(7392):62–68.
11. Vermaercke B, Op de Beeck HP. A multivariate approach reveals the behavioral templates underlying visual discrimination in rats. *Curr Biol*. 2011.

12. Witten IB, Steinberg EE, Lee SY, et al. Recombinase-driver rat lines: tools, techniques, and optogenetic application to dopamine-mediated reinforcement. *Neuron*. 2011;72(5):721–733.
13. Desai M, Kahn I, Knoblich U, et al. Mapping brain networks in awake mice using combined optical neural control and fMRI. *J Neurophysiol*. 2011;105(3):1393–1405.
14. Huberman AD, Niell CM. What can mice tell us about how vision works? *Trends Neurosci*. 2011.
15. Cruz-Martín A, Huberman AD. Visual cognition: rats compare shapes among the crowd. *Curr Biol*. 2012;22(1):R18–R20.
16. Ramon y Cajal S. *The Structure of the Retina* [Thorpe SA, Glickstein M, Trans. CC Thomas 1972]: Springfield, Illinois. 1892.
17. Schmidt TM, Chen SK, Hattar S. Intrinsically photosensitive retinal ganglion cells: many subtypes, diverse functions. *Trends Neurosci*. 2011.
18. Wässle H. Parallel processing in the mammalian retina. *Nat Rev Neurosci*. 2004;5(10):747–757.
19. Gastinger MJ, Tian N, Horvath T, Marshak DW. Retinopetal axons in mammals: emphasis on histamine and serotonin. *Curr Eye Res*. 2006;31(7–8):655–667.
20. Schwartz G, Harris R, Shrom D, Berry MJ. Detection and prediction of periodic patterns by the retina. *Nat Neurosci*. 2007;10(5):552–554.
21. Gollisch T, Meister M. Eye smarter than scientists believed: neural computations in circuits of the retina. *Neuron*. 2010; 65(2):150–164.
22. Hendry SHC, Reid RC. The koniocellular pathway in primate vision. *Annu Rev Neurosci*. 2000;23(1):127–153.
23. McAlonan K, Cavanaugh J, Wurtz RH. Guarding the gateway to cortex with attention in visual thalamus. *Nature*. 2008;456(7220): 391–394.
24. O'Connor DH, Fukui MM, Pinsk MA, Kastner S. Attention modulates responses in the human lateral geniculate nucleus. *Nat Neurosci*. 2002;5(11):1203–1209.
25. Saalmann YB, Kastner S. Cognitive and perceptual functions of the visual thalamus. *Neuron*. 2011;71(2):209–223.
26. Huguenard J. Low-threshold calcium currents in central nervous system neurons. *Annu Rev Physiol*. 1996;58(1):329–348.
27. Guido W, Weyand T. Burst responses in thalamic relay cells of the awake behaving cat. *J Neurophysiol*. 1995;74(4):1782–1786.
28. Alonso JM, Usrey WM, Reid RC. Precisely correlated firing in cells of the lateral geniculate nucleus. *Nature*. 1996;383(6603): 815–819.
29. May PJ. The mammalian superior colliculus: laminar structure and connections. *Prog Brain Res*. 2006;151:321–378.
30. Hofbauer A, Dräger UC. Depth segregation of retinal ganglion cells projecting to mouse superior colliculus. *J Comp Neurol*. 1985;234(4):465–474.
31. Wässle H, Illing RB. The retinal projection to the superior colliculus in the cat: a quantitative study with HRP. *J Comp Neurol*. 1980;190(2):333–356.
32. Perry V, Cowey A. Retinal ganglion cells that project to the superior colliculus and pretectum in the macaque monkey. *Neuroscience*. 1984;12(4):1125–1137.
33. Pegna AJ, Khateb A, Lazeyras F, Seghier ML. Discriminating emotional faces without primary visual cortices involves the right amygdala. *Nat Neurosci*. 2004;8(1):24–25.
34. Van den Stock J, Tamietto M, Sorger B, Pichon S, Grézes J, de Gelder B. Cortico-subcortical visual, somatosensory, and motor activations for perceiving dynamic whole-body emotional expressions with and without striate cortex (V1). *Proc Natl Acad Sci USA*. 2011;108(39):16188–16193.
35. Berman RA, Wurtz RH. Functional identification of a pulvinar path from superior colliculus to cortical area MT. *J Neurosci*. 2010;30(18):6342–6354.
36. Lyon DC, Nassi JJ, Callaway EM. A disynaptic relay from superior colliculus to dorsal stream visual cortex in macaque monkey. *Neuron*. 2010;65(2):270–279.
37. Kaas JH, Lyon DC. Pulvinar contributions to the dorsal and ventral streams of visual processing in primates. *Brain Res Rev*. 2007;55(2):285–296.
38. Wurtz RH. Neuronal mechanisms of visual stability. *Vision Res*. 2008;48(20):2070–2089.
39. Wurtz RH, McAlonan K, Cavanaugh J, Berman RA. Thalamic pathways for active vision. *Trends Cogn Sci*. 2011.
40. Fitzpatrick D, Diamond IT, Raczkowski D. Cholinergic and monoaminergic innervation of the cat's thalamus: comparison of the lateral geniculate nucleus with other principal sensory nuclei. *J Comp Neurol*. 1989;288(4):647–675.
41. Ward R, Danziger S, Owen V, Rafal R. Deficits in spatial coding and feature binding following damage to spatiotopic maps in the human pulvinar. *Nat Neurosci*. 2002;5(2):99–100.
42. Danziger S, Ward R, Owen V, Rafal R. Contributions of the human pulvinar to linking vision and action. *Cogn Affect Behav Neurosci*. 2004;4(1):89–99.
43. Snow JC, Allen HA, Rafal RD, Humphreys GW. Impaired attentional selection following lesions to human pulvinar: evidence for homology between human and monkey. *Proc Natl Acad Sci USA*. 2009;106(10):4054.
44. Wilke M, Turchi J, Smith K, Mishkin M, Leopold DA. Pulvinar inactivation disrupts selection of movement plans. *J Neurosci*. 2010;30(25):8650–8659.
45. Karnath HO, Himmelbach M, Rorden C. The subcortical anatomy of human spatial neglect: putamen, caudate nucleus and pulvinar. *Brain*. 2002;125(2):350–360.
46. Tootell RB, Silverman MS, Switkes E, De Valois RL. Deoxyglucose analysis of retinotopic organization in primate striate cortex. *Science*. 1982;218(4575):902–904.
47. Felleman DJ, Van Essen DC. Distributed hierarchical processing in the primate cerebral cortex. *Cereb Cortex*. 1991;1(1):1–47.
48. Hubel DH, Wiesel TN. Receptive fields of single neurones in the cat's striate cortex. *J Physiol*. 1959;148(3):574–591.
49. Hubel DH, Wiesel TN. Receptive fields and functional architecture of monkey striate cortex. *J Physiol*. 1968;195(1):215–243.
50. Pack CC, Livingstone MS, Duffy KR, Born RT. End-stopping and the aperture problem: two-dimensional motion signals in macaque V1. *Neuron*. 2003;39(4):671–680.
51. Kagan I, Gur M, Snodderly DM. Spatial organization of receptive fields of V1 neurons of alert monkeys: comparison with responses to gratings. *J Neurophysiol*. 2002;88(5):2557–2574.
52. Livingstone MS, Hubel DH. Anatomy and physiology of a color system in the primate visual cortex. *J Neurosci*. 1984;4(1): 309–356.
53. Chen Y, Geisler WS, Seidemann E. Optimal decoding of correlated neural population responses in the primate visual cortex. *Nat Neurosci*. 2006;9(11):1412–1420.
54. Ringach DL, Hawken MJ, Shapley R. Dynamics of orientation tuning in macaque primary visual cortex. *Nature*. 1997;387(6630): 281–284.
55. Callaway EM. Local circuits in primary visual cortex of the macaque monkey. *Annu Rev Neurosci*. 1998;21(1):47–74.
56. Poggio GF, Gonzalez F, Krause F. Stereoscopic mechanisms in monkey visual cortex: binocular correlation and disparity selectivity. *J Neurosci*. 1988;8(12):4531–4550.
57. Barlow HB, Blakemore C, Pettigrew J. The neural mechanism of binocular depth discrimination. *J Physiol*. 1967;193(2):327.
58. Mishkin M, Ungerleider LG, Macko KA. Object vision and spatial vision: two cortical pathways. *Trends Neurosci*. 1983;6:414–417.
59. Goodale MA, Milner AD. Separate visual pathways for perception and action. *Trends Neurosci*. 1992;15(1):20–25.

60. Orban GA. Higher order visual processing in macaque extrastriate cortex. *Physiol Rev.* 2008;88(1):59–89.
61. Wang Q, Sporns O, Burkhalter A. Network analysis of corticocortical connections reveals ventral and dorsal processing streams in mouse visual cortex. *J Neurosci.* 2012;32(13):4386–4399.
62. Van Essen DC, Anderson CH, Felleman DJ. Information processing in the primate visual system: an integrated systems perspective. *Science.* 1992;255(5043):419.
63. Maunsell JHR, Newsome WT. Visual processing in monkey extrastriate cortex. *Annu Rev Neurosci.* 1987;10(1):363–401.
64. Perrett D, Rolls E, Caan W. Visual neurones responsive to faces in the monkey temporal cortex. *Exp Brain Res.* 1982;47(3):329–342.
65. Orban GA, Janssen P, Vogels R. Extracting 3D structure from disparity. *Trends Neurosci.* 2006;29(8):466–473.
66. Brincat SL, Connor CE. Underlying principles of visual shape selectivity in posterior inferotemporal cortex. *Nat Neurosci.* 2004;7(8):880–886.
67. Heywood C, Gadotti A, Cowey A. Cortical area V4 and its role in the perception of color. *J Neurosci.* 1992;12(10):4056–4065.
68. Pasupathy A, Connor CE. Responses to contour features in macaque area V4. *J Neurophysiol.* 1999;82(5):2490–2502.
69. Desimone R, Schein SJ. Visual properties of neurons in area V4 of the macaque: sensitivity to stimulus form. *J Neurophysiol.* 1987;57(3):835–868.
70. Mazer JA, Gallant JL. Goal-related activity in V4 during free viewing visual search: evidence for a ventral stream visual salience map. *Neuron.* 2003;40(6):1241–1250.
71. Reynolds JH, Pasternak T, Desimone R. Attention increases sensitivity of V4 neurons. *Neuron.* 2000;26(3):703–714.
72. Roe AW, Chelazzi L, Connor CE, et al. Toward a unified theory of visual area V4. *Neuron.* 2012;74(1):12–29.
73. Inouye T. *Visual Disturbances following Gunshot Wounds of the Cortical Visual Area* [Glickestein M, Fahle M, Trans. Oxford: Oxford University Press, *Brain.* 2000;123(Suppl.):1–101]. Oxford University Press; 1909.
74. Holmes G. Disturbances of vision by cerebral lesions. *Br J Ophthalmol.* 1918;2(7):353–384.
75. Komatsu H. The neural mechanisms of perceptual filling-in. *Nat Rev Neurosci.* 2006;7(3):220–231.
76. Ramachandran VS, Gregory RL. Perceptual filling in of artificially induced scotomas in human vision. *Nature.* 1991;350(6320):699–702.
77. Cowey A, Stoerig P. The neurobiology of blindsight. *Trends Neurosci.* 1991;14(4):140–145.
78. Weiskrantz L. *Blindsight: A Case Study and Implications.* Vol. 12. USA: Oxford University Press; 1990.
79. Stoerig P, Cowey A. Wavelength discrimination in blindsight. *Brain.* 1992;115(2):425–444.
80. Stoerig P, Barth E. Low-level phenomenal vision despite unilateral destruction of primary visual cortex. *Conscious Cogn.* 2001;10(4):574–587.
81. Barbur JL, Watson J, Frackowiak RSJ, Zeki S. Conscious visual perception without VI. *Brain.* 1993;116(6):1293–1302.
82. Riddoch G. Dissociation of visual perceptions due to occipital injuries, with especial reference to appreciation of movement. *Brain.* 1917;40(1):15–57.
83. Zeki S. The primary visual cortex, and feedback to it, are not necessary for conscious vision. *Brain.* 2011;134(1):247–257.
84. Mohler CW, Wurtz RH. Role of striate cortex and superior colliculus in visual guidance of saccadic eye movements in monkeys. *J Neurophysiol.* 1977;40(1):74–94.
85. Schmid MC, Mrowka SW, Turchi J, et al. Blindsight depends on the lateral geniculate nucleus. *Nature.* 2010;466(7304):373–377.
86. Sacks OW, Olennick N. *An Anthropologist on Mars.* Taylor & Francis; 1996.
87. Haarmeier T, Thier P, Repnow M, Petersen D. False perception of motion in a patient who cannot compensate for eye movements. *Nature.* 1997;389(6653):849–851.
88. Merigan WH, Nealey TA, Maunsell J. Visual effects of lesions of cortical area V2 in macaques. *J Neurosci.* 1993;13(7):3180–3191.
89. Zihl J, Von Cramon D, Mai N. Selective disturbance of movement vision after bilateral brain damage. *Brain.* 1983;106(2):313–340.
90. Zihl J, Von Cramon D, Mai N, Schmid C. Disturbance of movement vision after bilateral posterior brain damage: further evidence and follow up observations. *Brain.* 1991;114(5):2235–2252.
91. Plant GT, Laxer KD, Barbaro NM, Schiffman JS, Nakayama K. Impaired visual motion perception in the contralateral hemifield following unilateral posterior cerebral lesions in humans. *Brain.* 1993;116(6):1303–1335.
92. Zeki S. A century of cerebral achromatopsia. *Brain.* 1990;113(6):1721–1777.
93. Hadjikhani N, Liu AK, Dale AM, Cavanagh P, Tootell RBH. Retinotopy and color sensitivity in human visual cortical area V8. *Nat Neurosci.* 1998;1(3):235–241.
94. Gross CG. How inferior temporal cortex became a visual area. *Cereb Cortex.* 1994;4(5):455–469.
95. Meadows J. The anatomical basis of prosopagnosia. *J Neurol Neurosurg Psychiatry.* 1974;37(5):489–501.
96. Vallar G, Perani D. The anatomy of unilateral neglect after right-hemisphere stroke lesions. A clinical/CT-scan correlation study in man. *Neuropsychologia.* 1986;24(5):609–622.
97. Karnath HO, Ferber S, Himmelbach M. Spatial awareness is a function of the temporal not the posterior parietal lobe. *Nature.* 2001;411(6840):950–952.
98. Bálint R, Harvey M. Psychic paralysis of gaze, optic ataxia, and spatial disorder of attention. *Cogn Neuropsychol.* 1995;12(3):265–281.
99. Gur M, Snodderly D. A dissociation between brain activity and perception: chromatically opponent cortical neurons signal chromatic flicker that is not perceived. *Vision Res.* 1997;37(4):377–382.
100. Crick F, Koch C. Are we aware of neural activity in primary visual cortex? *Nature.* 1995;375(6527):121–123.
101. Tong F. Primary visual cortex and visual awareness. *Nat Rev Neurosci.* 2003;4(3):219–230.
102. Von Helmholtz H. *Handbook of Physiological Optics* [Southhall JPC, Trans.]. Rochester, NY: Optical Society of America; 1866.
103. Furman M, Gur M. And yet it moves: perceptual illusions and neural mechanisms of pursuit compensation during smooth pursuit eye movements. *Neurosci Biobehav Rev.* 2011.
104. Lindner A, Thier P, Kircher TTJ, Haarmeier T, Leube DT. Disorders of agency in schizophrenia correlate with an inability to compensate for the sensory consequences of actions. *Curr Biol.* 2005;15(12):1119–1124.
105. Leopold DA, Logothetis NK. Multistable phenomena: changing views in perception. *Trends Cogn Sci.* 1999;3(7):254–264.
106. Sterzer P, Kleinschmidt A, Rees G. The neural bases of multistable perception. *Trends Cogn Sci.* 2009;13(7):310–318.
107. Polonsky A, Blake R, Braun J, Heeger DJ. Neuronal activity in human primary visual cortex correlates with perception during binocular rivalry. *Nat Neurosci.* 2000;3:1153–1159.
108. Tong F, Meng M, Blake R. Neural bases of binocular rivalry. *Trends Cogn Sci.* 2006;10(11):502–511.
109. Wilke M, Logothetis NK, Leopold DA. Local field potential reflects perceptual suppression in monkey visual cortex. *Proc Natl Acad Sci USA.* 2006;103(46):17507–17512.
110. Logothetis NK, Pauls J, Augath M, Trinath T, Oeltermann A. Neurophysiological investigation of the basis of the fMRI signal. *Nature.* 2001;412(6843):150–157.

111. Rees G. Neural correlates of the contents of visual awareness in humans. *Philos Trans R Soc Lond B Biol Sci.* 2007;362(1481):877–886.
112. Jiang Y, He S. Cortical responses to invisible faces: dissociating subsystems for facial-information processing. *Curr Biol.* 2006;16(20):2023–2029.
113. Williams MA, Morris AP, McGlone F, Abbott DF, Mattingley JB. Amygdala responses to fearful and happy facial expressions under conditions of binocular suppression. *J Neurosci.* 2004;24(12):2898–2904.
114. Plum F, Posner JB. *The Diagnosis of Stupor and Coma.* Vol. 19. USA: Oxford University Press; 1982.

CHAPTER

20

Auditory Neuronal Networks and Chronic Tinnitus

Thomas J. Brozoski, Carol A. Bauer

Division of Otolaryngology, Head and Neck Surgery, Southern Illinois University School of Medicine, Springfield, IL, USA

TINNITUS PHENOMENOLOGY AND EPIDEMIOLOGY

Tinnitus, commonly known as "ringing in the ears", is somewhat misnamed. A heterogeneous disorder, its most common form is subjective tinnitus, in which there are no acoustic correlates. Tinnitus is noted in the writings of Hippocrates and Galen, and its symptoms are well described in the Babylonian Talmud.[1] Although the subjective sensation of tinnitus may be projected as originating from an ear, the condition clearly arises from processes in the central nervous system. It has been shown, for example, that complete transection of the auditory nerve in the course of tumor surgery most often fails to diminish the sensation and may make it worse.[2,3] Although the range of sensations comprising tinnitus can be quite broad, it is typically described as a simple ringing tone, or a buzzing or hissing sound. While the sensory features of tinnitus are usually simple, the physiological underpinning of tinnitus is quite subtle, to date having eluded a definitive description. It is probably for this reason that no generally effective treatment or standard of care has been established. Another complicating factor is that tinnitus most likely is a heterogeneous disorder in the human population.[4] Estimates of chronic tinnitus prevalence vary from 10% to somewhat greater than 50%, while the prevalence of severe and bothersome tinnitus varies between 4% and 14%, depending upon population demographics and tinnitus definition.[5] The single greatest risk factor for tinnitus is hearing loss,[6] with evidence that high-level sound exposure in young adults, either voluntarily (e.g. from listening to loud music[7]) or involuntarily (e.g. in military environments[8]), is increasing the incidence of tinnitus.

PROCESSING ACOUSTIC INFORMATION: THE AUDITORY PATHWAY

The mammalian auditory system has evolved to detect and process sound. For terrestrial species, sound travels as airborne compression waves. The compression waves are transduced to mechanical motion by the tympanic membrane (Figure 20.1(A)) and transmitted to the cochlea (Figure 20.1(B)) via the middle ear ossicles, the chain of small bones (visible in Figure 20.1) linking the tympanic membrane to the cochlea. The cochlea is an elongated fluid-filled compartment coiled like a snail shell around the spiral nerve ganglion, which is the distal aspect of the auditory nerve. Traveling pressure waves in the cochlea deflect the basilar membrane that longitudinally bisects the cochlea. This motion disturbs hair cells situated in four rows along the length of the basilar membrane. The hair cells of the innermost row are responsible for transducing basilar membrane motion into bioelectric potentials. They also release neurotransmitters, the most important of which is glutamate. Glutamate excites spiral ganglion neurons, thereby driving activity in the auditory nerve (Figure 20.1(C)).

The analysis of sound begins in the cochlea, although the geometry of the external ear and mechanics of the middle ear significantly alter features of the sound, for example damping out some frequencies and enhancing others. Generally, sound amplitude is coded by the number of action potentials and the number of nerve cells driven by the sound. The psychological correlate is loudness. Louder sounds are coded by increased neural firing in a larger number of auditory neurons. Sometimes, this is called a "rate code", although it does have spatial aspects. It is important to note that in the absence

Neuronal Networks in Brain Function, CNS Disorders, and Therapeutics
http://dx.doi.org/10.1016/B978-0-12-415804-7.00020-4

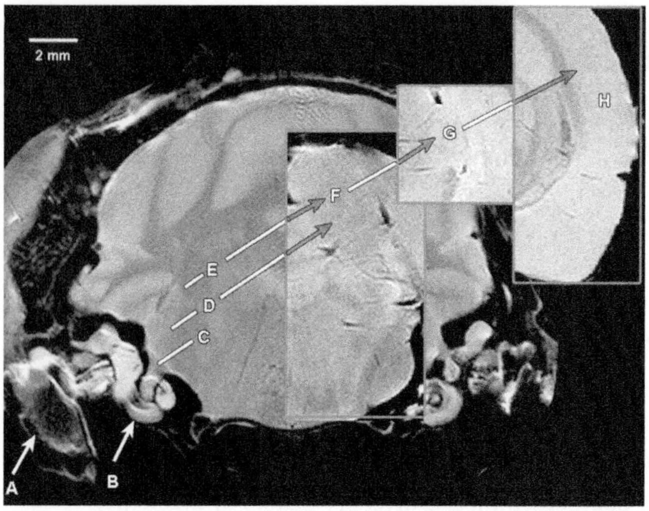

FIGURE 20.1 High-resolution MRI scan of an adult Long-Evans rat, showing major features of the auditory system. Inset structures are in more rostral image planes than the ear and auditory nerve. Aspects of the pathway, from the auditory nerve (C) to the auditory cortex (H), have been implicated in chronic tinnitus. Information flow and interactions at many levels in the system are both ascending and descending, despite the unidirectional arrows indicating afferent flow. Pathological processes responsible for tinnitus appear to be distributed across several levels. Key: (A) tympanic membrane, (B) cochlea, (C) auditory nerve, (D) ventral cochlear nucleus, (E) dorsal cochlear nucleus, (F) contralateral inferior colliculus (inset), (G) contralateral medial geniculate body (inset), and (H) primary auditory cortex. (For color version of this figure, the reader is referred to the online version of this book.)

of acoustic stimulation, healthy auditory primary fibers are nevertheless spontaneously active, and in a normal-hearing system the spontaneous activity is heard as silence.

In contrast to sound level, sound frequency is coded primarily by the locus of hair cells stimulated by the maximum of the traveling pressure wave in the cochlea. This scheme is often called a "place code". The transduction of low to high frequencies along the length of the basilar membrane, from base to apex, is called tonotopic organization. The psychological correlate of sound frequency is pitch. In general, tonotopic layout (i.e. the tonotopic map), first evident in the cochlea, is preserved across neurons throughout the primary auditory pathway (also known as the lemniscal pathway), from the cochlear nuclei in the brainstem (Figure 20.1(D) and (E)) to the primary auditory cortex (Figure 20.1(H)). A complexity is that frequencies below a certain level appear to be rate coded; moreover, parallel auxiliary pathways, comprising the extralemniscal system, are not tonotopically well organized.

Most auditory nerve fibers synapse with second-order neurons in the ipsilateral cochlear nuclei. In mammals, there are three cochlear nuclei: the anterior and posterior ventral cochlear nucleus (AVCN and PVCN, respectively) and the dorsal cochlear nucleus (DCN). All three are tonotopically organized, and all three receive parallel input from the auditory nerve. Understanding signal processing at different levels of the auditory system is a work in progress. Typically, signal processing is explained in terms of ascending neural codes. Much less well understood, although not necessarily less important, is how descending neural activity modifies ascending activity (i.e. contributes to the neural code). The ventral cochlear nuclei appear primarily engaged in improving signal temporal features. Meaningful aspects of sound are commonly present in temporal features. Examples would be repetitive alarm cries, or the stream of lexical units comprising human speech. Bushy cells, second-order units in the rat AVCN, have been shown to respond with greater temporal precision to low frequencies[9] such as those composing vowel sounds, and all four types of AVCN neurons respond with greater fidelity to amplitude-modulated tones (i.e. a twitter) than primary afferents.[10] Modeling studies have shown that cellular properties, such as membrane capacitance, and network properties, such as dendritic filtering, can account for aspects of cochlear nucleus temporal processing.[11] AVCN and DCN neurons also significantly contribute to broadening the dynamic range of auditory neurons. For example, DCN fusiform cells display a greater response compression to sound levels than primary auditory neurons. This means they can effectively code a broader range of sound levels (i.e. from soft to loud) than individual neurons in the auditory nerve. Finally, it is clear that the DCN and PVCN receive modulatory inputs from the somatosensory system. These inputs enable the auditory system to use head and ear position to improve sound localization. Information about body movement is also useful in distinguishing self-generated sounds from those of external origin.

Sound information ascends from the cochlear nuclei via the lateral lemniscus to the contralateral inferior colliculus (IC) (Figure 20.1(F)), with the majority of synapses in the central nucleus, or core, of the IC. The IC is the major integrative station of the rostral auditory brainstem, with substantial bilateral connections as well as descending inputs. The IC is typically divided into either two or three zones. In the bipartite scheme, there is the core, which is dominated by synapses of ascending fibers, and the shell, which has a more heterogeneous mixture of ascending and descending inputs. In the tripartite scheme, the shell is divided into a dorsal cortex and lateral nucleus. In general, the frequency selectivity of postsynaptic neurons in the IC is greater than that of input neurons, and their tuning can be improved by repeated exposure to tonal stimuli.[12] IC neurons have also been shown to be highly sensitive to potentially meaningful species-specific vocal sounds, with selectivity improved by application of gamma-aminobutyric acid (GABA) agonists that enhance neural inhibition.[13] In summary, the IC continues to further signal processing, particularly with respect to experiential and species-relevant features.

Globally, the medial geniculate body (MGB) (Figure 20.1(G)) of the thalamus functions as a sophisticated router between the auditory brainstem and auditory cortex, as well as other "nonauditory" structures such as the amygdala. The MGB receives massive input from the ipsilateral IC and, in turn, sends massive outputs to the primary auditory cortex (A1). Most often, the mammalian MGB is depicted as a tripartite structure. Of the three subdivisions, the ventral MGB (MGBv) has the most clearly defined tonotopic organization, with fast-conducting connections to layers 3 and 4 of A1 via a glutamatergic pathway.[14,15] The MGB receives reciprocal descending input from A1, primarily from neurons located in layer 6.[16] The role played by corticothalamic connections in perceptual processes such as selective attention must be profound, although current understanding is incomplete. Thalmocortical oscillatory rhythms are reciprocal interactions between the thalamus and cortex, typically measured as periodic field potentials. They have been hypothesized to reflect variations in attention and arousal that accompany signal processing.

The auditory cortex (Figure 20.1(H)), like other cortical areas, carries out tasks of higher order signal analysis and multimodal integration. Cortical function is strongly influenced by environmental and intrinsic motivational factors. As noted in this section, auditory information arrives in layers 3 and 4 from the MGBv. The tonotopic organization of A1 can be dramatically influenced by alterations in the acoustic environment, including those produced by partial deafening,[17] and it is particularly dramatic when combined with stimulation of the ascending cholinergic system.[18] Acetylcholinesterase staining shows that A1 and its surrounding belt regions are densely enervated by cholinergic fibers.[19] The auditory cortex not only receives inputs from all sensory modalities but also, via descending tracts, modulates the function of lower auditory structures, extending to the cochlea.[20] A1 has been characterized as an adaptive control system for signal processing and event modeling. It is driven by environmental and species-specific factors. A clear example of this was shown in experiments where A1 was surgically removed. Cats without A1 could accurately discriminate tones and even correctly orient to them, but they could not learn to actually approach a sound source to feed themselves.[21] In other words, the animals could not effectively use auditory information about their environment.

DE-AFFERENTATION AND HOMEOSTATIC COMPENSATION

It is well known that exposure to high-level sound produces a long-term decrease in auditory nerve sensitivity as a consequence of cochlear damage.[22] Moderate-level sound exposure (octave-band noise, centered at 16 kHz, 110 dB sound pressure level (SPL), for 1 h) has been shown to produce tinnitus in animals (animal models are discussed in more detail in this chapter) with low levels of cochlear damage and no long-term elevation in hearing threshold.[23] A significant correlation ($r = +0.91$), however, has been established between psychophysically defined tinnitus and the loss of primary afferent dendrites of large diameter.[23] These cochlear nerve fibers are characterized by high spontaneous firing rates and low thresholds. Loss of this subpopulation of afferents may initiate a cascade of compensatory changes in the central auditory pathway. The large-diameter fibers are the dominant input to small cells within the DCN.[24] These target cells are characterized by a seemingly paradoxical profile that includes low spontaneous activity and high thresholds, and morphologically includes a mixture of cell types, including interneurons and vertical cells that provide inhibitory input to DCN fusiform cells via their basal dendrites[25] (Figure 20.2). Increased compensatory gain following de-afferentation may depend upon several homeostatic mechanisms.[27] Tinnitus likely arises as an undesirable consequence of one or more of these compensatory processes being set in motion by de-afferentation. Understanding details of these mechanisms constitutes the core of contemporary tinnitus research.

An early compensatory hypothesis was that inhibition, perhaps that mediated by GABA or glycine, down-regulates in one or more areas in the auditory pathway, such as the DCN or IC. A good deal of evidence now supports this loss-of-inhibition hypothesis.[28] Following peripheral de-afferentation, often a consequence of high-level sound exposure, aspects of glycinergic transmission have been found to decrease in the cochlear nucleus of the auditory brainstem.[29,30] Similarly, GABA function has been shown to decrease in the IC following high-level sound exposure,[31,32] and decreases in GABA levels have been found in the auditory thalamus (i.e. MGB) in rats with psychophysical evidence of tinnitus.[33] Blocking GABA receptors in the DCN has been shown to exacerbate an autofluorescent marker of elevated neural activity in mice with behavioral evidence of tinnitus.[34] In addition, systemic treatment with GABA agonists, such as vigabatrin, a GABA transaminase inhibitor, and taurine, an extrasynaptic GABA receptor agonist, has been shown to effectively, and reversibly, alleviate tinnitus in a rat model.[35–37]

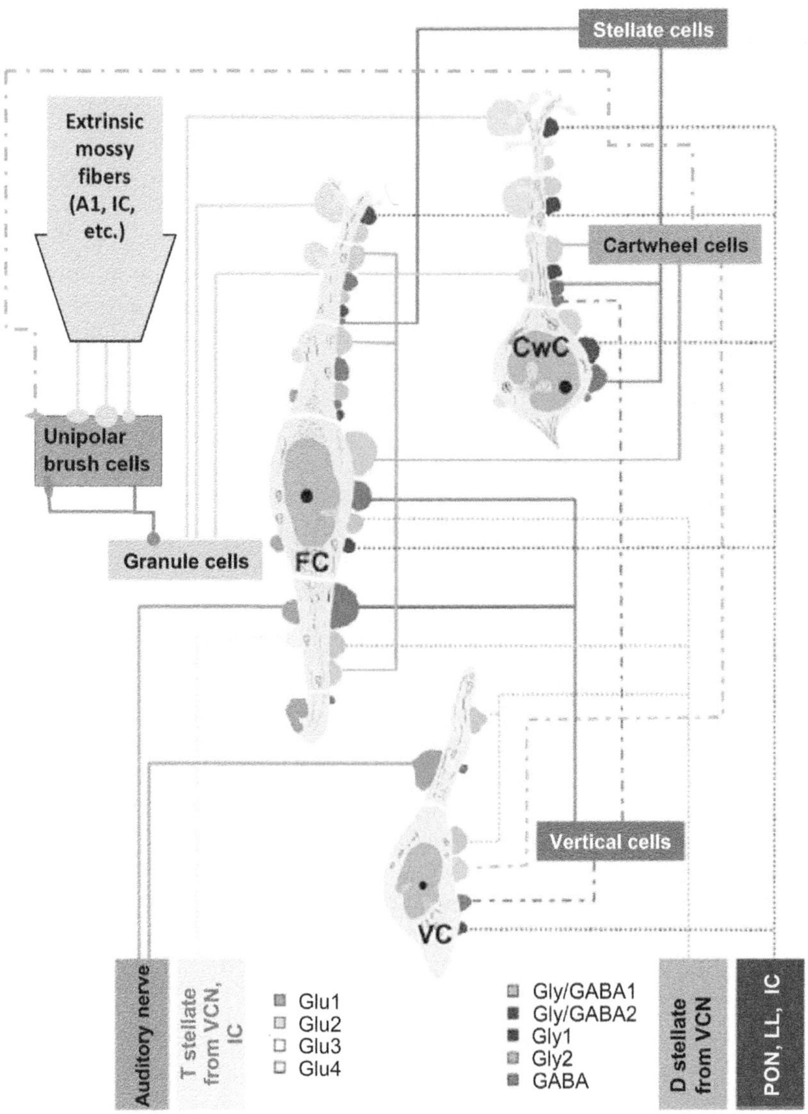

FIGURE 20.2 A summary of the neurotransmitter connections in the dorsal cochlear nucleus of the rat, adapted from Rubio.[26] It has been hypothesized that, following damage to the auditory periphery, there is a compensatory downregulation of inhibitory interneurons, particularly vertical cells, and an upregulation of excitatory interneurons, particularly unipolar brush cells. Also note that unipolar brush cells, via their descending mossy fiber inputs, comprise an excitatory positive feedback loop. (*Source: Reprinted with permission Ref. 26.*) (The figure is reproduced in color section.)

In addition to loss of inhibition, tinnitus may also be mediated by an increase in excitatory neurotransmission, which may or may not be dependent on inhibitory downregulation. The potential role of the excitatory glutamate system has been investigated, primarily using animal models. Guitton[38] showed that salicylate-induced tinnitus in rats was dependent upon cochlear glutamatergic *N*-methyl-D-aspartate (NMDA) receptors. Zhou[39] demonstrated that compensatory mechanisms in the brainstem cochlear nucleus were mediated by an increase in glutamatergic transmission, as indicated by upregulation of the glutamate transporter, vglut2. Further glutamatergic involvement in controlling spontaneous neural activity in the IC has been shown in sound-exposed mice. IC spontaneous activity was mediated by a balance of type I and type II metabotropic glutamate receptors.[40] Long-term potentiation and long-term depression of neural excitability reflect synaptic mechanisms of neural plasticity. Both have been demonstrated in vitro to be mediated by glutamatergic NMDA receptors located on the principal output (fusiform) cells of the DCN.[41] Elevated glutamate levels in the DCN, and possibly the primary auditory cortex (A1), have been found in rats with psychophysical evidence of tinnitus.[33] Rats with acoustic trauma-induced tinnitus have been shown to have an elevated marker of neuroplasticity (doublecortin (DCX)) in unipolar brush cells (UBCs) (Figure 20.2), glutamatergic interneurons in their DCN, and ventral cerebellar cortex.[42] In the same study, microquantities of glutamatergic antagonists infused directly into the cerebellar paraflocculus (PFL) effectively and reversibly decreased tinnitus, while direct infusion of glutamatergic agonists temporarily induced tinnitus-like symptoms in normal-hearing rats. In summary, excitatory glutamatergic neurotransmission appears to mediate aspects of chronic tinnitus, at least in animal models.

ANIMAL MODELS

Understanding the neuronal underpinnings of tinnitus has been significantly advanced by animal models. As a sensation of meaningless background sound, tinnitus most likely reflects primitive alterations in auditory processing. These alterations do not require higher order functions, such as language. It is therefore likely that most mammalian species, including rodents, have the capacity to experience tinnitus. Since many relatively simple events can cause tinnitus, such as high-level sound exposure, ototoxicity, and presbycusis, induction of tinnitus in animals is not difficult. Objectively measuring tinnitus, however, requires care. Current animal models derive from the pioneering experiments of Jastreboff.[43] Two features of the Jastreboff model have been incorporated in one form or another into all subsequent models: (1) use of a behavioral response to indicate the sensation of sound, and (2) reliance on the contrast between tinnitus and silence, since tinnitus must, by definition, be something other than silence. In order to be convincing, animal models must include controls to distinguish between hearing loss and tinnitus, since hearing loss is often associated with tinnitus. Behavioral measurement is required because tinnitus does not have universally agreed upon anatomical or physiological correlates. Therefore, direct systemic, cellular, or biochemical markers are unavailable. However, well-developed psychophysical methods are available for determining the sensory capacity of animals,[44] and a number have been adapted to objectively indicate tinnitus. Comprehensive reviews of animal tinnitus models have been published.[45–47] Current understanding of tinnitus pathophysiology derives significantly from animal research.

Two exemplary models may be used to illustrate the range of procedural variation in current animal models. In both of the following models, tinnitus is induced by a single unilateral exposure to high-level sound for 1 h. Exposure parameters may vary, depending upon the species and experiment, but for rats, band-limited noise with a peak level of 116 dB centered at 16 kHz would be typical. The "Bauer" conditioned suppression model[48] derives most directly from that of Jastreboff et al.[43] In this model, conditioned suppression of lever pressing for food is used to indicate the perception of sound. Animals are tested in individual operant chambers with a lever, food pellet dispenser, and overhead speaker. Low-level ambient sound (60 dB SPL, broad-band noise) is present throughout test sessions, and it is interrupted at random intervals by 1 min test periods. Test periods are characterized by either the speakers being turned off (i.e. a silent interval), or by the substitution of different tones at different levels. Lever pressing during any silent period results in a 1 s mild (0.5 mA) foot shock at the end of the silent period. Lever pressing during any sound presentation, including the background sound, never leads to a foot shock. Rodents learn very quickly, typically within two sessions, to stop lever pressing during silent periods. They also generalize their suppression to anything else that is perceived as similar to a silent period. The twist, of course, is that silent periods are perceived differently by normal-hearing animals than they are by animals with tinnitus. This difference can be objectively indicated by psychophysical discrimination functions for sounds that resemble the tinnitus. Animals with tinnitus suppress more in the presence of tinnitus-similar sounds than normal-hearing controls without tinnitus. This model has been used successfully with both rats and chinchillas. The data indicate that chronic tinnitus develops from 1 to 3 months after exposure in most, but not all, animals; the tinnitus is typically tonal, and it persists for the duration of the animal's life span.[45] Tinnitus, as reflected by this model, is indicated by a shift in psychophysical discrimination functions, as depicted in Figure 20.3.

A rapid behavioral tinnitus assay, of contrasting design, has been developed by Turner.[49] The Turner method derives from the acoustic startle reflex and its sensitivity to prepulse inhibition. A brief high-level sound pulse (e.g. broad-band noise, 115 dB SPL, 20 ms) is used to produce a startle reflex, which can be measured in a test chamber resting on an accelerometer. When the startle sound is preceded 50–100 ms by another low-level sound pulse (e.g. a 10 kHz tone at 60 dB SPL), the startle amplitude is decreased. This is prepulse inhibition. A silent gap (e.g. 50 ms in duration), imbedded in a low-level sound envelope (e.g. 10 kHz tone at 60 dB SPL), will produce a similar inhibitory effect (Figure 20.4(A)). This is sound gap inhibition. Varying the frequency envelope and the depth of the sound gap enables the method to detect tinnitus. Tinnitus fills in the sound gap, thereby decreasing the inhibition of startle (Figure 20.4(B)). That is to say, tinnitus is objectively indicated by a return to uninhibited levels of startle. The Turner model, which requires no special training or modulation of motivational states, both has face validity and has been cross-validated with the Bauer model. It has been successfully used with a variety of rodent species.[50]

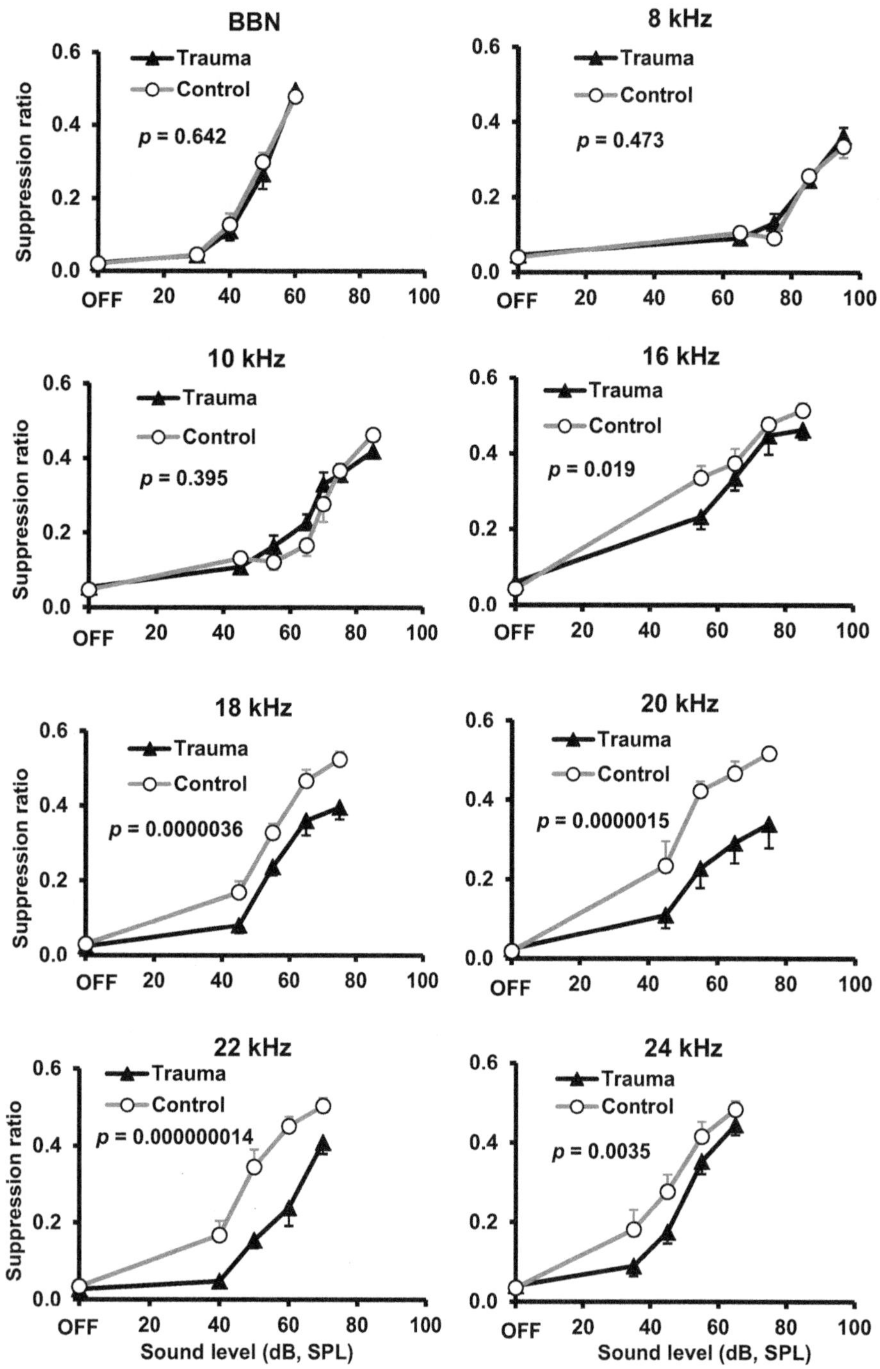

FIGURE 20.3 Auditory discrimination functions of two groups of rats, with one group having been exposed once unilaterally, for 1 h, to 116 dB band limited noise centered at 16 kHz. The exposure (i.e. "Trauma") was more than 3 months prior to data collection. The two groups were tested with the range of sounds indicated in the panel captions. Test presentations were 1 min each, randomly imbedded in a 1 h session of low-level broadband noise (BBN). Other test sounds were pure tones at the labeled frequencies. Psychophysical performance was quantified as the suppression of lever pressing for food pellets (i.e. suppression ratio) during test stimuli (plotted on the *y*-axis). The suppression ratio depicts performance relative to baseline, and varies from 0 to 1, with a value of 0.5 indicative of performance equal to baseline. The stimulus level is indicated on the *x*-axis (dB, sound pressure level re 20 μPa), with "OFF" indicating no sound. The functions slope upward from the origin because the animals have been conditioned to not lever press for food during "speaker off" periods, but to lever press for food under any other sound condition. The functions separate between groups when the animals are challenged with tones resembling their sensation during speaker off periods, which for trauma animals is their tinnitus. Maximum separation at 20–22 kHz indicates the region of tinnitus.

COMPENSATION AND OVERCOMPENSATION IN THE BRAINSTEM

A working hypothesis shared by many tinnitus researchers is that loss of afferent input to the auditory system, such as that caused by acoustic trauma or aging, leads to compensatory increases in system gain, and that this ultimately produces the sensation of tinnitus.[27,47] The engine that drives the compensatory gain most often has been attributed to a loss inhibition mediated by GABA or glycine.[28] As schematized in Figure 20.2, feedforward inhibitory circuits are prominent in the DCN. Compensatory gain may be reflected as an increase in the spontaneous activity of individual neurons[51] as well as an increase in the

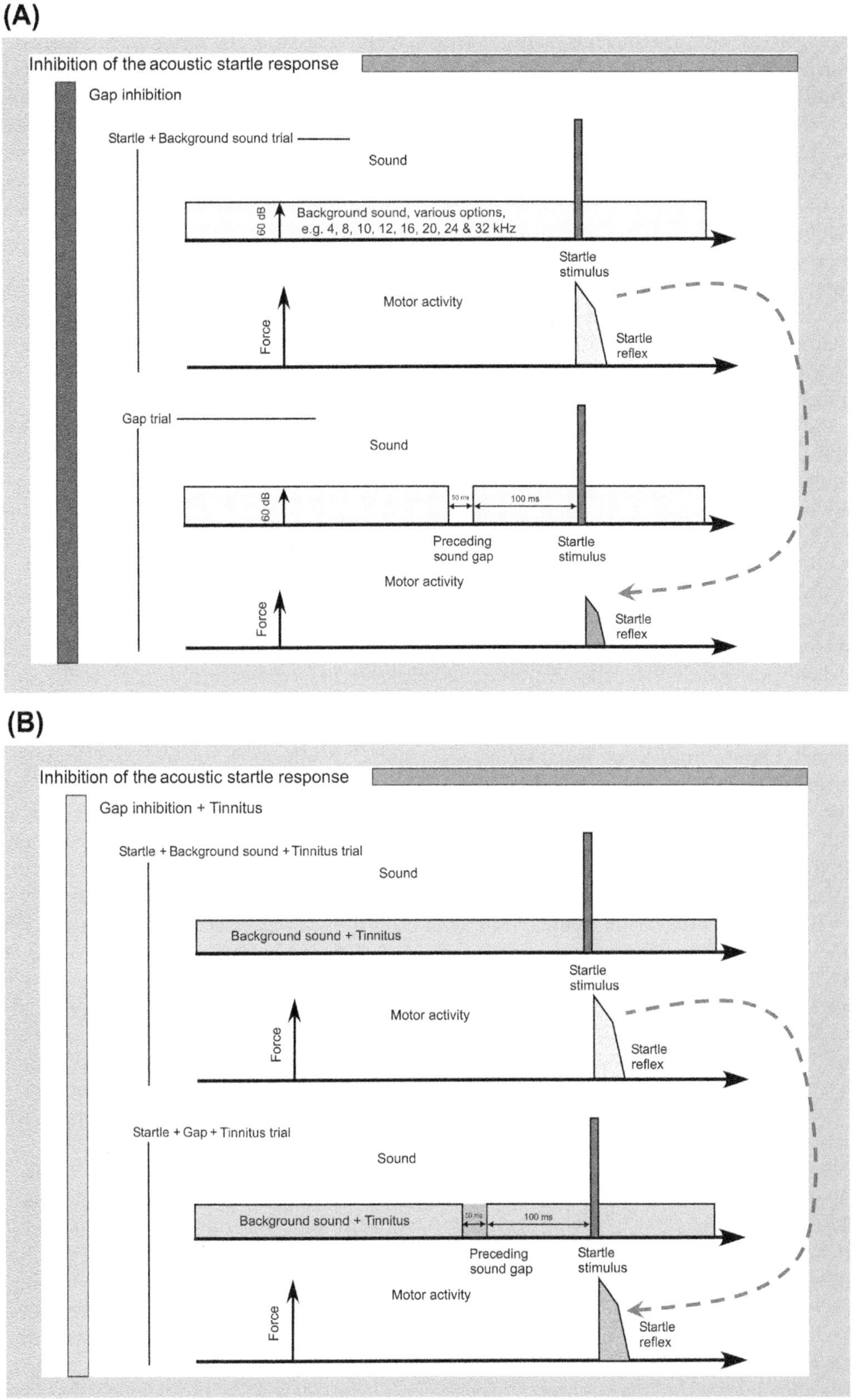

FIGURE 20.4 The Turner gap inhibition rapid assay for tinnitus. (A) The acoustic startle reflex, schematized on the motor activity line, is attenuated when preceded by a gap in low-level background sound. This gap inhibition of startle occurs somewhat independently of the frequency makeup of the background sound. (B) Animals with tinnitus do not show the expected level of gap inhibition for specific background frequencies. The interpretation is that their tinnitus masks, or "fills in" the gap when the background sound is qualitatively and quantitatively similar to their tinnitus. (For color version of this figure, the reader is referred to the online version of this book.)

number of spontaneously active neurons.[28] Also evident may be an increase in stimulus-driven activity,[51,52] increased regularity of firing in single neurons,[53] and increased synchrony of activity across a population of neurons.[47] These alterations in neuronal activity appear to be expressed differentially across different levels of the auditory system.

Exposure to high-level sound has been shown to *decrease* the sensitivity of the peripheral auditory system, as reflected by a significantly decreased response of primary auditory afferents[54] to sound. Interestingly, dramatic loss of peripheral sensitivity is evident even when cochlear hair cells, the sensory transducers, appear to be morphologically intact.[55] Although peripheral sensitivity decreases following traumatic sound exposure, central neurons show significant increases.[56,57] The expression of the increase appears to vary, depending upon the brain area and level. Kaltenbach and colleagues have extensively investigated the brainstem DCN of hamsters, following acoustic insults[58,59] and in conjunction with tinnitus.[60] They report multiunit spontaneous activity increases of at least an order of magnitude. The increase appeared within 5 days of exposure, but not immediately afterward, and it persisted for at least 180 days post insult.[61] Further experiments from the same group demonstrated a tonotopic distribution of the increased spontaneous activity that was biased toward high-to midrange frequencies, as would be expected of tinnitus.[52] Elevated DCN spontaneous activity may be independent of cochlear input,[62] although other research indicates that spontaneous hyperactivity in the IC, immediately rostral to the DCN, may be dependent upon spontaneously active cochlear afferents.[63] This issue remains to be clarified.

Understanding the normal function of the DCN is a focus of considerable research effort. The cytoarchitecture of the DCN shares many features in common with the cerebellum,[64] suggesting that a global function may be that of an adaptive sensory modeling system and mismatch comparator. The parallel fiber network in the DCN displays both long-term potentiation and long-term depression, with the outcome balanced by spike timing convergent on the principal output neurons of the DCN, the fusiform cells.[41] DCN fusiform cells have pyramidal soma with apical dendrites that receive excitatory parallel fiber synapses from granule cells (Figure 20.2). DCN fusiform cells also receive multiple interneuron inputs, including those from cartwheel cells, which use a retrograde cannabinoid receptor to mediate presynaptic long-term depression.[41] These synaptic engines of the DCN appear to drive adaptive signal processing, and they are dependent upon glutamatergic NMDA and AMPA (α-amino-3-hydroxy-5-methylisoxazole-4-propionate) receptors, since they are subject to disruption, at least in vitro, by an AMPA antagonist and an NMDA antagonist.[41,65] UBCs are glutamatergic interneurons that indirectly excite DCN fusiform cells. They may constitute important feedback as well as feedforward connections that enable a compensatory response to loss of peripheral input. Recently, UBCs have been shown to upregulate in animals with tinnitus.[42] Overcompensation could set in motion a physiological cascade that is responsible for tinnitus.

An important category of sensory integration mediated by the DCN involves somatosensory and auditory afferents, which may be relevant to tinnitus neuropathy. The somatosensory trigeminal nerve sends numerous terminals to the DCN.[66] The DCN may use body positional information to compensate for sound spectral shifts associated with head and ear orientation.[64] Somatosensory information may also be used to reduce the intrusion of self-generated sounds, such as vocalization, into an analysis of the auditory scene. Shore and colleagues showed that somatosensory excitatory input to the DCN was enhanced after noise-induced hearing loss,[67] and that spontaneous and sound-driven DCN output was enhanced in guinea pigs that experienced an acute period (2 h) of moderately high-level (96 dB root mean square SPL) noise in conjunction with trigeminal nerve stimulation.[68] A subset of the exposed animals also displayed evidence of tinnitus using the gap inhibition startle method. Their general conclusion was that acoustic damage to the DCN facilitates a compensatory increase in somatosensory excitation in that nucleus. Opening this somatosensory gate may, therefore, be a source of the tinnitus signal. Clinically, "somatosensory tinnitus" is a well-recognized subcategory. It is seen in patients who can modulate the loudness or quality of their tinnitus with eye movement or oro-facial and head position maneuvers.[69–71] Although not rare, these patients nevertheless constitute a minority of those who present symptoms of chronic tinnitus. Therefore, the general significance of somatosensory factors in tinnitus needs to be further defined.

Whether the DCN serves as a necessary generator of tinnitus is still uncertain. It has been shown, for example, that rats with chronic tinnitus continue to display psychophysical evidence of tinnitus even after bilateral DCN ablation.[72] This finding supports the contention of many tinnitus researchers that tinnitus neuropathy is likely to be a distributed phenomenon involving more than one brain area, including areas not considered to be part of the classical auditory pathway.[73,74] In addition, tinnitus may not simply be the experiential correlate of elevated spontaneous or stimulus-driven activity. It is important to note that, clinically, tinnitus is often very difficult, and in some cases impossible, to mask using external sound.[75] This aspect of tinnitus would be very unlikely if its neuronal underpinning was simply elevated spontaneous neural activity in the DCN or elsewhere. Nevertheless, involvement of the DCN does appear to be obligatory for the induction of tinnitus. Bilateral, but not unilateral, DCN lesions in rats have been reported to prevent the induction of tinnitus via traumatic sound exposure.[76] It has been suggested that there may be distinct tinnitus trigger zones as well as distinct tinnitus generator areas for tinnitus.

The IC, located in the rostral brainstem, is not only the primary target of DCN fusiform cells but also a large area of convergence and integration, where descending pathways from the auditory cortex converge directly on tonotopically organized auditory afferents (the lemniscal pathway) as well as on diffusely organized afferents (the extralemniscal pathway). Human imaging studies[77] and animal studies[53,78] have identified altered activity in the IC of individuals with tinnitus or tinnitus in association with hyperacusis. While some evidence suggests that IC spontaneous activity may be elevated in animals with evidence of tinnitus,[78,79] other evidence indicates that alterations in neuronal activity patterns may more directly reflect the signature of tinnitus pathology. Bauer et al.[53] reported that chinchillas, with tinnitus caused by either acoustic or ototoxic insult, displayed a triad of neural activity changes. The triad was characterized by decreased interspike-interval variance and a clustering of spikes into bursts with high-peak discharge frequencies, similar to the psychophysically defined frequency of the animal's tinnitus. This triad, which was found in about 50% of the units sampled in the IC, was evident bilaterally (although the tinnitus-inducing auditory insult was unilateral) and was not focal to any tonotopic region of the IC. It has long been thought that an important aspect of central neuropathy underpinning tinnitus is an "edge effect" and that this might be particularly important in the IC, where lateral inhibition is a feature of signal processing.[80] An edge effect would be characterized by an area where tonotopic organization was distorted. The distortion would appear primarily at the border of a zone where cochlear damaged resulted in a focal loss of afferents. Decreased lateral inhibition at the edge of the loss zone would therefore enable frequencies adjoining the zone to be overrepresented, or overly active. While this is mechanistically an attractive hypothesis, at least as an explanation of tonal tinnitus, it has not received much empirical support.[81] The IC study of Bauer et al.[53] did not find an overrepresentation or elevated driven activity of single units tuned at or near the psychophysically defined tinnitus frequency. The current weight of evidence is that tinnitus neuropathy may be rather diffusely distributed and involve a number of different mechanisms.[47]

LOSS OF INHIBITION

A prominent feature of normal auditory processing is dynamic range compression. Ten logarithmic units of sound-level variation are typically coded in individual auditory neurons by two logarithmic units of action potential frequency variation. This compression is clearly evident in the nonmonotonic rate-level functions of fusiform cells that comprise the major output pathway of the DCN.[82] As stimulus levels increase, most fusiform cells follow with increasing spike rates up to a maximum, and above that level, they continue to follow stimulus increases with decreased spike rates. In vivo iontophoretic application of GABA antagonists, such a bicuculline, alters the nonmonotonic leg of unit rate functions, making units follow stimulus increases more linearly.[83] Therefore, GABA release in the DCN underpins compression coding and limits neuron output. Decreased GABA-mediated inhibition may be the mechanism behind increased spontaneous and stimulus-driven activity in the DCN observed in tinnitus. GABA inputs to excitatory neurons are known to be mediators of homeostatic neuroplasticity.[84] A chronic decrease in system input has been shown to downregulate the density of postsynaptic $GABA_A$ receptors ($GABA_A$-R). Brain-derived neurotrophic growth factor (BDNF), a component of an intracellular signaling system known to be sensitive to neural activity, may mediate this homeostatic receptor response.[84] Acoustic overexposure may have an additional negative impact on auditory GABA. High-level sound exposure has been shown to have a long-term depression effect on glutamic acid decarboxylase (GAD) in the IC.[85] GAD_{67} is responsible for synthesizing GABA from its substrate, glutamic acid (Glu). The net long-term effect of system overstimulation would therefore be a loss of GABA-mediated inhibition via two mechanisms: postsynaptic receptor loss and presynaptic transmitter loss. In support, it has been shown that rats with tinnitus, when administered vigabatrin, an inhibitor of the GABA catabolic enzyme GABA transaminase, show rather complete alleviation of their tinnitus.[36,37] The therapeutic effect of vigabatrin was evident when the drug was present, and it was washed out when the drug was removed. Facilitating central inhibitory circuits using GABA agonists, therefore, provides a potential therapeutic avenue for treating chronic tinnitus and provides empirical support for loss-of-inhibition hypotheses.

AUDITORY CORTEX AND AMYGDALA

It is likely that related cortical activity would have to be present to be aware of tinnitus. This should be no less true of an animal than a human. In animals, awareness can be demonstrated when the animal is competent in using the tinnitus signal to direct a voluntary response such as selecting a drinking spout[86] or making a lever press.[48] Eggermont and colleagues have shown several near-term changes in anesthetized cat auditory cortex following exposure to high-level sound. The alterations were observed in multiunit activity and were generally more pronounced a few hours after exposure than immediately afterward. The changes included increased spontaneous activity, increased interunit synchrony, increased bursting (see Chapter 9), and distorted frequency representation.[87,88] The alterations were not mutually exclusive, being coevident in given samples of neurons, and all have been suggested to be potential neural correlates of tinnitus. The most dramatic cortical correlate of tinnitus may be tonotopic frequency map reorganization. This, of course, is a variant of the edge effect. Eggermont and colleagues have shown that not only does long-term tonotopic reorganization of the auditory cortex in cats follow traumatic sound exposure, but also therapeutic reversal can be obtained by exposure to well-chosen underrepresented sound frequencies.[17] However, these results must be interpreted with caution, because although the animals in the Eggermont experiments were exposed to high-level sound likely to produce tinnitus, tinnitus was not independently confirmed in any of the subjects. Nevertheless, confirmation was reported by Yang et al.,[37] who found that rats with acoustic-exposure-induced tinnitus had significantly distorted tonotopic representation in their primary auditory cortex. The distortion was characterized by a "vacant" zone interposed between low-frequency and high-frequency regions, in the approximate location of the traumatizing frequency. In addition, the high-frequency region was found to be deficient in inhibitory postsynaptic potentials, as determined in vitro. Finally, systemic treatment with the antagonist of GABA catabolism, vigabatrin, was able to alleviate psychophysical evidence of tinnitus, as indicated by the gap inhibition method.[37] If tonotopic reorganization contributes to the perception of tinnitus, then strategies for correcting the distortion may provide therapeutic relief. Engineer et al.[89] reported success in alleviating tinnitus in rats by pairing vagus nerve stimulation with presentation of tones in the traumatic vacant zone, over the course of 10 days. Vagus nerve stimulation has been shown in other studies to increase the release of acetylcholine in the nucleus basalis and to facilitate forebrain neuroplasticity.[18] Caution, however, is still in order. A recent functional imaging study using human subjects and state-of-the-art methods for optimizing spatial resolution failed to find evidence of cortical tonotopic reorganization in tinnitus patients compared to matched nontinnitus controls.[81] Therefore, the status of tonotopic reorganization in tinnitus remains, at present, in limbo. However, the same research group, using diffusion tensor imaging, reported enhanced cortico-amygdaloid and cortico-collicular connectivity in tinnitus patients, again compared to hearing-level-matched controls.[90] Diffusion tensor analysis permits quantification of coordinated regional activity in the brain. The cortico-amygdaloid connection was of particular interest because a limbic system component of tinnitus has been hypothesized for more than two decades[74,91] to account for the emotionally disturbing aspect of tinnitus seen in about 5% of the human tinnitus population. Magnetic resonance imaging morphometry has also shown structurally enlarged connections between the auditory cortex and multimodal cortical areas such as the medial prefrontal cortex, which have a role in regulating the emotional tone of behavior.[73] The weight of the evidence, therefore, points to alterations in cortical auditory processing accompanying tinnitus, and connections to other brain systems, such as the limbic system. Features of those alterations and connections (and, most importantly, their causal status) are still uncertain.

NONAUDITORY BRAIN AREAS

Hippocampus

For more than two decades, circumstantial evidence suggested involvement of the limbic areas in tinnitus neuropathy. Therefore, it is not surprising that limbic areas beyond the amygdala have been investigated. The hippocampus is a limbic area that bridges emotional, cognitive, and sensory functions. Attention was drawn to a hippocampal role in sensory gating by clinical electroencephalography studies showing attentional deficits in schizophrenic patients.[92] Well-defined auditory-evoked potentials have been recorded directly from the hippocampus in human volunteers with deep electrodes placed for control of epileptic seizures.[93] Single-unit as well as field potentials, evoked by auditory stimuli, have been recorded from the hippocampal CA3 region in awake behaving rats.[94] In rats tested with paired auditory click stimuli, separated by 500 ms, attenuation of the hippocampal response evoked by the second stimulus was clearly evident.[94] This demonstrates dynamic sensory gating in the hippocampus. Recently, it has been reported that bilateral moderate-level (4 kHz tones at 104 dB SPL) sound exposure (for 40 min), which might be expected to induce acute tinnitus, altered the spatial tuning of place cells (CA1 pyramidal cells that display spatial-location-specific responses) in the hippocampus of rats, for up to 24 h after sound exposure.[95] In this study, the sound-induced shift in unit place activity was more pronounced 24 h after exposure than immediately afterward. The significance for tinnitus is that sound exposure that produces tinnitus may shift the selectivity of hippocampal cells that in turn modify attention. The most clinically relevant feature of tinnitus in persons bothered by their condition is that they fail to habituate to the meaningless background sensation that is tinnitus. This could be construed as a failure of selective attention. Using a rat model of tinnitus, Kraus et al.[96] showed that unilateral sound exposure capable of producing tinnitus also significantly interfered with neurogenesis in the hippocampus. Hippocampal neurogenesis is a normal feature of adult mammalian brain function. Unfortunately, Kraus et al.[96] were not able to show that the interference with neurogenesis was directly tied to tinnitus, because traumatic-sound-exposed rats both with and without tinnitus, as indicated by gap inhibition of startle, displayed equal neurogenesis inhibition. Nevertheless, this result corresponds well with recent findings[97,98] that reported that rats with psychophysical evidence of tinnitus were not negatively impacted on spatial learning tasks such as radial maze learning or the Morris water maze. Hippocampal function has been traditionally linked to spatial learning tasks. However, animals with tinnitus were shown to be significantly worse at inhibiting impulsive behavior.[98] In conclusion, there is evidence supporting the hypothesis that hippocampal function may be compromised in animals exposed to tinnitus-inducing events, and that attention-related deficits may be a consequence.

Cerebellum

In addition to the hippocampus, recent experiments also suggest that the cerebellum, in particular the PFL, may significantly contribute to generation of the tinnitus signal. As discussed in this chapter, the DCN and cerebellum comprise similar neuronal networks. Functional imaging using manganese-enhanced magnetic resonance imaging (MEMRI) has identified the PFL to have significantly elevated activity in rats with evidence of tinnitus.[79] Increased uptake Mn^{2+} primarily at synaptic Ca^{2+} channels, while evident in rats with chronic tinnitus, was not evident in normal control rats exposed to an external 90 dB SPL tinnitus-like sound. These observations suggest that the PFL may play a unique role in processing auditory information and the pathology of tinnitus. Although the data are limited, acoustically responsive neurons in the PFL have been identified.[99–101] There is both descending acoustic input to the PFL from the secondary auditory cortex, via the pons, and direct ascending input to the flocculus from the cochlea.[100,102–104] As noted by Ito, differentiation between an internally generated event and one produced by an external stimulus may be based on the successful cancellation of self-produced sensations mediated by an internal cerebellar modeling process.[105] Following auditory damage, a cerebellar comparator may be fed conflicting information from a damaged periphery, with attendant decreased eighth nerve activity,[106] combined with enhanced activity in a trigger zone such as the DCN.[51,60] In this scenario, with a mismatch between externally and internally generated sensations, the cerebellar cancellation process could be distorted so that external silent conditions are no longer accurately represented. In support of the role of the PFL as a tinnitus generator, Bauer et al.[107] showed that PFL ablation eliminated established chronic tinnitus in rats, although identical ablations failed to protect against the development of tinnitus after exposure to high-level sound. It was also shown in complementary experiments that deactivating the PFL ipsilateral to the trauma-exposed ear with locally infused local anesthetic (4% lidocaine) reversibly eliminated established tinnitus, similar to the effect of ablations.[108] As expected, with lidocaine infusion the tinnitus was eliminated gradually over the 14-day course of treatment, and it reappeared once the lidocaine washed out. Therefore, the PFL appeared to serve as a generator site but not necessarily an obligatory one, nor did it appear to serve as a trigger zone.

Interestingly, there is also clinical evidence that the cerebellum may be serving as a tinnitus generator. Several functional imaging studies in humans have reported cerebellar involvement in tinnitus. Activation of the cerebellum in association with severely disturbing tinnitus was first noted by Shulman using single-photon emission computerized tomography (SPECT) measuring regional cerebral perfusion. Ten patients with severe tinnitus displayed significantly increased blood flow in their right and left cerebellum compared with nontinnitus controls.[109] Mirz et al. studied 12 patients with severely disturbing tinnitus using positron emission tomography (PET) imaging co-registered with MRI. Participants were imaged while listening to their tinnitus and under conditions of tinnitus suppression using masking sounds and lidocaine infusion. The structure with the largest difference in regional cerebral blood flow between baseline and masking with sound and lidocaine was in the cerebellum.[110] Osaki et al.[111] compared regional cerebral blood flow, using PET, in volunteers with bilateral tinnitus and in normal-hearing control subjects without tinnitus. The tinnitus participants were notable in that their tinnitus was completely inhibited when their cochlear implants were turned on, and the inhibition persisted for a time after the implants were again turned off (residual inhibition). The tinnitus patients were imaged while listening to their tinnitus with implants turned off and again after 15 min of cochlear implant stimulation and induction of residual inhibition. Control volunteers were imaged while listening to 75 dB noise and again during silence. Two tinnitus-related central sites were identified in the cochlear implant participants. Regional blood flow was significantly increased in the right cerebellum during tinnitus perception. During the period of residual inhibition of the tinnitus, there was enhanced blood flow in the right anterior temporal lobe. These clinical investigations strengthen the hypothesis of a cerebellar tinnitus generator site.

A CELLULAR COMPONENT OF TINNITUS

A unique cell type, the UBC, located in the PFL and DCN[112] may play an important role in the pathology of tinnitus. In the cerebellum, the UBC is an excitatory glutamatergic interneuron that receives mossy fiber inputs from vestibular, reticular, and somatosensory sources, and it synapses onto granule cells, other UBCs, and Purkinje cells.[113] UBC circuits in the DCN are similar to those in the cerebellum, although they additionally receive indirect (i.e. second- or third-order) auditory inputs and, most interestingly, modulatory input from auditory cortex[114] (Figure 20.2). The primary function of UBC networks appears to be feedforward amplification and fan-out integration, and in the DCN there exists the possibility of positive feedback from a cortical loop.[114,115] Anatomically, the largest density of UBCs is found in the transition zone between the PFL and the flocculus, as well as in the dorsomedial DCN. Although UBCs in the DCN do not receive direct inputs from the cochlea,[114] they do receive secondary inputs from brainstem auditory areas and probably comprise a positive feedforward circuit. Recently, using point-resolved magnetic resonance spectroscopy, it was shown that glutamate levels in the DCN were elevated in rats with tinnitus, compared to nontinnitus controls.[33] A further intriguing aspect of UBC function is their notable plasticity in the fully adult cerebellum and DCN. Baizer and colleagues[116] used a DCX stain to quantify postmitotic neurons, morphologically identified as UBCs, in the cerebellum and DCN of 3–16-month-old rats. DCX is a microtubule-associated protein that is highly elevated in recent postmitotic neurons. At present, the function of these emergent UBCs is not known, but they could develop in response to auditory insult and provide a source of homeostatic compensation for de-afferentation. In many instances, tinnitus does not emerge immediately after acoustic trauma, but it slowly develops over a few days[61] or for up to several months.[49] The UBC network might provide an attractive target for developing novel tinnitus therapeutics. Furthermore, a dual approach of targeting glutamatergic as well as GABAergic mechanisms might be more effective than targeting just one transmitter system.

CONCLUSIONS

Tinnitus pathology derives from abnormal activity in a distributed central network involving both traditionally defined auditory areas and nonauditory areas. This condition appears to characterize tinnitus clinically as well as experimentally in animal models, where causal conditions are singular and well controlled. At lower levels of the auditory system, most notably the DCN, elevated spontaneous activity may constitute the neuronal correlate of tinnitus. Loss of inhibition, particularly that mediated by GABA, appears to be partly responsible. Elevated excitation in glutamatergic circuits, perhaps mediated by local feedforward driving by UBCs, may also be involved. At levels above the cochlear nuclei, elevated spontaneous activity may be less relevant than other features of neuronal activity, such as activity pattern changes. Bursting and increased regularity of spiking have been found at the level of the IC and primary auditory cortex. At the level of the auditory cortex, tonotopic reorganization may additionally be relevant. It also seems likely, at least in acoustic-trauma-induced tinnitus, that some brain areas, such as the DCN, serve as necessary trigger zones, while other areas, such as the IC and PFL, serve as nonobigatory generator sites for the tinnitus signal.

Acknowledgment

Supported by the National Institute on Deafness and Other Communication Disorders #1R01DC009669-01.

References

1. Dan B. Titus's tinnitus. *J Hist Neurosci*. 2005;14(3):210–213.
2. Berliner KI, Shelton C, Hitselberger WE, Luxford WM. Acoustic tumors: effect of surgical removal on tinnitus. *Am J Otol*. 1992;13(1):13–17.
3. Kameda K, Shono T, Hashiguchi K, Yoshida F, Sasaki T. Effect of tumor removal on tinnitus in patients with vestibular schwannoma. *J Neurosurg*. 2010;112(1):152–157.
4. Tyler RS, Erlandsson S. Management of the tinnitus patient. In: Luxon LM, Furman JM, Martini A, Stephens SDG, eds. *Textbook of Audiological Medicine*. London: Martin Dunitz; 2002:571–578.
5. Hoffman HJ, Reed GW. Epidemiology of tinnitus. In: Snow Jr JB, ed. *Tinnitus: Theory and Management*. Hamilton, ON: B.C. Decker; 2004:16–42.

6. Dobie RA. Overview: suffering from tinnitus. In: Snow JB, ed. *Tinnitus: Theory and Management*. Hamilton, ON: B.C. Decker; 2004:1–7.
7. Figueiredo RR, Azevedo AA, Oliveira PM, Amorim SP, Rios AG, Baptista V. Incidence of tinnitus in mp3 player users. *Braz J Otorhinolaryngol*. 2011;77(3):293–298.
8. Muhr P, Rosenhall U. The influence of military service on auditory health and the efficacy of a Hearing Conservation Program. *Noise Health*. 2011;13(53):320–327.
9. Moller AR. Unit responses in the cochlear nucleus of the rat to pure tones. *Acta Physiol Scand*. 1969;75(4):530–541.
10. Frisina RD, Smith RL, Chamberlain SC. Encoding of amplitude modulation in the gerbil cochlear nucleus: I. A hierarchy of enhancement. *Hear Res*. 1990;44(2–3):99–122.
11. Arle JE, Kim DO. Neural modeling of intrinsic and spike-discharge properties of cochlear nucleus neurons. *Biol Cybern*. 1991;64(4):273–283.
12. Miyakawa A, Gibboni R, Bao S. Repeated exposure to a tone transiently alters spectral tuning bandwidth of neurons in the central nucleus of inferior colliculus in juvenile rats. *Neuroscience*. 2013;230:114–120.
13. Mayko ZM, Roberts PD, Portfors CV. Inhibition shapes selectivity to vocalizations in the inferior colliculus of awake mice. *Front Neural Circuits*. 2012;6:73.
14. Hackett TA, Barkat TR, O'Brien BM, Hensch TK, Polley DB. Linking topography to tonotopy in the mouse auditory thalamocortical circuit. *J Neurosci*. 2011;31(8):2983–2995.
15. de la Mothe LA, Blumell S, Kajikawa Y, Hackett TA. Thalamic connections of the auditory cortex in marmoset monkeys: core and medial belt regions. *J Comp Neurol*. 2006;496(1):72–96.
16. Winer JA. Decoding the auditory corticofugal systems. *Hear Res*. 2005;207(1–2):1–9.
17. Norena AJ, Eggermont JJ. Enriched acoustic environment after noise trauma reduces hearing loss and prevents cortical map reorganization. *J Neurosci*. 2005;25(3):699–705.
18. Kilgard MP, Merzenich MM. Cortical map reorganization enabled by nucleus basalis activity. *Science*. 1998;279(5357):1714–1718.
19. Hackett TA. Information flow in the auditory cortical network. *Hear Res*. 2011;271(1–2):133–146.
20. Winer JA, Lee CC. The distributed auditory cortex. *Hear Res*. 2007;229(1–2):3–13.
21. Masterton RB. Role of the mammalian forebrain in hearing. In: Syka J, ed. *International Symposium on Acoustical Signal Processing in the Central Auditory System*. Prague, Czech Republic: Plenum Press; 1996:1–17.
22. Liberman MC, Kiang NY. Acoustic trauma in cats. Cochlear pathology and auditory-nerve activity. *Acta Otolaryngol Suppl*. 1978;358:1–63.
23. Bauer CA, Brozoski TJ, Myers K. Primary afferent dendrite degeneration as a cause of tinnitus. *J Neurosci Res*. 2007;85(7):1489–1498.
24. Liberman MC. Central projections of auditory nerve fibers of differing spontaneous rate, II: posteroventral and dorsal cochlear nuclei. *J Comp Neurol*. 1993;327(1):17–36.
25. Young ED, Voigt HF. Response properties of type II and type III units in dorsal cochlear nucleus. *Hear Res*. 1982;6(2):153–169.
26. Rubio ME. Differential distribution of synaptic endings containing glutamate, glycine, and GABA in the rat dorsal cochlear nucleus. *J. Comp. Neurol*. 2004:253–272.
27. Norena AJ. An integrative model of tinnitus based on a central gain controlling neural sensitivity. *Neurosci Biobehav Rev*. 2011;35(5):1089–1109.
28. Wang H, Brozoski TJ, Caspary DM. Inhibitory neurotransmission in animal models of tinnitus: maladaptive plasticity. *Hear Res*. 2011;279(1–2):111–117.
29. Suneja SK, Potashner SJ, Benson CG. Plastic changes in glycine and GABA release and uptake in adult brain stem auditory nuclei after unilateral middle ear ossicle removal and cochlear ablation. *Exp Neurol*. 1998;151(2):273–288.
30. Wang H, Brozoski TJ, Turner JG, et al. Plasticity at glycinergic synapses in dorsal cochlear nucleus of rats with behavioral evidence of tinnitus. *Neuroscience*. 2009;164(2):747–759.
31. Caspary DM, Holder TM, Hughes LF, Milbrandt JC, McKernan RM, Naritoku DK. Age-related changes in $GABA_A$ receptor subunit composition and function in rat auditory system. *Neuroscience*. 1999;93(1):307–312.
32. Milbrandt JC, Holder TM, Wilson MC, Salvi RJ, Caspary DM. GAD levels and muscimol binding in rat inferior colliculus following acoustic trauma. *Hear Res*. 2000;147:251–260.
33. Brozoski T, Odintsov B, Bauer C. Gamma-aminobutyric acid and glutamic acid levels in the auditory pathway of rats with chronic tinnitus: a direct determination using high resolution point-resolved proton magnetic resonance spectroscopy (H-MRS). *Front Syst Neurosci*. 2012;6:9.
34. Middleton JW, Kiritani T, Pedersen C, Turner JG, Shepherd GM, Tzounopoulos T. Mice with behavioral evidence of tinnitus exhibit dorsal cochlear nucleus hyperactivity because of decreased GABAergic inhibition. *Proc Natl Acad Sci USA*. 2011;108(18):7601–7606.
35. Brozoski TJ, Caspary DM, Bauer CA, Richardson BD. The effect of supplemental dietary taurine on tinnitus and auditory discrimination in an animal model. *Hear Res*. 2010;270(1–2):71–80.
36. Brozoski TJ, Spires TJ, Bauer CA. Vigabatrin, a GABA transaminase inhibitor, reversibly eliminates tinnitus in an animal model. *J Assoc Res Otolaryngol*. 2007;8(1):105–118.
37. Yang S, Weiner BD, Zhang LS, Cho SJ, Bao S. Homeostatic plasticity drives tinnitus perception in an animal model. *Proc Natl Acad Sci USA*. 2011;108(36):14974–14979.
38. Guitton MJ, Dudai Y. Blockade of cochlear NMDA receptors prevents long-term tinnitus during a brief consolidation window after acoustic trauma. *Neural Plast*. 2007;2007:80904.
39. Zhou J, Zeng C, Cui Y, Shore S. Vesicular glutamate transporter 2 is associated with the cochlear nucleus commissural pathway. *J Assoc Res Otolaryngol*. 2010;11(4):675–687.
40. Voytenko SV, Galazyuk AV. mGluRs modulate neuronal firing in the auditory midbrain. *Neurosci Lett*. Apr 4, 2011;492(3):145–149.
41. Tzounopoulos T, Rubio ME, Keen JE, Trussell LO. Coactivation of pre- and postsynaptic signaling mechanisms determines cell-specific spike-timing-dependent plasticity. *Neuron*. Apr 19, 2007;54(2):291–301.
42. Bauer CA, Wisner KW, Baizer JS, Brozoski TJ. Tinnitus, unipolar brush cells, and cerebellar glutamatergic function in an animal model. *PLoS One*. 2013;8(6):e64726. http://dx.doi.org/10.1371/journal.pone.0064726.
43. Jastreboff PJ, Brennan JF, Coleman JK, Sasaki CT. Phantom auditory sensation in rats: an animal model for tinnitus. *Behav Neurosci*. 1988;102(6):811–822.
44. Stebbins W. *Animal Psychophysics*. New York: Appleton, Century, Crofts; 1970.
45. Brozoski TJ, Bauer CA. Learning about tinnitus from an animal model. *Semin Hear*. 2008;29(3):242–258.
46. Eggermont JJ. Hearing loss, hyperacusis, or tinnitus: what is modeled in animal research? *Hear Res*. 2012;295:140–149.
47. Roberts LE, Eggermont JJ, Caspary DM, Shore SE, Melcher JR, Kaltenbach JA. Ringing ears: the neuroscience of tinnitus. *J Neurosci*. 2010;30(45):14972–14979.

48. Bauer CA, Brozoski TJ. Assessing tinnitus and prospective tinnitus therapeutics using a psychophysical animal model. *J Assoc Res Otolaryngol*. 2001;2(1):54–64.
49. Turner JG, Brozoski TJ, Bauer CA, et al. Gap detection deficits in rats with tinnitus: a potential novel screening tool. *Behav Neurosci*. 2006;120(1):188–195.
50. Turner J, Larsen D, Hughes L, Moechars D, Shore S. Time course of tinnitus development following noise exposure in mice. *J Neurosci Res*. 2012;90:1480–1488.
51. Brozoski TJ, Bauer CA, Caspary DM. Elevated fusiform cell activity in the dorsal cochlear nucleus of chinchillas with psychophysical evidence of tinnitus. *J Neurosci*. 2002; 22(6):2383–2390.
52. Kaltenbach JA, Afman CE. Hyperactivity in the dorsal cochlear nucleus after intense sound exposure and its resemblance to tone-evoked activity: a physiological model for tinnitus. *Hear Res*. 2000;140(1–2):165–172.
53. Bauer CA, Turner JG, Caspary DM, Myers KS, Brozoski TJ. Tinnitus and inferior colliculus activity in chinchillas related to three distinct patterns of cochlear trauma. *J Neurosci Res*. 2008;86(11):2564–2578.
54. Salvi R, Perry J, Hamernik RP, Henderson D. *Relationships between Cochlear Pathologies and Auditory Nerve and Behavioral Responses following Acoustic Trauma*. New York: Raven Press; 1982.
55. Liberman MC, Beil DG. Hair cell condition and auditory nerve response in normal and noise-damaged cochleas. *Acta Otolaryngol*. 1979;88(3–4):161–176.
56. Syka J, Rybalko N. Threshold shifts and enhancement of cortical evoked responses after noise exposure in rats. *Hear Res*. 2000;139(1–2):59–68.
57. Syka J, Rybalko N, Popelar J. Enhancement of the auditory cortex evoked responses in awake guinea pigs after noise exposure. *Hear Res*. 1994;78(2):158–168.
58. Kaltenbach JA. Summary of evidence pointing to a role of the dorsal cochlear nucleus in the etiology of tinnitus. *Acta Otolaryngol Suppl*. 2006;556:20–26.
59. Kaltenbach JA. The dorsal cochlear nucleus as a participant in the auditory, attentional and emotional components of tinnitus. *Hear Res*. 2006;216–217:224–234.
60. Kaltenbach JA, Zacharek MA, Zhang J, Frederick S. Activity in the dorsal cochlear nucleus of hamsters previously tested for tinnitus following intense tone exposure. *Neurosci Lett*. 2004;355(1–2):121–125.
61. Kaltenbach JA, Zhang J, Afman CE. Plasticity of spontaneous neural activity in the dorsal cochlear nucleus after intense sound exposure. *Hear Res*. 2000;147(1–2):282–292.
62. Zhang JS, Kaltenbach JA, Godfrey DA, Wang J. Origin of hyperactivity in the hamster dorsal cochlear nucleus following intense sound exposure. *J Neurosci Res*. 2006;84(4):819–831.
63. Mulders WH, Robertson D. Hyperactivity in the auditory midbrain after acoustic trauma: dependence on cochlear activity. *Neuroscience*. 2009;164(2):733–746.
64. Oertel D, Young ED. What's a cerebellar circuit doing in the auditory system? *Trends Neurosci*. 2004;27(2):104–110.
65. Manis PB, Molitor SC. *N*-methyl-D-aspartate receptors at parallel fiber synapses in the dorsal cochlear nucleus. *J Neurophysiol*. 1996;76(3):1639–1656.
66. Shore SE, Zhou J. Somatosensory influence on the cochlear nucleus and beyond. *Hear Res*. 2006;216–217:90–99.
67. Shore SE, Koehler S, Oldakowski M, Hughes LF, Syed S. Dorsal cochlear nucleus responses to somatosensory stimulation are enhanced after noise-induced hearing loss. *Eur J Neurosci*. 2008;27(1):155–168.
68. Dehmel S, Pradhan S, Koehler S, Bledsoe S, Shore S. Noise overexposure alters long-term somatosensory-auditory processing in the dorsal cochlear nucleus – possible basis for tinnitus-related hyperactivity? *J Neurosci*. 2012;32(5):1660–1671.
69. Coad ML, Lockwood A, Salvi R, Burkard R. Characteristics of patients with gaze-evoked tinnitus. *Otol Neurotol*. 2001;22(5):650–654.
70. Levine RA, Abel M, Cheng H. CNS somatosensory-auditory interactions elicit or modulate tinnitus. *Exp Brain Res*. 2003;153(4):643–648.
71. Lockwood AH, Wack DS, Burkard RF, et al. The functional anatomy of gaze-evoked tinnitus and sustained lateral gaze. *Neurology*. 2001;56(4):472–480.
72. Brozoski TJ, Bauer CA. The effect of dorsal cochlear nucleus ablation on tinnitus in rats. *Hear Res*. 2005;206(1–2):227–236.
73. Leaver AM, Seydell-Greenwald A, Turesky TK, Morgan S, Kim HJ, Rauschecker JP. Cortico-limbic morphology separates tinnitus from tinnitus distress. *Front Syst Neurosci*. 2012;6:21.
74. Rauschecker JP, Leaver AM, Muhlau M. Tuning out the noise: limbic-auditory interactions in tinnitus. *Neuron*. 2010;66(6):819–826.
75. Penner MJ. Judgments and measurements of the loudness of tinnitus before and after masking. *J Speech Hear Res*. 1988;31(4):582–587.
76. Brozoski TJ, Wisner KW, Sybert LT, Bauer CA. Bilateral dorsal cochlear nucleus lesions prevent acoustic-trauma induced tinnitus in an animal model. *J Assoc Res Otolaryngol*. 2012;13(1):55–66.
77. Gu JW, Halpin CF, Nam EC, Levine RA, Melcher JR. Tinnitus, diminished sound-level tolerance, and elevated auditory activity in humans with clinically normal hearing sensitivity. *J Neurophysiol*. 2010;104(6):3361–3370.
78. Holt AG, Bissig D, Mirza N, Rajah G, Berkowitz B. Evidence of key tinnitus-related brain regions documented by a unique combination of manganese-enhanced MRI and acoustic startle reflex testing. *PLoS One*. 2010;5(12):e14260.
79. Brozoski TJ, Ciobanu L, Bauer CA. Central neural activity in rats with tinnitus evaluated with manganese-enhanced magnetic resonance imaging (MEMRI). *Hear Res*. 2007;228(1–2): 168–179.
80. Gerken GM. Central tinnitus and lateral inhibition: an auditory brainstem model. *Hear Res*. 1996;97(1–2):75–83.
81. Langers DR, de Kleine E, van Dijk P. Tinnitus does not require macroscopic tonotopic map reorganization. *Front Syst Neurosci*. 2012;6:2.
82. Joris PX. Response classes in the dorsal cochlear nucleus and its output tract in the chloralose-anesthetized cat. *J Neurosci*. 1998;18(10):3955–3966.
83. Backoff PM, Palombi PS, Caspary DM. Glycinergic and GABAergic inputs affect short-term suppression in the cochlear nucleus. *Hear Res*. 1997;110(1–2):155–163.
84. Wenner P. Mechanisms of GABAergic homeostatic plasticity. *Neural Plast*. 2011;2011:489470.
85. Abbott SD, Hughes LF, Bauer CA, Salvi R, Caspary DM. Detection of glutamate decarboxylase isoforms in rat inferior colliculus following acoustic exposure. *Neuroscience*. 1999;93(4):1375–1381.
86. Heffner HE, Harrington IA. Tinnitus in hamsters following exposure to intense sound. *Hear Res*. 2002;170(1–2):83–95.
87. Norena AJ, Tomita M, Eggermont JJ. Neural changes in cat auditory cortex after a transient pure-tone trauma. *J Neurophysiol*. 2003;90(4):2387–2401.
88. Seki S, Eggermont JJ. Changes in cat primary auditory cortex after minor-to-moderate pure-tone induced hearing loss. *Hear Res*. 2002;173(1–2):172–186.
89. Engineer ND, Riley JR, Seale JD, et al. Reversing pathological neural activity using targeted plasticity. *Nature*. Feb 3, 2011;470(7332):101–104.

90. Crippa A, Lanting CP, van Dijk P, Roerdink JB. A diffusion tensor imaging study on the auditory system and tinnitus. *Open Neuroimag J*. 2010;4:16–25.
91. Jastreboff PJ. Phantom auditory perception (tinnitus): mechanisms of generation and perception. *Neurosci Res (N Y)*. 1990;8(4):221–254.
92. Cromwell HC, Mears RP, Wan L, Boutros NN. Sensory gating: a translational effort from basic to clinical science. *Clin EEG Neurosci*. 2008;39(2):69–72.
93. Boutros NN, Brockhaus-Dumke A, Gjini K, et al. Sensory-gating deficit of the N100 mid-latency auditory evoked potential in medicated schizophrenia patients. *Schizophr Res*. 2009;113(2–3):339–346.
94. Moxon KA, Gerhardt GA, Bickford PC, et al. Multiple single units and population responses during inhibitory gating of hippocampal auditory response in freely-moving rats. *Brain Res*. 1999;825(1–2):75–85.
95. Goble TJ, Moller AR, Thompson LT. Acute high-intensity sound exposure alters responses of place cells in hippocampus. *Hear Res*. 2009;253(1–2):52–59.
96. Kraus KS, Mitra S, Jimenez Z, et al. Noise trauma impairs neurogenesis in the rat hippocampus. *Neuroscience*. 2010;167(4):1216–1226.
97. Zheng Y, Hamilton E, Begum S, Smith PF, Darlington CL. The effects of acoustic trauma that can cause tinnitus on spatial performance in rats. *Neuroscience*. 2011;186:48–56.
98. Zheng Y, Hamilton E, Stiles L, et al. Acoustic trauma that can cause tinnitus impairs impulsive control but not performance accuracy in the 5-choice serial reaction time task in rats. *Neuroscience*. 2011;180:75–84.
99. Azizi SA, Woodward DJ. Interactions of visual and auditory mossy fiber inputs in the paraflocculus of the rat: a gating action of multimodal inputs. *Brain Res*. 1990;533(2):255–262.
100. Azizi SA, Burne RA, Woodward DJ. The auditory corticopontocerebellar projection in the rat: inputs to the paraflocculus and midvermis. An anatomical and physiological study. *Exp Brain Res*. 1985;59(1):36–49.
101. Mortimer JA. Cerebellar responses to teleceptive stimuli in alert monkeys. *Brain Res*. 1975;83(3):369–390.
102. Morest DK, Kim J, Bohne BA. Neuronal and transneuronal degeneration of auditory axons in the brainstem after cochlear lesions in the chinchilla: cochleotopic and non-cochleotopic patterns. *Hear Res*. 1997;103(1–2):151–168.
103. Rasmussen G. Remarks on the cochleo-cerebellar connections. 1990; No. Notebook 3: 1–42. Located at: Research Notebooks, History of Medicine Division, National Library of Medicine, Washington, DC.
104. Eisenman LM. Pontocerebellar projections to the paraflocculus in the rat. *Brain Res*. 1980;188(2):550–554.
105. Ito M. Control of mental activities by internal models in the cerebellum. *Nat Rev Neurosci*. 2008;9(4):304–313.
106. Salvi R, Perry J, Hamerink RP, Henderson D. Relationships between cochlear pathologies and auditory nerve and behavioral responses following acoustic trauma. In: Hamerink RP, Henderson D, Salvi R, eds. *New Perspective on Noise-Induced Hearing Loss*. New York: Raven Press; 1982:165–188.
107. Bauer CA, Kurt W, Sybert LT, Brozoski TJ. The cerebellum as a novel tinnitus generator. *Hear Res*. 2013;295:130–139.
108. Bauer C, Wisner K, Sybert LT, Brozoski TJ. The cerebellum as a novel tinnitus generator. *Hear Res*. 2012;295:130–139.
109. Shulman A, Strashun A. Descending auditory system/cerebellum/tinnitus. *Int Tinnitus J*. 1999;5(2):92–106.
110. Mirz F, Pedersen B, Ishizu K, et al. Positron emission tomography of cortical centers of tinnitus. *Hear Res*. 1999;134(1–2): 133–144.
111. Osaki Y, Nishimura H, Takasawa M, et al. Neural mechanism of residual inhibition of tinnitus in cochlear implant users. *Neuroreport*. 2005;16(15):1625–1628.
112. Mugnaini E, Floris A. The unipolar brush cell: a neglected neuron of the mammalian cerebellar cortex. *J Comp Neurol*. 1994;339(2):174–180.
113. Dino MR, Schuerger RJ, Liu Y, Slater NT, Mugnaini E. Unipolar brush cell: a potential feedforward excitatory interneuron of the cerebellum. *Neuroscience*. 2000;98(4):625–636.
114. Dino MR, Mugnaini E. Distribution and phenotypes of unipolar brush cells in relation to the granule cell system of the rat cochlear nucleus. *Neuroscience*. 2008;154(1):29–50.
115. Mugnaini E, Sekerkova G, Martina M. The unipolar brush cell: a remarkable neuron finally receiving deserved attention. *Brain Res Rev*. 2011;66(1–2):220–245.
116. Manohar S, Paolone NA, Bleichfeld M, Hayes SH, Salvi RJ, Baizer JS. Expression of doublecortin, a neuronal migration protein, in unipolar brush cells of the vestibulocerebellum and dorsal cochlear nucleus of the adult rat. *Neuroscience*. Jan 27, 2012;202:169–183.

CHAPTER

21

Consciousness and Subcortical Arousal Systems

Joshua Motelow [1], Hal Blumenfeld [1,2,3]

[1]Department of Neurology, Yale University School of Medicine, New Haven, CT, USA,
[2]Department of Neurosurgery, Yale University School of Medicine, New Haven, CT, USA,
[3]Department of Neurobiology, Yale University School of Medicine, New Haven, CT, USA

INTRODUCTION

To begin discussing arousal or consciousness, we must understand both the associated behaviors as well as the electrographic patterns observed with neuroscience techniques. To understand the behaviors of consciousness, Plum and Posner[1,2] classically proposed the *content of consciousness* and the *level of consciousness*. The *content* comprises those things of which we are aware, including sensory and motor systems, memory, and emotions—in short, our experience. The content of consciousness is the subject matter of most studies in neuroscience. The *level* refers to the degree to which we are able to process the *content* and depends on our general wakefulness, attentiveness, and awareness. A general discussion of all aspects of consciousness is outside of the scope of this chapter. Instead, we focus on cellular mechanisms and brain systems that regulate the *level* of consciousness. In analogy to other specialized brain networks such as the motor, somatosensory, and limbic systems, we refer to the structures and pathways controlling the level of consciousness as the "consciousness system" (Figure 21.1).[3,4] More specifically, we focus on the phylogenetically older subcortical components of the brainstem, thalamus, hypothalamus, and basal forebrain (BF), which determine the *level of consciousness*, while leaving the specific functions of cortical structures for a separate discussion.

High levels of wakefulness correlate closely with certain neuronal firing patterns and electrographic signatures. This correlation is not perfect and may represent a continuum.[5] The cortical electroencephalogram (EEG) rhythms most commonly associated with wakefulness are known as "low-voltage high-frequency", "cortical activation", or "desynchronous cortical activity", and these represent rhythms above 4 Hz (Figure 21.2). This is opposed to "synchronous", slow (0.5–1 Hz), or delta (1–4 Hz) on EEG or Up and Down states on multiunit activity[7,8] seen in sleep,[9] coma,[10] anesthesia,[11] or even seizure components, during which consciousness is lost.[12–14] For the purposes of this discussion, we consider three cortical states: (1) non-REM (NREM) sleep, which is characterized by sleep spindles (7–15 Hz), delta waves (1–4 Hz), and slow oscillations (0.5–1.0 Hz); (2) REM sleep; and (3) wakefulness (Figure 21.2). Discussions of the detailed circuit and cellular basis of these rhythms are outside of the scope of this chapter.[15] The modulation of subcortical networks in controlling sleep states is discussed in Chapter 22, but it is important to establish these rhythms as epochs during which the activity levels of subcortical structures may play a role in the generation of cortical EEG.

The goal of this chapter is to discuss the contribution of subcortical structures to consciousness and wakeful cortical states, although the cortex may also contribute to arousal (e.g. NREM-active cortical neurons[16]). The regulation of these subcortical arousal systems as well as the regions controlling transitions in sleep and wake states are discussed in Chapter 22.

Broadly, there are at least seven modulatory neurotransmitters that are thought to contribute to arousal, including acetylcholine, norepinephrine (NE), histamine, serotonin, orexin, glutamate, and dopamine[3,9] (Figure 21.3). These neurotransmitters have overlapping functions,[18] making it difficult to declare the singular importance of one over another. New stimulation and suppression methods may help disentangle these overlaps,[19] while new methods of high-frequency neurotransmitter sampling may help to tighten the correlation between local electrophysiological recordings and neurotransmitter levels.[20,21]

Superb science from the last 100 years has clarified how these neurotransmitter systems interact. We discuss

Neuronal Networks in Brain Function, CNS Disorders, and Therapeutics
http://dx.doi.org/10.1016/B978-0-12-415804-7.00021-6

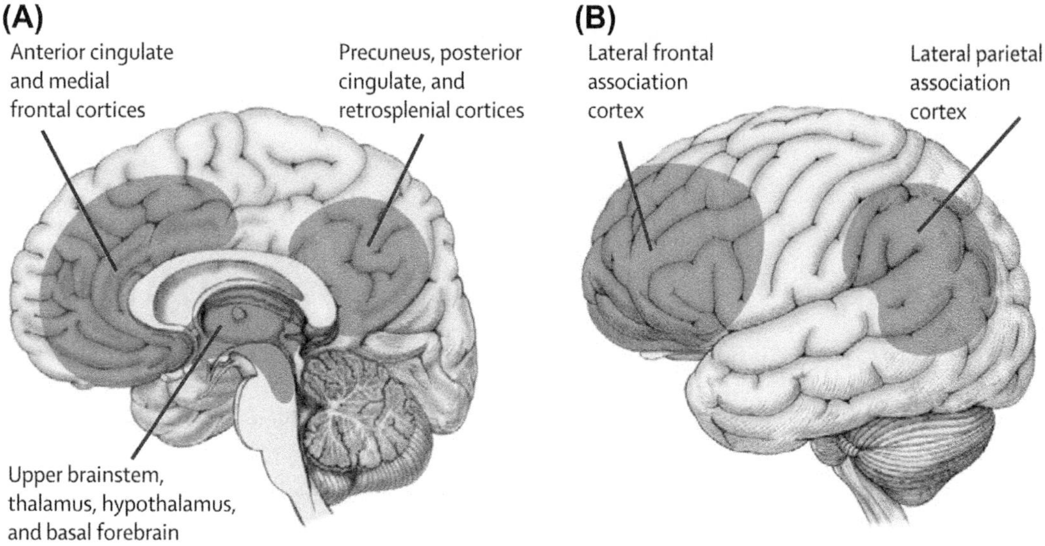

FIGURE 21.1 **The consciousness system.** (A) Medial view. (B) Lateral view. Cortical and subcortical components of the consciousness system responsible for controlling the overall *level* of consciousness. Additional specialized cortical-subcortical networks carry out specific functions comprising the *content* of consciousness (e.g. sensory processing, language, motor control, memory, emotions, etc.). (*Source: Reproduced with permission from Ref. 3.*) (For color version of this figure, the reader is referred to the online version of this book.)

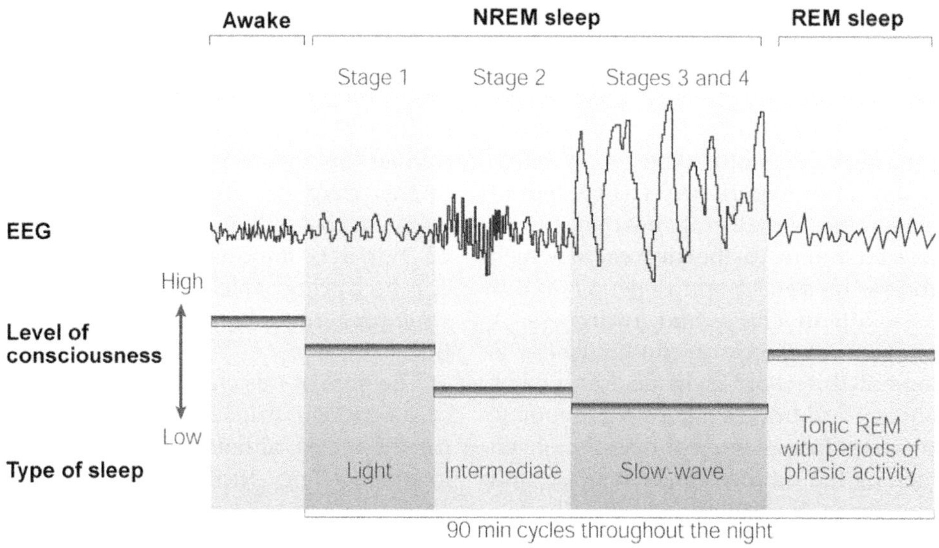

FIGURE 21.2 **Cortical EEG of human sleep stages.** Cortical EEG transitions from low-voltage, high-frequency activity during wakefulness to high-voltage, low-frequency activity during slow-wave non–rapid eye movement (NREM) sleep. Newer standards combine stage N4 into stage N3. The cortical EEG of REM sleep resembles wakefulness more than NREM sleep. (*Source: Reproduced with permission from Ref. 6.*) (For color version of this figure, the reader is referred to the online version of this book.)

the important arousal nuclei organized by their defining neurotransmitters. The focus is on the cell types contained within these sometimes heterogeneous networks, the structural connectivity through which the cortical effects can be understood, the firing patterns of these areas across behavioral states, and finally the direct effects of the arousal neurotransmitters on their targets. This chapter aims to summarize the subcortical structures that have the greatest effects on the level of consciousness.

ACETYLCHOLINE

Acetylcholine has long been implicated in the transition from cortical slow activity to cortical fast activity by both direct and indirect mechanisms.[22] Steriade described acetylcholine's role as twofold: (1) to abolish thalamocortical rhythms that mark NREM sleep, and (2) to convert cortical slow oscillations into cortical fast activity.[22] There is significant evidence that acetylcholine is important for these two functions, although some

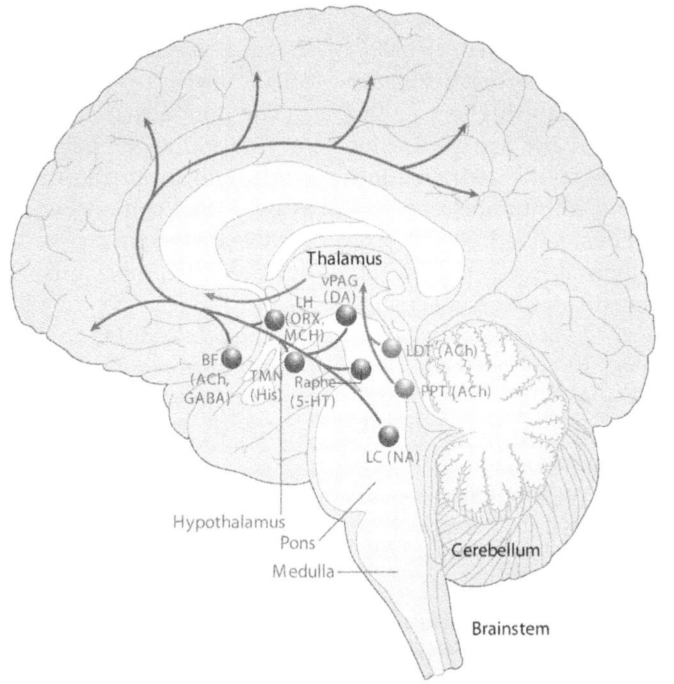

FIGURE 21.3 **Neurotransmitter systems modulating consciousness.** The anatomy of subcortical structures influencing thalamic (yellow) and cortical (red) arousal. Subcortical glutamatergic projections to the cortex, thalamus, and basal forebrain may also play an important role; they are not shown. 5-HT: serotonin neurons; ACh: cholinergic neurons; BF: basal forebrain; DA: dopamine; GABA: γ-aminobutyric acid; His: histamine; LDT: laterodorsal tegmental nucleus; LC: locus coeruleus; LH: lateral hypothalamus; MCH: melanin-concentrating hormone neurons; NA: noradrenergic neurons; ORX: orexin neurons; PPT: pedunculopontine tegmental nucleus; TMN: tuberomamillary nucleus. (*Source: Reproduced with permission from Ref. 17.*) (For interpretation of the references to color in this figure legend, the reader is referred to the online version of this book.)

evidence exists to the contrary. The major source of acetylcholine to the cortex originates from the nucleus basalis of Meynert (NBM) and surrounding areas, whereas the major cholinergic input to the thalamus is from the brainstem. Both have been implicated in arousal, and their effect is likely additive.[23] Each area is discussed separately throughout the rest of this section.

BF Anatomy (Chapter 4) and Connections

There are multiple cholinergic nuclei,[24–27] but three areas are particularly important in any discussion of arousal. Chapter 4, which contains the NBM and substantia innominata (SI) with extensions into the globus pallidus and preoptic magnocellular nucleus, provides the majority of the cholinergic input directly to the neocortex[28,29] (Figure 21.3). The cholinergic BF contains cholinergic neurons, glutamatergic neurons, as well as parvalbumin- and neuropeptide Y–containing gamma-aminobutyric acid (GABA) neurons, among other cell types.[30,31]

The BF provides the major cholinergic input to the neocortex[28,29] but also innervates some nuclei in the thalamus (in cat, monkey, and human), including the reticular thalamic nucleus, mediodorsal nucleus, anteroventral and anteromedial nuclei, and ventromedial nucleus.[32–34] The GABAergic neurons of the BF have both ascending and descending connections, allowing them to play important modulatory roles.[35–38] Efferent connections also extend to the amygdala.[39,40] The hippocampus, however, receives cholinergic inputs mainly from the medial septum (MS) and nucleus of the diagonal band (Chapters 1–3).[28]

Afferent connections to Chapter 4 include noncholinergic input from the cholinergic brainstem nuclei.[41–43] Inputs also arise from numerous other brainstem arousal nuclei, including the ventral tegmental area (VTA) and substantia nigra (SN), dorsal raphe nucleus (DRN), and locus coeruleus (LC).[42] Inputs also exist from the hypothalamus[44] and specifically the tuberomamillary nucleus (TMN).[45] The glutamatergic neurons of the parabrachial nucleus have been implicated in activation of the cholinergic BF.[46,47] GABAergic input arises from the amygdala.[48,49]

The Role of Basal Forebrain Cholinergic Projections in Arousal

The cholinergic system appears best correlated with the desynchronous EEG, because its neuronal firing patterns are increased during both wakefulness and REM; these neurons are mostly silent during NREM.[50] The majority of cholinergic input to the cortex originates in the BF,[29] and acetylcholine levels are highest in the cortex during wakefulness and REM and lowest during NREM.[51] Juxtacellular recordings allow extracellular unit activity to be recorded from immunohistochemically identified cells.[52] Under anesthetized conditions, cholinergic neurons increase their firing rates during desynchronous activity induced by somatosensory stimulation.[53,54]

When including all subtypes, BF neurons demonstrate a complex firing pattern across the sleep–wake cycle, with some neurons appearing to promote desynchronous activity and others promoting synchronous cortical oscillations.[50] GABAergic neurons in the BF have heterogeneous firing patterns with respect to cortical activation and sleep–wake cycles.[55–57] Parvalbumin-containing neurons are associated with cortical desynchrony, while neuropeptide Y–containing cells have the opposite correlation.[30,53] Anatomical evidence suggests that GABAergic neurons might promote arousal by projecting to cortical inhibitory interneurons.[38]

If cholinergic (and possibly noncholinergic) neurons in BF promote arousal, then stimulation should induce arousal and reduce sleep. Stimulation of the NBM leads to a cholinergic-mediated increase in desynchronous activity and a decrease in synchronous activity.[58–60] BF stimulation can also induce inhibition, suggesting that noncholinergic neurons may play a variable role in arousal, and the effects varied in different cortical regions, depending on the area of stimulation.[60] Optogenetics has allowed more selective stimulation of individual populations within heterogeneous nuclei. Stimulation of cholinergic terminals at the neocortex leads to cortical desynchrony.[61]

If the NBM is central to arousal, then lesions of the NBM should promote sleep and reduce wakefulness. Lesion of the NBM leads to an increase in cortical delta activity not seen with thalamic lesions,[46,62] although saporin-induced lesion of BF did not dramatically change the sleep–wake cycle.[63,64] Whether the NBM is necessary and/or sufficient for cortical desynchrony was questioned in one study that induced cortical desynchrony with pedunculopontine tegmental nucleus (PPT) stimulation while blocking the increase in cortical acetylcholine.[65]

Because the cholinergic BF is the primary source of cortical acetylcholine, local application of cortical cholinergic agonists and antagonists might reflect the actions of cholinergic BF neuronal activity. Local pharmacological application of cholinergic agonists abolishes slow activity and increases fast activity, while cholinergic antagonists have the opposite effect.[66] Systemic injection of cholinergic antagonists increases cortical delta activity.[62] In vitro, acetylcholine increased spiking in neocortical cells.[18]

The notion that cortical acetylcholine is either necessary or sufficient for arousal has been questioned by work with local pharmacological antagonists[67] as well as by a dissociation between cortical acetylcholine and cortical desynchrony.[65,68] Acetylcholine may have negative feedback mechanisms, because it has a hyperpolarizing effect on cholinergic BF and brainstem neurons.[69] Regulation of BF neurons may come from multiple sources, including parabrachial neurons, which also fire preferentially during wakefulness and REM, similar to cholinergic neurons.[70]

Cholinergic Brainstem Anatomy (Chapters 5 and 6) and Connections

Chapter 5, which contains the PPT, and Chapter 6, which contains the laterodorsal tegmental nucleus (LDT), provide the major cholinergic input to the thalamus (reviewed in this section). The PPT is one of the two main brainstem cholinergic nuclei[24] (Figure 21.3). It is composed of cholinergic, GABAergic, and glutamatergic neurons, and coexpression is rare.[71] Further subdivisions based on calcium-binding proteins are being developed.[72] The PPT stretches from the caudal midbrain to the rostral pons.[73,74] The rostral border of PPT is the caudal part of the SN *pars* reticulata, and it extends dorsocaudally toward the superior cerebellar peduncle.[73]

The PPT contains a rostral-caudal gradient of increasing cholinergic and decreasing GABAergic neurons.[71] Overall, 20–30% of neurons are cholinergic.[71] Rostral PPT, with its sparse cholinergic population, is referred to as *pars dissipata*, while the more densely cholinergic caudal region is known as *pars compacta*.[74,75] Cholinergic (choline acetyltransferase positive, or ChAT-positive) neurons have been consistently reported to be larger than ChAT-negative neurons.[74–77] ChAT-positive cells include polygonal, fusiform, and oval morphologies.[74,75]

Cholinergic LDT (Chapter 6) neurons are contained within the periventricular gray.[24] Cholinergic neurons are again intermixed with small noncholinergic neurons.[24] The other neurons in the LDT are mainly GABAergic and glutamatergic.[71]

Efferent connections from the PPT and LDT provide large cholinergic inputs into the thalamus, the brainstem, forebrain structures, and limited areas of the cortex.[32,43,78–82] Cholinergic PPT neurons have both ascending and descending projections as well as extensive local connectivity.[77] The putative arousal effects of the PPT and LDT are thought to rely upon both the cholinergic projections to the thalamus and the noncholinergic projections to Chapter 4.[65,68,83] There are important connections with the SN and basal ganglia.[77,84,85] There are some differences between the efferent connections of the PPT and LDT.[81,86]

Afferent connections to the PPT and LDT include ascending input from the spinal cord and cranial nerves, which is reviewed in Ref. 15. Projections from the thalamus arise from intralaminar, reticular, and zona incerta nuclei.[87,88] Hypothalamic input,[88] especially from the posterior hypothalamus,[89] and preoptic input are also seen.[90] Some input arises from the suprachiasmic nucleus.[91] Inputs to the LDT come from the midbrain reticular formation, medial preoptic area, anterior hypothalamus, lateral hypothalamus (LH), nucleus of the diagonal band, and medial prefrontal cortex, among others.[81] BF neurons innervate PPT as well, although these neurons are not primarily cholinergic.[33,92] Brainstem cholinergic nuclei have reciprocal connections with the amygdala.[93] Some neocortical input also exists.[94] An important inhibitory input arises from the SN, although this input may preferentially target noncholinergic cells.[95,96]

The Role of the PPT, the LDT, and Brainstem Cholinergic Projections in Arousal

The main role proposed for brainstem cholinergic neurons is to convert thalamic neurons from the firing patterns seen in NREM sleep to the firing patterns observed in wakefulness and REM[22] (Figure 21.4). Like the cholinergic BF neurons discussed here, brainstem cholinergic neurons fire most during wakefulness and REM while decreasing during NREM sleep, although some neurons fire specifically during REM and not wakefulness.[97,98] There is evidence that LDT and PPT neurons behave similarly across the sleep–wake cycle.[98] Increased firing rates in these structures are associated with increased excitability in the thalamus[98] and a change in thalamic firing patterns[99–101] (Figure 21.4).

Decreases in firing in the PPT and LDT precede cortical synchrony, and increases in firing precede cortical desynchrony.[98] PPT and LDT burst firing is very uncommon.[98] Under urethane anesthesia, PPT and LDT cholinergic neuronal firing is positively correlated with tail-pinch-induced desynchronous activity,

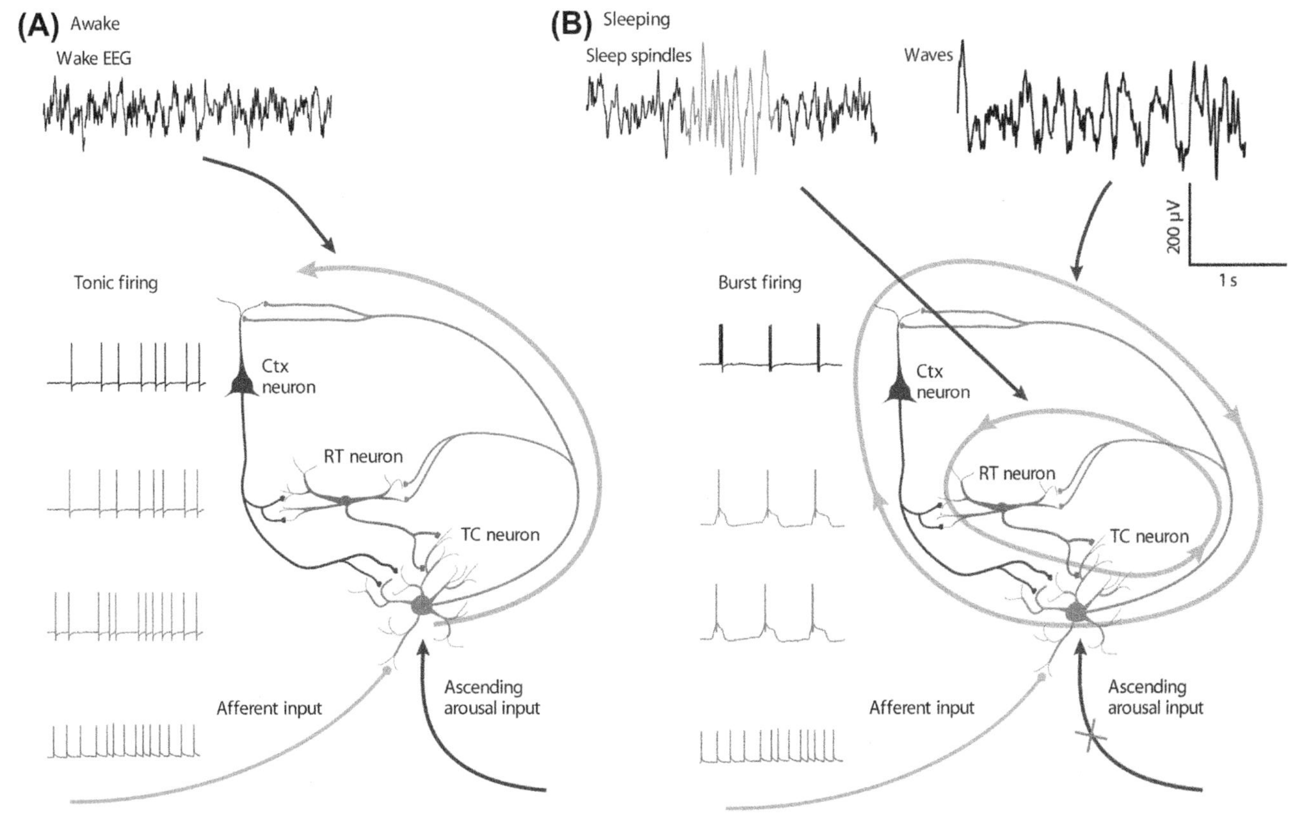

FIGURE 21.4 **Neuromodulators alter thalamic firing.** (A) During wakefulness, excitatory ascending input to the thalamus depolarizes thalamic intralaminar and relay neurons. This allows a tonic firing mode and faithful transmission of afferent sensory input. (B) During sleep, the thalamus is hyperpolarized due to withdrawal of excitatory ascending input. As a result, the tonic fires in bursts and does not relay afferent sensory input. *(Source: Reproduced with permission from Ref. 11.)* (The figure is reproduced in color section.)

whereas noncholinergic cells were both negatively and positively correlated.[76] PPT cholinergic neurons increase their firing rate when the cortex spontaneously transitions to a desynchronous state from synchronous activity as well as when the transition is due to sensory stimulation.[77] There is also evidence that cholinergic brainstem firing is related to the gamma oscillations found in cortical "Up" states.[77] Finally, the majority of cholinergic input into the thalamus originates from the brainstem, and thalamic extracellular acetylcholine levels are high during wakefulness and REM and lower during NREM.[102]

REM sleep provides an interesting separation of behavior and electrophysiology because the cortical EEG resembles the EEG of wakefulness. Some PPT and LDT neurons fire maximally during REM.[98,103] Lesions that induce destruction of brainstem cholinergic neurons lead to a large decrease in REM sleep.[104] Infusion of cholinergic agonists into the cholinergic brainstem nuclei initiates REM in animal models.[105]

Stimulation of the PPT and LDT dates back to classic experiments by Moruzzi and Magoun (Figure 21.5).[106] Multiple investigators have stimulated PPT in order to induce cortical desynchrony.[66,83,107] Because PPT projects to the cortex in only a limited manner, its arousal-promoting effects are thought to be mediated by both cholinergic projections to the thalamus and noncholinergic projections to the NBM.[22,83] Some investigators report that an NBM lesion does not change the stimulating effects of PPT,[83] while other investigators report that pharmacological inactivation of the NBM prior to PPT stimulation prevents acetylcholine release as well as cortical desynchrony.[68] The same group reported that glutamate receptor antagonists in the NBM prevented acetylcholine release in the cortex, but did not prevent cortical desynchrony.[65] This suggests that PPT may be able to induce desynchrony through either of its parallel ascending projections to the thalamus or cholinergic BF. PPT lesions disrupt sleep architecture, although they do not cause a coma-like appearance,[104,108,109] which is likely due to the parallel and overlapping arousal systems discussed throughout this chapter.

Local PPT application of cholinergic agonists suppresses firing in some, but not all, neurons.[110] However, the addition of cholinergic agonists induced increased cortical gamma activity at low concentrations, and at high concentrations it increased cortical gamma and decreased delta activity,[77] which is the same pattern that is induced by PPT stimulation (discussed in this section). Local application of monoamines in the PPT has mixed effects.[111] Local injection of histamine induced cortical desynchrony.[112] Cholinergic agonists can be used to stimulate the LC (discussed in this chapter), another arousal-promoting nucleus.[113]

NOREPINEPHRINE

NE plays a central role in arousal.[114,115] Like acetylcholine, it is proposed to have effects at both the cortical and subcortical levels.

Locus Coeruleus Anatomy and Connections

The arousal-promoting effects of NE-containing neurons are usually attributed to the LC, located in the pons and medulla close to the fourth ventricle[116,117] (Figure 21.3).

Projections from the LC reach numerous cortical and subcortical areas, including the thalamus, hypothalamus, and neocortex.[117–119] The efferent topography of LC neurons is reviewed in Ref. 120. As opposed to cholinergic innervation (discussed in this chapter), the noradrenergic innervation of the thalamus varies by nucleus and species.[121] In addition to the thalamic and cortical projections, potential arousal-promoting targets include the MS, medial preoptic nucleus, and cholinergic BF.[122] There are a small number of efferent connections from the LC to orexin neurons in the LH.[123]

Afferent connections to the LC arise from the nucleus paragigantocellularis, nucleus prepositus hypoglossus,

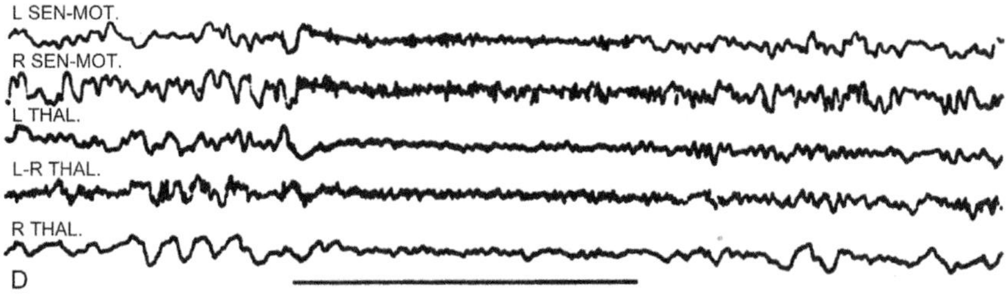

FIGURE 21.5 **Brainstem stimulation induces cortical activation.** Classic experiment from Moruzzi and Magoun showing stimulation of the left reticular formation in an anesthetized cat leading to low-voltage fast activity in the bilateral cortex and thalamus. Horizontal bar at the bottom indicates the time of stimulation. (*Source: Reproduced with permission from Ref. 106.*)

dorsal raphe (DR), LH, and prefrontal cortex, among other regions.[120,124–127]

The Role of the Locus Coeruleus and NE in Arousal

LC cells fire most during arousal, less during NREM, and least during REM.[66,128–130] Cortical levels of NE are related to LC firing.[113] During wakefulness, LC firing increases with periods of wakeful desynchronous EEG,[131] although NE levels and cortical activation are not perfectly correlated.[113] NE neurons in LC fire in relation to specific sensory stimuli.[131–135] Therefore, NE may enhance processing of external stimuli[136] or possibly arousal related to noxious stimuli.[135] There is evidence that NE can depolarize thalamic neurons leading to a transition to tonic firing from burst firing[137–139] (Figure 21.4). The LC has been implicated in circadian rhythms as well[140] (see Chapter 14).

Bilateral inactivation of the LC in halothane-anesthetized rats leads to an increase in low-frequency EEG power.[141] Saporin-induced lesions of the LC do not have dramatic effects on the sleep–wake cycle.[63,142] Removing cortical innervation by NE-containing neurons reduces wakefulness-dependent gene expression.[143] Mice lacking NE neurons demonstrated decreased sleep latency following stress.[144]

Electrical stimulation of LC converts cortical slow activity to fast, although it requires a higher intensity stimulus than that needed for PPT stimulation.[83] Optogenetic manipulation of the LC is difficult to interpret.[145] Photoinhibition of the LC appears to decrease wakefulness over the course of its 1 h suppression. Photostimulation decreases low-frequency power. These effects are significant but not dramatic. Interestingly, high-frequency stimulation actually leads to decreased cortical NE and behavioral arrest.[145]

Pharmacological activation of the LC using cholinergic agonists could also induce high-frequency, low-voltage EEG, although this effect may be delayed by as much as 30 s.[146] Cortical application of NE antagonists blocked "Up" states.[67] Application of NE receptor agonists in the MS and medial preoptic area, but not SI, increased arousal.[147,148] However, the arousal-promoting effects of NE may act through the cholinergic BF, where in vivo application of NE induced wakefulness,[149,150] or through the thalamus, where NE exerts a depolarizing effect on these neurons.[137] Systemic pharmacological manipulation of NE receptors may increase or decrease arousal depending on the receptor type.[151–153] Local injection of clonidine, an α-2 adrenergic agonist, directly into the LC suppresses arousal, while control injections of equal drug concentrations into other arousal regions do not.[152] A proposed mechanism of the anesthetic agent dexmedetomidine, a selective α-2-adrenergic agonist, is hyperpolarization at LC neurons.[154,155] In vitro, NE increased spiking in neocortical cells.[18]

HISTAMINE

The arousal-promoting effects of histamine[156,157] are well known to anyone who has ever taken a medication that contains a first-generation H_1 histamine antagonist.[158] The response to histamine is receptor dependent (H_1-receptor agonists induce sleep, as discussed in this section).

Histamine Anatomy and Connections

Most of the histaminergic neurons responsible for arousal are contained in the tuberomamillary area (Figure 21.3) located in the posterior hypothalamus.[159]

Histamine fibers project throughout the brain, including the cortex and brainstem.[160,161] Ascending projection targets include the hypothalamus, diagonal band, septum, thalamus, hippocampus, amygdala, and forebrain structures, among many others, while the descending pathway innervates the brainstem, including the brainstem cholinergic nuclei, LC, SN, and VTA as well as the spinal cord.[112,156]

Input to the TMN arises from the infralimbic division of the prefrontal cortex, lateral septum, and preoptic region.[162–165] The TMN is innervated by GABAergic and galaninergic neurons from the ventrolateral preoptic nucleus (VLPO)[166,167] as well as orexinergic neurons from the LH.[168,169] Afferent connections from the brainstem are widespread and include serotonergic, noradrenergic, and possibly cholinergic inputs among others.[163,170]

The Role of the TMN and Histamine in Arousal

Histamine release is circadian,[171] although there are shorter fluctuations as well.[172] Firing patterns in identified histamine neurons are active in arousal and suppressed in NREM and REM sleep[173,174] although there are reports of some putatively histaminergic neurons with increased firing during REM.[175]

The firing of histaminergic neurons has also been implicated in feeding-related motivational behavior.[176] Histamine may exert its arousal-promoting effects via actions on other hypothalamic nuclei.[156] Other possibilities include potentiating cholinergic mechanisms via the BF.[177,178] Histamine is capable of converting thalamus to tonic firing mode in an overlapping fashion with NE[139] (Figure 21.4), and stimulating the TMN induces an increase in processing of visual information.[179]

Inactivating histaminergic signaling has often yielded conflicting results. Injection of the $GABA_A$ agonist, muscimol, into the posterior hypothalamus induces hypersomnia,[180] while saporin-induced lesion of histaminergic neurons did not change daily levels of wakefulness.[63,181] H_1-receptor knockout mice have normal amounts of sleep and wakefulness but demonstrate fewer episodes of brief awakenings, longer episodes of NREM sleep, and fewer transitions between NREM and wakefulness. These mice also lack the normal wakeful response to H_3R-antagonists.[182] This evidence indicates that histamine has a role in initiating wakeful states via its H_1-receptor. Histidine decarboxylase knockout mice, which do not produce histamine, demonstrate increased REM, decreased NREM, decreased sleep latencies, decreased wakefulness in states requiring high vigilance, and decreased responsiveness to motor challenge.[183,184]

Pharmacological manipulation of histamine and its receptors generally increases arousal. H_1-receptor agonists increased wakefulness and decreased NREM and REM, while H_1-receptor antagonists had the opposite effect on wakefulness and NREM.[185] A histamine H_1-inhibitor increased NREM sleep and decreased wakefulness.[186] The same study found that administration of histamine and inhibition of histamine catabolism increased wakefulness and decreased NREM and REM.[186] Removing histaminergic input into the preoptic hypothalamus induced increases in REM and NREM and decreases in wakefulness,[187] although removing neocortical or hippocampal innervation does not have an effect.[188] Histamine depletion induces increased NREM and REM sleep,[189] and it may do so specifically during the dark phase of the circadian rhythm in rats.[190] Histamine is implicated in shifting circadian rhythms,[191] and it may have a direct effect on the suprachiasmatic nucleus.[192] Cortical desynchrony induced by brainstem stimulation was blocked by H_1-receptor antagonism.[193]

Histamine may act through subcortical arousal nuclei as well as directly at the cortex. Direct infusion of histamine into the preoptic hypothalamus induces wakefulness.[187] Infusion of histamine or an H_1-receptor agonist into brainstem cholinergic nuclei suppressed cortical slow activity and induced wakeful neocortical EEG.[112,194] Histamine depolarizes BF cholinergic neurons and induces cortical activation.[45,177] Histamine appears to suppress DR serotonin neurons[195,196] but excites NE neurons.[197] Direct application of histamine to the cortex induces suppression of delta power under urethane anesthesia.[178] In vitro, histamine increased spiking in neocortical cells.[18]

While H_1-receptors increase wakefulness, H_3-receptor agonists decrease wakefulness,[198] and H_3-receptor antagonists increase wakefulness likely due to the fact that H_3-receptors decrease histamine release.[182,198,199]

SEROTONIN

Serotonin has both sleep-promoting and arousal-promoting functions.[18,200,201] The serotonergic system is well situated with respect to other arousal systems to play a central role in maintaining consciousness.[202]

Serotonin Anatomy and Connections

The primary nuclei of serotonergic neurons associated with arousal are the raphe dorsalis and raphe medianus[203,204] (Figure 21.3). There is an incredible diversity of serotonin receptors,[205] making it difficult to declare a global statement regarding a singular role for serotonin.[206,207] The DRN also contains GABAergic neurons[208] and dopaminergic neurons.[209]

Arousal-promoting regions innervated by the DR include the VTA, periventricular gray matter, diagonal band of broca, intralaminar thalamus, amygdala, SI, PPT, and widespread cortical regions, among others.[210–213]

Inputs to the raphe nuclei arise from the SN, lateral habenula,[214] TMN,[159,215] orexinergic,[216] noradrenergic,[215,217,218] glutamatergic,[219] and cholinergic systems.[220,221]

The Role of the Raphe Nuclei and Serotonin in Arousal

Firing rates in the DR increase during wakefulness, decrease during NREM, and decrease more so during REM,[222–225] which reflects extracellular serotonin levels,[226] although there may exist subpopulations that behave differently.[227] "Typical" DR neurons fire slowly (1–6 Hz) and regularly.[204] These neurons have a long action potential duration, cease firing during REM, and are inhibited by $5\text{-}HT_{1A}$ agonists.[204,228] "Atypical" neurons exist as well,[229–231] including fast-firing cells in the DR, which were characterized with extracellular recordings.[232] Initially, three types of neurons were defined in the DR,[233] but this number has grown and has been reviewed.[234]

Serotonin contributes not only to arousal but also to thermoregulation, mood, and sexual function, among other roles. Serotonin knockout mice are not aroused when subjected to hypercapnia, suggesting that serotonin neurons promote arousal via chemosensitivity.[235] Some studies report limited response of serotonergic neurons to increased ambient temperature or pyrogen-induced fever,[236] which is supported by microdialysis measurements.[237] Serotonin knockout mice demonstrate increased wakefulness and decreased sleep at cool temperatures during the lights-off period as measured by 24 h sleep–wake recordings. This is due to increased movement as a compensatory response to the loss of other heat-generating activities at low temperatures.[235] Suppression of serotonin synthesis via intraperitoneal injection of *para*-chlorophenylalanine induces total insomnia, while microinjection of the serotonin precursor L-5-hydroxytryptophan into the anterior hypothalamus induces both NREM and REM sleep.[238]

Some authors have suggested that suppression of serotonergic DR neurons may play a role in REM genesis by disinhibiting brainstem REM-on neurons. The evidence is reviewed in Refs 15,234. However, the evidence that inhibiting DR neurons increases REM is mixed.[228,239] Application of serotonin has little effect on cholinergic brainstem neurons, which have a putatively causative role in REM sleep.[111,240] Arguing that serotonergic neurons inhibit REM but promote desynchronous EEG during wakefulness may be paradoxical because the cortical EEG of wakefulness and REM is similar. Therefore, the neuromodulator effect of serotonin on the cortical EEG appears to be "wake promoting" by producing cortical EEG desynchrony, yet "sleep promoting" by inhibiting brainstem cholinergic neurons, which are traditionally thought to produce wakeful cortical EEG,[69,241] although this may be species dependent.[240] In addition, in vitro application of serotonin onto NBM cholinergic neurons leads to hyperpolarization, conversion from tonic firing to low-threshold bursting, and suppression of rebound bursts following a hyperpolarizing pulse.[242] Furthermore, direct in vivo application of serotonin to the cholinergic forebrain induced a decrease in high-frequency cortical EEG, although no effect on sleep–wake states was seen.[149]

In vitro application of serotonin onto orexinergic neurons causes hyperpolarization.[243] However, in vivo antagonism of 5-HT_{1A} causes decreased locomotion via an orexin-dependent mechanism, decreased Fos-immunoreactivity in orexin neurons, and decreased spiking in putative orexinergic neurons.[243,244]

Serotonin hyperpolarizes thalamocortical neurons, decreases their discharge frequency, decreases their response to electrically evoked activity, and inhibits their tonic firing mode[138,245] (Figure 21.4), supporting the possibility that it is sleep promoting in the thalamus.

Agonists for various serotonin receptors increase wakefulness,[246,247] while antagonists are potential sleep aids.[248] Antidepressants increasing extracellular serotonin levels may also affect the sleep cycle.[249]

OREXIN

Orexin (or hypocretin) is the newest addition to the field of arousal neurotransmitters.[17,250–252]

Orexin Anatomy and Connections

mRNA for prepro-orexin, the precursor protein for orexin-A and orexin-B, is localized to the perifornical, lateral, and posterior hypothalamus[168,251] (Figure 21.3). Many of these neurons coexpress dynorphin[253] or glutamate.[169]

Orexinergic neurons project extensively throughout the brain and to multiple arousal nuclei. Arousal-promoting structures include the DR, LC, TMN, brainstem cholinergic nuclei, BF, intralaminar thalamus, parabrachial area, amygdala, and cortex.[168,254]

Afferents to orexinergic nuclei originate in many arousal nuclei, including the LC, DR, and PB. Input to orexinergic nuclei also arises from the lateral septum, hypothalamus, and periaqueductal gray area; from limited neocortical areas and limited cholinergic forebrain areas; and sparsely throughout the brainstem.[123]

The Role of the Lateral Hypothalamus and Orexin in Arousal

Orexinergic neurons fire during exploratory behavior and gradually decrease their activity during quiet wakefulness and NREM and REM sleep,[255,256] although orexin levels measured in cholinergic BF are greater in REM than in NREM.[257] Orexin levels have both a circadian and noncircadian component related to wakefulness.[258–260] Intermingled GABA neurons are more correlated with sleep than wakefulness.[261]

Orexin application onto LC slices causes NE neurons to increase their firing rate,[126,262,263] although the arousal-promoting mechanism may also involve histamine.[264] The effect may be presynaptic or postsynaptic,[265] and orexin may work through cation channels.[263,266] Orexin injection into the ventricles induces wakefulness and reduces NREM and REM sleep.[262,267] Orexin receptor activation directly in the LC increased LC neuronal activity, suppressed REM, and increased wakefulness.[268] Orexinergic activation of the cholinergic BF also results in increased wakefulness.[267] This finding combined with the microdialysis data indicating increased orexin during REM and wakefulness,[257] which both exhibit desynchronous EEG patterns, suggest that orexin may contribute indirectly to the desynchronous cortical EEG via the NBM. Finally, orexin excites GABAergic neurons in the SN and VTA, while its effect on dopaminergic neurons is mixed.[269,270] Orexinergic neurons may be inhibited by adenosine.[271]

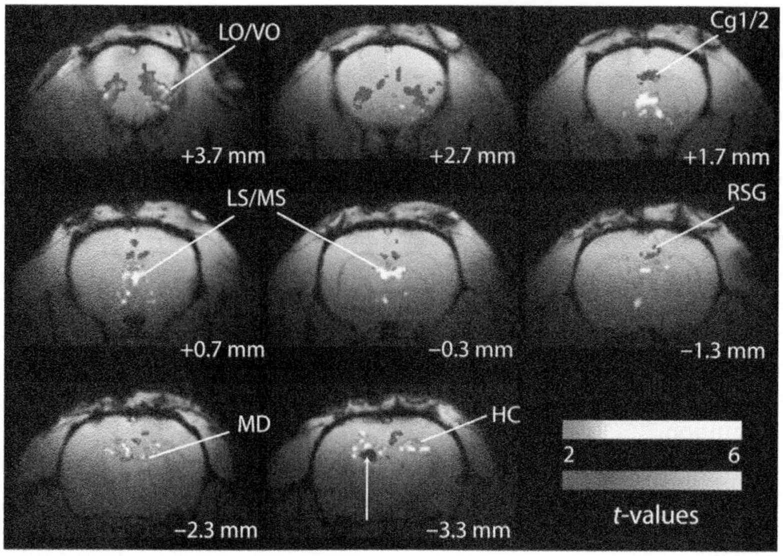

FIGURE 21.6 **Neuroimaging reveals consciousness networks.** Blood oxygen level dependent (BOLD) fMRI during a rodent model of complex partial seizures demonstrates coordinated cortical and subcortical changes. Seizures are induced by hippocampal stimulation (arrow indicates electrode), which leads to seizure activity (and an increased BOLD signal) in the hippocampus and septal nuclei, which causes slow oscillations (and a decreased BOLD signal) in the orbital frontal cortex. Limbic seizures of this kind are associated with behavioral arrest and decreased responsiveness in both animal models and human patients with temporal lobe epilepsy. Cg1/2: anterior cingulate cortex; HC: hippocampus; LO/VO: lateral and ventral orbital frontal cortex; LS/MS: lateral and medial septal nuclei; MD: mediodorsal thalamus; RSG: retrosplenial granular cortex. (*Source: Reproduced with permission from Ref. 345.*) (The figure is reproduced in color section.)

depolarize the relay nuclei of the thalamus, allowing faithful transmission of multiple sensory and other inputs to the cortex, which is a large component of the *content of consciousness*. Modulation of activity in the rostral thalamic intralaminar and paralaminar regions and direct modulation of cortical activity are crucial for cortical arousal, or a high *level of consciousness*. Because electrophysiology provides information from no more than a few areas at one time, it is not necessarily ideal for capturing large-scale networks. Neuroimaging has the power to visualize remote brain areas working in concert (see Figure 21.6). Imaging during changes in consciousness states, whether attention,[307] anesthesia,[346] or sleep,[347] reveals the coordination of cortical and subcortical changes. Although difficult, the imaging of central nervous system disorders involving changing consciousness states, such as epilepsy, provides unique insights into subcortical network changes[14,345,348–350] (Figure 21.6). The specific contribution of each individual neurotransmitter to specific cellular membrane potential changes or local field potentials is still being uncovered. Even more difficult, the unique role of each system in governing specific behaviors remains uncertain. Not all brainstem lesions prohibit cortical arousal,[351] although brainstem lesions often underlie coma in patients.[352] Finally, taking these findings from animal models and making conclusions regarding human behavior can be a difficult transition. Still, an understanding of the subcortical control of consciousness is vital for appreciating both normal arousal function and the complex sequelae of neurological disease.

LIST OF ABBREVIATIONS

BF Basal forebrain
ChAT Choline acetyltransferase
DRN Dorsal raphe nucleus
EEG Electroencephalogram
LC Locus coeruleus
LDT Laterodorsal tegmental nucleus
LH Lateral hypothalamus
MS Medial septum
NBM Nucleus basalis of Meynert
NE Norepinephrine
NREM Non–rapid eye movement sleep
PPT Pedunculopontine tegmental nucleus
SI Substantia innominata
SN Substantia nigra
TMN Tuberomamillary nucleus
VTA Ventral tegmental area

Acknowledgments

This work was supported by NIH 5F30NS071628-03 and MSTP TG T32GM07205 (JEM); and by NIH R01NS055829, R01NS066974, R01MH67528, R01HL059619, P30NS052519, and U01NS045911, a Donaghue Foundation Investigator Award, and the Betsy and Jonathan Blattmachr Family (HB).

References

1. Posner JB, Saper CB, Schiff ND, Plum F. *Plum and Posner's Diagnosis of Stupor and Coma*. 4th ed. USA: Oxford University Press; 2007.
2. Plum F, Posner JB. *Diagnosis of Stupor and Coma*. 3rd ed. Philadelphia, PA: FA Davis Company; 1980.
3. Blumenfeld H. *Neuroanatomy through Clinical Cases*. 2nd ed. Sunderland, MA: Sinauer Associates Publishing Company; 2010.
4. Blumenfeld H. Impaired consciousness in epilepsy. *Lancet Neurol*. 2012. In review.
5. Vyazovskiy VV, Olcese U, Hanlon EC, Nir Y, Cirelli C, Tononi G. Local sleep in awake rats. *Nature*. 2011;472(7344):443–447.
6. Bryant PA, Trinder J, Curtis N. Sick and tired: does sleep have a vital role in the immune system? *Nat Rev Immunol*. 2004;4(6):457–467.
7. Timofeev I, Grenier F, Bazhenov M, Sejnowski TJ, Steriade M. Origin of slow cortical oscillations in deafferented cortical slabs. *Cereb Cortex*. 2000;10(12):1185–1199.
8. Steriade M, Nuñez A, Amzica F. A novel slow (<1 Hz) oscillation of neocortical neurons in vivo: depolarizing and hyperpolarizing components. *J Neurosci*. 1993;13(8):3252–3265.
9. España RA, Scammell TE. Sleep neurobiology from a clinical perspective. *Sleep*. 2011;34(7):845–858.
10. Brown EN, Lydic R, Schiff ND. General anesthesia, sleep, and coma. *N Engl J Med*. 2010;363(27):2638–2650.
11. Franks NP. General anaesthesia: from molecular targets to neuronal pathways of sleep and arousal. *Nat Rev Neurosci*. 2008;9(5):370–386.
12. Norden AD, Blumenfeld H. The role of subcortical structures in human epilepsy. *Epilepsy Behav*. 2002;3(3):219–231.
13. Englot DJ, Yang L, Hamid H, et al. Impaired consciousness in temporal lobe seizures: role of cortical slow activity. *Brain*. 2010;133(12):3764–3777.
14. Englot DJ, Mishra AM, Mansuripur PK, Herman P, Hyder F, Blumenfeld H. Remote effects of focal hippocampal seizures on the rat neocortex. *J Neurosci*. 2008;28(36):9066–9081.
15. Steriade M, McCarley RW. *Brain Control of Wakefulness and Sleep*. 2nd ed. New York: Kluwer Academic/Plenum Publishers; 2005.
16. Gerashchenko D, Wisor JP, Burns D, et al. Identification of a population of sleep-active cerebral cortex neurons. *Proc Natl Acad Sci USA*. 2008;105(29):10227–10232.
17. Saper CB, Scammell TE, Lu J. Hypothalamic regulation of sleep and circadian rhythms. *Nature*. 2005;437(7063):1257–1263.
18. McCormick DA, Williamson A. Convergence and divergence of neurotransmitter action in human cerebral cortex. *Proc Natl Acad Sci USA*. 1989;86(20):8098–8102.
19. Boyden ES, Zhang F, Bamberg E, Nagel G, Deisseroth K. Millisecond-timescale, genetically targeted optical control of neural activity. *Nat Neurosci*. 2005;8(9):1263–1268.
20. Parikh V, Pomerieau F, Huettl P, Gerhardt GA, Sarter M, Bruno JP. Rapid assessment of in vivo cholinergic transmission by amperometric detection of changes in extracellular choline levels. *Eur J Neurosci*. 2004;20(6):1545–1554.
21. Parikh V, Man K, Decker MW, Sarter M. Glutamatergic contributions to nicotinic acetylcholine receptor agonist-evoked cholinergic transients in the prefrontal cortex. *J Neurosci*. 2008;28(14):3769–3780.
22. Steriade M. Acetylcholine systems and rhythmic activities during the waking-sleep cycle. *Prog Brain Res*. 2004;145:179–196.
23. Dringenberg HC, Olmstead MC. Integrated contributions of basal forebrain and thalamus to neocortical activation elicited by pedunculopontine tegmental stimulation in urethane-anesthetized rats. *Neuroscience*. 2003;119(3):839–853.
24. Mesulam MM, Mufson EJ, Wainer BH, Levey AI. Central cholinergic pathways in the rat: an overview based on an alternative nomenclature (Ch1–Ch6). *Neuroscience*. 1983;10(4):1185–1201.
25. Mufson EJ, Martin TL, Mash DC, Wainer BH, Mesulam MM. Cholinergic projections from the parabigeminal nucleus (Ch8) to the superior colliculus in the mouse: a combined analysis of horseradish peroxidase transport and choline acetyltransferase immunohistochemistry. *Brain Res*. 1986;370(1):144–148.
26. Vincent SR, Reiner PB. The immunohistochemical localization of choline acetyltransferase in the cat brain. *Brain Res Bull*. 1987;18(3):371–415.
27. Mesulam MM, Mufson EJ, Levey AI, Wainer BH. Atlas of cholinergic neurons in the forebrain and upper brainstem of the macaque based on monoclonal choline acetyltransferase immunohistochemistry and acetylcholinesterase histochemistry. *Neuroscience*. 1984;12(3):669–686.
28. Rye DB, Wainer BH, Mesulam MM, Mufson EJ, Saper CB. Cortical projections arising from the basal forebrain: a study of cholinergic and noncholinergic components employing combined retrograde tracing and immunohistochemical localization of choline acetyltransferase. *Neuroscience*. 1984;13(3):627–643.
29. Mesulam M, Mufson EJ, Levey AI, Wainer BH. Cholinergic innervation of cortex by the basal forebrain: cytochemistry and cortical connections of the septal area, diagonal band nuclei, nucleus basalis (substantia innominata), and hypothalamus in the rhesus monkey. *J Comp Neurol*. 1983;214(2):170–197.
30. Duque A, Tepper JM, Detari L, Ascoli GA, Zaborszky L. Morphological characterization of electrophysiologically and immunohistochemically identified basal forebrain cholinergic and neuropeptide Y-containing neurons. *Brain Struct Funct*. 2007;212(1):55–73.
31. Brashear HR, Zaborszky L, Heimer L. Distribution of GABAergic and cholinergic neurons in the rat diagonal band. *Neuroscience*. 1986;17(2):439–451.
32. Heckers S, Geula C, Mesulam MM. Cholinergic innervation of the human thalamus: dual origin and differential nuclear distribution. *J Comp Neurol*. 1992;325(1):68–82.
33. Parent A, Pare D, Smith Y, Steriade M. Basal forebrain cholinergic and noncholinergic projections to the thalamus and brainstem in cats and monkeys. *J Comp Neurol*. 1988;277(2):281–301.
34. Steriade M, Parent A, Pare D, Smith Y. Cholinergic and non-cholinergic neurons of cat basal forebrain project to reticular and mediodorsal thalamic nuclei. *Brain Res*. 1987; 408(1–2):372–376.
35. Gritti I, Mainville L, Mancia M, Jones BE. GABAergic and other noncholinergic basal forebrain neurons, together with cholinergic neurons, project to the mesocortex and isocortex in the rat. *J Comp Neurol*. 1997;383(2):163–177.
36. Gritti I, Mainville L, Jones BE. Projections of GABAergic and cholinergic basal forebrain and GABAergic preoptic-anterior hypothalamic neurons to the posterior lateral hypothalamus of the rat. *J Comp Neurol*. 1994;339(2):251–268.
37. Henny P, Jones BE. Projections from basal forebrain to prefrontal cortex comprise cholinergic, GABAergic and glutamatergic inputs to pyramidal cells or interneurons. *Eur J Neurosci*. 2008;27(3):654–670.
38. Freund TF, Meskenaite V. Gamma-aminobutyric acid-containing basal forebrain neurons innervate inhibitory interneurons in the neocortex. *Proc Natl Acad Sci USA*. 1992;89(2):738–742.
39. Kitt CA, Mitchell SJ, DeLong MR, Wainer BH, Price DL. Fiber pathways of basal forebrain cholinergic neurons in monkeys. *Brain Res*. 1987;406(1–2):192–206.
40. Russchen FT, Bakst I, Amaral DG, Price JL. The amygdalostriatal projections in the monkey. An anterograde tracing study. *Brain Res*. 1985;329(1–2):241–257.

41. Jones EG, Burton H, Saper CB, Swanson LW. Midbrain, diencephalic and cortical relationships of the basal nucleus of Meynert and associated structures in primates. *J Comp Neurol.* 1976;167(4):385–419.
42. Jones BE, Cuello AC. Afferents to the basal forebrain cholinergic cell area from pontomesencephalic–catecholamine, serotonin, and acetylcholine–neurons. *Neuroscience.* 1989;31(1):37–61.
43. Hallanger AE, Wainer BH. Ascending projections from the pedunculopontine tegmental nucleus and the adjacent mesopontine tegmentum in the rat. *J Comp Neurol.* 1988; 274(4):483–515.
44. Cullinan WE, Zaborszky L. Organization of ascending hypothalamic projections to the rostral forebrain with special reference to the innervation of cholinergic projection neurons. *J Comp Neurol.* 1991;306(4):631–667.
45. Khateb A, Fort P, Pegna A, Jones BE, Muhlethaler M. Cholinergic nucleus basalis neurons are excited by histamine in vitro. *Neuroscience.* 1995;69(2):495–506.
46. Fuller PM, Sherman D, Pedersen NP, Saper CB, Lu J. Reassessment of the structural basis of the ascending arousal system. *J Comp Neurol.* 2011;519(5):933–956.
47. Lu J, Sherman D, Devor M, Saper CB. A putative flip-flop switch for control of REM sleep. *Nature.* 2006;441(7093):589–594.
48. Zaborszky L, Heimer L, Eckenstein F, Leranth C. GABAergic input to cholinergic forebrain neurons: an ultrastructural study using retrograde tracing of HRP and double immunolabeling. *J Comp Neurol.* 1986;250(3):282–295.
49. Russchen FT, Amaral DG, Price JL. The afferent connections of the substantia innominata in the monkey, *Macaca fascicularis*. *J Comp Neurol.* 1985;242(1):1–27.
50. Lee MG, Manns ID, Alonso A, Jones BE. Sleep–wake related discharge properties of basal forebrain neurons recorded with micropipettes in head-fixed rats. *J Neurophysiol.* 2004; 92(2):1182–1198.
51. Marrosu F, Portas C, Mascia MS, et al. Microdialysis measurement of cortical and hippocampal acetylcholine release during sleep–wake cycle in freely moving cats. *Brain Res.* 1995;671(2):329–332.
52. Pinault D. A novel single-cell staining procedure performed in vivo under electrophysiological control: morpho-functional features of juxtacellularly labeled thalamic cells and other central neurons with biocytin or Neurobiotin. *J Neurosci Methods.* 1996;65(2):113–136.
53. Duque A, Balatoni B, Detari L, Zaborszky L. EEG correlation of the discharge properties of identified neurons in the basal forebrain. *J Neurophysiol.* 2000;84(3):1627–1635.
54. Manns ID, Alonso A, Jones BE. Discharge properties of juxtacellularly labeled and immunohistochemically identified cholinergic basal forebrain neurons recorded in association with the electroencephalogram in anesthetized rats. *J Neurosci.* 2000;20(4):1505–1518.
55. Manns ID, Alonso A, Jones BE. Discharge profiles of juxtacellularly labeled and immunohistochemically identified GABAergic basal forebrain neurons recorded in association with the electroencephalogram in anesthetized rats. *J Neurosci.* 2000;20(24):9252–9263.
56. Hassani OK, Lee MG, Henny P, Jones BE. Discharge profiles of identified GABAergic in comparison to cholinergic and putative glutamatergic basal forebrain neurons across the sleep–wake cycle. *J Neurosci.* 2009;29(38):11828–11840.
57. Jones BE. Activity, modulation and role of basal forebrain cholinergic neurons innervating the cerebral cortex. *Prog Brain Res.* 2004;145:157–169.
58. Metherate R, Cox CL, Ashe JH. Cellular bases of neocortical activation: modulation of neural oscillations by the nucleus basalis and endogenous acetylcholine. *J Neurosci.* 1992;12(12): 4701–4711.
59. Metherate R, Ashe JH. Basal forebrain stimulation modifies auditory cortex responsiveness by an action at muscarinic receptors. *Brain Res.* 1991;559(1):163–167.
60. Jiménez-Capdeville ME, Dykes RW, Myasnikov AA. Differential control of cortical activity by the basal forebrain in rats: a role for both cholinergic and inhibitory influences. *J Comp Neurol.* 1997; 381(1):53–67.
61. Kalmbach A, Hedrick T, Waters J. Selective optogenetic stimulation of cholinergic axons in neocortex. *J Neurophysiol.* Apr 2012;107(7):2008–2019.
62. Buzsaki G, Bickford RG, Ponomareff G, Thal LJ, Mandel R, Gage FH. Nucleus basalis and thalamic control of neocortical activity in the freely moving rat. *J Neurosci.* 1988;8(11):4007–4026.
63. Blanco-Centurion C, Gerashchenko D, Shiromani PJ. Effects of saporin-induced lesions of three arousal populations on daily levels of sleep and wake. *J Neurosci.* 2007;27(51):14041–14048.
64. Blanco-Centurion CA, Shiromani A, Winston E, Shiromani PJ. Effects of hypocretin-1 in 192-IgG-saporin-lesioned rats. *Eur J Neurosci.* 2006;24(7):2084–2088.
65. Rasmusson DD, Szerb IC, Jordan JL. Differential effects of alpha-amino-3-hydroxy-5-methyl-4-isoxazole propionic acid and *N*-methyl-D-aspartate receptor antagonists applied to the basal forebrain on cortical acetylcholine release and electroencephalogram desynchronization. *Neuroscience.* 1996;72(2):419–427.
66. Spehlmann R, Norcross K. Cholinergic mechanisms in the production of focal cortical slow waves. *Experientia.* 1982; 38(1):109–111.
67. Constantinople CM, Bruno Randy M. Effects and mechanisms of wakefulness on local cortical networks. *Neuron.* 2011;69(6): 1061–1068.
68. Rasmusson DD, Clow K, Szerb JC. Modification of neocortical acetylcholine release and electroencephalogram desynchronization due to brainstem stimulation by drugs applied to the basal forebrain. *Neuroscience.* 1994;60(3):665–677.
69. Leonard CS, Llinás R. Serotonergic and cholinergic inhibition of mesopontine cholinergic neurons controlling rem sleep: an in vitro electrophysiological study. *Neuroscience.* 1994;59(2):309–330.
70. Saito H, Sakai K, Jouvet M. Discharge patterns of the nucleus parabrachialis lateralis neurons of the cat during sleep and waking. *Brain Res.* 1977;134(1):59–72.
71. Wang H-L, Morales M. Pedunculopontine and laterodorsal tegmental nuclei contain distinct populations of cholinergic, glutamatergic and GABAergic neurons in the rat. *Eur J Neurosci.* 2009;29(2):340–358.
72. Martinez-Gonzalez C, Bolam JP, Mena-Segovia J. Topographical organization of the pedunculopontine nucleus. *Front Neuroanat.* 2012;5:22.
73. Mena-Segovia J, Micklem BR, Nair-Roberts RG, Ungless MA, Bolam JP. GABAergic neuron distribution in the pedunculopontine nucleus defines functional subterritories. *J Comp Neurol.* 2009;515(4):397–408.
74. Rye DB, Saper CB, Lee HJ, Wainer BH. Pedunculopontine tegmental nucleus of the rat: cytoarchitecture, cytochemistry, and some extrapyramidal connections of the mesopontine tegmentum. *J Comp Neurol.* 1987;259(4):483–528.
75. Honda T, Semba K. An ultrastructural study of cholinergic and non-cholinergic neurons in the laterodorsal and pedunculopontine tegmental nuclei in the rat. *Neuroscience.* 1995;68(3):837–853.
76. Boucetta S, Jones BE. Activity profiles of cholinergic and intermingled GABAergic and putative glutamatergic neurons in the pontomesencephalic tegmentum of urethane-anesthetized rats. *J Neurosci.* 2009;29(14):4664–4674.

77. Mena-Segovia J, Sims HM, Magill PJ, Bolam JP. Cholinergic brainstem neurons modulate cortical gamma activity during slow oscillations. *J Physiol.* 2008;586(12):2947–2960.
78. Hallanger AE, Levey AI, Lee HJ, Rye DB, Wainer BH. The origins of cholinergic and other subcortical afferents to the thalamus in the rat. *J Comp Neurol.* 1987;262(1):105–124.
79. Jones BE, Webster HH. Neurotoxic lesions of the dorsolateral pontomesencephalic tegmentum-cholinergic cell area in the cat. I. Effects upon the cholinergic innervation of the brain. *Brain Res.* 1988;451(1–2):13–32.
80. Beninato M, Spencer RF. A cholinergic projection to the rat substantia nigra from the pedunculopontine tegmental nucleus. *Brain Res.* 1987;412(1):169–174.
81. Satoh K, Fibiger HC. Cholinergic neurons of the laterodorsal tegmental nucleus: efferent and afferent connections. *J Comp Neurol.* 1986;253(3):277–302.
82. Cornwall J, Cooper JD, Phillipson OT. Afferent and efferent connections of the laterodorsal tegmental nucleus in the rat. *Brain Res Bull.* 1990;25(2):271–284.
83. Steriade M, Amzica F, Nuñez A. Cholinergic and noradrenergic modulation of the slow (approximately 0.3 Hz) oscillation in neocortical cells. *J Neurophysiol.* 1993;70(4):1385–1400.
84. Inglis WL, Winn P. The pedunculopontine tegmental nucleus: where the striatum meets the reticular formation. *Prog Neurobiol.* 1995;47(1):1–29.
85. Mena-Segovia J, Bolam JP, Magill PJ. Pedunculopontine nucleus and basal ganglia: distant relatives or part of the same family? *Trends Neurosci.* 2004;27(10):585–588.
86. Woolf NJ, Butcher LL. Cholinergic systems in the rat brain: III. Projections from the pontomesencephalic tegmentum to the thalamus, tectum, basal ganglia, and basal forebrain. *Brain Res Bull.* 1986;16(5):603–637.
87. Parent A, Steriade M. Afferents from the periaqueductal gray, medial hypothalamus and medial thalamus to the midbrain reticular core. *Brain Res Bull.* 1981;7(4):411–418.
88. Steriade M, Parent A, Ropert N, Kitsikis A. Zona incerta and lateral hypothalamic afferents to the midbrain reticular core of cat—HRP and electrophysiological study. *Brain Res.* 1982;238(1):13–28.
89. Pare D, Smith Y, Parent A, Steriade M. Neuronal activity of identified posterior hypothalamic neurons projecting to the brainstem peribrachial area of the cat. *Neurosci Lett.* 1989;107(1–3):145–150.
90. Swanson LW, Mogenson GJ, Simerly RB, Wu M. Anatomical and electrophysiological evidence for a projection from the medial preoptic area to the 'mesencephalic and subthalamic locomotor regions' in the rat. *Brain Res.* 1987;405(1):108–122.
91. Kucera P, Favrod P. Suprachiasmatic nucleus projection to mesencephalic central grey in the woodmouse (*Apodemus sylvaticus* L.). *Neuroscience.* 1979;4(11):1705–1716.
92. Swanson LW, Mogenson GJ, Gerfen CR, Robinson P. Evidence for a projection from the lateral preoptic area and substantia innominata to the 'mesencephalic locomotor region' in the rat. *Brain Res.* 1984;295(1):161–178.
93. Takeuchi Y, McLean JH, Hopkins DA. Reciprocal connections between the amygdala and parabrachial nuclei: ultrastructural demonstration by degeneration and axonal transport of horseradish peroxidase in the cat. *Brain Res.* 1982;239(2):583–588.
94. Catsman-Berrevoets CE, Kuypers HG. A search for corticospinal collaterals to thalamus and mesencephalon by means of multiple retrograde fluorescent tracers in cat and rat. *Brain Res.* 1981;218(1–2):15–33.
95. Grofova I, Zhou M. Nigral innervation of cholinergic and glutamatergic cells in the rat mesopontine tegmentum: light and electron microscopic anterograde tracing and immunohistochemical studies. *J Comp Neurol.* 1998;395(3):359–379.
96. Scarnati E, Proia A, Di Loreto S, Pacitti C. The reciprocal electrophysiological influence between the nucleus tegmenti pedunculopontinus and the substantia nigra in normal and decorticated rats. *Brain Res.* 1987;423(1–2):116–124.
97. el Mansari M, Sakai K, Jouvet M. Unitary characteristics of presumptive cholinergic tegmental neurons during the sleep-waking cycle in freely moving cats. *Exp Brain Res.* 1989;76(3):519–529.
98. Steriade M, Datta S, Pare D, Oakson G, Curró Dossi RC. Neuronal activities in brain-stem cholinergic nuclei related to tonic activation processes in thalamocortical systems. *J Neurosci.* 1990;10(8):2541–2559.
99. Steriade M. The corticothalamic system in sleep. *Front Biosci.* 2003;8(1–3).
100. McCormick DA, Prince DA. Actions of acetylcholine in the guinea-pig and cat medial and lateral geniculate nuclei, in vitro. *J Physiol.* 1987;392:147–165.
101. Curro Dossi R, Pare D, Steriade M. Short-lasting nicotinic and long-lasting muscarinic depolarizing responses of thalamocortical neurons to stimulation of mesopontine cholinergic nuclei. *J Neurophysiol.* 1991;65(3):393–406.
102. Williams JA, Comisarow J, Day J, Fibiger HC, Reiner PB. State-dependent release of acetylcholine in rat thalamus measured by in vivo microdialysis. *J Neurosci.* 1994;14(9):5236–5242.
103. Kayama Y, Ohta M, Jodo E. Firing of 'possibly' cholinergic neurons in the rat laterodorsal tegmental nucleus during sleep and wakefulness. *Brain Res.* 1992;569(2):210–220.
104. Webster HH, Jones BE. Neurotoxic lesions of the dorsolateral pontomesencephalic tegmentum-cholinergic cell area in the cat. II. Effects upon sleep-waking states. *Brain Res.* 1988;458(2):285–302.
105. Velazquez-Moctezuma J, Gillin JC, Shiromani PJ. Effect of specific M1, M2 muscarinic receptor agonists on REM sleep generation. *Brain Res.* 1989;503(1):128–131.
106. Moruzzi G, Magoun H. Brain stem reticular formation and activation of the EEG. *Electroencephalogr Clin Neurophysiol.* 1949;1(4):455–473.
107. Munk MH, Roelfsema PR, Konig P, Engel AK, Singer W. Role of reticular activation in the modulation of intracortical synchronization. *Science.* 1996;272(5259):271–274.
108. Hernandez-Chan NG, Gongora-Alfaro JL, Alvarez-Cervera FJ, Solis-Rodriguez FA, Heredia-Lopez FJ, Arankowsky-Sandoval G. Quinolinic acid lesions of the pedunculopontine nucleus impair sleep architecture, but not locomotion, exploration, emotionality or working memory in the rat. *Behav Brain Res.* 2011;225(2):482–490.
109. Shouse MN, Siegel JM. Pontine regulation of REM sleep components in cats: integrity of the pedunculopontine tegmentum (PPT) is important for phasic events but unnecessary for atonia during REM sleep. *Brain Res.* 1992;571(1):50–63.
110. el Mansari M, Sakai K, Jouvet M. Responses of presumed cholinergic mesopontine tegmental neurons to carbachol microinjections in freely moving cats. *Exp Brain Res.* 1990;83(1):115–123.
111. Crochet S, Sakai K. Effects of microdialysis application of monoamines on the EEG and behavioural states in the cat mesopontine tegmentum. *Eur J Neurosci.* 1999;11(10):3738–3752.
112. Lin JS, Hou Y, Sakai K, Jouvet M. Histaminergic descending inputs to the mesopontine tegmentum and their role in the control of cortical activation and wakefulness in the cat. *J Neurosci.* 1996;16(4):1523–1537.
113. Berridge CW, Abercrombie ED. Relationship between locus coeruleus discharge rates and rates of norepinephrine release within neocortex as assessed by in vivo microdialysis. *Neuroscience.* 1999;93(4):1263–1270.

114. Berridge CW, Schmeichel BE, España RA. Noradrenergic modulation of wakefulness/arousal. *Sleep Med Rev.* 2012;16(2):187–197.
115. Berridge CW. Noradrenergic modulation of arousal. *Brain Res Rev.* 2008;58(1):1–17.
116. Swanson LW. The locus coeruleus: a cytoarchitectonic, Golgi and immunohistochemical study in the albino rat. *Brain Res.* 1976;110(1):39–56.
117. Foote SL, Bloom FE, Aston-Jones G. Nucleus locus ceruleus: new evidence of anatomical and physiological specificity. *Physiol Rev.* 1983;63(3):844–914.
118. Pickel VM, Segal M, Bloom FE. A radioautographic study of the efferent pathways of the nucleus locus coeruleus. *J Comp Neurol.* 1974;155(1):15–42.
119. Morrison JH, Molliver ME, Grzanna R, Coyle JT. The intracortical trajectory of the coeruleo-cortical projection in the rat: a tangentially organized cortical afferent. *Neuroscience.* 1981;6(2): 139–158.
120. Berridge CW, Waterhouse BD. The locus coeruleus-noradrenergic system: modulation of behavioral state and state-dependent cognitive processes. *Brain Res Brain Res Rev.* 2003;42(1):33–84.
121. Morrison JH, Foote SL. Noradrenergic and serotoninergic innervation of cortical, thalamic, and tectal visual structures in Old and New World monkeys. *J Comp Neurol.* 1986;243(1): 117–138.
122. Zaborszky L, Cullinan WE. Direct catecholaminergic-cholinergic interactions in the basal forebrain. I. Dopamine-beta-hydroxylase- and tyrosine hydroxylase input to cholinergic neurons. *J Comp Neurol.* 1996;374(4):535–554.
123. Yoshida K, McCormack S, España RA, Crocker A, Scammell TE. Afferents to the orexin neurons of the rat brain. *J Comp Neurol.* 2006;494(5):845–861.
124. Aston-Jones G, Ennis M, Pieribone VA, Nickell WT, Shipley MT. The brain nucleus locus coeruleus: restricted afferent control of a broad efferent network. *Science.* 1986;234(4777):734–737.
125. Arnsten AF, Goldman-Rakic PS. Selective prefrontal cortical projections to the region of the locus coeruleus and raphe nuclei in the rhesus monkey. *Brain Res.* 1984;306(1–2):9–18.
126. Horvath TL, Peyron C, Diano S, et al. Hypocretin (orexin) activation and synaptic innervation of the locus coeruleus noradrenergic system. *J Comp Neurol.* 1999;415(2):145–159.
127. Cedarbaum JM, Aghajanian GK. Afferent projections to the rat locus coeruleus as determined by a retrograde tracing technique. *J Comp Neurol.* 1978;178(1):1–16.
128. Aston-Jones G, Bloom FE. Activity of norepinephrine-containing locus coeruleus neurons in behaving rats anticipates fluctuations in the sleep-waking cycle. *J Neurosci.* 1981;1(8):876–886.
129. Takahashi K, Kayama Y, Lin JS, Sakai K. Locus coeruleus neuronal activity during the sleep-waking cycle in mice. *Neuroscience.* 2010;169(3):1115–1126.
130. Chu N, Bloom FE. Norepinephrine-containing neurons: changes in spontaneous discharge patterns during sleeping and waking. *Science.* 1973;179(4076):908–910.
131. Foote SL, Aston-Jones G, Bloom FE. Impulse activity of locus coeruleus neurons in awake rats and monkeys is a function of sensory stimulation and arousal. *Proc Natl Acad Sci USA.* 1980;77(5):3033.
132. Aston-Jones G, Rajkowski J, Kubiak P, Alexinsky T. Locus coeruleus neurons in monkey are selectively activated by attended cues in a vigilance task. *J Neurosci.* 1994;14(7): 4467–4480.
133. Aston-Jones G, Cohen JD. An integrative theory of locus coeruleus-norepinephrine function: adaptive gain and optimal performance. *Annu Rev Neurosci.* 2005;28:403–450.
134. Gompf HS, Mathai C, Fuller PM, et al. Locus ceruleus and anterior cingulate cortex sustain wakefulness in a novel environment. *J Neurosci.* 2010;30(43):14543–14551.
135. Rasmussen K, Morilak DA, Jacobs BL. Single unit activity of locus coeruleus neurons in the freely moving cat. I. During naturalistic behaviors and in response to simple and complex stimuli. *Brain Res.* 1986;371(2):324–334.
136. Aston-Jones G, Bloom FE. Nonrepinephrine-containing locus coeruleus neurons in behaving rats exhibit pronounced responses to non-noxious environmental stimuli. *J Neurosci.* 1981;1(8):887.
137. McCormick DA, Prince DA. Noradrenergic modulation of firing pattern in guinea pig and cat thalamic neurons, in vitro. *J Neurophysiol.* 1988;59(3):978–996.
138. Rogawski MA, Aghajanian GK. Norepinephrine and serotonin: opposite effects on the activity of lateral geniculate neurons evoked by optic pathway stimulation. *Exp Neurol.* 1980;69(3):678–694.
139. McCormick DA, Williamson A. Modulation of neuronal firing mode in cat and guinea pig LGNd by histamine: possible cellular mechanisms of histaminergic control of arousal. *J Neurosci.* 1991;11(10):3188–3199.
140. Aston-Jones G, Chen S, Zhu Y, Oshinsky ML. A neural circuit for circadian regulation of arousal. *Nat Neurosci.* 2001;4(7):732–738.
141. Berridge CW, Page ME, Valentino RJ, Foote SL. Effects of locus coeruleus inactivation on electroencephalographic activity in neocortex and hippocampus. *Neuroscience.* 1993;55(2): 381–393.
142. Blanco-Centurion C, Gerashchenko D, Salin-Pascual RJ, Shiromani PJ. Effects of hypocretin2-saporin and antidopamine-beta-hydroxylase-saporin neurotoxic lesions of the dorsolateral pons on sleep and muscle tone. *Eur J Neurosci.* 2004;19(10): 2741–2752.
143. Cirelli C, Tononi G. Locus ceruleus control of state-dependent gene expression. *J Neurosci.* 2004;24(23):5410–5419.
144. Hunsley MS, Palmiter RD. Norepinephrine-deficient mice exhibit normal sleep–wake states but have shorter sleep latency after mild stress and low doses of amphetamine. *Sleep.* 2003;26(5): 521–526.
145. Carter ME, Yizhar O, Chikahisa S, et al. Tuning arousal with optogenetic modulation of locus coeruleus neurons. *Nat Neurosci.* 2010;13(12):1526–1533.
146. Berridge CW, Foote SL. Effects of locus coeruleus activation on electroencephalographic activity in neocortex and hippocampus. *J Neurosci.* 1991;11(10):3135–3145.
147. Berridge CW, Foote SL. Enhancement of behavioral and electroencephalographic indices of waking following stimulation of noradrenergic beta-receptors within the medial septal region of the basal forebrain. *J Neurosci.* 1996;16(21):6999–7009.
148. Berridge CW, O'Neill J. Differential sensitivity to the wake-promoting actions of norepinephrine within the medial preoptic area and the substantia innominata. *Behav Neurosci.* 2001;115(1):165–174.
149. Cape EG, Jones BE. Differential modulation of high-frequency gamma-electroencephalogram activity and sleep–wake state by noradrenaline and serotonin microinjections into the region of cholinergic basalis neurons. *J Neurosci.* 1998;18(7): 2653–2666.
150. Fort P, Khateb A, Pegna A, Muhlethaler M, Jones BE. Noradrenergic modulation of cholinergic nucleus basalis neurons demonstrated by in vitro pharmacological and immunohistochemical evidence in the guinea-pig brain. *Eur J Neurosci.* 1995;7(7):1502–1511.
151. Berridge CW, Isaac SO, España RA. Additive wake-promoting actions of medial basal forebrain noradrenergic

alpha1- and beta-receptor stimulation. *Behav Neurosci.* 2003;117(2):350–359.
152. De Sarro GB, Ascioti C, Froio F, Libri V, Nistico G. Evidence that locus coeruleus is the site where clonidine and drugs acting at alpha 1- and alpha 2-adrenoceptors affect sleep and arousal mechanisms. *Br J Pharmacol.* 1987;90(4):675–685.
153. Berridge CW, España RA. Synergistic sedative effects of noradrenergic α_1- and β-receptor blockade on forebrain electroencephalographic and behavioral indices. *Neuroscience.* 2000;99(3):495–505.
154. Scheinin M, Schwinn DA. The locus coeruleus. Site of hypnotic actions of alpha 2-adrenoceptor agonists? *Anesthesiology.* 1992;76(6):873–875.
155. Correa-Sales C, Rabin BC, Maze M. A hypnotic response to dexmedetomidine, an alpha 2 agonist, is mediated in the locus coeruleus in rats. *Anesthesiology.* 1992;76(6):948–952.
156. Brown RE, Stevens DR, Haas HL. The physiology of brain histamine. *Prog Neurobiol.* 2001;63(6):637–672.
157. Haas HL, Sergeeva OA, Selbach O. Histamine in the nervous system. *Physiol Rev.* 2008;88(3):1183–1241.
158. White JM, Rumbold GR. Behavioural effects of histamine and its antagonists: a review. *Psychopharmacology (Berl).* 1988;95(1):1–14.
159. Panula P, Yang HY, Costa E. Histamine-containing neurons in the rat hypothalamus. *Proc Natl Acad Sci USA.* 1984;81(8):2572–2576.
160. Panula P, Pirvola U, Auvinen S, Airaksinen MS. Histamine-immunoreactive nerve fibers in the rat brain. *Neuroscience.* 1989;28(3):585–610.
161. Hong EY, Lee HS. Retrograde study of projections from the tuberomammillary nucleus to the mesopontine cholinergic complex in the rat. *Brain Res.* 2011;1383:169–178.
162. Wouterlood FG, Steinbusch HW, Luiten PG, Bol JG. Projection from the prefrontal cortex to histaminergic cell groups in the posterior hypothalamic region of the rat. Anterograde tracing with *Phaseolus vulgaris* leucoagglutinin combined with immunocytochemistry of histidine decarboxylase. *Brain Res.* 1987;406(1–2):330–336.
163. Ericson H, Blomqvist A, Kohler C. Origin of neuronal inputs to the region of the tuberomammillary nucleus of the rat brain. *J Comp Neurol.* 1991;311(1):45–64.
164. Wouterlood FG, Gaykema RP. Innervation of histaminergic neurons in the posterior hypothalamic region by medial preoptic neurons. Anterograde tracing with *Phaseolus vulgaris* leucoagglutinin combined with immunocytochemistry of histidine decarboxylase in the rat. *Brain Res.* 1988;455(1):170–176.
165. Wouterlood FG, Gaykema RP, Steinbusch HW, Watanabe T, Wada H. The connections between the septum-diagonal band complex and histaminergic neurons in the posterior hypothalamus of the rat. Anterograde tracing with *Phaseolus vulgaris*-leucoagglutinin combined with immunocytochemistry of histidine decarboxylase. *Neuroscience.* 1988;26(3):827–845.
166. Sherin JE, Shiromani PJ, McCarley RW, Saper CB. Activation of ventrolateral preoptic neurons during sleep. *Science.* 1996; 271(5246):216–219.
167. Sherin JE, Elmquist JK, Torrealba F, Saper CB. Innervation of histaminergic tuberomammillary neurons by GABAergic and galaninergic neurons in the ventrolateral preoptic nucleus of the rat. *J Neurosci.* 1998;18(12):4705–4721.
168. Peyron C, Tighe DK, van den Pol AN, et al. Neurons containing hypocretin (orexin) project to multiple neuronal systems. *J Neurosci.* 1998;18(23):9996–10015.
169. Torrealba F, Yanagisawa M, Saper CB. Colocalization of orexin A and glutamate immunoreactivity in axon terminals in the tuberomammillary nucleus in rats. *Neuroscience.* 2003;119(4): 1033–1044.
170. Ericson H, Blomqvist A, Kohler C. Brainstem afferents to the tuberomammillary nucleus in the rat brain with special reference to monoaminergic innervation. *J Comp Neurol.* 1989;281(2): 169–192.
171. Mochizuki T, Yamatodani A, Okakura K, Horii A, Inagaki N, Wada H. Circadian rhythm of histamine release from the hypothalamus of freely moving rats. *Physiol Behav.* 1992;51(2):391–394.
172. Philippu A, Prast H. Patterns of histamine release in the brain. *Agents Actions.* 1991;33(1–2):124–125.
173. Takahashi K, Lin JS, Sakai K. Neuronal activity of histaminergic tuberomammillary neurons during wake–sleep states in the mouse. *J Neurosci.* 2006;26(40):10292–10298.
174. Szymusiak R, Iriye T, McGinty D. Sleep-waking discharge of neurons in the posterior lateral hypothalamic area of cats. *Brain Res Bull.* 1989;23(1–2):111–120.
175. Steininger TL, Alam MN, Gong H, Szymusiak R, McGinty D. Sleep-waking discharge of neurons in the posterior lateral hypothalamus of the albino rat. *Brain Res.* 1999;840(1–2):138–147.
176. Valdes JL, Farias P, Ocampo-Garces A, Cortes N, Seron-Ferre M, Torrealba F. Arousal and differential Fos expression in histaminergic neurons of the ascending arousal system during a feeding-related motivated behaviour. *Eur J Neurosci.* 2005; 21(7):1931–1942.
177. Zant JC, Rozov S, Wigren HK, Panula P, Porkka-Heiskanen T. Histamine release in the basal forebrain mediates cortical activation through cholinergic neurons. *J Neurosci.* 2012; 32(38):13244–13254.
178. Dringenberg HC, Kuo MC. Histaminergic facilitation of electrocorticographic activation: role of basal forebrain, thalamus, and neocortex. *Eur J Neurosci.* 2003;18(8):2285–2291.
179. Uhlrich DJ, Manning KA, Xue JT. Effects of activation of the histaminergic tuberomammillary nucleus on visual responses of neurons in the dorsal lateral geniculate nucleus. *J Neurosci.* 2002;22(3):1098–1107.
180. Lin JS, Sakai K, Vanni-Mercier G, Jouvet M. A critical role of the posterior hypothalamus in the mechanisms of wakefulness determined by microinjection of muscimol in freely moving cats. *Brain Res.* 1989;479(2):225–240.
181. Gerashchenko D, Chou TC, Blanco-Centurion CA, Saper CB, Shiromani PJ. Effects of lesions of the histaminergic tuberomammillary nucleus on spontaneous sleep in rats. *Sleep.* 2004;27(7):1275–1281.
182. Huang ZL, Mochizuki T, Qu WM, et al. Altered sleep–wake characteristics and lack of arousal response to H_3 receptor antagonist in histamine H_1 receptor knockout mice. *Proc Natl Acad Sci USA.* 2006;103(12):4687–4692.
183. Anaclet C, Parmentier R, Ouk K, et al. Orexin/hypocretin and histamine: distinct roles in the control of wakefulness demonstrated using knock-out mouse models. *J Neurosci.* 2009;29(46): 14423–14438.
184. Parmentier R, Ohtsu H, Djebbara-Hannas Z, Valatx JL, Watanabe T, Lin JS. Anatomical, physiological, and pharmacological characteristics of histidine decarboxylase knock-out mice: evidence for the role of brain histamine in behavioral and sleep–wake control. *J Neurosci.* 2002;22(17):7695–7711.
185. Monti JM, Pellejero T, Jantos H. Effects of H_1- and H_2-histamine receptor agonists and antagonists on sleep and wakefulness in the rat. *J Neural Transm.* 1986;66(1):1–11.
186. Lin JS, Sakai K, Jouvet M. Evidence for histaminergic arousal mechanisms in the hypothalamus of cat. *Neuropharmacology.* 1988;27(2):111–122.
187. Lin JS, Sakai K, Jouvet M. Hypothalamo-preoptic histaminergic projections in sleep–wake control in the cat. *Eur J Neurosci.* 1994;6(4):618–625.

188. Servos P, Barke KE, Hough LB, Vanderwolf CH. Histamine does not play an essential role in electrocortical activation during waking behavior. *Brain Res.* 1994;636(1):98–102.
189. Monti JM, D'Angelo L, Jantos H, Pazos S. Effects of a-fluoromethylhistidine on sleep and wakefulness in the rat. Short note. *J Neural Transm.* 1988;72(2):141–145.
190. Itowi N, Yamatodani A, Kiyono S, Hiraiwa ML, Wada H. Effect of histamine depletion on the circadian amplitude of the sleep-wakefulness cycle. *Physiol Behav.* 1991;49(3):643–646.
191. Itowi N, Yamatodani A, Mochizuki T, Wada H. Effects of intracerebroventricular histamine injection on circadian activity phase entrainment during rapid illumination changes. *Neurosci Lett.* 1991;123(1):53–56.
192. Cote NK, Harrington ME. Histamine phase shifts the circadian clock in a manner similar to light. *Brain Res.* 1993;613(1): 149–151.
193. Tasaka K, Chung YH, Sawada K, Mio M. Excitatory effect of histamine on the arousal system and its inhibition by H_1 blockers. *Brain Res Bull.* 1989;22(2):271–275.
194. Khateb A, Serafin M, Muhlethaler M. Histamine excites pedunculopontine neurones in guinea pig brainstem slices. *Neurosci Lett.* 1990;112(2–3):257–262.
195. Lakoski JM, Aghajanian GK. Effects of histamine, H_1- and H_2-receptor antagonists on the activity of serotonergic neurons in the dorsal raphe nucleus. *J Pharmacol Exp Ther.* 1983;227(2): 517–523.
196. Lakoski JM, Gallager DW, Aghajanian GK. Histamine-induced depression of serotoninergic dorsal raphe neurons: antagonism by cimetidine, a reevaluation. *Eur J Pharmacol.* 1984; 103(1–2):153–156.
197. Korotkova TM, Sergeeva OA, Ponomarenko AA, Haas HL. Histamine excites noradrenergic neurons in locus coeruleus in rats. *Neuropharmacology.* 2005;49(1):129–134.
198. Lin JS, Sakai K, Vanni-Mercier G, et al. Involvement of histaminergic neurons in arousal mechanisms demonstrated with H_3-receptor ligands in the cat. *Brain Res.* 1990;523(2):325–330.
199. Valjakka A, Vartiainen J, Kosunen H, et al. Histaminergic modulation of neocortical spindling and slow-wave activity in freely behaving rats. *J Neural Transm.* 1996;103(11):1265–1280.
200. Jacobs BL, Fornal C. Brain serotonergic neuronal activity in behaving cats. In: Monti JM, Pandi-Perumal SR, Jacobs BL, Nutt DJ, eds. *Serotonin and Sleep: Molecular, Functional and Clinical Aspects.* Basel: Birkhauser Verlag; 2008:185–204.
201. Monti JM, Pandi-Perumal SR, Jacobs BL, Nutt DJ, eds. *Serotonin and Sleep: Molecular, Functional and Clinical Aspects.* Basel: Birkhauser Verlag; 2008.
202. Brown RE, Sergeeva OA, Eriksson KS, Haas HL. Convergent excitation of dorsal raphe serotonin neurons by multiple arousal systems (orexin/hypocretin, histamine and noradrenaline). *J Neurosci.* 2002;22(20):8850–8859.
203. Wiklund L, Leger L, Persson M. Monoamine cell distribution in the cat brain stem. A fluorescence histochemical study with quantification of indolaminergic and locus coeruleus cell groups. *J Comp Neurol.* 1981;203(4):613–647.
204. Jacobs BL, Azmitia EC. Structure and function of the brain serotonin system. *Physiol Rev.* 1992;72(1):165–229.
205. Hannon J, Hoyer D. Molecular biology of 5-HT receptors. In: Monti JM, Pandi-Perumal SR, Jacobs BL, Nutt DJ, eds. *Serotonin and Sleep: Molecular, Functional and Clinical Aspects.* Basel: Birkhauser Verlag; 2008:155–182.
206. Monti JM, Jantos H. Effects of the serotonin $5\text{-}HT_{2A/2C}$ receptor agonist DOI and of the selective $5\text{-}HT_{2A}$ or $5\text{-}HT_{2C}$ receptor antagonists EMD 281014 and SB-243213, respectively, on sleep and waking in the rat. *Eur J Pharmacol.* 2006;553(1–3):163–170.
207. Monti JM, Jantos H. Effects of the $5\text{-}HT_7$ receptor antagonist SB-269970 microinjected into the dorsal raphe nucleus on REM sleep in the rat. *Behav Brain Res.* 2006;167(2):245–250.
208. Belin MF, Aguera M, Tappaz M, McRae-Degueurce A, Bobillier P, Pujol JF. GABA-accumulating neurons in the nucleus raphe dorsalis and periaqueductal gray in the rat: a biochemical and radioautographic study. *Brain Res.* 1979;170(2):279–297.
209. Descarries L, Berthelet F, Garcia S, Beaudet A. Dopaminergic projection from nucleus raphe dorsalis to neostriatum in the rat. *J Comp Neurol.* 1986;249(4):511–520, 484–485.
210. Vertes RP. A PHA-L analysis of ascending projections of the dorsal raphe nucleus in the rat. *J Comp Neurol.* 1991;313(4):643–668.
211. Parent A, Descarries L, Beaudet A. Organization of ascending serotonin systems in the adult rat brain. A radioautographic study after intraventricular administration of [3H]5-hydroxytryptamine. *Neuroscience.* 1981;6(2):115–138.
212. Crunelli V, Segal M. An electrophysiological study of neurones in the rat median raphe and their projections to septum and hippocampus. *Neuroscience.* 1985;15(1):47–60.
213. Consolazione A, Priestley JV, Cuello AC. Serotonin-containing projections to the thalamus in the rat revealed by a horseradish peroxidase and peroxidase antiperoxidase double-staining technique. *Brain Res.* 1984;322(2):233–243.
214. Sakai K, Salvert D, Touret M, Jouvet M. Afferent connections of the nucleus raphe dorsalis in the cat as visualized by the horseradish peroxidase technique. *Brain Res.* 1977;137(1):11–35.
215. Lee HS, Lee BY, Waterhouse BD. Retrograde study of projections from the tuberomammillary nucleus to the dorsal raphe and the locus coeruleus in the rat. *Brain Res.* 2005;1043(1–2):65–75.
216. Lee HS, Park SH, Song WC, Waterhouse BD. Retrograde study of hypocretin-1 (orexin-A) projections to subdivisions of the dorsal raphe nucleus in the rat. *Brain Res.* 2005;1059(1):35–45.
217. Kim MA, Lee HS, Lee BY, Waterhouse BD. Reciprocal connections between subdivisions of the dorsal raphe and the nuclear core of the locus coeruleus in the rat. *Brain Res.* 2004;1026(1):56–67.
218. Baraban JM, Aghajanian GK. Noradrenergic innervation of serotonergic neurons in the dorsal raphe: demonstration by electron microscopic autoradiography. *Brain Res.* 1981; 204(1):1–11.
219. Lee HS, Kim MA, Valentino RJ, Waterhouse BD. Glutamatergic afferent projections to the dorsal raphe nucleus of the rat. *Brain Res.* 2003;963(1–2):57–71.
220. Behzadi G, Kalen P, Parvopassu F, Wiklund L. Afferents to the median raphe nucleus of the rat: retrograde cholera toxin and wheat germ conjugated horseradish peroxidase tracing, and selective D-[^{3}H]aspartate labelling of possible excitatory amino acid inputs. *Neuroscience.* 1990;37(1):77–100.
221. Woolf NJ, Butcher LL. Cholinergic systems in the rat brain: IV. Descending projections of the pontomesencephalic tegmentum. *Brain Res Bull.* 1989;23(6):519–540.
222. Trulson ME, Jacobs BL. Raphe unit activity in freely moving cats: correlation with level of behavioral arousal. *Brain Res.* 1979;163(1):135–150.
223. McGinty DJ, Harper RM. Dorsal raphe neurons: depression of firing during sleep in cats. *Brain Res.* 1976;101(3):569–575.
224. Rasmussen K, Heym J, Jacobs BL. Activity of serotonin-containing neurons in nucleus centralis superior of freely moving cats. *Exp Neurol.* 1984;83(2):302–317.
225. Fornal C, Auerbach S, Jacobs BL. Activity of serotonin-containing neurons in nucleus raphe magnus in freely moving cats. *Exp Neurol.* 1985;88(3):590–608.

226. Portas CM, Bjorvatn B, Fagerland S, et al. On-line detection of extracellular levels of serotonin in dorsal raphe nucleus and frontal cortex over the sleep/wake cycle in the freely moving rat. *Neuroscience.* 1998;83(3):807–814.
227. Kocsis B, Varga V, Dahan L, Sik A. Serotonergic neuron diversity: identification of raphe neurons with discharges time-locked to the hippocampal theta rhythm. *Proc Natl Acad Sci USA.* 2006;103(4):1059–1064.
228. Sakai K, Crochet S. Role of dorsal raphe neurons in paradoxical sleep generation in the cat: no evidence for a serotonergic mechanism. *Eur J Neurosci.* 2001;13(1):103–112.
229. Hajos M, Gartside SE, Villa AE, Sharp T. Evidence for a repetitive (burst) firing pattern in a sub-population of 5-hydroxytryptamine neurons in the dorsal and median raphe nuclei of the rat. *Neuroscience.* 1995;69(1):189–197.
230. Urbain N, Creamer K, Debonnel G. Electrophysiological diversity of the dorsal raphe cells across the sleep–wake cycle of the rat. *J Physiol.* 2006;573(Pt 3):679–695.
231. Sakai K, Crochet S. Differentiation of presumed serotonergic dorsal raphe neurons in relation to behavior and wake–sleep states. *Neuroscience.* 2001;104(4):1141–1155.
232. Park MR. Intracellular horseradish peroxidase labeling of rapidly firing dorsal raphe projection neurons. *Brain Res.* 1987;402(1):117–130.
233. Aghajanian GK, Wang RY, Baraban J. Serotonergic and non-serotonergic neurons of the dorsal raphe: reciprocal changes in firing induced by peripheral nerve stimulation. *Brain Res.* 1978;153(1):169–175.
234. Sakai K. Electrophysiological studies on serotonergic neurons and sleep. In: Monti JM, Pandi-Perumal SR, Jacobs BL, Nutt DJ, eds. *Serotonin and Sleep: Molecular, Functional and Clinical Aspects.* Basel: Birkhauser Verlag; 2008:205–236.
235. Buchanan GF, Richerson GB. Central serotonin neurons are required for arousal to CO_2. *Proc Natl Acad Sci USA.* 2010;107(37):16354–16359.
236. Fornal CA, Litto WJ, Morilak DA, Jacobs BL. Single-unit responses of serotonergic dorsal raphe nucleus neurons to environmental heating and pyrogen administration in freely moving cats. *Exp Neurol.* 1987;98(2):388–403.
237. Wilkinson LO, Auerbach SB, Jacobs BL. Extracellular serotonin levels change with behavioral state but not with pyrogen-induced hyperthermia. *J Neurosci.* 1991;11(9):2732–2741.
238. Denoyer M, Sallanon M, Kitahama K, Aubert C, Jouvet M. Reversibility of para-chlorophenylalanine-induced insomnia by intrahypothalamic microinjection of L-5-hydroxytryptophan. *Neuroscience.* 1989;28(1):83–94.
239. Nitz D, Siegel J. GABA release in the dorsal raphe nucleus: role in the control of REM sleep. *Am J Physiol.* 1997;273(1 Pt 2): R451–R455.
240. Koyama Y, Sakai K. Modulation of presumed cholinergic mesopontine tegmental neurons by acetylcholine and monoamines applied iontophoretically in unanesthetized cats. *Neuroscience.* 2000;96(4):723–733.
241. Luebke JI, Greene RW, Semba K, Kamondi A, McCarley RW, Reiner PB. Serotonin hyperpolarizes cholinergic low-threshold burst neurons in the rat laterodorsal tegmental nucleus in vitro. *Proc Natl Acad Sci USA.* 1992;89(2):743–747.
242. Khateb A, Fort P, Alonso A, Jones BE, Muhlethaler M. Pharmacological and immunohistochemical evidence for serotonergic modulation of cholinergic nucleus basalis neurons. *Eur J Neurosci.* 1993;5(5):541–547.
243. Muraki Y, Yamanaka A, Tsujino N, Kilduff TS, Goto K, Sakurai T. Serotonergic regulation of the orexin/hypocretin neurons through the $5\text{-}HT_{1A}$ receptor. *J Neurosci.* 2004;24(32): 7159–7166.
244. Kumar S, Szymusiak R, Bashir T, Rai S, McGinty D, Alam MN. Effects of serotonin on perifornical-lateral hypothalamic area neurons in rat. *Eur J Neurosci.* 2007;25(1):201–212.
245. Monckton JE, McCormick DA. Neuromodulatory role of serotonin in the ferret thalamus. *J Neurophysiol.* 2002;87(4):2124–2136.
246. Dzoljic MR, Ukponmwan OE, Saxena PR. $5\text{-}HT_1$-like receptor agonists enhance wakefulness. *Neuropharmacology.* 1992;31(7): 623–633.
247. Dugovic C, Wauquier A, Leysen JE, Marrannes R, Janssen PA. Functional role of $5\text{-}HT_2$ receptors in the regulation of sleep and wakefulness in the rat. *Psychopharmacology (Berl).* 1989;97(4): 436–442.
248. Lemoine P, Guilleminault C, Alvarez E. Improvement in subjective sleep in major depressive disorder with a novel antidepressant, agomelatine: randomized, double-blind comparison with venlafaxine. *J Clin Psychiatry.* Nov 2007;68(11):1723–1732.
249. Maudhuit C, Jolas T, Lainey E, Hamon M, Adrien J. Effects of acute and chronic treatment with amoxapine and cericlamine on the sleep-wakefulness cycle in the rat. *Neuropharmacology.* 1994;33(8):1017–1025.
250. de Lecea L, Kilduff TS, Peyron C, et al. The hypocretins: hypothalamus-specific peptides with neuroexcitatory activity. *Proc Natl Acad Sci USA.* 1998;95(1):322–327.
251. Sakurai T, Amemiya A, Ishii M, et al. Orexins and orexin receptors: a family of hypothalamic neuropeptides and G protein-coupled receptors that regulate feeding behavior. *Cell.* 1998;92(5), 1 page following 696.
252. Saper CB, Fuller PM, Pedersen NP, Lu J, Scammell TE. Sleep state switching. *Neuron.* 2010;68(6):1023–1042.
253. Chou TC, Lee CE, Lu J, et al. Orexin (hypocretin) neurons contain dynorphin. *J Neurosci.* 2001;21(19):RC168.
254. Chemelli RM, Willie JT, Sinton CM, et al. Narcolepsy in orexin knockout mice: molecular genetics of sleep regulation. *Cell.* 1999;98(4):437–451.
255. Mileykovskiy BY, Kiyashchenko LI, Siegel JM. Behavioral correlates of activity in identified hypocretin/orexin neurons. *Neuron.* 2005;46(5):787–798.
256. Lee MG, Hassani OK, Jones BE. Discharge of identified orexin/hypocretin neurons across the sleep-waking cycle. *J Neurosci.* 2005;25(28):6716–6720.
257. Kiyashchenko LI, Mileykovskiy BY, Maidment N, et al. Release of hypocretin (orexin) during waking and sleep states. *J Neurosci.* 2002;22(13):5282–5286.
258. Zeitzer JM, Buckmaster CL, Parker KJ, Hauck CM, Lyons DM, Mignot E. Circadian and homeostatic regulation of hypocretin in a primate model: implications for the consolidation of wakefulness. *J Neurosci.* 2003;23(8):3555–3560.
259. Taheri S, Sunter D, Dakin C, et al. Diurnal variation in orexin A immunoreactivity and prepro-orexin mRNA in the rat central nervous system. *Neurosci Lett.* 2000;279(2):109–112.
260. Yoshida Y, Fujiki N, Nakajima T, et al. Fluctuation of extracellular hypocretin-1 (orexin A) levels in the rat in relation to the light–dark cycle and sleep–wake activities. *Eur J Neurosci.* 2001;14(7):1075–1081.
261. Hassani OK, Henny P, Lee MG, Jones BE. GABAergic neurons intermingled with orexin and MCH neurons in the lateral hypothalamus discharge maximally during sleep. *Eur J Neurosci.* 2010;32(3):448–457.
262. Hagan JJ, Leslie RA, Patel S, et al. Orexin A activates locus coeruleus cell firing and increases arousal in the rat. *Proc Natl Acad Sci USA.* 1999;96(19):10911–10916.
263. van den Pol AN, Ghosh PK, Liu R-j, Li Y, Aghajanian GK, Gao X-B. Hypocretin (orexin) enhances neuron activity and cell synchrony in developing mouse GFP-expressing locus coeruleus. *J Physiol.* 2002;541(1):169–185.

264. Eriksson KS, Sergeeva O, Brown RE, Haas HL. Orexin/hypocretin excites the histaminergic neurons of the tuberomammillary nucleus. *J Neurosci*. 2001;21(23):9273–9279.
265. van den Pol AN, Gao XB, Obrietan K, Kilduff TS, Belousov AB. Presynaptic and postsynaptic actions and modulation of neuroendocrine neurons by a new hypothalamic peptide, hypocretin/orexin. *J Neurosci*. 1998;18(19):7962–7971.
266. Hoang QV, Bajic D, Yanagisawa M, Nakajima S, Nakajima Y. Effects of orexin (hypocretin) on GIRK channels. *J Neurophysiol*. 2003;90(2):693–702.
267. España RA, Baldo BA, Kelley AE, Berridge CW. Wake-promoting and sleep-suppressing actions of hypocretin (orexin): basal forebrain sites of action. *Neuroscience*. 2001;106(4):699–715.
268. Bourgin P, Huitrón-Reséndiz S, Spier AD, et al. Hypocretin-1 modulates rapid eye movement sleep through activation of locus coeruleus neurons. *J Neurosci*. 2000;20(20):7760–7765.
269. Korotkova TM, Eriksson KS, Haas HL, Brown RE. Selective excitation of GABAergic neurons in the substantia nigra of the rat by orexin/hypocretin in vitro. *Regul Pept*. 2002;104(1–3):83–89.
270. Korotkova TM, Sergeeva OA, Eriksson KS, Haas HL, Brown RE. Excitation of ventral tegmental area dopaminergic and non-dopaminergic neurons by orexins/hypocretins. *J Neurosci*. 2003;23(1):7–11.
271. Liu ZW, Gao XB. Adenosine inhibits activity of hypocretin/orexin neurons by the A_1 receptor in the lateral hypothalamus: a possible sleep-promoting effect. *J Neurophysiol*. 2007;97(1):837–848.
272. Brisbare-Roch C, Dingemanse J, Koberstein R, et al. Promotion of sleep by targeting the orexin system in rats, dogs and humans. *Nat Med*. 2007;13(2):150–155.
273. Dugovic C, Shelton JE, Aluisio LE, et al. Blockade of orexin-1 receptors attenuates orexin-2 receptor antagonism-induced sleep promotion in the rat. *J Pharmacol Exp Ther*. 2009;330(1):142–151.
274. Moriguchi T, Sakurai T, Nambu T, Yanagisawa M, Goto K. Neurons containing orexin in the lateral hypothalamic area of the adult rat brain are activated by insulin-induced acute hypoglycemia. *Neurosci Lett*. 1999;264(1–3):101–104.
275. Adamantidis AR, Zhang F, Aravanis AM, Deisseroth K, de Lecea L. Neural substrates of awakening probed with optogenetic control of hypocretin neurons. *Nature*. 2007;450(7168):420–424.
276. Carter ME, Adamantidis A, Ohtsu H, Deisseroth K, de Lecea L. Sleep homeostasis modulates hypocretin-mediated sleep-to-wake transitions. *J Neurosci*. 2009;29(35):10939–10949.
277. Tsunematsu T, Kilduff TS, Boyden ES, Takahashi S, Tominaga M, Yamanaka A. Acute optogenetic silencing of orexin/hypocretin neurons induces slow-wave sleep in mice. *J Neurosci*. 2011;31(29):10529–10539.
278. Nishino S, Ripley B, Overeem S, Lammers GJ, Mignot E. Hypocretin (orexin) deficiency in human narcolepsy. *Lancet*. 2000;355(9197):39–40.
279. Peyron C, Faraco J, Rogers W, et al. A mutation in a case of early onset narcolepsy and a generalized absence of hypocretin peptides in human narcoleptic brains. *Nat Med*. 2000;6(9):991–997.
280. Thannickal TC, Moore RY, Nienhuis R, et al. Reduced number of hypocretin neurons in human narcolepsy. *Neuron*. 2000;27(3):469–474.
281. Hara J, Beuckmann CT, Nambu T, et al. Genetic ablation of orexin neurons in mice results in narcolepsy, hypophagia, and obesity. *Neuron*. 2001;30(2):345–354.
282. Gerashchenko D, Blanco-Centurion C, Greco MA, Shiromani PJ. Effects of lateral hypothalamic lesion with the neurotoxin hypocretin-2-saporin on sleep in Long-Evans rats. *Neuroscience*. 2003;116(1):223–235.
283. Lin L, Faraco J, Li R, et al. The sleep disorder canine narcolepsy is caused by a mutation in the hypocretin (orexin) receptor 2 gene. *Cell*. 1999;98(3):365–376.
284. Jones EG, Leavitt RY. Demonstration of thalamo-cortical connectivity in the cat somato-sensory system by retrograde axonal transport of horseradish peroxidase. *Brain Res*. 1973;63:414–418.
285. McCormick DA, Bal T. Sleep and arousal: thalamocortical mechanisms. *Annu Rev Neurosci*. 1997;20:185–215.
286. Steriade M, Glenn LL. Neocortical and caudate projections of intralaminar thalamic neurons and their synaptic excitation from midbrain reticular core. *J Neurophysiol*. 1982;48(2):352–371.
287. Scannell JW, Burns GA, Hilgetag CC, O'Neil MA, Young MP. The connectional organization of the cortico-thalamic system of the cat. *Cereb Cortex*. 1999;9(3):277–299.
288. Endo K, Araki T, Ito K. Short latency EPSPs and incrementing PSPs of pyramidal tract cells evoked by stimulation of the nucleus centralis lateralis of the thalamus. *Brain Res*. 1977;132(3):541–546.
289. Van der Werf YD, Witter MP, Groenewegen HJ. The intralaminar and midline nuclei of the thalamus. Anatomical and functional evidence for participation in processes of arousal and awareness. *Brain Res Brain Res Rev*. 2002;39(2–3):107–140.
290. Krout KE, Belzer RE, Loewy AD. Brainstem projections to midline and intralaminar thalamic nuclei of the rat. *J Comp Neurol*. 2002;448(1):53–101.
291. Hubel DH. Single unit activity in lateral geniculate body and optic tract of unrestrained cats. *J Physiol*. 1960;150:91–104.
292. Hirsch JC, Fourment A, Marc ME. Sleep-related variations of membrane potential in the lateral geniculate body relay neurons of the cat. *Brain Res*. 1983;259(2):308–312.
293. McCarley RW, Benoit O, Barrionuevo G. Lateral geniculate nucleus unitary discharge in sleep and waking: state- and rate-specific aspects. *J Neurophysiol*. 1983;50(4):798–818.
294. Jahnsen H, Llinas R. Electrophysiological properties of guinea-pig thalamic neurones: an in vitro study. *J Physiol*. 1984;349:205–226.
295. Landisman CE, Connors BW. VPM and PoM nuclei of the rat somatosensory thalamus: intrinsic neuronal properties and corticothalamic feedback. *Cereb Cortex*. 2007;17(12):2853–2865.
296. Domich L, Oakson G, Steriade M. Thalamic burst patterns in the naturally sleeping cat: a comparison between cortically projecting and reticularis neurones. *J Physiol*. 1986;379:429–449.
297. Lee J, Kim D, Shin HS. Lack of delta waves and sleep disturbances during non-rapid eye movement sleep in mice lacking alpha1G-subunit of T-type calcium channels. *Proc Natl Acad Sci USA*. 2004;101(52):18195–18199.
298. Glenn LL, Steriade M. Discharge rate and excitability of cortically projecting intralaminar thalamic neurons during waking and sleep states. *J Neurosci*. 1982;2(10):1387–1404.
299. Schiff ND. Central thalamic contributions to arousal regulation and neurological disorders of consciousness. *Ann N Y Acad Sci*. 2008;1129:105–118.
300. Steriade M, Curró Dossi RC, Contreras D. Electrophysiological properties of intralaminar thalamocortical cells discharging rhythmic (approximately 40 HZ) spike-bursts at approximately 1000 HZ during waking and rapid eye movement sleep. *Neuroscience*. 1993;56(1):1–9.
301. Sukov W, Barth DS. Cellular mechanisms of thalamically evoked gamma oscillations in auditory cortex. *J Neurophysiol*. 2001;85(3):1235–1245.
302. Schiff ND, Giacino JT, Kalmar K, et al. Behavioural improvements with thalamic stimulation after severe traumatic brain injury. *Nature*. 2007;448(7153):600–603.

303. Schiff ND. Recovery of consciousness after brain injury: a mesocircuit hypothesis. *Trends Neurosci.* 2010;33(1):1–9.
304. Poulet JFA, Fernandez LMJ, Crochet S, Petersen CCH. Thalamic control of cortical states. *Nat Neurosci.* 2012;15(3):370–372.
305. Lee JH, Durand R, Gradinaru V, et al. Global and local fMRI signals driven by neurons defined optogenetically by type and wiring. *Nature.* 2010;465(7299):788–792.
306. Rigas P, Castro-Alamancos MA. Thalamocortical Up states: differential effects of intrinsic and extrinsic cortical inputs on persistent activity. *J Neurosci.* 2007;27(16):4261–4272.
307. Kinomura S, Larsson J, Gulyas B, Roland PE. Activation by attention of the human reticular formation and thalamic intralaminar nuclei. *Science.* 1996;271(5248):512–515.
308. Vanderwolf CH, Stewart DJ. Thalamic control of neocortical activation: a critical re-evaluation. *Brain Res Bull.* 1988;20(4):529–538.
309. Kinney HC, Samuels MA. Neuropathology of the persistent vegetative state. A review. *J Neuropathol Exp Neurol.* 1994;53(6):548–558.
310. Adams JH, Graham DI, Jennett B. The neuropathology of the vegetative state after an acute brain insult. *Brain.* 2000; 123(Pt 7):1327–1338.
311. Maxwell WL, MacKinnon MA, Smith DH, McIntosh TK, Graham DI. Thalamic nuclei after human blunt head injury. *J Neuropathol Exp Neurol.* 2006;65(5):478–488.
312. Castaigne P, Lhermitte F, Buge A, Escourolle R, Hauw JJ, Lyon-Caen O. Paramedian thalamic and midbrain infarct: clinical and neuropathological study. *Ann Neurol.* 1981;10(2):127–148.
313. Kinney HC, Korein J, Panigrahy A, Dikkes P, Goode R. Neuropathological findings in the brain of Karen Ann Quinlan. The role of the thalamus in the persistent vegetative state. *N Engl J Med.* 1994;330(21):1469–1475.
314. Schiff ND, Plum F. The role of arousal and "gating" systems in the neurology of impaired consciousness. *J Clin Neurophysiol.* 2000;17(5):438–452.
315. Reilly M, Connolly S, Stack J, Martin EA, Hutchinson M. Bilateral paramedian thalamic infarction: a distinct but poorly recognized stroke syndrome. *Q J Med.* 1992;82(297):63–70.
316. Schmahmann JD. Vascular syndromes of the thalamus. *Stroke.* 2003;34(9):2264–2278.
317. Palmiter RD. Dopamine signaling as a neural correlate of consciousness. *Neuroscience.* 2011;198:213–220.
318. Dahlstrom A, Fuxe K. Localization of monoamines in the lower brain stem. *Experientia.* 1964;20(7):398–399.
319. Geffard M, Buijs RM, Seguela P, Pool CW, Le Moal M. First demonstration of highly specific and sensitive antibodies against dopamine. *Brain Res.* 1984;294(1):161–165.
320. Arsenault MY, Parent A, Seguela P, Descarries L. Distribution and morphological characteristics of dopamine-immunoreactive neurons in the midbrain of the squirrel monkey (*Saimiri sciureus*). *J Comp Neurol.* 1988;267(4):489–506.
321. Matsuda W, Furuta T, Nakamura KC, et al. Single nigrostriatal dopaminergic neurons form widely spread and highly dense axonal arborizations in the neostriatum. *J Neurosci.* 2009;29(2):444–453.
322. Fallon JH. Collateralization of monoamine neurons: mesotelencephalic dopamine projections to caudate, septum, and frontal cortex. *J Neurosci.* 1981;1(12):1361–1368.
323. Oades RD, Halliday GM. Ventral tegmental (A10) system: neurobiology. 1. Anatomy and connectivity. *Brain Res.* 1987;434(2):117–165.
324. Lu J, Jhou TC, Saper CB. Identification of wake-active dopaminergic neurons in the ventral periaqueductal gray matter. *J Neurosci.* 2006;26(1):193–202.
325. Sanchez-Gonzalez MA, Garcia-Cabezas MA, Rico B, Cavada C. The primate thalamus is a key target for brain dopamine. *J Neurosci.* 2005;25(26):6076–6083.
326. Garcia-Cabezas MA, Martinez-Sanchez P, Sanchez-Gonzalez MA, Garzon M, Cavada C. Dopamine innervation in the thalamus: monkey versus rat. *Cereb Cortex.* 2009;19(2):424–434.
327. Groenewegen HJ. Organization of the afferent connections of the mediodorsal thalamic nucleus in the rat, related to the mediodorsal-prefrontal topography. *Neuroscience.* 1988;24(2): 379–431.
328. Zahm DS, Cheng AY, Lee TJ, et al. Inputs to the midbrain dopaminergic complex in the rat, with emphasis on extended amygdala-recipient sectors. *J Comp Neurol.* 2011;519(16): 3159–3188.
329. Phillipson OT. Afferent projections to the ventral tegmental area of Tsai and interfascicular nucleus: a horseradish peroxidase study in the rat. *J Comp Neurol.* 1979;187(1):117–143.
330. Trulson ME. Simultaneous recording of substantia nigra neurons and voltammetric release of dopamine in the caudate of behaving cats. *Brain Res Bull.* 1985;15(2):221–223.
331. Trulson ME, Preussler DW. Dopamine-containing ventral tegmental area neurons in freely moving cats: activity during the sleep-waking cycle and effects of stress. *Exp Neurol.* 1984;83(2):367–377.
332. Deutch AY, Goldstein M, Roth RH. Activation of the locus coeruleus induced by selective stimulation of the ventral tegmental area. *Brain Res.* 1986;363(2):307–314.
333. Neylan TC, van Kammen DP, Kelley ME, Peters JL. Sleep in schizophrenic patients on and off haloperidol therapy. Clinically stable vs relapsed patients. *Arch Gen Psychiatry.* 1992;49(8):643–649.
334. Volkow ND, Fowler JS, Logan J, et al. Effects of modafinil on dopamine and dopamine transporters in the male human brain: clinical implications. *JAMA.* 2009;301(11):1148–1154.
335. Qu WM, Huang ZL, Xu XH, Matsumoto N, Urade Y. Dopaminergic D_1 and D_2 receptors are essential for the arousal effect of modafinil. *J Neurosci.* 2008;28(34):8462–8469.
336. Ongini E, Bonizzoni E, Ferri N, Milani S, Trampus M. Differential effects of dopamine D-1 and D-2 receptor antagonist antipsychotics on sleep–wake patterns in the rat. *J Pharmacol Exp Ther.* 1993;266(2):726–731.
337. Paus S, Brecht HM, Koster J, Seeger G, Klockgether T, Wullner U. Sleep attacks, daytime sleepiness, and dopamine agonists in Parkinson's disease. *Mov Disord.* 2003;18(6):659–667.
338. Kitaoka K, Shimizu M, Shimizu N, et al. Retinoic acid receptor antagonist LE540 attenuates wakefulness via the dopamine D_1 receptor in mice. *Brain Res.* 2011;1423:10–16.
339. Shang Y, Haynes P, Pírez N, et al. Imaging analysis of clock neurons reveals light buffers the wake-promoting effect of dopamine. *Nat Neurosci.* 2011;14(7):889–895.
340. Zant JC, Leenaars CH, Kostin A, Van Someren EJ, Porkka-Heiskanen T. Increases in extracellular serotonin and dopamine metabolite levels in the basal forebrain during sleep deprivation. *Brain Res.* 2011;1399:40–48.
341. Lavin A, Grace AA. Dopamine modulates the responsivity of mediodorsal thalamic cells recorded in vitro. *J Neurosci.* 1998;18(24):10566–10578.
342. Govindaiah G, Wang Y, Cox CL. Dopamine enhances the excitability of somatosensory thalamocortical neurons. *Neuroscience.* 2010;170(4):981–991.
343. Penit-Soria J, Audinat E, Crepel F. Excitation of rat prefrontal cortical neurons by dopamine: an in vitro electrophysiological study. *Brain Res.* 1987;425(2):263–274.
344. Bandyopadhyay S, Hablitz JJ. Dopaminergic modulation of local network activity in rat prefrontal cortex. *J Neurophysiol.* 2007;97(6):4120–4128.
345. Englot DJ, Modi B, Mishra AM, DeSalvo M, Hyder F, Blumenfeld H. Cortical deactivation induced by subcortical

network dysfunction in limbic seizures. *J Neurosci.* 2009;29(41):13006–13018.

346. Langsjo JW, Alkire MT, Kaskinoro K, et al. Returning from oblivion: imaging the neural core of consciousness. *J Neurosci.* 2012;32(14):4935–4943.
347. Boly M, Perlbarg V, Marrelec G, et al. Hierarchical clustering of brain activity during human nonrapid eye movement sleep. *Proc Natl Acad Sci USA.* 2012;109(15):5856–5861.
348. Motelow JE, Blumenfeld H. Functional neuroimaging of spike-wave seizures. *Dyn Brain Imaging.* 2009:189–209.
349. Blumenfeld H, Varghese GI, Purcaro MJ, et al. Cortical and subcortical networks in human secondarily generalized tonic-clonic seizures. *Brain.* 2009;132(4):999–1012.
350. Danielson NB, Guo JN, Blumenfeld H. The default mode network and altered consciousness in epilepsy. *Behav Neurol.* 2011;24(1):55–65.
351. Adametz JH. Rate of recovery of functioning in cats with rostral reticular lesions; an experimental study. *J Neurosurg.* 1959;16(1):85–97 discussion 97–88.
352. Parvizi J, Damasio AR. Neuroanatomical correlates of brainstem coma. *Brain.* 2003;126(Pt 7):1524–1536.

CHAPTER

22

Networks of Normal and Disordered Sleep

Pierre-Hervé Luppi, Patrice Fort

INSERM, U1028, CNRS, UMR5292, Lyon Neuroscience Research Center, Team "Physiopathologie des réseaux neuronaux responsables du cycle veille-sommeil", Lyon, France and University Lyon 1, Lyon, France

INTRODUCTION

In most mammals, there are three vigilance states, which are characterized by clear differences in electroencephalogram (EEG), electromyogram (EMG), and electro-oculogram (EOG) recordings. The waking state (W) is characterized by high-frequency, low-amplitude (desynchronized) activity on the EEG, and sustained EMG activity and ocular movements; non–rapid eye movement (non-REM, or NREM) sleep, also named slow-wave sleep (SWS) (synchronized), is characterized by low-frequency, high-amplitude delta oscillations on the EEG, low muscular activity on the EMG, and no ocular movement; and rapid eye movement (REM), also called paradoxical sleep (PS), is characterized by an activated low-amplitude EEG similar to the waking EEG, but with complete disappearance of postural muscle tone and the occurrence of rapid eye movements and muscle twitches.

A wealth of neuropathological evidence dating back to the nineteenth century indicated that altered states of vigilance can be induced by focal brain lesions and that different neurochemical mechanisms are responsible for the succession of the three vigilance states across the 24 h day.[1] However, the mechanisms underlying the switch of cortical activity from an activated (desynchronized) state during waking to a synchronized state during deep SWS and then to the activated state of PS have not yet been precisely described. This chapter examines the possible neuronal networks and mechanisms responsible for the switch from waking to SWS and PS.

MECHANISMS INVOLVED IN WAKING (FIGURE 22.1)

The activated cortical state during waking is induced by the activity of multiple waking neurochemical systems. Some of these belong to the ascending reticular activating system (ARAS)[2] (see Chapter 21). These neurochemical systems include the serotonergic neurons, which are mainly localized in the dorsal raphe nucleus; the noradrenergic neurons located in the locus coeruleus (LC); the cholinergic neurons in the pontine brainstem; and other systems that are located more rostrally in the forebrain. These systems include the cholinergic neurons in the basal forebrain, the histaminergic neurons localized in the tuberomammillary nucleus (TMN), and the orexin (hypocretin) system in the tuberal hypothalamus.[1]

Altogether, these systems control arousal characterized by high-frequency, low-amplitude cortical activation[3] and widely project to the thalamus and/or the neocortex. When these waking systems are inactivated, the thalamo-cortical network oscillates in the delta range (i.e. the slow-wave mode of activity typical of SWS).[1]

During sleep, it is believed that these waking systems are all inhibited by gamma-aminobutyric acid (GABA), the main inhibitory neurotransmitter in the brain. Indeed, it has been shown that the serotonergic neurons of the dorsal raphe nucleus and the noradrenergic neurons of the LC are inhibited by GABA during SWS and PS.[4,5] However, the role of GABAergic inhibition is yet to be demonstrated for the other waking systems.

We demonstrated that the unit activity of a single serotonergic neuron shows activity during waking, decreases its activity until it is nearly silent during SWS sleep, and is completely silent during PS sleep.[5] Furthermore, by the localized application of bicuculline, a competitive antagonist of $GABA_A$ receptors, we demonstrated that these neurons cease or decrease firing during sleep because GABA tonically inhibits them. Indeed, application of bicuculline during SWS and PS restores the waking activity of the neurons. Similar results have been obtained for the noradrenergic neurons of the LC.[4]

Neuronal Networks in Brain Function, CNS Disorders, and Therapeutics
http://dx.doi.org/10.1016/B978-0-12-415804-7.00022-8

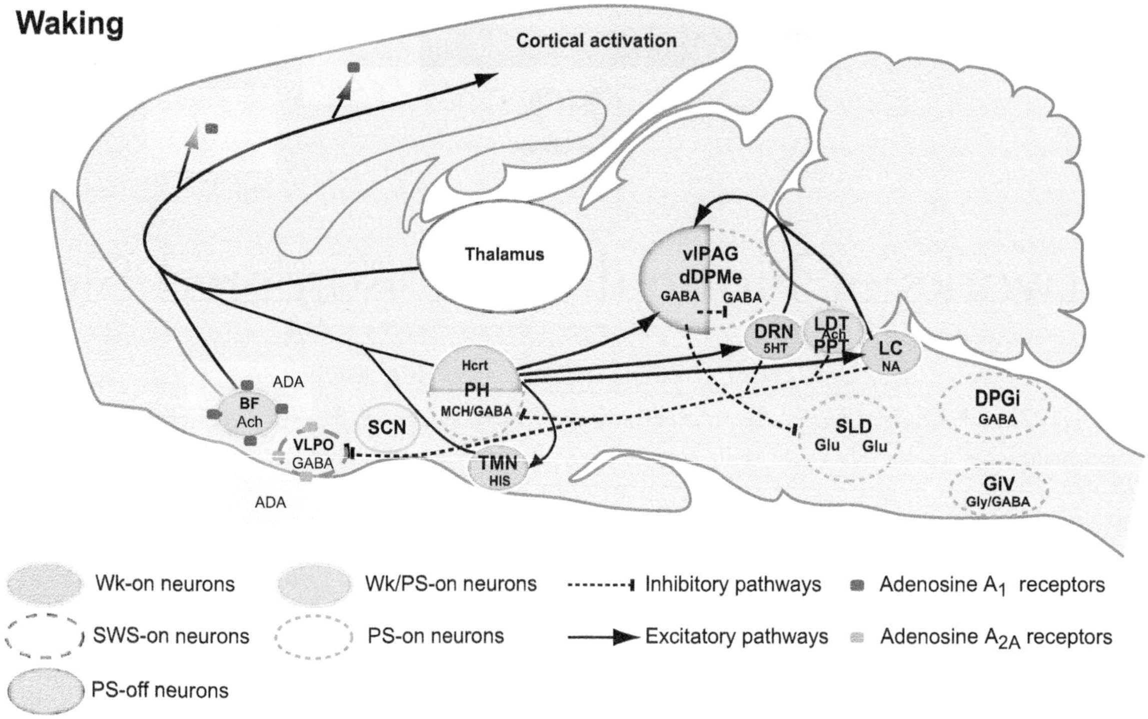

FIGURE 22.1 **Neuronal networks responsible for waking.** At sleep–wake transitions, the hypocretin neurons would be the first to start firing, exciting all the other waking systems (histaminergic, monoaminergic, and cholinergic). In turn, these waking systems activate the thalamus and/or the cortex, leading to cortical activation and, importantly, inhibiting the GABAergic SWS (non-REM, or NREM, sleep)-active neurons of the VLPO and MnPn. Abbreviations: 5HT, 5-hydroxytryptamine (serotonin); Ach, acetylcholine; ADA, adenosine; BF, basal forebrain; DPGi, dorsal paragigantocellular reticular nucleus; dDPMe, deep mesencephalic reticular nucleus; DRN, dorsal raphe nucleus; GABA, gamma-aminobutyric acid; GiV, ventral gigantocellular reticular nucleus; Gly, glycine; Hcrt, hypocretin (orexin)-containing neurons; His, histamine; LC, locus coeruleus; LDT, laterodorsal tegmental nucleus; MCH, neurons containing melanin-concentrating hormone; NA, noradrenaline; PH, posterior hypothalamus; PPT, pedunculopontine tegmental nucleus; PS, paradoxical sleep; RT, reticular thalamic neurons; SCN, suprachiasmatic nucleus; SLD, sublaterodorsal nucleus; SWS, slow-wave sleep; TMN, tuberomamillary nucleus; vlPAG, ventrolateral periaqueductal gray; VLPO, ventrolateral preoptic nucleus; W, waking. (The figure is reproduced in color section.)

MECHANISMS INVOLVED IN NREM (SWS) INDUCTION AND MAINTENANCE (FIGURE 22.2)

The Forebrain (Preoptic) Sleep Center

Following studies of patients with postinfluenza encephalitis, the neuropathologist von Economo reported that inflammatory lesions of the preoptic area (POA) were often associated with insomnia and therefore proposed that the POA was critical for the production of normal sleep.[6] Then, Ranson in monkeys, Nauta in rats, and McGinty in cats showed that POA lesions induce a profound and persistent insomnia.[7–9] It was later shown in cats that POA electrical stimulation induces EEG slow-wave activity and SWS.[10] Finally, putative sleep-promoting neurons displaying an elevated discharge rate during SWS compared to W, diffusely distributed within a large region encompassing the horizontal limb of the diagonal bands of Broca and the lateral POA–substantia innominata, were recorded in freely moving cats.[11] Altogether, these studies indicate that the POA is a unique brain structure containing neurons that directly promote sleep.

This simplicity greatly contrasts with the complex network responsible for W, involving redundant neurotransmitter systems with populations of neurons disseminated from the upper brainstem to the caudal hypothalamus and basal forebrain, such as neurons containing acetylcholine, noradrenaline (NA), serotonin, histamine, and hypocretin (orexin) (Figure 22.1). During the transition to sleep, the hypnogenic center would inhibit the multiple arousal systems of the ARAS via a sustained and coordinated inhibition (Figure 22.2).

Then, researchers identified specific sleep-active neurons by using expression of an immediate early gene, Fos, as a marker of neuronal activation in rats that had slept for a long period before sacrifice.[12] These neurons are distributed diffusely in the POA but are more densely packed in the median preoptic nucleus (MnPn) and the ventrolateral preoptic nucleus

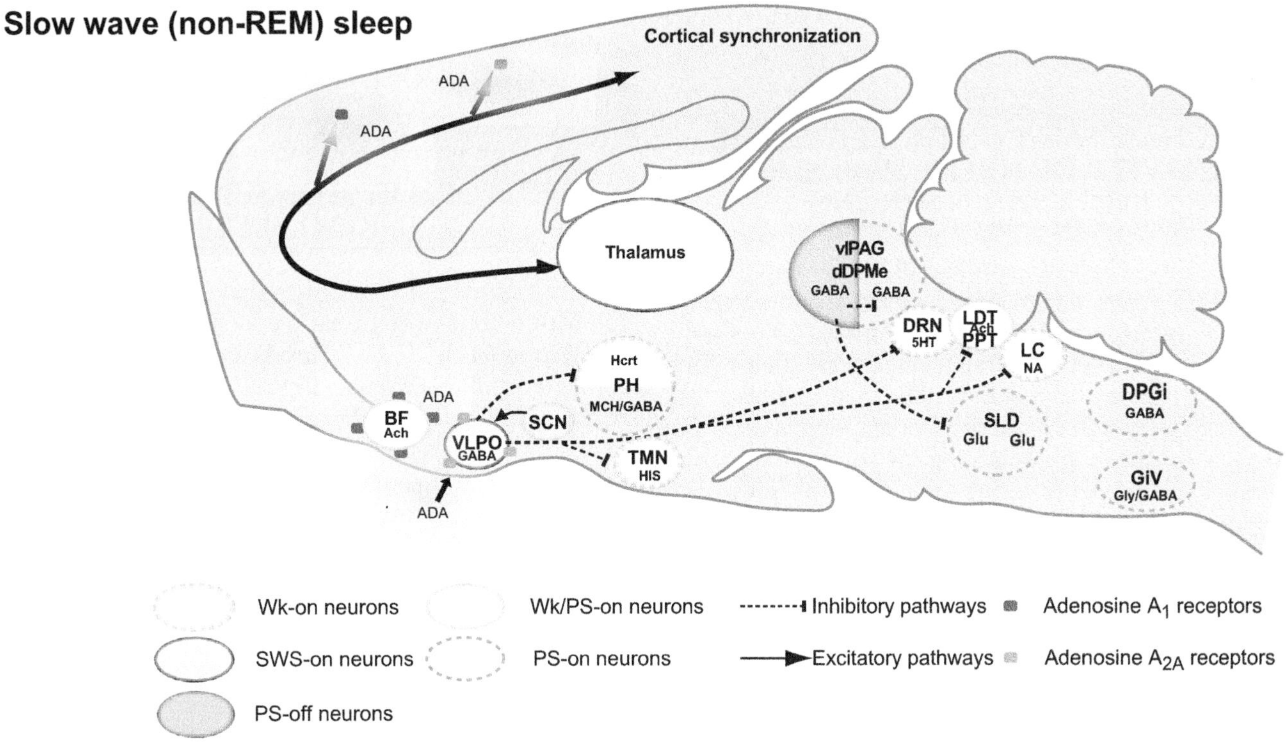

FIGURE 22.2 **Neuronal networks responsible for slow-wave (NREM) sleep.** VLPO and MnPo GABAergic neurons would be inhibited by noradrenergic and cholinergic inputs during waking. The majority of them would start firing at sleep onset (drowsiness) in response to excitatory, homeostatic (adenosine), and circadian drives (suprachiasmatic input). These activated neurons, through the reciprocal GABAergic inhibition of all wake-promoting systems, would be in a position to suddenly unbalance the "flip-flop" network, as required for switching from W (drowsiness) to a consolidation of SWS sleep. Conversely, the slow removal of excitatory influences would result in a progressive firing decrease in VLPO neurons and therefore an activation of wake-promoting systems leading to the awakening event. (The figure is reproduced in color section.)

(VLPO). These studies showed that the number of Fos-immunoreactive neurons in the VLPO and MnPn positively correlated with sleep quantity and sleep consolidation during the last hour preceding sacrifice. Numerous Fos-positive neurons were also observed in sleep-deprived rats in the MnPn but not in the VLPO.[12,13] It appears, therefore, that VLPO neurons would be primarily responsible for the induction of sleep, while MnPn neurons may also have a homeostatic role in sleep control. It was later demonstrated that the VLPO and the suprachiasmatic nucleus (SCN), a critical site in the circadian rhythm network (Chapter 14), have synchronized activity.[14] Considering that both areas are interconnected and receive inputs from the retinal ganglion cells, it is thus possible that circadian- and photic-linked information may be conveyed to modulate VLPO activity[1] (Figure 22.2).

Electrophysiology experiments in behaving rats have shown that neurons recorded in the VLPO and MnPn are active during SWS, generally anticipating its onset by several seconds. Further, their firing rate is positively correlated with sleep depth and duration. Some of these neurons are also active during PS, with a higher firing frequency than during the preceding SWS.[15] In addition, VLPO and MnPn neurons display a firing pattern reciprocal to the wake-active neurons (discussed in this chapter). Functionally, bilateral neurotoxic destruction of the VLPO is followed by a profound and long-lasting insomnia in rats.[16] Retrograde and anterograde tract-tracing studies indicate that VLPO and MnPn neurons are reciprocally connected with wake-active neurons such as those containing histamine in the TMN, hypocretin in the perifornical hypothalamic area (PeF), serotonin in the dorsal raphe nuclei (DRN), NA in the LC, and acetylcholine in the pontine (laterodorsal tegmental (LDT) and pedunculopontine tegmental (PPT)) and basal forebrain nuclei. In these wake-promoting areas, extracellular levels of GABA increase during SWS compared to W. It has also been shown that Fos-positive neurons in the VLPO express galanin mRNA, and 80% of VLPO neurons projecting to the TMN contain both galanin and glutamic acid decarboxylase (GAD), the GABA-synthesizing enzyme. Finally, electrical stimulation of the VLPO area evokes a GABA-mediated inhibition of TMN neurons, suggesting that VLPO and MnPn efferents to the wake-promoting systems are inhibitory.[1]

MECHANISMS CONTROLLING THE ACTIVITY OF NREM (SWS) SLEEP-INDUCING NEURONS

Electrophysiological recordings of VLPO neurons in rat brain slices showed that they contain a homogeneous neuronal group with specific intrinsic membrane properties, a clear-cut chemomorphology, and an inhibitory response to the major waking neurotransmitters. Their high proportion matching that of cells active during sleep and their pharmacological profile represent convincing arguments about their status as presumed sleep-promoting (PSP) neurons.[17] It was further shown that PSP neurons are GABAergic and galaninergic in nature, are multipolar triangular shaped, and exhibit a potent low-threshold calcium potential. These neurons are always inhibited by NA, via postsynaptic alpha2-adrenoceptors. The wake-promoting drug modafinil was shown to increase the NA-mediated inhibition of VLPO neurons, perhaps by blocking NA reuptake by local noradrenergic terminals.[18] Interestingly, NA-inhibited neurons are also inhibited by acetylcholine through muscarinic postsynaptic and nicotinic presynaptic actions on noradrenergic terminals. In contrast, histamine and hypocretin did not modulate PSP neurons.[17,19] Finally, serotonin showed complex effects, inducing either excitation (50%, Type 2) or inhibition (50%, Type 1) of the PSP neurons.[1,20]

Among processes that are likely to modulate the activity of PSP neurons, homeostatic mechanisms, involving natural sleep-promoting factors accumulating during waking, had long been thought to play a crucial role in triggering sleep. Among these factors, prostaglandin D2 and adenosine have been functionally implicated in sleep, although their neuronal targets and mechanisms of action remain largely unknown. In this context, we showed that application of an adenosine A_{2A} receptor ($A_{2A}R$) agonist evoked direct excitatory effects specifically in Type 2 PSP neurons that are also activated by serotonin.[1,20] Other results also suggested that adenosine may directly activate VLPO neurons at sleep onset via an action on postsynaptic $A_{2A}R$. Indeed, infusion of an $A_{2A}R$ agonist into the subarachnoid space rostral to the VLPO increases SWS and induces Fos expression in VLPO neurons[21] (Figure 22.2).

In contrast, a number of studies showed that adenosine A_1 receptors (A_1R) promote sleep through inhibition of the wake-promoting neurons, in particular cholinergic and hypocretin neurons.[22,23] However, transgenic mice that lack A_1R exhibit normal homeostatic regulation of sleep. In contrast, the lack of $A_{2A}R$ prevents normal sleep regulation and blocks the wake-inducing effect of caffeine, suggesting that the activation of $A_{2A}R$ is crucial in SWS.[24–26]

OVERVIEW OF THE NEURONAL NETWORK RESPONSIBLE FOR SWS (NREM) SLEEP

A line of evidence indicates that both the VLPO and the MnPn contain neurons responsible for sleep onset and maintenance. These neurons are inhibited by noradrenergic and cholinergic inputs during waking. The majority of them start firing at sleep onset (drowsiness) in response to excitatory, homeostatic (adenosine and serotonin), and circadian drives (suprachiasmatic input). These activated neurons, through the reciprocal GABAergic inhibition of all wake-promoting systems, would be in a position to suddenly unbalance the "flip-flop" network, as required for switching from W or drowsiness to SWS. Conversely, the slow removal of excitatory influences would result in a progressive firing decrease in VLPO neurons and, therefore, active wake-promoting systems leading to awakening.[20,27]

MECHANISMS INVOLVED IN PARADOXICAL (REM) SLEEP GENESIS (FIGURE 22.3)

The Localization of the Neurons Generating PS in the Pontine Reticular Formation

It was first shown that a state characterized by muscle atonia and REM persists following decortication, cerebellar ablation, or brainstem transections rostral to the pons and in the "pontine cat", a preparation in which all the structures rostral to the pons have been removed.[28] These results indicated that brainstem structures are necessary and sufficient to trigger and maintain the state of PS. Electrolytic and chemical lesions showed that the dorsal part of the pontis oralis (PnO) and caudalis (PnC) nuclei, also named the peri-locus coeruleus α (peri-LCα), pontine inhibitory area (PIA), and subcoeruleus nucleus (SubC), contains the neurons responsible for PS onset.[28] More recently, a corresponding area has been identified in rats and named the sublaterodorsal tegmental nucleus (SLD). It was also shown that a bilateral injection in cats of a cholinergic agonist, carbachol, into the PnO and PnC dramatically increases PS quantities in cats.[29,30] In addition, the PnO and PnC and the adjacent LDT and PPT cholinergic nuclei contain many neurons that show a tonic firing selective to PS (called "PS-on" neurons).[31,32] From these results, it was thought for more than 40 years that the PS-on neurons generating PS were cholinoceptive and cholinergic.

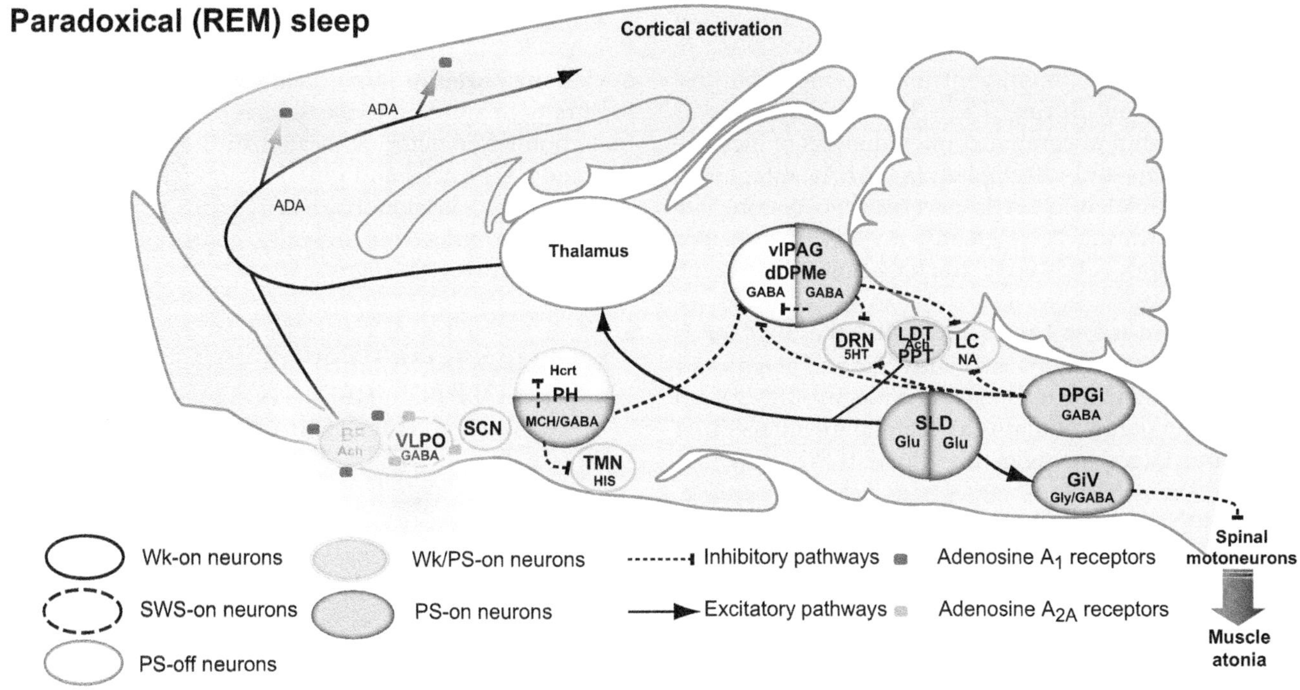

FIGURE 22.3 **Neuronal networks responsible for paradoxical (PS; also called REM) sleep.** PS onset would be due to the activation of glutamatergic PS-on neurons localized in the sublaterodorsal tegmental nucleus (SLD). During waking (W) and SWS (NREM) sleep, these PS-on neurons would be inhibited by a tonic inhibitory GABAergic tone originating from PS-off neurons localized in the ventrolateral periaqueductal gray (vlPAG) and the dorsal deep mesencephalic nucleus (dDPMe). These neurons would be activated during W by the hypocretin (Hcrt) neurons and the monoaminergic neurons. The onset of PS would be due to the activation by intrinsic mechanisms of PS-on GABAergic neurons localized in the posterior lateral hypothalamic area, the dorsal paragigantocellular reticular nucleus (DPGi), and the vlPAG. These neurons would also inactivate the PS-off monoaminergic neurons during PS. The disinhibited ascending SLD PS-on neurons would in turn induce cortical activation via their projections to intralaminar thalamic relay neurons in collaboration with W/PS-on cholinergic and glutamatergic neurons from the LDT and PPT, mesencephalic and pontine reticular nuclei, and basal forebrain. Descending PS-on SLD neurons would induce muscle atonia via their excitatory projections to glycinergic premotoneurons localized in the alpha and ventral gigantocellular reticular nuclei (GiA and GiV, respectively). The exit from PS would be due to the activation of waking systems since PS episodes are almost always terminated by an arousal. The waking systems would inhibit the GABAergic PS-on neurons localized in the DPGi and vlPAG. Since the duration of PS is negatively coupled with the metabolic rate, we propose that the activity of the waking systems is triggered to end PS to restore competing physiological parameters like thermoregulation. (The figure is reproduced in color section.)

PARADOXICAL (REM) SLEEP-GENERATING NEURONS: THE SWITCH FROM ACETYLCHOLINE TO GLUTAMATE

However, in contrast to cats, carbachol iontophoresis into the rat SLD failed to induce a significant increase in PS quantities.[33] Furthermore, only a few cholinergic neurons were immunostained for c-Fos in the LDT, PPT, and SLD after PS hypersomnia.[34,35] Finally, neurochemical lesions in rats of both the LDT and PPT induced no effect on PS and cortical activation.[36] Then, Lu et al.[36] reported for the first time the presence of neurons expressing a specific marker of glutamatergic neurons, the vesicular glutamate transporter 2 (vGlut2) in the SLD. We recently further demonstrated that most of the Fos-labeled neurons localized in the SLD after PS recovery express vGlut2.[37] Altogether, these results obtained in rats indicate that the PS-on SLD neurons triggering PS are glutamatergic.

A number of recent results further suggest that PS-on glutamatergic neurons located in the SLD generate muscle atonia via descending projections to PS-on GABA and glycinergic premotoneurons located at the medullary level rather than directly in the spinal cord. First, by means of intracellular recordings during PS, it has been shown that trigeminal, hypoglossal and spinal motoneurons are tonically hyperpolarized by large inhibitory postsynaptic potentials (IPSPs) during PS. Furthermore, when these recordings were combined with local iontophoretic application of strychnine (a specific antagonist of the inhibitory neurotransmitter, glycine), motoneuron hyperpolarization strongly decreased, indicating that they are tonically inhibited by glycinergic neurons during PS.[38–40] It has then been shown that the levels of glycine but also those of

GABA increase within hypoglossal and spinal motor pools during PS-like atonia, suggesting that GABA, in addition to glycine, might contribute to motoneurons' hyperpolarization during PS.[41] Furthermore, it was recently shown that combined microdialysis of bicuculline, strychnine, and phaclophen (a $GABA_B$ antagonist) in the trigeminal nucleus is necessary to restore jaw muscle tone during PS.[42] Finally, mice with impaired glycinergic and GABAergic transmissions display PS without atonia.[43]

In addition, it has been shown that the SLD sends direct efferent projections to GABAergic and glycinergic neurons located in the nucleus raphe magnus (RMg) and the ventral gigantocellular (GiV), alpha gigantocellular (GiA), and lateral paragigantocellular (LPGi) reticular nuclei.[33,44] Furthermore, glutamate release increases specifically during PS in the GiA and GiV.[45] In addition, injection of non-NMDA glutamate agonists in these nuclei suppresses muscle tone, while an increased tonus is seen during PS in cats with GiA and GiV cytotoxic lesion.[46,47] In addition, it was previously shown in cats using antidromic activation that SLD PS-on neurons directly project to the ventral medulla but not to the spinal cord, whereas SLD neurons with a firing rate unrelated to PS display spinal cord projections.[31] Besides, GABAergic and glycinergic neurons of the GiA, GiV, LPGi, and RMg express c-Fos after induction of PS by bicuculline (Bic, a $GABA_A$ antagonist) injection in the SLD.[33] In addition, nearly all Fos-labeled neurons localized in these nuclei after 3 h of PS recovery following 72 h of PS deprivation express GAD67 mRNA.[48] At variance with these results, it has been shown by combining retrograde tracing with vglut2 labeling that some of the glutamatergic neurons located in the SLD directly project to the spinal cord.[36] Furthermore, it was shown that 10% of these neurons are Fos-labeled during PS enhanced by dark conditions. It was also recently shown that inactivation in mice of the glutamatergic but not of the GABAergic and glycinergic neurons of the GiV region induced an increased motor activity during PS.[49] However, inactivation of GABAergic and glycinergic transmissions in the spinal cord induced only the occurrence of small phasic movements during PS sleep in contrast to medullary lesions, suggesting that spinal cord GABAergic and glycinergic interneurons might play a minor role compared to medullary ones.[50]

In view of all these results, we propose that the SLD glutamatergic PS-on neurons induce muscle atonia during PS by means of direct projections to medullary RMg, GiA, GiV, and LPGi, and, to a minor extent, spinal GABAergic and glycinergic PS-on neurons. These neurons hyperpolarize motoneurons mainly using glycine but also, to a minor extent, GABA acting on $GABA_A$ and $GABA_B$ receptors.

It has also been shown that a subpopulation of SLD PS-on neurons projects to the intralaminar thalamic nuclei, the posterior hypothalamus (PH), and the basal forebrain. In addition to the SLD, it has also been shown that cholinergic neurons located in the pedunculopontine and LDT nuclei and glutamatergic neurons located in the reticular formation are active during both waking and PS and, projecting rostrally, contribute to cortical activation during PS sleep.[1,33]

MECHANISMS RESPONSIBLE FOR SLD PS-ON NEURON ACTIVATION DURING PS

In cats and rats, microdialysis administration in the SLD of kainic acid, a glutamate agonist, induces a PS-like state.[33,51] A long-lasting PS-like hypersomnia can also be pharmacologically induced with a short latency in head-restrained unanesthetized rats by iontophoretic application into the SLD of bicuculline or gabazine, two $GABA_A$ receptor antagonists.[33] Furthermore, application of kynurenate, a glutamate antagonist, reverses the PS-like state induced by bicuculline.[33] In the head-restrained rat, we also recorded neurons within the SLD that were specifically active during PS and excited following bicuculline or gabazine iontophoresis.[52] Taken together, these data indicate that the activation of SLD PS-on neurons is mainly due to the removal during PS of a tonic GABAergic tone present during W and SWS combined with the continuous presence of a glutamatergic input. Combining retrograde tracing with cholera toxin b subunit (CTb) injected in SLD and glutamate decarboxylase 67 (GAD67) immunohistochemistry or Fos immunohistochemistry with GAD67 mRNA "in situ hybridization" after 72 h of PS deprivation, we recently demonstrated that the ventrolateral periaqueductal gray (vlPAG) and the adjacent dorsal deep mesencephalic nucleus (dDPMe) are the only ponto-medullary structures containing a large number of GABAergic neurons activated during PS deprivation projecting to the SLD.[48] Furthermore, injection of muscimol in the vlPAG and/or the dDPMe induces strong increases in PS quantities in cats[53] and rats.[48] Finally, neurochemical lesion of these two structures induces profound increases in PS quantities.[36] These congruent experimental data led us to propose that PS-off GABAergic neurons within the vlPAG and the dDPMe are gating PS by tonically inhibiting PS-on neurons of the SLD during W and SWS. Our results indicate that these GABAergic neurons are crucial to gate PS, although they do not rule out a secondary role for monoaminergic neurons, because increases in monoaminergic transmission by either reuptake blockers or agonists are well known to inhibit PS.[54]

The targets of monoaminergic neurons responsible for their inhibitory effects remain to be defined. They can either excite PS-off neurons or inhibit PS-on neurons. One possibility is that the monoaminergic neurons are exciting the GABAergic PS-off neurons during waking to preclude PS onset.

NEURONS INHIBITING THE GABAERGIC AND MONOAMINERGIC PS-OFF NEURONS AT THE ONSET OF AND DURING PS

We previously reported that bicuculline application on serotonergic and noradrenergic neurons during SWS or PS restores a tonic firing pattern in both types of neurons.[4,5,55] These results strongly suggest that an increased GABA release is responsible for the PS-selective inactivation of monoaminergic neurons. This hypothesis is well supported by microdialysis experiments in cats, which measured a significant increase in GABA release in the DRN and LC during PS as compared to W and SWS but no detectable changes in glycine concentration.[56,57]

By combining retrograde tracing with CTb and GAD immunohistochemistry in rats, we found that the vlPAG and the dorsal paragigantocellular reticular nucleus (DPGi)[5,58] contained numerous GABAergic neurons projecting to both the DRN and LC. We then demonstrated, by combining c-Fos and retrograde labeling, that both nuclei contain numerous LC-projecting neurons that are selectively activated during PS rebound following PS deprivation.[59,60] Furthermore, we found that the DPGi contains numerous PS-on neurons that are increasing their activity specifically during PS.[61] Taken together, these data highly suggest that the DPGi contains the neurons responsible for the inactivation of LC noradrenergic neurons during PS.[61] A contribution from the vlPAG in the inhibition during PS of LC noradrenergic and dorsal raphe serotonergic neurons is also likely. Indeed, an increase in c-Fos and GAD immunoreactive neurons has been reported in the vlPAG after a PS rebound following deprivation in rats.[35,48] In summary, a large body of data indicates that GABAergic PS-on neurons localized in the vlPAG and the DPGi hyperpolarize the monoaminergic neurons during PS.

We first proposed that these neurons might be also responsible for the inhibition of the dDPMe and vlPAG PS-off GABAergic neurons during PS. To test this hypothesis, we recently localized the neurons active during PS hypersomnia projecting to the dDPMe and vlPAG PS-off GABAergic neurons.[62] We found out that the vlPAG and the DPGi, respectively, contained a substantial and a small number of CTb and Fos double-labeled neurons in PS hypersomniac rats. Although the GABAergic nature of these neurons remains to be demonstrated, our results indicate that the vlPAG and DPGi might contain PS-on GABAergic neurons inhibiting the vlPAG and dDPMe PS-off GABAergic neurons at the onset of and during PS. However, we also demonstrated that the lateral hypothalamic area (LH) is the only brain structure containing a very large number of neurons activated during PS hypersomnia and projecting to the VLPAG and dDPMe. We further demonstrated that 44% of these neurons express the neuropeptide melanin-concentrating hormone (MCH). These results indicate that LH hypothalamic neurons might play a crucial role in PS onset and maintenance by means of descending projections to the vlPAG and dDPMe PS-off GABAergic neurons. They confirmed previous data, discussed in the "Role of the MCH and GABAergic Neurons" section, indicating that the PH contains neurons implicated in PS control.

ROLE OF THE MCH AND GABAERGIC NEURONS OF THE LATERAL HYPOTHALAMIC AREA IN PS CONTROL

To localize all brain areas activated during PS, we extensively mapped the distribution of c-Fos-positive neurons in control rats, rats selectively deprived of PS for 72 h, and rats allowed to recover from such deprivation.[60,63] Surprisingly, we observed a very large number of c-Fos-positive cells in the PH, including the zona incerta (ZI), PeF, and LH. Only a few experimental results already supported the notion that the PH contributes to PS regulation. Bilateral injection of muscimol in the cat mammillary and tuberal hypothalamus induced a drastic inhibition of PS.[64] Furthermore, neurons specifically active during PS were recorded in the PH of cats[65–67] or head-restrained rats.[68] By using double immunostaining, we further showed that around 75% of PH cells labeled for c-Fos after PS rebound express GAD67 mRNA and are therefore GABAergic.[69] One-third of these GABAergic neurons were also immunoreactive for the neuropeptide MCH. Almost 60% of all of the MCH-immunoreactive neurons counted in PeF, ZI, and LHA were c-Fos-positive.[63,70] We recently further demonstrated that these neurons co-contain Nesfatin, another recently discovered peptide.[71] In support of our Fos data, it has recently been shown in head-restrained rats that MCH neurons fire exclusively during PS.[72] Importantly, MCH neurons start to fire simultaneously with the onset of PS and, therefore, can play a role in PS maintenance but not in PS induction. Nevertheless, rats receiving intracerebroventricular (ICV) administration of MCH showed a strong dose-dependent increase in PS and, to a minor extent, SWS quantities, due to an increased number of PS bouts.[63] Further, subcutaneous injection of an MCH antagonist decreases SWS and PS quantities[73] and mice with genetically inactivated MCH signaling exhibit altered vigilance state architecture and sleep homeostasis.[74,75] In addition, disruption of Nesfatin-1 signaling by ICV administration of Nesfatin-1 antiserum or antisense against the nucleobindin2 (NUCB2) prohormone suppressed PS. Further, the infusion of Nesfatin-1 antiserum after selective PS deprivation precluded PS recovery.[71] Finally, it was recently shown that optogenetic stimulation of MCH neurons increased total time in SWS and PS at night.[76]

In agreement with our results showing that MCH neurons constitute only one-third of the GABAergic neurons activated during PS hypersomnia, it was recently shown that a large population of GABAergic neurons without MCH localized in the LH discharge maximally during PS.[77] These neurons are mostly silent during active W with high muscle tone, and they progressively increase their discharge from quiet W through SWS to be maximally active during PS. Since these neurons anticipate PS onset, they can play a role in triggering the state.

To determine the function of the LH MCH+/GABA+ and MCH−/GABA+ neurons in PS control, we inactivated all LH neurons with muscimol (a $GABA_A$ agonist) or only those bearing alpha-2 adrenergic receptors using clonidine. We found that muscimol and, to a lesser degree, clonidine bilateral injections in the LH induce an inhibition of PS with or without an increase in SWS quantities, respectively. We further showed that after muscimol injection in the LH, the vlPAG and dDPMe regions contain a large number of c-FOS−GAD67+ and c-FOS−CTb+ neurons in animals with a CTb injection in the SLD. Our results indicate that the activation of PS-on MCH and GABAergic neurons localized in the LH is a necessary step for PS to occur. They further suggest that MCH and GABAergic PS-on neurons of the LH control PS onset and maintenance by means of a direct inhibitory projection to vlPAG and dDPMe PS-off GABAergic neurons. From our results, it can be proposed that MCH and GABAergic neurons of the LH constitute a master generator of PS, which controls a slave generator located in the brainstem. At variance with this hypothesis, it is well accepted that the brainstem is necessary and sufficient to generate a state characterized by muscle atonia and REM.[28] To reconcile these and our results, we therefore propose that after removal of the forebrain, the brainstem generator is sufficient to induce a state with muscle atonia and REM by means of a reorganization of the brainstem systems generating PS. However, the brainstem generator would be under the control of the LH generator in intact animals.

In addition to the descending pathway to the PS-off GABAergic neurons, the MCH and GABAergic PS-on neurons might also promote PS by means of other pathways to the histaminergic neurons, the monoaminergic PS-off neurons, and the hypocretinergic neurons.[33,78,79]

The mechanisms at the origin of the activation of the MCH and GABAergic neurons of the LH at the entrance into PS remain to be identified. A large number of studies indicate that MCH neurons also play a key role in metabolism control.[80] Therefore, the activation of these neurons at the onset and during PS could be influenced by the metabolic state. In addition, we propose that yet-undiscovered endogenous cellular or molecular clock-like mechanisms may play a role in their activation.

The cessation of activity of the MCH and GABAergic PS-on neurons and, more largely of all, the PS-on neurons at the end of PS episodes is certainly due to a completely different mechanism than the entrance into the state. Indeed, animals are entering PS slowly from SWS, while in contrast they exit from it abruptly by a microarousal.[81] This indicates that the end of PS is induced by the activation of the W systems like the monoaminergic, hypocretin, or histaminergic neurons. The mechanisms responsible for their activation remain to be identified.

CONCLUSION

A Network Model for PS Onset and Maintenance

The onset of PS would be due to the activation by intrinsic and extrinsic factors of PS-on MCH and GABAergic neurons localized in the LH. These neurons would inhibit, at the onset of and during PS, the PS-off GABAergic neurons localized in the vlPAG and dDPMe tonically inhibiting during W and SWS the glutamatergic PS-on neurons from the SLD. The disinhibited ascending glutamatergic SLD PS-on neurons would in turn induce cortical activation via their projections to intralaminar thalamic relay neurons in collaboration with W PS-on cholinergic and glutamatergic neurons from the LDT and PPT, mesencephalic and pontine reticular nuclei, and basal forebrain. Descending glutamatergic PS-on SLD neurons would induce muscle atonia via their excitatory projections to GABAergic and glycinergic premotoneurons localized in the RMg, GiA, and GiV. PS-on GABAergic neurons localized in the LH, DPGi, and vlPAG would also inactivate the PS-off orexin (hypocretin) and monoaminergic neurons during PS. The exit from PS would be due to the activation of waking systems since PS episodes are almost always terminated by an arousal. The waking systems would reciprocally inhibit the GABAergic PS-on neurons localized in the LH, vlPAG, and DPGi. Since the duration of PS is negatively coupled with the metabolic rate, we propose that the activity of the waking systems is triggered to end PS to restore crucial physiological parameters like thermoregulation.

Dysfunctions of the Network Responsible for Narcolepsy

Narcolepsy–cataplexy is characterized by two major symptoms, excessive daytime sleepiness (EDS) and cataplexy, and by two auxiliary symptoms, hypnagogic hallucinations and sleep paralysis. EDS occurs daily and is characterized by sleep episodes with a premature onset of REM sleep. A sudden drop of muscle tone triggered by emotional factors, most often positive, characterizes cataplexy. It can affect all striated muscles or be limited to facial muscles or to the upper or lower limbs. The monosynaptic H-reflex is suppressed, like during PS. Patients remain fully conscious during cataplexy.[82] All of these symptoms suggest that PS is disinhibited in narcoleptic patients. It has then been shown that disruption of type 2 hypocretin receptor induces narcolepsy in dogs and mice.[83,84] No mutation was found in human narcoleptics.[85] Instead, a marked reduction in the quantities of the peptide Hcrt 1 was found in their cerebrospinal fluid, and a disappearance of Hcrt staining was observed in the hypothalamus of postmortem brain tissues.[85] Importantly, it has been shown that Hcrt neurons are specifically active during W and increase their activity during muscle activation.[86,87] They are silent during SWS or PS, excepting during phasic twitches during which they can fire in burst. Interestingly, they start to fire several seconds before the onset of W at the end of PS episodes.[72] Hcrt neurons, like the monoaminergic neurons, send projections throughout the brain, from the olfactory bulb, cerebral cortex, and thalamus to the brainstem and the spinal cord.[88,89] It is therefore difficult to determine, based solely on the projections of the Hcrt neurons, which missing pathway(s) is (are) responsible for the four symptoms of narcolepsy. It has been proposed that the absence of dense Hcrt projections to the histaminergic and noradrenergic LC neurons might be responsible for narcolepsy symptoms.[90] Indeed, ICV administration or local injection of Hcrt in the noradrenergic LC or the histaminergic TMN neurons induces W and inhibits PS.[91–93] Furthermore, administration of selective NA reuptake inhibitors and alpha-1 adrenergic agonists specifically suppresses cataplexy.[82] Besides, the absence of the hypocretin input on serotonin neurons could also play a role, since selective serotonin reuptake inhibitors are effective in treating cataplexy, at least in humans.[82] Finally, a missing hypocretin projection to GABAergic PS-off neurons might be implicated, since the most recent treatment for cataplexy, gamma-hydroxybutyrate (GHB), may act through increased $GABA_B$ transmission.[94] This is an attractive hypothesis in view of our recent finding that GABAergic PS-off neurons localized in the vlPAG and dDPMe region gate the onset of PS by means of their tonic inhibition of the SLD neurons during W and SWS. Furthermore, we found that inactivating neurons in the vlPAG and dDPMe region by means of muscimol induced not only an increase in PS quantities but also an increase in sleep-onset PS.[48] It thus can be hypothesized that, during emotions in healthy subjects, there is a phasic increase in hypocretin release on GABAergic PS-off neurons. Since the hypocretin neurons also project to monoaminergic neurons, they would excite these neurons, which in turn would reinforce the activation of the GABAergic PS-off neurons via direct projections (Figure 22.1). The phasic increase of inhibition by GABAergic PS-off neurons would counterbalance an increased glutamatergic excitation of SLD neurons arising in the central amygdala. We indeed demonstrated that non-GABAergic neurons of the central amygdala project to the SLD.[95] Furthermore, neurons increasing their activity during W and/or PS or prior to and during cataplexy were recorded in the central amygdala.[96,97] In short, cataplexy would be due to a phasic activation of SLD neurons by central amygdala neurons, normally counterbalanced by an increased phasic GABAergic inhibition from vlPAG and dDPMe neurons. Importantly, our hypothesis implies that the projection from central amygdala neurons is specific to the PS-on SLD neurons responsible for muscle atonia projecting to GABAergic and glycinergic premotoneurons and not to those responsible for PS itself or the EEG activation. Indeed, in such a case, a full PS episode would be induced. Cataplexy would be inhibited in narcoleptic patients treated with serotonin and noradrenergic reuptake inhibitors or alpha-1 adrenergic agonists by means of increased excitation of the GABAergic PS-off neurons. EDS, sleep paralysis, and hypnagogic hallucinations suggest that the Hcrt neurons might inhibit and delay the onset of PS and strongly contribute to the abrupt end of PS episodes, in line with their increase in firing before the end of a PS episode.[72] In their absence, the onset of PS could occur more quickly and the end of PS might take more time, leading to hypnagogic hallucinations and sleep paralysis, respectively. The inhibition of PS by hypocretin neurons would be direct by means of excitation of the PS-off GABAergic and monoaminergic neurons but also indirect via direct excitation of the motor system, including the motoneurons that express hypocretin type 2 receptors.[98]

Acknowledgments

This work was supported by Centre National de la Recherche Scientifique, Université de Lyon, and Université Lyon 1. The authors have no conflicts of interest to declare.

References

1. Fort P, Bassetti CL, Luppi PH. Alternating vigilance states: new insights regarding neuronal networks and mechanisms. *Eur J Neurosci.* 2009;29(9):1741–1753.
2. Moruzzi G, Magoun HW. Brain stem reticular formation and activation of the EEG. *J Neuropsychiatry Clin Neurosci JID – 8911344.* 1949;7(2):251–267.
3. Jones BE. Basic mechanisms of sleep–wake states. In: Kryger MH, Roth T, Dement WC, eds. *Principles and Practice of Sleep Medicine.* Philadelphia: Saunders W.B.; 1994:145–162.
4. Gervasoni D, Darracq L, Fort P, Souliere F, Chouvet G, Luppi PH. Electrophysiological evidence that noradrenergic neurons of the rat locus coeruleus are tonically inhibited by GABA during sleep. *Eur J Neurosci.* 1998;10(3):964–970.
5. Gervasoni D, Peyron C, Rampon C, et al. Role and origin of the GABAergic innervation of dorsal raphe serotonergic neurons. *J Neurosci.* 2000;20(11):4217–4225.
6. von Economo C. In: Von Bethe A, Bergman GV, Embden G, Ellinger UA, eds. *Die Pathologie des Schlafes. Handbuch des Normalen und Pathologischen Physiologie.* Berlin: Springer; 1926:591–610.
7. McGinty DJ, Sterman MB. Sleep suppression after basal forebrain lesions in the cat. *Science.* 1968;160(833):1253–1255.
8. Nauta W. Hypothalamic regulation of sleep in rats. An experimental study. *J Neurophysiol.* 1946;9:285–316.
9. Ranson SW. Somnolence caused by hypothalamic lesions in the monkey. *Arch Neurol Psychiatry.* 1939;41:1–23.
10. Sterman MB, Clemente CD. Forebrain inhibitory mechanisms: cortical synchronization induced by basal forebrain stimulation. *Exp Neurol.* 1962;6:91–102.
11. Szymusiak R, McGinty D. Sleep-related neuronal discharge in the basal forebrain of cats. *Brain Res.* 1986;370(1):82–92.
12. Sherin JE, Shiromani PJ, McCarley RW, Saper CB. Activation of ventrolateral preoptic neurons during sleep. *Science.* 1996;271(5246):216–219.
13. Gvilia I, Turner A, McGinty D, Szymusiak R. Preoptic area neurons and the homeostatic regulation of rapid eye movement sleep. *J Neurosci.* 2006;26(11):3037–3044.
14. Novak CM, Nunez AA. Daily rhythms in Fos activity in the rat ventrolateral preoptic area and midline thalamic nuclei. *Am J Physiol JID – 0370511.* 1998;275(5 Pt 2):R1620–R1626.
15. Szymusiak R, Alam N, Steininger TL, McGinty D. Sleep-waking discharge patterns of ventrolateral preoptic/anterior hypothalamic neurons in rats. *Brain Res.* 1998;803(1–2):178–188.
16. Lu J, Greco MA, Shiromani P, Saper CB. Effect of lesions of the ventrolateral preoptic nucleus on NREM and REM sleep. *J Neurosci.* 2000;20(10):3830–3842.
17. Gallopin T, Fort P, Eggermann E, et al. Identification of sleep-promoting neurons in vitro. *Nature.* 2000;404(6781): 992–995.
18. Gallopin T, Luppi PH, Rambert FA, Frydman A, Fort P. Effect of the wake-promoting agent modafinil on sleep-promoting neurons from the ventrolateral preoptic nucleus: an in vitro pharmacologic study. *Sleep.* 2004;27(1):19–25.
19. Eggermann E, Serafin M, Bayer L, et al. Orexins/hypocretins excite basal forebrain cholinergic neurones. *Neuroscience.* 2001;108(2):177–181.
20. Gallopin T, Luppi PH, Cauli B, et al. The endogenous somnogen adenosine excites a subset of sleep-promoting neurons via A_{2A} receptors in the ventrolateral preoptic nucleus. *Neuroscience.* 2005;134(4):1377–1390.
21. Scammell TE, Gerashchenko DY, Mochizuki T, et al. An adenosine A_{2a} agonist increases sleep and induces Fos in ventrolateral preoptic neurons. *Neuroscience.* 2001;107(4):653–663.
22. Porkka-Heiskanen T, Strecker RE, McCarley RW. Brain site-specificity of extracellular adenosine concentration changes during sleep deprivation and spontaneous sleep: an in vivo microdialysis study. *Neuroscience JID – 7605074.* 2000;99(3): 507–517.
23. Rainnie DG, Grunze HC, McCarley RW, Greene RW. Adenosine inhibition of mesopontine cholinergic neurons: implications for EEG arousal. *Science.* 1994;263(5147):689–692.
24. Stenberg D, Litonius E, Halldner L, Johansson B, Fredholm BB, Porkka-Heiskanen T. Sleep and its homeostatic regulation in mice lacking the adenosine A_1 receptor. *J Sleep Res.* 2003; 12(4):283–290.
25. Urade Y, Eguchi N, Qu WM, et al. Minireview: sleep regulation in adenosine A_{2A} receptor-deficient mice. *Neurology.* 2003;61(11 Suppl. 6):S94–S96.
26. Huang ZL, Qu WM, Eguchi N, et al. Adenosine A_{2A}, but not A_1, receptors mediate the arousal effect of caffeine. *Nat Neurosci.* 2005;8(7):858–859.
27. Fort P, Luppi PH, Gallopin T. In vitro identification of the presumed sleep-promoting neurons of the ventrolateral preoptic nucleus (VLPO). In: Luppi PH, ed. *Sleep: Circuits and Functions.* CRC Press; 2005:43–64.
28. Jouvet M. Recherches sur les structures nerveuses et les mécanismes responsables des différentes phases du sommeil physiologique. *Arch Ital Biol.* 1962;100:125–206.
29. George R, Haslett WL, Jenden DJ. A cholinergic mechanism in the brainstem reticular formation: induction of paradoxical sleep. *Int J Neuropharmacol.* 1964;3:541–552.
30. Vanni-Mercier G, Sakai K, Lin JS, Jouvet M. Mapping of cholinoceptive brainstem structures responsible for the generation of paradoxical sleep in the cat. *Arch Ital Biol.* 1989; 127(3):133–164.
31. Sakai K. Neurons responsible for paradoxical sleep. In: Wauquier A, Janssen Research Foundation, eds. *Sleep: Neurotransmitters and Neuromodulators.* New York: Raven Press; 1985:29–42.
32. Sakai K, Koyama Y. Are there cholinergic and non-cholinergic paradoxical sleep-on neurones in the pons? *Neuroreport.* 1996;7(15–17):2449–2453.
33. Boissard R, Gervasoni D, Schmidt MH, Barbagli B, Fort P, Luppi PH. The rat ponto-medullary network responsible for paradoxical sleep onset and maintenance: a combined microinjection and functional neuroanatomical study. *Eur J Neurosci.* 2002;16(10):1959–1973.
34. Verret L, Leger L, Fort P, Luppi PH. Cholinergic and noncholinergic brainstem neurons expressing Fos after paradoxical (REM) sleep deprivation and recovery. *Eur J Neurosci.* 2005;21(9):2488–2504.
35. Maloney KJ, Mainville L, Jones BE. Differential c-Fos expression in cholinergic, monoaminergic, and GABAergic cell groups of the pontomesencephalic tegmentum after paradoxical sleep deprivation and recovery. *J Neurosci.* 1999;19(8):3057–3072.
36. Lu J, Sherman D, Devor M, Saper CB. A putative flip-flop switch for control of REM sleep. *Nature.* 2006;441(7093):589–594.
37. Clement O, Sapin E, Berod A, Fort P, Luppi PH. Evidence that neurons of the sublaterodorsal tegmental nucleus triggering paradoxical (REM) sleep are glutamatergic. *Sleep.* 2011;34(4): 419–423.

38. Chase MH, Soja PJ, Morales FR. Evidence that glycine mediates the postsynaptic potentials that inhibit lumbar motoneurons during the atonia of active sleep. *J Neurosci.* 1989;9(3):743–751.
39. Soja PJ, Lopez-Rodriguez F, Morales FR, Chase MH. The postsynaptic inhibitory control of lumbar motoneurons during the atonia of active sleep: effect of strychnine on motoneuron properties. *J Neurosci.* 1991;11(9):2804–2811.
40. Yamuy J, Fung SJ, Xi M, Morales FR, Chase MH. Hypoglossal motoneurons are postsynaptically inhibited during carbachol-induced rapid eye movement sleep. *Neuroscience.* 1999;94(1): 11–15.
41. Kodama T, Lai YY, Siegel JM. Changes in inhibitory amino acid release linked to pontine-induced atonia: an in vivo microdialysis study. *J Neurosci.* 2003;23(4):1548–1554.
42. Brooks PL, Peever JH. Identification of the transmitter and receptor mechanisms responsible for REM sleep paralysis. *J Neurosci.* 2012;32(29):9785–9795.
43. Brooks PL, Peever JH. Impaired GABA and glycine transmission triggers cardinal features of rapid eye movement sleep behavior disorder in mice. *J Neurosci.* 2011;31(19):7111–7121.
44. Sirieix C, Gervasoni D, Luppi PH, Leger L. Role of the lateral paragigantocellular nucleus in the network of paradoxical (REM) sleep: an electrophysiological and anatomical study in the rat. *PLoS One.* 2012;7(1):e28724.
45. Kodama T, Lai YY, Siegel JM. Enhanced glutamate release during REM sleep in the rostromedial medulla as measured by in vivo microdialysis. *Brain Res.* 1998;780(1):178–181.
46. Lai YY, Siegel JM. Pontomedullary glutamate receptors mediating locomotion and muscle tone suppression. *J Neurosci.* 1991;11(9):2931–2937.
47. Holmes CJ, Jones BE. Importance of cholinergic, GABAergic, serotonergic and other neurons in the medial medullary reticular formation for sleep–wake states studied by cytotoxic lesions in the cat. *Neuroscience.* 1994;62(4):1179–1200.
48. Sapin E, Lapray D, Berod A, et al. Localization of the brainstem GABAergic neurons controlling paradoxical (REM) sleep. *PLoS One.* 2009;4(1):e4272.
49. Vetrivelan R, Fuller PM, Tong Q, Lu J. Medullary circuitry regulating rapid eye movement sleep and motor atonia. *J Neurosci.* 2009;29(29):9361–9369.
50. Krenzer M, Anaclet C, Vetrivelan R, et al. Brainstem and spinal cord circuitry regulating REM sleep and muscle atonia. *PLoS One.* 2011;6(10):e24998.
51. Onoe H, Sakai K. Kainate receptors: a novel mechanism in paradoxical (REM) sleep generation. *Neuroreport.* 1995;6(2):353–356.
52. Boissard R, Gervasoni D, Fort P, Henninot V, Barbagli B, Luppi PH. Neuronal networks responsible for paradoxical sleep onset and maintenance in rats: a new hypothesis. *Sleep.* 2000;23(Suppl.):107.
53. Sastre JP, Buda C, Kitahama K, Jouvet M. Importance of the ventrolateral region of the periaqueductal gray and adjacent tegmentum in the control of paradoxical sleep as studied by muscimol microinjections in the cat. *Neuroscience.* 1996;74(2):415–426.
54. Luppi PH, Clement O, Sapin E, et al. The neuronal network responsible for paradoxical sleep and its dysfunctions causing narcolepsy and rapid eye movement (REM) behavior disorder. *Sleep Med Rev.* 2011;15(3):153–163.
55. Darracq L, Gervasoni D, Souliere F, et al. Effect of strychnine on rat locus coeruleus neurones during sleep and wakefulness. *Neuroreport.* 1996;8(1):351–355.
56. Nitz D, Siegel J. GABA release in the dorsal raphe nucleus: role in the control of REM sleep. *Am J Physiol.* 1997;273(1 Pt 2): R451–R455.
57. Nitz D, Siegel JM. GABA release in the locus coeruleus as a function of sleep/wake state. *Neuroscience.* 1997;78(3):795–801.
58. Luppi PH, Peyron C, Rampon C, et al. Inhibitory mechanisms in the dorsal raphe nucleus and locus coeruleus during sleep. In: Lydic R, Baghdoyan HA, eds. *Handbook of Behavioral State Control.* CRC Press; 1999:195–211.
59. Verret L, Fort P, Luppi PH. Localization of the neurons responsible for the inhibition of locus coeruleus noradrenergic neurons during paradoxical sleep in the rat. *Sleep.* 2003;26:69.
60. Verret L, Fort P, Gervasoni D, Leger L, Luppi PH. Localization of the neurons active during paradoxical (REM) sleep and projecting to the locus coeruleus noradrenergic neurons in the rat. *J Comp Neurol.* 2006;495(5):573–586.
61. Goutagny R, Luppi PH, Salvert D, Lapray D, Gervasoni D, Fort P. Role of the dorsal paragigantocellular reticular nucleus in paradoxical (rapid eye movement) sleep generation: a combined electrophysiological and anatomical study in the rat. *Neuroscience.* 2008;152(3):849–857.
62. Clement O, Sapin E, Libourel PA, et al. The lateral hypothalamic area controls paradoxical (REM) sleep by means of descending projections to brainstem GABAergic neurons. *J Neurosci.* 2012;32(47):16763–16774.
63. Verret L, Goutagny R, Fort P, et al. A role of melanin-concentrating hormone producing neurons in the central regulation of paradoxical sleep. *BMC Neurosci.* 2003;4(1):19.
64. Lin JS, Sakai K, Vanni-Mercier G, Jouvet M. A critical role of the posterior hypothalamus in the mechanisms of wakefulness determined by microinjection of muscimol in freely moving cats. *Brain Res.* 1989;479(2):225–240.
65. Alam MN, Gong H, Alam T, Jaganath R, McGinty D, Szymusiak R. Sleep-waking discharge patterns of neurons recorded in the rat perifornical lateral hypothalamic area. *J Physiol.* 2002;538(Pt 2):619–631.
66. Koyama Y, Takahashi K, Kodama T, Kayama Y. State-dependent activity of neurons in the perifornical hypothalamic area during sleep and waking. *Neuroscience.* 2003;119(4):1209–1219.
67. Steininger TL, Alam MN, Gong H, Szymusiak R, McGinty D. Sleep-waking discharge of neurons in the posterior lateral hypothalamus of the albino rat. *Brain Res.* 1999;840(1–2): 138–147.
68. Goutagny R, Luppi PH, Salvert D, Gervasoni D, Fort P. GABAergic control of hypothalamic melanin-concentrating hormone-containing neurons across the sleep-waking cycle. *Neuroreport.* 2005;16(10):1069–1073.
69. Sapin E, Berod A, Leger L, Herman PA, Luppi PH, Peyron C. A very large number of GABAergic neurons are activated in the tuberal hypothalamus during paradoxical (REM) sleep hypersomnia. *PLoS One.* 2010;5(7):e11766.
70. Hanriot L, Camargo N, Courau AC, Leger L, Luppi PH, Peyron C. Characterization of the melanin-concentrating hormone neurons activated during paradoxical sleep hypersomnia in rats. *J Comp Neurol.* 2007;505(2):147–157.
71. Jego S, Salvert D, Renouard L, et al. Tuberal hypothalamic neurons secreting the satiety molecule Nesfatin-1 are critically involved in paradoxical (REM) sleep homeostasis. *PLoS One.* 2012;7(12):e52525.
72. Hassani OK, Lee MG, Jones BE. Melanin-concentrating hormone neurons discharge in a reciprocal manner to orexin neurons across the sleep–wake cycle. *Proc Natl Acad Sci USA.* 2009;106(7):2418–2422.
73. Ahnaou A, Drinkenburg WH, Bouwknecht JA, Alcazar J, Steckler T, Dautzenberg FM. Blocking melanin-concentrating hormone MCH_1 receptor affects rat sleep–wake architecture. *Eur J Pharmacol.* 2008;579(1–3):177–188.

74. Adamantidis A, Salvert D, Goutagny R, et al. Sleep architecture of the melanin-concentrating hormone receptor 1-knockout mice. *Eur J Neurosci.* 2008;27(7):1793–1800.
75. Willie JT, Sinton CM, Maratos-Flier E, Yanagisawa M. Abnormal response of melanin-concentrating hormone deficient mice to fasting: hyperactivity and rapid eye movement sleep suppression. *Neuroscience.* 2008;156(4):819–829.
76. Konadhode RR, Pelluru D, Blanco-Centurion C, et al. Optogenetic stimulation of MCH neurons increases sleep. *J Neurosci.* 2013;33(25):10257–10263.
77. Hassani OK, Henny P, Lee MG, Jones BE. GABAergic neurons intermingled with orexin and MCH neurons in the lateral hypothalamus discharge maximally during sleep. *Eur J Neurosci.* 2010.
78. Luppi PH, Boissard R, Gervasoni D, et al. The network responsible for paradoxical sleep onset and maintenance: a new theory based on the head-restrained rat model. In: Luppi PH, ed. *Sleep: Circuits and Function.* CRC Press; 2004:272.
79. Luppi PH, Gervasoni D, Verret L, et al. Paradoxical (REM) sleep genesis: the switch from an aminergic-cholinergic to a GABAergic-glutamatergic hypothesis. *J Physiol Paris.* 2006;100(5–6):271–283.
80. Qu D, Ludwig DS, Gammeltoft S, et al. A role for melanin-concentrating hormone in the central regulation of feeding behaviour. *Nature.* 1996;380(6571):243–247.
81. Gervasoni D, Lin SC, Ribeiro S, Soares ES, Pantoja J, Nicolelis MA. Global forebrain dynamics predict rat behavioral states and their transitions. *J Neurosci.* 2004;24(49):11137–11147.
82. Dauvilliers Y, Billiard M, Montplaisir J. Clinical aspects and pathophysiology of narcolepsy. *Clin Neurophysiol.* 2003;114(11):2000–2017.
83. Lin L, Faraco J, Li R, et al. The sleep disorder canine narcolepsy is caused by a mutation in the hypocretin (orexin) receptor 2 gene. *Cell.* 1999;98(3):365–376.
84. Chemelli RM, Willie JT, Sinton CM, et al. Narcolepsy in orexin knockout mice: molecular genetics of sleep regulation. *Cell.* 1999;98(4):437–451.
85. Peyron C, Faraco J, Rogers W, et al. A mutation in a case of early onset narcolepsy and a generalized absence of hypocretin peptides in human narcoleptic brains. *Nat Med.* 2000; 6(9):991–997.
86. Mileykovskiy BY, Kiyashchenko LI, Siegel JM. Behavioral correlates of activity in identified hypocretin/orexin neurons. *Neuron.* 2005;46(5):787–798.
87. Lee MG, Hassani OK, Jones BE. Discharge of identified orexin/hypocretin neurons across the sleep-waking cycle. *J Neurosci.* 2005;25(28):6716–6720.
88. van den Pol AN. Hypothalamic hypocretin (orexin): robust innervation of the spinal cord. *J Neurosci.* 1999;19(8):3171–3182.
89. Peyron C, Tighe DK, van den Pol AN, et al. Neurons containing hypocretin (orexin) project to multiple neuronal systems. *J Neurosci.* 1998;18(23):9996–10015.
90. Taheri S, Zeitzer JM, Mignot E. The role of hypocretins (orexins) in sleep regulation and narcolepsy. *Annu Rev Neurosci.* 2002;25:283–313.
91. Espana RA, Baldo BA, Kelley AE, Berridge CW. Wake-promoting and sleep-suppressing actions of hypocretin (orexin): basal forebrain sites of action. *Neuroscience.* 2001;106(4):699–715.
92. Huang ZL, Qu WM, Li WD, et al. Arousal effect of orexin A depends on activation of the histaminergic system. *Proc Natl Acad Sci USA.* 2001;98(17):9965–9970.
93. Hagan JJ, Leslie RA, Patel S, et al. Orexin A activates locus coeruleus cell firing and increases arousal in the rat. *Proc Natl Acad Sci USA.* 1999;96(19):10911–10916.
94. van Nieuwenhuijzen PS, McGregor IS, Hunt GE. The distribution of gamma-hydroxybutyrate-induced Fos expression in rat brain: comparison with baclofen. *Neuroscience.* 2009; 158(2):441–455.
95. Boissard R, Fort P, Gervasoni D, Barbagli B, Luppi PH. Localization of the GABAergic and non-GABAergic neurons projecting to the sublaterodorsal nucleus and potentially gating paradoxical sleep onset. *Eur J Neurosci.* 2003;18(6):1627–1639.
96. Jha SK, Ross RJ, Morrison AR. Sleep-related neurons in the central nucleus of the amygdala of rats and their modulation by the dorsal raphe nucleus. *Physiol Behav.* 2005;86(4):415–426.
97. Gulyani S, Wu MF, Nienhuis R, John J, Siegel JM. Cataplexy-related neurons in the amygdala of the narcoleptic dog. *Neuroscience.* 2002;112(2):355–365.
98. Marcus JN, Aschkenasi CJ, Lee CE, et al. Differential expression of orexin receptors 1 and 2 in the rat brain. *J Comp Neurol.* 2001;435(1):6–25.

CHAPTER

23

Networks for the Modulation of Acute and Chronic Pain

Inna Sukhotinsky [1], *Marshall Devor* [2]

[1]Gonda Multidisciplinary Brain Research Center, Bar-Ilan University, Ramat-Gan, Israel,

[2]Department of Cell and Developmental Biology, Silberman Institute of Life Sciences and the Center for Research on Pain, The Hebrew University of Jerusalem, Jerusalem, Israel

INTRODUCTION

Pain, although seemingly unwanted, is the sentinel that protects our bodies from potential harm. It provides protection through rapid, adaptive, and automatic reflexive responses and also by conveying an alarm message about noxious stimuli to our conscious awareness. The importance of pain is highlighted in disorders in which pain sensation is absent. This may occur, for example, due to lack or dysfunction of peripheral nociceptive neurons or impaired signal transduction in them. Such conditions include congenital insensitivity to pain due to channelopathies or the failure of nociceptors to survive during development, and acquired nerve injury such as in leprosy. Individuals with these conditions can sustain major bodily harm without even being aware of it. Normally, pain sensation prevents such damage from happening. It is of crucial importance for an organism's survival and functioning. The protective function of pain is present in various forms in a wide range of organisms. In the most primitive ones, it is represented by cellular chemo-, thermo-, or mechano-taxis. The response is automatic and reflexive. In organisms with a well-developed nervous system, reflex "nocifensive" responses are augmented by conscious pain awareness. The pain system is complex and interconnected with various other networks in the brain that modulate its activity depending on the environment and the situation.

Pain sensation is not fixed, delivering exactly the same signal each time in response to a given level of stimulus. Rather, it is dynamic. Pain experience and response depend significantly on expectation, attention, stress, affect, arousal state, and hormonal levels.[1–5] A classic example of pain modulation is stress-induced analgesia (e.g. during combat), where a soldier may not even notice an otherwise painful injury due to the stressful situation. He will feel pain sensation only later on, when the danger is over.

Pain sensation and modulation are normal and necessary. But in some circumstances, a chronic, abnormal condition can develop where the amount of pain felt is disproportionate to the stimulus, or pain may occur spontaneously without a stimulus. In these cases, the nociceptive system is altered on the peripheral and/or central levels, resulting in persistent and unbearable pain conditions. Examples include chronic inflammatory and neuropathic pain states. Neuronal networks processing and modulating noxious input, and changes in these networks in chronic pain states, will be reviewed in this chapter. Among the modulatory systems, we will consider a recently discovered brainstem locus named the MPTA (mesopontine tegmental anesthesia area), where microinjection of general anesthetics that act at the $GABA_A$-R produces a general anesthesia-like state.[6] MPTA connectivity with pain, arousal, and motor control structures suggests that it plays an important role as an integrative node for control of networks that produce the constellation of effects constituting the general anesthetic state.

PAIN-PROCESSING PATHWAYS

Pain Signalling

Under normal circumstances, nociception or transmission of information on specific noxious stimuli starts at the

Neuronal Networks in Brain Function, CNS Disorders, and Therapeutics
http://dx.doi.org/10.1016/B978-0-12-415804-7.00023-X

periphery with the process of transduction. Highly specialized, small-diameter sensory fibers, which are characterized by a high threshold to applied stimuli, convey noxious information from their peripheral terminals to the central nervous system (CNS). In terms of the morphological characteristics of their axons, nociceptors are classified into unmyelinated C afferent fibers and thinly myelinated Aδ afferent fibers. These innervate all body tissues, including the skin, muscles, joints, and viscera. They belong to the broader category of primary sensory neurons, whose cell bodies reside in the dorsal root and cranial ganglia. The axon bifurcates into two branches: peripheral, innervating the target tissues or organs, and central, projecting to the spinal cord or sensory nuclei of the brainstem. Nociceptors are sensitive to different kinds of stimuli, and many of them respond to multiple modalities, such as mechanical, heat, cold, and chemical stimuli. C-mechano-heat sensitive fibers that also respond to irritant chemicals are referred to as polymodal nociceptors. The threshold of nociceptive fibers is high; therefore, noxious stimuli are needed to activate them. In all of them, the intensity of the noxious stimulus is encoded by the rate of firing of action potentials. The resulting sensation (pain) matches the stimulus (noxious), producing normal or "nociceptive" pain.

The central branches of primary sensory neurons terminate on dorsal horn neurons in the spinal cord with a high level of anatomical organization. The equivalent for the craniofacial region is the spinal portion of the trigeminal nuclear complex in the medulla and upper cervical cord, which is analogous to the dorsal horn in the trigeminal system. High-threshold C and Aδ nociceptors terminate predominantly in lamina I and II of the dorsal horn (substantia gelatinosa) and have some contribution to lamina V. Neurons residing deep to laminae I and II receive innocuous input, and many are multimodal. The location of the receptive field on the body surface is encoded by medio-lateral and rostro-caudal terminal locations, creating a somatotopic map.[7]

Nociceptive information is relayed from the spinal cord to the brain via long projecting axons. There are also propriospinal neurons, which transfer information between the segments of the spinal cord, and spinal interneurons that are local and send projections over only short distances. Direct ascending pathways carry the information to higher brain structures: sensory relay nuclei of the thalamus, as well as the cerebellum, and homeostatic control regions of the reticular brainstem, hypothalamus, and ventral forebrain. Cranial and facial regions are represented in a way similar to the rest of the body by ascending projection pathways originating in trigeminal sensory nuclei. In addition, pain-related information is also relayed by postsynaptic neurons of the dorsal column system. This pathway originates primarily in laminae IV–V and projects to the dorsal column nuclei (gracile and cuneate), from which the signal is relayed to the thalamus via the medial lemniscus. The dorsal column–medial lemniscus pathway predominantly carries low-threshold tactile information, but it was shown to convey nociceptive information as well.[8–11]

The projections most closely associated with pain are the direct spinothalamic and trigeminothalamic pathways, originating in the most superficial aspect of the dorsal horn (laminae I and II), laminae IV–V, and the intermediate and medial ventral horn (laminae VI–VIII).[11] The majority of the projection fibers cross to the contralateral side within one or two segments rostral to the cell body and ascend in the lateral and anterior (ventral) funiculi with coarse somatotopic organization. Axons from the caudal parts of the spinal cord ascend superficially in the spinal white matter, and axons from more rostral parts are located more deeply (medially) in the white matter. The spinothalamic fibers ascend through the brainstem to the thalamus and terminate in the ventral posterior nuclei (VP)—the main somatosensory relay nuclei. The VP also relays lemniscal input from the dorsal column system and the principal trigeminal nuclei to the somatosensory cortex. The posterior portion of the ventral medial nucleus (a thalamocortical relay that receives much of its input from neurons of lamina I[11,12]), the ventral lateral nucleus, the ventral caudal portion of the medial dorsal nucleus, as well as intralaminar nuclei (the central lateral nucleus and parafascicular nucleus) also relay spinothalamic input to the cortex.[11,13–16]

Additional components of the spinal nociceptive pathway include significant bulbar projections, notably to the parabrachial nuclei and periaqueductal gray (PAG); hypothalamic projections; as well as projections to subcortical forebrain structures such as the septal nuclei, pallidum, amygdala, and elsewhere. The distribution of spinal cells of origin that project to these various nonthalamic structures is largely overlapping. Often, the same neuron gives off collaterals to several of these structures, with various percentages of fibers sending collateral projections to different structures, depending on the lamina of origin and projection targets.[11,17–20] Among the regions receiving dense spinal nociceptive input are the brainstem areas involved in pain regulation: the PAG, dorsolateral pons, locus coeruleus, parabrachial nuclei, ventrolateral medulla (VLM), and reticular formation.[11,21–23] These structures participate in pain modulation and control, and they project in turn to additional pain modulation areas, such as the anterior and lateral hypothalamus, thalamus, and amygdala.[11,24–26] Spinobulbar relay projections provide a major indirect source of communication to forebrain structures, including the cerebral cortex.

Among the cortical areas activated by pain-provoking stimuli, the most consistent are the primary and secondary somatosensory cortices (S1 and S2), anterior cingulate cortex (ACC), and insular and prefrontal cortices, as evidenced by functional imaging studies.[27,28] Others are less consistent. The entire set of cortical activations evoked by painful stimuli is often called the "pain matrix". Activation of S1 and S2 is mostly associated with sensory-discriminative aspects of pain, although S2 is likely to have additional affective and cognitive functions. The ACC and insula are thought to be involved in affectivel, attentional and certain cognitive dimensions of pain processing. The prefrontal cortex is usually assigned pain's motivational and cognitive aspects.[2,28–30] However, imaging studies show complex patterns of brain activation and connectivity in association with painful stimuli, which vary with context, presumably due to the state of intrinsic pain-modulating systems. It is clearly sophomoric to assign a specific component of pain experience to a specific brain region. This approach is little more than a stopgap until a more sophisticated model emerges of how brain activity maps onto conscious experience.

Pain Modulation Network

The existence of specific endogenous pain modulatory systems was first postulated by Melzack and Wall (the "Gate Control Theory" of pain[31,32]; see Chapter 29). The first demonstration of selective supraspinal modulation of pain came from studies showing that electrical stimulation of the midbrain PAG in rats produces analgesia.[33,34] Corresponding deep brain stimulation in patients evokes the same phenomenon in humans[35,36] (see Chapter 31).

Follow-up research revealed that the PAG is a central junction of a larger pain-modulating network that receives inputs from several forebrain structures and controls nociceptive input at the spinal level via its descending projections, notably by way of a major relay station in the rostral ventromedial medulla (RVM).[32,37] Electrical or opioid stimulation in the PAG or RVM produces analgesia, inhibits nociceptive responses of dorsal horn neurons, and suppresses nocifensive behavior. This effect is attenuated by lesions to these areas or by cutting connections descending in the spinal dorsolateral funiculus (DLF).[32,38–44]

The RVM consists of the midline raphe nuclei and the adjacent reticular formation, i.e. the magnocellular field just dorsal to the pyramids, called the gigantocellular reticular nucleus pars alpha (GiA), also known as the nucleus reticularis magnocellularis (NRMC). The PAG, especially its lateral and ventrolateral parts, and the adjacent MPTA (discussed further in this chapter) are the major sources of its input.[45–49] The RVM, in turn, constitutes the major relay station from the PAG to the spinal cord. This relay is also presumably used by the MPTA. Direct spinal dorsal horn projections of the PAG are minimal, although the nearby MPTA does project spinally and could provide additional modulation of spinal nociceptive input. The most dense terminations of the RVM are in target regions of nociceptive primary afferent input—the substantia gelatinosa (laminae I and II) and lamina V.[32,50]

The pain-modulating RVM neuron population is heterogeneous in terms of neurotransmitter content and sensitivity, as well as physiological effects mediated. "ON cells" are activated by nociceptive stimulation and fire just before a pain-evoked response, while "OFF cells" are inhibitory and appear to suppress nocifensive responses. They are inhibited by nociceptive stimulation and show decreased firing right before nociceptive responses.[51–56] The activation mode of ON and OFF cells is influenced by the arousal state, suggesting a more complex role in pain modulation than originally thought.[57] "Neutral cells" exhibit no consistent change in activity upon noxious stimulation. ON, OFF, and neutral neurons, like those in the RVM, have also been shown to exist in the PAG and the dorsolateral pontine tegmentum (DLPT).[58,59]

The DLPT is an additional important relay area of the pain-modulating system. It includes the dorsolateral area of the pontine tegmentum adjacent to the ventrolateral PAG, the subcoerulear and parabrachial regions, and the brainstem noradrenergic neurons that project to the RVM and spinal cord, such as the locus coeruleus and the A5 and A7 groups.[32,60,61] The DLPT is reciprocally connected with the RVM and participates in relaying RVM-induced analgesia. Its effects are partially blocked by noradrenergic antagonists.[32,62,63]

The analgesia produced by the PAG–RVM–spinal pain modulation network under natural conditions is mediated in large part by endogenous opioid peptides on the grounds that it is blocked by the μ-opioid receptor antagonist, naloxone. This system can also be activated by opioid microinjection into its elements (e.g. PAG, RVM, and amygdala)[32,64–66] and by systemic opiates. All three major opioid receptor types (μ, δ, and κ) are present throughout the pain-modulating network. Agonists of μ-opioid receptors (e.g. morphine) are the most effective in inducing analgesia, both after systemic administration and after direct microinjection into nodal points in the pain-modulating network.[32,67–69] An additional receptor, which shares sequence homology with opioid receptors and is involved in pain modulation, is the opioid receptor-like 1 (ORL1) receptor.[70]

There are numerous endogenous opioid receptor agonists, including the enkephalin, endorphin, dynorphin, and endomorphin peptide families, as well as orphanin FQ(nociceptin), the putative ligand of the ORL1 receptor. These endogenous peptides have different distributions across the pain-modulating network. β-endorphin-containing neuronal cell bodies, for example, occur largely in the ventromedial hypothalamus, while enkephalin and dynorphin-containing neurons are more widely distributed, including in the PAG, RVM, hypothalamus, and amygdala.[32,71–75] Nociceptin has an overlapping distribution with the other endogenous opioid peptides, but apparently it is not co-localized with them.[73] Terminal distribution is more widespread, and it often overlaps with that of the opioid receptors through which the specific endogenous opioid predominantly acts.

Major sources of input to the PAG are the prefrontal, anterior cingulate, and insular cortices, the amygdala, and the hypothalamus.[2,76] These forebrain structures interact with the pain-processing system, and they modulate nociceptive transmission in a variety of behavioral and psychological contexts such as expectation, attention, stress, emotional state, and arousal.[2,76] The observation that placebo analgesia, at least under some circumstances, is blocked by naloxone led to the hypothesis that it is also mediated by the endogenous descending pain-modulating network. A significant body of evidence confirming this has accumulated, although nonopioid mechanisms have been shown to contribute as well.[2,77–79] Imaging studies have shown that top-down influences occur along the pain modulation pathway during opioid and placebo analgesia. These originate in forebrain structures such as the ACC, with the results eventually exerted upon spinal cord nociceptive processing circuitry.[80–82]

The organization of the descending pain modulation network, with principal nodes that have a high level of interconnectivity with other networks, allows the integration of input from multiple systems, and modulation of pain perception by a variety of internal and external factors. This confers upon the pain-processing system a high level of regulatory flexibility. By the same token, it renders it capable of dynamic plastic readjustments depending on the received input and the context in which the input is generated. This plasticity can also lead to maladaptive changes. In the case of neuropathy and related pain disorders, plastic changes in the pain-processing system may cause abnormal and sustained neural activity, leading to the development and maintenance of chronic pain.[2,30]

PROCESSING CHANGES IN CHRONIC PAIN

Pain sensation arising as an immediate consequence of injury, and pain caused by inflammation, are physiological (nociceptive) in nature. In these kinds of pain, the system detects and conveys nociceptive information related to the noxious stimuli occurring in peripheral organs or tissues by sending neuronal impulses from peripheral sensory endings.

Pain following an injury or disease that persists beyond the healing phase is chronic pain, as defined by the International Association for the Study of Pain (IASP).[83] Chronic pain may involve both peripheral and central processes in its development. In instances in which the pain is caused by a lesion or disease of the somatosensory nervous system, it is referred to as "neuropathic pain" (Resources/IASP Taxonomy, http://www.iasp-pain.org/). In the presence of neuropathy, pain may be unrelated to the presence of noxious stimuli. It can be of central or peripheral origin, depending on the location of the primary damage sustained. Often, neuropathic pain is induced by a disease process (e.g. in painful diabetic neuropathy or postherpetic neuralgia) that causes a cascade of events leading to peripheral nerve damage and the triggering of chronic neuropathic pain. In the case of "central pain", the lesion is usually a result of spinal cord injury, stroke, or multiple sclerosis. Experimental evidence based on animal models of neuropathic and inflammatory pain, as well as human studies, shows that persistent pain results from nervous system reorganization at peripheral and central levels. Central changes are often triggered and maintained by input from the periphery.[84–87] The result is a change in the way the nervous system responds to stimuli. The resulting pain sensation does not necessarily match the stimulus, and it may occur spontaneously, without stimulation.

Peripheral and Spinal Changes

When tissue or nerve damage is sustained in the periphery, many changes take place. Responses start with disruption in the normal flow of neurotrophic signaling molecules between the peripheral endings of the primary sensory neuron and the cell body. Intracellular signal transduction pathways within the sensory ending are also modified by inflammatory mediators in the tissue. Both neuropathy and inflammation cause changes in gene expression that result in upregulation and downregulation of literally thousands of molecules in the peripheral nervous system (PNS) and CNS (including many Na^+ and K^+ channels). This causes numerous significant changes in neuronal function.[88–92] This section is a description, far from exhaustive, of some of the processes that take place in chronic pain.

Multiple changes in the functioning of nociceptors and other primary afferents are triggered by peripheral nerve injury. These include (1) disruption in the trafficking of signaling molecules, resulting in accumulation or depletion of ion channels and transducers at the site of axonal injury (e.g. neuroma and sites of demyelination); (2) changes in expression levels of ion channels and neurotransmitter receptors in afferent neuron somata; (3) changes in levels of ion channels, receptors, and neurotransmitter receptors in peripheral afferent neuron ends and their central terminals; (4) the appearance of pro-inflammatory cytokines; and (5) structural changes such as demyelination, the formation of neuromas, and peripheral and central terminal sprouting.[89,90,93,94] An important consequence of these changes is that many afferent neurons develop a tendency to excess generation of electrical impulses (hyperexcitability). This occurs not only at sensory endings but also at ectopic impulse generation sites (pacemaker sites), locations that are normally incapable of sustained impulse generation, such as midnerve injury sites and sensory ganglia. Ectopic electrogenesis at these sites often occurs spontaneously at resting membrane potential.[95–97] Spontaneous ectopically generated discharge drives central pain-signaling neurons and gives rise to abnormal pain sensations that are characteristic of neuropathic pain. There is abundant evidence of ectopia in animal models of neuropathic pain and in human patients.[94,98–100]

Peripheral changes, notably ectopia in nociceptors, also cause modifications of afferent signal processing in the spinal cord. This results in abnormal signal amplification ("central sensitization"). Our knowledge of how these central changes are induced and maintained is less developed than for peripheral processes. Among the potential contributors is the fact that the ongoing barrage of ectopic activity causes the resting potential of the postsynaptic neuron to depolarize and come closer to the spike threshold. Activity of postsynaptic neurons is also modulated by molecules released from the central afferent terminals. These molecules include neurotransmitters and trophic factors. Other central factors associated with the afferent neuron are increased membrane excitability, facilitation of synaptic strength, decrease of inhibitory influences from dorsal horn interneurons, and structural changes that alter synaptic function.[85,101] There are also changes in spinal postsynaptic neurons. Spinal cord neurons show induction of activity-regulated immediate early genes and regulation of transcription factors, which may affect downstream genes. This can activate signaling cascades in the postsynaptic neuron, resulting in altered neurotransmitter content, upregulated Na^+ channels, depleted μ-opiate receptors, recruitment of *N*-methyl-D-aspartate (NMDA)-type glutamate receptors to the cell membrane, increased spinal content of pro-inflammatory cytokines, activation of dorsal horn astrocytes and microglia, and degeneration of spinal inhibitory neurons (probably because of glutamate-mediated excitotoxicity sustained by ectopic discharge).[94,101–104] Remarkably, in the presence of central sensitization, impulses carried by low-threshold Aβ afferents can yield a sensation of pain (tactile allodynia, or "Aβ pain"). Normally, these afferents evoke a sensation of touch. Impulses carried by nociceptors (C, Aδ) can produce more pain than they normally would (hyperalgesia).[101,105]

Additional important modifications occur in neurons of the sympathetic nervous system and in the sensory neurons with which they interact. Normally, nociceptor activity induces an increase in sympathetic discharge, not vice versa. But in some patients with inflammatory and neuropathic pain conditions, sympathetic-sensory coupling develops. In these cases, nociceptors develop catecholamine sensitivity. Noradrenaline released from sympathetic terminals during sympathetic discharge then elicits pain. Following nerve injury, sympathetic fibers begin to sprout within the neuroma, the associated dorsal root ganglia, and also the distal partially denervated skin.[106–108] Sympathetically maintained pain is mediated by both α_1 and α_2 adrenergic receptors[109] and is relieved by sympathetic block, sympathectomy, α-adrenergic receptor antagonists, and inhibition of noradrenaline release from sympathetic terminals.[110,111]

Supraspinal Changes

A significant amount of our current knowledge about central responses in chronic pain conditions comes from imaging studies of changes in cerebral activity in patients in response to acute stimuli. Overall, it is evident from these studies that pain processing in chronic pain patients differs significantly from that in normal individuals.[112] Paradoxically, structures that are activated during acute noxious stimulus processing in healthy subjects sometimes show a *decreased* activation pattern in patients with rheumatoid arthritis and other chronic pain conditions.[113,114] Reduction in thalamic activity was also demonstrated in neuropathic pain.[115,116] Such reductions might represent inhibitory compensation, learning-associated plasticity, or even neuronal atrophy (discussed further in this chapter). Patients with some chronic pain syndromes such as back pain, fibromyalgia, and irritable bowel syndrome demonstrate higher pain ratings and *enhanced* stimulus-evoked cortical activations.[27] The direction of change (hypo- or hyperresponsiveness) might be affected by the imaging method, the experimental paradigm, the stimuli used, the specific pain condition involved, or its stage. These and additional factors contribute to the variability across the studies.

Imaging studies also reveal thalamic and cortical "atrophy", as indicated, for example, by significant reductions in gray matter density in the prefrontal cortex in patients with chronic back pain, chronic headache, and other conditions. A decrease in gray matter was also found in the brainstem and somatosensory cortex.[117–120] The meaning of these imaging changes is uncertain. They are unlikely to reflect neurodegeneration as at least some are reversible when pain is relieved.[112,121–123]

Changes in descending pain control systems have also been documented in chronic pain conditions. There is a decrease in tonic inhibition, as well as active descending facilitation. These pro-nociceptive actions are relayed by the PAG, RVM, and dorsal reticular nucleus.[124–126] The activation of supraspinal structures involved in pain processing (the S1, ACC, insula, prefrontal cortex, ventral striatum, and PAG) is increased in chronic pain patients during pain anticipation and contributes to an altered pain-evoked response.[27,28,127–129] Biochemical changes in supraspinal pain-modulating circuitry have also been documented. Reduced opioid-receptor agonist binding was found in key nociceptive processing regions in central poststroke pain patients.[130,131]

Plastic changes that occur in chronic pain conditions alter the interplay between various parts of the nociceptive transmission system and its modulation by other networks. This process is manifested in modified and abnormal pain experience. Brainstem nuclei are important convergence and integration loci of these numerous pathways. In addition to the nuclei already known (reviewed above in this chapter), a new locus has been discovered recently that potentially plays an important role in controlling pain circuitry and other functions. This is discussed next.

THE MESOPONTINE TEGMENTAL ANESTHESIA AREA (MPTA)

Interesting new information on central networks that could participate in pain control comes from the Devor laboratory.[6] The initial motivation was to investigate the mechanisms underlying general anesthesia as the basis for pain-free surgery. The emergence of general anesthesia as a clinical tool is usually marked as William Morton's demonstration of ether for surgical anesthesia at the Massachusetts General Hospital in 1846.[132] Ever since then, it has been an indispensable clinical tool. A large number of surgical procedures and other methodologies used in modern medicine would be impossible to carry out without it. But despite the unique importance of general anesthesia for permitting pain-free surgery for over 160 years, our understanding of the specific underlying neural mechanisms remains extremely limited. Here, we review in some detail a recently discovered brainstem locus involved in general anesthesia, the mesopontine tegmental anesthesia area (MPTA), and discuss mechanisms whereby it could control neural systems involved in pain regulation.

Research on anesthetic mechanisms tends to fall into two largely separate areas: (1) molecular properties of anesthetic agents and their receptors, and (2) neural systems affected by anesthetics. The former area is well developed, but not the latter. The correlation of anesthetic agents' potency with their oil–water partition (the Overton–Meyer correlation) suggests that general anesthetics act in a lipid domain, presumably the nerve cell membrane. Today, it is largely accepted that these agents act on transmembrane proteins. The leading target candidates are ion channels, especially the $GABA_A$-R and its chloride channel complex, although there are new candidates (especially for volatile anesthetics), including the KCNK 2-p domain K^+ channels. The list is constantly growing.[133–144] Since the discovery of the Overton–Meyer correlation, it has been widely believed that anesthetic agents act in a distributed manner in the CNS, or at least in the cortex, via cellular mechanisms that are similar at all locations. This is reflected by the fact that research on the molecular targets of anesthetics is done without much regard for the source of the cells tested.

Compared to the considerable advances in our knowledge of the molecular pharmacological basis of anesthetic action, little is known about the neural systems upon which anesthetics act. The anesthetic state is multifaceted. It involves several effects, including analgesia, atonia, amnesia, and loss of consciousness. This suggests that anesthetics influence widely distributed CNS locations (e.g. the spinal cord, hippocampus, neocortex etc) to generate the various general anesthesia components. This distributed model is consistent with the ubiquity of the candidate anesthetic-binding sites, and with the fact that anesthetics suppress cerebral metabolism globally.[145,146] These facts provide a basis for the hypothesis that anesthetics distribute in the systemic circulation and act ubiquitously and directly throughout the CNS by generalized neural suppression and the decoupling of transmission in and between the spinal cord, thalamus, and cortex.[147,148]

On the other hand, several lines of evidence argue against the distributed anesthetic action hypothesis. Among them is the fact that minimal alveolar concentration (MAC) for volatile anesthetics is not affected by cortical lesions or precollicular decerebration,[149–151] and the observation that anesthesia has only relatively subtle effects on receptive fields and somatotopy in the primary sensory cortex. Substantial cortical processing, at least in primary processing areas, persists in the presence of anesthesia as evidenced by cortical recordings carried out in anesthetized animals.[152,153] This implies that effects might not be due primarily to a generalized cortical suppression by anesthetics, but rather to their selective network action.[6,149,154,155]

Similarly, there is evidence for supraspinal versus exclusively direct spinal involvement in anesthetic suppression of motor function and pain. For example, (1) spinal cord injury decreases the ability of systemic barbiturates and ketamine to suppress spinal nociceptive transmission; (2) selective anesthetic application to the brain can induce depression of nocifensive responses or anesthesia (although at higher concentrations), and it reduces MAC for inhaled anesthetics; and (3) lesions in the pontomesencephalic tegmentum alter MAC for halothane and cyclopropane.[156–164]

Work pointing toward the involvement of specific neuronal networks in general anesthesia stems from classic experiments conducted by Moruzzi and Magoun in cats. Those studies revealed the critical role of the brainstem reticular formation in maintaining cortical arousal in the context of sleep–wake transitions (the "reticular activating system", or RAS) and demonstrated that barbiturate anesthetics could selectively switch off arousal by acting on the brainstem reticular formation[149,165] (Chapters 21 and 22). Accordingly, damage (e.g. stroke) or experimental lesions to the brainstem reticular formation can cause cortical synchronization and result in a comatose state.[166–168] These findings indicate that the midbrain–pontine junction contains an important node for arousal regulation. Such a node could be modulated by drug binding and exert its effects on the rest of the brain via distributed neuronal networks.

DISCOVERY OF THE MPTA

Indeed, a systematic mapping survey in which the barbiturate anesthetic pentobarbital was stereotaxically microinjected into a matrix of bilaterally symmetrical locations in the rat brain demonstrated such a locus. Specifically, microinjection induced a consistent, rapid, and fully reversible anesthesia-like state. The locus, a restricted part of the upper brainstem, was referred to as the mesopontine tegmental anesthesia area (MPTA).[6] Microinjections elsewhere had little effect. The minimal dose of pentobarbital sufficient to induce an anesthesia-like state was less than 1/1000th of the systemic dose. The effect was rapid in onset (and hence not caused by drug spread elsewhere), specific (the vehicle had no effect), and reproducible, and it lasted 20–40 min. This finding, independently verified by Voss and colleagues,[169] demonstrated for the first time that anesthesia can be elicited by drug action on a specific brain locus. Other agents that enhance $GABA_A$-R activation also work, including phenobarbital, muscimol, thiopentone, propofol, and alphathesin (a neurosteroid).[6,169]

The anesthesia induced by MPTA microinjection was accompanied by all the characteristic sensory and motor changes: analgesia (i.e. loss of response to sensory stimuli, including noxious pinch), loss of weight support, righting reflex, and atonia. Microinjection also produced a cortical electroencephalographic transition from the low-voltage high frequencies of wake to the high-voltage low frequencies of systemic anesthesia, and it suppressed baseline *c-fos* expression in the cortex, particularly in prefrontal areas. This mirrors the suppression of cortical neuron activity characteristic of systemic barbiturate anesthesia.[170,171] Interestingly, in the MPTA itself, *c-fos* expression is suppressed during systemic anesthesia. This implies that systemic general anesthetics may work at least in part by acting on MPTA neurons.

Lidocaine microinjection into the MPTA had an analgesic effect, but it did not induce sedation or anesthesia. This suggests that anesthetics that enhance the activation of $GABA_A$-Rs have a more complex network effect than simple nonselective block of MPTA neuron activity.[6] In addition to indiscriminate inactivation of neurons in the MPTA, lidocaine blocks fibers-of-passage. Pentobarbital, in contrast, acts selectively on $GABA_A$-R expressing neurons. GABAergic neurons, and neurons bearing $GABA_A$-Rs (GABAceptive), are plentiful in the MPTA as demonstrated by immunohistochemistry, providing a molecular basis for pentobarbital action in this locus.[172] Barbiturates act at a modulatory site on the $GABA_A$-R to increase Cl^- channel open probability. This enhances the response to endogenous GABA. Alternatively, at higher concentrations (>1 mM), pentobarbital can open the $GABA_A$-R channel directly. Both effects suppress activity in GABAceptive neurons.[173] MPTA neurons may be inhibited by agents that, when microinjected directly into the MPTA, enhance the action of GABA, or by such agents reaching the MPTA by volume transmission (Chapter 8) or via the systemic circulation.

The MPTA is a small locus, as demonstrated by the spatial selectivity for anesthetic induction. Injections only 1 mm outside its boundaries fail to produce the anesthesia-like state, indicating that the effect is mediated by a specific spatially confined cell population. The MPTA has no clear cytoarchitectonic borders. But, based on the effects of microinjection, it is delineated dorsally by the decussation of the superior cerebellar peduncle and the ventrolateral PAG, ventrally by the reticulotegmental nucleus of the pons, laterally by the rubrospinal tract and pedunculopontine tegmental nucleus, medially by the median and paramedian pontine raphe nuclei, anteriorly by the retrorubral field, and posteriorly by the caudal pontine reticular formation (Figure 23.1).[6]

Although connectivity of the reticular core of the brainstem has been studied in some detail,[46,174–180] the MPTA region per se received close attention only following the finding of the anesthesia-like effect it mediates.[45,170,181–184] MPTA neurons do not have extremely widespread and diffuse connectivity like the locus coeruleus. Instead, these neurons have specific ascending and descending connections, often reciprocal, to neural systems known to control modulation of pain, arousal, and motor functions. It is through these connections that the MPTA conveys the constellation of observed effects that add up to a general anesthesia-like state.

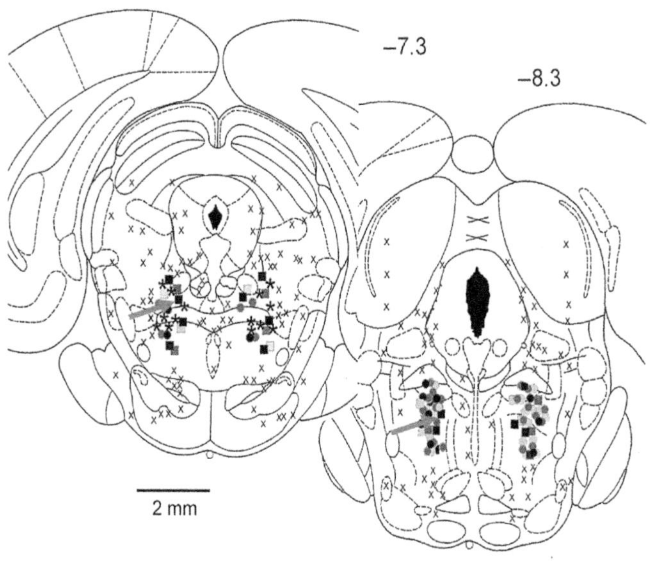

FIGURE 23.1 Solid symbols indicate loci at which bilaterally symmetrical microinjections of pentobarbital induced a general anesthesia-like state. These define the MPTA area (arrows). Each symbol represents a single microinjection experiment. Squares and circles represent microinjections in the initial brain survey that yielded moderate or deep anesthesia: scores of 11–13 and 14–16, respectively, in a total of 43 microinjections in 26 rats. Scores are a sum of sensory and motor deficit scales (each 0–8), as presented in detail in Devor and Zalkind.[6] Asterisks mark follow-up microinjections targeted to MPTA in experiments in which anesthesia was obtained using relatively low doses (10 or 20 μg, seven rats). Microinjections outside of the MPTA that were ineffective (score ≤ 5) are marked X. (*Source: Figure from Ref. 6, with permission of the International Association for the Study of Pain (IASP).*) (For color version of this figure, the reader is referred to the online version of this book.)

MPTA CONNECTIVITY: INTERRELATIONSHIPS WITH THE PAIN CONTROL NETWORK

Connections via Brainstem Relays

The MPTA projects strongly to several pontine regions, and even more strongly to particular medullary regions, that constitute parts of the descending pain modulation system. These include the PAG, dorsal raphe nucleus (DRN), DLPT, and RVM. The densest projections are to the RVM, including the GiA.[182] Indeed, the MPTA is no less a contributor to the RVM than is the PAG. This is confirmed by retrograde labeling experiments showing that microinjections into the RVM yield prominent labeling of neurons in both the PAG and the MPTA.[45,182] Although the MPTA-to-RVM pathway was known previously,[47,49] it had not been appreciated as a potential contributor to the descending pain modulatory system, possibly because opioid microinjections in the MPTA do not induce analgesia.[39] The connectivity of the MPTA with the RVM is bilateral and reciprocal, as shown by combined retrograde and anterograde tracing experiments. Thus, the MPTA also receives connections from the RVM and the adjacent gigantocellular reticular field. The observation of numerous close axonal appositions of RVM projecting MPTA neurons on neuronal cell bodies projecting back to the MPTA suggests the possibility of direct synaptic contacts between these neurons.[45,182]

As discussed in this chapter, the RVM is considered to be the major relay station of endogenous descending pain modulation.[32,44,76,185–187] It is possible that the analgesic component of general anesthesia is mediated by the MPTA via a relay in the RVM. In line with this, RVM neuron physiology is significantly altered by systemic barbiturates, and the volatile anesthetic, isoflurane, modulates RVM ON- and OFF-cell activity.[188–190] Also consistent with this hypothesis, combined anterograde tracing from the MPTA and retrograde tracing from the spinal cord showed at the light and electron microscopic levels that MPTA neurons frequently end synaptically on spinally projecting RVM neurons.[182] In the absence of reliable anatomical markers of ON- and OFF-cells, however, the identity of the RVM neurons that are targeted by the MPTA projection (ON, OFF, or neutral) is not known. In addition to its RVM connectivity, the MPTA could also modulate nociception indirectly via other brainstem relays, such as its projections to the PAG, the DRN, and the DLPT (Figure 23.2). These regions project, in turn, to the RVM, the spinal cord dorsal horn, or both.[32,60,61,183]

Direct support for the hypothesis that the MPTA modulates neuronal activity of spinal nociceptive circuitry by a descending bulbospinal pathway comes from a study conducted by Namjoshi and colleagues in isoflurane-anesthetized rats.[191] Microinjection of pentobarbital (but not vehicle) into the MPTA significantly suppressed both the spontaneous firing rate and nerve stimulation-evoked responses of lumbar spinothalamic tract neurons. This also demonstrates that the MPTA's descending control is exerted on ascending transmission through the spinothalamic tract, although other ascending tracts might also be affected. We conclude that the antinociception that occurs as part of the anesthesia-like state evoked by pentobarbital microinjections into the MPTA is due, at least in part, to direct and/or indirect descending inhibition of ascending spinothalamic tract neurons.

Several caudal medullary regions that participate in pain processing and modulation also receive MPTA projections. Compared to its RVM connectivity, the MPTA projects relatively sparsely to the VLM and to the dorsal reticular field of the medulla (DRt; MdD in the atlas of Paxinos and Watson, 1998). VLM neurons are probably also a source of tonic descending inhibition to dorsal horn nociceptive neurons, since electrical stimulation

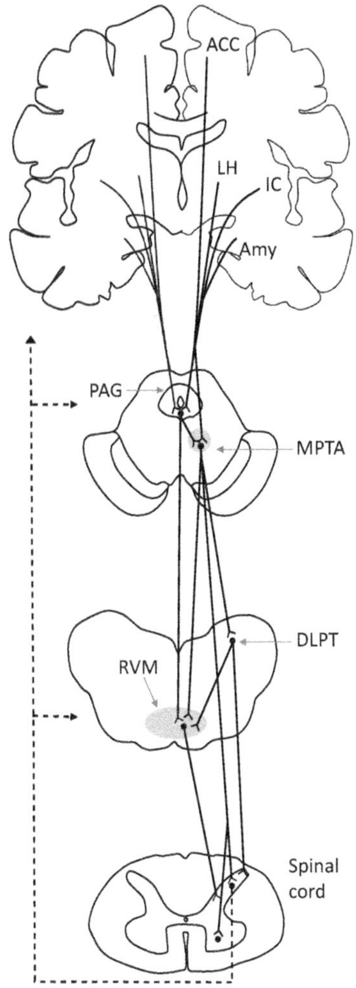

FIGURE 23.2 Schematic representation of MPTA connectivity illustrating the pathways through which pain modulation may occur. These include connections with nodal points in known endogenous pain control systems. The MPTA is shown unilaterally for the sake of clarity. ACC: anterior cingulate cortex; LH: lateral hypothalamus; IC: insular cortex; Amy: amygdala; DLPT: dorsolateral pontine tegmentum.

of the VLM inhibits them.[192–194] In contrast, the DRt is a pronociceptive relay of the endogenous pain-regulating system. Stimulating it *increases* the response of spinal neurons to noxious stimulation.[125,195–197] It has been suggested that in chronic pain conditions, the balance between descending inhibition and facilitation might tip toward sustained pain facilitation, driven by persistent and abnormal nociceptive input.[53,198]

Direct Spinal Connections

The MPTA also has direct projections to the trigeminal nuclear complex and to the spinal cord via the lateral and anterior funiculi. Most terminations are in the deep laminae of the dorsal horn and ventral horn, with superficial dorsal-horn terminations being relatively scarce. However, retrograde labeling from the superficial dorsal horn revealed that a substantial number of MPTA neurons with descending spinal projections have terminal arbors that reach laminae I and II. Indeed, it turns out that the MPTA contains the large majority of all neurons present at mesopontine levels that project spinally (about two-thirds). This suggests that in addition to the indirect modulatory pathways via the RVM and the other brainstem relays, direct spinal MPTA connections might also have functional importance in the modulation of nociception.[184]

Interestingly, double retrograde labeling with contrasting tracers showed that the MPTA neurons that project directly to the spinal cord and the ones that project to the RVM comprise, for the most part, separate and morphologically distinct cell populations. MPTA neurons that project directly to the spinal cord are larger than those projecting to the rostromedial medulla and differ in shape. Their roles are also likely to be different. For example, the ones that project to the spinal cord are much more likely to express $GABA_A$-Rs than the ones that project to the RVM.[183] This finding suggests that the direct spinal projections are the primary route for MPTA modulation of pain, although action via RVM relay is also likely.

Axons of individual descending MPTA (as well as RVM) neurons collateralize broadly in the spinal cord. The pattern of single and double labeling with contrasting retrograde tracers indicates that many of the spinally projecting neurons in both regions have a highly collateralized projection pattern across various spinal levels and to both dorsal and ventral spinal horns. However, collateralization across the midline is minimal. The majority of neurons project either ipsilaterally or contralaterally.[181,184] This pattern of connectivity suggests a system designed primarily to exert global modulation over the entire spinal neuraxis, rather than regionally or segmentally, but it retains a left-right selectivity. Thus, MPTA neurons are likely to play a generalized modulatory role across functional modalities, rather than specific topographically delimited roles.[181,184]

Ascending Connections

Ascending MPTA projections connect it with multiple structures that are potentially related to the regulation of pain. The most prominent projections are to the zona incerta and lateral hypothalamus with which the MPTA has robust reciprocal connectivity,[170,199–201] as well as to several forebrain structures known to modulate pain processing. The MPTA also projects to parts of the nigrostriatal system, including the basal ganglia,[20,202] and, less prominently, to the amygdala.[30,203–205] Finally, there is a modest direct projection from the MPTA to the frontal, rostral cingulate, and insular cortices, and retrograde tracing established that those cortices have reciprocal connections with the MPTA. The most prominent among them are the medial frontal and cingulate cortices.[170] These cortical areas are prominent parts of the "pain matrix". They are well placed to influence nociception via projections to the descending pain modulation system, especially the PAG, as discussed in this chapter.

The MPTA does not project to specific sensory relay nuclei of the thalamus. However, it projects strongly to the intralaminar thalamic nuclei. These nuclei, in turn, project diffusely to the cortex. This implies that the mechanism by which the MPTA exerts its control over higher cortical processes has less to do with the control of primary sensory information relayed to the cortex and more to do with effects on higher levels of processing and modulation within the cortex. Examples of these influences are modulation of arousal and possibly affective-emotional aspects of pain experience. The finding that both MPTA-mediated and systemically induced anesthesia suppress cortical activity similarly, as assessed by electroencephalography and *c-fos* expression, supports the hypothesis that cortical processing of sensations, including pain, is affected similarly by both modes of anesthesia. On the other hand, there are differences in the pattern of *subcortical* brain activity in the two modes.[171] Better understanding of the role of the MPTA in the regulation of pain, as well as other networks, could be achieved by selective block and lesion of its neuronal activity or interference with its connections, using surgical, pharmacological, or perhaps optogenetic approaches (as discussed below in this chapter).

NETWORK INTERACTIONS AND THERAPEUTIC IMPLICATIONS

Pain processing and modulatory pathways have several relay loci in which information from multiple structures is integrated. This allows for network flexibility in response to contextual circumstances. One of the important regions for network interaction is the brainstem. It contains several neuroanatomically interconnected loci that serve as important nodes of network regulation, such as the PAG, MPTA, RVM, and locus coeruleus. The brainstem reticular formation contains many neurons that possess conditional multireceptive (CMR) capabilities—a trait that enables brainstem nuclei to interact with multiple networks variably, depending on the arousal state, internal conditions, and input characteristics[206] (see Chapter 28). The location of the MPTA in a CMR-rich brainstem region, and its neuroanatomical connectivity, make this locus a prime candidate for such a control node of network interactions.

One of the important features of CMR regions is their sensitivity to modulation by convulsants and anticonvulsants, general anesthetics, and depressants. These drugs affect the animal's global responsiveness to stimuli. The overall excitability of neuronal networks has been proposed to be modulated by tonic inhibition by GABA (or glycine) acting via $GABA_A$ receptors.[206] GABAceptive neurons are ubiquitous in the MPTA region and provide a molecular substrate for general anesthetic action there. This supports the idea that the MPTA is a key node for network regulation.[172]

The RVM, the major pain modulation system relay, contains such state-modulated neurons as well. The activation of RVM neurons can generate either facilitation or inhibition of pain transmission under different conditions. Importantly, the pattern of RVM ON- and OFF-cell activity varies with the state of arousal[57] and other conditions. Depending on the circumstances, ON-cells or OFF-cells dominate, resulting in a tendency to either pronociceptive or antinociceptive processing modes. Prolonged nociceptive input or opioid agonist administration, for example, can tip the system toward pronociceptive or antinociceptive states.[57,76] Additional structures participating in pain modulation, such as the amygdala and association areas of the cerebral cortex, also contain significant populations of CMR neurons. This provides a basis for their state-dependent role in pain regulation.[30,206]

Multiple changes take place in chronic pain, making it challenging to treat. The variety of nuclei and underlying mechanisms involved suggests many molecular targets that could be addressed. Various chronic pain conditions and components are sensitive to different agents. In the case of neuropathic pain, the most effective treatments are drugs that reduce membrane excitability by affecting ion channels, and hence inhibit ectopic discharge in the periphery.[99,207] Central pain-modulating networks may provide alternative therapeutic targets for direct intervention as well. Opiate action in the PAG and RVM is a prime example. Drugs that alter the excitability of other brainstem network modulation nodes also show efficacy in certain pain conditions, such as some antiepileptic drugs (AEDs), anesthetics, and CNS depressants that enhance $GABA_A$-R activation. Modulation of the excitability state of pain-regulating brainstem regions could be one of the mechanisms by which antiepileptic drugs affect neuropathic pain.[206,208,209]

The main problem with all agents affecting excitability, whether they act synaptically or on membrane excitability (e.g. by opening or blocking ion channels), is their undesired central side effects. Fine tuning of pharmacological selectivity is a possibility. $GABA_A$-Rs, for example, exhibit considerable subunit heterogeneity. Drugs are being developed that act selectively on specific $GABA_A$-Rs subtypes, including those that mediate tonic inhibition.[210,211] To address the fundamental problem of universal distribution of the CNS targets, local selective targeting of the therapeutic agent may prove to be a viable strategy. One of the exciting new approaches for highly selective control of specific brain regions is optogenetics. By transducing selected neuronal populations with light-sensitive channels and pumps, it is possible to manipulate their activity with light with fine spatial and temporal resolution.[212,213] Clinical application of this approach might be closer to implementation than it seems given recent advances in the development of viral vectors that are safe for human use, ongoing clinical trials of such viral vectors in the nervous system, and the ease of light delivery.[214,215] Focal optogenetic manipulation (excitation or inhibition) of specific locally transformed neurons in pain-regulating networks could provide a promising and powerful therapeutic approach, overcoming one of the major disadvantages of current pharmacological treatments—adverse side effects.

SUMMARY

Nociceptive information is conveyed from the periphery to higher brain structures, and processing gains in complexity as the signal proceeds toward pain experience. Pain perception is modulated endogenously by intrinsic circuitry. The processing and regulation of pain signals involve complex orchestration of multiple interacting networks. These, in turn, depend on a variety of factors, including modulation of afferent input and cognitive and emotional context. Environmental- and state-dependent influences on network interplay provide a basis for flexibility of regulation and adaptation of the organism. However, network interplay can lead to maladaptive plastic changes, resulting in the development of chronic pain when injury is sustained by the system. Input convergence and interconnectivity of specific brainstem reticular formation nodes provide them with the integrative capabilities necessary for control of interactions between networks. These features play a key role in pain modulation and possibly in the modulation of additional CNS functions. They are pregnant subjects for further research, and promising therapeutic targets for intervention in the treatment of chronic pain.

Acknowledgments

Professor Devor's work on the topic of this chapter is supported by the Israel Ministry of Health and the Hebrew University's Center for Research on Pain. Dr. Sukhotinsky is supported by the I-CORE Program of the Planning and Budgeting Committee and The Israel Science Foundation (grant No. 51/11).

References

1. Smith YR, Stohler CS, Nichols TE, Bueller JA, Koeppe RA, Zubieta JK. Pronociceptive and antinociceptive effects of estradiol through endogenous opioid neurotransmission in women. *J Neurosci.* 2006;26(21):5777–5785.
2. Tracey I, Mantyh PW. The cerebral signature for pain perception and its modulation. *Neuron.* 2007;55(3):377–391.
3. Teepker M, Peters M, Vedder H, Schepelmann K, Lautenbacher S. Menstrual variation in experimental pain: correlation with gonadal hormones. *Neuropsychobiology.* 2010;61(3):131–140.
4. Mogil JS. Sex differences in pain and pain inhibition: multiple explanations of a controversial phenomenon. *Nat Rev Neurosci.* 2012;13(12):859–866.
5. Bushnell MC, Ceko M, Low LA. Cognitive and emotional control of pain and its disruption in chronic pain. *Nat Rev Neurosci.* 2013;14(7):502–511.
6. Devor M, Zalkind V. Reversible analgesia, atonia, and loss of consciousness on bilateral intracerebral microinjection of pentobarbital. *Pain.* 2001;94(1):101–112.
7. Doubell TP, Mannion RJ, Woolf CJ. The dorsal horn: state-dependent sensory processing, plasticity and the generation of pain. In: Wall PD, Melzack R, eds. *Textbook of Pain.* 4th ed. Churchill Livingstone; 1999:165–181.
8. Ferrington DG, Downie JW, Willis Jr WD. Primate nucleus gracilis neurons: responses to innocuous and noxious stimuli. *J Neurophysiol.* 1988;59(3):886–907.
9. Willis WD, Al-Chaer ED, Quast MJ, Westlund KN. A visceral pain pathway in the dorsal column of the spinal cord. *Proc Natl Acad Sci USA.* 1999;96(14):7675–7679.
10. Al-Chaer ED, Feng Y, Willis WD. A role for the dorsal column in nociceptive visceral input into the thalamus of primates. *J Neurophysiol.* 1998;79(6):3143–3150.
11. Craig AD, Dostrovsky JO. Medulla to thalamus. In: Wall PD, Melzack R, eds. *Textbook of Pain.* 4th ed. Churchill Livingstone; 1999:183–214.
12. Craig AD, Bushnell MC, Zhang ET, Blomqvist A. A thalamic nucleus specific for pain and temperature sensation. *Nature.* 1994;372(6508):770–773.
13. Craig AD. Distribution of trigeminothalamic and spinothalamic lamina I terminations in the macaque monkey. *J Comp Neurol.* 2004;477(2):119–148.
14. Boivie J. An anatomical reinvestigation of the termination of the spinothalamic tract in the monkey. *J Comp Neurol.* 1979;186(3):343–369.
15. Apkarian AV, Hodge CJ. Primate spinothalamic pathways: III. Thalamic terminations of the dorsolateral and ventral spinothalamic pathways. *J Comp Neurol.* 1989;288(3):493–511.
16. Craig AD. Distribution of trigeminothalamic and spinothalamic lamina I terminations in the cat. *Somatosens Mot Res.* 2003;20(3–4):209–222.
17. Kevetter GA, Willis WD. Collaterals of spinothalamic cells in the rat. *J Comp Neurol.* 1983;215(4):453–464.
18. Hylden JL, Anton F, Nahin RL. Spinal lamina I projection neurons in the rat: collateral innervation of parabrachial area and thalamus. *Neuroscience.* 1989;28(1):27–37.
19. Zhang DX, Carlton SM, Sorkin LS, Willis WD. Collaterals of primate spinothalamic tract neurons to the periaqueductal gray. *J Comp Neurol.* 1990;296(2):277–290.
20. Braz JM, Nassar MA, Wood JN, Basbaum AI. Parallel "pain" pathways arise from subpopulations of primary afferent nociceptor. *Neuron.* 2005;47(6):787–793.
21. Westlund KN, Craig AD. Association of spinal lamina I projections with brainstem catecholamine neurons in the monkey. *Exp Brain Res.* 1996;110(2):151–162.

22. Wiberg M, Blomqvist A. The spinomesencephalic tract in the cat: its cells of origin and termination pattern as demonstrated by the intraaxonal transport method. *Brain Res.* 1984;291(1):1–18.
23. Craig AD. Distribution of brainstem projections from spinal lamina I neurons in the cat and the monkey. *J Comp Neurol.* 1995;361(2):225–248.
24. Mantyh PW. Connections of midbrain periaqueductal gray in the monkey. I. Ascending efferent projections. *J Neurophysiol.* 1983; 49(3):567–581.
25. Reichling DB, Basbaum AI. Collateralization of periaqueductal gray neurons to forebrain or diencephalon and to the medullary nucleus raphe magnus in the rat. *Neuroscience.* 1991;42(1): 183–200.
26. Cameron AA, Khan IA, Westlund KN, Cliffer KD, Willis WD. The efferent projections of the periaqueductal gray in the rat: a *Phaseolus vulgaris*-leucoagglutinin study. I. Ascending projections. *J Comp Neurol.* 1995;351(4):568–584.
27. Schweinhardt P, Bushnell MC. Pain imaging in health and disease—how far have we come? *J Clin Invest.* 2010;120(11): 3788–3797.
28. Apkarian AV, Bushnell MC, Treede RD, Zubieta JK. Human brain mechanisms of pain perception and regulation in health and disease. *Eur J Pain.* 2005;9(4):463–484.
29. Moisset X, Bouhassira D. Brain imaging of neuropathic pain. *Neuroimage.* 2007;37(Suppl. 1):S80–S88.
30. Neugebauer V, Galhardo V, Maione S, Mackey SC. Forebrain pain mechanisms. *Brain Res Rev.* 2009;60(1):226–242.
31. Melzack R, Wall PD. Pain mechanisms: a new theory. *Science.* 1965;150(3699):971–979.
32. Fields HL, Basbaum AI. Central nervous system mechanisms of pain modulation. In: Wall PD, Melzack R, eds. *Textbook of Pain.* 4th ed. Churchill Livingstone; 1999:309–329.
33. Mayer D, Wolfle T, Akil H, Carder B, Liebeskind J. Analgesia from electrical stimulation in the brainstem of the rat. *Science.* 1971;174(16):1351–1354.
34. Reynolds DV. Surgery in the rat during electrical analgesia induced by focal brain stimulation. *Science.* 1969;164(878): 444–445.
35. Boivie J, Meyerson BA. A correlative anatomical and clinical study of pain suppression by deep brain stimulation. *Pain.* 1982;13(2):113–126.
36. Baskin DS, Mehler WR, Hosobuchi Y, Richardson DE, Adams JE, Flitter MA. Autopsy analysis of the safety, efficacy and cartography of electrical stimulation of the central gray in humans. *Brain Res.* 1986;371(2):231–236.
37. Basbaum A, Fields H. Endogenous pain control mechanisms: review and hypothesis. *Ann Neurol.* 1978;4(5):451–462.
38. Basbaum AI, Clanton CH, Fields HL. Opiate and stimulus-produced analgesia: functional anatomy of a medullospinal pathway. *Proc Natl Acad Sci USA.* 1976;73(12):4685–4688.
39. Yaksh TL, Yeung JC, Rudy TA. Systematic examination in the rat of brain sites sensitive to the direct application of morphine: observation of differential effects within the periaqueductal gray. *Brain Res.* 1976;114(1):83–103.
40. Basbaum A, Marley N, O'Keefe J, Clanton C. Reversal of morphine and stimulus-produced analgesia by subtotal spinal cord lesions. *Pain.* 1977;3(1):43–56.
41. Fields HL, Basbaum AI, Clanton CH, Anderson SD. Nucleus raphe magnus inhibition of spinal cord dorsal horn neurons. *Brain Res.* 1977;126(3):441–453.
42. Yaksh T, Plant R, Rudy T. Studies on the antagonism by raphe lesions of the antinociceptive action of systemic morphine. *Eur J Pharmacol.* 1977;41(4):399–408.
43. Bryant RM, Olley JE, Tyers MB. Involvement of the median raphe nucleus in antinociception induced by morphine, buprenorphine and tilidine in the rat. *Br J Pharmacol.* 1982;77(4):615–624.
44. Jones S, Gebhart G. Inhibition of spinal nociceptive transmission from the midbrain, pons and medulla in the rat: activation of descending inhibition by morphine, glutamate and electrical stimulation. *Brain Res.* 1988;460(2):281–296.
45. Sukhotinsky I, Hopkins DA, Lu J, Saper CB, Devor M. Movement suppression during anesthesia: neural projections from the mesopontine tegmentum to areas involved in motor control. *J Comp Neurol.* 2005;489(4):425–448.
46. Rye D, Lee H, Saper C, Wainer B. Medullary and spinal efferents of the pedunculopontine tegmental nucleus and adjacent mesopontine tegmentum in the rat. *J Comp Neurol.* 1988;269(3):315–341.
47. Lai Y, Clements J, Wu X, et al. Brainstem projections to the ventromedial medulla in cat: retrograde transport horseradish peroxidase and immunohistochemical studies. *J Comp Neurol.* 1999;408:419–436.
48. Abols I, Basbaum A. Afferent connections of the rostral medulla of the cat: a neural substrate for midbrain-medullary interactions in the modulation of pain. *J Comp Neurol.* 1981;201:285–297.
49. Wang H, Wessendorf M. μ- and δ-opioid receptor mRNAs are expressed in periaqueductal gray neurons projecting to the rostral ventromedial medulla. *Neuroscience.* 2002;109(3):619–634.
50. Basbaum AI, Clanton CH, Fields HL. Three bulbospinal pathways from the rostral medulla of the cat: an autoradiographic study of pain modulating systems. *J Comp Neurol.* 1978;178(2): 209–224.
51. Fields H, Bry J, Hentall I, Zorman G. The activity of neurons in the rostral medulla of the rat during withdrawal from noxious heat. *J Neurosci.* 1983;3(12):2545–2552.
52. Mason P. Central mechanisms of pain modulation. *Curr Opin Neurobiol.* 1999;9(4):436–441.
53. Porreca F, Ossipov M, Gebhart G. Chronic pain and medullary descending facilitation. *Trends Neurosci.* 2002;25(6):319–325.
54. Foo H, Mason P. Discharge of raphe magnus ON and OFF cells is predictive of the motor facilitation evoked by repeated laser stimulation. *J Neurosci.* 2003;23(5):1933–1940.
55. Neubert M, Kincaid W, Heinricher M. Nociceptive facilitating neurons in the rostral ventromedial medulla. *Pain.* 2004;110(1–2): 158–165.
56. Fields H, Heinricher M. Anatomy and physiology of a nociceptive modulatory system. *Philos Trans R Soc Lond B Biol Sci.* 1985;308(1136):361–374.
57. Mason P. Contributions of the medullary raphe and ventromedial reticular region to pain modulation and other homeostatic functions. *Annu Rev Neurosci.* 2001;24:737–777.
58. Heinricher MM, Cheng ZF, Fields HL. Evidence for two classes of nociceptive modulating neurons in the periaqueductal gray. *J Neurosci.* 1987;7(1):271–278.
59. Haws CM, Williamson AM, Fields HL. Putative nociceptive modulatory neurons in the dorsolateral pontomesencephalic reticular formation. *Brain Res.* 1989;483(2):272–282.
60. Kwiat GC, Basbaum AI. The origin of brainstem noradrenergic and serotonergic projections to the spinal cord dorsal horn in the rat. *Somatosens Mot Res.* 1992;9(2):157–173.
61. Clark FM, Proudfit HK. The projection of noradrenergic neurons in the A7 catecholamine cell group to the spinal cord in the rat demonstrated by anterograde tracing combined with immunocytochemistry. *Brain Res.* 1991;547(2):279–288.
62. Yaksh TL. Direct evidence that spinal serotonin and noradrenaline terminals mediate the spinal antinociceptive effects of morphine in the periaqueductal gray. *Brain Res.* 1979;160(1):180–185.

63. Barbaro NM, Hammond DL, Fields HL. Effects of intrathecally administered methysergide and yohimbine on microstimulation-produced antinociception in the rat. *Brain Res*. 1985;343(2):223–229.
64. Yeung JC, Yaksh TL, Rudy TA. Concurrent mapping of brain sites for sensitivity to the direct application of morphine and focal electrical stimulation in the production of antinociception in the rat. *Pain*. 1977;4(1):23–40.
65. Helmstetter FJ, Tershner SA, Poore LH, Bellgowan PS. Antinociception following opioid stimulation of the basolateral amygdala is expressed through the periaqueductal gray and rostral ventromedial medulla. *Brain Res*. 1998; 779(1–2):104–118.
66. Fang FG, Haws CM, Drasner K, Williamson A, Fields HL. Opioid peptides (DAGO-enkephalin, dynorphin A(1–13), BAM 22P) microinjected into the rat brainstem: comparison of their antinociceptive effect and their effect on neuronal firing in the rostral ventromedial medulla. *Brain Res*. 1989;501(1):116–128.
67. Akil H, Owens C, Gutstein H, Taylor L, Curran E, Watson S. Endogenous opioids: overview and current issues. *Drug Alcohol Depend*. 1998;51(1–2):127–140.
68. Mansour A, Fox CA, Akil H, Watson SJ. Opioid-receptor mRNA expression in the rat CNS: anatomical and functional implications. *Trends Neurosci*. 1995;18(1):22–29.
69. Snyder SH, Pasternak GW. Historical review: opioid receptors. *Trends Pharmacol Sci*. 2003;24(4):198–205.
70. Anton B, Fein J, To T, Li X, Silberstein L, Evans CJ. Immunohistochemical localization of ORL-1 in the central nervous system of the rat. *J Comp Neurol*. 1996;368(2):229–251.
71. Finley JC, Maderdrut JL, Petrusz P. The immunocytochemical localization of enkephalin in the central nervous system of the rat. *J Comp Neurol*. 1981;198(4):541–565.
72. Weber E, Barchas JD. Immunohistochemical distribution of dynorphin B in rat brain: relation to dynorphin A and alpha-neo-endorphin systems. *Proc Natl Acad Sci USA*. 1983;80(4): 1125–1129.
73. Schulz S, Schreff M, Nuss D, Gramsch C, Hollt V. Nociceptin/orphanin FQ and opioid peptides show overlapping distribution but not co-localization in pain-modulatory brain regions. *Neuroreport*. 1996;7(18):3021–3025.
74. Meunier JC. Nociceptin/orphanin FQ and the opioid receptor-like ORL1 receptor. *Eur J Pharmacol*. 1997;340(1):1–15.
75. Burke MC, Letts PA, Krajewski SJ, Rance NE. Coexpression of dynorphin and neurokinin B immunoreactivity in the rat hypothalamus: morphologic evidence of interrelated function within the arcuate nucleus. *J Comp Neurol*. 2006;498(5):712–726.
76. Fields H. State-dependent opioid control of pain. *Nat Rev Neurosci*. 2004;5(7):565–575.
77. Levine JD, Gordon NC, Fields HL. The mechanism of placebo analgesia. *Lancet*. 1978;2(8091):654–657.
78. Benedetti F, Mayberg HS, Wager TD, Stohler CS, Zubieta JK. Neurobiological mechanisms of the placebo effect. *J Neurosci*. 2005;25(45):10390–10402.
79. Benedetti F, Amanzio M, Rosato R, Blanchard C. Nonopioid placebo analgesia is mediated by CB1 cannabinoid receptors. *Nat Med*. 2011;17(10):1228–1230.
80. Petrovic P, Kalso E, Petersson KM, Ingvar M. Placebo and opioid analgesia—imaging a shared neuronal network. *Science*. 2002;295(5560):1737–1740.
81. Eippert F, Finsterbusch J, Bingel U, Buchel C. Direct evidence for spinal cord involvement in placebo analgesia. *Science*. 2009;326(5951):404.
82. Wager TD, Rilling JK, Smith EE, et al. Placebo-induced changes in FMRI in the anticipation and experience of pain. *Science*. 2004;303(5661):1162–1167.
83. Merskey H, Bogduk N, eds. *Classification of Chronic Pain*. 2nd ed. IASP Press; 1994.
84. Woolf CJ. Central sensitization: implications for the diagnosis and treatment of pain. *Pain*. 2011;152(3 Suppl.):S2–S15.
85. Latremoliere A, Woolf CJ. Central sensitization: a generator of pain hypersensitivity by central neural plasticity. *J Pain*. 2009; 10(9):895–926.
86. Flor H, Braun C, Elbert T, Birbaumer N. Extensive reorganization of primary somatosensory cortex in chronic back pain patients. *Neurosci Lett*. 1997;224(1):5–8.
87. Flor H, Elbert T, Knecht S, et al. Phantom-limb pain as a perceptual correlate of cortical reorganization following arm amputation. *Nature*. 1995;375(6531):482–484.
88. Boucher TJ, McMahon SB. Neurotrophic factors and neuropathic pain. *Curr Opin Pharmacol*. 2001;1(1):66–72.
89. Costigan M, Befort K, Karchewski L, et al. Replicate high-density rat genome oligonucleotide microarrays reveal hundreds of regulated genes in the dorsal root ganglion after peripheral nerve injury. *BMC Neurosci*. 2002;3:16.
90. Xiao HS, Huang QH, Zhang FX, et al. Identification of gene expression profile of dorsal root ganglion in the rat peripheral axotomy model of neuropathic pain. *Proc Natl Acad Sci USA*. 2002;99(12):8360–8365.
91. Devor M. Peripheral neuropathic pain. In: Willis W, Schmidt R, eds. *Encyclopedia of Pain*. Springer; 2007.
92. Persson AK, Gebauer M, Jordan S, et al. Correlational analysis for identifying genes whose regulation contributes to chronic neuropathic pain. *Mol Pain*. 2009;5:7.
93. Waxman SG, Cummins TR, Dib-Hajj SD, Black JA. Voltage-gated sodium channels and the molecular pathogenesis of pain: a review. *J Rehabil Res Dev*. 2000;37(5):517–528.
94. Costigan M, Scholz J, Woolf CJ. Neuropathic pain: a maladaptive response of the nervous system to damage. *Annu Rev Neurosci*. 2009;32:1–32.
95. Devor M, Govrin-Lippmann R, Angelides K. Na^+ channel immunolocalization in peripheral mammalian axons and changes following nerve injury and neuroma formation. *J Neurosci*. 1993;13(5):1976–1992.
96. Devor M. Sodium channels and mechanisms of neuropathic pain. *J Pain*. 2006;7(1 Suppl. 1):S3–S12.
97. Amir R, Michaelis M, Devor M. Membrane potential oscillations in dorsal root ganglion neurons: role in normal electrogenesis and neuropathic pain. *J Neurosci*. 1999;19(19):8589–8596.
98. Nordin M, Nystrom B, Wallin U, Hagbarth KE. Ectopic sensory discharges and paresthesiae in patients with disorders of peripheral nerves, dorsal roots and dorsal columns. *Pain*. 1984;20(3): 231–245.
99. Devor M. Peripheral nerve generators of neuropathic pain. In: Campbell JN, Basbaum AI, Dray A, Dubner R, Dworkin RH, Sang CN, eds. *Emerging Strategies for the Treatment of Neuropathic Pain*. Seattle: IASP Press; 2006:37–68.
100. Serra J, Bostock H, Sola R, et al. Microneurographic identification of spontaneous activity in C-nociceptors in neuropathic pain states in humans and rats. *Pain*. 2012;153(1):42–55.
101. Devor M. Central changes after peripheral nerve injury. In: Willis W, Schmidt R, eds. *Encyclopedia of Pain*. Springer; 2007: 306–311.
102. McMahon SB, Cafferty WB, Marchand F. Immune and glial cell factors as pain mediators and modulators. *Exp Neurol*. 2005; 192(2):444–462.
103. Scholz J, Broom DC, Youn DH, et al. Blocking caspase activity prevents transsynaptic neuronal apoptosis and the loss of inhibition in lamina II of the dorsal horn after peripheral nerve injury. *J Neurosci*. 2005;25(32):7317–7323.

104. Whiteside GT, Munglani R. Cell death in the superficial dorsal horn in a model of neuropathic pain. *J Neurosci Res*. 2001;64(2):168–173.
105. Devor M. Ectopic generators. In: Basbaum AI, Kaneko A, Shepherd GM, Westheimer G, eds. *The Senses: A Comprehensive Reference*. San Diego: Academic Press; 2008:83–88. Basbaum AI, Bushnell CM, eds. Pain; Vol. 5.
106. Devor M, Janig W. Activation of myelinated afferents ending in a neuroma by stimulation of the sympathetic supply in the rat. *Neurosci Lett*. 1981;24(1):43–47.
107. Devor M, Janig W, Michaelis M. Modulation of activity in dorsal root ganglion neurons by sympathetic activation in nerve-injured rats. *J Neurophysiol*. 1994;71(1):38–47.
108. Shinder V, Govrin-Lippmann R, Cohen S, et al. Structural basis of sympathetic-sensory coupling in rat and human dorsal root ganglia following peripheral nerve injury. *J Neurocytol*. 1999;28(9):743–761.
109. Chen Y, Michaelis M, Janig W, Devor M. Adrenoreceptor subtype mediating sympathetic-sensory coupling in injured sensory neurons. *J Neurophysiol*. 1996;76(6):3721–3730.
110. Raja SN, Meyer RA, Ringkamp M, Campbell JN. Peripheral neural mechanisms of nociception. In: Wall PD, Melzack R, eds. *Textbook of Pain*. 4th ed. Churchill Livingstone; 1999:11–57.
111. Devor M, Seltzer Z. Pathophysiology of damaged nerves in relation to chronic pain. In: Wall PD, Melzack R, eds. *Textbook of Pain*. 4th ed. Churchill Livingstone; 1999:129–164.
112. Baliki MN, Schnitzer TJ, Bauer WR, Apkarian AV. Brain morphological signatures for chronic pain. *PLoS One*. 2011;6(10):e26010.
113. Jones AK, Derbyshire SW. Reduced cortical responses to noxious heat in patients with rheumatoid arthritis. *Ann Rheum Dis*. 1997;56(10):601–607.
114. Derbyshire SW. Meta-analysis of thirty-four independent samples studied using PET reveals a significantly attenuated central response to noxious stimulation in clinical pain patients. *Curr Rev Pain*. 1999;3(4):265–280.
115. Hsieh JC, Belfrage M, Stone-Elander S, Hansson P, Ingvar M. Central representation of chronic ongoing neuropathic pain studied by positron emission tomography. *Pain*. 1995;63(2):225–236.
116. Iadarola MJ, Max MB, Berman KF, et al. Unilateral decrease in thalamic activity observed with positron emission tomography in patients with chronic neuropathic pain. *Pain*. 1995;63(1):55–64.
117. Apkarian AV, Sosa Y, Sonty S, et al. Chronic back pain is associated with decreased prefrontal and thalamic gray matter density. *J Neurosci*. 2004;24(46):10410–10415.
118. Schmidt-Wilcke T, Leinisch E, Straube A, et al. Gray matter decrease in patients with chronic tension type headache. *Neurology*. 2005;65(9):1483–1486.
119. Kuchinad A, Schweinhardt P, Seminowicz DA, Wood PB, Chizh BA, Bushnell MC. Accelerated brain gray matter loss in fibromyalgia patients: premature aging of the brain? *J Neurosci*. 2007;27(15):4004–4007.
120. Schmidt-Wilcke T, Leinisch E, Ganssbauer S, et al. Affective components and intensity of pain correlate with structural differences in gray matter in chronic back pain patients. *Pain*. 2006;125(1–2):89–97.
121. Rodriguez-Raecke R, Niemeier A, Ihle K, Ruether W, May A. Brain gray matter decrease in chronic pain is the consequence and not the cause of pain. *J Neurosci*. 2009;29(44):13746–13750.
122. Seminowicz DA, Wideman TH, Naso L, et al. Effective treatment of chronic low back pain in humans reverses abnormal brain anatomy and function. *J Neurosci*. 2011;31(20):7540–7550.
123. Obermann M, Nebel K, Schumann C, et al. Gray matter changes related to chronic posttraumatic headache. *Neurology*. 2009;73(12):978–983.
124. Vera-Portocarrero LP, Zhang ET, Ossipov MH, et al. Descending facilitation from the rostral ventromedial medulla maintains nerve injury-induced central sensitization. *Neuroscience*. 2006;140(4):1311–1320.
125. Lima D, Almeida A. The medullary dorsal reticular nucleus as a pronociceptive centre of the pain control system. *Prog Neurobiol*. 2002;66(2):81–108.
126. Rahman W, D'Mello R, Dickenson AH. Peripheral nerve injury-induced changes in spinal α_2-adrenoceptor-mediated modulation of mechanically evoked dorsal horn neuronal responses. *J Pain*. 2008;9(4):350–359.
127. Fairhurst M, Wiech K, Dunckley P, Tracey I. Anticipatory brainstem activity predicts neural processing of pain in humans. *Pain*. 2007;128(1–2):101–110.
128. Song GH, Venkatraman V, Ho KY, Chee MW, Yeoh KG, Wilder-Smith CH. Cortical effects of anticipation and endogenous modulation of visceral pain assessed by functional brain MRI in irritable bowel syndrome patients and healthy controls. *Pain*. 2006;126(1–3):79–90.
129. May A. Chronic pain may change the structure of the brain. *Pain*. 2008;137(1):7–15.
130. Willoch F, Schindler F, Wester HJ, et al. Central poststroke pain and reduced opioid receptor binding within pain processing circuitries: a [^{11}C]diprenorphine PET study. *Pain*. 2004;108(3):213–220.
131. Jones AK, Watabe H, Cunningham VJ, Jones T. Cerebral decreases in opioid receptor binding in patients with central neuropathic pain measured by [^{11}C]diprenorphine binding and PET. *Eur J Pain*. 2004;8(5):479–485.
132. Brown WM. The conquest of pain. *Ulster Med J*. 1959;28:101–117.
133. Franks NP, Lieb WR. Molecular and cellular mechanisms of general anaesthesia. *Nature*. 1994;367(6464):607–614.
134. Eckenhoff RG, Johansson JS. Molecular interactions between inhaled anesthetics and proteins. *Pharmacol Rev*. 1997;49(4):343–367.
135. Patel AJ, Honore E, Lesage F, Fink M, Romey G, Lazdunski M. Inhalational anesthetics activate two-pore-domain background K^+ channels. *Nat Neurosci*. 1999;2(5):422–426.
136. Solt K, Forman SA. Correlating the clinical actions and molecular mechanisms of general anesthetics. *Curr Opin Anaesthesiol*. 2007;20(4):300–306.
137. Urban BW, Bleckwenn M, Barann M. Interactions of anesthetics with their targets: non-specific, specific or both? *Pharmacol Ther*. 2006;111(3):729–770.
138. Daniels S, Roberts RJ. Post-synaptic inhibitory mechanisms of anaesthesia; glycine receptors. *Toxicol Lett*. 1998;100–101:71–76.
139. Mehta AK, Ticku MK. An update on $GABA_A$ receptors. *Brain Res Brain Res Rev*. 1999;29(2–3):196–217.
140. Cheng G, Kendig JJ. Enflurane directly depresses glutamate AMPA and NMDA currents in mouse spinal cord motor neurons independent of actions on $GABA_A$ or glycine receptors. *Anesthesiology*. 2000;93(4):1075–1084.
141. Arias HR, Kem WR, Trudell JR, Blanton MP. Unique general anesthetic binding sites within distinct conformational states of the nicotinic acetylcholine receptor. *Int Rev Neurobiol*. 2003;54:1–50.
142. Gomez RS, Guatimosim C. Mechanism of action of volatile anesthetics: involvement of intracellular calcium signaling. *Curr Drug Targets CNS Neurol Disord*. 2003;2(2):123–129.
143. Yost CS. Update on tandem pore (2P) domain K^+ channels. *Curr Drug Targets*. 2003;4(4):347–351.
144. Franks NP. General anaesthesia: from molecular targets to neuronal pathways of sleep and arousal. *Nat Rev Neurosci*. 2008;9(5):370–386.
145. Alkire M, Haier R, Barker S, et al. Toward a unified theory of narcosis: brain imaging evidence for a thalamocortical switch as

the neurophysiological basis of anaesthetic-induced unconsciousness. *Conscious Cogn*. 2000;9:370–386.
146. Fiset P, Paus T, Daloze T, et al. Brain mechanisms of propofol-induced loss of consciousness in humans: a positron emission tomographic study. *J Neurosci*. 1999;19(13):5506–5513.
147. Antkowiak B. How do general anaesthetics work? *Naturwissenschaften*. 2001;88:201–213.
148. Grasshoff C, Rudolph U, Antkowiak B. Molecular and systemic mechanisms of general anaesthesia: the 'multi-site and multiple mechanisms' concept. *Curr Opin Anaesthesiol*. 2005;18(4):386–391.
149. Magni F, Moruzzi G, Rossi G, Zanchetti A. EEG arousal following inactivation of the lower brain stem by selective injection of barbiturate into the vertebral circulation. *Arch Ital Biol*. 1959;97:33–41.
150. Rampil I, Mason P, Singh H. Anesthetic potency (MAC) is independent of forebrain structures in the rat. *Anesthesiology*. 1993; 78(4):707–712.
151. Todd MM, Weeks JB, Warner DS. A focal cryogenic brain lesion does not reduce the minimum alveolar concentration for halothane in rats. *Anesthesiology*. 1993;79(1):139–143.
152. Livingstone MS, Hubel DH. Effects of sleep and arousal on the processing of visual information in the cat. *Nature*. 1981; 291(5816):554–561.
153. Stryker MP, Jenkins WM, Merzenich MM. Anesthetic state does not affect the map of the hand representation within area 3b somatosensory cortex in owl monkey. *J Comp Neurol*. 1987;258(2): 297–303.
154. Saper CB, Chou TC, Scammell TE. The sleep switch: hypothalamic control of sleep and wakefulness. *Trends Neurosci*. 2001; 24(12):726–731.
155. Nelson L, Guo T, Lu J, Saper C, Franks N, Maze M. The sedative component of anesthesia is mediated by $GABA_A$ receptors in an endogenous sleep pathway. *Nat Neurosci*. 2002;5(10):979–984.
156. D'Aquili EG, Chambers WW, Liu CN, McCouch GP. Reflex resistance to anesthesia in partially denervated neurons. *Exp Neurol*. 1966;16(3):307–315.
157. Jugovac I, Imas O, Hudetz AG. Supraspinal anesthesia: behavioral and electroencephalographic effects of intracerebroventricularly infused pentobarbital, propofol, fentanyl, and midazolam. *Anesthesiology*. 2006;105(4):764–778.
158. Tomemori N, Komatsu T, Shingu K, Urabe N, Seo N, Mori K. Activation of the supraspinal pain inhibition system by ketamine hydrochloride. *Acta Anaesthesiol Scand*. 1981;25:355–359.
159. Stabernack C, Zhang Y, Sonner JM, Laster M, Eger 2nd EI. Thiopental produces immobility primarily by supraspinal actions in rats. *Anesth Analg*. 2005;100(1):128–136.
160. Jinks S, Antognini JF, Carstens E, Buzin V, Simons C. Isoflurane can indirectly depress lumbar dorsal horn activity in the goat via action within the brain. *Br J Anaesth*. 1999;82(2):244–249.
161. Borges M, Antognini JF. Does the brain influence somatic responses to noxious stimuli during isoflurane anesthesia? *Anesthesiology*. 1994;81(6):1511–1515.
162. Antognini J, Carstens E, Atherley R. Does the immobilizing effect of thiopental in brain exceed that of halothane? *Anesthesiology*. 2002;96(4):980–986.
163. Antognini J, Schwartz K. Exaggerated anesthetic requirements in the preferentially anesthetized brain. *Anesthesiology*. 1993;79: 1244–1249.
164. Roizen MF, White PF, Eger 2nd EI, Brownstein M. Effects of ablation of serotonin or norepinephrine brain-stem areas on halothane and cyclopropane MACs in rats. *Anesthesiology*. 1978; 49(4):252–255.
165. Moruzzi G, Magoun H. Brain stem reticular formation and activation of the EEG. *Electroencephalogr Clin Neurophysiol*. 1949;1: 455–473.
166. Lindsley DB, Schreiner LH, Knowles WB, Magoun HW. Behavioral and EEG changes following chronic brain stem lesions in the cat. *Electroencephalogr Clin Neurophysiol*. 1950;2(4):483–498.
167. Plum F, Posner J. *The Diagnosis of Stupor and Coma*. Philadelphia: Davis; 1980.
168. Parvizi J, Damasio AR. Neuroanatomical correlates of brainstem coma. *Brain*. 2003;126(Pt 7):1524–1536.
169. Voss LJ, Young BJ, Barnards JP, Sleigh J. Differential anaesthetic effects following microinjection of thiopentone and propofol into the pons of adult rats: a pilot study. *Anaesth Intensive Care*. 2005;33(3):373–380.
170. Sukhotinsky I, Zalkind V, Lu J, Hopkins DA, Saper CB, Devor M. Neural pathways associated with loss of consciousness caused by intracerebral microinjection of $GABA_A$-active anesthetics. *Eur J Neurosci*. 2007;25(5):1417–1436.
171. Abulafia R, Zalkind V, Devor M. Cerebral activity during the anesthesia-like state induced by mesopontine microinjection of pentobarbital. *J Neurosci*. 2009;29(21):7053–7064.
172. Sukhotinsky I, Zalkind V, Devor M. Anesthetic effect of barbiturates microinjected into the brainstem: neuroanatomy. In: Dostrovsky J, Carr D, Koltzenburg M, eds. *Proceedings of the 10th World Congress on Pain*. Vol. 24. Seattle: IASP Press; 2003:305–313.
173. Lim M, Lindquist C, Birnir B. Effects of pentobarbital on GABA-activated currents in acutely-isolated rat dentate gyrus granule neurons. *Neurosci Lett*. 2003;353(2):139–142.
174. Woolf NJ, Butcher LL. Cholinergic systems in the rat brain: III. Projections from the pontomesencephalic tegmentum to the thalamus, tectum, basal ganglia, and basal forebrain. *Brain Res Bull*. 1986;16(5):603–637.
175. Jones B. Reticular formation: cytoarchitecture, transmitters and projections. In: Paxinos G, ed. *The Rat Nervous System*. 2nd ed. San Diego: Academic Press; 1995:155–171.
176. Shammah-Lagnado S, Negrao N, Silva B, Ricardo J. Afferent connections of the nuclei reticularis pontis oralis and caudalis: a horseradish peroxidase study in the rat. *Neuroscience*. 1987;20(3): 961–989.
177. Jones B, Yang T. The efferent projections from the reticular formation and the locus coeruleus studied by anterograde and retrograde axonal transport in the rat. *J Comp Neurol*. 1985;242:56–92.
178. Ford B, Holmes C, Mainville L, Jones B. GABAergic neurons in the rat pontomesencephalic tegmentum: codistribution with cholinergic and other tegmental neurons projecting to the posterior lateral hypothalamus. *J Comp Neurol*. 1995;363(2):177–196.
179. Newman DB, Ginsberg CY. Brainstem reticular nuclei that project to the thalamus in rats: a retrograde tracer study. *Brain Behav Evol*. 1994;44(1):1–39.
180. Semba K, Fibiger HC. Afferent connections of the laterodorsal and the pedunculopontine tegmental nuclei in the rat: a retro- and antero-grade transport and immunohistochemical study. *J Comp Neurol*. 1992;323(3):387–410.
181. Lefler Y, Arzi A, Reiner K, Sukhotinsky I, Devor M. Bulbospinal neurons of the rat rostromedial medulla are highly collateralized. *J Comp Neurol*. 2008;506(6):960–978.
182. Sukhotinsky I, Reiner K, Govrin-Lippmann R, et al. Projections from the mesopontine tegmental anesthesia area to regions involved in pain modulation. *J Chem Neuroanat*. 2006;32(2–4):159–178.
183. Reiner K, Sukhotinsky I, Devor M. Mesopontine tegmental anesthesia area projects independently to the rostromedial medulla and to the spinal cord. *Neuroscience*. 2007;146(3):1355–1370.
184. Reiner K, Sukhotinsky I, Devor M. Bulbospinal neurons implicated in mesopontine-induced anesthesia are substantially collateralized. *J Comp Neurol*. 2008;508(3):418–436.
185. Hajnik T, Lai Y, Siegel J. Atonia-related regions in the rodent pons and medulla. *J Neurophysiol*. 2000;84(4):1942–1948.

186. Liebeskind J, Guilbaud G, Besson J, Oliveras J. Analgesia from electrical stimulation of the periaqueductal gray matter in the cat: behavioral observations and inhibitory effects on spinal cord interneurons. *Brain Res.* 1973;50(2):441–446.
187. Carstens E, Watkins L. Inhibition of the responses of neurons in the rat spinal cord to noxious skin heating by stimulation in midbrain periaqueductal gray or lateral reticular formation. *Brain Res.* 1986;382(2):266–277.
188. Jinks S, Carstens E, Antognini J. Isoflurane differentially modulates medullary on and off neurons while suppressing hind-limb motor withdrawals. *Anesthesiology.* 2004;100(5):1224–1234.
189. Oliveras J, Montagne-Clavel J, Martin G. Drastic changes of ventromedial medulla neuronal properties induced by barbiturate anesthesia. I. Comparison of the single-unit types in the same awake and pentobarbital-treated rats. *Brain Res.* 1991;563(1–2):241–250.
190. Leung CG, Mason P. Physiological properties of raphe magnus neurons during sleep and waking. *J Neurophysiol.* 1999;81(2): 584–595.
191. Namjoshi DR, McErlane SA, Taepavarapruk N, Soja PJ. Network actions of pentobarbital in the rat mesopontine tegmentum on sensory inflow through the spinothalamic tract. *J Neurophysiol.* 2009;102(2):700–713.
192. Tavares I, Lima D. The caudal ventrolateral medulla as an important inhibitory modulator of pain transmission in the spinal cord. *J Pain.* 2002;3(5):337–346.
193. Gebhart G, Ossipov M. Characterization of inhibition of the spinal nociceptive tail-flick reflex in the rat from the medullary lateral reticular nucleus. *J Neurosci.* 1986;6(3):701–713.
194. Hall J, Duggan A, Morton C, Johnson S. The location of brainstem neurones tonically inhibiting dorsal horn neurones of the cat. *Brain Res.* 1982;244(2):215–222.
195. Almeida A, Storkson R, Lima D, Hole K, Tjolsen A. The medullary dorsal reticular nucleus facilitates pain behaviour induced by formalin in the rat. *Eur J Neurosci.* 1999;11(1):110–122.
196. Monconduit L, Desbois C, Villanueva L. The integrative role of the rat medullary subnucleus reticularis dorsalis in nociception. *Eur J Neurosci.* 2002;16(5):937–944.
197. Dugast C, Almeida A, Lima D. The medullary dorsal reticular nucleus enhances the responsiveness of spinal nociceptive neurons to peripheral stimulation in the rat. *Eur J Neurosci.* 2003;18(3):580–588.
198. Suzuki R, Rygh LJ, Dickenson AH. Bad news from the brain: descending 5-HT pathways that control spinal pain processing. *Trends Pharmacol Sci.* 2004;25(12):613–617.
199. Dafny N, Dong W, Prieto-Gomez C, Reyes-Vazquez C, Stanford J, Qiao J. Lateral hypothalamus: site involved in pain modulation. *Neuroscience.* 1996;70(2):449–460.
200. Franco A, Prado W. Antinociceptive effects of stimulation of discrete sites in the rat hypothalamus: evidence for the participation of the lateral hypothalamus area in descending pain suppression mechanisms. *Braz J Med Biol Res.* 1996;29(11):1531–1541.
201. Okada N, Matsumoto N, Kitada Y. Responses of diencephalic nociceptive neurones to orofacial stimuli and effects of internal capsule stimulation in the rat. *Arch Oral Biol.* 2002;47(12): 815–829.
202. Jaaskelainen SK, Rinne JO, Forssell H, et al. Role of the dopaminergic system in chronic pain – a fluorodopa-PET study. *Pain.* 2001;90(3):257–260.
203. Butler RK, Nilsson-Todd L, Cleren C, Lena I, Garcia R, Finn DP. Molecular and electrophysiological changes in the prefrontal cortex–amygdala–dorsal periaqueductal grey pathway during persistent pain state and fear-conditioned analgesia. *Physiol Behav.* 2011;104(5):1075–1081.
204. Neugebauer V, Li W, Bird GC, Han JS. The amygdala and persistent pain. *Neuroscientist.* 2004;10(3):221–234.
205. Bourbia N, Ansah OB, Pertovaara A. Corticotropin-releasing factor in the rat amygdala differentially influences sensory-discriminative and emotional-like pain response in peripheral neuropathy. *J Pain.* 2010;11(12):1461–1471.
206. Faingold CL. Electrical stimulation therapies for CNS disorders and pain are mediated by competition between different neuronal networks in the brain. *Med Hypotheses.* 2008;71(5): 668–681.
207. Sukhotinsky I, Ben-Dor E, Raber P, Devor M. Key role of the dorsal root ganglion in neuropathic tactile hypersensibility. *Eur J Pain.* 2004;8(2):135–143.
208. Iannetti GD, Zambreanu L, Wise RG, et al. Pharmacological modulation of pain-related brain activity during normal and central sensitization states in humans. *Proc Natl Acad Sci USA.* 2005;102(50):18195–18200.
209. Gale K. Subcortical structures and pathways involved in convulsive seizure generation. *J Clin Neurophysiol.* 1992;9(2): 264–277.
210. Belelli D, Harrison NL, Maguire J, Macdonald RL, Walker MC, Cope DW. Extrasynaptic $GABA_A$ receptors: form, pharmacology, and function. *J Neurosci.* 2009;29(41):12757–12763.
211. Vithlani M, Terunuma M, Moss SJ. The dynamic modulation of $GABA_A$ receptor trafficking and its role in regulating the plasticity of inhibitory synapses. *Physiol Rev.* 2011;91(3):1009–1022.
212. Deisseroth K. Optogenetics. *Nat Methods.* 2011;8(1):26–29.
213. Sukhotinsky I, Chan AM, Ahmed OJ, et al. Optogenetic delay of status epilepticus onset in an in vivo rodent epilepsy model. *PLoS One.* 2013;8(4):e62013.
214. Costantini LC, Bakowska JC, Breakefield XO, Isacson O. Gene therapy in the CNS. *Gene Ther.* 2000;7(2):93–109.
215. Mandel RJ, Burger C. Clinical trials in neurological disorders using AAV vectors: promises and challenges. *Curr Opin Mol Ther.* 2004;6(5):482–490.
216 Paxinos G, Watson C. *The rat brain in stereotaxic coordinates.* 4th ed. Academic Press; 1998.

CHAPTER

24

Networks in Mood and Anxiety Disorders

Hamada Hamid [1,2]

[1]Departments of Psychiatry and Neurology, Yale University, New Haven, CT, USA,
[2]Connecticut Veterans Administration Health Care System, West Haven, CT, USA

Discoveries in structural and functional networks involved in emotional processing have been among the most exciting developments in neuroscience. Emotional processing affects interpersonal relationships, determines the capacity to sympathize, provides a warning to aversive exposures, and shapes interpsychic homeostasis. Although highly debated, emotion is not simply a cognitive label to what is good or bad and happy or sad, but it is an independent process that provides valence to environmental stimuli.[1] While cognitive appraisal influences and is, at times, a component of emotional processing, people feel emotions independent of and, sometimes, prior to thoughts. Furthermore, people suffer from emotional distress independent of cognitive impairment or cognitive distortions.[2] Our modern understanding of the functional networks involved in emotional processes began with describing behavioral correlates to neurological lesions; developing experimental animal models in fear conditioning, learned helplessness, and psychiatric diseases; and demonstrating differences in brain activity (with or without specific tasks) in functional neuroimaging of various emotions' states and traits.

The clinical application of functional networks in the management of psychiatric disease is most apparent in the potential of deep brain stimulation (see Chapter 31) for the treatment of mood disorders,[3] obsessive-compulsive disorder,[4] and even Alzheimer dementia.[5] As more is learned about the mechanisms of emotional processing and clinical correlates to dysfunctional neural networks, psychiatric disease will be redefined, incorporating neuroanatomical changes to establish diagnoses and treatment interventions. The current *Diagnostic and Statistical Manual of Mental Disorders* (DSM) and *International Classification of Diseases* (ICD) model of diagnosing psychiatric disease relies on narrowly based phenomenological definitions of psychopathology: a cluster of signs and symptoms determines the current criteria of each psychiatric disease. For many psychiatric illnesses, there is a significant overlap in these signs and symptoms. Some suggest that the high comorbidity of psychiatric illnesses demonstrates the imprecision of psychiatric diagnosis.[6] Conversely, shared symptoms may be a result of common networks shared across disease states.[7] Across psychiatric states, symptoms such as difficulty with sleep, psychomotor agitation, and negative thoughts involve circadian circuits, subcortical structures, and prefrontal regions, respectively, regardless of the mental illness. For instance, difficulty sleeping involves dysfunction in circadian circuits (see Chapter 14) regardless of whether a person suffers from a mood or anxiety disorder. People who attempt suicide, whether diagnosed with major depressive disorder, bipolar disorder, or an anxiety disorder, demonstrate similar changes in neural networks involved in impulse control, emotional regulation, decision making, and reward processing. Interventions that target specific symptoms and their respective networks may be more effective in treating psychiatric disease.[8] Due to the limited space, this chapter will focus on neural networks of mood and anxiety disorders and demonstrate how these models are reshaping how psychiatric illness is conceptualized and treated. To begin to understand the networks involved in mood and anxiety, first the individual components, or nodes, of these networks will be reviewed.

AMYGDALA

The amygdala establishes the emotional tone of the neuronal network. Amygdalar function and circuits have been extensively reviewed[1,9,10] and may be summarized as playing a central role in fear conditioning and extinction, emotional regulation, consolidation of emotional memories, and interpretation of emotional cues. The amygdala may be divided into 12 different nuclei; however, the primary nuclei involved in

Neuronal Networks in Brain Function, CNS Disorders, and Therapeutics
http://dx.doi.org/10.1016/B978-0-12-415804-7.00024-1

emotional processing are the lateral (LA), basal (B), accessory basal (AB), and central (CE) nuclei. Structural networks, based on rodent and primate models, show that afferent projections to the amygdala arrive from the orbital and mesial prefrontal cortex and appear to modulate fear learning (Figure 24.1). Afferent pathways from the primary auditory cortex, auditory association cortex, and medial geniculate body process aversive auditory and sensory stimuli and terminate in the LA.[11] When the LA is lesioned, fear learning in response to auditory stimuli is prevented. The amygdala, particularly the CE, projects to neurons in the hypothalamus that mediate autonomic responses, such as increased heart rate and blood pressure, sweating, and piloerection. Efferent projections to the basal ganglia mediate behavioral responses such as avoidance and freezing when faced with threat.

The central role of amygdalar circuits in fear learning has been delineated using Pavlov's classical conditioning model in rodent and primate models. The model pairs innately fearful exposures as unconditioned stimuli (US) with emotionally neutral conditioned stimuli (CS), resulting in development of a fearful reaction to the CS (see Chapter 13). Since classical conditioning is modulated by the amygdala and is independent of the hippocampi and frontal regions, fear may develop unconsciously or through subliminal stimuli. In contrast, explicit fear memories are processed through pathways linking the ventral hippocampus to B and AB.[12,13] Rodents may be conditioned in an environmental context with lights, sounds, and smells when these are paired with electric shocks in a chamber. Rodents with intact amygdala and hippocampal connections will freeze when returned to the chamber that they were previously conditioned to fear. However, when hippocampal connections to the amygdala are lesioned, freezing behavior no longer occurs. Even with hippocampal lesions, rodents continue to freeze when exposed to the US (whether it is light, sound, or smell). This suggests that the amygdala is the central component to fear learning; however, the hippocampus plays a primary role in contextualizing fear memories.

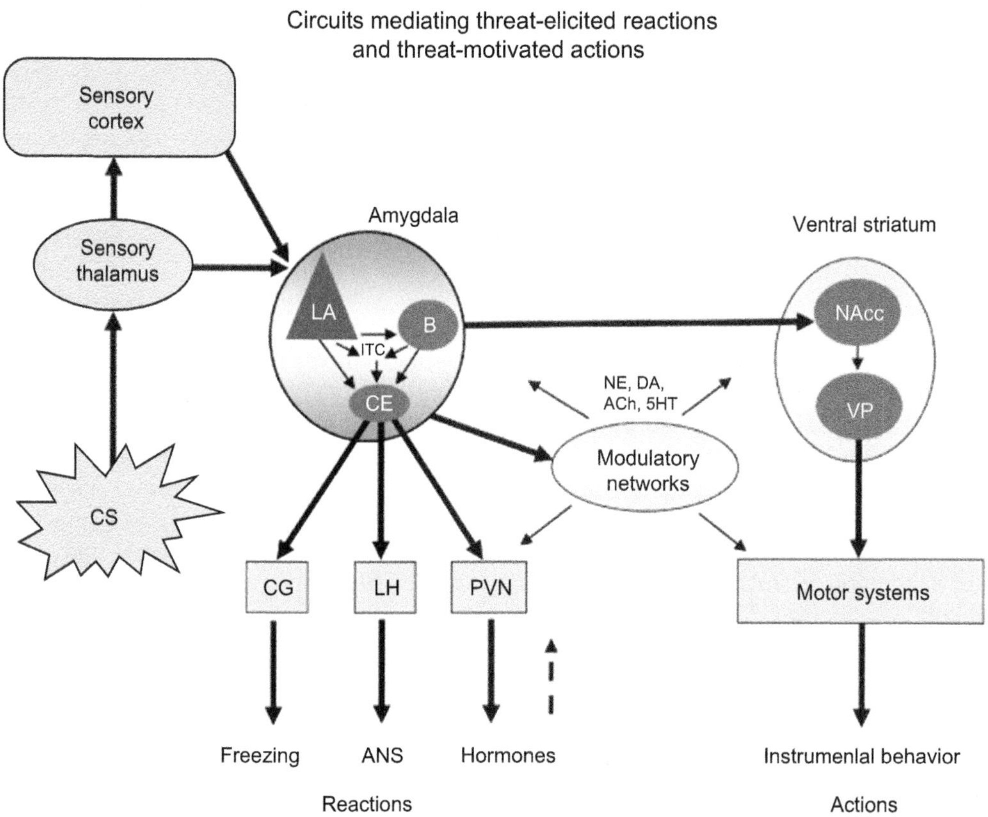

FIGURE 24.1 This model demonstrates the central role of the amygdala in the emotional memory network. Condition stimulus (CS) when paired with unconditioned stimulus (US) induces synaptic plasticity within the lateral nucleus of the amygdala (LA). With emotional stimulation the central nucleus (CE) activates neural modulators such as norepinephrine (NE), dopamine (DA), acetylcholine (Ach), and serotonin (5HT). Neural modulators stimulate the paraventricular nucleus of the hypothalamus (PVN) releasing hormones; central grey of the periaqueductal grey (CG) mediates freezing behavior during fear; the lateral hypothalamus (LH) mediates the autonomic nervous system's (ANS) response to fear. (*Source: LeDoux J. Evolution of Human Brain Emotion in "Evolution of the Primate Brain, Volume 195: From Neuron to Behavior (Progress in Brain Research)" Eds Hofman MA & Falk D. page 437 with permission from Elsevier.*)

The role of the amygdala in anxiety disorders, such as generalized anxiety disorders and panic attacks, is clear when considering fear learning and the classical conditioning model. Social phobias and generalized anxiety disorders are likely a consequence of fear conditioning through amygdalar pathways. Functional imaging studies of people with anxiety disorders demonstrate heightened amygdalar activity,[14–16] whereas structural imaging has in large part failed to show significant volumetric changes in the amygdala, with a few exceptions in the case of people with posttraumatic stress disorder (PTSD).[14,17] Functional imaging studies have consistently shown overactivity of the amygdala in a variety of tasks. Increased amygdalar responsiveness has been demonstrated in a variety of paradigms in subjects with PTSD, including traumatic narratives,[18–20] combat sounds,[21,22] combat pictures,[23] and words.[24] Amygdalar hyperactivity has also been shown in people with PTSD during resting state[25] and with neutral tasks.[26,27] Two treatment studies have demonstrated suppression of amygdalar hyperactivity with successful cognitive-behavioral therapy.[28,29]

The amygdala's role in mood disorders has been demonstrated through emotional-processing paradigms.[30] People with major depressive disorder attend to negative faces more than neutral or happy faces.[30,31] People with depression tend to assign negative interpretations to neutral words and recall sad words more than neutral or happy ones.[32,33] Multiple resting-state functional imaging studies have shown increased left amygdala activity in depressed subjects compared to healthy controls. Functional neuroimaging studies demonstrate increased amygdalar activity in people with depression compared to healthy controls when they are presented with sad faces or fearful faces. Furthermore, increased amygdalar activity is suppressed with successful antidepressant therapy[34,35] and cognitive-behavioral therapy.[36,37]

F-fluoro-2-deoxy-D-glucose (F-FDG) positron emission tomography (PET) imaging has shown amygdala overactivity in subjects with bipolar depression; however, the role of laterality is inconsistent.[38,39] Drevets et al.[40] also showed that amygdalar activity remained elevated in spite of depression remission and that activity was suppressed in patients in remission who were taking mood stabilizers.[40] Several functional magnetic resonance imaging (fMRI) studies demonstrated increased amygdalar activity with emotional facial tasks in bipolar depression. One study demonstrated that increased activity amygdala was suppressed with mood-stabilizing agents in bipolar depression.[40,41]

HIPPOCAMPUS

The primary function of the hippocampi is to consolidate semantic memory. The left and right hippocampi encode verbal and visual-spatial memories, respectively. Memories encoded by the hippocampus include aversive and negative memories, and the hippocampus is likely involved in contextualizing negative appraisals to environmental stimuli. As described in this chapter, in fear learning the hippocampus plays a central role in contextualizing fearful stimuli, including modulating explicit memories of fearful events. More recent research suggests that components of the hippocampus have

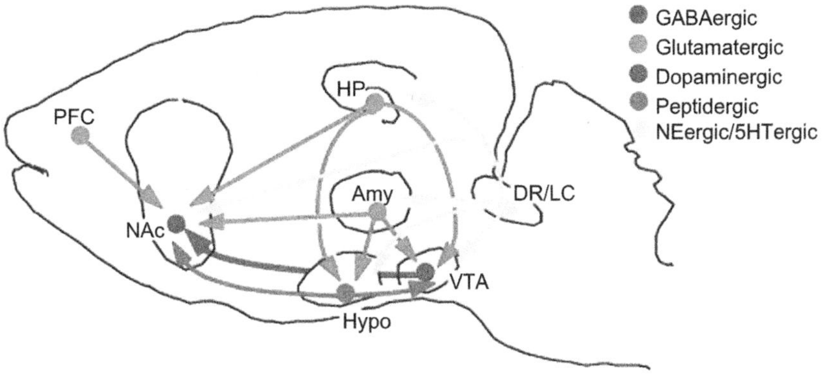

FIGURE 24.2 The figure offers a simplified model of neural circuits involved in processing mood. While the hippocampus (HP) and the amygdala (Amy) play a central role in processing emotion, they are regulated by the prefrontal cortex (PFC). The nucleus accumbens (NAc) and hypothalamus (Hypo) play a large role in reward, fear, and motivation. Not discussed extensively in this chapter, but alluded to here, is the role of neurotransmitters in these networks. The ventral tegmental area (VTA) provides dopaminergic input to the NAc; inputs to most of the other brain areas are not shown in the figure. Norepinephrine (NE, from the locus coeruleus or LC) and serotonin (5HT from the dorsal raphe and other raphe nuclei) innervate all of the regions shown in the figure. In addition, strong connections between the hypothalamus and VTA-NAc pathway have been established in recent years. GABA, gamma-aminobutyric acid; DR, dorsal raphe. (*Source: Reprinted from Nestler EJ & Carlezon WA. Mesolimbic Dopamine Reward Circuit in Depression; Biological Psychiatry, 2008; 59 (12) 111–1159 with permission from Elsevier.*) (The figure is reproduced in color section.)

specialized roles in emotional processing.[42,43] The dorsal (posterior) portion of the hippocampus (DH) is more highly connected to the frontal cortex and is involved in encoding spatial memory, while the ventral (anterior) portion (VH) is involved in emotional processing (Figure 24.2). In water and food maze paradigms, rodents with DH lesions, but not VH lesions, have difficulty returning to the newly learned locations. VH-lesioned rodents show decreased anxiety and fear-related behavior, such as decreased cold or restraint stress ulcers and decreased defecation in brightly lit chambers.[12,44]

The ability of the DH to help navigate and encode spatial information is due to its extensive projections to the subiculum, mammillary nuclei, and anterior thalamic complex. In rats and monkeys, the VH projects extensively to the olfactory bulb, olfactory cortical regions, ventral subiculum, amygdalar nuclei, and bed nuclei of the stria terminalis (BST). The BST projects to the periventricular (PVN) and medial nuclei of the hypothalamus, modulating neuroendocrine functions. The BST sends direct neural projection to corticotropin-releasing hormone (CRH). CRH is the central factor that releases stress hormones, such as glucocorticoids, and modulates the stress response system. The hippocampus inhibits secretion of CRH by the PVN, and damage leads to elevated secretion of CRH and glucocorticoids.[45,46] Chronic elevated levels of glucocorticoids are associated with increased fear and anxiety, enhanced consolidation of aversive memories, and impaired extinction to fear.[12] Furthermore, chronic stress models and elevated glucocorticoids in rodent and primate models cause neuronal loss, inhibit adult neurogenesis and neuroplasticity, and lead to hippocampal atrophy.[47] This stress model has been implicated in the pathogenesis of mood and anxiety disorders.[48]

Hippocampal atrophy is the most common structural finding seen in mood disorders. In a meta-analysis of magnetic resonance imaging (MRI) studies of depressive disorders, subjects in general had an average of 8% decrease in left hippocampal volume and a 10% decrease in right volume.[49] In particular, the extent of the length of time of untreated depression correlates strongly with hippocampal volume loss.[50] Hippocampal volume loss associated with major depression is also associated with executive dysfunction and memory impairment.[51,52]

Hippocampal atrophy is also commonly seen in people with PTSD. Several meta-analyses have shown decreased hippocampal volumes bilaterally among those with PTSD, approximately 6–7% smaller than controls.[53] However, one study showed that identical twins of combat veterans with PTSD had decreased hippocampi volumes compared to combat veterans without PTSD,[54] suggesting that hippocampi volumes may serve as a risk factor rather than a consequence of PTSD.

PREFRONTAL CORTEX

The prefrontal cortex may be roughly divided into the orbitofrontal cortex ((Brodmann Area [BA]) 11, 12, and 13), medial prefrontal cortex ((Brodmann Area [BA]) 24, 25, 32, and mesial portions of 10), and dorsolateral cortex ((Brodmann Area [BA]) 8, 9, and 46). Each region has a distinct cytoarchitecture and function as well as distinct connections, the details of which are beyond the scope of this chapter. Briefly, the orbitofrontal cortex is involved in decision making, processing award and punishment; the dorsolateral cortex is involved in planning and processing working memory; and the medial prefrontal cortex, particularly the anterior cingulate cortex, mediates emotional monitoring and self-regulation.

The orbitofrontal cortex has bidirectional connections to the medial temporal cortex, including the entorhinal cortex and perirhinal cortex, which may modulate the encoding of emotionally laden memories. The medial prefrontal region and orbitofrontal regions project extensively to the amygdala and are thought to be critical in "top-down" regulation of fear learning and extinction of fear response. Orbitofrontal circuits play a particularly important role in sensory processing and anticipating award, while the medial network is more involved in directing tasks, self-reflection, emotional monitoring, and self-regulation.[55,56]

The anterior cingulate is thought to integrate ventral (emotional) and dorsal (cognitive) streams of the brain.[57] The subgenual prefrontal cortex (SGPFC), BA25, has also been implicated in monitoring and regulating emotions.

Decreased prefrontal gray matter, particularly the ventral prefrontal regions, is reduced in people with mood disorders compared to healthy controls. Bifrontal hypometabolism in resting-state functional neuroimaging is the most common finding in people with a mood disorder.[58,59] Human functional imaging studies have shown decreased amygdalar activity and increased medial prefrontal cortex activity when emotions are controlled[3,60–62] (Figure 24.3).

Several structural neuroimaging studies have demonstrated decreased anterior cingulate volume in people with PTSD,[14] suggesting that frontal pathways that normally inhibit amygdalar driven fear are impaired in PTSD.[16] Functional neuroimaging has also demonstrated less activation in the medial prefrontal cortex and rostral anterior cingulate cortex when people with PTSD are exposed to trauma-related stimuli.[63–66]

BASAL GANGLIA

Although the motor function of the basal ganglia is well described, the extent to which the basal ganglia impacts mood and anxiety is still unclear. Marchand[67]

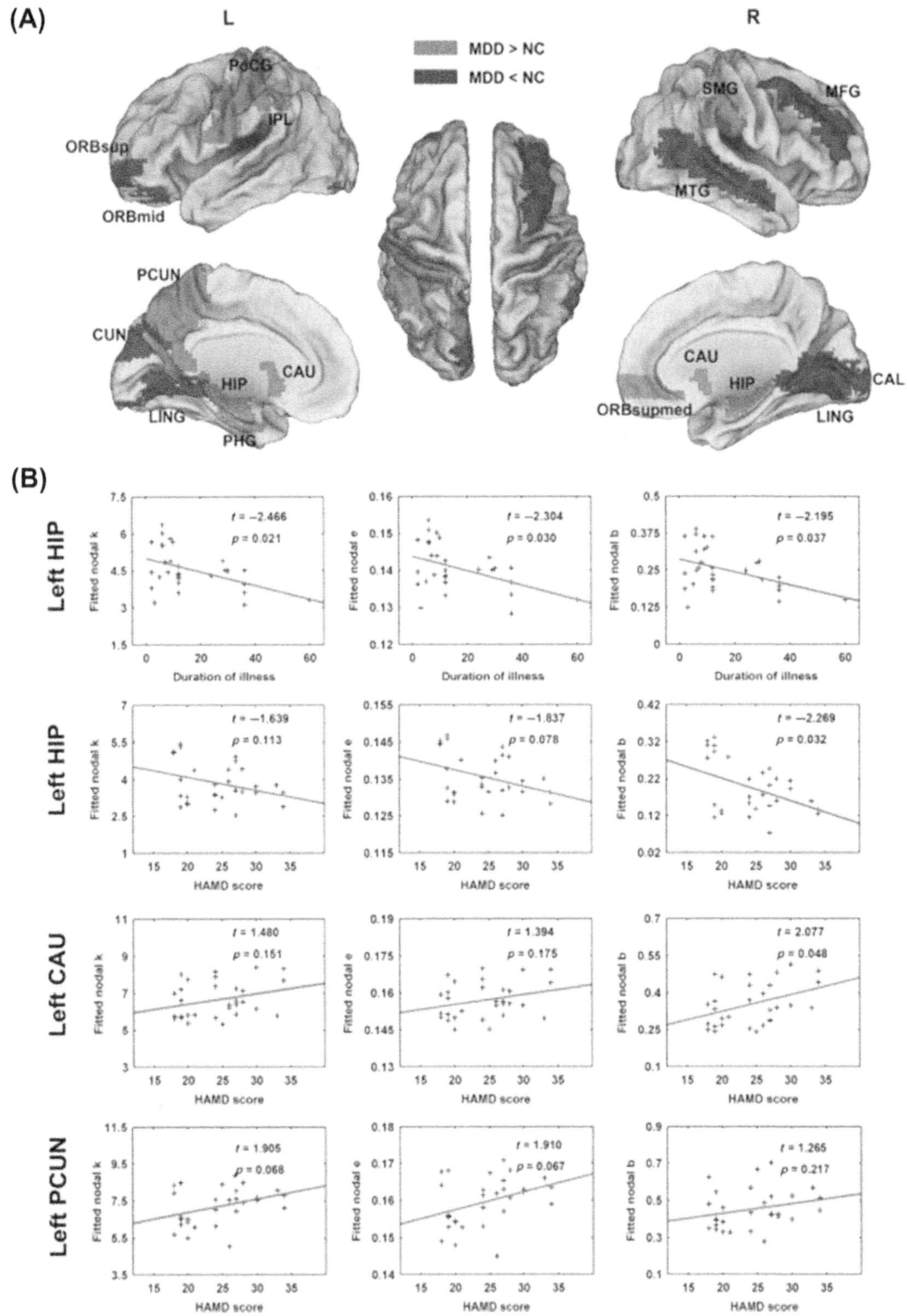

FIGURE 24.3 This study demonstrates the multiple cortical regions associated with depressed mood in medication naïve, first episode of Major Mood Disorder (MDD). Brain regions showing abnormal nodes in brain functional networks and their relationships with clinical variables in MDD patients. (A) Regions with abnormal nodes in MDD patients include: CAL, calcarine fissure and surrounding cortex; CAU, caudate nucleus; CUN, cuneus; HIP, hippocampus; MFG, middle frontal gyrus; ORBmid, middle frontal gyrus, orbital part; ORBsup, superior frontal gyrus, orbital part; ORBsupmed, superior frontal gyrus, medial orbital; PCUN, precuneus; PHG, parahippocampal gyrus; PoCG, postcentral gyrus; R, right hemisphere; SMG, supramarginal gyrus.MTG, middle temporal gyrus; IPL, inferior parietal, but supramarginal and angular gyri; L, left hemisphere; LING, lingual gyrus. (B) Scatter plots of nodal metrics against disease duration and HAMD scores which rate depressive symptoms (the higher the score the greater the depression). HAMD, Hamilton Depression Rating Scale; MDD, major depressive disorder; NC, normal control subjects. (*Source: Reprinted from Zhang J et al. Disrupted Brain Connectivity Networks in Drug-Naïve, First Episode Major Depressive Disorder; 2011, 70 (4) 334–342 with permission from Elsevier.*) (The figure is reproduced in color section.)

51. O'Brien JT, Lloyd A, McKeith I, Gholkar A, Ferrier N. A longitudinal study of hippocampal volume, cortisol levels, and cognition in older depressed subjects. *Am J Psychiatry.* 2004; 161(11):2081–2090.
52. Frodl T, Schaub A, Banac S, et al. Reduced hippocampal volume correlates with executive dysfunctioning in major depression. *J Psychiatry Neurosci.* 2006;31(5):316–323.
53. Smith ME. Bilateral hippocampal volume reduction in adults with post-traumatic stress disorder: a meta-analysis of structural MRI studies. *Hippocampus.* 2005;15(6):798–807.
54. Gilbertson MW, Shenton ME, Ciszewski A, et al. Smaller hippocampal volume predicts pathologic vulnerability to psychological trauma. *Nat Neurosci.* 2002;5(11):1242–1247.
55. Ongur D, Price JL. The organization of networks within the orbital and medial prefrontal cortex of rats, monkeys and humans. *Cereb Cortex.* 2000;10(3):206–219.
56. Price JL, Drevets WC. Neurocircuitry of mood disorders. *Neuropsychopharmacology.* 2010;35(1):192–216.
57. Devinsky O, Morrell MJ, Vogt BA. Contributions of anterior cingulate cortex to behaviour. *Brain.* 1995;118(Pt 1):279–306.
58. Baxter Jr LR, Schwartz JM, Phelps ME, et al. Reduction of prefrontal cortex glucose metabolism common to three types of depression. *Arch Gen Psychiatry.* 1989;46(3):243–250.
59. Bench CJ, Friston KJ, Brown RG, Scott LC, Frackowiak RS, Dolan RJ. The anatomy of melancholia—focal abnormalities of cerebral blood flow in major depression. *Psychol Med.* 1992;22(3):607–615.
60. Kennedy SH, Konarski JZ, Segal ZV, et al. Differences in brain glucose metabolism between responders to CBT and venlafaxine in a 16-week randomized controlled trial. *Am J Psychiatry.* 2007;164(5):778–788.
61. Mayberg HS, Liotti M, Brannan SK, et al. Reciprocal limbic-cortical function and negative mood: converging PET findings in depression and normal sadness. *Am J Psychiatry.* 1999;156(5):675–682.
62. Brody AL, Saxena S, Stoessel P, et al. Regional brain metabolic changes in patients with major depression treated with either paroxetine or interpersonal therapy: preliminary findings. *Arch Gen Psychiatry.* 2001;58(7):631–640.
63. Shin LM, Whalen PJ, Pitman RK, et al. An fMRI study of anterior cingulate function in posttraumatic stress disorder. *Biol Psychiatry.* 2001;50(12):932–942.
64. Shin LM, Wright CI, Cannistraro PA, et al. A functional magnetic resonance imaging study of amygdala and medial prefrontal cortex responses to overtly presented fearful faces in posttraumatic stress disorder. *Arch Gen Psychiatry.* 2005; 62(3):273–281.
65. Bremner JD, Staib LH, Kaloupek D, Southwick SM, Soufer R, Charney DS. Neural correlates of exposure to traumatic pictures and sound in Vietnam combat veterans with and without posttraumatic stress disorder: a positron emission tomography study. *Biol Psychiatry.* 1999; 45(7):806–816.
66. Bremner JD, Vermetten E, Vythilingam M, et al. Neural correlates of the classic color and emotional stroop in women with abuse-related posttraumatic stress disorder. *Biol Psychiatry.* 2004;55(6):612–620.
67. Marchand WR. Cortico-basal ganglia circuitry: a review of key research and implications for functional connectivity studies of mood and anxiety disorders. *Brain Struct Funct.* 2010;215(2):73–96.
68. Price JL, Drevets WC. Neural circuits underlying the pathophysiology of mood disorders. *Trends Cogn Sci.* 2012;16(1): 61–71.
69. Treadway MT, Zald DH. Reconsidering anhedonia in depression: lessons from translational neuroscience. *Neurosci Biobehav Rev.* 2011;35(3):537–555.
70. Wacker J, Dillon DG, Pizzagalli DA. The role of the nucleus accumbens and rostral anterior cingulate cortex in anhedonia: integration of resting EEG, fMRI, and volumetric techniques. *Neuroimage.* 2009;46(1):327–337.
71. Mayberg HS. Limbic-cortical dysregulation: a proposed model of depression. *J Neuropsychiatry Clin Neurosci.* 1997;9(3):471–481.
72. Krishnan V, Nestler EJ. Linking molecules to mood: new insight into the biology of depression. *Am J Psychiatry.* 2010;167(11): 1305–1320.
73. Delaveau P, Jabourian M, Lemogne C, Guionnet S, Bergouignan L, Fossati P. Brain effects of antidepressants in major depression: a meta-analysis of emotional processing studies. *J Affect Disord.* 2011;130(1–2):66–74.
74. Rush AJ, Trivedi MH, Wisniewski SR, et al. Acute and longer-term outcomes in depressed outpatients requiring one or several treatment steps: a STAR*D report. *Am J Psychiatry.* 2006;163(11):1905–1917.

CHAPTER

25

Neuronal Networks and Therapeutics in Neurodegenerative Disorders

Amanda-Amrita D. Lakraj, Bahman Jabbari, Duarte G. Machado

Department of Neurology, Yale University School of Medicine, New Haven, CT, USA

INTRODUCTION

Neurodegenerative disorders are a group of disabling and often fatal conditions that arise from the progressive loss of neurons, ultimately leading to dysfunction of the nervous system. Many models and ideas have been thoroughly researched over the years in an effort to construct the exact pathophysiology and mechanisms of neurodegeneration in these diseases. These constructs range from studies of metabolic disturbances to those studying protein aggregates, enzymes, and patterns of spread between neurons. Fortunately, our understanding of these diseases has greatly improved over recent decades. Although a definitive cure is yet to be discovered for any of these diseases, for some we now have effective symptomatic treatment.

This chapter will describe the neuronal networks involved in the symptomatology of neurodegenerative disorders, and it will discuss the importance of these networks in relation to both pharmacologic and nonpharmacologic treatment. We have chosen Parkinson's disease (PD), essential tremor (ET), primary torsion dystonia, Tourette's syndrome (TS), Huntington's disease (HD), and Alzheimer's disease (AD) as examples. It is important to note that the neuronal networks involved in the aforementioned neurodegenerative disorders affect both cortical and subcortical structures. Since the core of the subcortical networks for a majority of these disorders is the basal ganglia, a brief description of the basal ganglia and their neuronal circuits is provided.

BASAL GANGLIA

The basal ganglia are a group of four distinct subcortical nuclei. These include the striatum (the caudate, putamen, and ventral striatum), globus pallidus (both the internal (GPi) and external (GPe) parts), subthalamic nucleus (STN), and substantia nigra (both the pars reticulata (SNr) and pars compacta (SNc)). These nuclei are major components of large cortical-subcortical reentrant circuits linking the thalamus to the cortex (Figure 25.1). Primary input comes from the cortex, and output goes to the thalamus and back to the cortex. Information from cortical areas, which is processed in basal ganglia territories, is mostly nonoverlapping and functions in five distinct loops that are segregated both structurally and functionally.[1,2]

Striatum

The striatum is the major basal ganglia recipient of the cortex and all other inputs to basal ganglia. It consists of the caudate and putamen (which together are known as the neostriatum) and the ventral striatum; the latter includes the nucleus accumbens. The striatum is both anatomically and functionally heterogeneous, and it consists of two separate parts: the matrix and striosome. These two components are different both histochemically and in their receptors. The striosome compartment receives its major input from the limbic cortex and projects primarily to the SNc. Of striatal cell types, 90–95% are gamma-aminobutyric acid (GABA)-ergic medium-spiny projection neurons.[1] These cells are the target of cortical input and the only source of output. Studies performed in primates have shown that these cells may be further divided into two subgroups with different projections. Projections to the external pallidum express the neuropeptides enkephalin and neurotensin (in addition to GABA), while projections to the major output basal ganglia structures (GPi and SNr) express substance P and dynorphin. GABAergic medium-spiny projection neurons are active during

Neuronal Networks in Brain Function, CNS Disorders, and Therapeutics
http://dx.doi.org/10.1016/B978-0-12-415804-7.00025-3

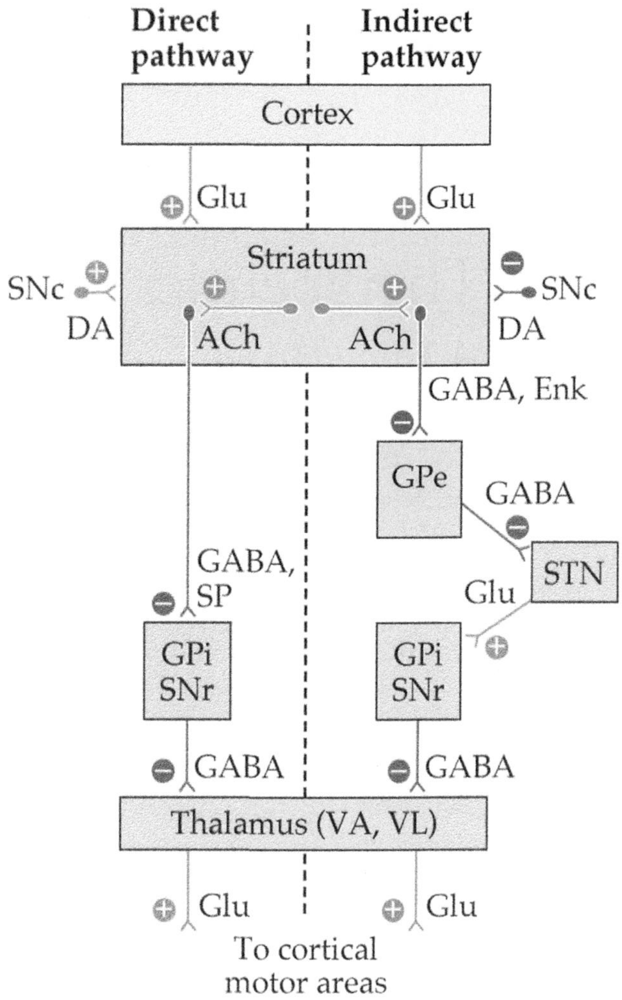

FIGURE 25.1 Network commonly used for understanding basal ganglia function in normal conditions and neurodegenerative movement disorders. (*Source: Reproduced with permission from Blumenfeld H. Neuroanatomy through Clinical Cases. 2nd ed. Sunderland, MA: Sinauer Associates, Inc.; 2010.*) (For color version of this figure, the reader is referred to the online version of this book.)

movement and in response to peripheral stimuli. The striatum further contains local inhibitory neurons. The large cell type contains acetylcholine, and the smaller type contains somatostatin, neuropeptide Y, or nitric oxide synthase. Both cell types have extensive axon collaterals that reduce the activity of the striatal output neurons, and, although they are few in quantity, they are responsible for most of the tonic activity occurring in the striatum.

Globus Pallidus and Substantia Nigra

Neurons of the striatum project to the two major output basal ganglia structures, the GPi and SNr. These two nuclei, which are morphologically very similar, together create the major output projections from basal ganglia. Both GPi and substantia nigra use GABA as a neurotransmitter.[1] GPe receives GABAergic input from the putamen and projects to the STN via GABAergic fibers. Its role is further described in the "Basal Ganglia Internal Circuitry: Direct and Indirect Pathways" section. The SNc contains dopaminergic neurons that project to the striatum. The ventral tegmental area is an extension of the SNc.

Subthalamic Nucleus

The STN is a unique structure in the basal ganglia. It is the only neural aggregate in the basal ganglia that has glutamatergic projections (to the GPi). It receives GABAergic input from the GPe and glutamatergic input from the cortex.

Normal Circuitry of the Basal Ganglia

There are five main circuits that have been proposed, based on known functions of cortical areas, from which the individual circuits originate: the motor, anterior cingulate (limbic), oculomotor, dorsolateral prefrontal associative, and lateral orbitofrontal circuits. Each circuit originates in a specific area of the cortex and engages different portions of the basal ganglia and the thalamus, which then projects back to the cortical area from which the circuit was originally derived. Projections from the cortex to discrete regions of striatum occur in a highly topographical manner such that sensorimotor areas project to the putamen, association areas project to the caudate and rostral putamen, and limbic areas project to the ventral striatum and olfactory tubercle. It is known that structural convergence and functional integration may occur within, instead of between, the five identified basal ganglia circuits. There is some anatomical evidence that the circuits converge to some degree in the SNr.[1]

While many models describing basal ganglia focus on its relation to the cortex, basal ganglia also project to the pedunculopontine nucleus (PPN) and the superior colliculus (SC) of the brainstem. These projections may have specific roles: for example, the GPi-to-PPN projection may have a role in locomotion,[1] and the SNr-to-SC projection may have a role in control of eye and head movements.[1] Since more is known about the motor circuit, and it is the motor circuit that is mainly involved in most of the neurodegenerative disorders discussed in this chapter, we describe it in more detail in the "Motor Circuit and Skeletomotor Circuit" section.

Motor Circuit and Skeletomotor Circuit

Cortical motor areas project to the postcommissural putamen. To be more specific, it is the primary motor, premotor, and arcuate premotor areas as well as somatosensory areas 3a, 1, 2, and 5. While the cortical motor areas send their projections in a highly topographical manner, somatosensory projections are overlapping and project mainly to the motor portions of the putamen.[1] Topographically specific projections result in somatotopic organization of movement-related neurons in the putamen, so that, for example, the leg is represented in the dorsolateral zone, the orofacial region in the ventromedial zone, and the arm in the zone that lies between these two. For this reason, the putamen is an important site for the integration of both motor and somatosensory feedback information specific to movement. The postcommissural putamen then sends efferents to the ventrolateral GPi and the caudolateral SNr, both of which have motor areas. Output projections to caudoventral and caudolateral portions of the pallidum and SNr, respectively, are also highly topographical. The motor areas of the GPi and SNr send projections to the ventral anterior, ventrolateral, and centromedian portions of the thalamus. Finally, these thalamic regions return output to the supplementary motor area, with lesser projections to premotor and motor cortices, thus completing the loop. While increased basal ganglia output leads to less movement through the inhibition of thalamocortical projection neurons, reduced basal ganglia output could translate to increased movements via the disinhibition of thalamic neurons. Throughout this circuit, neuronal specificity and somatotopy are maintained, as there are separate pathways for control of leg, arm, and orofacial movements.[1,2] Although the input from the GPi reaches a region distinct from that of cerebellar afferents, namely, the ventralis intermedius nucleus (ViM), there is recent evidence that the two may share part of a circuit by cerebellar inputs projecting to the striatum through the thalamus and some of the output from the STN reaching the cerebellum.[3] A feedback loop connects the thalamus to basal ganglia through the parafascicular and ventralis oralis anterior (VoA) nuclei.

Basal Ganglia Internal Circuitry: Direct and Indirect Pathways

The striatum receives excitatory glutaminergic projections from all areas of the cortex, excitatory glutamatergic inputs from intralaminar nuclei of the thalamus, dopaminergic projections from the midbrain, and/or serotonergic input from the raphe nuclei. The striatum projects output nuclei via indirect and direct interbasal ganglia pathways.

Direct and indirect pathways have different origins. Together, they can be seen as parallel pathways to output nuclei, which serve to modulate inhibitory output. The neurons in both these nuclei are tonically active and discharge at high frequencies. Except for the STN projections, which are glutamatergic, all intrinsic and output projections of the basal ganglia are GABAergic and inhibitory in nature. Activity in indirect and direct pathways and corticostriatal synapses is regulated by striatal dopamine. Striatal dopamine comes from the nigrostriatal projections from the SNc. Dopamine acts differently upon dopamine (D)1 (direct pathway) and D2 (indirect pathway) receptors. It excites D1 receptors and inhibits D2 receptors, which translates into increased GABAergic activity upon the GPi in the direct pathway, and decreased GABAergic activity upon the GPe in the first arm of the indirect pathway. The net effect of both pathways over the GPi is inhibitory, with a resultant increase in thalamic and thalamocortical activity (inhibiting the GPi and decreasing its inhibitory effect upon the thalamus, hence facilitation of movement). For this reason, lack of dopamine, for example in PD, leads to overactivity of the GPi (more inhibition of the thalamus) and inhibition or impairment of movement. In this way, lack of dopaminergic input to the striatum will lead to a failure of the striatum to exert its normal, inhibitory, GABAergic effects, ultimately leading to increased output. Increased output further inhibits the thalamocortical neurons necessary to initiate movement, leading to impairment of movement.

The presence of dopaminergic neurons at locations other than the striatum, for example in the pallidum, substantia nigra, and STN, has led to the suggestion that dopaminergic activity at these other sites and in the cortex could play a role in mediating actions from the striatum to the indirect and direct pathways. Anatomic studies show extensive collaterals between the direct and indirect pathways.

Mesolimbic-Cortical Circuitry

The mesolimbic circuitry originates in the ventral tegmental area. It gives innervations mainly to the nucleus accumbens and the olfactory tubercle. It is also involved in arousal, locomotion, motivational, and affective states. The mesolimbic-cortical pathway, on the other hand, gives innervations to the septum, hippocampus, amygdala, and several important cortical regions such as the prefrontal and cingulate cortices. It is mainly important in higher cortical functions.[4]

PARKINSON'S DISEASE

PD is a predominantly hypokinetic disorder characterized by loss of spontaneous movement, akinesia (trouble initiating movement), bradykinesia (reduced velocity and amplitude of voluntary movement), and muscle rigidity. Approximately 80% of the patients also manifest a resting tremor at some time during the course of the disease. In addition to motor symptoms, PD patients also exhibit a number of nonmotor symptoms, such as autonomic dysfunction, depression, and dementia.

The role of dopamine in PD began with Arvid Carlson's discovery that 80% of the brain's dopamine is located in the basal ganglia, and the discovery of Oleh Horynekiewicz, who revealed that the brains of patients who had died from PD were dopamine deficient in the striatum, and more specifically in the putamen. Eventually, in the 1960s, it was shown that PD is the result of degeneration of dopaminergic neurons in the SNc. Another discovery showed that the environmental toxin 1-methyl-4-phenyl-1,2,3,6-tetrahydropyridine (MPTP) can also cause depletion of dopamine, resulting in a profound Parkinsonian state. The working model for the pathophysiology of PD suggests that loss of dopaminergic input from the SNc to the striatum via altered activity of D1 and D2 receptors causes less inhibition of GPi. The overactive GPi inhibits thalamic neurons and leads to less excitation of the cortex via thalamic neurons and hence the development of hypokinesia, the cardinal symptom of PD.

Pharmacological Treatment

Motor symptoms of PD are treated with both dopaminergic drugs and dopamine-enhancing drugs to improve the loss of dopamine in the neuronal network of the basal ganglia. Levodopa replenishes the lost dopamine in the striatum and is the strongest drug available for treatment of PD (starting dose 300–400 mg/day). It is not, however, the drug of choice in young patients with PD due to a high incidence of dyskinesias after long-term treatment. Since these effects of levodopa are not seen in normal patients or patients in the early treatment phases of PD, it is thought that this phenomenon is the result of receptor regulation, supersensitivity, and altered gene expression caused by prolonged administration of the drug.[1] Dopamine agonists, such as pramipexole, ropinirole, and rotigotine, mimic the effect of dopamine upon dopamine receptors and are used often as firstline treatment for younger PD patients. Another firstline option is enzyme inhibitors that prevent the degradation of dopamine. While rasagiline and selegiline inhibit monoamine oxidase B (MAO-B), entacapone and tolcapone inhibit cathecol-o-methyltransferase (COMT). Amantadine is an antiviral agent that most likely exerts its therapeutic action in PD through inhibition of *N*-methyl-D-aspartate (NMDA) receptors. It too can be used as a firstline drug for treatment of PD (100 mg two to three times daily) or for treatment of dopamine-induced dyskinesias. Anticholinergic drugs, such as trihexyphnidyl and benztropine, are also effective against all symptoms of PD. However, they are not favored due to common side effects of memory loss, blurring of vision, dry mouth, and poor tolerance in the elderly population. PD patients with a refractory tremor that is poorly responsive to levodopa may respond to trihexyphenidyl. Advanced PD often requires combination drug therapy.

Nonmotor Symptoms of PD

Although a great deal of attention is given to the nigrostriatal dopaminergic circuit and hypokinetic symptoms of PD, there are also other equally debilitating nonmotor symptoms in PD patients, including cognitive deficits (dementia), depression, apathy, sleep disorders, constipation, orthostatic hypotension, and erectile dysfunction. Some of these symptoms can be explained via neural degeneration in other pathways, for example nigral projections to the ventral striatum, including the mesocortical and mesolimbic dopamine pathways.[5–7] It cannot be overlooked that these ascending dopamine pathways also play a role in supporting the function of many of the corticostriatal circuits. Some of these circuits, such as loops going from the prefrontal and limbic cortices, are proposed to support cognitive and motivational responses, respectively.[8,9] In this section, we discuss the mesolimbic dopamine system and cognitive circuits in more detail. It is important to consider, while reviewing these pathways, that the role of dopaminergic drugs may have great implications in treating nonmotor symptoms of PD. It has been suggested that dopamine deficiency involving the limbic areas may be the cause of apathy in PD.[10] PD patients may exhibit clinical signs of depression starting even before the onset of classic PD symptoms. While the exact origin is still not understood, dopamine loss in the mesolimbic system has been associated with symptoms such as anhedonia, which is also a primary sign of depression. Interference in systems involved in motivation and decision making could be due to altered synaptic plasticity in the nucleus accumbens.[11]

Cognitive Circuits

It is estimated that between 15 and 20% of PD patients develop frank dementia.[12] Less severe patterns of cognitive impairment seen in the early stages of PD are well recognized and are thought to play a role in predicting quality of life.[13,14] Patterns of cognitive impairment seen in PD patients closely resemble those resulting from frontal lobe lesions and thus mainly include deficits in executive function.[15] It is important to note that equivalence between executive dysfunction and the prefrontal cortex cannot be assumed, and this is especially true for patients with PD, where executive dysfunction has been shown to be extremely sensitive to the effects of controlled levodopa withdrawal.[16,17] Neuroimaging studies have investigated the origin of executive defects in PD and give evidence for roles of disruption in both the nigrostriatal and mesocortical pathways, with the mesocortical pathway having less importance.[6,18–20] Early changes in cognition in PD patients might involve the caudate and corticostriatal pathways,[21] and cortical loss of dopamine is a cause of cognitive deterioration in PD.[22] Changes in dopamine uptake and metabolism in cortical-striatal dopaminergic fibers have been reported in the literature.[23,24] Specific studies of the basal ganglia in primates, which investigated sequence learning, suggested that while the caudate nucleus may be particularly important in the acquisition of new sequence memories, the putamen may have a greater role in the performance of learned sequences.[25] This point is important considering that cognitive difficulty in PD is mostly difficulty with procedural learning, specifically sequence learning.[26]

DEEP BRAIN STIMULATION AND PD

Among the treatment modalities employed in neurodegenerative disorders, no modality takes greater advantage of our current knowledge of neuronal networks than deep brain stimulation (DBS) (see Chapter 31). It has been shown convincingly that electrical stimulation of a certain neuronal aggregate within a defined network can improve both motor and nonmotor symptoms in neurodegenerative disorders. DBS is now an established treatment for symptoms of PD. All three cardinal symptoms of PD—hypokinesia, rigidity, and tremor—can improve significantly after DBS. DBS also significantly reduces levodopa-induced dyskinesias. The results are not only the management of symptoms but also the provision of an opportunity to reduce anti-Parkinson medications. In the elderly, less medication is always favored due to the higher incidence of drug-induced side effects and drug–drug interactions. This is important, as many patients with PD are elderly. Indications for DBS include patients who failed pharmacotherapy (usually beyond 2 years), or those who suffer from persistent symptoms and side effects secondary to poor anti-PD drug tolerance. Severe depression or dementias are contraindications to this procedure. The procedure has two steps. During the first step, the stimulating electrode is implanted into the target after microelectrode recording from the surface to the depth. Each stimulating electrode has four contacts. The patient is sedated but awake and is tested in the operating room to see how the symptoms of hypokinesia, rigidity, and tremor are affected by the stimulation. A week later, a DBS stimulator is inserted into the ipsilateral chest wall under generalized anesthesia and connected to the intracranial electrode. The patient then visits the clinic after 2–3 weeks when DBS parameters (voltage, pulse width, range, contact connections, etc.) are set for an optimum response.

Microelectrode recordings in primate models of PD demonstrate hyperactivity of the GPi and STN.[27] In humans, loss of dopamine (which excites D1 receptors) leads to increased activity of the GPi (due to decreased GABAergic inhibition of the GPi). Since dopamine inhibits D2 receptors, its loss decreases GPe inhibition and ultimately decreases STN inhibition, which results in overactive STN and again overactivity of GPi. In patients with PD, microelectrode recording clearly shows increased activity of GPi and STN neurons. Taking advantage of knowledge learned from lesional studies that improved PD symptoms, Benabid et al. pioneered the use of DBS in the treatment of PD.[28] These investigators reported that the unilateral high-frequency stimulation of the STN (130/s) caused remarkable reductions of hypokinesia (in the limb contralateral to the stimulation) in 51 patients with PD.[28] STN and GPi locations are depicted by measurements from the middle of the antero-posterior commissural line (AC-PC line), using magnetic resonance imaging (MRI). Currently, both the STN and GPi are used for DBS treatment of PD, although most centers prefer STN stimulation. In a recent, blinded, multicenter study that compared STN and GPi locations, improvement of motor symptoms of PD and quality of life occurred equally for both locations.[29] Patients with STN stimulation were able to reduce their PD medications after DBS, but GPi patients did not. Side effects were slightly more common in the STN group.[29] The exact mechanism of how DBS ameliorates symptoms of PD is not yet defined. It may be related to "jamming" increased electrical activity in the target by a high-frequency stimulus, enhancement of inhibitory transmitters, and yet other unknown mechanisms. Postural instability, a late development in PD, does not respond to DBS targeted to the STN or GPi. Stefani et al. reported significant improvement of gait in six patients after combined stimulation of the STN with PPN.[30] PPN stimulation was carried out with the slow rate of 25 Hz. In a double-blind study of a small number of patients with PD, unilateral PPN–DBS reduced falls in advanced PD.[31] Further studies are necessary to explore the importance of PPN–DBS in improvement of gait and prevention of falls in PD.

ESSENTIAL TREMOR

ET is the most common movement disorder of adults, with a prevalence of 5%. It is defined as a bilateral action tremor that predominantly involves the hands and head, with no other neurologic problems except for a slight problem with gait. Some 60–70% of the patients respond with reduced symptoms to alcohol.[32] ET, unlike PD tremor, is best seen during postural positioning with both hands stretched out and held against gravity. The frequency of this tremor is faster than a PD tremor, and it is usually at 5–8 Hz. Family history is often present with an autosomal dominant pattern.

Pharmacological Treatment

Propranolol and primidone are the most effective medications to decrease ET.[33] Alprazolam, topiramate, and gabapentin are often used as adjunctive therapy. Up to 50% of the patients, however, are not satisfied with the level of control.[34]

Deep Brain Stimulation

It is currently believed that ET results from self-sustained oscillations in an extensive neuronal network that encompasses olivo-cerebellar pathways, the cerebellum itself, cerebello-thalamic projections, the thalamus, and corticothalamic projections. In recent years, the presence of these oscillations was confirmed by magnetoencephalography and, more recently, by electroencephalography–electromyography coherence and coherence source analysis.[35] In the diencephalon, the source of tremor is believed to be thalamic due to the proximity of the source to the thalamus. When ET patients were compared to those with PD, the source in ET was more posterior in location. This agrees with the anatomical information that suggests that input ends in Vim (part of the ventrolateral complex), which is posterior to VoA, which receives the input from basal ganglia. The oscillations were bidirectional in the thalamocortical network in both ET and PD, in contrast to the unilateral oscillations that are demonstrated in voluntary tremor. Bidirectionality of oscillations seems to correlate with the pathological nature of the tremor and its sustainability. It has been shown now that the tremors of ET and PD both have two different frequency peaks. For ET, the second frequency peak is exactly double the basic frequency, and the source for the two frequencies is in the same anatomical region.[35]

In DBS of Vim, the stimulating electrode and stimulator implantation procedures are similar to those for PD. The stimulating frequency, like that for PD, is in a high-frequency range (130–185 Hz). Recently, Nazzaro et al. reported on the long-term follow-up of 91 patients with ET who had unilateral DBS of the STN.[36] Unilateral DBS significantly improved quality of life and tremor for at least 7 years.

PRIMARY TORSION DYSTONIA

Primary torsion dystonia is a progressive neurodegenerative disease that starts in childhood. The dystonic distortions usually start in one lower limb and gradually affect others. Most children are disabled by their late teens, and many are confined to a wheelchair. Several abnormal genes have been described. The most common is dystonic locus 1 (DYT1), which is seen predominantly in the Ashkenazi Jewish population. Unlike PD, the neurochemistry of primary torsion dystonia is not yet elucidated, and the pathophysiology of it is poorly understood.

Pharmacological Treatment

Treatment is focused on reducing the cholinergic activity and enhancing the GABAergic activity in the basal ganglia. In this regard, anticholinergic drugs and the $GABA_B$ agonist baclofen are the drugs of choice for treatment of generalized primary dystonia in childhood. Although both treatments are effective, often high doses are required and tolerance is poor in adults.

Deep Brain Stimulation

It has been known for decades that inducing lesions in the globus pallidus (pallidotomy) alleviates severe dystonic posturing of primary torsion dystonia.[37] High-frequency stimulation of GPi does not improve dystonia, but low-frequency stimulation at 60 Hz results in marked improvement of movements and of ambulation.[38] In fact, improvement of ambulation is sometimes remarkable, with nonambulatory or poorly ambulatory patients being able to walk without difficulty. The best response is seen in patients with DTY1 gene abnormality. Recently, Cif et al. described the results of a 10-year follow-up in 26 patients with DYT1 dystonia.[37] Marked improvements of dystonia (using the Burke–Fahn Scale) and quality of life were sustained over the follow-up period.

TOURETTE'S SYNDROME

TS is a chronic and disabling disorder characterized by motor and phonic tics as well as behavioral disorders at an early age (mean age of onset 5–7 years old), and it has male predominance (3:1). Definite diagnosis of TS requires the presence of motor and phonic tics. Approximately 90% of children with TS have behavioral disorders, which include obsessive compulsive disorder (OCD), attention deficit hyperactivity disorder (ADHD), depression, and anxiety. The prevalence may be as high as 50/10,000.[39] Symptoms may improve or remit with the passage of years, usually after age 20.

The pathophysiology of TS is still not well understood. Impaired modulation of neuronal networks that contribute to behavioral inhibition has been proposed based on functional MRI (fMRI) findings. The neurophysiological theory suggests that TS results from disinhibition of thalamic afferents or blockade of cortical inhibition, whereas a neurochemical theory attributes it to dopaminergic sensitivity, a presynaptic abnormality, or second mediator abnormalities.[40] Anatomic striatal abnormalities are also suspected in TS.

Pharmaceutical treatment of motor tics in TS includes alpha-2 adrenergic agonists, such as clonidine and guanfacine, as well as typical and atypical neuroleptics; this treatment is done in conjunction with behavioral modification protocols. Unfortunately, a sizeable number of patients fail to respond well to treatment, with a small number suffering from severe tics that cause self-injury.

Neuronal Networks in TS

Recently, Wang and colleagues explored the neuronal circuits in TS with fMRI, comparing the activity during motor tics of TS with voluntary mimicked tics.[41] During the premonitory sensory urges of TS, fMRI activity was significantly increased in the substantia nigra, nigrostriatal pathways, putamen, thalamocortical projection, somatosensory and supplementary motor cortices, and corticothalamic projections. This was interpreted as increased dopaminergic activity in TS, with hyperactivity of the putamen leading to disinhibition of the thalamus, which enhances glutamergic thalamocortical activity leading to the emergence of motor tics. Enhanced activity of thalamocortical projection, which is also glutamatergic, further promotes the putamen's overactivity. In contrast, the caudate and anterior cingulate, which are known as cognitive regions, demonstrated decreased activity in fMRI. This was attributed to hypofunctioning of these two regions, which modulate and control unwanted behavior. Furthermore, hyperactivity of the amygdala denotes the enhanced emotional component of TS symptoms.

Anatomical and physiological studies indicate that the centromedian–parafascicular (CM–pf) nuclear complex of the thalamus exerts significant influence over striatal neurons via widespread inhibitory feedback. This complex is a part of the intralaminar nucleus of the thalamus involved in the sensory motor basal ganglia network. The intralaminar nuclei send sensory motor signals to the striatum and are involved in attention and arousal. The neurons of this nuclear complex project as follows: (1) the rostral third projects to the nucleus accumbens (the limbic cortex), (2) the caudal two-thirds project to the caudate (the cognitive striatum), (3) the dorsolateral projects to the anterior putamen (the associative stratum), (4) the medial two-thirds of the CM project to the sensory motor putamen (the postcommissural segment), and (5) the lateral two-thirds of the CM project to the primary motor cortex. The CM–pf neurons also project heavily to striatal interneurons, which by and large contain acetylcholine and GABA. CM–pf neurons also project to both sensorimotor and limbic segments of the STN.[42] In primates, electrical stimulation of CM and pf neurons results in inhibition of all aforementioned targets. Some of the major afferents to the CM–pf complex come from the PPN, SNr, and brainstem reticular formation. The significant and widespread inhibitory influence of the CM–pf nucleus raised interest in this nucleus complex for electrical stimulation studies in TS.

Deep Brain Stimulation

Successful treatment of intractable tics with DBS was first reported by Vandewalle et al. in 1999.[43] Since then, a number of investigators reported success with DBS in TS. Although the overall number of treated patients is still small, the reports are consistent in the efficacy of DBS against motor tics and behavioral symptoms. In the largest number of patients reported to date, Porta et al. studied 18 patients with DBS stimulation of CM–pf and reported the results at 2 years follow-up.[44] After 2 years, careful rating of the symptoms showed marked reductions of motor tics, depressive and anxiety scores (for all $P = 0.001$), obsessive compulsive symptoms ($P = 0.009$), and patient perception of quality of life ($P = 0.002$). Two years after surgery, there was 76% improvement of the Yale–Brown Obsessive Compulsive Scale. Using the same target and 2-year follow-up, we also documented a marked reduction of very frequent and severe motor tics (rapid flexion and extension of the neck) with improvement of quality of life in a patient disabled by motor tics.[45] More recently, Ackermans et al. reported on a double-blind study conducted on six patients with TS with a minimal Yale Global Tourette Severity Scale (YGTSS Leckman, 1989).[46] At 1 year after DBS, there was significant improvement of YGTSS and reduced frequency of both motor and vocal tics. In fact, vocal tics improved more than motor tics.

The final choice of optimum target is not still settled for DBS in TS as other investigators reported success with other targets such as GPi, VoA, anterior limb of internal capsule, and STN. Very recently, Saleh et al. reviewed the world literature on the subject of DBS in TS and OCD.[47] Of 88 patients reported, 43 had thalamic DBS, 12 patients had GPi DBS, and a few patients had DBS of the nucleus accumbens and anterior limb of internal capsule and STN. Several patients had multiple-target DBS. The results of thalamic DBS and Gpi DBS were comparable regarding the improvement of motor tics and improvement of quality of life.

Obsessive compulsive behavior occurs in approximately 50% of the patients with TS. Pharmacological treatment usually employs one of the selective serotonin reuptake inhibitors alone or in combination with clomipramine. DBS of nucleus accumbens is shown to improve OCD significantly.[48] Huff et al. conducted a double-blind study in 10 patients with recalcitrant OCD. DBS stimulation of the right nucleus accumbens produced at least partial improvement in OCD symptoms in five of 10 patients after the first year. Quality of life was also improved.[49]

The nucleus accumbens modulates the activity of the neuronal network that composes the amygdaloid-prefrontal cortex circuitry. The activity of nucleus accumbens neurons is, in turn, modulated by dopamine since its cells have large numbers of D1 and D3 receptors. Alternatively, DBS stimulation of the nonmotor part of the STN also leads to marked improvement of OCD.[50] A recent positron emission tomography (PET) study shows that stimulation of the STN decreases the metabolism of the prefrontal cortex in TS.[51] The US Food and Drug Administration (FDA) approved the use of DBS for recalcitrant OCD in the United States in April 2012.

HUNTINGTON'S DISEASE

HD is the most commonly known heritable hyperkinetic neurodegenerative disorder affecting the basal ganglia and is also one of the first complex human disorders to be traced to a single gene. HD is a trinucleotide repeat disorder of the CAG sequence, which codes for the amino acid glutamine. An individual must have more than 40 copies of this CAG repeat to have the disease, and there is a direct correlation between disease severity and number of repeats. HD is inherited in an autosomal dominant pattern and also displays the genetic phenomenon known as anticipation. Affecting men and women equally, Huntington's commonly occurs in the third to fifth decade of life and is characterized by five main features: heritability, chorea, psychiatric or behavioral disturbances, gait disturbance, and cognitive impairment, which presents as dementia. Although there are many different models that focus on various aspects possibly leading to the pathogenesis of HD, this section will focus on the pathophysiology from a neuronal network point of view.

Current models for neuronal networking in HD are still evolving. Mutant huntingtin proteins made of multiple intranuclear inclusions were expressed in mice and found to sufficiently cause a progressive neurologic phenotype.[52] Accumulation of huntingtin protein and thus CAG glutamate repeats is correlated with the onset of neuronal degeneration. The continued expansion of CAG repeats causes polyglutamine stretches in the huntingtin protein. These polyglutamine stretches eventually induce progressive neurodegeneration.[53] Ultimately, it is the length of the repeat as well as the nuclear localization of the huntingtin protein that dictate the onset and severity of neuronal degeneration. The highest levels of huntingtin protein in the whole body can be found in the testis and the brain; in the brain itself, the highest levels are found in the cortex, striatum, and hippocampus.[54,55] This finding correlates with the mechanism and location of HD pathophysiology.

Cortical Striatal Processing Deficits Preclude Neurodegeneration

The pattern of neuronal loss in HD begins in the striatum, with severe cell loss and atrophy in the caudate and putamen, and ultimately progresses to widespread loss of neurons in the brain. After the striatum, the second most affected area is the cortex, and it is mainly the neurons in layers IV and V of the cortex that are affected as they have projections to the striatum.[56] This is confirmed by patient autopsies, which indicate massive cell loss in the striatum and cerebral cortex.[57] Recent studies using transgenic animal models indicate that corticostriatal neuronal processing is altered much earlier in relation to the onset of neuronal death and neurodegeneration and, in fact, appears to be the primary driver of the HD behavioral phenotype. Dysregulation of the excitatory amino acid glutamate, which is released by the corticostriatal pathway, is believed to play a critical role in the disruption of corticostriatal processing.[57] Evidence shows that this dysregulation of glutamate is due to mutant huntingtin protein, which interferes with the activity of proteins involved in glutamate transmission, and subsequent decrease in the activity of glutamate trasporter 1 (GLT1), which is an astrocytic protein responsible for the bulk of glutamate uptake. This may suggest a role of GLT1 and its expression in astrocytes as a possible therapeutic target.[57]

More support for the occurrence of corticostriatal processing before neurodegeneration is offered by functional neuroimaging studies done on pre-HD patients with near-onset HD. In this study, lower activation of the right frontostriatal regions during phasic alertness, decreased striatal activity, and lower functional connectivity of the motor regions were observed in patients with pre-HD when compared to both healthy individuals and pre-HD individuals far from the time of onset. The overall data suggested that, although alertness-related performance remained normal, the underlying frontostriatal activity and motor cortex connectivity declined when approaching the onset of unequivocal signs of HD.[58]

Neurodegeneration

Cellular models to study the effects of gene-induced neurodegeneration itself have been formed by transfecting cultured striatal neurons with the mutant Huntington's gene. It was found that gene-induced neurodegeneration occurs by an apoptotic mechanism, specifically in the nucleus. When nuclear localization was blocked, the ability of the huntingtin protein to both form intranuclear inclusions and induce apoptosis was inhibited. However, it was also noted that there was no correlation between apoptosis and intranuclear inclusion formation, thus suggesting that intranuclear inclusions may not have an important role in leading to mutant huntingtin-induced death. This notion was supported by the observation that full-length huntingtin only very rarely is associated with the formation of inclusions, and when transfected striatal neurons were exposed to conditions that suppressed the formation of intranuclear inclusion, there was an increase in huntingtin-induced death. This leads to the idea that mutant huntingtin alone may be the cause of neurodegeneration in the nucleus, and instead, intranuclear inclusions themselves may be protective.[56]

Cognitive Deficits and Depression

Hippocampal atrophy is commonly seen in patients with HD. It can be correlated with the cognitive deficits and depression observed in HD patients.[59,60]

Chorea

The leading hypothesis for choreiform movements, which comprise the major symptom in early HD, is as follows: striatal neurons giving rise to the indirect pathway are lost, leading to a disinhibition of the neurons in the external pallidum. This disinhibition, or excitation of the GPe, then causes excessive discharge of neurons and inhibition of the STN neurons. This is known as a "functional inactivation" of the STN and is thought to explain why choreiform symptoms, which occur in the disease, actually resemble hemiballism.[1]

While choreiform movements are related to overactivity of GPe and inhibition of STN, rigidity and akinesia are associated with a loss of striatal neurons that project to the GPi. In this case, loss of inhibition on the GPi results in increased firing of GPi neurons.

PHARMACOLOGIC TREATMENT

Tetrabenazine (TBZ) is the only drug approved for the treatment of HD and is mainly used for chorea. It works as a specific inhibitor of vesicular monoamine transporters. First introduced for the use of schizophrenia in the 1950s, TBZ was first used for dyskinesias in the 1980s. It was only in 2008 when TBZ was finally approved by the FDA for the treatment of chorea.[61] The mechanism by which TBZ exerts antichoreic effects is by decreasing the amount of dopamine in the brain by two different mechanisms.[62] The first and best-known mechanism is by the avid bind of TBZ to specialized proteins known as vesicular monoamine transporters (VMATs). The normal role of VMATs is to facilitate neurotransmitter transport into vesicles. When VMATs are bound by TBZ, neurotransmitters (e.g. dopamine) cannot be stored in vesicles and secondarily cannot be released into synapses. This results in both prevention of dopamine release and inhibition of monoamine uptake. Conveniently, the highest binding densities of TBZ are in the caudate nucleus, the putamen, and the nucleus accumbens.[63,64] These areas are also the locations of most HD pathology.

The second mechanism by which TBZ reduces dopamine is by directly blocking dopamine receptors, as evidenced by in vitro studies.[65,66] Once TBZ binds to receptors on a receiving nerve cell surface, dopamine can no longer pass on its message. While of less importance, this mechanism may also be responsible for the acute dystonic reactions that can sometimes be reported as an adverse effect associated with TBZ.[67] Neuroleptic medications, through blocking dopamine receptors and decreasing dopamine activity in the striatum, can improve chorea. Until recently, neuroleptics such as haloperidol have been the drug of choice for treatment of disabling chorea. Significant side effects, in particular the emergence of tardive dyskinesia (TD), limit their use. The antichorea effect of atypical neuroleptics (e.g. quetiapine) is weaker, but they induce a much lower incidence of TD. Other medications that can be used include amantadine (300–400 mg/day) or riluzole (200 mg/day), which offer varying degrees of benefit.[68]

DEEP BRAIN STIMULATION IN HD

The literature on DBS in HD is so far limited to a few case reports. The chosen target is the GPi, which is most extensively studied electrophysiologically. Surprisingly, microelectrode recording of the GPi in two patients with HD and 14 patients with PD showed similar pattern of increased activity, with comparable frequency rates of discharges in both, but the pattern of neuronal activity was less burst-like and more regular in HD.[69] Bilateral DBS with both 40 Hz and 130 Hz in the GPi of a patient with HD improved chorea. The 40 Hz stimulation did not worsen bradykinesia and also demonstrated increased blood flow (measured by PET) during decision-making tasks.[70] Recently, Kang et al. reported long-term (beyond 2 years) effects of DBS in two patients with HD.[71] They showed that chorea remained improved over time (using the Unified Huntington Disease Chorea Scale) despite progressive cognitive decline.

ALZHEIMER'S DISEASE

AD is the sixth leading cause of death and most common form of dementia and cognitive impairment.[72–74] Symptoms of AD include progressive decline and memory loss as well as an inability to perform routine daily activities.[75] While AD is very common, the neuronal network in AD is the least understood. Although its progression has been demonstrated to involve very intricate alterations of complex protein networks, more information about these networks is needed.[66] Genetic studies have provided an explanation for inherited forms of AD; however, the majority of AD cases are sporadic and lack a simple genetic cause.[75]

Interestingly, just as accumulation of CAG repeats seems to be the inciting factor for the cascade of destructive events and neurodegeneration occurring in HD, similarly, accumulation of beta amyloid (Aβ) is considered pivotal for the development of AD.[76] Accumulation of Aβ seems to be the cause of the phosphorylation of tau, which in turn leads to the formation of neurofibrillary tangles.[77] Initial events triggering the accumulation and plaque formation of Aβ are unknown, and thus to date there are no treatments that may stop this specific event.[77] Recent research has identified this phenomenon of biomarkers, such as brain amyloid deposition and cerebral spinal fluid tau and amyloid, as a "predromal period" that can be found in asymptomatic patients before the onset of cognitive decline.[78–80] During this predromal period, amyloid pathology is surprisingly *not* occurring in the medial temporal lobe itself but, rather, in regions comprising what is known as a "default mode network".[79,81] This default mode network is composed of functionally interconnected cortical areas, including the posterior cingulate, inferior parietal lobule, lateral temporal cortex, and centromedial and dorsomedial prefrontal cortices. The default network heavily sends projections to the medial temporal lobe and precedes cell death in the hippocampus by years.[82]

While early-onset AD is predominantly in a distributed cortical pattern, late-age-onset AD follows a hippocampal-predominant pattern.[77,83] Also, for reasons that are still not yet understood, early AD pathology is found to frequently target large-scale neuroanatomical networks for episodic memory before targeting other networks that are known to subserve language, attention, executive functions, and visuospatial abilities.[84] This initial disruption of the neuronal network critical for episodic memory is the reason for circumscribed memory deficits in the early stages of disease and the clinical hallmark of AD: anterograde amnesia.[84–87] As pathology spreads to other neocortical regions with time, the full dementia syndrome is fully expressed.[88–90] For example, defects in language and semantic knowledge, which occur later, are thought to be the result of the encroachment of AD neuropathology on the temporal, frontal, and parietal association cortices.[91] Overall, clinical deficits are found to be consistent with the anatomical locus of impact.[92–95]

This impact of anatomical specificity of a pathology on the disruption of neocortical networks is best exemplified by direct relations between specific AD clinical findings and AD neuropathology.[84] Deficits in executive functioning are hypothesized to be secondary to the burden of neurofibrillary tangles in the prefrontal cortex, as evidenced by profound prefrontal cortex pathology in a subset of patients with predominant executive dysfunction.[96,97] Deficits in visuospatial abilities, which may occur early in the disease or even in preclinical stages, are thought to arise from loss of effective interactions between distinct and relatively intact cortical information-processing systems.[98]

In accordance with the described anatomical network, there is increasing evidence that suggests that pathology may begin in certain vulnerable locations of the brain known as "hubs", which are further defined as central nodules within the target network's architecture (see Chapter 1). Recent studies using various imaging techniques, including task-free fMRI and graph studies, have been performed in an effort to obtain a better understanding of the pathophysiology of AD. These studies suggest that the angular gyrus may serve as the key heteromodal association hub from which information flows in the posterior unimodal and polymodal association cortices to modules specialized for memory, visuospatial, language, and praxis functions, which are lost in patients with AD.[99] It is further suspected that since AD pathology is more closely related to tau neurofibrillary tangles than to amyloid plaque pathology, the connectivity–vulnerability findings in AD greatly reflect tau pathology within posterior elements of a large-scale network (default mode network).[100] It is thought that this hub-like nature of the angular gyrus may produce activity-dependent wear and tear or increased amyloid production, thus increasing its early vulnerability to amyloid deposition.[101]

Role of Cholinergic Pathways

Since the early 1980s, cholinergic pathways in AD have been studied, and over time what is known as the "cholinergic hypothesis" has been established. According to this cholinergic hypothesis, disruption of cholinergic pathways in the basal forebrain portion of the central nervous system leads to a cognitive decline in individuals with AD.[102] A loss of cholinergic input into the areas of the cerebral neocortex and hippocampus leads to a decline in the level of acetylcholine, a key neuromodulator of synaptic plasticity for learning and memory.[103,104]

Pharmacological Treatment

The cholinesterase inhibitors donepezil, galantamine, and rivastigmine are the mainstays of pharmacological therapy in AD. A meta-analysis of cholinesterase inhibitors used for at least 6 months showed mild improvement in cognition, daily function, and behavior.[105] An NMDA antagonist, memantine, is also available for treatment of moderate to severe AD. When memantine is added to a cholinesterase inhibitor in patients with moderate to severe impairment, an improvement may be seen in behavior.[106]

Deep Brain Stimulation in AD

Very limited information is available to date on this subject. Laxton et al. conducted a phase I DBS study in six patients with AD with continuous stimulation of the Meynert nucleus and fornix for 12 months. An early and dramatic reversal of parietal and temporal hypometabolism in deoxyglucose PET was noted after DBS treatment. At 12 months, the effects on memory and cognition were modest, suggesting improvement.[107]

CONCLUSION

The past decade has led to greater understanding of the dysfunction that occurs in neuronal networks with major neurodegenerative disorders. This, in turn, has resulted in new therapeutic approaches of these disorders from both pharmacological and surgical perspectives. Yet there are currently many unanswered questions about treatments for PD and other neurodegenerative disorders, and more research is needed. For example, future options for surgery in PD may be aimed at replacing and/or restoring the dying dopamine cells through implantation of fetal brain tissue and/or infusion of growth factors, respectively. These approaches currently remain experimental and need to be addressed in further clinical trials. Understanding neuronal networks in neurodegenerative diseases will allow for the generation of more comprehensive disease pathogenesis models so that the interface between disease protein aggregation and selective, network-driven neuronal vulnerability can be achieved.

References

1. DeLong MR. The basal ganglia. In: Kandel ER, Schwartz JH, Jessell TM, eds. *Principles of Neural Science*. 4th ed. New York: McGraw-Hill; 2000:853–867.
2. DeLong M, Wichmann T. Update on models of basal ganglia function and dysfunction. *Parkinsonism Relat Disord*. 2009;15(Suppl. 3):S237–S240.
3. Bostan AC, Dum RP, Strick PL. The basal ganglia communicate with the cerebellum. *Proc Natl Acad Sci USA*. 2010;107:8452–8456.
4. Ebadi M, Pfeiffer RF, eds. *Parkinson's Disease*. (568). Boca Raton: CRC Press; 2005.
5. Ito K, Nagano-Saito A, Kato T, et al. Striatal and extrastriatal dysfunction in Parkinson's disease with dementia: a 6-[^{18}F] fluoro-L-dopa PET study. *Brain*. 2002;125:1358–1365.
6. Mattay VS, Tessitore A, Callicott JH, et al. Dopaminergic modulation of cortical function in patients with Parkinson's disease. *Ann Neurol*. 2002;51:156–164.
7. Chaudhuri KR, Schapira AH. Non-motor symptoms of Parkinson's disease: dopaminergic pathophysiology and treatment. *Lancet Neurol*. 2009;8:464–474.
8. Shore DM, Rafal R, Parkinson JA. Appetitive motivational deficits in individuals with Parkinson's disease. *Mov Disord*. 2011; 26:1887–1892.
9. Alexander GE, Crutcher MD. Functional architecture of basal ganglia circuits – neural substrates of parallel processing. *Trends Neurosci*. 1990;13:266–271.
10. Czernecki V, Schupbach M, Yaici S, et al. Apathy following subthalamic stimulation in Parkinson's disease: a dopamine responsive syndrome. *Mov Disord*. 2008;23:964–969.
11. Grace AA. Anatomy and physiology of limbic system dysfunction in Parkinson's disease. In: Olanow CW, Stocchi F, Lang AE, eds. *Parkinson's Disease: Non-motor and Non-dopaminergic Features*. Oxford, UK: Blackwell Publishing Ltd; 2011. http://dx.doi.org/10.1002/9781444397970.ch6.
12. Brown RG, Marsden CD. How common is dementia in Parkinson's disease? *Lancet*. 1984;2:1262–1265.
13. Karlsen KH, Larsen JP, Tandberg E, Maland JG. Quality of life measurements in patients with Parkinson's disease: a community based study. *Eur J Neurol*. 1998;5:443–450.
14. Schrag A, Jahanshahi M, Quinn N. What contributes to quality of life in patients with Parkinson's disease? *J Neurol Neurosurg Psychiatry*. 2000;69:308–312.
15. Owen A. Cognitive dysfunction in Parkinson's disease: the role of frontostriatal circuitry. *Neuroscientist*. 2004;10:525–535.
16. Morris RG, Downes JJ, Robbins TW. The nature of the dysexecutive syndrome in Parkinson's disease. In: Gilhooly KJ, Keane MTG, Logie RH, Erdos G, eds. *Lines of Thinking: Reflections on the Psychology of Thought*. Vol. 2. New York: Wiley; 1990, 247–258.
17. Lange KW, Robbins TW, Marsden CD, James M, Owen AM, Paul GM. L-dopa withdrawal in Parkinson's disease selectively impairs cognitive performance in tests sensitive to frontal lobe dysfunction. *Psychopharmacology (Berl)*. 1992;107:394–404.
18. Owen AM, Doyon J, Dagher A, Sadikot A, Evans AC. Abnormal basal ganglia outflow in Parkinson's disease identified with PET: implications for higher cortical functions. *Brain*. 1998; 121:949–965.
19. Dagher A, Owen AM, Boecker H, Brooks DJ. The role of the striatum and hippocampus in planning: a PET activation study in Parkinson's disease. *Brain*. 2001;124:1020–1032.
20. Cools R, Stefanova E, Barker RA, Robbins TW, Owen AM. Dopaminergic modulation of high-level cognition in Parkinson's disease: the role of the prefrontal cortex revealed by PET. *Brain*. 2002;125:584–594.
21. Emre M. What causes mental dysfunction in Parkinson's disease? *Mov Disord*. 2003;18:S63–S71.
22. Parkinson JA, Dalley JW, Cardinal RN, et al. Nucleus accumbens dopamine depletion impairs both acquisition and performance of appetitive Pavlovian approach behaviour: implications for

mesoaccumbens dopamine function. *Behav Brain Res.* 2002;137: 149–163.
23. Lewis S, Dove A, Robbins T, Barker R, Owen A. Cognitive impairments in early Parkinson's disease are accompanied by reductions in activity in frontostriatal neural circuitry. *J Neurosci.* 2003;23:6351–6356.
24. Rinne J, Portin R, Ruottinen H, et al. Cognitive impairment and the brain dopaminergic system in Parkinson disease—[F-18] fluorodopa positron emission tomographic study. *Arch Neurol.* 2000;57:470–475.
25. Nakamura T, Ghilardi MF, Mentis M, et al. Functional networks in motor sequence learning: abnormal topographies in Parkinson's disease. *Hum Brain Mapp.* 2001;12:42–60.
26. Miyachi S, Hikosaka O, Miyashita K, et al. Differential roles of monkey striatum in learning of sequential hand movement. *Exp Brain Res.* 1997;115:1–5.
27. Wichmann T, DeLong MR, Guridi J. Milestones in research on pathophysiology of Parkinson's disease. *Mov Disord.* 2011;26: 1032–1041.
28. Benabid AL, Pollak P, Gross C, et al. Acute and long-term effects of subthalamic nucleus stimulation in Parkinson's disease. *Stereotact Funct Neurosurg.* 1994;62:76–84.
29. Moro E, Lozano AM, Pollak P, et al. Long-term results of a multicenter study on subthalamic and pallidal stimulation in Parkinson's disease. *Mov Disord.* 2010;15:578–586.
30. Stefani A, Lozano AM, Peppe A, et al. Bilateral deep brain stimulation of the pedunculopontine and subthalamic nuclei in severe Parkinson's disease. *Brain.* 2007;130:1596–1607.
31. Moro E, Hamani C, Poon YY, et al. Unilateral pedunculopontine stimulation improves falls in Parkinson's disease. *Brain.* 2010; 133:215–224.
32. Raethjen J, Deuschl G. The oscillating central network of Essential tremor. *Clin Neurophysiol.* 2012;123:61–64.
33. Zesiewicz TA, Elble RJ, Louis ED, et al. Evidence-based guideline update: treatment of essential tremor: report of the Quality Standards subcommittee of the American Academy of Neurology. *Neurology.* Nov 8, 2011;77(19):1752–1755. Epub 2011 Oct 19.
34. Lyons KE, Pahwa R, Comella CL, et al. Benefits and risks of pharmacological treatments for essential tremor. *Drug Saf.* 2003;26:461–481.
35. Muthuraman M, Heute U, Arning K, et al. Oscillating central motor networks in pathological tremors and voluntary movements. What makes the difference? *Neuroimage.* 2012; 60:1331–1339.
36. Cif L, Vasques X, Gonzalez V, et al. Long-term follow-up of DYT1 dystonia patients treated by deep brain stimulation: an open-label study. *Mov Disord.* 2010;25:289–299.
37. Vitek JL, Zhang J, Evatt M, et al. GPi pallidotomy for dystonia: clinical outcome and neuronal activity. *Adv Neurol.* 1998; 78:209–211.
38. Alterman RL, Miravite J, Weisz D, Shils JL, Bressman SB, Tagliati M. Sixty hertz pallidal deep brain stimulation for primary torsion dystonia. *Neurology.* 2007;69:681–688.
39. Leckman J. Tourette syndrome. *Lancet.* 2002;360:1577–1586.
40. Singer HS, Minzer K. Neurobiology of Tourette syndrome: concept of neuroanatomic localization and neurochemical abnormalities. *Brain Dev.* 2003;25(Suppl. 1):S70–S84.
41. Wang Z, Malia TV, Marsh R, Colibazzi T, Gerber A, Petersen BS. The neural circuits that generate tics in Tourette syndrome. *Am J Psychiatry.* 2011;168:1326–1337.
42. Smith Y, Galvan A, Raju D, Wichmann T. Anatomical and functional organization of the thalamostriatal systems. In: *Handbook of Basal Ganglia Structure and Function.* Elsevier Publisher; 2010.
43. Vandewalle V, Van der Linden C, et al. Stereotactic treatment of Gille de la Tourette syndrome by high frequency stimulation of thalamus. *Lancet.* 1999;353:724.
44. Porta M, Brambilla A, Cavanna AE, et al. Thalamic deep brain stimulation for treatment-refractory Tourette syndrome: two-year outcome. *Neurology.* 2009;73:1375–1380.
45. Bajwa RJ, de Lotbinière AJ, King RA, et al. Deep brain stimulation in Tourette's syndrome. *Mov Disord.* 2007;22:1346–1350.
46. Ackermans L, Duits A, van der Linden C, et al. Double-blind clinical trial of thalamic stimulation in patients with Tourette syndrome. *Brain.* 2011;134:832–844.
47. Saleh C, Gonzalez V, Cif L, Coubes P. Deep brain stimulation of the globus pallidus internus and Gilles de la Tourette syndrome: toward multiple networks modulation. *Surg Neurol Int.* 2012;3(Suppl. 2):S127–S142. Epub 2012.
48. Sturm V, Lenartz D, Koulousakis A, et al. The nucleus accumbens: a target for deep brain stimulation in obsessive-compulsive- and anxiety-disorders. *J. Chem Neuroanat.* 2003;26:293–299.
49. Huff W, Lenartz D, Schormann M, et al. Unilateral deep brain stimulation of the nucleus accumbens in patients with treatment-resistant obsessive-compulsive disorder: outcomes after one year. *Clin Neurol Neurosurg.* 2010;112:137–143.
50. Chabardès S, Polosan M, Krack P, et al. Deep brain stimulation for obsessive-compulsive disorder: subthalamic nucleus target. *World Neurosurg.* 2012. Epub ahead of print.
51. Le Jeune F, Vérin M, N'Diaye K, et al. French Stimulation dans le trouble obsessionnel compulsif (STOC) study group. Decrease of prefrontal metabolism after subthalamic stimulation in obsessive-compulsive disorder: a positron emission tomography study. *Biol Psychiatry.* 2010;68:1016–1022. Epub 2010.
52. Mangiarini L, Sathasivam K, Seller M, et al. Exon I of the HD gene with an expanded CAG repeat is sufficient to cause a progressive neurological phenotype in transgenic mice. *Cell.* 1996;87(3):493–506.
53. Walker FO. Huntington's disease. *Lancet.* 2007;369(9557): 218–228.
54. Schmitt I, Bachner D, Megow D, et al. Expression of the Huntington disease gene in rodents: cloning the rat homologue and evidence for downregulation in non-neuronal tissues during development. *Hum Mol Genet.* 1995;4(7): 1173–1182.
55. Landwehrmeyer GB, McNeil SM, Dure LS, et al. Huntington's disease gene: regional and cellular expression in brain of normal and affected individuals. *Ann Neurol.* 1995;37(2):218–230.
56. Kandasamy M, Reilmann R, Winkler J, Bogdahn U, Aigner L. Transforming growth factor-beta signaling in the neural stem cell niche: a therapeutic target for Huntington's disease. *Neurol Res Int.* 2011;2011:124256.
57. Estrada-Sánchez AM, Rebec GV. Corticostriatal dysfunction and glutamate transporter 1 (GLT1) in Huntington's disease: interactions between neurons and astrocytes. *Basal Ganglia.* Jul 2012;2(2):57–66.
58. Wolf RC, Grön G, Sambataro F, et al. Brain activation and functional connectivity in premanifest Huntington's disease during states of intrinsic and phasic alertness. *Hum Brain Mapp.* 2012;33:2161–2173.
59. Chesselet MF, Delfs JM, Mackenzie L. Dopamine control of gene expression in basal ganglia nuclei: striatal and nonstriatal mechanisms. *Adv Pharmacol.* 1998;42:674–677.
60. Rosas HD, Koroshetz WJ, Chen YI, et al. Evidence for more widespread cerebral pathology in early HD: an MRI based morphometric analysis. *Neurology.* 2003;60(10):1615–1620.

61. de Tommaso M, Serpino C, Sciruicchio V. Management of Huntington's disease: role of tetrabenazine. *Ther Clin Risk Manag.* 2011;7:123–129. Epub 2011 Mar 21.
62. Scherman D, Jaudon P, Henry JP. Characterization of the monoamine carrier of chromaffin granule membrane by binding of [2-^{3}H]dihydrotetrabenazine. *Proc Natl Acad Sci USA.* 1983; 80:584–588.
63. Mehvar R, Jamali F. Concentration-effect relationships of tetrabenazine and dihydrotetrabenazine in the rat. *J Pharm Sci.* 1987;76:461–465.
64. Thibaut F, Faucheux BA, Marquez J, et al. Regional distribution of monoamine vesicular uptake sites in the mesencephalon of control subjects and patients with Parkinson's disease: a postmortem study using tritated tetrabenazine. *Brain Res.* 1995; 692:233–243.
65. Login IS, Cronin MJ, MacLeod RM. Tetrabenazine has properties of a dopamine receptor antagonist. *Ann Neurol.* 1982;12:257–262.
66. Reches A, Burke RE, Kuhn CM, et al. Tetrabenazine, an amine-depleting drug, also blocks dopamine receptors in rat brain. *J Pharmacol Exp Ther.* 1983;225:515–521.
67. Burke RE, Reches A, Traub MM, et al. Tetrabenazine induces acute dystonic reactions. *Ann Neurol.* 1985;17:200–202.
68. Armstrong MJ, Miyasaki JM. Evidence-based guideline: pharmacologic treatment of chorea in Huntington disease: report of the Guideline Development Subcommittee of the American Academy of Neurology. *Neurology.* Aug 7, 2012;79(6):597–603. Epub 2012 Jul 18.
69. Tang JK, Moro E, Lozano AM, et al. Firing rates of pallidal neurons are similar in Huntington's and Parkinson's disease patients. *Exp Brain Res.* 2005;166:230–236.
70. Moro E, Lang AE, Strafella AP, et al. Bilateral globus pallidus stimulation for Huntington's disease. *Ann Neurol.* 2004;56:290–294.
71. Kang GA, Heath S, Rothlind J, Starr PA. Long-term follow-up of pallidal deep brain stimulation in two cases of Huntington's disease. *J Neurol Neurosurg Psychiatry.* 2011;82:272–277.
72. Hebert LE, Scherr PA, Bienias JL, Bennett BD, Evans DA. Alzheimer's disease in the US population. *Arch Neurol.* 2003;60: 1119–1122.
73. Ashford JW. APOE genotype effects on Alzheimer's disease onset and epidemiology. *J Mol Neurosci.* 2004;23:157–165.
74. Mattson MP, Maudsley S, Martin B. BDNF and 5-HT: a dynamic duo in age-related neuronal plasticity and neurodegenerative disorders. *Trends Neurosci.* 2004;27:589–594.
75. Cai H, Cong W, Ji S, Rothman S, Maudsley S, Martin B. Metabolic dysfunction in Alzheimer's disease and related neurodegenerative disorders. *Curr Alzheimer Res.* 2012;9(1):5–17.
76. Hardy J, Selkoe DJ. The amyloid hypothesis of Alzheimer's disease: progress and problems on the road to therapeutics. *Science.* 2002;297:353–356.
77. Yates D. *Nat Rev Neurosci.* May 18, 2012;13(5):288–289.
78. Perrin RJ, Fagan AM, Holtzman DM. Multimodal techniques for diagnosis and prognosis of Alzheimer's disease. *Nature.* 2009; 461:916–922.
79. Sperling RA, Laviolette PS, O'Keefe K, et al. Amyloid deposition is associated with impaired default network function in older persons without dementia. *Neuron.* 2009;63:178–188.
80. Jack Jr CR, Knopman DS, Jagust WJ, et al. Hypothetical model of dynamic biomarkers of the Alzheimer's pathological cascade. *Lancet Neurol.* 2010;9:119–128.
81. Buckner RL, Snyder AZ, Shannon BJ, et al. Molecular, structural, and functional characterization of Alzheimer's disease: evidence for a relationship between default activity, amyloid, and memory. *J Neurosci.* 2005;25:7709–7717.
82. Buckner RL, Andrews-Hanna JR, Schacter DL. The brain's default network: anatomy, function, and relevance to disease. *Ann N Y Acad Sci.* 2008;1124:1–38.
83. Kim EJ, Cho SS, Jeong Y, et al. Glucose metabolism in early onset versus late onset Alzheimer's disease: an SPM analysis of 120 patients. *Brain.* 2005;128:1790–1801.
84. Weintraub S, Wicklund AH, Salmon DP. The neuropsychological profile of Alzheimer disease. *Cold Spring Harb Perspect Med.* 2012;2:a006171.
85. Braak H, Braak E. Neuropathological staging of Alzheimer-related changes. *Acta Neuropathol (Berl).* 1991;82:239–259.
86. Jack Jr CR, Petersen RC, Xu YC, et al. Medial temporal atrophy on MRI in normal aging and very mild Alzheimer's disease. *Neurology.* 1997;49:786–794.
87. de Toledo-Morrell L, Goncharova I, Dickerson B, Wilson RS, Bennett DA. From healthy aging to early Alzheimer's disease: in vivo detection of entorhinal cortex atrophy. *Ann N Y Acad Sci.* 2000;911:240–253.
88. Braak H, Braak E. Development of Alzheimer-related neurofibrillary changes in the neocortex inversely recapitulates cortical myelogenesis. *Acta Neuropathol (Berl).* 1996;92:197–201.
89. Braak E, Arai K, Braak H. Cerebellar involvement in Pick's disease: affliction of mossy fibers, monodendritic brush cells, and dentate projection neurons. *Exp Neurol.* 1999;159:153–163.
90. Jack Jr CR, Petersen RC, Xu Y, et al. Rates of hippocampal atrophy correlate with change in clinical status in aging and AD. *Neurology.* 2000;55:484–489.
91. Hodges JR, Patterson K. Is semantic memory consistently impaired early in the course of Alzheimer's disease? Neuroanatomical and diagnostic implications. *Neuropsychologia.* 1995; 33:441–459.
92. Weintraub S, Mesulam M. Four neuropsychological profiles of dementia. In: Boller F, Grafman J, eds. *Handbook of Neuropsychology.* Amsterdam: Elsevier; 1993.
93. Weintraub S, Mesulam M-M. From neuronal networks to dementia: four clinical profiles. In: Fôret F, Christen Y, Boller F, eds. *La demence: Pourquoi?* Paris: Foundation Nationale de Gerontologie; 1996:75–97.
94. Weintraub S, Mesulam M. With or without FUS, it is the anatomy that dictates the dementia phenotype. *Brain.* 2009;132:2906–2908.
95. Seeley WW, Crawford RK, Zhou J, Miller BL, Greicius MD. Neurodegenerative diseases target large-scale human brain networks. *Neuron.* 2009;62:42–52.
96. Johnson JK, Head E, Kim R, Starr A, Cotman CW. Clinical and pathological evidence for a frontal variant of Alzheimer disease. *Arch Neurol.* 1999;56:1233–1239.
97. Waltz JA, Knowlton BJ, Holyoak KJ, et al. Relational integration and executive function in Alzheimer's disease. *Neuropsychology.* 2004;18:296–305.
98. Morrison JH, Hof PR, Bouras C. An anatomic substrate for visual disconnection in Alzheimer's disease. *Ann N Y Acad Sci.* 1991;640:36–43.
99. Zhou J, Gennatas ED, Kramer JH, Miller BL, Seeley WW. Predicting regional neurodegeneration from the healthy brain functional connectome. *Neuron.* Mar 22, 2012;73(6):1216–1227.
100. Greicius MD, Krasnow B, Reiss AL, Menon V. Functional connectivity in the resting brain: a network analysis of the default mode hypothesis. *Proc Natl Acad Sci USA.* 2003;100: 253–258.
101. Buckner RL, Sepulcre J, Talukdar T, et al. Cortical hubs revealed by intrinsic functional connectivity: mapping, assessment of stability, and relation to Alzheimer's disease. *J Neurosci.* 2009; 29:1860–1873.

102. Bartus RT, Dean III RL, Beer B, Lippa AS. The cholinergic hypothesis of geriatric memory dysfunction. *Science*. 1982;217:408–414.
103. Buccafusco JJ, Terry Jr AV. Multiple central nervous system targets for eliciting beneficial effects on memory and cognition. *J Pharmacol Exp Ther*. 2000;295:438–446.
104. Terry Jr AV, Buccafusco JJ. The cholinergic hypothesis of age and Alzheimer's disease-related cognitive deficits: recent challenges and their implications for novel drug development. *J Pharmacol Exp Ther*. 2003;306:821–827.
105. Birks J. Cholinesterase inhibitors for Alzheimer's disease. *Cochrane Database Syst Rev*. Jan 25, 2006;1:CD005593.
106. Cummings J, Schneider L, Tariot E, Graham PN, Graham SM. Memantine MEM-MD-02 Study Group. Behavioral effect of memantine in Alzheimer disease patients receiving donepezil treatment. *Neurology*. 2006;44:2308–2314.
107. Laxton AW, Tang-Wai DF, McAndrews MP, et al. A phase I trial of deep brain stimulation of memory circuits in Alzheimer's disease. *Ann Neurol*. 2010;68:521–534.

CHAPTER

26

Neuronal Networks in Epilepsy: Comparative Audiogenic Seizure Networks

Carl L. Faingold[1], *Manish Raisinghani*[2], *Prosper N'Gouemo*[3]

[1]Departments of Pharmacology and Neurology, Division of Neurosurgery, Southern Illinois University School of Medicine, Springfield, IL, USA, [2]P2ALS Foundation, Columbia University Medical Center, New York, NY, USA, [3]Department of Pediatrics, Georgetown University Medical Center, Washington, DC, USA

INTRODUCTION

As noted in Chapter 1, the study of epilepsy is one of the major driving forces behind research into neuronal networks of the brain, especially interactions between different networks, since these disorders are a "window into the brain" that provides a lens through which these network interactions have come into sharp focus. The large number of network-related studies that have been done in epilepsy ranges from neuronal cultures through animal models to human epilepsy. As discussed in Chapter 1, there are various reasons why epilepsy research has involved network approaches so prominently. Historically, evaluation of brain activity began in epileptic patients and animal models of epilepsy, and it continues to this day; these approaches have been joined by in vitro and ex vivo approaches as well as computational approaches.

The epilepsies are a heterogeneous group of brain disorders characterized by abnormal firing patterns of neurons within neuronal networks that are specific to the class of epilepsy being studied. Two major classes of epilepsy have been identified, partial (focal) or "generalized", based on the pattern of onset of the seizures, strongly implicating major network differences between these classes. This dichotomy has been quite useful clinically, but experimentally this difference is less clear, in part because partial seizures can become secondarily generalized after the onset of the seizure. Recent evidence indicates that additional brain structures become involved in the seizure network during secondary generalization.[1] In addition, partial or focal epilepsy does not involve only a small, anatomically isolated "focus" of neurons, as was once thought; rather, it has been established that these forms of epilepsy also involve more widespread neuronal networks.[2–4] In fact, there is good evidence that all of the epilepsies are caused by abnormal neuronal network activity, as was suggested over 20 years ago.[5] In addition, it was once thought that the network for generalized seizures involved the entire brain or at least the entire cortex. However, more recent studies have made it clear that, although the epileptic neuronal networks for generalized seizures involve a large number of cerebral neurons, many other neurons and brain regions do not become involved.[6] Critical brain sites or "hubs" within networks have been identified,[7] and experimental studies on specific seizure models have identified many of the hubs in these networks (e.g. Ref. 8). Thus, extensive research on epilepsy networks has been done in animal models and more recently in human epilepsy with the advent of noninvasive imaging techniques.

Different types of epilepsy models have allowed the elucidation of potential comparative network mechanisms. From the beginning of modern epilepsy research, field potentials in the form of the electroencephalogram (EEG) recorded from the cortex via scalp or surface electrodes and localized field potentials from specific subcortical brain structures in invasive studies have provided important insights into epilepsy mechanisms. These were originally done using polygraph machines with mechanical pen outputs onto paper. These methods have important limitations, especially with respect to faithfully recording higher frequency activity. More recently, using newer equipment, higher frequencies have been detected and quantified, leading to additional insights into epileptiform mechanisms. For example,

Neuronal Networks in Brain Function, CNS Disorders, and Therapeutics
http://dx.doi.org/10.1016/B978-0-12-415804-7.00026-5

higher frequency (gamma frequency) oscillations (>40 Hz) have been proposed to be an indicator for seizure onset, and the simultaneous occurrence of these frequencies in different brain regions suggests the existence of a long-range synchronizing mechanism at seizure onset.[9]

DEVELOPMENTAL EPILEPSY NETWORKS

In a developmental epilepsy model, in which certain hippocampal neurons act as network "hubs" that are critical in this synchronizing mechanism, elimination of certain of these neurons abolishes the epileptiform activity and prevents the development of the epileptic state.[9] Recent studies in another developmental seizure model indicate that early-life seizures result in alterations of short-term plasticity in the prefrontal cortex, which involve network interaction changes between specific layers of the cortex. These alterations include plasticity changes within these networks, and these changes are proposed to lead to the cognitive deficits seen in human developmental epilepsy.[10,11] Thus, developmental models are illuminating the role of critical network hubs and neuroplastic changes in network function, but the diverse nature of developmental network models does not allow close comparisons of network mechanisms.

NETWORKS FOR ABSENCE EPILEPSY MODELS

A common form of "generalized-onset" human epilepsy is called absence (petit mal) epilepsy, and network mechanisms for both human and animal models have been evaluated. Thalamocortical pathways are known to be critical to all of these networks. Abnormal neurotransmitter activity in this network, including $GABA_A$ receptor-mediated neurotransmission, is implicated in mediation of this disorder. For example, in genetic absence epilepsy rats, $GABA_A$ receptor-mediated inhibitory postsynaptic potentials in thalamic reticular neurons were abnormally large, especially at the EEG frequencies that occur during the absence seizures.[12] $GABA_B$ receptors are also implicated in other genetic models of absence seizures; $GABA_B$ receptor agonists exacerbate, while $GABA_B$ antagonists suppress, seizures in these models. $GABA_B$ receptor abnormalities within specific sites in the thalamus are proposed to be a key element in this network.[13] Thus, gamma-aminobutyric acid (GABA) receptor abnormalities are implicated in the thalamocortical networks, but the nature of the involvement appears to differ, depending on the model examined.

NETWORKS FOR EPILEPSY KINDLING MODELS

Electrical kindling models of temporal lobe epilepsy are induced by repeated (often daily) stimulation pulses in limbic structures, most commonly in the amygdala, which result in the gradual induction of limbic system seizures, allowing the evaluation of network mechanisms. The network structures that are recruited in these forms of limbic seizures in animals include piriform, perirhinal, and entorhinal areas, based on studies utilizing in vitro and in vivo electrophysiological recording and radioactive 2-deoxyglucose (2-DG) uptake as well as the behavioral effects of lesions within this network.[14,15] As noted in this chapter, partial seizures, including temporal lobe seizures, can often result in "secondary" generalization, during which consciousness is lost. The loss of consciousness implicates network mechanisms beyond the limbic sites into subcortical structures involved in maintaining consciousness. In an animal model of temporal lobe seizures, increased neuronal activity and cerebral blood flow were observed in subcortical structures, while decreases in these activities occurred in cortical structures. These changes were abolished by transecting the major pathways to the subcortical structures, showing the importance of subcortical structures in the seizure-induced depression of consciousness.[16]

Other recent studies on network mechanisms in limbic kindling have also implicated basal ganglia structures in this temporal lobe epilepsy model. Thus, histological and neurochemical changes in the striatum of amygdala-kindled rats were examined, as well as in vivo neuronal recording, which showed an increased irregularity of firing in and increased spontaneous activity of striatal projection neurons within the sensorimotor subregion of the striatum. This activity appears to represent a kindling-induced functional reorganization of this network, which either facilitates epileptic discharge propagation or is a compensatory network to prevent the propagation of seizure activity.[17] Thus, subcortical structures appear to become involved in these forms of kindling-induced seizures, but different subcortical sites are implicated, depending on the kindling techniques used.

STATUS EPILEPTICUS NETWORKS

Status epilepticus is an acute and often life-threatening event in human epilepsy, consisting of repeated or continuous seizures. Network mechanisms in a chemically induced (kainate) status epilepticus model involve changes in the firing properties of hippocampal neurons that interact with field potential oscillations and project bilaterally to the cortex.[18] In another drug-induced status model, induced by pilocarpine, the network changes involved in the transition between the interictal and ictal states in the hippocampus were evaluated with neuronal recordings during the development of these drug-induced seizures in vivo. The preictal state was characterized by an early desynchronization phase in the hippocampus, which correlated with decreasing neuronal firing, leading to a late resynchronization phase in which the synchronization of neuronal firing within the network increased. During seizures, individual neurons firing and interneuronal synchronization increased further.[19] Experiments on subcortical structures in the network for status epilepticus induced by 4-aminopyridine have implicated impairment of the pontine reticular formation (PRF) in this status model. "Dark" neurons consistent with cellular injury were consistently found in the PRF of animals in the later phases of status epilepticus simultaneous with the presence of slow oscillations, suggesting that the PRF may become involved importantly in the network for status epilepticus as the syndrome progresses.[20] Electrical stimulation–induced status epilepticus resulted in spontaneous field depolarizations, population spikes, and epileptiform discharges in hippocampal granule cells prior to each generalized behavioral seizure, which was coincident with initial neuron loss. The authors proposed that the entorhinal cortex within this seizure network caused disrupted function and synchronous discharges that project to the dentate gyrus and contribute importantly to generation of the seizure behavior.[21] Thus, the different status models show a considerable amount of network variability, depending on the method used to induce the status.

NETWORKS FOR GENERALIZED HUMAN EPILEPSY

Loss of consciousness is observed in human and animal models of epilepsy that begin or proceed to seizure "generalization". Under normal conditions, a "default mode" network is proposed to be activated during the resting state and deactivated during engagement with task, which primarily involves specific cortical areas (see Ref. 22). This network has been shown to be selectively impaired during epileptic seizures associated with loss of consciousness. Neuroimaging and electrophysiological methods have shown decreased activity in the default-mode network during complex partial, generalized tonic-clonic, and absence seizures.[22] It has been proposed that the specific mechanisms of onset and propagation of these seizure types are due to active inhibition of subcortical arousal systems, including those that maintain default-mode network activity. These findings support a general "network inhibition hypothesis", during which active inhibition of arousal systems by seizures in certain cortical regions leads to cortical deactivation in other cortical areas.[22,23] Human absence seizures are a form of generalized seizures with transient loss of consciousness and generalized spike wave discharges in the EEG, which result from highly synchronized activity in the thalamocortical network,[24] like that seen in the absence models discussed in this chapter. EEG and imaging data in human absence seizures indicate blood oxygenation level–dependent (BOLD) magnetic resonance imaging activation in the thalamus, the frontomesial cortex, and the cerebellum, and they also show BOLD deactivation in default-mode areas during the seizures, which returned to normal network patterns between seizures.[24] Thus, the network involved in human absence epilepsy involves both inactivation of certain intracortical circuits and activation of thalamocortical circuits.

One of the problems with much of the network-related information in the foregoing seizure model data and much of human epilepsy is that the actual seizure onset is unpredictable, so the hierarchical elements are difficult to determine. That is, what is the actual triggering site for the seizure, and how does it progress from this site within the network as the different behavioral phases are expressed during the course of the seizure? However, there are several animal models and certain forms of human epilepsy that are triggered by an external stimulus that can be controlled experimentally; these are termed "reflex" epilepsy.[25] In humans, the most common epilepsy trigger is sensory, usually a visual stimulus such as a flashing light.[26] However, animal models of visually evoked seizures are uncommon [e.g. in a genetic baboon model (*Papio papio*) and an epileptic avian model].[27,28] In many types of rodents and rarely in people,[29] the trigger for seizure onset is an acoustic stimulus. The vast majority of sensory-induced seizure models in animals are induced by auditory stimuli, and these are called audiogenic seizures (AGS).[30,31] The main reason why reflex epilepsy models are of great experimental value is that induction of the seizure is under the direct and reliable control of the experimenter. These reflex epilepsy models are often genetic, like much of human epilepsy. The stimulus is external and does not require prior invasive brain surgery or the administration of exogenous chemicals to normal animals, as do many of the other experimental epilepsy models discussed in this chapter. Genetic animal models of reflex epilepsy also allow the modeling of the many forms of human epilepsy that involve a genetic component.[32,33]

There have been a number of network studies in different inherited and acquired forms of AGS that provide a rare insight into the similarities and differences between closely related networks, which will be considered in detail in this chapter. Hopefully, these "variations on a theme" will be instructive for understanding human brain disorders that are closely related but have clear, individualized behavioral differences. These include temporal lobe epilepsy, many cases of which exhibit different constellations of behaviors, and anxiety disorders that exhibit overlapping but distinguishably different symptoms.

As will be discussed in detail in this chapter, in essence the prototypical AGS network consists of the auditory network [up to the level of the inferior colliculus (IC); see Chapter 20]. The auditory network interacts with the brainstem elements of the locomotor network (see Chapter 17). Proprioceptive feedback also appears to be a critical element in AGS,[34] since reversible (pharmacological) paralysis can prevent seizures emanating from the brainstem.[35] The IC is the consensus seizure initiation site in all AGS models in which this issue has been examined (as discussed in this chapter). The exact nature of the involvement of specific network nuclei appears to differ somewhat in the different AGS forms, in part due to the behavioral differences and to the mechanism(s) responsible for seizure susceptibility. Thus, in many of the inherited forms, including genetically epilepsy-prone rats (GEPRs), the involvement of partial auditory deafferentation (hearing loss) early in development appears to contribute to the primary role of brainstem structures. On the other hand, in the adult-onset induced forms, such as ethanol withdrawal (ETX), the network appears to be more widespread, since systemically administered ethanol exerts effects throughout the brain, as discussed in the "Alcohol Withdrawal (ETX)-induced AGS Susceptibility" section.

FORMS OF AGS

A number of different forms of AGS have been observed in rodents, and this type of "reflex epilepsy" is very commonly seen in genetic models and is also easily inducible in previously normal rodents.

GENETIC FORMS OF AGS SUSCEPTIBILITY

Inherited susceptibility to AGS, which has proven to be extensive and robust in rodents, has been reported at least as far back as 1924.[36] Because the cerebral cortex was once considered to be the crucial site in the generation of epilepsy, AGS was not accepted as a valid form of epilepsy by certain epilepsy researchers (Naquet, public communication, 1989; Kelly, public communication, 2004), since the cortex is not a required element of most AGS networks.[8,37,38] However, a more recent authoritative review has made it clear that, although the cortex is the primary element in human epileptic seizure generation, seizures can also originate in the brainstem.[39] In addition, it should be noted that all drugs with anticonvulsant properties that have been tested will effectively block AGS, including one clinically useful drug that was not effective in the standard drug-screening models.[40,41] New and experimental drugs often utilize these models for anticonvulsant screening. Neuronal network investigations have been carried out in several forms of rat AGS. Among the most widely studied inherited forms of AGS in rats are the two strains of GEPR derived from the Sprague–Dawley strain, the severe seizure strain (GEPR-9s) and the moderately severe seizure strain (GEPR-3s). These substrains each exhibit a consistent pattern of convulsive behavior during AGS, and it consistently differs between the two strains.[42–47] There are also AGS-susceptible rats derived from the Wistar rat strain, including the Wistar audiogenic rats (WARs), Strasbourg Wistar rats (Wistar AGS-susceptible rats from Strasbourg, France), Krushinski–Molodkina (KM) rat strain, and P77PMC rats.[48–53] There are also over a dozen different inbred mouse strains that exhibit AGS, including the DBA/2, DBA/1, and Frings mice,[54–56] as well as genetically epilepsy-prone hamsters.[57] DBA/2 and DBA/1 mice are known to exhibit very severe seizures that culminate in the death of many of the animals, which is due to respiratory arrest. These mice are a current model for sudden unexpected death that occurs in patients[58–60] (see Chapter 29).

A number of strains of genetically modified mice also exhibit AGS susceptibility, including fragile X mice, 5-HT_{2C} receptor knockout mice, dopamine betahydroxylase null mutant mice, Fynkinase-deficient mice, thyroid hormone receptor beta mutant mice, interleukin 6 (IL-6)-deficient mice, mice lacking exons 2–4 of Vlgr1 gene, NB-2 knockout mice (a contactin subgroup in the immunoglobulin superfamily), as well as Alzheimer disease and Down syndrome mouse models. Other mouse forms of AGS include mutations of the leucine-rich glioma-inactivated 1 gene, GAIP interacting protein, and C terminus-3 gene.[55,61–72]

INDUCED FORMS OF AGS

Developmentally related AGS susceptibility can be induced in previously normal rodents, including young rats or mice, in which AGS susceptibility can be produced by inducing a hearing deficit during the critical period for hearing development.[73,74] Forms of AGS that are induced in early development include neonatal thyroid deficiency, intense acoustic stimulation (priming), and administration of ototoxic drugs such as kanamycin.[74–79] There is evidence that each of these latter models has a component of cochlear damage–induced hearing deficits (partial deafferentation) as a mechanism for AGS susceptibility.

THYROID-DEFICIENT FORM OF AGS SUSCEPTIBILITY

Organisms that are thyroid deficient (THX) early in development exhibit susceptibility to seizures, and, in rodents, AGS susceptibility is commonly observed, which is likely due to compensatory mechanisms for the induction of cochlear damage and the resultant hearing deficits.[79–88] In our studies discussed in this chapter, AGS susceptibility was induced in normal neonatal Sprague–Dawley rats by producing THX in their dams by administering propylthiouracil (PTU; 0.0075%) in the drinking water on the day of birth and for 19 days thereafter, which results in subnormal T4 thyroid levels of their pups throughout nursing.[88–90]

AGS susceptibility can also be induced in adult rodents without an accompanying detectable hearing deficit; techniques include the induction of a magnesium deficiency or a postischemia syndrome, and systemic administration of several pharmacological agents, including metaphit, which is thought to be mediated by an action on glutamate receptors.[91–95] These latter forms of AGS, with the exception of the ischemia model, are often temporary, in contrast to the chronic susceptibility seen in most of the genetic forms.

ISCHEMIA-INDUCED FORM OF AGS SUSCEPTIBILITY

Animals, including humans, that suffer from brain ischemia often exhibit elevated susceptibility to seizures. In rodent models of ischemia, susceptibility to AGS occurs in animals that were not susceptible to AGS prior to the induction of ischemia.[93,96–99] Human stroke patients show a significantly higher relative risk of seizures as compared with the general population.[100] Ischemic attacks, which increase with age, may be a major causative factor in the increased incidence of human epilepsy seen with aging.[101–105] The rat ischemia model of AGS[93] was examined in our lab, as discussed in this chapter. When these AGS-susceptible animals were treated with a GABA uptake inhibitor (tiagabine), or an uncompetitive *N*-methyl-D-aspartate (NMDA) antagonist (MK-801), the severity of seizures was significantly decreased and in many cases completely blocked, which was similar to the effect seen with these agents in GEPR-9s.[106,107]

ALCOHOL WITHDRAWAL (ETX)-INDUCED AGS SUSCEPTIBILITY

AGS susceptibility is also seen during the withdrawal syndrome after continued administration of depressant drugs, including ethanol.[108–110] When ethanol is ingested repeatedly (binge protocol) for a sufficient duration and then withdrawn abruptly, most species, including humans, will exhibit convulsive seizures; in rodents, these convulsive seizures are commonly AGS.[108,111–115] Alcohol is known to enhance the inhibitory action of GABA as well as block the action of glutamate at NMDA receptors.[116–118] The ETX-induced AGS susceptibility in previously normal rodents is thought to be due to $GABA_A$ receptor downregulation and/or desensitization or due to NMDA receptor upregulation.[119–123]

AGS SEVERITY

A standard Jobe seizure severity scale (from 1 to 9) for AGS in the GEPR[44] evaluates the appearance of three behaviors [wild running, clonus (generalized), and tonus], which are followed by a period of postictal depression during which consciousness is lost. Generalized clonus consists of a rapid succession of alternating contractions and relaxations that are a common behavior seen in human convulsions and in AGS, which is thought to be related to the locomotor network that mediates the wild-running behavior that precedes it, as discussed in this chapter. This contrasts with another type of clonus called facial and forelimb (F&F) clonus, in which the alternating contractions and relaxations occur in the forelimbs and in the facial muscles, but do not involve the hind limbs. The neuronal network for F&F clonus, which is seen in other seizure models, is thought to be driven by a very different (forebrain) neuronal network[124–126] (see Chapter 27). Tonus is a state of continuous contraction of the muscles in all four limbs, which is seen in generalized convulsive human epilepsy and some forms of AGS (e.g. GEPR-9s and DBA/2 mice). Tonus usually begins as tonic flexion and, in the most severe AGS, proceeds to tonic extension (stiffening), which is the key sign of the most severe AGS (a score of 9 on the Jobe scale). These seizures are considered to result from auditory network interaction with an excessive activation of the midbrain locomotor network (Chapter 29).[8,127] This idea is based on the fact that AGS begin with a locomotor activity (running), and the movements during these convulsions are bilaterally symmetrical; it is further supported by the finding that the neuronal network nuclei for AGS include brainstem nuclei that are major elements of the midbrain locomotor network (see Chapter 17).

Two strains of GEPR have been developed. The GEPR-9s exhibit a score of 9 and have the most severe seizure, ending in tonic hind limb extension. The other GEPR strain is the moderate-severity seizure strain (GEPR-3s), which exhibits a score of 3, characterized by seizures that end with generalized clonus. This severity scale was developed based on the effects of anticonvulsant drugs on AGS in GEPR-9s wherein the increasing doses of these drugs reduced the severity along the Jobe scale. In addition, electrical stimulation of the spinal cord, which is the actual source of the motor behaviors (see Chapter 17), will reproduce this pattern of seizure severity as the intensity of the stimulus is increased.[128] Other rat forms of AGS have utilized a somewhat different seizure severity scale,[129] but the Jobe scale or the specific AGS behavior will be used throughout the remainder of this chapter. Some forms of AGS consistently exhibit generalized clonic seizures, while others consistently exhibit tonic seizures. Thus, tonic seizures are the final convulsive behavior in GEPR-9s (tonic extension) and Strasbourg Wistar rats (tonic flexion). GEPR-3s exhibit generalized clonic seizures. AGS associated with ETX tend to be more variable, but in the studies discussed here, most ETX rats exhibit varying severities of AGS, most often ending in generalized clonic seizures.[130,131] The other genetic forms of AGS-susceptible rats, including WAG/Rij and KM Wistar, exhibit behaviors during seizure that are similar to those of GEPRs and ETX rats.[31,132–134] Extensive evidence suggests that there are many similarities in the AGS networks of these closely related seizure forms, but data have been accumulating that suggest that there are also certain surprising differences, as discussed in this chapter.

NEURONAL NETWORKS IN AGS

As described in several other chapters of this book, a number of different approaches are utilized to evaluate the identities of the brain nuclei involved in specific neuronal networks.

Anatomical Techniques

The nuclei involved in neuronal networks can be determined initially using anatomical approaches, including various forms of imaging and immunohistological mapping in many cases. Subsequently, lesion and ablation as well as reversible local blockade techniques in a specific brain site and local stimulation techniques in that brain site are evaluated, which often involve evaluation of neurotransmitter involvement in the specific site. Electrophysiological techniques, including recordings of neuronal firing in awake, behaving animals, are then employed, if feasible. Electrophysiological studies in awake, behaving animals allow evaluation of the activity changes dynamically during the actual seizures. The EEG has also been evaluated in several models but has been less than instructive, since the most common EEG finding in both WARs and GEPR-9s is a reduced-amplitude (electrodecremental) cortical EEG, unlike the EEG changes seen during most human epilepsies. Recent findings suggest that in certain models of epilepsy and forms of human epilepsies, the electrodecrement is actually associated with rhythmic, high-frequency, ripple-like events that are not detectable when using conventional EEG recording techniques.[135,136] However, at AGS onset, epileptiform EEG activity in brainstem structures, particularly in the IC, has been reported during the tonic phase of seizure in WARs and GEPR-9s.[137,138] The electrographic technique of EEG does not indicate how the neurons are actually firing during these events, since it is only an indirect and often unreliable indicator of neuronal firing. However, the temporal resolution of EEG events is roughly 100 times longer, making it difficult to correlate with the rapid and often brief changes in neuronal firing that occur during AGS. Neuronal recordings in many AGS network sites in GEPR-9s have been accomplished over a several-year period in a series of studies, as discussed here.

AGS in most studies are induced using a broad-spectrum, mixed-frequency, high-intensity acoustic stimulus (e.g., electrical bell). However, acoustic stimulation in neuronal recording studies in GEPRs and ETX rats (described in this chapter) involved sculptured bursts of pure tone at 12 kHz (100 ms duration), which is the most effective frequency for AGS induction in GEPR-9s. This stimulus is also effective in GEPR-3s and ETX rats and does not produce the electrical interference that is seen with electrical bells.[139–141] This stimulus allows the pathophysiological neuronal mechanisms responsible for seizure initiation to be evaluated at stimulus intensities below and at the threshold for AGS induction in awake, unanesthetized, and behaving animals, allowing the simultaneous correlation of changes in behavior pattern with neuronal firing.[8,42] Since the intensity of the acoustic stimulus can be readily controlled with a simple auditory attenuator, the neuronal response to the 12 kHz stimulus can be evaluated below the threshold for AGS induction. This allows an extensive evaluation of the input–output relationship of neuronal firing and also allows comparison with the firing patterns of neurons in the same brain structure in normal animals. In addition, when the stimulus intensity is increased to a level that exceeds the seizure threshold, the neuronal firing pattern changes during the actual seizure can be evaluated in real time. Neuronal network studies have been performed in several of these AGS models, and this review will compare the similarities and differences of these networks. Considerable experimental evidence has localized the seizure initiation site in all these models in a midbrain auditory site, the IC (as discussed in the next section), but involvement of specific brain nuclei efferent to the IC appears to vary among the different AGS forms.

AGS NEURONAL NETWORK STUDIES

Role of the IC in AGS Networks

The IC is a major midbrain nucleus in the auditory pathway (see Chapter 20). Imaging studies strongly support the critical involvement of the IC in AGS networks. These studies utilized radiolabeled 2-DG, an indicator of increases in metabolic activity and immunohistological methods, evaluating the expression of the immediate early gene c-Fos in several AGS models, including GEPR-9s and Strasbourg Wistar rats, but to a lesser extent in GEPR-3s.[142–144] c-Fos changes in IC are also seen in other genetic AGS models, including DBA/2 mice,[31,145,146] and in AGS susceptibility induced by ototoxic drugs and priming (high-intensity acoustic stimulation early in development).[147–149]

It has become clear that the initiating event—the acoustic stimulus, which enters from the ear—is transmitted to the cochlea and ascends via the primary auditory network that begins in the cochlear nucleus (see Chapter 20). However, not all nuclei of the auditory network are required for AGS. Thus, the neuronal network that is required in the tonic form of AGS in GEPR-9s is confined exclusively to the brainstem, including the lower brainstem primary auditory structures (the cochlear nucleus, superior olivary complex, and nuclei of the lateral lemniscus) (see Figure 26.1). However, various forms of stimulation of the auditory nuclei below or above the level of the IC are not consistently able to trigger susceptibility to AGS or mimic AGS in normal rats, while several different forms of stimulation in the IC can readily trigger susceptibility to AGS or AGS-like seizure behaviors, as discussed here. The IC contains several subnuclei, including the inferior colliculus central nucleus (ICc), which contains the principal cells for the primary auditory pathway of this midbrain structure (Chapter 20), as well as the dorsal cortex (ICd)

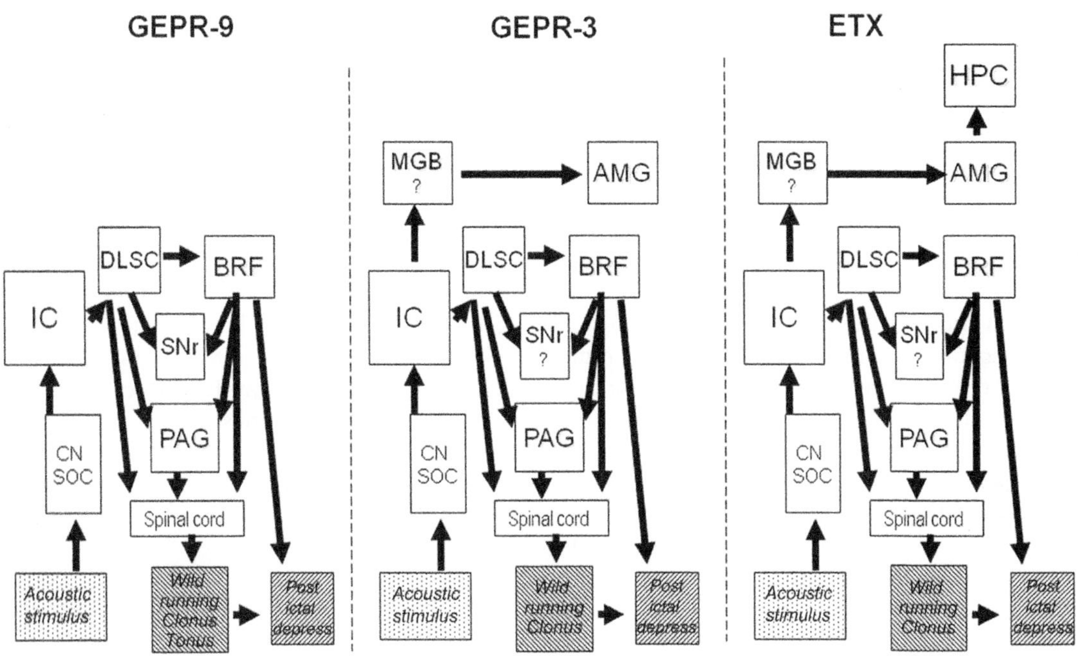

FIGURE 26.1 Comparative network diagrams in three forms of audiogenic seizures: GEPR-9s (left panel), GEPR-3s (middle panel), and ETX rats (right panel). The required network structures in all three models begins in the auditory network [the cochlear nucleus (CN) and superior olivary complex (SOC)], which project to the critical hub in the inferior colliculus (IC). The IC projects to the deep layers of the superior colliculus (DLSC) and brainstem conditional multireceptive regions, including the (pontine) brainstem reticular formation (BRF) and ventrolateral periaqueductal gray (PAG) and substantia nigra reticulata (SNr). These structures project to the spinal cord, which generates the wild-running and tonic seizures, which end in tonic extension of the hind limbs in GEPR-9s and which end in forelimb clonus in GEPR-3s and ETX rats (with some variability). However, in the GEPR-3s and ETX rats, the amygdala (AMG) is also involved in the network, and the medial geniculate body (MGB) is implicated, since this structure is the likely pathway from the IC to the AMG. The hippocampus (HPC) is implicated in the network for ETX. The cortex is not involved in either GEPR-9s or GEPR-3s unless further intervention occurs (see Chapter 27).

and external cortex (ICx), and each of these subnuclei is implicated in AGS.

The centrality of the IC in the AGS network is based, in part, on the defects of GABA-mediated inhibition that have been identified in this structure and the extensive connections from the IC to nuclei in the midbrain locomotor network that mediates the motor convulsions of these seizures.[30,31,42,108,139,141,154–158] Neurotransmitter-mediated excitation induced by focal microinjection into the IC of a $GABA_A$ receptor antagonist or an NMDA receptor agonist can consistently induce susceptibility to AGS, but this is not the case with any of the other nuclei in the AGS network.[159–161] Withdrawal after chronic bilateral infusion of GABA or an NMDA antagonist into the IC also results in AGS susceptibility.[162] Electrical stimulation of the IC induces a seizure pattern closely resembling AGS, including tonic seizures, after the first stimulation.[163] Focal blockade of the IC, using lesioning and focal microinjection techniques, has consistently established the critical role of the IC as the initiation site for AGS, as discussed in detail here. There is no other site in the brain that plays as critical a role in AGS as the IC.[161,164] However, the auditory pathway has little in the way of direct motor connections that would allow it to produce the behavioral seizures, which are mediated by cross-network interactions (see Chapter 29), as discussed in this chapter.

IC Focal Microinjections

Focal microinjection of inhibitors of neuronal firing into the IC blocks AGS in several AGS forms, including GEPR-9s, GEPR-3s, and acoustically primed, thyroid-deficient, ischemia-induced, and ETX rats, as well as in several AGS forms in mice.[31,42,78,108,139,141,145,147,149,154,155,158,162,165–168] The agents utilized in most of these focal blockade studies include GABA receptor agonists or NMDA receptor antagonists based on the importance of GABA and glutamate in normal neurotransmission in the IC and changes in the activity of these neurotransmitters associated with changes in AGS susceptibility.[151,160,167,169–172]

The major ascending auditory network nuclei that project to the IC (the cochlear nucleus and superior olivary complex) (see Chapter 20) are absolutely required (requisite) for the auditory stimulus to induce AGS, since focal blockade in these nuclei completely blocks the seizures.[42,108] Focal infusion of NMDA into the IC produced susceptibility to AGS without causing non-AGS. However, AGS alone were never induced by infusions of NMDA into the cochlear nucleus or the auditory nucleus rostral to the IC (the medial geniculate body) or by other nonauditory structures in the AGS network rostral to the IC.[160,164] These data further confirm that the IC is the most critical AGS network nucleus for seizure initiation.

TABLE 26.1 Comparative Doses of NMDA Receptor Antagonist (AP7) in AGS Models: Bilateral Microinjection of AP7 in AGS Network Sites

Drug dose nMol/side	GEPR-9s	GEPR-3s	ETX	THX	Compress
Inferior colliculus	0.1	0.5	8.0[a]	25	1.0
Pontine reticular formation	5.0	7.5	20[a]		
Periaqueductal gray	1.0	1.0	5.0		
Deep layers of the superior colliculus	2.0	2.0	5.0		

[a]*Comparable dose of a different NMDA receptor antagonist.*
AP7 = 2-amino-7-phosphonoheptanoate; Compress = cardiac compression model of AGS; ETX: ethanol withdrawal (rats); GEPR-9s: genetically epilepsy-prone rats, severe strain; GEPR-3s: genetically epilepsy-prone rats, moderate-severity strain; THX = thyroid deficient model of AGS (rats).

BLOCKADE STUDIES OF THE IC IN INDUCED AGS MODELS

IC in THX Rats

There is also evidence suggesting a role for glutamate in the IC in AGS susceptibility in neonatal THX rats.[79,89] THX-induced AGS susceptibility was induced in neonatal Sprague–Dawley rats in our lab by administering PTU, as described in this chapter.[88–90] AGS susceptibility was induced (>90% incidence), and the seizure behaviors consisted of wild running followed by generalized clonus.[173] In the THX model of AGS, focal microinjection of a competitive NMDA antagonist reversibly attenuated AGS, with complete block at the highest dose (Table 26.1). Similar effects have been observed in the THX model in other labs.[174] Bilateral microinjection of the $GABA_B$ agonist baclofen (28 nmol/side) or the $GABA_A$ agonist THIP (68 nmol/side) into the IC of THX rats also significantly reduced the incidence of AGS.[173] The doses of these agents are 5–250 times the doses required to suppress AGS in GEPR-9s,[159,175] indicating major sensitivity differences between the different AGS forms.

BLOCKADE OF THE IC IN THE ISCHEMIA MODEL

As noted here, compression of the chest of an anesthetized animal until a complete loss of blood pressure was induced resulted in chronic susceptibility to generalized clonic AGS upon recovery.[93] There is some histological evidence of cellular damage in the IC and several other brain regions in this model.[96,98] In our lab, focal bilateral microinjection of a competitive

NMDA receptor antagonist into the IC of ischemic rats also completely blocked AGS susceptibility 30 min after the microinjection but with a dose 10 times that required in GEPR-9s (Table 26.1), and AGS susceptibility returned after 3 h. Thus, focal blockade of the IC in the GEPR-9, GEPR-3, ETX, THX, and ischemia-induced forms of AGS blocked AGS susceptibility reversibly. These data support the importance of this AGS network structure in initiation of all of these various forms of AGS but with varying degrees of sensitivity. The comparison of doses between the various models indicates that AGS in GEPR-9s are blocked by the lowest dose, while the dose required in THX rats was 250 times that dose (Table 26.1). The sensitivity of three other sites [the deep layers of the superior colliculus (DLSC), PRF, and periaqueductal gray (PAG)] to bilateral 2-amino-7-phosphonoheptanoate (AP7) microinjection was evaluated in GEPR-9s, GEPR-3s, and ETX rats. Differential sensitivities were seen, with similarities in the amounts needed to block AGS in both strains of GEPR and considerably higher doses of NMDA antagonist required in ETX rats in several network nuclei (Table 26.1), which may be related to the antagonistic effects of ethanol on NMDA receptors.[176]

Neuronal Recording Studies

Extracellular action potentials (APs) provide a clear understanding of the neuronal mechanisms of seizure that cause the behavior changes in epilepsy models as well as human epileptics.[177,178] It is, however, vital that these studies be carried out in the absence of drugs that are sedative or anesthetic, since these agents exert profound effects on the functions of networks (see Chapter 32).[179] Neuronal recording studies have been carried out in the IC in three AGS models—GEPR-9s, GEPR-3s, and ETX rats—using chronically implanted microwire electrodes in freely moving animals (see Chapter 4 for methods).

IC Neuronal Firing and AGS

The threshold acoustic intensity required to consistently evoke neuronal firing was significantly elevated in awake, behaving GEPR-9s, as compared to normal Sprague–Dawley rats (Figure 26.6). Neurons in the ICc and ICx in GEPR-9s exhibit tremendous auditory-evoked increases in firing just prior to and during the onset of AGS [Figure 26.2(A) and (B)], and the acoustically evoked firing below the seizure threshold was significantly increased as compared to normal rats at the same intensity (Figure 26.5). Since the IC is the consensus site for AGS initiation, as noted in this chapter, these elevated firing patterns are the critical AGS-initiating event that triggers the participation of the rostral nuclei of the seizure network to propagate the seizure. Since the acoustic stimulus that triggers AGS can be delivered at sub–AGS threshold intensities, changes in auditory responsiveness as well as differences in the subthreshold auditory responses can be evaluated. This allows the determination of whether elevated neuronal responsiveness to the stimulus is occurring prior to seizure induction in the IC and the other AGS network nuclei (see Figures 26.5 and 26.6).

As noted here, the key pathophysiological mechanism responsible for the critical role of the IC in AGS initiation is the defect in GABA-mediated inhibition in GEPR-9s. This defect makes a very important contribution to the excitability of this structure, because this form of acoustically evoked inhibition in IC (central) neurons is normally pervasive. Thus, most IC neurons in normal rats exhibit several forms of GABA-mediated inhibition (evoked in response to acoustic stimulation) that play a role in sensory coding. Iontophoretic application of GABA onto IC neurons produces significant inhibition of neuronal firing [Figure 26.3(D)],[30] as shown by the example in Figure 26.3(D) in a normal ICc neuron. The "dosage" of GABA required to produce 20% inhibition was significantly lower in normal rats than in GEPR-9s, as shown by the bar graphs in Figure 26.3(D). A similar significant decrease in directly applied GABA effectiveness is also seen in ETX rats.[30,157] This reduced efficacy of exogenously applied GABA is also seen in several other brain loci in GEPR-9s and ETX rats.[157,180–183]

The incidence and effectiveness of several forms of GABA-mediated, acoustically evoked inhibition are significantly reduced in AGS-susceptible GEPR-9s in vivo and in vitro.[30,139,151,155,171,184] These acoustically evoked inhibitory responses of IC neurons include binaural inhibition that occurs when the sound is presented to both ears (Figure 26.3), which is mediated largely by GABAergic input from the contralateral dorsal nucleus of the lateral lemniscus[170,171,184–189] (see Chapter 7, Figure 7.2). As shown in the examples in Figure 26.3(A), the inhibitory response to binaural stimulation in many IC neurons is considerably lower in GEPR-9s as compared to normal rats, and this form of inhibition can be blocked by direct application of a $GABA_A$ antagonist onto IC neurons.[151] High-intensity-induced inhibition (nonmonotonic rate intensity response) [Figure 26.3(B)] is another form of GABA-mediated inhibition induced in many normal IC neurons when the intensity of the acoustic stimulus is increased. This inhibition can also be blocked by application of a $GABA_A$ antagonist directly onto these neurons [Figure 26.3(B)]. Failure of this form of inhibition occurred significantly more often in GEPR-9s than normal rats [Figure 26.3(A) and (B)]. Another

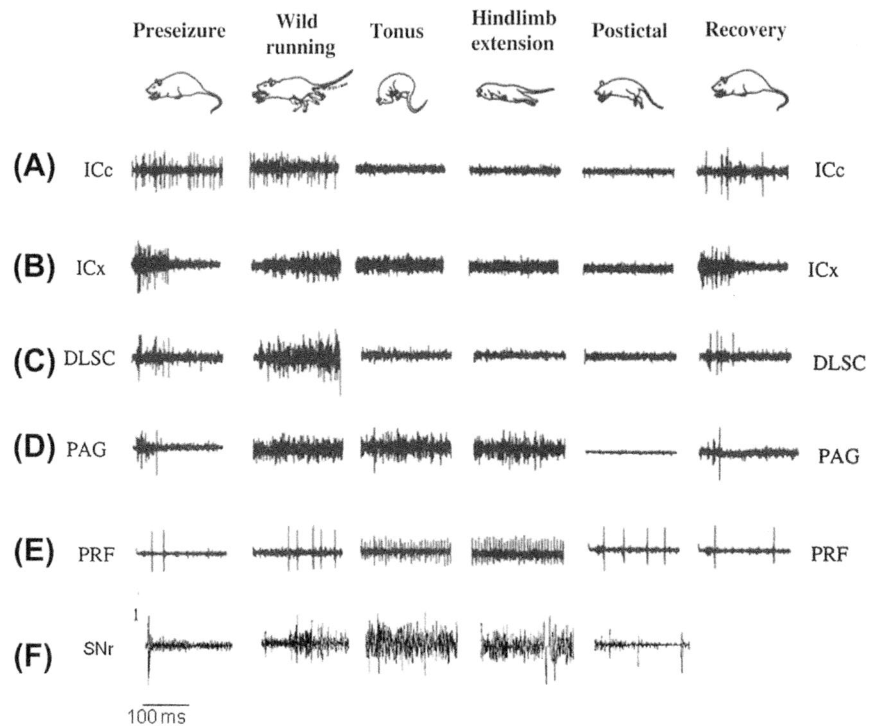

FIGURE 26.2 Composite behavioral activity in GEPR-9s and concurrent typical examples of neuronal firing in the major network nuclei for AGS seen during each seizure behavior. The structures include the (A) inferior colliculus central (ICc) nucleus; (B) inferior colliculus external (ICx) nucleus; (C) deep layers of the superior colliculus (DLSC); (D) periaqueductal gray (PAG); (E) pontine brainstem reticular formation (PRF); and (F) substantia nigra reticulata (SNr). Thus, ICc and ICx firing is greatest during AGS initiation, while the greatest increase in DLSC neuronal firing occurs at the onset of wild running. The greatest increases in PAG, SNr, and PRF neuronal firing occur during the tonus and tonic hindlimb extension phases of AGS. The PRF and SNr are the only areas active during postictal depression of consciousness. Note: Recovery of SNr firing occurred but was not recorded in the example in (F). Acoustic stimulus parameters: 12 kHz tone burst, 100 ms duration, 5 ms rise-fall, 100 dB SPL, 2–4 Hz repetition rate. Each row is from the same rat. *(Source: Drawings courtesy of Naritoku et al.[150] From Faingold[8] by permission.)*

GABA-mediated form of inhibition—offset inhibition—occurs at the end of an acoustic stimulus and prevents the appearance of an offset response, but when a $GABA_A$ antagonist is applied directly onto many normal IC neurons, this can allow an offset peak to appear [Figure 26.3(C)]. Offset inhibition is mediated largely by the superior periolivary nucleus, which is a nucleus in the primary auditory network that contains a high percentage of GABAergic neurons.[190,191] The offset peak was observed significantly more commonly in GEPR-9s than normal rats [Figure 26.3(C)] and may be a form of after-discharge. Other forms of inhibition, including "pauser" responses and tonic inhibition, are also observed in IC neurons.[192–194] Thus, IC neurons exhibit significant decreases in both endogenous acoustically evoked, GABA-mediated inhibition, and the effectiveness of exogenously applied GABA is reduced in both genetic and induced forms of AGS.[139,152,155,157,195] Other agents that enhance or block the action of GABA will increase or reduce, respectively, inhibition in IC neurons that is acoustically evoked or tonic in nature.[30,170,171,184,196–201]

These inhibition deficits in IC neurons from GEPR-9s and ETX rats have been confirmed and extended in intracellular recordings in brain slices.[152,153,156,202] IC neuronal input resistance was abnormally high, and the threshold for repetitive firing was abnormally low, in neurons from GEPR-9s and ETX rats. Electrical stimulation of the commissure of the IC caused paired-pulse inhibition in normal IC neurons, which is known to be GABA mediated in the IC and in a number of other brain sites.[153,203,204] However, the incidence of this form of inhibition was significantly reduced in IC neurons from ETX rats and GEPR-9s. Inhibitory postsynaptic potentials (IPSPs) in IC neurons evoked by stimulation of the commissure of the IC also displayed a significantly greater sensitivity to a $GABA_A$ antagonist, bicuculline, in ETX rats and GEPR-9s.[30,156,205] Paired-pulse facilitation was frequently observed in IC neurons from GEPR-9s and ETX rats, but it was not seen in IC neurons from normal rats (Figure 26.4).[153,205]

Stimulation of the IC commissure also resulted in a high incidence of large epileptiform depolarizing events in the IC neurons of GEPR-9s and in ETX, but

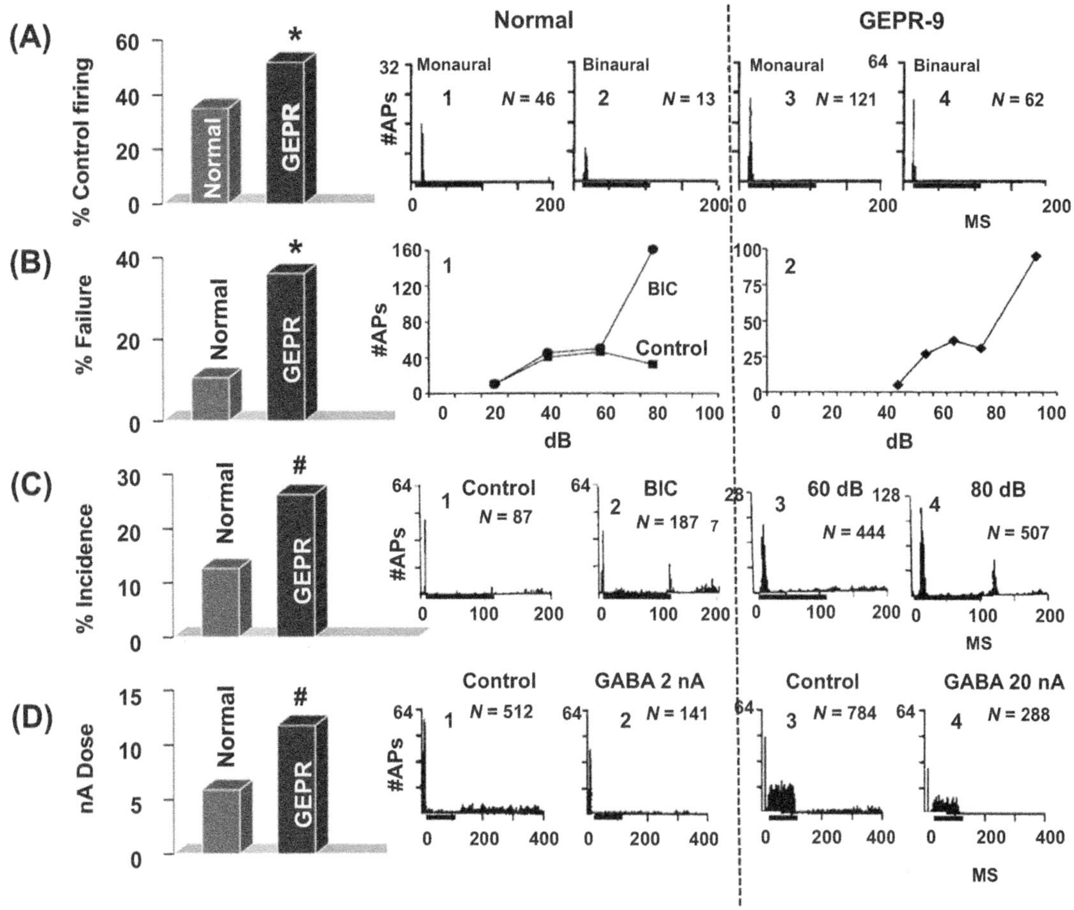

FIGURE 26.3 GABA-mediated inhibition defects in GEPR-9s: GABAergic neurotransmission normally plays a critical role in determining the responses of the inferior colliculus (IC) to acoustic stimulation, and defects in specific forms of inhibition are key causative factors in audiogenic seizure initiation. Line (A) illustrates binaural inhibition common in ICc neurons. In the poststimulus time histogram (PSTH) example in line (A) ("Normal" column), binaural presentation of the stimulus results in a greatly reduced number of action potentials (*N*), as compared to the response to the same stimulus to one ear (monaurally to the contralateral ear). In GEPR-9 ICc neurons, the effect of binaural inhibition is significantly reduced, as shown in this example by the comparison of the line (A) ("GEPR-9" column) example when the sound is presented to both ears (binaural). This difference in effectiveness of GABA-mediated inhibition was significant, as shown by the bar graphs in line (A), illustrating the mean normal versus GEPR IC data. This form of inhibition can be blocked by direct application of a $GABA_A$ antagonist onto ICc neurons.[151] Line (B) illustrates examples of high-intensity-induced inhibition (a nonmonotonic rate intensity response), which is a form of inhibition seen in many normal ICc neurons when the intensity of the acoustic stimulus is increased, as shown by the rate–intensity curve in line (B) ("Normal" column), and this inhibition can be blocked by application of a $GABA_A$ antagonist, bicuculline (BIC), directly onto these neurons, as also shown by the example in 3B ("Normal" column). An example of the failure of this form of inhibition in the GEPR is shown in line (B) ("GEPR-9" column), and the significant mean difference in the normal versus GEPR comparison is shown by the bar graph in line (B). A form of inhibition that occurs at the end of a finite acoustic stimulus is called the offset response and is seen in a small percentage of normal ICc neurons, but it is often hard to detect [line (C), "Control" column]. However, when BIC is applied directly onto many ICc neurons, this can cause an offset peak to appear by blocking offset inhibition [line (C), "Normal" column, right panel]. In GEPR-9s, the incidence of failure of offset inhibition allowing the appearance of the offset response are often induced by increasing the sound intensity [line (C), "GEPR-9" column, right panel]. The incidence of neurons showing the offset peak was significantly greater in GEPR-9s as compared to normal rats, as shown by the bar graphs in line (C). Direct iontophoretic application of GABA onto ICc neurons produces significant inhibition in acoustically evoked firing [line (D), "Normal" panel, right versus left panel at 2 nA of GABA]. In GEPR-9s, the effectiveness of iontophoretically applied GABA was significantly reduced [line (D), "GEPR-9" column, right versus left panel, 20 nA of GABA], despite the fact that this was applied using the same electrode in both rats. The mean difference in GABA effectiveness was significant, as shown by the bar graphs in line (D). PSTH parameters = 25 or 50 stimulus presentations at 2/s of 100 ms 12 kHz tone bursts (100 ms duration denoted by the heavy line beneath each PSTH; 5 ms rise-fall). N = number of action potentials per PSTH. * Significantly different at $p < 0.05$; # significantly different at $p < 0.02$. (For color version of this figure, the reader is referred to the online version of this book.)

these were not seen in slices from normal rats.[156] A reduced degree of spike-firing adaptation and an increased incidence of anode-break firing were also seen in IC neurons in brain slices during ETX, similar to the offset response seen in vivo. These abnormal IC membrane and synaptic properties in AGS-susceptible rats likely make a major contribution to the IC hyperexcitability that subserves AGS initiation.

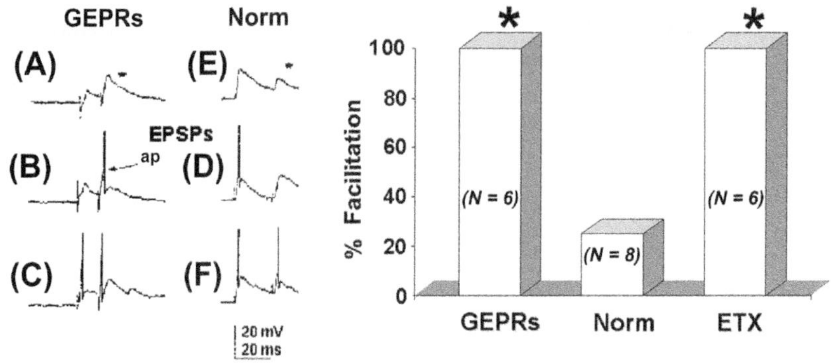

FIGURE 26.4 In animals susceptible to AGS (in GEPRs and during ETX), paired-pulse inhibition in inferior colliculus dorsal nucleus (ICd) neurons (in vitro) is replaced by facilitation as compared to responses in normal ICd neurons. Paired-pulse inhibition was seen in normal (Norm) ICd neurons [(D) low intensity; (E) moderate intensity; (F) high intensity] in response to increasing stimulus intensity in the IC commissure. In GEPRs, paired-pulse facilitation was observed [(A) low intensity; (B) moderate intensity; (C) high intensity]. A similar effect was seen in ICd neurons during ETX, as shown by the significant differences in the mean incidence of facilitation shown in the bar graphs in the right panel. *(Source: Based on Refs 152,153.)* * $p < 0.05$: Significantly different from normal controls (Student's *t*-test). *(Source: Reprinted from Faingold,[30] with permission.)*

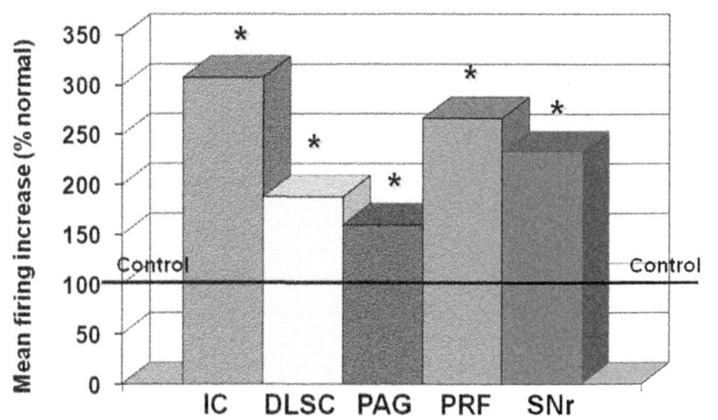

FIGURE 26.5 Compilation of mean acoustically evoked neuronal firing in GEPR-9s as a percentage, with normal Sprague–Dawley rats as control (100%). The acoustic stimuli (12 kHz 100 ms tone burst) was at 90 dB (SPL Re 0.0002 dyn/cm^2). Five AGS network sites are compared: the inferior colliculus (IC), deep layers of the superior colliculus (DLSC), periaqueductal gray (PAG), pontine reticular formation (PRF), and substantia nigra reticulata (SNr). The mean neuronal firing percentages were increased in all the network structures with the greatest increase in the consensus AGS initiation site in the IC. Significantly different from control at * $p < 0.05$ (Student's *t*-test). (For color version of this figure, the reader is referred to the online version of this book.)

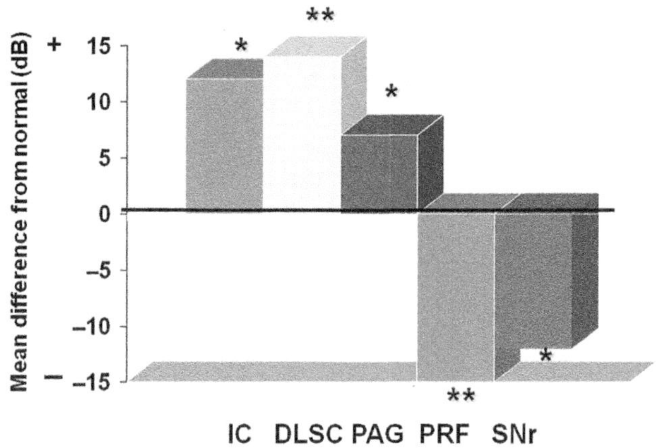

FIGURE 26.6 Compilation of mean acoustic response threshold differences between GEPR-9s and normal Sprague–Dawley rats. Five AGS network sites are compared: the inferior colliculus (IC), deep layers of the superior colliculus (DLSC), periaqueductal gray (PAG), pontine reticular formation (PRF), and substantia nigra reticulata (SNr). In the IC, DLSC, and PAG, the response thresholds are significantly above those of normal rats, consistent with the known hearing deficit in these rats. However, in the PRF and SNr, the neuronal response threshold is significantly below that of the neurons in the same structures in normal rats. Significantly different from control at * $p < 0.05$ and ** $p < 0.01$ (Student's *t*-test). (For color version of this figure, the reader is referred to the online version of this book.)

The projection pathways of these abnormal firing patterns from the IC have been evaluated in several AGS models. The ICx is proposed as the crucial site for the outflow from the ICc to the DLSC and PRF, which are also requisite network hubs for the AGS network in GEPR-9s; the IC also projects to the next, more rostral site in the auditory network, the medial geniculate body (see Chapter 20), but this structure is not a requisite hub in this network, at least in GEPR-9s.[143,206–208]

THE DLSC IN AGS NETWORKS

The DLSC are implicated in the AGS networks of several forms of AGS.[143,160,209] The DLSC has important motor connections that play a critical role in triggering the wild-running phase, which is the initial behavior of AGS.[143,162,210] Thus, c-Fos-related immunoreactivity has implicated the DLSC in the AGS network in GEPR-9s and Strasbourg Wistar rats and in priming-induced AGS.[143,144,147,211] In Strasbourg Wistar rats, local cerebral blood flow increases were induced in DLSC.[212]

In addition, surgical ablation of or inhibitory microinjection into DLSC in WARs abolished AGS.[129,213] Focal microinjection of the NMDA receptor antagonist AP7 was able to completely block AGS in GEPR-9s, GEPR-3s, and ETX rats.[141,162,214] The doses of the NMDA antagonist AP7 that were required to completely block AGS in DLSC were comparable in GEPR-3s and GEPR-9s (Table 26.1), but considerably higher doses were required in ETX. These data support a critical role of the DLSC in the AGS networks in these models, and the higher dose requirement in ETX rats may involve NMDA receptor upregulation caused by sustained blockade of these receptors by ethanol.[176]

DLSC Neurons and AGS

DLSC neuronal firing in awake, behaving GEPR-9s showed an abrupt onset of acoustically evoked firing at approximately 80–90 dB, which was significantly above the threshold in normal rats (Figure 26.6), but the neurons were more responsive to the high-intensity acoustic stimuli than in normal rats (Figure 26.5). DLSC neurons exhibited rapid tonic and burst firing just prior (1–2 s) to the onset of the wild-running behavior that begins AGS. As the tonic behavioral phase of the seizure began, DLSC firing completely ceased, and firing returned towards normal as postictal depression ended [Figure 26.2(C)]. By contrast, in ETX-induced AGS, acoustically evoked DLSC firing was significantly suppressed during ETX. However, DLSC neurons began to fire tonically 1–2 s before the onset of the wild-running behavior of ETX-induced AGS. Acoustically evoked DLSC firing was suppressed during postictal depression, with recovery beginning as the righting reflex returned. These data support a requisite role of the DLSC in AGS during ETX seizures as well, but not prior to AGS. The neuronal firing changes in GEPR-9s and ETX rats suggest an important role of DLSC neurons in generation of the wild-running phase of AGS, which may be a general pathophysiological mechanism and a critical event in the initiation of the wild-running phase of AGS.[162,210] A dichotomy is observed between the effects of ETX on c-Fos and neuronal firing during AGS in the DLSC,[215] where little change in c-Fos occurs and the spontaneous and auditory-evoked activity of DLSC neurons is reduced.[162] However, during AGS, the firing of DLSC neurons is quite intense, suggesting that the extensive projections from the highly active sites of neuronal firing, such as the IC, appear to drive the DLSC neurons as the ETX seizure proceeds in this AGS model.[166] As the AGS behaviors progress and the tonic phase of the seizure begins, DLSC firing ceases, and it returns to normal only following postictal depression. These neuronal mechanisms may be relevant to other seizure models in which the DLSC is implicated. The temporal pattern of neuronal firing during AGS is specific to DLSC and differs markedly from those observed elsewhere in the AGS neuronal network. The DLSC project to the spinal cord directly and via the PRF and ventrolateral PAG.[141,162,216]

ROLE OF THE PAG IN AGS NETWORKS

Imaging studies using Fos-like immunoreactivity have implicated the PAG in the AGS network in Wistar AGS rats, GEPR-3s, GEPR-9s, and ETX rats.[142–144,211,215] Microinjection studies also support the role of the PAG in GEPR-3s, GEPR-9s, and ETX rats.[141,217,218] The dose of NMDA antagonist required to completely block seizures in the PAG was similar in GEPR-3s and GEPR-9s (Table 26.1). However, the duration of action was shorter in the GEPR-3s (full recovery in 24 h, as compared to 48 h in the GEPR-9s). The PAG is also implicated in initiation of the clonic phase of AGS.[147,216,218,219] The PAG receives input from the DLSC and projects directly and indirectly to the spinal cord.[220–222]

PAG Neurons and AGS

PAG neurons in awake, behaving GEPR-9s also exhibited a distinctly different pattern of firing from other network sites leading up to and during AGS [Figure 26.2(D)].[216,219] The mean threshold of acoustically evoked neuronal firing of short-latency neurons in the PAG was significantly higher than normal in GEPR-9s (Figure 26.6). Acoustically evoked neuronal firing in the PAG was significantly elevated in GEPR-9s, particularly at the highest stimulus intensities (Figure 26.5). PAG neurons, which had diminished firing rates due to habituation, exhibited a tonic firing pattern during wild-running and tonic seizures in GEPR-9s (Figure 26.3). Immediately (1–5 s) prior to the onset of tonic convulsive behaviors, an increase in the rate of PAG tonic firing was observed, which suggests that PAG neurons may contribute to the generation of the tonic seizure behavioral component of AGS.[216] During ETX, when the animals were susceptible to AGS, significant increases in spontaneous and acoustically evoked PAG neuronal firing occurred. PAG neurons exhibited burst firing 2–4 s prior to the tonic-clonic phase of AGS and tonic repetitive firing during this seizure phase, which ceased during postictal depression.[218]

Brain slice studies indicate that the properties of ventrolateral PAG neurons exhibit abnormal membrane and synaptic properties in animals that are susceptible to AGS.[219,223] The depolarizing current needed to generate an AP was significantly less in ETX rats than in control rats. PAG neurons in ETX rat slices had significantly enhanced spike-firing tendencies and significantly increased firing compared to PAG neurons of normal rats. Stimulation in the dorsolateral PAG evoked a fast excitatory postsynaptic potential (EPSP), and the stimulus intensities required to evoke EPSPs were significantly lower than control in neurons during ETX. Epileptiform firing in PAG neurons was observed commonly in ETX rats but was never seen in control rats. In control rats, paired-pulse responses evoked paired-pulse inhibition in PAG neurons to a significantly greater extent than in ETX rats, but paired-pulse facilitation was significantly more common in ETX rats. PAG hyperexcitability during ETX results from alterations of both NMDA and AMPA receptor-mediated neurotransmission, which may contribute importantly to ETX seizures. The hyperexcitability observed in PAG neurons in vivo may make a major contribution to propagating seizures occurring during ETX in intact animals.[219] These results differ from previous in vitro findings in the seizure-initiating site for ETX seizures in the IC, where NMDA receptor-mediated mechanisms dominate excitability increases during ETX, which may be related to the different roles played by the IC and PAG in the ETX seizure network.[224]

THE PRF IN AGS NETWORKS

Fos-like immunoreactivity studies have implicated areas in the brainstem reticular formation, including the PRF, in the AGS network in Wistar AGS rats and GEPR-9s as well as in ETX.[144,211,225] In Strasbourg Wistar rats, local cerebral blood flow increases were induced in the AGS network, with extensive increases in the reticular formation.[212]

The amount of NMDA antagonist required to block AGS and the duration of effect on the AGS in the PRF were similar in GEPR-3s and GEPR-9s (Table 26.1), while higher amounts were required in the ETX rats. The PRF is implicated in triggering the final phase of AGS in GEPR-9s and GEPR-3s.[113,141,226] The DLSC project to the PRF and the substantia nigra reticulata (SNr). The postictal depression period appears to be dominated by the PRF, since it and the SNr are the only network nuclei that are active during this behavior, at least in GEPR-9s and ETX rats.[8,42,226] This activity in the PRF may be related to maintenance of respiration and cardiovascular function, in which other nuclei of the brainstem reticular formation have long been implicated (see Chapter 18). The PRF is implicated in AGS and several other forms of generalized seizures.[161,227] The PRF exerts a powerful excitatory influence on spinal cord neurons via the reticulospinal pathway.[228,229]

Reticular Formation Neuronal Firing and AGS

In awake, behaving GEPR-9s, PRF neurons exhibit precipitous intensity-evoked increases at a significantly lower ($\sim$15 dB SPL) intensity than that seen in normal Sprague–Dawley rats (Figure 26.6). These findings indicate that the PRF in GEPR-9s is more responsive to acoustic stimuli than in normal rats, which is diametrically opposite of that seen in the other brain structures discussed in this chapter. PRF neurons in the GEPR-9 also exhibit increased firing rates to acoustic stimuli below the seizure threshold (Figure 26.5) and auditory response latencies as compared to normal rats. At the onset of AGS (wild running), the firing rate of PRF neurons increased somewhat, but the rate of PRF firing increased dramatically as the tonic phases of the seizure began [Figure 26.2(E)]. During postictal depression, the rate of PRF neuronal firing slowed but did not stop, and then it gradually returned to normal. This pattern of PRF peri-seizural neuronal-firing changes differs dramatically in pattern and temporal characteristics from those in other AGS network sites (as discussed earlier in this chapter). These changes in PRF neuronal-firing pattern suggest that the PRF may play a major role in the generation of the tonic phase of AGS. This is further supported by the finding that anticonvulsant drug doses that blocked only the tonic component of AGS in GEPR-9s blocked the firing change in the PRF but not in the PAG.[230] The premature onset of the precipitous rise in PRF neuronal firing suggests that the influence of the IC on PRF neurons may be magnified in association with AGS susceptibility.[226] The PRF is also a requisite AGS neuronal network site in GEPR-3s. AGS in GEPR-3s culminate in generalized clonus, and PRF neuronal responses to acoustic stimuli (12 kHz) in this AGS model exhibited onset responses. Tonic and burst firing of PRF neurons occurred during generalized clonus in GEPR-3s. During postictal depression, PRF neurons in GEPR-3s did not fire for a variable period until the rats exhibited the righting reflex.[46] This firing pattern during postictal depression was in marked contrast with the continued firing seen during the same period in GEPR-9s, as discussed in this chapter. Since the responses of PRF neurons to sensory stimuli are normally very labile (conditional multireceptive), sensory transmission via this pathway has the potential to increase dramatically, as seen in AGS (Chapter 28). PRF neurons are also a key element in the neuronal network for the acoustic startle response (Chapter 28).[231–233]

ROLE OF THE SUBSTANTIA NIGRA RETICULATA IN AGS NETWORKS

The involvement of the SNr in AGS networks has been controversial, and both positive and negative data have been reported, depending on the seizure model, age, and sex of the animal as well as the location within the SNr that was investigated (see Chapter 11). In Strasbourg Wistar rats, local cerebral blood flow increases were induced in the AGS network, with extensive increases in the substantia nigra.[212] The SNr is also implicated in control of seizures, including AGS in GEPR-9s. Increased 2-DG uptake was seen in the SNr of GEPR-9s and GEPR-3s, although these changes were not accompanied by increased c-Fos expression in this brain region.[142]

In the Strasbourg Wistar rat AGS model, bilateral injection of the $GABA_A$ agonist muscimol into the substantia nigra had no effect. In AGS kindling in these rats, the effect of blockade of the SNr was to suppress only the clonic seizure behavior in these rats.[234] However, focal blockade by microinjection of an NMDA receptor antagonist into the SNr blocks AGS in GEPR-9s.[161] Microinjections of a GABA agonist into the SNr in the Wistar AGS rats have yielded mixed results, with suppression of clonic but not tonic seizures.[234] Lesions of the SNr actually resulted in increased sensitivity to AGS in previously resistant rats,[235] but bilateral lesions of the SNr attenuate AGS in GEPR-9s.[236] These inconsistencies of effect may be related to the further subdivision of SNr into anterior and posterior regions that exert differential effects in other seizure models[237] (see Chapter 11).

SNr Neuronal Firing and AGS

Acoustically evoked SNr neuronal firing in awake, normal rats was not detectable except at very high intensities, but the threshold for acoustically evoked neuronal firing in awake, behaving GEPR-9s was significantly lower than in normal rats (Figure 26.6), which was also seen in the PRF, as noted here. SNr neuronal responsiveness to acoustic stimuli in GEPR-9s was also significantly greater as compared to normal rats (Figure 26.5). SNr neuronal firing during AGS in GEPR-9s showed enhanced rapid firing [Figure 26.2(F)]. The SNr neurons showed occasional APs during postictal depression.[8]

In awake, behaving GEPR-9s, mean neuronal responses to auditory stimuli were significantly increased in neurons in all of the AGS network structures evaluated (Figure 26.5). There were differing degrees of firing increase, with the IC showing the greatest increase (>300% of normal), while the PAG showed the smallest increase (<200%). The stimuli were at 90 dB, which is the most intense stimulus presented that was consistently below the threshold for inducing AGS. However, the auditory threshold for consistently evoking neuronal firing in these AGS network sites showed a different pattern. GEPR-9s are known to suffer from hearing loss.[75] This is reflected in the elevated threshold seen for IC neurons in these animals as compared to normal rats (Figure 26.6). Elevated thresholds are also seen in the DLSC and PAG. However, aberrant threshold differences were seen in PRF and SNr neurons, which actually showed auditory response thresholds in those nuclei that are lower than those in normal rats (Figure 26.6). This may be related to the relatively high threshold for acoustic responses seen in these structures in normal rats. The cause for the threshold decreases in these nuclei may be due to the greater acoustically evoked neuronal firing in GEPR-9s and ETX rats, particularly in the IC. This results in greater output from these structures to the PRF and SNr once the thresholds in the IC and other projecting nuclei are reached. These findings infer that once a critical network site (hub) such as the IC is activated, its projections to the next nuclei in the network may result in greater activation due to the elevated input, causing certain (but not all) projection sites to respond at lower stimulus (acoustic) intensities and to a greater degree.

FOREBRAIN STRUCTURES IN AGS

Role of the Amygdala in AGS Networks

The role of forebrain structures above the level of the IC in the AGS network appears to vary considerably among different forms of AGS.[42,141,154,158,238] There is evidence suggesting that limbic structures, including the amygdala and hippocampus, are implicated in the AGS network during ETX[239–241] and in the moderate-severity AGS of GEPR-3s. However, these limbic structures are not critically involved in two other well-studied genetic forms of AGS.[144,242,243] The differences among the AGS networks for the GEPR-9s, GEPR-3s, and ETX rats are illustrated in Figure 26.1. The amygdala in GEPR-3s displayed intense seizure-related c-Fos labeling, but there were no detectable increases in 2-DG uptake during AGS.[142] During ETX, c-Fos was induced most prominently in forebrain areas, including the amygdala.[215]

Microinjection of a competitive NMDA receptor antagonist into the lateral amygdala (LA) of GEPR-9s had no effect on AGS susceptibility until the dose reached 20 times that which was effective in the IC.[242] These data suggest that the amygdala does not play a requisite role in the neuronal network for AGS in GEPR-9s unless the microinjection dose reaches excessive levels, which are likely to affect other parts of the brain via volume transmission mechanisms (see Chapter 8).

In GEPR-3s, by contrast, microinjection of a competitive NMDA receptor antagonist into the LA in doses only three times that which was effective in the IC and comparable to other network sites was able to block

AGS reversibly. These data support a critical role for the LA in clonic AGS modulation in GEPR-3s, suggesting important network differences between clonic and tonic forms of inherited AGS. In ETX-induced AGS induced with the binge protocol,[112] bilateral focal microinjection of AP7 into the LA significantly reduced AGS, suggesting that the LA participates in the network that mediates ETX-induced AGS susceptibility.[140] As noted in this section, the amygdala is not a requisite structure in the AGS network for GEPR-9s, but abnormal firing patterns in LA neurons were observed in this structure during AGS in GEPR-9s. Thus, sporadic tonic and phasic firing of LA neurons occurred during the tonus and tonic hind limb extension phases of AGS, indicating that neurons in this structure are active during AGS. However, this activity is not required to produce AGS in GEPR-9s,[244] indicating that the LA is an ancillary structure in the AGS network in this AGS model (see Chapter 33).

As noted here, the LA is involved in the requisite AGS network in GEPR-3s, and LA neurons in awake, behaving GEPR-9s exhibited only onset-type neuronal responses to the acoustic stimuli, unlike LA neurons in normal rats. During AGS in GEPR-3s, burst firing occurred in the LA during wild running and generalized clonic behaviors. These findings indicate the nature of the critical role that LA neurons play in the neuronal network for generalized clonus in GEPR-3s, which contrasts markedly with the lack of important role that LA neurons play in tonic AGS in GEPR-9s.[47]

In ETX-induced AGS susceptibility induced using the binge protocol,[112] LA neurons consistently exhibited rapid tonic firing during the generalized tonic convulsions of AGS. These findings support a critical role of the amygdala in the ETX seizure network in generating tonic convulsions during AGS in this model.[140]

Role of the Hippocampus in AGS

The hippocampus is a major limbic site associated with seizure susceptibility, and ethanol is known to exert important effects on hippocampal neurons.[118] In ETX, prominent c-Fos-related immunoreactivity was observed in the hippocampus,[215] but this structure is not implicated in the neuronal network for AGS in GEPR-3s or GEPR-9s. The role of the dentate gyrus (DG) of the hippocampus in ETX seizures was examined using focal microinjection into the DG of an NMDA receptor antagonist. Using the binge protocol described here,[112] ETX induced AGS susceptibility in >95% of rats. An NMDA antagonist bilaterally microinjected into the DG produced a significant blockade ($p < 0.001$) of ETX seizures lasting from 0.5 to 5 h, depending on the dose. During ETX, DG neuronal firing remained depressed, unlike certain other sites in the ETX seizure network (discussed here). However, during ETX seizures, DG neurons exhibited repetitive firing patterns. These data indicate that DG neuronal firing was elevated during seizure, suggesting that the DG may not play a role in seizure initiation but may play an important role in the propagation of ETX-induced AGS.[245]

A number of drugs with anticonvulsant properties have been administered systemically to more than one of the AGS models. Although these drugs were able to block seizures, the doses were often quite different between the models. Thus, the uncompetitive NMDA receptor antagonist MK-801 blocked AGS in GEPR-9s at a dose of 0.05 mg/kg, while the dose required in THX and ETX rats was 10 times that (0.5 mg/kg).[106,246] The larger doses of this NMDA antagonist in the THX and ETX models are consistent with the higher doses of NMDA antagonist required by microinjection in these models (Table 26.1). On the other hand, tiagabine, an anticonvulsant that inhibits GABA uptake, blocked AGS in similar doses in GEPR-9s and the ischemia model (30 mg/kg, intraperitoneal).[107]

HIERARCHICAL ORGANIZATION OF THE AGS NETWORK

The mechanisms that produce the firing changes in these network nuclei have not been examined in these models in all of these sites as yet. Excitatory amino acid receptors, which mediate normal excitatory neurotransmission in the IC, also contribute to AGS susceptibility in ETX and both GEPR substrains.[42,167,170,172,247] Both $GABA_A$ deficits and excessive excitatory amino acid neurotransmitter-based mechanisms result in abnormally intense neuronal output from the IC at high stimulus intensities, which is critical to the initiation of AGS.[208,209,242,248] Since chemical or electrical stimulation in the IC can produce AGS susceptibility or seizures that closely resemble AGS, respectively, in normal rats,[160,163,249,250] the transmitter-based IC excitability increases are strongly implicated as the critical AGS-initiating mechanisms. However, the IC must ultimately project to nuclei that produce motor behaviors by projections to the spinal cord that are required to produce the convulsive motor behaviors seen in AGS. Brainstem projections to the spinal cord are known to be present in the DLSC, the PAG and particularly the PRF. Networks that project from the brainstem reticular formation (to which the PRF belongs) to the spinal cord are a critical network component for normal locomotion (Chapter 17).[251–254] Brainstem neurons are subject to extensive interconnectivity within the reticular formation and have a multiplicity of projections to and from essentially all primary sensory and motor systems, allowing this structure to become a critical network component of potential seizure networks, including those in AGS (see Chapter 28).

Different Nuclei are Dominant during Each AGS Phase

The dominance of each component in an operating neuronal network is known to change temporally during the phases of a multistage behavioral convulsive pattern. Thus, dominance shifts within the brain are seen as major driving forces in elaboration of the sleep states in the sleep—wakefulness cycle (Chapters 21 and 22).[255] The neuronal recording evidence indicates that the dominance of each component of the neuronal network also changes temporally during the behavioral phases of convulsion during AGS. The seizure behaviors in GEPR-9s are stereotyped and occur in a highly predictable sequence.[128] This predictability allows comparisons of neuronal firing in different recording sites in different animals, based on the temporal relationship between each behavior change and the change in neuronal patterns of firing in each network nucleus. Temporal shifts in hierarchical dominance are seen in both genetic and ETX-induced AGS.[8,108,256] The ability to examine neuronal firing in behaving animals using chronically implanted microwire electrodes (Figure 26.2) allowed for these dominance shifts to be observed as the different seizure behaviors proceeded.[195,218,226] A composite of behavioral activity in GEPR-9s and concurrent neuronal firing in the major network nuclei for AGS seen during each seizure behavior is shown in Figure 26.2. Tonic- and especially burst-firing patterns are highly indicative of maximal activation of neurons in a network site (see Chapter 9). These patterns occur in neurons in different sites within the network as the temporal evolution of each behavioral phase of AGS proceeds. Therefore, we propose the following network hierarchical activation process during which the dominant site shifts temporally. During the AGS initiation phase, IC neurons are dominant, since these neurons become most active just prior to and during the onset of the seizure. During the wild-running phase, DLSC neurons are dominant, since these neurons fire most intensely at the onset of and during this behavior. During the tonus and the hind limb extension phases, the PRF, PAG, and SNr are dominant due to the major neuronal firing increases in these sites, while neurons in the other sites are quiescent. The PRF and SNr are the only areas that are active during the postictal depression of consciousness, and this may be related to maintenance of respiration and cardiac activities, the control of which resides primarily in the lower reticular formation, these brainstem activities are necessary to prevent death during postictal depression (see Chapters 18 and 29).

Variations in Requisite Network Nuclei among Different AGS Forms

As discussed in this chapter, the neuronal network for *tonic* forms of AGS in GEPR-9s and Strasbourg Wistar rats resides exclusively in brainstem nuclei (Figure 26.1). However, focal blockade studies in GEPR-3s and ETX rats indicate that the amygdala appears to be a requisite element for these *clonic* forms of AGS.[141,257] Thus, participation of the amygdala as a requisite AGS network structure is strikingly different from the role of this structure in the two other well-studied *tonic* forms of AGS where the amygdala is not a required element of the neuronal network for AGS, as discussed here. However, a complete and reversible block of AGS was seen in nonkindled GEPR-3s and ETX rats by focal blockade of the amygdala.[141,257] Single-unit studies indicate that tonic neuronal firing in the amygdala was observed during ETX seizures,[240] and burst firing during wild running and clonus was seen in the amygdala of GEPR-3s.[47] This was the first neuronal-firing evidence that a forebrain structure is a requisite component of the AGS neuronal network before AGS kindling (see Chapter 27). The requisite role of the amygdala in the generation of generalized clonic AGS offers a new insight into the underlying neuronal networks driving these seizures. Thus, despite the extensive similarities of AGS network nuclei in clonic and tonic forms of AGS, these data indicate that there is at least one major difference in the network components required for these closely related seizure models. The mechanistic differences that are operating in these different forms of AGS require further study to be better understood.

The AGS networks discussed here are dynamic entities, and seizure repetition can induce neuroplastic changes that result in prolongation of the seizures and expansion of the networks in several of these AGS forms, as discussed in Chapter 27. The actions of several anticonvulsant drugs on the AGS network during ETX and in GEPR-9s indicate that relatively selective actions on neurons in different parts of the network are observed (Chapter 32).[258]

CONCLUSIONS

The data discussed in this chapter on AGS paint a clear picture of the important anatomical elements (hubs) of the network for AGS. The data on all the models, taken together, reemphasize the importance of the IC as the critical consensus site for the ability of the auditory stimulus to initiate AGS. This site is the most rostral requisite nucleus of the auditory network in GEPR-9s and is a critical hub in all the other forms of AGS. The specific brainstem areas involved in the motor output (wild running and convulsions) lie primarily in the midbrain locomotor network further reinforcing the network interaction that subserves this epilepsy model (see Chapter 29). The variations on this theme in the several AGS models discussed in this chapter show that other brain nuclei, such as the amygdala, can also be required nuclei in the AGS network in the GEPR-3 and ETX forms of AGS. In addition, AGS in GEPR-3s and ETX rats culminate in generalized (four-limb) clonus, while AGS in GEPR-9s end in a more severe tonic extension seizure.[44,166] Reasons for these variations may be related to several different mechanisms, including the greater degree of hearing loss in GEPR-3s as compared to GEPR-9s.[75] In addition, the fact that ETX rats are treated systemically with ethanol means that the drug exerts a widespread action throughout the brain but does not cause the hearing impairment seen in many other AGS models. All of these forms of AGS are similarly affected by the systemic injection of drugs with anticonvulsant properties, including glutamate antagonists, suggesting important common sites of drug action within these networks. Further research is required to establish a more complete picture of how these AGS network differences produce clonic versus tonic seizures. Despite the fact that all of these AGS forms begin with the same motor behavior—wild running—identification of the network mechanisms behind the difference between clonic and tonic AGS requires further research. Finally, the involvement of the same network hub (the IC) for seizure initiation in all of these rat models, as well as the many genetic and induced mouse models, indicates that the similar abnormal patterns of behavior are likely to have a common origin within the network and possibly a common mechanism. The mechanisms responsible for the excessive excitation in IC neurons are related to specific reductions of the effectiveness of GABA-mediated inhibition in the models in which this has been examined. The idea that similar abnormal patterns of behavior are likely to have a common origin within a general seizure network for that seizure type may be applicable to other forms of epilepsy such as the kindling and status epilepticus models. This concept may also be applicable to human forms of temporal lobe epilepsy, since many of these forms exhibit overlapping spectrums but not identical patterns of behaviors. Application of this idea to other brain disorders would suggest a general concept. Thus, a common mechanism and hub may be responsible for the critical elements in related networks for chronic pain (Chapter 23) or related networks for mood disorders and anxiety disorders that exhibit overlapping but distinguishably different symptoms (Chapter 24). Specific drug actions on the emergent properties of neurons (see Chapters 30 and 32) in these hubs may be the key to establishing the most effective therapeutic measures for a class of closely related varieties of these disorders. These concepts will require extensive future research to validate.

Acknowledgments

The authors gratefully acknowledge the technical assistance of Marcus Randall, Dareea Patrick Paiva, and Doris Casebeer, and the involvement of Dr. Joni Clark in the thyroid deficiency–related and ischemia-related experiments discussed in this chapter. The authors were supported by NIH, NINDS, and NIAAA during these experiments, and we acknowledge the assistance of Gayle Stauffer in preparing this manuscript and Professor Ronald Browning for comments on the manuscript.

References

1. Cavanna AE, Rickards H, Ali F. What makes a simple partial seizure complex? *Epilepsy Behav.* 2011;22(4):651–658.
2. Bertram EH. Neuronal circuits in epilepsy: do they matter? *Exp Neurol.* Feb 8, 2012 (Epub ahead of print).
3. Fahoum F, Lopes R, Pittau F, Dubeau F, Gotman J. Widespread epileptic networks in focal epilepsies: EEG–fMRI study. *Epilepsia.* 2012;53(9):1618–1627.
4. Tatum WO. Mesial temporal lobe epilepsy. *J Clin Neurophysiol.* 2012;29(5):356–365.
5. Faingold CL, Fromm GH. *Drugs for Control of Epilepsy: Actions on Neuronal Networks Involved in Seizure Disorders.* Boca Raton, FL: CRC Press; 1992.
6. Blumenfeld H. Cellular and network mechanisms of spike-wave seizures. *Epilepsia.* 2005;46(Suppl. 9):21–33.
7. Bullmore E, Sporns O. Complex brain networks: graph theoretical analysis of structural and functional systems. *Nat Rev Neurosci.* 2009;10(3):186–198.
8. Faingold CL. Brainstem networks: reticulocortical synchronization in generalized convulsive seizures. In: Noebels JL, Avoli M, Rogawski MA, Olsen RW, Delgado-Escueta AV, eds. *Jasper's Basic Mechanisms of the Epilepsies.* 4th ed. New York, NY: Oxford University Press; 2012:257–271.
9. Quilichini PP, Le Van Quyen M, Ivanov A, et al. Hub GABA neurons mediate gamma-frequency oscillations at ictal-like event onset in the immature hippocampus. *Neuron.* 2012;74(1):57–64.
10. Graef JD, Godwin DW. Intrinsic plasticity in acquired epilepsy: too much of a good thing? *Neuroscientist.* 2010;16(5):487–495.
11. Hernan AE, Holmes GL, Isaev D, Scott RC, Isaeva E. Altered short-term plasticity in the prefrontal cortex after early life seizures. *Neurobiol Dis.* 2013;50:120–126.
12. Toth TI, Bessaih T, Leresche N, Crunelli V. The properties of reticular thalamic neuron $GABA_A$ IPSCs of absence epilepsy rats lead to enhanced network excitability. *Eur J Neurosci.* 2007;26(7):1832–1844.
13. Han HA, Cortez MA, Snead III OC. $GABA_B$ receptor and absence epilepsy. In: Noebels JL, Avoli M, Rogawski MA, Olsen RW, Delgado-Escueta AV, eds. *Jasper's Basic Mechanisms of the Epilepsies.* 4th ed. New York, NY: Oxford University Press; 2012:242–256.
14. Blume WT. The progression of epilepsy. *Epilepsia.* 2006;47(Suppl. 1):71–78.
15. McIntyre DC, Gilby KL. Mapping seizure pathways in the temporal lobe. *Epilepsia.* 2008;49(Suppl. 3):23–30.
16. Englot DJ, Modi B, Mishra AM, DeSalvo M, Hyder F, Blumenfeld H. Cortical deactivation induced by subcortical network dysfunction in limbic seizures. *J Neurosci.* 2009;29(41):13006–13018.

17. Kucker S, Tollner K, Piechotta M, Gernert M. Kindling as a model of temporal lobe epilepsy induces bilateral changes in spontaneous striatal activity. *Neurobiol Dis*. 2010;37(3):661–672.
18. Karunakaran S, Grasse DW, Moxon KA. Changes in network dynamics during status epilepticus. *Exp Neurol*. 2012;234(2):454–465.
19. Cymerblit-Sabba A, Schiller Y. Network dynamics during development of pharmacologically induced epileptic seizures in rats in vivo. *J Neurosci*. 2010;30(5):1619–1630.
20. Baracskay P, Kiglics V, Kekesi KA, Juhasz G, Czurko A. Status epilepticus affects the gigantocellular network of the pontine reticular formation. *BMC Neurosci*. 2009;10:133.
21. Sloviter RS, Bumanglag AV, Schwarcz R, Frotscher M. Abnormal dentate gyrus network circuitry in temporal lobe epilepsy. In: Noebels JL, Avoli M, Rogawski MA, Olsen RW, Delgado-Escueta AV, eds. *Jasper's Basic Mechanisms of the Epilepsies*. 4th ed. New York, NY: Oxford University Press; 2012:454–469.
22. Danielson NB, Guo JN, Blumenfeld H. The default mode network and altered consciousness in epilepsy. *Behav Neurol*. 2011;24(1): 55–65.
23. Blumenfeld H, Varghese GI, Purcaro MJ, et al. Cortical and subcortical networks in human secondarily generalized tonic-clonic seizures. *Brain*. 2009;132(Pt 4):999–1012.
24. Moeller F, Maneshi M, Pittau F, et al. Functional connectivity in patients with idiopathic generalized epilepsy. *Epilepsia*. 2011;52(3):515–522.
25. Kasteleijn-Nolst Trenite DG. Provoked and reflex seizures: surprising or common? *Epilepsia*. 2012;53(Suppl. 4):105–113.
26. Kasteleijn-Nolst Trenite D, Rubboli G, Hirsch E, et al. Methodology of photic stimulation revisited: updated European algorithm for visual stimulation in the EEG laboratory. *Epilepsia*. 2012;53(1):16–24.
27. Batini C, Teillet MA, Naquet R. An avian model of genetic reflex epilepsy. *Arch Ital Biol*. 2004;142(3):297–312.
28. Brailowsky S. GABA and epilepsy in the photosensitive baboon *Papio papio*. *Proc West Pharmacol Soc*. 1996;39:71–75.
29. Grosso S, Farnetani MA, Bernardoni E, Morgese G, Balestri P. Intractable reflex audiogenic seizures in Aicardi syndrome. *Brain Dev*. 2007;29(4):243–246.
30. Faingold CL. Role of GABA abnormalities in the inferior colliculus pathophysiology – audiogenic seizures. *Hear Res*. 2002;168(1–2):223–237.
31. Garcia-Cairasco N. A critical review on the participation of inferior colliculus in acoustic-motor and acoustic-limbic networks involved in the expression of acute and kindled audiogenic seizures. *Hear Res*. 2002;168(1–2):208–222.
32. Noh GJ, Jane Tavyev Asher Y, Graham Jr JM. Clinical review of genetic epileptic encephalopathies. *Eur J Med Genet*. 2012;55(5): 281–298.
33. Pandolfo M. Genetics of epilepsy. *Semin Neurol*. 2011;31(5): 506–518.
34. Rossignol S, Barriere G, Frigon A, et al. Plasticity of locomotor sensorimotor interactions after peripheral and/or spinal lesions. *Brain Res Rev*. 2008;57(1):228–240.
35. Maton B, Vergnes M, Hirsch E, Marescaux C. Involvement of proprioceptive feedback in brainstem-triggered convulsions. *Epilepsia*. 1997;38(5):509–515.
36. Jobe PC. Pharmacology of audiogenic seizures. In: Brown RD, ed. *Pharmacology of Hearing: Experimental Clinical Bases*. New York, NY: John Wiley & Sons, Inc.; 1981:271–304.
37. Browning RA, Wang C, Nelson DK, Jobe PC. Effect of precollicular transection on audiogenic seizures in genetically epilepsy-prone rats. *Exp Neurol*. 1999;155(2):295–301.
38. Jobe PC, Browning RA. From brainstem to forebrain in generalized animal models of seizures and epilepsies. In: Hirsch E, Andermann F, Chauvel P, Engel J, Lopes da Silva F, Luders H, eds. *Progress in Epileptic Disorders: Generalized Seizures: From Clinical Phenomenology to Underlying Systems and Networks*. Montrouge: John Libbey Eurotext; 2006:33–52.
39. Fisher RS, van Emde Boas W, Blume W, et al. Epileptic seizures and epilepsy: definitions proposed by the International League Against Epilepsy (ILAE) and the International Bureau for Epilepsy (IBE). *Epilepsia*. 2005;46(4):470–472.
40. Gower AJ, Noyer M, Verloes R, Gobert J, Wulfert E. ucb L059, a novel anti-convulsant drug: pharmacological profile in animals. *Eur J Pharmacol*. 1992;222(2–3):193–203.
41. Kaminski RM, Gillard M, Klitgaard H. Targeting SV2A for discovery of antiepileptic drugs. In: Noebels JL, Avoli M, Rogawski MA, Olsen RW, Delgado-Escueta AV, eds. *Jasper's Basic Mechanisms of the Epilepsies*. 4th ed. New York, NY: Oxford University Press; 2012:974–983.
42. Faingold CL. Neuronal networks in the genetically epilepsy-prone rat. *Adv Neurol*. 1999;79:311–321.
43. Faingold CL, Naritoku DK. The genetically epilepsy-prone rat: neuronal networks and actions of amino acid neurotransmitters. In: Faingold CL, Fromm GH, eds. *Drugs for Control of Epilepsy: Actions on Neuronal Networks Involved in Seizure Disorders*. Boca Raton, FL: CRC Press; 1992:277–308.
44. Jobe PC, Picchioni AL, Chin L. Role of brain norepinephrine in audiogenic seizure in the rat. *J Pharmacol Exp Ther*. 1973;184(1):1–10.
45. Jobe PC, Mishra PK, Dailey JW. Genetically epilepsy-prone rats: actions of antiepileptic drugs and monoaminergic neurotransmitters. In: Faingold CL, Fromm GH, eds. *Drugs for Control of Epilepsy, Actions on Neuronal Networks Involved in Seizure Disorders*. Boca Raton, FL: CRC Press; 1992:253–275.
46. Raisinghani M, Faingold CL. Pontine reticular formation neurons are implicated in the neuronal network for generalized clonic seizures which is intensified by audiogenic kindling. *Brain Res*. 2005;1064(1–2):90–97.
47. Raisinghani M, Faingold CL. Neurons in the amygdala play an important role in the neuronal network mediating a clonic form of audiogenic seizures both before and after audiogenic kindling. *Brain Res*. 2005;1032(1–2):131–140.
48. Garcia-Cairasco N, Oliveira JA, Wakamatsu H, Bueno ST, Guimaraes FS. Reduced exploratory activity of audiogenic seizures susceptible Wistar rats. *Physiol Behav*. 1998;64:671–674.
49. Onodera K, Tuomisto L, Tacke U, Airaksinen M. Strain differences in regional brain histamine levels between genetically epilepsy-prone and resistant rats. *Methods Find Exp Clin Pharmacol*. 1992;14:13–16.
50. Shan W, Wu X, Zhang G, Zhang Y, Liang Y, Wang Z. Effects of antisense oligodeoxynucleotides to NR1 on suppression of seizures and protection of cortical neurons from excitotoxicity in vivo and in vitro. *Chin Med J (Engl Ed)*. 1997;110:579–583.
51. Simler S, Vergnes M, Marescaux C. Spatial and temporal relationships between C-Fos expression and kindling of audiogenic seizures in Wistar rats. *Exp Neurol*. 1999;157(1):106–119.
52. Surina NM, Kalinina TS, Volkova AV, et al. Anxiety and predisposition to audiogenic epilepsy in rats of different genotypes. *Bull Exp Biol Med*. 2011;151(1):47–50.
53. Yechikhov S, Morenkov E, Chulanova T, Godukhin O, Shchipakina T. Involvement of cAMP- and Ca^{2+}/calmodulin-dependent neuronal protein phosphorylation in mechanisms underlying genetic predisposition to audiogenic seizures in rats. *Epilepsy Res*. 2001;46:15–25.
54. Fuller JL, Sjursen Jr FH. Audiogenic seizures in eleven mouse strains. *J Hered*. 1967;58:135–140.
55. The Jackson Laboratory. *Mouse Phenome Database Web Site*. Bar Harbor, ME, USA: The Jackson Laboratory; Mar 2013. http://phenome.jax.org.

56. Seyfried TN, Todorova MT, Poderycki MJ. Experimental models of multifactorial epilepsies: the EL mouse and mice susceptible to audiogenic seizures. *Adv Neurol.* 1999;79:279–290.
57. Fuentes-Santamaria V, Alvarado JC, Herranz AS, Garcia-Atares N, Lopez DE. Morphologic and neurochemical alterations in the superior colliculus of the genetically epilepsy-prone hamster (GPG/Vall). *Epilepsy Res.* 2007;75(2–3):206–219.
58. Faingold CL, Randall M, Tupal S. DBA/1 mice exhibit chronic susceptibility to audiogenic seizures followed by sudden death associated with respiratory arrest. *Epilepsy Behav.* 2010;17(4): 436–440.
59. Tupal S, Faingold CL. Evidence supporting a role of serotonin in modulation of sudden death induced by seizures in DBA/2 mice. *Epilepsia.* 2006;47(1):21–26.
60. Venit EL, Shepard BD, Seyfried TN. Oxygenation prevents sudden death in seizure-prone mice. *Epilepsia.* 2004;45(8):993–996.
61. Baulac S, Ishida S, Mashimo T, et al. A rat model for LGI1-related epilepsies. *Hum Mol Genet.* 2012;21(16):3546–3557.
62. Brennan TJ, Seeley WW, Kilgard M, Schreiner CE, Tecott LH. Sound-induced seizures in serotonin 5-HT_{2c} receptor mutant mice. *Nat Genet.* 1997;16:387–390.
63. Charizopoulou N, Lelli A, Schraders M, et al. Gipc3 mutations associated with audiogenic seizures and sensorineural hearing loss in mouse and human. *Nat Commun.* 2011;2:201.
64. Chen L, Toth M. Fragile X mice develop sensory hyper-reactivity to auditory stimuli. *Neuroscience.* 2001;103(4):1043–1050.
65. De Luca G, Di Giorgio RM, Macaione S, et al. Susceptibility to audiogenic seizure and neurotransmitter amino acid levels in different brain areas of IL-6-deficient mice. *Pharmacol Biochem Behav.* 2004;78(1):75–81.
66. Goebel-Goody SM, Wilson-Wallis ED, Royston S, Tagliatela SM, Naegele JR, Lombroso PJ. Genetic manipulation of STEP reverses behavioral abnormalities in a fragile X syndrome mouse model. *Genes Brain Behav.* 2012;11(5):586–600.
67. Li H, Takeda Y, Niki H, et al. Aberrant responses to acoustic stimuli in mice deficient for neural recognition molecule NB-2. *Eur J Neurosci.* 2003;17(5):929–936.
68. Miyakawa T, Yagi T, Taniguchi M, Matsuura H, Tateishi K, Niki H. Enhanced susceptibility of audiogenic seizures in Fyn-kinase deficient mice. *Brain Res Mol Brain Res.* 1995;28:349–352.
69. Szot P, Weinshenker D, White SS, et al. Norepinephrine-deficient mice have increased susceptibility to seizure-inducing stimuli. *J Neurosci.* 1999;19:10985–10992.
70. Tecott LH, Sun LM, Akana SF, et al. Eating disorder and epilepsy in mice lacking 5-HT_{2c} serotonin receptors. *Nature.* 1995;374: 542–546.
71. Westmark CJ, Westmark PR, Malter JS. Alzheimer's disease and Down syndrome rodent models exhibit audiogenic seizures. *J Alzheimers Dis.* 2010;20(4):1009–1013.
72. Yagi H, Takamura Y, Yoneda T, et al. Vlgr1 knockout mice show audiogenic seizure susceptibility. *J Neurochem.* 2005;92(1): 191–202.
73. Kai N, Niki H. Altered tone-induced Fos expression in the mouse inferior colliculus after early exposure to intense noise. *Neurosci Res.* 2002;44(3):305–313.
74. Ross KC, Coleman JR, Jones LS. Anti-epileptiform effects of audiogenic seizure printing on in vitro kindling in rat hippocampus. *Neurosci Lett.* 2001;299:234–238.
75. Faingold CL, Walsh EJ, Maxwell JK, Randall ME. Audiogenic seizure severity and hearing deficits in the genetically epilepsy-prone rat. *Exp Neurol.* 1990;108(1):55–60.
76. Pierson M, Li D. Cochlear integrity in rats with experimentally induced audiogenic seizure susceptibility. *Hear Res.* 1996;101: 7–13.
77. Reid HM, Collins RL. Lateralized audiogenic seizure: motor asymmetries exhibited and the effects of interrupted stimulation. *Behav Neural Biol.* 1986;46:424–431.
78. Sakamoto T, Niki H. Acoustic priming lowers the threshold for electrically induced seizures in mice inferior colliculus, but not in the deep layers of superior colliculus. *Brain Res.* 2001;898(2):358–363.
79. Yasuda S, Ishida N, Higashiyama A, Morinobu S, Kato N. Characterization of audiogenic-like seizures in naïve rats evoked by activation of AMPA and NMDA receptors in the inferior colliculus. *Exp Neurol.* 2000;164:396–406.
80. Deol MS. The role of thyroxine in the differentiation of the organ of Corti. *Acta Otolaryngol.* 1976;81(5–6):429–435.
81. Hebert R, Langlois JM, Dussault JH. Permanent defects in rat peripheral auditory function following perinatal hypothyroidism: determination of a critical period. *Brain Res.* 1985;355(2): 161–170.
82. Meyerhoff WL. Hypothyroidism and the ear: electrophysiological, morphological, and chemical considerations. *Laryngoscope.* 1979;89(10 Pt 2 Suppl. 19):1–25.
83. Sprenkle PM, McGee J, Bertoni JM, Walsh EJ. Consequences of hypothyroidism on auditory system function in Tshr mutant (hyt) mice. *J Assoc Res Otolaryngol.* 2001;2(4):312–329.
84. Sprenkle PM, McGee J, Bertoni JM, Walsh EJ. Development of auditory brainstem responses (ABRs) in Tshr mutant mice derived from euthyroid and hypothyroid dams. *J Assoc Res Otolaryngol.* 2001;2(4):330–347.
85. Sprenkle PM, McGee J, Bertoni JM, Walsh EJ. Prevention of auditory dysfunction in hypothyroid Tshr mutant mice by thyroxin treatment during development. *J Assoc Res Otolaryngol.* 2001;2(4):348–361.
86. Uziel A, Gabrion J, Ohresser M, Legrand C. Effects of hypothyroidism on the structural development of the organ of Corti in the rat. *Acta Otolaryngol.* 1981;92(5–6):469–480.
87. Uziel A, Legrand C, Ohresser M, Marot M. Maturational and degenerative processes in the organ of Corti after neonatal hypothyroidism. *Hear Res.* 1983;11(2):203–218.
88. Van Middlesworth L, Norris CH. Audiogenic seizures and cochlear damage in rats after perinatal antithyroid treatment. *Endocrinology.* 1980;106(6):1686–1690.
89. Patrick DL, Faingold CL. Sensitivity differences to blockade of audiogenic seizures (AGS) in thyroid deficient (THX) or genetically epilepsy-prone rats (GEPRs): microinjection into brainstem auditory nuclei. Program No. 16.785. In: *1990 Neuroscience Meeting Planner.* St. Louis, MO: Society for Neuroscience; 1990.
90. Schalock RL, Brown WJ, Smith RL. Long-term effects of propylthiouracil-induced neonatal hypothyroidism. *Dev Psychobiol.* 1979;12(3):187–199.
91. Bac P, Maurois P, Dupont C, et al. Magnesium deficiency-dependent audiogenic seizures (MDDASs) in adult mice: a nutritional model for discriminatory screening of anticonvulsant drugs and original assessment of neuroprotection properties. *J Neurosci.* 1998;18:4363–4373.
92. Chung SH, Johnson MS. Studies on sound-induced epilepsy in mice. *Proc R Soc Lond B Biol Sci.* 1984;221:145–168.
93. Reid KH, Young C, Schurr A, et al. Audiogenic seizures following global ischemia induced by chest compression in Long-Evans rats. *Epilepsy Res.* 1996;23(3):195–209.
94. Stanojlovic O, Zivanovic D, Susic V. Potentiation of metaphit-induced audiogenic epilepsy with *N*-methyl-D-aspartate in rats. *Srp Arh Celok Lek.* 2000;128:316–321.
95. Wada JA. Susceptibility to audiogenic seizure induced by thiosemicarbazide. *Electroencephalogr Clin Neurophysiol.* 1970;28:100.
96. Kawai K, Penix LP, Kawahara N, Ruetzler CA, Klatzo I. Development of susceptibility to audiogenic seizures following cardiac

arrest cerebral ischemia in rats. *J Cereb Blood Flow Metab.* 1995;15(2):248–258.

97. Ross DT, Duhaime AC. Degeneration of neurons in the thalamic reticular nucleus following transient ischemia due to raised intracranial pressure: excitotoxic degeneration mediated via non-NMDA receptors? *Brain Res.* 1989;501(1):129–143.
98. Vanicky I, Cizkova D, Prosbova T, Marsala M. Audiogenic seizures after neck tourniquet-induced cerebral ischemia in the rat. *Brain Res.* 1997;766(1–2):262–265.
99. Voll CL, Auer RN. Postischemic seizures and necrotizing ischemic brain damage: neuroprotective effect of postischemic diazepam and insulin. *Neurology.* 1991;41(3):423–428.
100. Burn J, Dennis M, Bamford J, Sandercock P, Wade D, Warlow C. Epileptic seizures after a first stroke: the Oxfordshire Community Stroke Project. *BMJ.* 1997;315(7122):1582–1587.
101. De La Court A, Breteler MM, Meinardi H, Hauser WA, Hofman A. Prevalence of epilepsy in the elderly: the Rotterdam Study. *Epilepsia.* 1996;37(2):141–147.
102. Freeman WD, Dawson SB, Flemming KD. The ABC's of stroke complications. *Semin Neurol.* 2010;30(5):501–510.
103. Stolarek IH, Brodie AF, Brodie MJ. Management of seizures in the elderly: a survey of UK geriatricians. *J R Soc Med.* 1995;88(12): 686–689.
104. Thomas SV, Pradeep KS, Rajmohan SJ. First ever seizures in the elderly: a seven-year follow-up study. *Seizure.* 1997;6(2): 107–110.
105. Willmore LJ. Management of epilepsy in the elderly. *Epilepsia.* 1996;37(Suppl. 6):S23–S33.
106. Faingold CL, Randall ME, Naritoku DK, Boersma Anderson CA. Noncompetitive and competitive NMDA antagonists exert anticonvulsant effects by actions on different sites within the neuronal network for audiogenic seizures. *Exp Neurol.* 1993; 119(2):198–204.
107. Faingold CL, Randall ME, Anderson CA. Blockade of GABA uptake with tiagabine inhibits audiogenic seizures and reduces neuronal firing in the inferior colliculus of the genetically epilepsy-prone rat. *Exp Neurol.* 1994;126(2):225–232.
108. Faingold CL, N'Gouemo P, Riaz A. Ethanol and neurotransmitter interactions—from molecular to integrative effects. *Prog Neurobiol.* 1998;55:509–535.
109. Nath C, Gupta MB. Role of central histaminergic system in lorazepam withdrawal syndrome in rats. *Pharmacol Biochem Behav.* 2001;68:777–782.
110. Oh S, Ho IK. Changes of [^{3}H]muscimol binding and $GABA_A$ receptor beta2-subunit mRNA level by tolerance to and withdrawal from pentobarbital in rats. *Neurochem Res.* 1999;24(12): 1603–1609.
111. Atkins AL, Rustay NR, Crabbe JC. Anxiety and sensitivity to ethanol and pentobarbital in alcohol withdrawal seizure-prone and withdrawal seizure-resistant mice. *Alcohol Clin Exp Res.* 2000;24(12):1743–1749.
112. Faingold CL. The Majchrowicz binge alcohol protocol: an intubation technique to study alcohol dependence in rats. *Curr Protoc Neurosci.* 2008;44:9.28.1–9.28.12.
113. Faingold CL, Riaz A. Increased responsiveness of pontine reticular formation neurons associated with audiogenic seizure susceptibility during ethanol withdrawal. *Brain Res.* 1994;663:69–76.
114. Koob GF. Animal models of craving for ethanol. *Addiction.* 2000;95(Suppl. 2):S73–S81.
115. Majchrowicz E. Induction of physical dependence upon ethanol and the associated behavioral changes in rats. *Psychopharmacologia.* 1975;43:245–254.
116. Dopico AM, Lovinger DM. Acute alcohol action and desensitization of ligand-gated ion channels. *Pharmacol Rev.* 2009;61(1): 98–114.
117. Kumar S, Porcu P, Werner DF, et al. The role of $GABA_A$ receptors in the acute and chronic effects of ethanol: a decade of progress. *Psychopharmacology (Berl).* 2009;205(4):529–564.
118. Moykkynen T, Korpi ER. Acute effects of ethanol on glutamate receptors. *Basic Clin Pharmacol Toxicol.* 2012;111(1):4–13.
119. Bianchi MT, Macdonald RL. Slow phases of $GABA_A$ receptor desensitization: structural determinants and possible relevance for synaptic function. *J Physiol.* 2002;544(Pt 1):3–18.
120. Chang Y, Ghansah E, Chen Y, Ye J, Weiss DS, Chang Y. Desensitization mechanism of GABA receptors revealed by single oocyte binding and receptor function. *J Neurosci.* 2002;22(18):7982–7990.
121. Chen G, Cuzon Carlson VC, Wang J, et al. Striatal involvement in human alcoholism and alcohol consumption, and withdrawal in animal models. *Alcohol Clin Exp Res.* 2011;35(10):1739–1748.
122. Clapp P, Gibson ES, Dell'acqua ML, Hoffman PL. Phosphorylation regulates removal of synaptic *N*-methyl-D-aspartate receptors after withdrawal from chronic ethanol exposure. *J Pharmacol Exp Ther.* 2010;332(3):720–729.
123. Mozrzymas JW, Barberis A, Mercik K, Zarnowska ED. Binding sites, singly bound states, and conformation coupling shape GABA-evoked currents. *J Neurophysiol.* 2003;89(2):871–883.
124. Marescaux C, Vergnes M, Kiesmann M, Depaulis A, Micheletti G, Warter JM. Kindling of audiogenic seizures in Wistar rats: an EEG study. *Exp Neurol.* 1987;97(1):160–168.
125. Merrill MA, Clough RW, Jobe PC, Browning RA. Brainstem seizure severity regulates forebrain seizure expression in the audiogenic kindling model. *Epilepsia.* 2005;46(9):1380–1388.
126. Reigel CE, Dailey JW, Jobe PC. The genetically epilepsy-prone rat: an overview of seizure-prone characteristics and responsiveness to anticonvulsant drugs. *Life Sci.* 1986;39(9):763–774.
127. Faingold CL. Locomotor behaviors in generalized convulsions are hierarchically driven from specific brain-stem nuclei in the network subserving audiogenic seizure. *Ann N Y Acad Sci.* 1998;860:566–569.
128. Jobe PC. Spinal seizures induced by electrical stimulation. In: Fromm GH, Faingold CL, Browning RA, Burnham WM, eds. *Epilepsy and the Reticular Formation: The Role of the Reticular Core in Convulsive Seizures.* New York, NY: Alan R. Liss; 1987:81–91.
129. Doretto MC, Cortes-de-Oliveira JA, Rossetti F, Garcia-Cairasco N. Role of the superior colliculus in the expression of acute and kindled audiogenic seizures in Wistar audiogenic rats. *Epilepsia.* 2009;50(12):2563–2574.
130. Gonzalez LP, Czachura JF, Brewer KW. Spontaneous versus elicited seizures following ethanol withdrawal: differential time course. *Alcohol.* 1989;6(6):481–487.
131. Riaz A, Faingold CL. Seizures during ethanol withdrawal are blocked by focal microinjection of excitant amino acid antagonists into the inferior colliculus and pontine reticular formation. *Alcohol Clin Exp Res.* 1994;18(6):1456–1462.
132. Ni H, Lu ZH, Wang SB, Tang M. A transient increase in CCK mRNA levels in hippocampus following audiogenic convulsions in audiogenic seizure-prone rats. *Acta Pharmacol Sin.* 2000;21(5):425–428.
133. Valjakka A, Jaakkola M, Vartiainen J, et al. The relationship between audiogenic seizure (AGS) susceptibility and forebrain tone-responsiveness in genetically AGS-prone Wistar rats. *Physiol Behav.* 2000;70(3–4):297–309.
134. Vinogradova LV, Shatskova AB. Lateral asymmetry of early seizure manifestations in experimental generalized epilepsy. *Neuroscience.* 2012;213:133–143.
135. Frost Jr JD, Lee CL, Hrachovy RA, Swann JW. High frequency EEG activity associated with ictal events in an animal model of infantile spasms. *Epilepsia.* 2011;52(1):53–62.
136. Stafstrom CE, Sasaki-Adams DM. NMDA-induced seizures in developing rats cause long-term learning impairment and increased seizure susceptibility. *Epilepsy Res.* 2003;53(1–2):129–137.

137. Dutra Moraes MF, Galvis-Alonso OY, Garcia-Cairasco N. Audiogenic kindling in the Wistar rat: a potential model for recruitment of limbic structures. *Epilepsy Res.* 2000;39(3):251–259.
138. Moraes MF, Mishra PK, Jobe PC, Garcia-Cairasco N. An electrographic analysis of the synchronous discharge patterns of GEPR-9s generalized seizures. *Brain Res.* 2005;1046(1–2):1–9.
139. Faingold CL, Travis MA, Gehlbach G, et al. Neuronal response abnormalities in the inferior colliculus of the genetically epilepsy-prone rat. *Electroencephalogr Clin Neurophysiol.* 1986; 63(3):296–305.
140. Feng HJ, Yang L, Faingold CL. Role of the amygdala in ethanol withdrawal seizures. *Brain Res.* 2007;1141:65–73.
141. Raisinghani M, Faingold CL. Identification of the requisite brain sites in the neuronal network subserving generalized clonic audiogenic seizures. *Brain Res.* 2003;967(1–2):113–122.
142. Eells JB, Clough RW, Miller JW, Jobe PC, Browning RA. Fos expression and 2-deoxyglucose uptake following seizures in developing genetically epilepsy-prone rats. *Brain Res Bull.* 2000;52(5):379–389.
143. Ribak CE, Manio AL, Navetta MS, Gall CM. In situ hybridization for c-fos mRNA reveals the involvement of the superior colliculus in the propagation of seizure activity in genetically epilepsy-prone rats. *Epilepsy Res.* 1997;26(3):397–406.
144. Simler S, Hirsch E, Danober L, Motte J, Vergnes M, Marescaux C. C-fos expression after single and kindled audiogenic seizures in Wistar rats. *Neurosci Lett.* 1994;175(1–2):58–62.
145. Klein BD, Fu YH, Ptacek LJ, White HS. c-Fos immunohistochemical mapping of the audiogenic seizure network and tonotopic neuronal hyperexcitability in the inferior colliculus of the Frings mouse. *Epilepsy Res.* 2004;62(1):13–25.
146. Le Gal La Salle G, Naquet R. Audiogenic seizures evoked in DBA/2 mice induce c-fos oncogene expression into subcortical auditory nuclei. *Brain Res.* 1990;518:308–312.
147. Ishida Y, Nakahara D, Hashiguchi H, et al. Fos expression in GABAergic cells and cells immunopositive for NMDA receptors in the inferior and superior colliculi following audiogenic seizures in rats. *Synapse.* 2002;46(2):100–107.
148. Pierson M, Snyder-Keller A. Development of frequency-selective domains in inferior colliculus of normal and neonatally noise-exposed rats. *Brain Res.* 1994;636(1):55–67.
149. Snyder-Keller AM, Pierson MG. Audiogenic seizures induce c-fos in a model of developmental epilepsy. *Neurosci Lett.* 1992;135(1):108–112.
150. Naritoku DK, Mecozzi LB, Aiello MT, Faingold CL. Repetition of audiogenic seizures in genetically epilepsy-prone rats induces cortical epileptiform activity and additional seizure behaviors. *Exp Neurol.* 1992;115(3):317–324.
151. Faingold CL, Gehlbach G, Caspary DM. On the role of GABA as an inhibitory neurotransmitter in inferior colliculus neurons: iontophoretic studies. *Brain Res.* 1989;500(1–2):302–312.
152. Li Y, Evans MS, Faingold CL. Inferior colliculus neuronal membrane and synaptic properties in genetically epilepsy-prone rats. *Brain Res.* 1994;660(2):232–240.
153. Evans MS, Li Y, Faingold C. Inferior colliculus intracellular response abnormalities in vitro associated with susceptibility to ethanol withdrawal seizures. *Alcohol Clin Exp Res.* 2000;24(8):1180–1186.
154. Browning RA. Anatomy of generalized convulsive seizures. In: Malafosse A, Genten P, Hirsch E, Marescaux C, Broglin D, Bernasconi R, eds. *Idiopathic Generalized Epilepsies: Clinical, Experimental and Genetic Aspects*. London: Libbey; 1994:399–413.
155. Faingold CL, Gehlbach G, Caspary DM. Decreased effectiveness of GABA-mediated inhibition in the inferior colliculus of the genetically epilepsy-prone rat. *Exp Neurol.* 1986;93:145–159.
156. Faingold C, Li Y, Evans MS. Decreased GABA and increased glutamate receptor-mediated activity on inferior colliculus neurons in vitro are associated with susceptibility to ethanol withdrawal seizures. *Brain Res.* 2000;868(2):287–295.
157. N'Gouemo P, Caspary DM, Faingold CL. Decreased GABA effectiveness in inferior colliculus neurons during ethanol withdrawal in rats susceptible to audiogenic seizures. *Brain Res.* 1996;724(2):200–204.
158. Ribak CE, Morin CL. The role of the inferior colliculus in a genetic model of audiogenic seizures. *Anat Embryol.* 1995;191:279–295.
159. Faingold CL, Millan MH, Boersma CA, Meldrum BS. Excitant amino acids and audiogenic seizures in the genetically epilepsy-prone rat. I. Afferent seizure initiation pathway. *Exp Neurol.* 1988;99(3):678–686.
160. Millan MH, Meldrum BS, Faingold CL. Induction of audiogenic seizure susceptibility by focal infusion of excitant amino acid or bicuculline into the inferior colliculus of normal rats. *Exp Neurol.* 1986;91(3):634–639.
161. Millan MH, Meldrum BS, Boersma CA, Faingold CL. Excitant amino acids and audiogenic seizures in the genetically epilepsy-prone rat. II. Efferent seizure propagating pathway. *Exp Neurol.* 1988;99(3):687–698.
162. Yang L, Long C, Faingold CL. Neurons in the deep layers of superior colliculus are a requisite component of the neuronal network for seizures during ethanol withdrawal. *Brain Res.* 2001;920(1–2):134–141.
163. McCown TJ, Greenwood RS, Frye GD, Breese GR. Electrically elicited seizures from the inferior colliculus: a potential site for the genesis of epilepsy? *Exp Neurol.* 1984;86(3):527–542.
164. Faingold CL, Millan MH, Boersma Anderson CA, Meldrum BS. Induction of audiogenic seizures in normal and genetically epilepsy-prone rats following focal microinjection of an excitant amino acid into reticular formation and auditory nuclei. *Epilepsy Res.* 1989;3:199–205.
165. Bagri A, Di Scala G, Sandner G. Myoclonic and tonic seizures elicited by microinjection of cholinergic drugs into the inferior colliculus. *Therapie.* 1999;54(5):589–594.
166. Faingold CL, Riaz A. Ethanol withdrawal induces increased firing in inferior colliculus neurons associated with audiogenic seizure susceptibility. *Exp Neurol.* 1995;132(1):91–98.
167. Faingold CL, Naritoku DK, Copley CA, et al. Glutamate in the inferior colliculus plays a critical role in audiogenic seizure initiation. *Epilepsy Res.* 1992;13:95–105.
168. Marchand MJ, Ward R, Moreau B. Different patterns of dendritic branching of posterior collicular neurons in two mouse strains are associated with a difference in audiogenic seizure susceptibility. *J Hirnforsch.* 1996;37:135–143.
169. Chapman AG. Regional changes in transmitter amino acids during focal and generalized seizures in rats. *J Neural Transm.* 1985;63(2):95–107.
170. Faingold CL, Hoffmann WE, Caspary DM. Effects of excitant amino acids on acoustic responses of inferior colliculus neurons. *Hear Res.* 1989;40(1–2):127–136.
171. Faingold CL, Boersma Anderson CA, Caspary DM. Involvement of GABA in acoustically-evoked inhibition in inferior colliculus neurons. *Hear Res.* 1991;52(1):201–216.
172. Ribak CE, Byun MY, Ruiz GT, Reiffenstein RJ. Increased levels of amino acid neurotransmitters in the inferior colliculus of the genetically epilepsy-prone rat. *Epilepsy Res.* 1988;2(1):9–13.
173. Patrick DL, Faingold CL. Auditory brainstem responses (ABRs) and effects of microinjection into inferior colliculus (IC) of an excitant amino acid (EAA) antagonist or GABA agonist on audiogenic seizures (AGS) in thyroid deficient (THX) or genetically epilepsy-prone rats (GEPRs). Program No. 15.46. In: *1989*

Neuroscience Meeting Planner. Phoenix, AZ: Society for Neuroscience; 1989.

174. Higashiyama A, Ishida N, Nishimura T, et al. NMDA receptors in the inferior colliculus are critically involved in audiogenic seizures in the adult rats with neonatal hypothyroidism. *Exp Neurol*. 1998;153(1):94–101.
175. Faingold CL, Marcinczyk MJ, Casebeer DJ, Randall ME, Arneric SP, Browning RA. GABA in the inferior colliculus plays a critical role in control of audiogenic seizures. *Brain Res*. 1994;640:40–47.
176. Krystal JH, Petrakis IL, Mason G, Trevisan L, D'Souza DC. N-methyl-D-aspartate glutamate receptors and alcoholism: reward, dependence, treatment, and vulnerability. *Pharmacol Ther*. 2003;99(1):79–94.
177. Tupal S, Faingold CL. The amygdala to periaqueductal gray pathway: plastic changes induced by audiogenic kindling and reversal by gabapentin. *Brain Res*. 2012;1475:71–79.
178. Worrell GA, Gardner AB, Stead SM, et al. High-frequency oscillations in human temporal lobe: simultaneous microwire and clinical macroelectrode recordings. *Brain*. 2008;131(Pt 4):928–937.
179. Samineni V, Premkumar L, Faingold C. Changes in periaqueductal gray neuronal responses to pain induced by barbiturate administration. *Anesthesiology*. in press.
180. Evans MS, Viola-McCabe KE, Caspary DM, Faingold CL. Loss of synaptic inhibition during repetitive stimulation in genetically epilepsy-prone rats (GEPR). *Epilepsy Res*. 1994;18:97–105.
181. Gould EM, Craig CR, Fleming WW, Taylor DA. Sensitivity of cerebellar Purkinje neurons to neurotransmitters in genetically epileptic rats. *J Pharmacol Exp Ther*. 1991;259:1008–1012.
182. Gould EM, Curto KA, Craig CR, Fleming WW, Taylor DA. The role of $GABA_A$ receptors in the subsensitivity of Purkinje neurons to GABA in genetic epilepsy prone rats. *Brain Res*. 1995;698:62–68.
183. Molnar LR, Fleming WW, Taylor DA. Alterations in neuronal gamma-aminobutyric $acid_A$ receptor responsiveness in genetic models of seizure susceptibility with different expression patterns. *J Pharmacol Exp Ther*. 2000;295:1258–1266.
184. Faingold CL, Gehlbach G, Caspary DM. Functional pharmacology of inferior colliculus neurons. In: Altschuler RA, ed. *Neurobiology of Hearing: The Central Auditory System*. New York, NY: Raven Press; 1991:223–251.
185. Burger RM, Pollak GD. Reversible inactivation of the dorsal nucleus of the lateral lemniscus reveals its role in the processing of multiple sound sources in the inferior colliculus of bats. *J Neurosci*. 2001;21(13):4830–4843.
186. Faingold CL, Boersma Anderson CA, Randall ME. Stimulation or blockade of the dorsal nucleus of the lateral lemniscus alters binaural and tonic inhibition in contralateral inferior colliculus neurons. *Hear Res*. 1993;69:98–106.
187. Gonzalez-Hernandez T, Mantolan-Sarmiento B, Gonzalez-Gonzalez B, Perez-Gonzalez H. Sources of GABAergic input to the inferior colliculus of the rat. *J Comp Neurol*. 1996;372:309–326.
188. Kelly JB, Li L. Two sources of inhibition affecting binaural evoked responses in the rat's inferior colliculus: the dorsal nucleus of the lateral lemniscus and the superior olivary complex. *Hear Res*. 1997;104(1–2):112–126.
189. Li L, Kelly JB. Inhibitory influence of the dorsal nucleus of the lateral lemniscus on binaural responses in the rat's inferior colliculus. *J Neurosci*. 1992;12:4530–4539.
190. Kulesza Jr RJ, Berrebi AS. Superior paraolivary nucleus of the rat is a GABAergic nucleus. *J Assoc Res Otolaryngol*. 2000;1(4):255–269.
191. Kulesza RJ, Vinuela A, Saldana E, Berrebi AS. Unbiased stereological estimates of neuron number in subcortical auditory nuclei of the rat. *Hear Res*. 2002;168(1–2):12–24.
192. Caird D. Processing in the colliculi. In: Altschuler RA, ed. *Neurobiology of Hearing: The Central Auditory System*. New York, NY: Raven Press; 1991:253–292.
193. Covey E, Casseday JH. Timing in the auditory system of the bat. *Annu Rev Physiol*. 1999;61:457–476.
194. Pedemonte M, Torterolo P, Velluti RA. In vivo intracellular characteristics of inferior colliculus neurons in guinea pigs. *Brain Res*. 1997;759:24–31.
195. Faingold CL, Boersma Anderson CA. Loss of intensity-induced inhibition in inferior colliculus neurons leads to audiogenic seizure susceptibility in behaving genetically epilepsy-prone rats. *Exp Neurol*. 1991;113:354–363.
196. Fuzessery ZM, Hall JC. Role of GABA in shaping frequency tuning and creating FM sweep selectivity in the inferior colliculus. *J Neurophysiol*. 1996;76:1059–1073.
197. Jen PH, Sun X, Chen QC. An electrophysiological study of neural pathways for corticofugally inhibited neurons in the central nucleus of the inferior colliculus of the big brown bat, *Eptesicus fuscus*. *Exp Brain Res*. 2001;137:292–302.
198. Le Beau FE, Rees A, Malmierca MS. Contribution of GABA- and glycine-mediated inhibition to the monaural temporal response properties of neurons in the inferior colliculus. *J Neurophysiol*. 1996;75:902–919.
199. Palombi PS, Caspary DM. GABA inputs control discharge rate primarily within frequency receptive fields of inferior colliculus neurons. *J Neurophysiol*. 1996;75:2211–2219.
200. Pollak GD. Roles of GABAergic inhibition for the binaural processing of multiple sound sources in the inferior colliculus. *Ann Otol Rhinol Laryngol Suppl*. 1997;168:44–54.
201. Vaughn MD, Pozza MF, Lingenhohl K. Excitatory acoustic responses in the inferior colliculus of the rat are increased by $GABA_B$ receptor blockade. *Neuropharmacology*. 1996;35:1761–1767.
202. Li Y, Evans MS, Faingold CL. Synaptic response patterns of neurons in the cortex of rat inferior colliculus. *Hear Res*. 1999;137(1–2):15–28.
203. Dalkara T. Nipecotic acid, an uptake blocker, prevents fading of the gamma-aminobutyric acid effect. *Brain Res*. 1986;366:314–319.
204. Margineanu DG, Wulfert E. Differential paired-pulse effects of gabazine and bicuculline in rat hippocampal CA3 area. *Brain Res Bull*. 2000;51:69–74.
205. Li Y. In vitro electrophysiological properties of inferior colliculus cortex neurons in genetically epilepsy prone rats and rats undergoing ethanol withdrawal (seizures). *Diss Abstr Int*. 1997;59-02(Sect. B):0548.
206. Aitkin L. *The Auditory Midbrain. Structure and Function in the Central Auditory Pathway*. Clifton, NJ: Humana Press; 1986.
207. Caicedo A, Herbert H. Topography of descending projections from the inferior colliculus to auditory brainstem nuclei in the rat. *J Comp Neurol*. 1993;328(3):377–392.
208. Ribak CE, Khurana V, Lien NT. The effect of midbrain collicular knife cuts on audiogenic seizure severity in the genetically epilepsy-prone rat. *J Hirnforsch*. 1994;35(2):303–311.
209. Merrill MA, Clough RW, Jobe PC, Browning RA. Role of the superior colliculus and the intercollicular nucleus in the brainstem seizure circuitry of the genetically epilepsy-prone rat. *Epilepsia*. 2003;44(3):305–314.
210. Faingold CL, Randall ME. Neurons in the deep layers of superior colliculus play a critical role in the neuronal network for audiogenic seizures: mechanisms for production of wild running behavior. *Brain Res*. 1999;815:250–258.
211. Clough RW, Eells JB, Browning RA, Jobe PC. Seizures and proto-oncogene expression of fos in the brain of adult genetically epilepsy-prone rats. *Exp Neurol*. 1997;146:341–353.
212. Nehlig A, Vergnes M, Hirsch E, Boyet S, Koziel V, Marescaux C. Mapping of cerebral blood flow changes during audiogenic

seizures in Wistar rats: effect of kindling. *J Cereb Blood Flow Metab.* 1995;15(2):259–269.

213. Rossetti F, Rodrigues MC, de Oliveira JA, Garcia-Cairasco N. Behavioral and EEG effects of GABAergic manipulation of the nigrotectal pathway in the Wistar audiogenic rat strain. *Epilepsy Behav.* 2011;22(2):191–199.
214. Faingold C, Casebeer D. Modulation of the audiogenic seizure network by noradrenergic and glutamatergic receptors of the deep layers of superior colliculus. *Brain Res.* 1999;821:392–399.
215. Knapp DJ, Duncan GE, Crews FT, Breese GR. Induction of Fos-like proteins and ultrasonic vocalizations during ethanol withdrawal: further evidence for withdrawal-induced anxiety. *Alcohol Clin Exp Res.* 1998;22(2):481–493.
216. N'Gouemo P, Faingold CL. Periaqueductal gray neurons exhibit increased responsiveness associated with audiogenic seizures in the genetically epilepsy-prone rat. *Neuroscience.* 1998;84:619–625.
217. N'Gouemo P, Faingold CL. The periaqueductal grey is a critical site in the neuronal network for audiogenic seizures: modulation by $GABA_A$, NMDA and opioid receptors. *Epilepsy Res.* 1999;35(1):39–46.
218. Yang L, Long C, Randall ME, Faingold CL. Neurons in the periaqueductal gray are critically involved in the neuronal network for audiogenic seizures during ethanol withdrawal. *Neuropharmacology.* 2003;44(2):275–281.
219. Yang L, Long C, Evans MS, Faingold CL. Ethanol withdrawal results in aberrant membrane properties and synaptic responses in periaqueductal gray neurons associated with seizure susceptibility. *Brain Res.* 2002;957(1):99–108.
220. Bajic D, Proudfit HK. Projections of neurons in the periaqueductal gray to pontine and medullary catecholamine cell groups involved in the modulation of nociception. *J Comp Neurol.* 1999;405(3):359–379.
221. Mouton LJ, Holstege G. The periaqueductal gray in the cat projects to lamina VIII and the medial part of lamina VII throughout the length of the spinal cord. *Exp Brain Res.* 1994;101(2):253–264.
222. Yang K, Ma WL, Feng YP, Dong YX, Li YQ. Origins of $GABA_B$ receptor-like immunoreactive terminals in the rat spinal dorsal horn. *Brain Res Bull.* 2002;58(5):499–507.
223. Long C, Yang L, Evans MS, Faingold CL. Alteration of GABA receptor-mediated inhibition in periaqueductal gray (PAG) neurons by ethanol withdrawal (ETX). Program No. 607.13. In: *2002 Neuroscience Meeting Planner.* Orlando, FL: Society for Neuroscience; 2002. Online.
224. Long C, Yang L, Faingold CL, Evans MS. Excitatory amino acid receptor-mediated responses in periaqueductal gray neurons are increased during ethanol withdrawal. *Neuropharmacology.* 2007;52(3):802–811.
225. Eckardt MJ, Campbell GA, Marietta CA, Majchrowicz E, Wixon HN, Weight FF. Cerebral 2-deoxyglucose uptake in rats during ethanol withdrawal and post-withdrawal. *Brain Res.* 1986;366:1–9.
226. Faingold CL, Randall ME. Pontine reticular formation neurons exhibit a premature and precipitous increase in acoustic responses prior to audiogenic seizures in genetically epilepsy-prone rats. *Brain Res.* 1995;704:218–226.
227. Faingold CL, Riaz A. Neuronal networks in convulsant drug-induced seizures. In: Faingold CL, Fromm GH, eds. *Drugs for Control of Epilepsy: Actions on Neuronal Networks Involved in Seizure Disorders.* Boca Raton, FL: CRC Press; 1992:213–251.
228. Baldissera F, Di Loreto S, Florio T, Scarnati E. Short-latency excitation of hindlimb motoneurons induced by electrical stimulation of the pontomesencephalic tegmentum in the rat. *Neurosci Lett.* 1994;169(1–2):13–16.
229. Lingenhöhl K, Friauf E. Giant neurons in the rat reticular formation: a sensorimotor interface in the elementary acoustic startle circuit? *J Neurosci.* 1994;14:1176–1194.
230. N'Gouemo P, Faingold CL. Phenytoin administration reveals a differential role of pontine reticular formation and periaqueductal gray neurons in generation of the convulsive behaviors of audiogenic seizures. *Brain Res.* 2000;859(2):311–317.
231. Koch M. The neurobiology of startle. *Prog Neurobiol.* 1999;59(2):107–128.
232. Leumann L, Sterchi D, Vollenweider F, Ludewig K, Fruh H. A neural network approach to the acoustic startle reflex and prepulse inhibition. *Brain Res Bull.* 2001;56(2):101–110.
233. Meloni EG, Davis M. GABA in the deep layers of the superior colliculus/mesencephalic reticular formation mediates the enhancement of startle by the dopamine D_1 receptor agonist SKF 82958 in rats. *J Neurosci.* 2000;20(14):5374–5381.
234. Deransart C, Le-Pham BT, Hirsch E, Marescaux C, Depaulis A. Inhibition of the substantia nigra suppresses absences and clonic seizures in audiogenic rats, but not tonic seizures: evidence for seizure specificity of the nigral control. *Neuroscience.* 2001;105(1):203–211.
235. Garcia-Cairasco N, Sabbatini RM. Possible interaction between the inferior colliculus and the substantia nigra in audiogenic seizures in Wistar rats. *Physiol Behav.* 1991;50(2):421–427.
236. Browning RA. Neuroanatomical localization of structures responsible for seizures in the GEPR: lesion studies. *Life Sci.* 1986;39(10):857–867.
237. Veliskova J, Moshe SL. Update on the role of substantia nigra pars reticulata in the regulation of seizures. *Epilepsy Curr.* 2006;6(3):83–87.
238. Faingold CL, Randall M. Involvement of the hippocampus in ethanol withdrawal seizures. *Alcohol Clin Exp Res.* 2005;29(5):95A.
239. Dahchour A, De Witte P. Effects of acamprosate on excitatory amino acids during multiple ethanol withdrawal periods. *Alcohol Clin Exp Res.* 2003;27(3):465–470.
240. Faingold CL, Feng HJ, Yang L. Focal blockade and neuronal recordings indicate that the amygdala is critical in the neuronal network for ethanol withdrawal seizures. *Alcohol Clin Exp Res.* 2003;27:99A.
241. Veatch LM, Gonzalez LP. Repeated ethanol withdrawal produces site-dependent increases in EEG spiking. *Alcohol Clin Exp Res.* 1996;20(2):262–267.
242. Chakravarty DN, Faingold CL. Differential roles in the neuronal network for audiogenic seizures are observed among the inferior colliculus subnuclei and the amygdala. *Exp Neurol.* 1999;157(1):135–141.
243. Hirsch E, Danober L, Simler S, et al. The amygdala is critical for seizure propagation from brainstem to forebrain. *Neuroscience.* 1997;77(4):975–984.
244. Feng HJ, Faingold CL. Repeated generalized audiogenic seizures induce plastic changes on acoustically evoked neuronal firing in the amygdala. *Brain Res.* 2002;932(1–2):61–69.
245. Faingold CL, Randall M. Ethanol withdrawal seizures – role of dentate gyrus neurons. *Alcohol Clin Exp Res.* 2006;30(6):78A.
246. Faingold CL, Patrick DL, Randall ME. Anticonvulsant effects of non-competitive excitant amino acid antagonists, dextromethorphan and MK-801, on audiogenic seizures. *Eur J Pharmacol.* 1990;183:952–953.
247. Chapman AG, Faingold CL, Hart GP, Bowker HM, Meldrum BS. Brain regional amino acid levels in seizure susceptible rats:

changes related to sound-induced seizures. *Neurochem Int.* 1986;8(2):273–279.

248. Chakravarty DN, Faingold CL. Aberrant neuronal responsiveness in the genetically epilepsy-prone rat: acoustic responses and influences of the central nucleus upon the external nucleus of inferior colliculus. *Brain Res.* 1997;761(2):263–270.
249. McCown TJ, Duncan GE, Johnson KB, Breese GR. Metabolic and functional mapping of the neural network subserving inferior collicular seizure generalization. *Brain Res.* 1995;701(1–2):117–128.
250. Sakamoto T, Mishina M, Niki H. Mutation of NMDA receptor subunit epsilon 1: effects on audiogenic-like seizures induced by electrical stimulation of the inferior colliculus in mice. *Brain Res Mol Brain Res.* 2002;102(1–2):113–117.
251. Cangiano L, Wallen P, Grillner S. Role of apamin-sensitive K_{Ca} channels for reticulospinal synaptic transmission to motoneuron and for the afterhyperpolarization. *J Neurophysiol.* 2002;88(1):289–299.
252. Grillner S, Parker D, el Manira A. Vertebrate locomotion-a lamprey perspective. *Ann N Y Acad Sci.* 1998;860:1–18.
253. Leonard JL. Network architectures and circuit function: testing alternative hypotheses in multifunctional networks. *Brain Behav Evol.* 2000;55:248–255.
254. Noga BR, Kriellaars DJ, Brownstone RM, Jordan LM. Mechanism for activation of locomotor centers in the spinal cord by stimulation of the mesencephalic locomotor region. *J Neurophysiol.* 2003;90(3):1464–1478.
255. Saper CB, Chou TC, Scammell TE. The sleep switch: hypothalamic control of sleep and wakefulness. *Trends Neurosci.* 2001;24(12):726–731.
256. Faingold CL. Neuronal networks, epilepsy and the action of antiepileptic drugs. In: Faingold CL, Fromm GH, eds. *Drugs for Control of Epilepsy: Actions on Neuronal Networks Involved in Seizure Disorders.* Boca Raton, FL: CRC Press; 1992:1–21.
257. Yang L, Faingold CL. The amygdala is a requisite nucleus in the neuronal network for ethanol withdrawal seizures. Program No. 607.1. In: *2002 Neuroscience Meeting Planner.* Orlando, FL: Society for Neuroscience; 2002. Online.
258. Faingold CL. Anticonvulsant drugs as neuronal network-modifying agents. In: Schwartzkroin PA, ed. *Encyclopedia of Basic Epilepsy Research.* Vol. 1.

CHAPTER

27

Physiological and Pathophysiological Expansion of Neuronal Networks

Prosper N'Gouemo[1], *Norberto Garcia-Cairasco*[2], *Carl L. Faingold*[3]

[1]Department of Pediatrics, Georgetown University Medical Center, Washington, DC, USA, [2]Department of Physiology, School of Medicine of Ribeirão Preto, University of São Paulo Ribeirão Preto, São Paulo, Brazil, [3]Department of Pharmacology, Southern Illinois University School of Medicine, Springfield, IL, USA

NEURONAL NETWORK EXPANSION MECHANISMS

Introduction

Long-lasting changes in the function of neuronal networks can be mediated by structural or functional alterations in the network and may involve single or, more commonly, repetitive experiences. Thus, behavioral-conditioning paradigms can produce long-lasting changes in the way that neurons, particularly conditional multireceptive (CMR) neurons (Chapter 28),[1] in intact and behaving animals respond to stimuli in several parts of the brain. Neurons that were minimally responsive to a stimulus before conditioning can become extensively responsive after the negative or positive conditioning process.[2–7] Thus, conditioning methods enabled the stimulus to expand the initial network or increase the responses of neurons that were receiving input from the circuit but were minimally or not directly involved in network operations until they were recruited by the novel behavioral situation.

Figure 27.1 shows a prototype diagram for network expansion involving interaction between two neuronal networks of the brain. Network 1 receives random input (1) from its "sensory" system, which causes the network to perform its function or behavior (Behavior 1). Network 1 has relatively minor anatomical connections to Network 2, which performs a different function (Behavior 2), but the interaction between the networks is relatively or completely inactive under basal conditions (Arrow A). Under conditions that induce network expansion, the interaction between the networks may undergo a major change in their interaction, as exemplified by Arrow B between the networks, and result in a new behavior (3). This could be due to repetitive stimulation of Input 1 or an intense activation of this input. The resultant change can be temporary, or it can be prolonged due to neuroplastic changes. This network interaction could be an enduring excitatory coupling of these networks, but in other cases the interaction could be inhibitory.

Prototypical mechanisms for these long-lasting interactions include long-term potentiation (LTP), a form of plasticity that results in facilitation of synaptic efficacy. In contrast, long-term depression (LTD) results in a long-lasting decrease in synaptic efficacy. Two mechanistic forms of LTD have been described: depotentiation, which refers to the reversal of LTP (LTP-D), and de novo LTD. LTP mechanisms contribute to functional and structural changes in brain networks that undergo sustained alterations due to repeated or intense experience, and LTD can alter network function as well (see Refs. 8–10 for a review). Figure 27.2 illustrates a simplified version of events that underlie LTP, LTD, LTP-D, and LTP block, which emphasizes common mechanisms. Major elements that contribute to the early phase of LTP include *N*-methyl-D-aspartate receptor (NMDAR) activation, which allows ionic calcium (Ca^{2+}) influx into postsynaptic neurons and activation of several Ca^{2+}-dependent messenger systems. Longer term changes include effects on α-amino-3-hydroxy-5-methyl-4-isoxazolepropionic acid receptor (AMPAR) trafficking, gene expression, and protein synthesis.[10]

LTD between elements of a network would tend to reduce rather than expand the network, but in a more complex circuit LTD could also contribute to network

Neuronal Networks in Brain Function, CNS Disorders, and Therapeutics
http://dx.doi.org/10.1016/B978-0-12-415804-7.00027-7

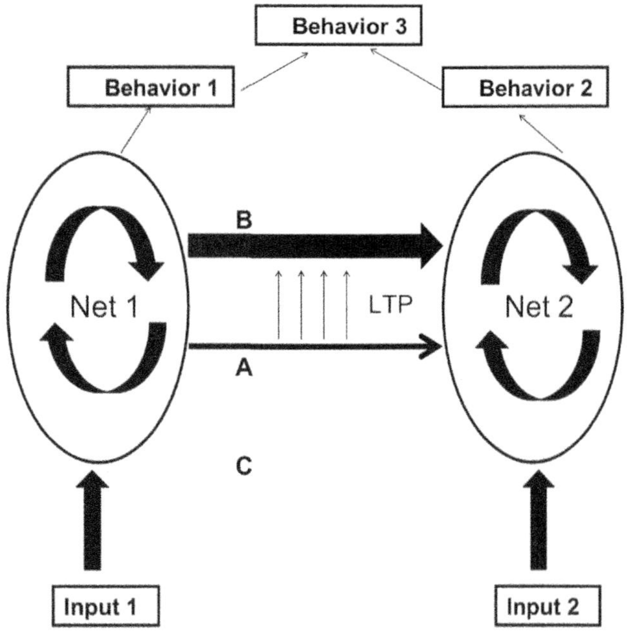

FIGURE 27.1 Simplified diagram for a theoretical network expansion involving interaction between two specific neuronal networks of the brain. Network 1 receives random input (1) from its "sensory" system, which causes the network to perform its function or behavior (Behavior 1). This network has the capability for self-organization, as illustrated by the dual semicircular arrows. An example of this might be the auditory network receiving a single acoustic stimulus, which results in the organism perceiving the stimulus but not otherwise reacting to it. Network 1 has anatomical connections with Network 2, which performs a different function (Behavior 2), but the interaction between the networks is relatively or completely inactive under basal conditions (Arrow A). An example of Network 2 may be the midbrain locomotor network, which is responsible for various organized movements of the organism. Alternatively, Network 2 may be involved in emotional behavior such as anxiety. Network 2 may or may not be receiving its own additional input (2) and produce its own behavior (2), and it is also capable of self-organization (as illustrated by the dual semicircular arrows). Under conditions that induce network expansion, the interaction between the networks may undergo a major change as exemplified by Arrow B between the networks, and results in a new behavior (3). This could be due to repetitive stimulation of Input 1 or an intense activation of this input. The resultant change can be temporary, or it can be long-lasting if the stimulus repetition triggers a neuroplastic process, such as long-term potentiation (LTP). This network interaction would be an enduring excitatory coupling of these networks, but in other cases the interaction could be inhibitory, such as long-term depression. Note: Multiple networks can also interact in a similar fashion.

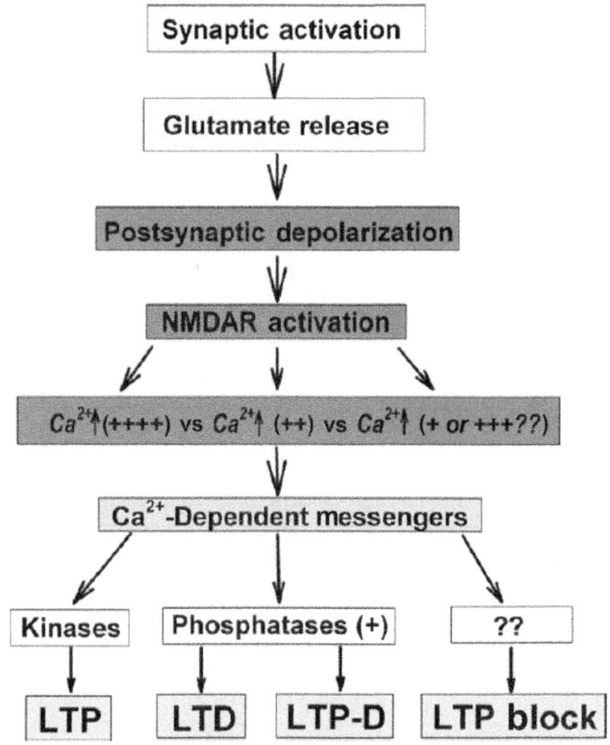

FIGURE 27.2 The diagram depicts a simplified scheme of early events underlying homosynaptic LTP, LTD, depotentiation (LTP-D), and LTP block (metaplasticity), highlighting commonalities. Key events include NMDAR activation that leads to calcium influx into postsynaptic neurons. The elevated intracellular Ca^{2+} can trigger Ca^{2+} release from Ca^{2+}-gated Ca^{2+} stores and activates different Ca^{2+}-dependent messengers. We have put LTD and LTP-D together because they share the involvement of phosphatases, but they are not necessarily the same process. Longer term changes include effects on AMPAR trafficking, gene expression, and protein synthesis (not depicted). (*Source: From Zorumski and Izumi*[10] *with permission.*)

expansion. The postsynaptic forms of LTP and LTD are known to regulate AMPARs in the hippocampus and are thought to apply to synapses in many other brain regions. However, differences in the mechanisms involving differential functional requirements for LTP have been observed, depending on the brain region.[11] LTP and LTD alter AMPAR-mediated fast synaptic transmission, and recent evidence indicates that NMDARs are also subject to activity-dependent long-term plasticity. NMDARs can significantly contribute to information transfer at synapses, particularly during periods of repetitive activity. NMDARs are, therefore, critical for generating the persistent activity of neural assemblies and have emerged as an important prototypical mechanism for encoding and storage of information in neuronal networks.[12]

Although LTP is a well-established mechanism for improving brain function through learning, this process can also result in network expansion that has negative consequences for the organism. Thus, LTP at synapses in the pain-processing networks can result in network expansion that results in increased sensitivity and chronic pain syndromes in response to trauma, inflammation, nerve injury, or opiate drug withdrawal.[13,14] LTP and LTD in the corticostriatal pathway are altered in Parkinson's disease and are thought to involve the imbalance between dopamine and acetylcholine activity in this network, which may contribute to the cognitive deficits that occur in patients with this brain disorder (see Chapter 25).[15]

Aging is associated with declines in learning and memory, and with altered neuroplastic mechanisms. These alterations are proposed to involve decreases in synaptic transmission and a reduced ability to induce LTP, as well as a shift in synaptic plasticity favoring LTD over LTP, both of which contribute to decreased synaptic transmission in aged animals (see Ref. 16 for a review). Repetitive seizures can lead to an expansion of the single-seizure neuronal network and also suppress LTP, which has been observed in mesial temporal lobe epilepsy in humans.[17,18] It is also possible that neuronal hyperexcitability resulting from repetitive seizures could be reduced by the induction of LTD. Thus, repetitive seizures can alter LTP and LTD by affecting their molecular mechanisms, and these alterations can contribute to an expansion of the seizure network.

Other forms of neuroplasticity can occur at nonglutamatergic synapses. Interestingly, it has become clear that the strength of GABAergic inhibitory synapses is also modulated by activity, and inhibitory neuronal plasticity has the capacity to alter the excitability and function of neuronal networks (see Ref. 19 for a review). The intracellular mechanisms involved in the induction and expression of inhibitory LTP differ among different brain regions. Thus, in the visual cortex, LTP of gamma-aminobutyric acid A ($GABA_A$) receptor-mediated inhibitory synaptic transmission requires the activation of $GABA_B$ receptors. Activation of postsynaptic $GABA_B$ receptors initiates LTP by potentiating α1-adrenoreceptor-mediated and serotonin ($5\text{-}HT_2$) receptor-mediated inositol triphosphate formation. In the hippocampus and visual cortex, Ca^{2+} release from intracellular Ca^{2+}-gated Ca^{2+} stores initiates a brain-derived neurotropic factor (BDNF)–Trkβ-mediated signaling cascade that modulates GABA release. In other brain sites such as the ventral tegmental area, inhibitory LTP requires a retrograde signaling via a nitric oxide–guanylate cyclase and protein kinase G pathway.

In the pathological disorder of epilepsy, repeated seizures can induce neurogenesis in susceptible network sites, causing structural and functional network expansion.[20–25] Although such structural changes can result in increased postsynaptic excitation and increased frequency of network bursts that are detectable in vitro,[26] there is considerable debate on how these newly born neurons and their insertion into the existing circuits contribute to hyperexcitability and epileptogenicity.[27–29] Moreover, neurogenesis results in clear-cut rearrangements of axonal[30,31] and dendritic processes[32–34] as a result of the insults that induce circuit neurodegeneration.[35–37] In general, whether repeated seizure-induced neurogenesis is reactive or compensatory, it tends to be strongly maladaptive. Interestingly, certain anticonvulsant drugs can suppress seizure-induced neurogenesis and restore normal axonal and dendritic processes.[38]

BDNF and other growth factors have been implicated in mechanisms for network expansion in learning as well as in epilepsy induced by seizure repetition.[39–41] Repetitive seizures increase BDNF mRNA and protein expression, and interfering with BDNF signal transduction in vivo inhibits epileptogenesis.[42,43] Expression of tissue-type plasminogen activator (tPA) is also seen in the brain during neuroplasticity, and it is reported to play a role in mediating the progression of kainate-induced seizures, which can be partially blocked with a tPA inhibitor.[44] Another recently described molecular mechanism for plasticity in the central nervous system is the change brought about by altering glutamate receptor subunits through the action of neuronal activity-related pentraxin (NARP). NARP is an immediate early-gene product that is induced by synaptic activity, which is proposed to be an extracellular aggregating factor for AMPARs and is implicated in mossy-fiber sprouting.[45] This mechanism has been reported to convert "silent" glutamatergic synapses to active ones via repeated activation.[46]

Network Expansion of Audiogenic Seizures

Audiogenic seizures (AGS) are generalized convulsive seizures that are induced, by a loud sound, in rodents in which susceptibility can occur genetically or be induced by a large variety of treatments (see Chapter 26). Repetition of AGS (AGS kindling), typically 14 seizures over a 7-day period, results in increases in the duration of seizures and significant alterations of convulsive behaviors in five different forms of AGS in rats.[47–51] In at least four forms of AGS kindling, this process induces expansion of the neuronal network from the brainstem to involve the cortex, amygdala, and hippocampus, but these forebrain structures participate in the neuronal network only after AGS kindling.[47–50,52,53] The changes in convulsive behavior induced by AGS kindling consist of a generalized clonic phase following the tonic phase (post-tonic clonus, or PTC) in the substrain of genetically epilepsy-prone rats (GEPR-9s) that exhibit the most severe AGS form, but they also consist of a different behavior, face and forelimb (F&F) clonus, in GEPR-3s that displayed moderate AGS severity.[50] These AGS kindling-induced behavior changes are quite substrain specific.[54] In the Strasbourg Wistar AGS-susceptible rats, the unkindled seizure behavior involves an episode of wild running followed by a tonic flexion phase, and AGS kindling (10–20 AGS) in this strain results in the emergence of F&F clonus.[55] In the case of the Wistar audiogenic rat (WAR) strain from Brazil, acutely evoked brainstem AGS also evolve to generalized limbic seizures due to AGS kindling[47,56] (details are discussed in this chapter).

Imaging Studies in AGS Kindling

The 2-deoxyglucose (2-DG) technique (see Chapter 3) was used to map the brain regions activated by AGS before and after AGS kindling. In naïve, unkindled Strasbourg Wistar AGS rats, significant increases in 2-DG activity were observed in the amygdala, perirhinal cortex, medial septum, and subthalamic and caudate nuclei as compared to nonepileptic controls. After AGS kindling in these rats, significant increases in 2-DG labeling were seen in the substantia nigra, the hippocampus, the basolateral amygdala, three thalamic nuclei, and the frontal motor and prefrontal cortices.[55] Immunoreactivity for immediate early-gene *c-fos* or the Fos protein has been used to help identify brain regions involved in various brain networks, including the AGS network of the Strasbourg Wistar AGS-susceptible rat strain. In rats that exhibited only sound-evoked wild running, a pattern of *c-fos* was observed similar to that seen resulting from complete AGS, supporting the epileptic nature of this initial behavior. AGS-induced *c-fos* labeling in the Strasbourg Wistar rats was seen in the brainstem auditory nuclei, and after AGS kindling, *c-fos* labeling also appeared in the amygdala and perirhinal cortex, followed by the frontoparietal cortex, the piriform cortex, and finally the hippocampus and entorhinal cortex. *c-fos* expression was no longer detected in these rats 24 h after AGS.[57]

Blockade and Microinjection Studies in AGS Kindling

As noted in the imaging chapters (e.g. Chapters 3 and 6), these methods are indirect measures of brain changes and don't indicate the nature of the involvement of a given brain structure in seizure production or whether the structure may be involved in compensatory mechanisms to limit seizure duration or spread. This is where focal microinjection to temporarily block a structure can then show the nature of the involvement of a structure identified by the imaging methods (Chapter 4). Application of focal blockade to AGS kindling in GEPR-9s showed that expansion of the seizure network from the brainstem into the forebrain structures, including the medial geniculate body (MGB) and amygdala. Focal and functional blockade of these nuclei reversibly blocked cortical epileptiform discharges and induced a temporary return of AGS to the prekindled pattern of convulsive behavior without completely blocking AGS.[49,57,58] AGS kindling in GEPR-3s results in F&F clonus, and this behavior could be blocked following bilateral microinjection of an NMDA antagonist (2-amino-7-phosphonoheptanoate, or AP7) without affecting the prekindling generalized clonus.[59,63] These findings suggest that NMDA receptors may play an important role in the generation of additional seizure behaviors following AGS kindling.

Neuronal-Recording Studies in AGS Kindling

Auditory Network Neuronal-Recording Studies in AGS Kindling

Neuronal responses in the inferior colliculus (IC), which is the consensus site of AGS initiation, during AGS kindling in GEPR-9s underwent modest changes that were observable soon after AGS kindling began.[60] Repeated AGS in GEPR-9s also resulted in reduced $GABA_A$ receptor function in the IC.[61] However, no further increase in IC firing was observed with seizures after day 4 of kindling, despite the fact that extensive increases in AGS kindling-induced seizure severity and PTC duration continued to occur as the kindling proceeded. These findings suggest that changes in IC neuronal excitability did not play a major role in generation of the PTC component of kindled AGS in GEPR-9s. MGB neuronal responses to acoustic stimuli in GEPR-9s were also enhanced during AGS kindling, and these changes were somewhat more extensive and continued to exhibit changes for a longer period during AGS kindling than those in IC.[62] Thus, an elevated number of action potentials was observed in the MGB neuronal responses after AGS kindling in GEPR-9s. This increase of MGB neuronal firing was associated with a reduction of response habituation and an increase in sustained acoustic responses. MGB neurons also exhibited rapid tonic firing during tonic seizures in behaving GEPR-9s, but MGB firing was silent during PTC, a behavior seen in GEPR-9s only after AGS repetition. This finding indicates that MGB, the first major synapse in the auditory network efferent to the IC, does not play a direct role in the generation of this convulsive behavior, and it suggests that mechanistic events in more rostral network nuclei may be more critical in the prolongation of seizure duration and additional seizure behavior (PTC) induced by AGS kindling. The AGS kindling-induced changes involve expansion of the neuronal network to involve the amygdala, which appears to be a major site for kindling-induced mechanistic changes, as discussed in this chapter.

Reticular Formation Neuronal-Firing Changes in AGS Kindling

Although the brainstem reticular formation (BRF) neuronal-firing changes induced by AGS kindling in GEPR-9s have not been evaluated, the changes in BRF firing induced by AGS kindling in GEPR-3s have been studied.[59,63] The pontine BRF also plays a critical part in the neuronal network for AGS in GEPR-9s and GEPR-3s.[59,64] AGS in unkindled GEPR-3s culminate in generalized clonus, but AGS kindling in GEPR-3s results in a different additional seizure behavior, F&F clonus, which is not seen prior to AGS kindling but is seen after kindling in several other AGS models.[48,50,52] After AGS kindling in GEPR-3s, BRF neuronal firing greatly increased. Tonic BRF neuronal firing (relatively high-rate continuous firing) occurred during generalized clonus, and it changed to burst firing (repeated short periods of very rapid firing followed by silent periods) after AGS-kindling (see Chapter 9). Burst firing in BRF neurons also occurred during F&F clonus.[59] Thus, increased neuronal firing and the change from tonic to burst firing suggest that AGS kindling involves increased BRF excitability. These data support an important role for BRF neurons in the generation of both generalized clonus and the F&F clonus induced by AGS kindling in GEPR-3s. Similar changes may also be induced in BRF neurons following AGS kindling in GEPR-9s. The origin of burst firing in BRF neurons may lie within the BRF itself or may result from an altered neuronal excitability in the other brain nuclei in the network that project to the BRF.

Periaqueductal Gray Neuronal-Firing Changes in AGS Kindling

AGS kindling in GEPR-9s also induces changes in periaqueductal gray (PAG) neuronal firing.[65] The PAG is implicated in generalized clonus initiation in unkindled GEPR-9s.[66] A pathway from the amygdala to PAG has been established.[67] PAG neurons in kindled GEPR-9s showed significantly elevated responses to acoustic stimuli at intensities below the threshold for evoking seizures, as compared to unkindled GEPR-9s. During the wild running and tonic hind-limb extension, PAG neurons display tonic firing. Burst firing is seen in the PAG during PTC that coincided temporally with expression of the PTC behavior in kindled GEPR-9s, which was never seen in unkindled GEPR-9s.[68] The presence of burst patterns of neuronal activity in the PAG suggests that neuroplastic changes may be occurring in this brain site or may originate in projections to the PAG, and that may contribute importantly to AGS kindling-associated epileptic network expansion and the emergence of PTC in GEPR-9s (see Chapters 7, 9, 28, and 30).

Amygdala Neuronal-Firing Changes in AGS Kindling

As noted in this chapter, the amygdala is recruited into the AGS neuronal network in GEPR-9s and Strasbourg Wistar AGS-susceptible rats after AGS kindling, as shown by the 2-DG, *c-fos*, and microinjection techniques.[48,54,57,58,69] Single-unit neuronal-firing pattern changes have also been observed in the lateral nucleus of the amygdala (LAMG) of GEPR-9s and GEPR-3s.[70–72] Thus, after AGS kindling in GEPR-9s, extensive synchronization of LAMG neuronal firing and dramatic (>500%) increases in acoustic responsiveness were seen in these neurons.[70] LAMG neurons fired tonically during tonic convulsions and exhibited burst firing during the PTC component of kindled AGS in GEPR-9s. These AGS kindling-induced LAMG neuronal-firing pattern changes appear to be critical mechanisms for mediating the behavioral and electroencephalography (EEG) changes induced by AGS kindling in GEPR-9s. The pathway, projecting the acoustic stimulus into the LAMG, undergoes considerable plasticity as a result of AGS kindling, as shown by increases in the efficacy of the thalamo-amygdala pathway after AGS kindling in GEPR-9s.[71]

Neuronal-recording studies in GEPR-3s have shown a somewhat different pattern from that in GEPR-9s, as might be predicted by the microinjection differences in these different AGS forms, as noted in this chapter. Thus, LAMG neurons in GEPR-3s exhibited only onset-type neuronal responses both before and after AGS kindling, unlike LAMG neurons in normal rats and in GEPR-9s. A significantly greater LAMG neuronal-firing rate occurred after AGS kindling at high acoustic intensities. The latency of LAMG neuronal firing increased significantly after AGS kindling. Burst firing occurred during wild running and generalized clonic behaviors before and after AGS kindling in GEPR-3s. Burst firing also occurred during F&F clonus after AGS kindling. These findings indicate that LAMG neurons play a critical role in the neuronal network for generalized clonus as well as F&F clonus in GEPR-3s, both before and after AGS kindling, which contrasts markedly with the role of LAMG in GEPR-9s.[70,72]

Plasticity in the Amygdala-to-PAG Pathway in AGS Kindling

As noted in the "Periaqueductal Gray" section, pathways from the amygdala to PAG are well documented, and the PTC behavior induced by AGS kindling in GEPR-9s may involve a reentry of AGS activity from the amygdala to PAG, as suggested by recent studies.[73] The pathway between the amygdala and PAG proceeds from input to the LAMG, which projects to the central amygdala (CeA), and the CeA is known to project to several brainstem sites, including the PAG. This amygdala-to-PAG pathway is implicated in several disorders, including pain and anxiety (Chapters 23 and 24), and is also implicated in the AGS network in GEPR-9s in AGS kindling. As noted in this chapter, increases in seizure duration and the emergence of PTC in GEPR-9s involves expansion of the localized brainstem AGS network to include the amygdala, which is a critical site in the expanded network. AGS kindling-induced changes in PAG extracellular action potentials evoked by electrical stimuli in CeA in awake, behaving GEPR-9s were evaluated. Electrical stimuli in CeA evoked consistent, short-latency, and intensity-dependent PAG neuronal-firing increases in unkindled GEPR-9s. However, in AGS-kindled GEPR-9s, these responses showed a precipitous firing increase with increasing stimulus intensity, as compared to unkindled GEPR-9s. These data suggest that neuroplastic changes in the amygdala-to-PAG pathway may be an important epileptogenic mechanism, mediating the emergence of the PTC behavior that is induced by AGS kindling.[73]

Cerebral Cortical Neuronal-Firing Changes in AGS Kindling

Cortical epileptiform activity is induced during AGS kindling in GEPR-9s and GEPR-3s; it is absent prior to AGS kindling.[50] Neuronal changes in the cortex induced by AGS kindling have not been evaluated in GEPR-9s, but perirhinal cortex neuronal-firing changes induced by AGS kindling in GEPR-3s were examined.[74] As noted in the "Network Expansion of Audiogenic Seizures" section, AGS kindling in GEPR-3s induces an additional behavior, F&F clonus, immediately following generalized clonus.[50] Focal bilateral blockade of the perirhinal cortex resulted in complete and reversible blockade of only the F&F clonic seizure behavior in AGS-kindled GEPR-3s, but it did not affect the generalized clonus seen both before and after AGS kindling.[74] Significant increases in perirhinal cortex neuronal responses to acoustic stimuli were also induced by AGS kindling in GEPR-3s.[74] During F&F clonus in GEPR-3s, these cortical neurons exhibited burst firing. These findings support a critical role of the perirhinal cortex in the neuronal network for AGS kindling in GEPR-3s associated with the emergence of epileptiform cortical EEG activity. Furthermore, these findings also suggest that the epileptiform EEG activity seen in the cortex of kindled GEPR-9s may involve neuronal firing changes that are similar to those seen in kindled GEPR-3s.

AGS Kindling-Induced Behavioral, EEG, and Structural Effects in WARs

In WARs, AGS kindling resulted in significant behavioral alterations, transforming the brainstem-driven tonic-clonic seizures to temporal lobe-like limbic seizures.[47,75,76] Those results confirmed and extended data from Marescaux et al.[48] on AGS kindling in Strasbourg audiogenic rats and from Naritoku et al.[50] on AGS kindling in GEPR-3s. In addition to the behavioral alterations in kindled WARs and GEPR-9s, EEG alterations were detected, initially only in the IC, which exhibited synchronous EEG spiking activity before AGS kindling. But as AGS kindling progressed, epileptiform EEG activity was seen in the cortex, amygdala, and hippocampus,[52,76–78] which strongly supports expansion of the brainstem network into the forebrain.

The structural sequelae of AGS kindling in the WARs share similarities with models of temporal lobe epilepsy.[35,37] However, in contrast with the pilocarpine model of temporal lobe epilepsy where both strong mossy-fiber sprouting and neurogenesis were detected,[79,80] AGS kindling in WARs resulted in neurogenesis in the absence of mossy-fiber sprouting.[47,75,76] These findings suggest that mossy-fiber sprouting is not necessary for the development of limbic seizures following AGS kindling in the WARs. Nevertheless, the role of mossy-fiber sprouting in the pathogenesis of limbic epilepsy remains unclear.

Molecular Mechanisms of AGS Kindling

The kindling-induced plasticity in the pathway to the amygdala in GEPR-9s may be due, in part, to an increase in NMDA receptor-mediated neurotransmission, since amygdala neuronal responses to acoustic stimuli are greatly suppressed by systemic administration of an uncompetitive NMDA antagonist.[70] The tonic firing of amygdala neurons observed during AGS in GEPR-9s suggests that the effect of repeated activation on this structure during tonic convulsions may be a key element in expansion of the seizure network induced by AGS kindling, as discussed in this chapter. Neurons in the presumptive input pathway to the amygdala (IC and MGB) showed a much lower degree of firing increase as compared to the amygdala. Therefore, the AGS kindling-induced neuroplastic changes, occurring in circuits of the expanded seizure network that project onto the amygdala, may be the locus of one of the most critical pathophysiological mechanisms subserving the additional seizure behaviors in AGS-kindled GEPR-9s.

AGS kindling and subsequent increased amygdala neuronal firing may initiate permanent pathophysiological alterations in the amygdala itself, in part by enhanced glutamate receptor-mediated excitation, since focal microinjection of NMDA into the amygdala of unkindled GEPR-9s or GEPR-3s induces a transient susceptibility to PTC in GEPR-9s and F&F clonus in GEPR-3s, which mimic AGS-kindling behaviors in both AGS models.[54] When a cyclic adenosine monophosphate (cAMP) activator is microinjected into the amygdala of unkindled GEPR-9s, seizures that mimic AGS kindling are also evocable; however, this effect lasts indefinitely.[81] Conversely, when an NMDA antagonist or inhibitor of cAMP synthesis was microinjected into the amygdala, the effects of AGS kindling were reversed, and the seizure pattern temporarily reverted to that seen prior to AGS kindling.[49,81] These data suggest that AGS kindling alters the expression and/or function of NMDA receptors as well as the phosphorylation state

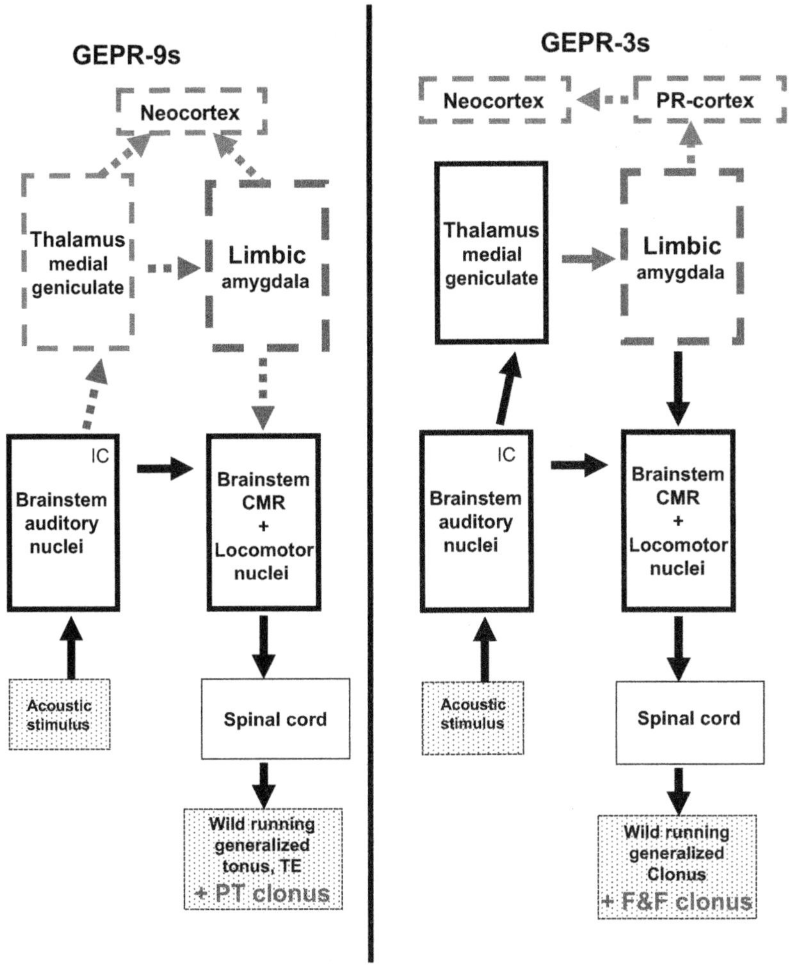

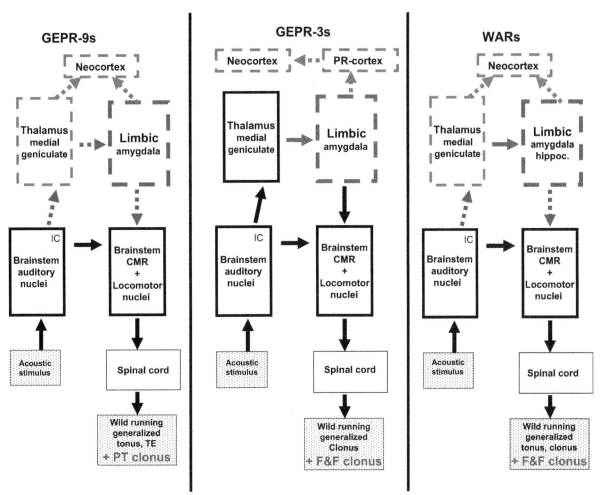

FIGURE 27.3 Comparative network expansion diagrams in three forms of audiogenic seizure kindling. Audiogenic kindling consists of daily or twice-daily audiogenic seizure repetition for 14–21 seizures, typically. The diagram for the severe seizure strain of genetically epilepsy-prone rats (GEPR-9s) is shown in the left panel. Prior to audiogenic kindling, the required network structures are confined to the brainstem, including the brainstem auditory nuclei up to the level of the inferior colliculus (IC), which projects to brainstem conditional multireceptive (CMR) regions, including the brainstem reticular formation (BRF) and periaqueductal gray (PAG), as well as midbrain locomotor network structures. These structures project to the spinal cord, which generates the wild running and tonic seizures, ending in tonic extension (TE) of the hind limbs of GEPR-9s. After audiogenic kindling, the network of GEPR-9s expands to include the medial geniculate body (MGB) of the thalamus, which projects to the limbic system, specifically the amygdala and then to the neocortex. This audiogenic seizure kindling-induced network expansion results in increased seizure duration due to an additional behavior, posttonic generalized clonus (PTC), and this emergent behavior is mediated by the thalamic and limbic structures, since blockade of these sites blocks PTC only. The diagram for the moderate seizure strain of genetically epilepsy-prone rats (GEPR-3s) is shown in the middle panel. Prior to audiogenic kindling, the network of GEPR-3s includes the brainstem auditory nuclei up to the IC, which projects to the brainstem CMR regions as well as midbrain locomotor network structures. The amygdala is also involved in the seizure network of GEPR-3s prior to audiogenic kindling. The brainstem structures project to the spinal cord, which generates the wild running and generalized clonic seizures of GEPR-3s. After audiogenic kindling, the role of the amygdala is increased, and the perirhinal cortex (PR-cortex) also becomes involved and then disseminates more widely to the rest of the neocortex. This audiogenic seizure-induced network expansion results in an increase in seizure duration due to an additional behavior, facial and forelimb (F&F) clonus. The right panel shows the network diagram for Wistar audiogenic rats (WARs). Prior to audiogenic kindling. the network is confined to the brainstem, including the brainstem auditory nuclei up to the level of the inferior colliculus (IC), which projects to the brainstem CMR brain regions and midbrain locomotor network structures. These structures project to the spinal cord, which generates the wild running and tonic seizures, ending in forelimb and hind limb extension of WARs. After audiogenic kindling, the network expands to include limbic sites (the amygdala and hippocampus) and the neocortex. This audiogenic seizure-induced network expansion results in an increase in seizure duration due to the mixing of the brainstem plus limbic seizures (see the text for details). Note: The dashed lines indicate the brain regions that are recruited into the requisite seizure network structures after audiogenic kindling-induced expansion. (For color version of this figure, the reader is referred to the online version of this book.)

of various voltage- and ligand-gated channels, including NMDA receptors within the amygdala. These changes may contribute to the permanent expansion of the neuronal network for AGS kindling in GEPR-9s.

In the WARs, AGS kindling induces increases in the expression of the GLUR2 flip isoform, as well as a down-regulation of the non-protein-coding RNA for BC1 in the hippocampus.[82,83] AGS-kindled WARs also exhibit upregulation of the hippocampal B1 and B2 bradykinin receptors,[84] hippocampal angiotensin 1 (AT1) receptor, and angiotensin-converting enzyme (ACE),[85] and administration of an AT1 receptor blocker or an ACE inhibitor exerted anticonvulsant effects. It is not clear if similar receptor changes occur in the other AGS-kindling models, and further research will be needed to clarify this issue.

Figure 27.3 shows diagrams for network expansion in three forms of AGS kindling. In GEPR-9s (left panel), prior to audiogenic kindling, the required network is confined to the brainstem, including the IC, which projects to brainstem CMR regions and midbrain locomotor pathway (see Chapter 28); these, in turn, project to the spinal cord that generates the wild running and tonic-clonic seizures, ending in tonic extension (TE) of the forelimbs and hind limbs of GEPR-9s. After AGS kindling, the network of GEPR-9s expands to include the MGB, the amygdala, and then the neocortex, based on neuronal-firing changes and epileptiform EEG changes, respectively. This kindling-induced network expansion results in increased seizure duration (PTC), which is mediated by the thalamic and limbic structures. The middle diagram of Figure 27.3 displays the network for AGS in GEPR-3s. Prior to AGS kindling, the network of GEPR-3s includes the brainstem auditory nuclei up to the IC, which projects to brainstem CMR regions and midbrain locomotor network structures, as well as the amygdala, which is presumed to involve the MGB. The brainstem structures project to the spinal cord, which generates the wild running and generalized clonic seizures of GEPR-3s. After AGS kindling, neuronal excitability is increased in the amygdala and the perirhinal cortex and then projects to the rest of the neocortex, based on epileptiform EEG changes. The network expansion results in an increase in seizure duration due to an additional behavior, the F&F clonus. The right panel shows the network diagram for WARs. Similar to the GEPR-9s, prior to audiogenic kindling, the network is confined to the brainstem, including the brainstem auditory nuclei up to the level of the IC, which projects to the brainstem sensorimotor brain regions and midbrain locomotor network structures. EEG and transection studies have shown that dorsal and external IC nuclei and deep layers of the superior colliculus are crucially involved in the sensorimotor integration necessary for the expression of AGS.[86] The sensorimotor structures project to the spinal cord, which generates the wild running and tonic seizures, ending in forelimb and hind limb extension. After AGS kindling, the network expands to include the amygdala, hippocampus, and cortex based on the appearance of epileptiform EEG patterns in these structures.[52,76] AGS kindling-induced network expansion results in an increase in seizure duration due to an additional clonic component, including F&F clonus.[52,77,78]

CONCLUSIONS

The AGS neuronal network in the various AGS models, which is mediated by interaction of the normal auditory network with the normal midbrain locomotor network, undergoes network expansion following repetitive seizures. This expansion involves clear evidence of recruitment of the limbic network in all of the AGS models. In each of these models, the role played by these structures is somewhat different. Thus, the "variations on the theme" seen in the different AGS-kindling models are extensive. The GEPR-9s show a very different behavioral result (the PTC component of kindled AGS) thought to be primarily of brainstem origin, which may be driven by the reentry of seizure activity from the amygdala to the PAG. By contrast, AGS kindling in the other models (GEPR-3s, WARs, and Strasbourg AGS rats) shows a very different form of clonus, F&F clonus, thought to be driven primarily from limbic circuitry via a currently unknown pathway. It is not clear why these circuit differences between AGS models exist, and further research is needed to understand these mechanistic differences. However, there is considerable evidence at the behavioral, electrophysiological, cellular, and molecular levels indicating that there is an interplay between changes in synaptic strength, neurodegeneration, neurogenesis, and synaptogenesis (see Chapter 7), which could explain the complex neuroplastic changes that accompany network expansion in these AGS-kindling models. AGS kindling can be considered an analog of repetitive seizures that occur in many epileptic patients and are known to contribute to negative effects on mood, behavior, and memory as well as long-term cognitive effects. Since the AGS kindling-induced network expansion results in limbic network involvement, this network expansion may provide a model of the neuronal circuitry to explain these behavioral comorbidities in patients. Identification of the specific sites of these network changes may also provide specific therapeutic targets for which drugs can be developed to prevent network expansion, which results in the worsening of these disorders of brain function. Finally, comparison of these similar types of network expansion may shed light on potential general mechanisms of network expansion and also provide evidence about the processes that are involved in network changes. Such changes occur in other brain disorders, such as chronic pain and affective and anxiety disorders, that often undergo increases in the severity of symptoms with repeated episodes of the disorder.

Acknowledgments

We thank Gayle Stauffer and Diana Smith for assistance with the manuscript. Support for P.N. is from NIH/NINDS grant NS047193. Support for N.G.C. is from the Brazilian foundations FAPESP, FAPESP-Cinapce, PROEX-CAPES and CNPq. Support for C.L.F. is from NINDS, Excellence in Academic Medicine, and Southern Illinois University School of Medicine.

References

1. Faingold CL. Electrical stimulation therapies for CNS disorders and pain are mediated by competition between different neuronal networks in the brain. *Med Hypotheses*. 2008;71(5):668–681.
2. Bryden DW, Johnson EE, Diao X, et al. Impact of expected value on neural activity in rat substantia nigra pars reticulata. *Eur J Neurosci*. 2011;33(12):2308–2317.
3. Gulley JM, Kosobud AE, Rebec GV. Amphetamine inhibits behavior-related neuronal responses in substantia nigra pars reticulata of rats working for sucrose reinforcement. *Neurosci Lett*. 2002;322(3):165–168.
4. Gulley JM, Kosobud AE, Rebec GV. Behavior-related modulation of substantia nigra pars reticulata neurons in rats performing a conditioned reinforcement task. *Neuroscience*. 2002;111(2):337–349.
5. Toyomitsu Y, Nishijo H, Uwano T, Kuratsu J, Ono T. Neuronal responses of the rat amygdala during extinction and reassociation learning in elementary and configural associative tasks. *Eur J Neurosci*. 2002;15(4):753–768.
6. Weldon DA, DiNieri JA, Silver MR, Thomas AA, Wright RE. Reward-related neuronal activity in the rat superior colliculus. *Behav Brain Res*. 2007;177(1):160–164.
7. Woody CD, Zotova E, Gruen E. Multiple representations of information in the primary auditory cortex of cats. I. Stability and change in slow components of unit activity after conditioning with a click conditioned stimulus. *Brain Res*. 2000;868(1):56–65.
8. Collingridge GL, Peineau S, Howland JG, Wang YT. Long-term depression in the CNS. *Nat Rev Neurosci*. 2010;11(7):459–473.
9. Glanzman DL. Common mechanisms of synaptic plasticity in vertebrates and invertebrates. *Curr Biol*. 2010;20(1):R31–R36.
10. Zorumski CF, Izumi Y. NMDA receptors and metaplasticity: mechanisms and possible roles in neuropsychiatric disorders. *Neurosci Biobehav Rev*. 2012;36(3):989–1000.
11. Lee HK, Kirkwood A. AMPA receptor regulation during synaptic plasticity in hippocampus and neocortex. *Semin Cell Dev Biol*. 2011;22(5):514–520.
12. Hunt DL, Castillo PE. Synaptic plasticity of NMDA receptors: mechanisms and functional implications. *Curr Opin Neurobiol*. 2012;22(3):496–508.
13. Kerchner GA, Li P, Zhuo M. Speaking out of turn: a role for silent synapses in pain. *IUBMB Life*. 1999;48(3):251–256.
14. Sandkühler J, Gruber-Schoffnegger D. Hyperalgesia by synaptic long-term potentiation (LTP): an update. *Curr Opin Pharmacol*. 2012;12(1):18–27.
15. Calabresi P, Galletti F, Saggese E, Ghiglieri V, Picconi B. Neuronal networks and synaptic plasticity in Parkinson's disease: beyond motor deficits. *Parkinsonism Relat Disord*. 2007;13(Suppl. 3):S259–S262.
16. Kumar A. Long-term potentiation at CA3–CA1 hippocampal synapses with special emphasis on aging, disease, and stress. *Front Aging Neurosci*. 2011;3:7.
17. Beck H, Goussakov IV, Lie A, Helmstaedter C, Elger CE. Synaptic plasticity in the human dentate gyrus. *J Neurosci*. 2000;20(18):7080–7086.
18. Leung LS, Wu C. Kindling suppresses prime-burst-induced long-term potentiation in hippocampal CA1. *Neuroreport*. 2003;14(2):211–214.
19. Maffei A. The many forms and functions of long term plasticity at GABAergic synapses. *Neural Plast*. 2011;2011:254724.
20. Lynch M, Sutula T. Recurrent excitatory connectivity in the dentate gyrus of kindled and kainic acid-treated rats. *J Neurophysiol*. 2000;83(2):693–704.
21. Lynch M, Sayin U, Bownds J, Janumpalli S, Sutula T. Long-term consequences of early postnatal seizures on hippocampal learning and plasticity. *Eur J Neurosci*. 2000;12(7):2252–2264.
22. Lynch M, Sayin U, Golarai G, Sutula T. NMDA receptor-dependent plasticity of granule cell spiking in the dentate gyrus of normal and epileptic rats. *J Neurophysiol*. 2000;84(6):2868–2879.
23. Parent JM, Lowenstein DH. Seizure-induced neurogenesis: are more new neurons good for an adult brain? *Prog Brain Res*. 2002;135:121–131.
24. Radley JJ, Jacobs BL. Pilocarpine-induced status epilepticus increases cell proliferation in the dentate gyrus of adult rats via a 5-HT_{1A} receptor-dependent mechanism. *Brain Res*. 2003;966(1):1–12.
25. Ribak CE, Dashtipour K. Neuroplasticity in the damaged dentate gyrus of the epileptic brain. *Prog Brain Res*. 2002;136:319–328.
26. Smith BN, Dudek FE. Network interactions mediated by new excitatory connections between CA1 pyramidal cells in rats with kainate-induced epilepsy. *J Neurophysiol*. 2002;87(3):1655–1658.
27. Murphy BL, Danzer SC. Somatic translocation: a novel mechanism of granule cell dendritic dysmorphogenesis and dispersion. *J Neurosci*. 2011;31(8):2959–2964.
28. Murphy BL, Pun RY, Yin H, Faulkner CR, Loepke AW, Danzer SC. Heterogeneous integration of adult-generated granule cells into the epileptic brain. *J Neurosci*. 2011;31(1):105–117.
29. Parent JM, Yu TW, Leibowitz RT, Geschwind DH, Sloviter RS, Lowenstein DH. Dentate granule cell neurogenesis is increased by seizures and contributes to aberrant network reorganization in the adult rat hippocampus. *J Neurosci*. 1997;17(10):3727–3738.
30. Nadler JV. The recurrent mossy fiber pathway of the epileptic brain. *Neurochem Res*. 2003;28(11):1649–1658.
31. Sutula T, Zhang P, Lynch M, Sayin U, Golarai G, Rod R. Synaptic and axonal remodeling of mossy fibers in the hilus and supragranular region of the dentate gyrus in kainate-treated rats. *J Comp Neurol*. 1998;390(4):578–594.
32. Arisi GM, Garcia-Cairasco N. Doublecortin-positive newly born granule cells of hippocampus have abnormal apical dendritic morphology in the pilocarpine model of temporal lobe epilepsy. *Brain Res*. 2007;1165:126–134.
33. Santos VR, de Castro OW, Pun RY, et al. Contributions of mature granule cells to structural plasticity in temporal lobe epilepsy. *Neuroscience*. 2011;197:348–573.
34. Shapiro LA, Ribak CE. Newly born dentate granule neurons after pilocarpine-induced epilepsy have hilar basal dendrites with immature synapses. *Epilepsy Res*. 2006;69(1):53–66.

35. Castro OW, Furtado MA, Tilelli CQ, Fernandes A, Pajolla GP, Garcia-Cairasco N. Comparative neuroanatomical and temporal characterization of FluoroJade-positive neurodegeneration after status epilepticus induced by systemic and intra-hippocampal pilocarpine in Wistar rats. *Brain Res.* 2011;1374:43–55.
36. Schmued LC, Albertson C, Slikker W. Fluoro-Jade: a novel fluorochrome for the sensitive and reliable histochemical localization of neuronal degeneration. *Brain Res.* 1997;751:37–46.
37. Turski L, Cavalheiro EA, Czuczwar SJ, Turski WA, Kleinrok Z. The seizures induced by pilocarpine: behavioral, electroencephalographic and neuropathological studies in rodents. *Pol J Pharmacol Pharm.* 1987;39:545–555.
38. Jessberger S, Nakashima K, Clemenson Jr GD, et al. Epigenetic modulation of seizure-induced neurogenesis and cognitive decline. *J Neurosci.* 2007;27(22):5967–5975.
39. Binder DK, Croll SD, Gall CM, Scharfman HE. BDNF and epilepsy: too much of a good thing? *Trends Neurosci.* 2001;24(1):47–53.
40. Meis S, Endres T, Lessmann V. Postsynaptic BDNF signaling regulates long-term potentiation at thalamo-amygdala afferents. *J Physiol.* 2012;590(Pt 1):193–208.
41. Ou LC, Yeh SH, Gean PW. Late expression of brain-derived neurotrophic factor in the amygdala is required for persistence of fear memory. *Neurobiol Learn Mem.* 2010;93(3):372–382.
42. Elmer E, Kokaia Z, Kokaia M, Carnahan J, Nawa H, Lindvall O. Dynamic change of brain derived neurotrophic factor protein levels in rat forebrain after single and recurring kindling-induced seizures. *Neuroscience.* 1998;83(2):351–362.
43. Kokaia M, Ernfors K, Kokaia Z, Elmer E, Jaenisch R, Lindvall O. Suppressed epileptogenesis in BNF mutant mice. *Exp Neurol.* 1995;133(2):215–224.
44. Yepes M, Sandkvist M, Coleman TA, et al. Regulation of seizure spreading by neuroserpin and tissue-type plasmi nogen activator is plasminogen-independent. *J Clin Invest.* 2002;109(12):1571–1578.
45. Reti IM, Reddy R, Worley PF, Baraban JM. Selective expression of Narp, a secreted neuronal pentraxin, in orexin neurons. *J Neurochem.* 2002;82(6):1561–1565.
46. Li SY, Xu DS, Jia HT. AGS-induced expression of Narp is concomitant with expression of AMPA receptor subunits GluR1 and GluR2 in hippocampus but not inferior colliculus of P77PMC rats. *Neurobiol Dis.* 2003;14(3):328–335.
47. Garcia-Cairasco N, Wakamatsu H, Oliveira JAC, Gomes L, Del-Bel EA, Mello LE. Neuroethological and morphological (NEO-TIMM staining) correlates of limbic recruitment during the development of audiogenic kindling in seizure susceptible Wistar rats. *Epilepsy Res.* 1996;26(1):177–192.
48. Marescaux C, Vergnes M, Kiesmann M, Depaulis A, Micheletti G, Warter JM. Kindling of audiogenic seizures in Wistar rats: an EEG study. *Exp Neurol.* 1987;97(1):160–168.
49. Naritoku D, Randall ME, Faingold CL. Microinfusion of GABA agonists and 2-APH into the amygdala reduce seizure duration and clonus in repeated audiogenic seizures of the genetically epilepsy-prone rat. *Epilepsia.* 1989;30(5):698.
50. Naritoku DK, Mecozzi LB, Aiello MT, Faingold CL. Repetition of audiogenic seizures in genetically epilepsy-prone rats induces cortical epileptiform activity and additional seizure behaviors. *Exp Neurol.* 1992;115:317–324.
51. Vinogradova LV, van Rijn CM. Anticonvulsive and antiepileptogenic effects of levetiracetam in the audiogenic kindling model. *Epilepsia.* 2008;49(7):1160–1168.
52. Dutra Moraes MF, Galvis-Alonso OY, Garcia-Cairasco N. Audiogenic kindling in the Wistar rat: a potential model for recruitment of limbic structures. *Epilepsy Res.* 2000;39(3):251–259.
53. Garcia-Cairasco N. A critical review on the participation of inferior colliculus in acoustic-motor and acoustic-limbic networks involved in the expression of acute and kindled audiogenic seizures. *Hear Res.* 2002;168(1–2):208–222.
54. Raisinghani M, Feng HJ, Faingold CL. Glutamatergic activation of the amygdala differentially mimics the effects of audiogenic seizure kindling in two sub-strains of genetically epilepsy-prone rats. *Exp Neurol.* 2003;183(2):516–522.
55. Pereira de Vasconcelos A, Vergnes M, Boyet S, Marescaux C, Nehlig A. Forebrain metabolic activation induced by the repetition of audiogenic seizures in Wistar rats. *Brain Res.* 1997;762(1–2):114–120.
56. Doretto MC, Fonseca CG, Lobo RB, Terra VC, Oliveira JAC, Garcia-Cairasco N. Quantitative study of the response to genetic selection of the Wistar audiogenic rat strain (WAR). *Behav Genet.* 2003;33(1):33–41.
57. Hirsch E, Danober L, Simler S, et al. The amygdala is critical for seizure propagation from brainstem to forebrain. *Neuroscience.* 1997;77(4):975–984.
58. Feng HJ, Naritoku DK, Randall ME, Faingold CL. Modulation of audiogenically kindled seizures by gamma-aminobutyric acid-related mechanisms in the amygdala. *Exp Neurol.* 2001;172:477–481.
59. Raisinghani M, Faingold CL. Pontine reticular formation neurons are implicated in the neuronal network for generalized clonic seizures which is intensified by audiogenic kindling. *Brain Res.* 2005;1064:90–97.
60. N'Gouemo P, Faingold CL. Repetitive audiogenic seizures cause an increased acoustic response in inferior colliculus neurons and additional convulsive behaviors in the genetically-epilepsy prone rat. *Brain Res.* 1996;710(1–2):92–96.
61. Evans MS, Cady CJ, Disney KE, Yang L, Laguardia JJ. Three brief epileptic seizures reduce inhibitory synaptic currents, $GABA_A$ currents, and $GABA_A$-receptor subunits. *Epilepsia.* 2006;47(10):1655–1664.
62. N'Gouemo P, Faingold CL. Audiogenic kindling increases neuronal responses to acoustic stimuli in neurons of the medial geniculate body of the genetically epilepsy-prone rat. *Brain Res.* 1997;761:217–224.
63. Raisinghani M, Faingold CL. Identification of the requisite brain sites in the neuronal network subserving generalized clonic audiogenic seizures. *Brain Res.* 2003;967(1–2):113–122.
64. Faingold CL, Randall ME. Pontine reticular formation neurons exhibit a premature and precipitous increase in acoustic responses prior to audiogenic seizures in genetically epilepsy-prone rats. *Brain Res.* 1995;704(2):218–226.
65. Tupal S, Faingold CL. Precipitous induction of audiogenic kindling by activation of adenylyl cyclase in the amygdala. *Epilepsia.* 2010;51(3):354–361.
66. N'Gouemo P, Faingold CL. Periaqueductal gray neurons exhibit increased responsiveness associated with audiogenic seizures in the genetically epilepsy-prone rat. *Neuroscience.* 1998;84:619–625.
67. da Costa Gomez TM, Behbehani NM. An electrophysiological characterization of the projection from the central nucleus of the amygdala to the periaqueductal gray of the rat: the role of opioid receptors. *Brain Res.* 1995;689:21–31.
68. Tupal S, Faingold CL. Audiogenic kindling induces plastic changes in the neuronal firing patterns in periaqueductal gray. *Brain Res.* 2011;1377:60–66.
69. Simler S, Vergnes M, Marescaux C. Spatial and temporal relationships between C-Fos expression and kindling of audiogenic seizures in Wistar rats. *Exp Neurol.* 1999;157:106–119.
70. Feng HJ, Faingold CL. Repeated generalized audiogenic seizures induce plastic changes on acoustically evoked neuronal firing in the amygdala. *Brain Res.* 2002;932(1–2):61–69.

71. Feng HJ, Faingold CL. Synaptic plasticity in the pathway from the medial geniculate body to the lateral amygdala is induced by seizure repetition. *Brain Res.* 2002;946:198–205.
72. Raisinghani M, Faingold CL. Neurons in the amygdala play an important role in the neuronal network mediating a clonic form of audiogenic seizures both before and after audiogenic kindling. *Brain Res.* 2005;1032(1–2):131–140.
73. Tupal S, Faingold CL. The amygdala to periaqueductal gray pathway: plastic changes induced by audiogenic kindling and reversal by gabapentin. *Brain Res.* 2012;1475:71–79.
74. Raisinghani M, Faingold CL. Evidence for the perirhinal cortex as a requisite component in the seizure network following seizure repetition in an inherited form of generalized clonic seizures. *Brain Res.* 2005;1048(1–2):193–201.
75. Galvis-Alonso OY, Oliveira JAC, Garcia-Cairasco N. Limbic epileptogenicity, cell loss and axonal reorganization induced by audiogenic and amygdala kindling in Wistar audiogenic rats (WAR strain). *Neuroscience.* 2004;3:787–802.
76. Romcy-Pereira RN, Garcia-Cairasco N. Hippocampal cell proliferation and epileptogenesis after audiogenic kindling are not accompanied by Mossy fiber sprouting or Fluoro-Jade staining. *Neuroscience.* 2003;119:533–546.
77. Moraes MFD, Chavali M, Jobe PC, Garcia-Cairasco N. A comprehensive electrographic and behavior analysis of generalized tonic-clonic seizures of GEPR-9s. *Brain Res.* 2005;1033:1–12.
78. Moraes MFD, Mishra PK, Jobe PC, Garcia-Cairasco N. An electrographic analysis of the synchronous discharge patterns of GEPR-9s generalized seizures. *Brain Res.* 2005;1046:1–9.
79. Furtado MA, Braga GK, Oliveira JAC, Vecchio FD, Garcia-Cairasco N. Behavioral, morphologic and electroencephalographic evaluation of seizures induced by intrahippocampal microinjections of pilocarpine. *Epilepsia (Copenhagen).* 2002;43(Suppl. 5):37–39.
80. Leite JP, Garcia-Cairasco N, Cavalheiro EA. New insights from the use of pilocarpine and kainate models. *Epilepsy Res.* 2002;50(1–2):93–103.
81. Tupal S, Faingold CL. Inhibition of adenylyl cyclase in amygdala blocks the effect of audiogenic seizure kindling in genetically epilepsy-prone rats. *Neuropharmacology.* 2010;59(1–2):107–111.
82. Gitaí DLG, Martinelli HN, Valente V, et al. Increased expression of GLUR2-flip in the hippocampus of the Wistar audiogenic rat strain after acute and kindled seizures. *Hippocampus.* 2010;19:413–506.
83. Gitaí DLG, Fachin AL, Mello SS, et al. The non-coding RNA BC1 is down-regulated in the hippocampus of Wistar audiogenic rat (WAR) strain after audiogenic kindling. *Brain Res.* 2011;1367:114–121.
84. Pereira MGAG, Gitaí DLG, Paçó-Larson ML, Pesquero JB, Garcia-Cairasco N, Costa Neto CM. Modulation of B_1 and B_2 kinin receptors expression levels in the hippocampus of rats after audiogenic kindling and with limbic recruitment, a model of temporal lobe epilepsy. *Int Immunopharmacol.* 2008;8:200–205.
85. Pereira MGAG, Becari C, Oliveira JAC, Salgado MC, Garcia-Cairasco N, Costa Neto CM. Inhibition of the renin angiotensin system prevents seizures in a rat model of epilepsy. *Clin Sci.* 2010;119(11):477–482.
86. Doretto MC, Cortes-de-Oliveira JA, Rossetti F, Garcia-Cairasco N. Role of the superior colliculus in the expression of acute and kindled audiogenic seizures in Wistar audiogenic rats. *Epilepsia.* 2009;50(12):2563–2574.

CHAPTER

28

Neuronal Network Plasticity and Network Interactions are Critically Dependent on Conditional Multireceptive (CMR) Brain Regions

Carl L. Faingold[1], *Awais Riaz*[2], *James D. Stittsworth, Jr.*[3]

[1]Departments of Pharmacology and Neurology, and Division of Neurosurgery, Southern Illinois University School of Medicine, Springfield, IL, USA, [2]Department of Neurology, University of Utah School of Medicine, Salt Lake City, UT, USA, [3]Florida State College at Jacksonville, Kent Campus, Jacksonville, FL, USA

INTRODUCTION

Many of the chapters in this volume clearly indicate that neuronal networks are the critical elements in control of normal brain function. Other chapters have shown that neuronal network alterations are also critical to central nervous system (CNS) disorders. Knowledge of the nature of these network alterations is the key to devising effective therapies for these CNS disorders (Chapters 31 and 32). As noted in Chapter 1, one of the major important ways that networks are initially identified is through the use of imaging techniques (Chapters 3 and 6). It should be noted, however, that these imaging techniques do not necessarily indicate the nature of functional changes, since both active excitation and active inhibition will result in blood flow increases. In addition, episodic neuronal firing patterns, such as the critically significant burst-firing patterns (Chapter 9), often cannot be detected by techniques such as functional magnetic resonance imaging (fMRI) because of temporal resolution limitations (Chapter 6). In humans in particular, these approaches can also rarely identify differential roles of specific subnuclei within a major brain structure because of spatial resolution limitations. Detailed investigations of the differential roles of these subnuclei in the function of a brain structure in specific networks are being evaluated by using invasive techniques, primarily in animals. Thus, for example, the role of the amygdala in fear conditioning (Chapter 13) has been evaluated, including differential roles played by specific amygdala subnuclei in this learning paradigm in rats. However, the role of the amygdala in pain networks is much less well understood. For vital functions, such as nociception, the involvement of amygdala subnuclei is difficult to differentiate, especially in human imaging studies,[1] and will also require further investigation in animal models.

A number of neuronal networks exhibit a high degree of both short-term and long-term neuroplasticity, which greatly complicates their identification and study. Neuroplasticity is also a critical process in the formation, control, and early development of neuronal networks. The development of many normal networks, including the locomotor network that occurs in altricial animals, which are unable to walk at birth and must learn this behavior, involves neuroplasticity that underlies this learning.[2] This is in contrast to precocial animals, which are born with locomotor ability shortly after birth.[3,4] CNS lesions that affect locomotion can cause the network to relearn this behavior if sufficient neuroplasticity remains in the neurons in the pathway.[5]

One of the major sources of CNS neuroplasticity is network nuclei, which we have termed conditional multireceptive (CMR) nuclei.[6] These CMR regions contain a large percentage of CMR neurons that respond in highly variable ways and exhibit extensive short-term and long-term experience-induced changes. The CMR neuronal responses are highly dependent on

Neuronal Networks in Brain Function, CNS Disorders, and Therapeutics
http://dx.doi.org/10.1016/B978-0-12-415804-7.00028-9

the conditions being experienced by the organism. Conditions that have major impact on the firing and responsiveness pattern of CMR neurons include external environmental factors, such as salient or exigent (potentially life-threatening) events, and internal factors, such as the state of vigilance. When the intact organism is experiencing resting (nonexigent) conditions, many CMR neurons and regions are in a state of negative nonlinearity with minimal neuronal responsiveness induced by input repetition (Figure 28.1). A prominent form of negative nonlinearity is discussed in this chapter under the topic of response habituation. However, under exigent conditions when the organism is experiencing a behaviorally imperative perturbation,

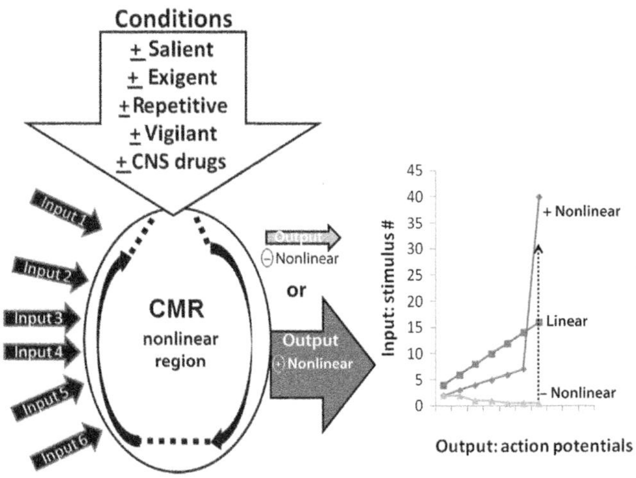

FIGURE 28.1 Input–output relationships of a prototypical conditional multireceptive (CMR) brain region, which is capable of a significant degree of self-organization, as shown by the paired semicircular arrows. This diagram illustrates the numerous inputs that the neurons in this CMR region receive from primary networks and other CMR networks. The output of neurons in the CMR nuclei is highly dependent on the conditions that the animal is experiencing, including salient, exigent, and repetitive conditions, and can also be governed by the animal's state of vigilance as well as centrally acting pharmacological agents. The output of CMR regions is subject to nonlinearity wherein CMR neuronal responsiveness to any input can change dramatically from nonresponsiveness to hyperresponsiveness, depending on the stimulus parameter type, strength, and repetition rate, as illustrated in the graph on the right. Under nonexigent (resting) conditions, many CMR neurons exhibit negative (−) nonlinearity with minimal responsiveness or even nonresponsiveness to the input, as seen in neurons that exhibit response habituation. The various exigent conditions can cause CMR neurons to exhibit hyperresponsiveness and exhibit positive (+) nonlinearity, which can result in massive output, activating the self-organization characteristics of the CMR network, and result in emergent properties of that network that range, for example, from startle responses to generalized seizures. CMR neurons that exhibit negative nonlinearity under resting conditions can convert to positive nonlinearity in response to exigent changes in the animal's behavioral state (dotted line). The nonlinear output characteristics of CMR brain regions contrast with the relatively linear responses seen in primary networks, such as sensory systems. (For color version of this figure, the reader is referred to the online version of this book.)

including appetitive, rewarding, aversive, painful, or fear-inducing conditions, the negative nonlinearity of CMR neurons and regions can reverse and become positive nonlinearity. In the latter situations, the output will be elevated considerably beyond that which is linearly related to the input. Thus, under exigent conditions, these CMR regions are a major source of positive nonlinearity in brain networks, which can lead to the expression of emergent properties at the mesoscopic (middle) level of brain function[7,8] (Chapter 30). An example of this positive nonlinearity occurs during the startle response, also discussed in this chapter.

As shown diagrammatically in Figure 28.1, regions high in CMR neurons receive a wide array of inputs from many primary networks and other CMR networks. A key feature of CMR neurons is that their responsiveness is highly dependent on the conditions that the animal is experiencing, such as potentially threatening or rewarding external environmental events. CMR neuronal responsiveness is also affected by conditions within the internal environment, including the state of vigilance and wake-sleep states, and is also greatly affected by circadian rhythms and CNS drugs (Chapters 14, 21, 22, and 32). Thus, CMR neuronal responsiveness to any given stimulus modality can change dramatically, depending on the stimulus parameter type, strength, and repetition rate. The extreme differences in CMR neuronal firing can range from nonresponsiveness to hyperresponsiveness. In the hyperresponsive mode, highly positive nonlinear outputs can occur, involving self-organization and resulting in emergent properties of the networks, which range from simple sensorimotor integration, as in the startle response, to the extreme of generalized convulsive seizures. This can be visualized in the graph in Figure 28.1 (right panel), which is a simplified illustration of the types of input–output relationships that occur in different brain neurons. A relatively linear pattern is often seen in primary sensory neurons in which the output, at least at physiological repetition rates, is often a linear function of the input within certain ranges. In CMR neurons, both negative and positive nonlinearity can occur. Negative nonlinearity is seen often in CMR neurons in which the neuron responds the first few times that a stimulus is presented but soon fails to respond or responds poorly or sporadically, as discussed in the "Habituation and Novelty" section. CMR neurons can also exhibit positive linearity, in which the output greatly exceeds the input. CMR neurons that initially exhibit negative nonlinearity can convert to positive nonlinearity due to a change in the conditions that the animal is experiencing.

CNS regions that contain a high proportion of CMR neurons include the brainstem reticular formation (BRF), periaqueductal gray (PAG), hippocampus, amygdala, cerebellum, and cortical association areas.[9–14]

These different CMR regions exhibit varying degrees of the CMR property and can respond differentially to environmental and internal conditions. Neurons that exhibit CMR properties are also seen in the spinal cord (see Chapter 17). Although most brain regions, including the primary sensory nuclei, such as the inferior colliculus (IC) (auditory network) and lateral geniculate body (visual network), contain some CMR neurons, these structures contain a considerably lower proportion of such neurons.[6] The prototypical CMR region we will emphasize is the BRF, which has been broadly defined as the tegmentum or netlike central core of the brainstem in the medulla, pons, and midbrain.[15] A previous functionally based term that included the BRF is the "ascending reticular activating system" (ARAS)[15] (Chapters 21 and 22). However, because of the complex neuroanatomical and physiological nature of the BRF, a prominent neuroanatomist once stated that this acronym actually stood for the "asinine ridiculously aggravating system" (Cowan WM, public communication, 1978). Computational approaches to the BRF, using graph-theoretic analysis, discussed in Chapter 1, have observed that the medial BRF is "configured" as a small-world network, which implies that this network possesses coherent rapid-processing capabilities, but it is not a scale-free network.[16]

Another important CMR region that is discussed here is the midbrain PAG, which is the central gray columns of neurons that surround the cerebral aqueduct. We will also consider the amygdala as a prototypical forebrain (limbic) CMR structure. The amygdala is an almond-shaped structure deep in the temporal lobe of the brain. As neuroscience research on these structures has advanced, subdivisions of these nuclei have been defined anatomically with different neurotransmitters and physiologies. However, for the overview purposes of this chapter, we will not emphasize these subdivisions. These three CMR structures will be used as exemplars in the remainder of the chapter. Other areas of the brain, including nuclei in primary sensory or motor nuclei, contain a much smaller percentage of CMR neurons, and these areas also show much smaller degrees of neuroplasticity, as discussed in this chapter.

The extensive response variability of neurons in CMR regions confers the capability for these neurons to exhibit extensively enhanced responses to multiple sources of external input. Thus, the responses of CMR regions to input from neuronal networks that mediate CNS disorders may result in recruitment of those regions into an expanded disease network that mediates this disorder (e.g. References 17,18, and see Chapter 27). In contrast, the same CMR region may also become responsive to externally controlled therapeutic stimulation, becoming a functional part of a therapeutic network that was previously dormant. This "newly" activated network is proposed to compete with the network that mediates the brain disorder for "control" of an overlapping population of CMR neurons, as discussed in this chapter (and see Chapter 31).

Several of the networks in other chapters have a "dedicated" function (Chapters 17–20) and consist largely of well-defined "primary" pathways. These primary networks interact with other networks (Chapter 29), but their main function is to help the organism breathe, hear, see, or move. CMR regions are generally considered to be "secondary" (or nonspecific) pathways that interact with the primary pathways, often in unpredictable ways. Under certain conditions, connections from other nuclei to CMR nuclei can activate dormant CMR networks that are not dedicated to a single function but have the ability to become involved in many different functions, due to their extensive interactions with other networks' primary and secondary pathways (see Chapter 29). These "nondedicated" CMR networks are harder to study for several reasons, including the sensitivity of CMR neurons to anesthetic drugs, and have been investigated to a much lesser degree than the dedicated ones.[6] The studies that have been performed on neurons in these networks reveal a rich complexity of response patterns and a high degree of both long- and short-term neuroplasticity.

As noted in this chapter, CMR brain regions are postulated to be very susceptible to being recruited into networks that mediate CNS disorders as well as networks that are activated by stimulation therapies (Chapter 31). This recruitability is due, in part, to the fact that the CMR neurons exhibit relatively weak, often subthreshold, responses to many inputs. Although CMR neurons in different brain regions share many characteristics, specific CMR regions appear to be involved in different aspects of brain function and are generally, though not exclusively, involved differentially in long-term versus short-term plasticity. Thus, CMR neurons in the BRF, which is strongly implicated in arousal, alertness, and response to salient conditions, such as startle responses, show a great degree of short-term plastic changes. CMR neurons in the PAG are associated largely with nociception-related events, including pain syndromes, while CMR neurons in the amygdala are associated with emotional states, such as mood disorders. However, these CMR neurons, because of their extensive highly variable response characteristics and diverse connections, have the potential to engage in both long-term and short-term neuroplasticity that can mediate interactions with other networks. In certain circumstances, these CMR regions can work together in even larger neuronal networks to play a major role in the genesis of certain CNS disorders, such as epilepsy (Chapter 27). These CMR network interactions also have the potential to become involved in therapy for these disorders, such as chronic pain therapies (Chapter 31). The BRF exhibits a high degree of neuroplastic change on a short-term basis, and the amygdala exhibits a high degree of neuroplastic change on a long-term basis. It has been suggested that the acute effects of the therapeutic stimulation paradigms may be due to activation of these short-term plastic CMR regions, while the effects of chronic stimulation therapies may be due to activation of CMR sites that exhibit a high degree of long-term plasticity[6] (Chapter 31).

Likewise, the development of CNS disorders in many cases, such as epilepsy, involves neuroplasticity of a pathological nature. Therapeutic stimulation paradigms for CNS disorders can also involve neuroplastic processes, as discussed in Chapter 31. Similarly, emergent properties of these CNS disorder networks induced via neuroplasticity are also the target of network-modifying drugs, such as anticonvulsants[19] (Chapter 32).

COMMON CHARACTERISTICS OF CMR NEURONS

Both long-term and short-term plastic changes can occur in CMR neurons. Short-term plasticity of the responses to external stimulation is a cardinal but often ignored feature of many CMR neurons, particularly in the BRF, although this can occur in a small minority of primary neurons as well. However, the incidence and degree of short-term plasticity in these primary neurons are significantly lower.[9,10,20–23]

Multisensory Responsiveness

Many of the neurons in CMR regions are responsive to stimuli in multiple modalities, including all sensory modalities in CMR neurons in the BRF. For example, in awake, behaving animals, multireceptive neurons are observed in the ventromedial medullary BRF, which respond to light touch and thermal noxious stimuli and auditory stimuli, and these neurons are thought to play a role in pain perception.[24] The majority of neurons in BRF sites, including several nuclei in the medulla, respond to more than one of the five inputs tested, including stimulation of the peripheral nerves, as well as somatic, auditory, and visual stimuli under chloralose anesthesia.[25] The responsiveness of these neurons may have been enhanced by this anesthetic, since it shares response enhancement properties with gamma-aminobutyric acid A ($GABA_A$) antagonists (see Reference 9), as discussed further in this chapter. However, many BRF neurons respond to multiple sensory inputs in the unanesthetized condition as well.[26–28] Amygdala neurons also respond to visual, auditory, and somatosensory stimuli.[29–35] PAG neurons respond to auditory and somatosensory stimuli as well.[36,37] Thus, these CMR neurons exhibit sensory convergence, which indicates that many of these CMR regions have connections to multiple primary sensory networks as well as other CMR networks. CMR neurons also send synaptic inputs to a whole host of other neuronal networks, which has important functional significance in the interaction of brain networks that occurs in normal functions and CNS disorders (Chapter 29). CMR neuronal responsiveness has been observed in several vertebrate and invertebrate species, as well.

Sensorimotor Integration

Neurons in many CMR regions are also involved in sensorimotor processes, as might be expected from the multiple connectivity of CMR neurons described here.[38,39] Thus, in addition to receiving many inputs, CMR regions also project to a number of other networks, including networks with motor functions.[40,41] Some CMR neurons in the BRF also exert motor functions. The reticulospinal tract has long been known to play a critical role in the initiation and control of locomotion via its extensive connections to spinal cord motor neurons (see Chapter 17). Descending axons from the BRF are the largest contingent of all descending axons and mediate a large percentage of motor function in mammals and other vertebrates.[40–42] BRF neurons in the pons are known to respond to auditory stimuli as well as provide output to vocalization muscles, and they may mediate audio-vocal sensorimotor integration.[43] Human functional imaging has provided evidence for hierarchical function of the network for postural control involving the "locomotor regions" in the midbrain and other brain regions. These regions initiate or modulate spinal stepping in animals that involves signals, which are transmitted from the midbrain to the spinal cord via the ponto-medullary BRF, with multisensory integration at several different levels (see Chapter 17).[44,45]

Salience

Salience is used to describe events or conditions, ranging from novelty to startle and fear to pain, that are important to the survival and well-being of the organism. An exigent condition is the most intense degree of salience during which the organism may experience a potentially existential threat. Salience can determine whether and to what extent a CMR neuron will respond and is a major source of short-term plasticity (e.g. References 46,47). Salience can be augmented by behavioral or pharmacological means. Behaviorally based salience is most easily seen in the case of a painful stimulus.

Another example of acute network alteration is seen with the acoustic startle response.[48] Pharmacologically, the administration of a drug that blocks GABAergic inhibition and brings the organism into a preseizure state can result in increased salience, as shown by neuronal response changes that occur under these conditions.[6] The ability to distinguish novel from familiar stimuli allows the brain to rapidly encode significant events following even a single exposure to a stimulus. This is often vital to the survival or well-being, and is thought to be important for many types of learning, which can greatly modify CMR neuronal responses. For example, saliency is proposed to be coded by neuronal (burst) firing in CMR neurons in the amygdala.[49]

Habituation and Novelty

A common feature of CMR neurons is the attenuation of responsiveness with stimulus repetition, called "habituation", which contributes to the variability of neuronal firing that is one of the hallmarks of CMR neurons. Habituation is a form of short-term neuroplasticity that can be viewed as a response to a novel stimulus that diminishes as the stimulus becomes less novel. As has been long known, the first time an organism experiences a stimulus in a given time period it is relatively novel, but when the stimulus is presented repeatedly it often loses its novelty and rarely evokes an action potential in neurons in many CMR regions, including the BRF, PAG, and amygdala.[50–55]

Thus, as shown by the example in Figure 28.2 (top panel), at a relatively slow repetition (0.5 Hz) rate, the acoustic stimulus-evoked firing in this CMR neuron in the BRF increased with increasing stimulus intensity. However, when the rate of stimulus repetition was increased, this neuron showed a decline in firing and was minimally responsive at the highest repetition rate, which in this case was 2 Hz. This is in stark contrast to most neurons in the brainstem nuclei of the primary auditory network, which respond quite consistently and do not show habituation at the 2 Hz repetition rate (e.g. Reference 57). Although habituation also occurs in primary neurons, the repetition rates at which this happens are much lower in CMR neurons than in primary neurons. This feature allows primary neurons to convey information with greater fidelity, while the CMR neurons detect novelty or lack thereof. The example in Figure 28.2 (top panel) also shows another aspect of CMR neuronal responsiveness, the lack of response to low-intensity stimuli; in this example from the BRF, responsiveness did not begin until relatively high-intensity stimuli were presented. This lack of response at low-stimulus intensities in CMR neurons is also a major contrast with the responsiveness seen commonly in primary auditory network neurons (e.g. Reference 57).

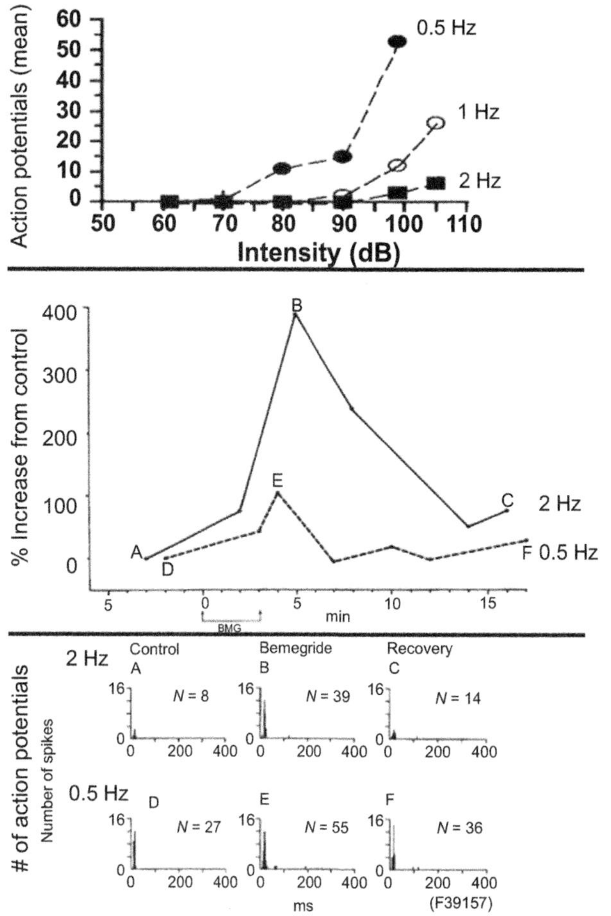

FIGURE 28.2 Top panel: Typical example of the BRF (pontine) neuronal response attenuation (habituation) produced by increasing the repetition rate of an acoustic stimulus (100 ms, 12 kHz tone burst) in a normal (Sprague–Dawley) awake, behaving rat. The BRF neuronal firing was decreased to less than 50% of the 0.5 Hz rate (closed circles) at both 1 Hz (open circles) and 2 Hz (square symbols). Bottom panels: Example of enhanced responsiveness induced by a $GABA_A$ receptor antagonist (bemegride, or BMG) in a CMR neuron in BRF at habituating versus nonhabituating rates of stimulus presentation. This figure shows the effects of bemegride on the responses to auditory stimuli (click, 95 dB (SPL), 25 presentations at (A–C) 2 Hz and (D–F) 0.5 Hz). The middle graph shows total action potentials per poststimulus time histogram (PSTH) as a percentage of predrug control for each of the two repetition rates. The PSTH is a summation of single neuron extracellular action potential in response to a constant number of repetitions, which are shown in the bottom panel. The letters on the PSTHs correspond to the points on the time course graphs in the middle panel. In the control column in the middle panel, this neuron responded well to the auditory stimulus at the 0.5 Hz repetition rate (D), as indicated by the consistent time-locked peak in the PSTH, but relatively little response was evoked at 2 Hz in control (A), which shows repetition-induced response attenuation ("habituation"). After BMG (1.8 mg/kg, intravenous) (see the "Bemegride" column), the number of action potentials in the PSTH is enhanced to a maximum of ~390% of control levels at 2 Hz (B), while at 0.5 Hz the percentage increase is ~100%. Recovery to near-control values is noted at 3 min following termination of BMG administration at 2 Hz and at about 14 min at 0.5 Hz (C). (*Source: From Reference 56 with permission.*) Stimulus onset is at 0 ms in each PSTH (PSTH parameters: 25 stimulus presentations, 1 ms bin width). Top-panel data were

Under certain circumstances, CMR response habituation can be reversed, including sudden increases in behavioral salience of the stimulus or administration of certain drugs that block inhibition, as discussed in this chapter. In addition, CMR neurons are also very sensitive to depressant drugs, often used as anesthetics, which render them essentially unresponsive to stimuli, as also detailed in this chapter. These factors often result in apparent unresponsiveness that is often observed in neurons in various CMR regions, especially when a low-intensity stimulus is presented repetitively. The physiological basis of habituation has been studied in nonmammalian and mammalian neurons. The initial stimulus may result in an action potential, but continuing repetition of the stimulus results in progressive reductions in the amplitude of excitatory postsynaptic potentials (EPSPs) until they become subthreshold.[52,58–64] This habituation process may involve reductions of excitatory neurotransmitter release probability,[65] as well as tonic inhibition. Tonic inhibition, mediated by extrasynaptic $GABA_A$ receptors, is proposed to modulate the overall excitability of many neuronal networks, and GABA-mediated tonic inhibition is known to occur extensively in CMR regions, including the BRF, PAG, and amygdala.[66–71] Drugs that block inhibition, such as $GABA_A$ receptor antagonists,[72,73] have been shown to enhance the responsiveness of CMR neurons in intact animals[6] and also enhance cognition.[74] These antagonists may allow previously subthreshold EPSPs to reach the threshold for eliciting action potentials by allowing the resting membrane potential to rise closer to the threshold. This phenomenon would result in consistent responsiveness of these CMR neurons to external stimuli, mediated by short-term plastic changes, as described in this chapter[6,10] (see Chapters 31 and 32).

Startle

The startle response is an extreme response to a highly novel and/or intense stimulus that carries potential major salience for the intact organism (Figure 28.3). The stimulus may be indicative of an exigent or life-threatening situation, and the intense response is often critical to the survival of an animal in its normal environment. Startle can be induced by any sensory stimulus, and the acoustically-evoked startle has been studied extensively. The input from the auditory network to the BRF neurons and then output to the locomotor network produces a rapid movement that appears to serve the purpose of triggering a flight response. Ponto-medullary BRF neurons are critically involved in the neuronal network that mediates the acoustically evoked startle response (Figure 28.3). Single low-intensity electrical stimuli in the BRF paired with a previously subthreshold acoustic stimulus will lower the threshold for an electrically-evoked startle response.[75] The initial rapid acoustic startle response occurs within a few milliseconds and is mediated by a small neuronal network, consisting of the cochlear nucleus and superior olivary complex and their projections to giant neurons in the caudal pontine reticular nucleus, which project to the spinal cord to trigger the initial motor movements of this reflex.[76–78] The acoustic startle response is also a prominent example of network interaction involving the auditory network, which receives the stimulus and interacts with the midbrain locomotor network to provide a motor output (Chapter 29). The acoustic startle response is subject to a considerable degree of plasticity, including habituation, sensitization, and prepulse inhibition,[79,80] which are mirrored in the responses of BRF neurons. There are additional behavioral components of the startle response, and a more extensive neuronal network, including the PAG and amygdala, is implicated in these later components, especially in fear-potentiated startle.[77,81,82] A more complete discussion of fear-potentiated startle is included in Chapter 29.

The tactile startle pathway involves a direct projection from the principal somatosensory nucleus to the

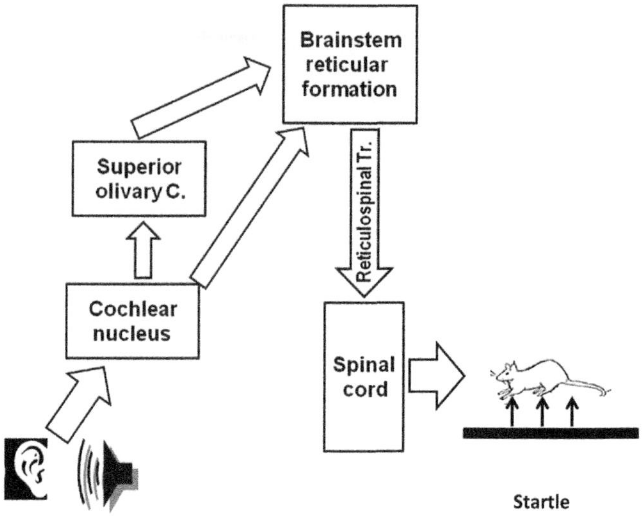

FIGURE 28.3 Diagram of the network that mediates the initial and shortest latency component of the acoustic startle response. The intense and unexpected acoustic stimulus is delivered to the ear and is transmitted via the cochlea to the primary auditory network, beginning with the cochlear nucleus, which projects to the superior olivary complex (C). Both of these primary auditory structures project to the brainstem (ponto-medullary) reticular formation, which projects via the reticulospinal tract to the spinal cord. This pathway produces the short-latency motor component of the startle response.

obtained with microwire electrodes in awake, behaving rats, and data in the lower panels were obtained from an unanesthetized cat with a glass microelectrode. *N* is the total number of action potentials in each PSTH. (*Source: Modified from References 17,56 with permission.*)

caudal pontine BRF neurons, which exhibit homosynaptic depression at low rates of stimulation, which may mediate habituation of the startle response.[83] These same BRF neurons also receive auditory input, suggesting that these two different sources of startle involve the same pathway. Thus, the startle response can be seen to be a classic example of CMR-mediated sensorimotor integration,[84] which is phylogenetically robust from simple organisms to humans. The unexpected intense stimulus triggers self-organization in the startle network, as emergent properties that are mediated by the interaction of this CMR network with the acoustic network (Chapters 29 and 30).

Pain

Pain is among the most intense stimuli that organisms experience, and CMR regions are extensively affected by nociceptive stimuli.[1,85–87] CMR neurons in the BRF, PAG, and amygdala are among the CNS regions that are important in pain networks (Chapter 23). CMR regions are also implicated in endogenous pain suppression mechanisms and pain therapies (including acupuncture) that exert major effects on these regions, particularly the PAG (see Chapter 31). There is considerable anatomical and functional evidence of extensive interconnections between these CMR regions in pain networks, as discussed in this chapter.

Brain State (Sleep State and UP State)

Sleep

The brain undergoes major changes in state associated with the sleep-waking cycle, and CMR regions are involved in the mechanisms of sleep cycle control in the sleep networks (Chapters 21 and 22). The pontine BRF has a major cholinergic component (pedunculopontine nucleus) along with nearby monoaminergic nuclei (locus coeruleus and dorsal raphe nucleus), which are strongly implicated as major elements in the network oscillations that subserve changes in the sleep-waking cycle (Chapters 21 and 22). In addition, CMR neurons in the BRF, PAG, and amygdala undergo periodic alterations in responsiveness, depending on the concurrent sleep state, and the PAG and BRF play roles in the sleep network[88–93] (Chapters 21 and 22).

Brain states have also been characterized based on the frequency of oscillation of large populations of neurons into "UP states", during which these neurons exhibit a state of subthreshold depolarization and are more likely to be responsive. UP states are contrasted with "DOWN states", during which neurons are hyperpolarized and less likely to be responsive. These states have been proposed to play important computational roles.[94] These brain states have been observed mostly in anesthetized and in vitro preparations, and those observed in unanesthetized animals exhibited a dependence on the behavioral (sleep) state.[94] Astrocytic networks recently have been implicated in determining these states.[95] Although these states have been observed primarily in cortical neurons, CMR neurons, at least in the amygdala, also exhibit these states. A foot shock delivered to an awake rat will cause transition to the UP state in amygdala neurons, which begins with an excitatory drive that is rapidly countered by inhibitory input, which reduces neuronal firing frequency, and then the UP state is maintained by a balance between excitation and inhibition. This pattern of changes differs from that in cortical neurons.[96]

CMR Neuronal Plastic Changes

A key feature of CMR neurons is their ability to exhibit a high degree of neuroplastic changes, in both the short term and long term. Neuroplasticity in CMR neurons can also be observed in their ability to undergo network switching, wherein the neurons can participate in one network and subsequently change their firing pattern to participate in an entirely different network. In addition, CMR neurons have a high capacity to change responsiveness due to behavioral conditioning and therapeutic stimulation, and CNS drugs can readily induce neuroplastic changes in many CMR neurons (Chapters 31 and 32). Subthreshold responsiveness is a key feature of CMR neurons that allows CMR regions to become readily involved in a wide variety of both active and previously dormant neuronal networks. CMR neuronal habituation and the startle response, during which CMR neurons undergo significant plasticity changes, as discussed in this chapter, are examples of short-term plastic changes in CMR regions. CMR neurons in all three of the exemplar CMR regions show these effects to a major degree, although not all to the same extent. Thus, BRF neurons exhibit a very high degree of neuroplastic changes on a short-term basis with relatively minor evidence for long-term plastic changes. Amygdala neurons exhibit some degree of short-term plasticity, but long-term plastic changes are very common in this structure, as discussed in this chapter. PAG neurons show mostly short-term changes, but long-term PAG changes also appear to occur in chronic pain networks. Synaptic mechanisms for long-term plastic changes in CMR responsiveness may involve persistent increases in synaptic strength (see Chapter 7), which may result from enhanced presynaptic activity (see Chapter 9). This process effectively magnifies the stimulation-induced input to these neurons.[97] Elevated neuronal firing increases the release of neuroactive substances, which can lead to long-term changes in network function that involve changes in synaptic strength, synaptogenesis, and even neurogenesis (see Chapters 7 and 16).

Network Switching

Many CMR neurons are responsive to inputs from multiple sources, as described here. However, under basal conditions where the organism is not being subjected to exigent conditions, the responsiveness is often very limited and is subject to extensive habituation (see the "Habituation and Novelty" section). Under exigent or appetitive conditions, many CMR neurons can participate prominently in more than one CNS network. This ability to undergo network switching has important precedents phylogenetically, including in invertebrate networks, such as those in crustacean stomatogastric ganglia, and in simple vertebrates. Certain identified neurons in these structures participate actively in a network that mediates a specific physiological function. However, when a network that mediates a different function becomes active, this same neuron can change its firing properties to become an integral part of the newly activated network.[98–101] Similarly, different modes of locomotion in lampreys can be mediated by overlapping groups of reticulospinal neurons.[39] Participation of CMR neurons in multiple networks can also be induced by certain stimulant drugs, as discussed in this chapter.

Conditioning

As discussed here, when "exigent" conditions (e.g. pain avoidance) or motivating conditions (e.g. a food reward) are experienced by the awake, behaving organism, the initiating stimuli acquire major salience, and the animals can undergo behavioral conditioning. Conditioning paradigms utilize existing neuronal networks, which may undergo expansion (Chapter 27), and/or dormant networks may be activated or accentuated by the process. Conditioning-induced changes in neuronal firing involve neuroplastic changes in many CNS neurons, and CMR neurons are often involved. Conditioning paradigms have been shown to induce neuronal firing changes in a number of CMR regions, including prominently hippocampal, cerebellar, and cortical areas as well as the exemplar CMR areas, especially neurons in the amygdala subnuclei. Thus, amygdala CMR neurons in several species, including humans, show extensive firing changes in association with various aspects of learning and conditioning. Amygdala (lateral) neurons show marked changes in both cue-induced neuronal firing and input-specific synaptic strength with the successful acquisition of a cue–reward association.[102] Chronic restraint stress causes neurons in the amygdala (lateral) to undergo hyperexcitability, as measured by increased spontaneous firing rates and lower thresholds for induction of firing by direct stimulation.[103] Amygdala (central) neuron activity in rats performing a reward task responded to the novelty of omitting the reward by increased firing selectively.[104] A fear-conditioning paradigm (Chapter 13) caused amygdala (central) neurons to increase their conditioned stimulus responsiveness, which diminished as extinction of the paradigm progressed.[105] Amygdala neuronal firing in an inhibitory avoidance task in rats showed consistent firing changes associated with shock.[106] Neurons in the human amygdala and hippocampus during single-trial learning show rapid plasticity, as shown by the finding of two consistent classes of responses. These neurons exhibit selective firing increases in response to either novel or "old" stimuli that had been presented within the previous 24 h period.[107] Memory improvement in humans during a learning task is associated with phase locking of single-neuron firing in the amygdala and hippocampus, with local electroencephalogram oscillations at theta frequencies, which previously have been associated with the induction of synaptic plasticity.[108]

CMR neurons in the PAG are also known to undergo conditioning in conjunction with amygdala neurons,[109] as discussed in the section on fear conditioning. PAG (ventrolateral) neurons showed response alteration in contextual conditioned fear and poststress recovery.[110] Behavioral-conditioning procedures have been reported to render some BRF neurons responsive to sensory stimuli to which they did not initially respond.[51,111] Neurons in the BRF in rats in a classical-conditioning paradigm and a spatial working memory task displayed long-lasting alterations of firing patterns.[112,113]

Seizure

Subseizure doses of convulsant drugs, many of which block $GABA_A$ receptors, induced neuroplastic changes in CMR neurons, including the transition from nonresponsiveness to avid responsiveness.[10] Responsiveness change in primary sensory neurons, such as those in the primary auditory network (the IC), is induced simultaneously by the same drugs.[114] On the other hand, IC neurons, which normally respond robustly to acoustic stimuli, can temporarily cease responding to these stimuli but instead be driven by a generalized seizure network when it becomes active.[6,115] Seizures can cause both acute and chronic neuroplasticity in CMR neurons, depending on their frequency and the number of seizure repetitions. For example, repetition of audiogenic seizures (AGS; also called audiogenic kindling) causes long-term neuronal plasticity changes and firing increases in the amygdala, PAG, and BRF neurons[18,37,116–118] (Chapter 27). Short-term plasticity in neurons in these same exemplar CMR regions is induced by convulsant drug treatments, as discussed in the "Therapeutic Approaches" section[10] (see Chapter 32). Thus, either long-term or short-term plasticity can be induced in the same CMR site, depending on the nature, duration, and number of repetitions of the treatment procedure, and this has been observed prominently in the amygdala and BRF.

Therapeutic Approaches—Effects of Drugs and Therapeutic Stimulation

DRUGS WITH CNS DEPRESSANT PROPERTIES

The responsiveness of many neurons in CMR brain regions varies extensively with pharmacological treatment, particularly with various types of drugs that affect the activation of $GABA_A$ receptors. Drugs with CNS depressant properties, including anesthetic agents, which enhance the activation of $GABA_A$ receptors, exert major effects on CMR neurons in the BRF, PAG, and amygdala.[9,18,87,119] Thus, most PAG (ventrolateral) neurons in awake, behaving rats respond to a nociceptive stimulus, and many of these responses are excitatory (Figure 28.4). However, when a low (subanesthetic) dose of an agent that enhances $GABA_A$-mediated inhibition (pentobarbital) is administered systemically, the spontaneous firing and nociceptive responses of these PAG neurons are significantly reduced, with recovery to predrug patterns by 30 min.[87] The extreme sensitivity of CMR neurons to barbiturates is in major contrast with the effect of these drugs on primary sensory neurons, including the IC, which respond to acoustic stimuli quite well in the presence of much higher (anesthetic) doses.[120] In fact, actions on CMR neurons in the BRF have long been proposed to be the mechanism of action of certain anesthetic agents, including barbiturates[24,121–123] (Chapters 23 and 32). The exquisite sensitivity of CMR neurons to these anesthetic agents has made it quite difficult to study these neurons except in unanesthetized animals. Thus, CMR neurons are affected greatly by depressant drugs, which is due, in part, to the ease with which CMR neuronal responses become subthreshold, as noted in the habituation discussion in this chapter. Thus, these depressant drugs will block the sensory responses of CMR neurons in the BRF, PAG, and amygdala, but the neuronal response of many primary sensory neurons is not detectably

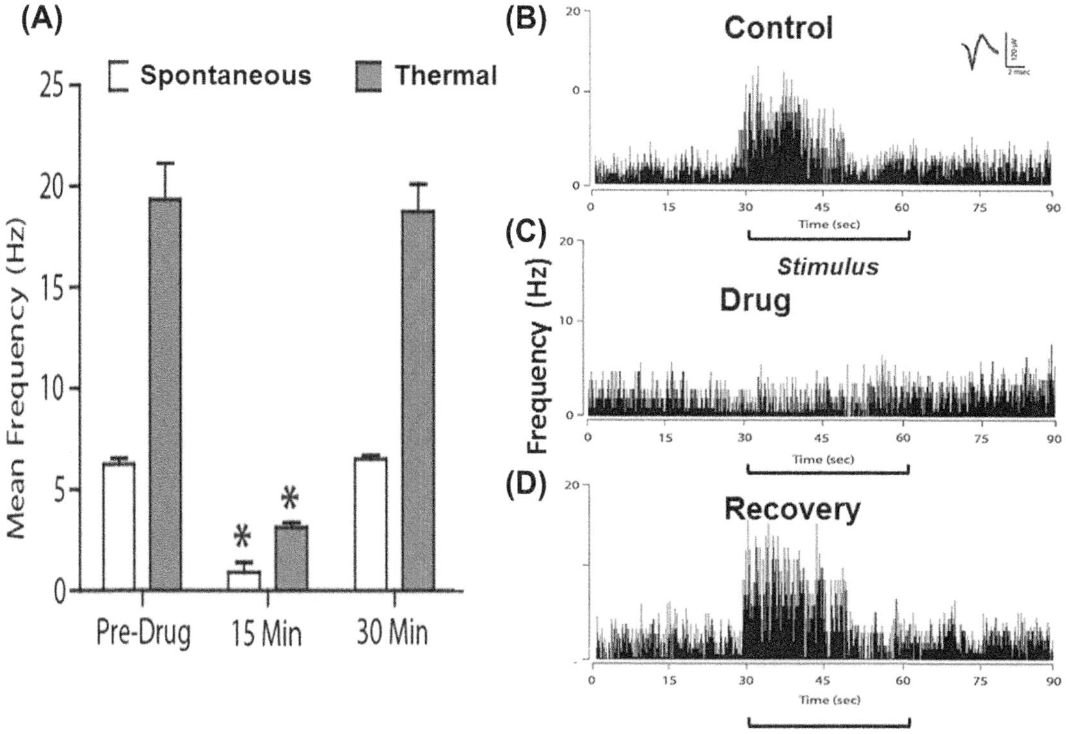

FIGURE 28.4 CNS depressant drugs, such as barbiturates, reduce CMR neuronal firing in the ventrolateral periaqueductal gray (PAG) at low doses. (A) The mean (±SEM) reduction of both spontaneous and thermally evoked firing by pentobarbital ($N = 18$ neurons) at 15 min after systemic (intraperitoneal, or i.p.) administration, with recovery by 30 min. (B–D) An example rate meter histogram analysis of a PAG neuronal spontaneous and evoked excitatory firing in response to a 30 s (bracket) noxious thermal stimulation (53 °C) before (B, "Control"), 15 min after pentobarbital (15 mg/kg i.p.) treatment (C, "Drug"), and during the subsequent recovery (at 30 min) (D, "Recovery"). Prior to pentobarbital, the majority (18/35) of PAG neurons increased firing in response to the thermal stimulus in this study. (Note that 10 mg/kg of pentobarbital had no significant effect on PAG neuronal firing, while 20 mg/kg produced greater depression of PAG firing than the 15 mg dose.) The action potential above the top histogram represents the waveform of the neuron being analyzed. The onset and duration of the thermal stimulus (Stim.) are illustrated by the bracket. Data from awake, behaving normal (Sprague–Dawley) rat. *Significance at $p < 0.01$ (repeated-measure ANOVA). (For color version of this figure, the reader is referred to the online version of this book.)

reduced by the same drugs in the same or even much higher doses.[9,18]

Neurons in CMR nuclei that are initially responsive to stimuli also readily lose responsiveness to the stimuli when a dissociative anesthetic is administered.[18,119] Many amygdala (lateral) neurons are clearly responsive to sensory stimuli in the unanesthetized state, but following administration of a low subanesthetic dose of a dissociative anesthetic (ketamine), the response is blocked. The neuroplastic effect of the drug is short term, and the responsiveness of the amygdala neurons returns (see Chapter 32). This dissociative anesthetic is highly depressant to the CMR neurons in the amygdala.[18,124] However, auditory neurons in the primary auditory nucleus (medial geniculate body), which is the major auditory input to the amygdala, respond well to acoustic stimuli with a much higher (anesthetic) dose of this same agent,[125] which is in stark contrast.

DRUGS WITH STIMULANT PROPERTIES

A number of different drugs with stimulant properties, especially $GABA_A$ receptor antagonists, also exert major effects on CMR neuronal firing, particularly in the BRF and amygdala (see Chapter 32). Blockade of CMR neuronal response habituation by these agents may play an important role in response enhancement, since administration of these agents is very effective in reversing such attenuation (Figure 28.2, middle and bottom panels). In this example (Figure 28.2, middle panel) a $GABA_A$ antagonist (bemegride) that binds at the barbiturate site[126] induces a much greater relative increase in firing at a higher rate of presentation (2 Hz) as compared to a lower presentation rate (0.5 Hz) in the same BRF neuron.[56] Thus, the relative degree of enhancement produced by the $GABA_A$ antagonists was often considerably more pronounced when the stimulus was presented at a rate that produced habituation in BRF neurons. The same BRF neuronal response is also illustrated in poststimulus time histogram (PSTH) analysis in the middle panels. The PSTH summates the number of single-neuron extracellular action potentials and their time of firing with respect to the onset of the stimulus in response to a constant number of repetitions of the same stimulus. The letters on the PSTHs correspond to the points on the time course plot (top panel). In the control column in the middle panel, this neuron responded well to the auditory stimulus at the 0.5 Hz repetition rate in the PSTH (D), as indicated by the consistent time-locked peak in the PSTH, but relatively little response was evoked at 2 Hz in the PSTH (A). However, after systemic administration of this $GABA_A$ antagonist (see the middle panel, "Bemegride" column), the same neuron responded intensively to the stimulus at both repetition rates, as shown by the increased peak and number of action potentials in each PSTH. This drug-induced responsiveness increase is short term, lasting from 10 to 30 min, and the response pattern gradually reverted to the pattern seen prior to the treatment (see the middle panels in the "Recovery" column). In addition, the effect of $GABA_A$ antagonists was often relatively greater at lower stimulus intensities than at higher intensities.[56]

As noted here, multisensory responsiveness of CMR neurons is another important characteristic of these neurons, and administration of $GABA_A$ antagonists will also accentuate this property and illuminate the degree to which it occurs. Thus, as shown in Figure 28.5, many BRF neurons were minimally responsive to repeated presentations of various stimuli, as illustrated in the PSTHs in the "Control" column. Figure 28.5 (panel A) illustrates the minimal response to visual stimuli in control, as indicated by the lack of a consistent time-locked peak in the PSTH and the sporadic firing pattern in the oscilloscope (raw) action potential data in the photograph above this PSTH. However, after systemic administration of a $GABA_A$ antagonist (pentylenetetrazol), the same neuron responded very intensively to the stimulus, as shown by the peak in the PSTH and the appearance of repetitive action potentials in the photograph above it [Figure 28.5(A), "Drug" column]. Similar effects were induced in a large percentage of CMR neurons in the BRF. Another CMR neuron in the BRF did not exhibit any consistent (time-locked) response to auditory, visual, or electrical stimuli in a primary auditory network site, as shown in the PSTHs in the "Control" column of Figure 28.5(B), the PSTH inset in this figure, and the PSTH in Figure 28.5(C), respectively. After systemic administration of the same $GABA_A$ antagonist, this neuron responded to all three stimuli (see Figure 28.5(B), inset and "C-Drug" column). This was a short-term effect, since it was reversible with time (20–30 min), as shown in the "Recovery" column. This same effect was also seen with direct (iontophoretic or pneumatic) application of another $GABA_A$ antagonist, bicuculline, onto CMR neurons in the BRF, as illustrated by the data in Figure 28.5(D). This effect was observed in both unanesthetized cats and rats. The convulsant drug-induced responsiveness with direct application onto CMR neurons in the BRF was shorter in duration, lasting from 2 to 10 min.[127] In many cases, BRF responsiveness to three or sometimes four sensory modalities was observed[10,114] (see Chapters 31 and 32).

A similar degree of pharmacologically induced neuronal response enhancement is also seen in neurons in other CMR regions, including the amygdala and pericruciate cortex. The response changes in CMR neurons in the amygdala or pericruciate were compared to BRF, in many cases simultaneously[128] (see Chapter 32). The degree of neuronal response enhancement induced by several different drugs with convulsant properties was extensive in all three areas. Most neurons exhibited

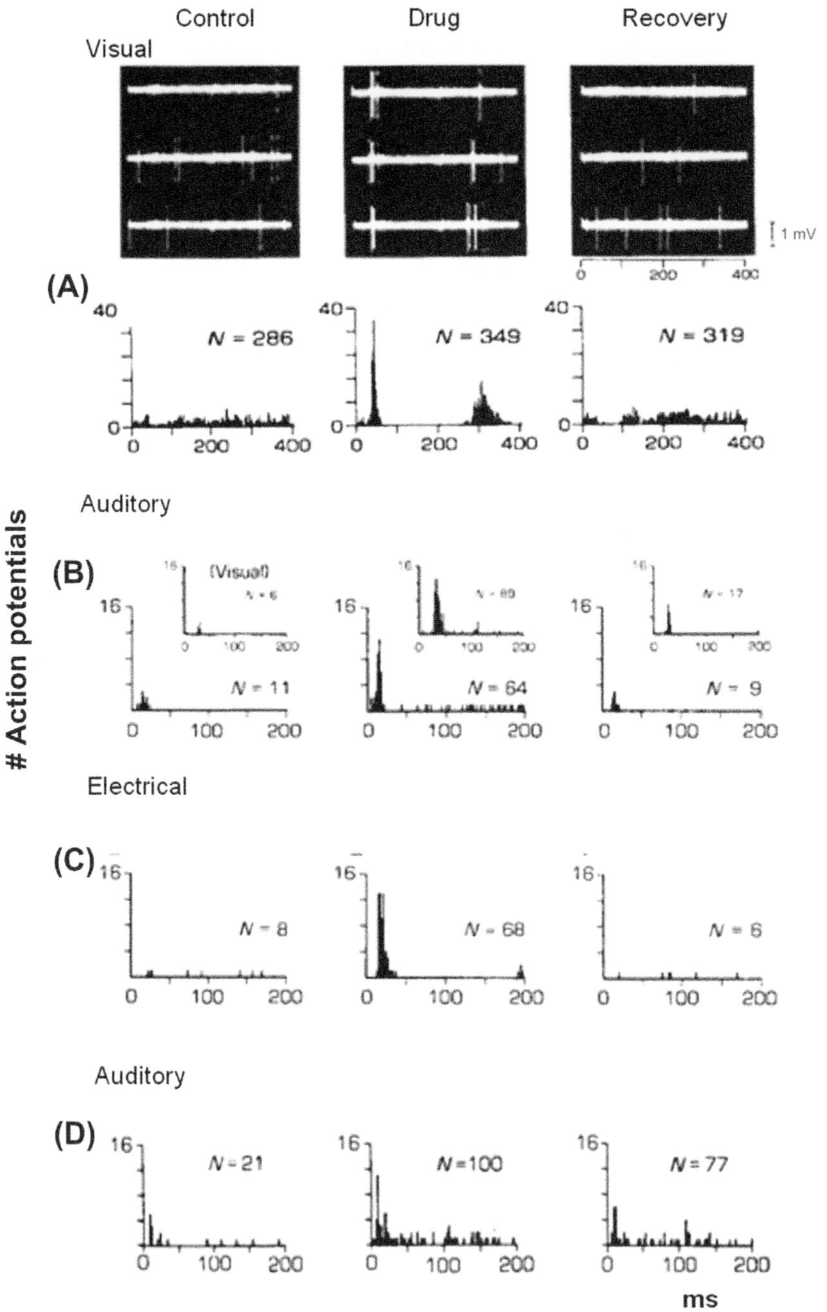

FIGURE 28.5 Induction of responsiveness in CMR neurons by $GABA_A$ receptor antagonists to stimuli in several stimulus modalities. This figure shows examples of brainstem (mesencephalic) reticular formation (BRF) neurons that were minimally responsive to stimuli before drug administration ("Control" column). However, after administration of $GABA_A$ antagonists, each of these neurons became responsive to the stimuli ("Drug" column) and recovered with time ("Recovery" column). (A) An example of poststimulus time histograms (PSTHs) of a BRF neuronal response to visual stimuli (duration: a 10 μs flash) and the response increase after administration of the $GABA_A$ antagonist pentylenetetrazol (PTZ, 12.5 mg/kg, i.v.). The photographs above each PSTH in line (A) illustrate three examples of the oscilloscope traces of action potentials from which the PSTH was constructed. (B) A different BRF neuronal response to auditory stimuli (95 dB clicks SPL) and the insets above each PSTH shows the PSTH of responses of the same neuron to visual stimuli. (C) The response of the same neuron in (B) to electrical stimuli (0.1 ms) in the primary auditory network (lateral lemniscus). This neuron became responsive to all three stimuli simultaneously following PTZ (7.5 mg/kg, i.v.). (D) An example of the effect of the $GABA_A$ antagonist, bicuculline, applied by iontophoresis (80 nA for 3 min) in another BRF neuron, which also induced a significant increase in responsiveness in this neuron. This effect was observed in unanesthetized cats (lines A–C) and rat (line D) (PSTH parameters: 50 stimulus presentations, 1 ms bin width, 0.5 Hz rate). *N* is the total number of action potentials in each PSTH. (Stimulus onset is at 0 ms in each PSTH.)

minimal responsiveness before convulsant administration, but they showed extensive responsiveness after drug administration, as discussed here.

The changes in responsiveness in non-CMR primary sensory neurons induced by administration of $GABA_A$ antagonists are relatively minor in comparison to the changes in CMR neurons in the BRF.[10] Thus, the bar graphs in Figure 28.6(A) illustrate a comparison of response changes induced by a $GABA_A$ antagonist in neurons in the IC, which is a requisite nucleus in the auditory network (Chapter 20), as compared to neurons in the BRF. The mean increase in IC neurons that showed a drug-induced firing increase was ~60%, while in the BRF, in many cases recorded simultaneously, the increase above control was >300% in these studies. An example of the effect on simultaneously recorded neurons in the BRF and IC is shown by the PSTHs in Figure 28.6(B) and (C). In Figure 28.6(B), minimal responsiveness was seen in the predrug control column in the BRF neuron, but clear responsiveness to the stimulus (auditory) was seen in the simultaneously recorded IC neurons [Figure 28.6(C)]. Systemic administration of

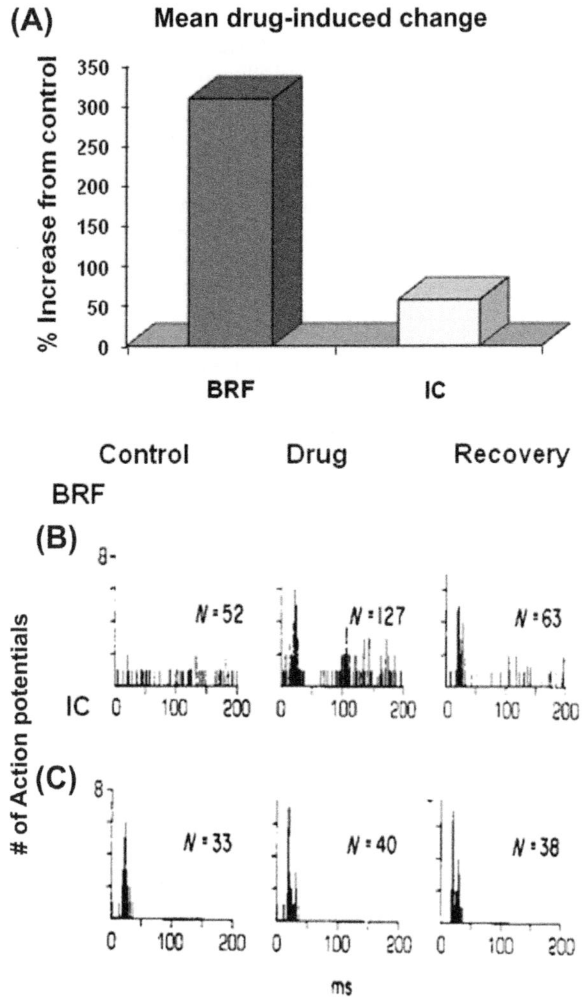

FIGURE 28.6 Effects of a $GABA_A$ antagonist on the responsiveness of CMR neurons in the BRF as compared to primary sensory neurons. This figure illustrates an example of the effects of the $GABA_A$ antagonist, pentylenetetrazol (PTZ), on the responses to auditory stimuli of primary auditory (inferior colliculus, or IC) and brainstem (mesencephalic) reticular formation (BRF). The bar graphs in panel A show the mean response increase from control (predrug) for each brain site, which was >300% in BRF neurons and ~60% in IC neurons in this series of studies. An example of the comparative effect on BRF neuronal response is shown by the poststimulus time histograms (PSTHs) in panel B, while the simultaneously recorded IC neuronal response is shown by the PSTHs in panel C. The control columns in panels B and C illustrate the responses of both neurons to the acoustic stimulus (prior to drug administration). The IC neuron was quite responsive, as shown by the consistent time-locked response (peak in the PSTH), while the BRF neuron was not clearly responsive. Following administration of PTZ (6 mg/kg, i.v.) (see the "Drug" column), the BRF neurons became very responsive to the stimulus, indicated by the emerging peak in the PSTH. At the same time, the IC neuron showed a minor firing increase. Recovery toward control firing patterns occurred in both neurons several minutes later ("Recovery" column). Increases greater than 10% were seen in 51% of IC neurons and 85% of BRF neurons in the same experimental series. Stimuli: 95 dB SPL re 0.002 $dyne/cm^2$, 0.1 ms clicks with onset at 0 time on each PSTH; PSTH parameters: 50 stimulus presentations, 1 ms bin width, 0.5 Hz rate. Data obtained from an unanesthetized cat with glass microelectrodes. *N* is the total number of action potentials in each PSTH. (*Source: Modified from Reference 114 with permission.*) (For color version of this figure, the reader is referred to the online version of this book.)

a $GABA_A$ antagonist (pentylenetetrazol) induced responsiveness to the stimulus in the CMR neurons in the BRF, while simultaneously the IC neurons showed only a minor firing increase (Figure 28.6, "Drug" column).[9,114] Likewise, primary visual neurons in the lateral geniculate nucleus also showed relatively minor firing increases (~40%) as compared with the BRF (medulla) (~200%) and midbrain (~300%). In many cases, the lateral geniculate and BRF neuronal changes were recorded simultaneously.[129] A comparison of this pharmacologically induced response enhancement over seven brain regions showed that the greatest percentage of neurons and the greatest degree of convulsant-induced firing increase occurred in the BRF, followed closely by two other CMR sites, the pericruciate cortex and amygdala (see References 6,10 for a review). Increased neuronal responsiveness was also seen in CMR neurons in conditioning paradigms.[130–133]

There is recent evidence that agents that reduce $GABA_A$ receptor-mediated inhibition, including pentylenetetrazol, are capable of enhancing cognition in an animal model of a cognitive disorder,[74,134] and the enhancement of CMR neuronal responsiveness, as discussed here, could be a potential mechanism for this effect. This potentially may be important in light of the finding that normal aging, which results in diminished activation of the primary cortex, simultaneously exhibits increased activation of CMR areas of the cortex.[135] The agents that reduce $GABA_A$ receptor activation and enhance CMR responsiveness could have the potential to improve cognition in normal aging and in CNS disorders of cognition, such as Alzheimer's disease. Interestingly, the prototypical centrally acting cholinesterase inhibitor (physostigmine), which acts by the same mechanism as most of the drugs that are approved therapies for Alzheimer's disease, also enhances the responses of CMR neurons in the BRF and amygdala[128] (see Chapter 32). Depressant drugs, including barbiturates, which exert agonist effects on the $GABA_A$ receptor, can reverse the effect of the $GABA_A$ antagonists (see Chapter 32). Thus, administration of a short-acting barbiturate or a benzodiazepine reversed the neuronal response enhancement.[9,10]

STIMULATION THERAPIES

It has been proposed that the acute effects of therapeutic stimulation paradigms may be due, in part, to induction of short-term neuroplasticity of neurons in CMR regions, while the effects of chronic stimulation therapies may be due to activation of CMR sites that exhibit a high degree of long-term plasticity[6] (Chapter 31).

Stimulation therapies have been evaluated, using human fMRI, and the involvement of several CMR regions, including the PAG, has been observed, for example in pain-relieving therapies (Chapter 31).

SPECIFIC CHARACTERISTICS AND COMPARISON OF NEURONS IN DIFFERENT CMR REGIONS

As noted in this chapter, a number of brain regions contain a high proportion of CMR neurons. Although CMR neurons in different brain CMR regions share many properties, there are also several important differential characteristics among the regions. Each of these regions often plays a role in different domains of brain and behavioral activity. These differences in domains can be seen by considering the three exemplar regions that have been emphasized in this chapter, which are discussed in more detail here.

BRF CMR Neurons

The domains in which BRF neurons are key elements include many of those that are fundamental to survival. Damage to the BRF that disrupts function is often fatal, while damage to other CMR regions, such as the amygdala, while behaviorally very disruptive, is seldom fatal. The reason for this difference may be due to the fact that the BRF contains brainstem circuits that control functions that are critical to survival, such as consciousness and respiration (see Chapters 18, 21, and 22). The relative importance of the BRF to survival is likely related to the fact that the brainstem is phylogenetically older than most other brain areas. Visual inspection of the brains of simpler vertebrates, such as the frog, indicates that the size of the brainstem is much larger relative to the cerebrum or even the cerebellum when compared to the human brain. The functions in which the brainstem is implicated in higher vertebrates, including humans, are obviously present in these simpler species. Thus, the frog brainstem, like that in humans, is the source of central control of "vegetative" functions, such as respiration and cardiac function. In addition, other important brain network activities, such as sleep, startle response, nociception, and even CNS disorders such as generalized seizures, in which the brainstem is strongly implicated in higher vertebrates, also occur or can be induced in these simpler species (see footnote below).[136–140] Therefore, plasticity is most often short term, because it may be important not to permanently alter the function of the BRF to avoid interfering with the important survival-related activities in brainstem networks. These include the startle response and nociception, as discussed here. However, long-term plasticity changes in BRF neuronal response, although less common, can also occur, as seen with seizure repetition,[116,141] discussed in this chapter[a].

Periaqueductal Gray

The midbrain PAG is involved in a number of neuronal networks, including those that mediate pain and analgesia, fear and anxiety, sleep, mood disorders, epilepsy, vocalization, lordosis, and respiratory and cardiovascular function[140,143–145] (see Chapters 18, 21, and 26). Neurons in the ventrolateral PAG respond to stimuli in multiple modalities, including nociceptive and auditory stimuli.[37,87] As with neurons in other CMR regions, PAG neurons exhibit a high degree of short-term plasticity, including habituation, with increases in the stimulus repetition rate.[37] Major long-term plasticity changes in PAG neuronal response are also seen with seizure repetition,[118] as discussed here.

Amygdala

As noted in this chapter, the amygdala also contains a high percentage of CMR neurons, but, unlike the BRF neurons, which most commonly exhibit short-term plasticity, amygdala neurons commonly show long-term neuroplasticity. These neuroplastic changes are associated with long-lasting behavior changes, including those that occur during learning.[102,103] The propensity for chronic neuroplasticity is due, in part, to the finding that robust activity of amygdala neurons can activate neurochemical events that lead to changes, such as long-term

[a]Kluge: The mammalian and, particularly, the human brain is often considered to be a "kluge", which is a derogatory engineering term that conjures up a "Rube Goldberg"-like device that only circuitously performs its function by utilizing a series of simpler devices that are strung together in a semirandom way. The kluge performs a function that it was not originally created to do and in a seemingly clumsy or haphazard way.[142] The kluge is the opposite of a purpose-built device, which is streamlined to perform a specific function. So, for example, a supercomputer works faster and has more storage capacity than the human brain that created it, but it has a limited capacity to repair itself. The main reason that a human brain is kluge-like is that it evolved from simpler brains while retaining all or most of the properties of neurons in simpler organisms. It includes many, if not all, of the circuitry and mechanisms from the simpler species, with additional mechanisms accumulated during evolution in a cumulative and seemingly haphazard process. This gives the brain and its neuronal networks a high degree of redundancy, which is an important feature for coping with the different milieus in which the organism finds itself. This redundancy also allows a tremendous robustness and resilience (antifragility) that underlie the ability to adapt and learn and have helped catapult humans to the top of the food chain.

potentiation, which involve increased intracellular Ca^{2+} levels mediated by N-methyl-D-aspartate (NMDA) receptor activation or related mechanisms in learning[146–148] (Chapters 7, 13, and 27). NMDA-receptor-mediated long-term neuroplastic changes were also seen in amygdala neurons in a seizure model induced by AGS kindling,[18,141,149] as discussed in the "Kindling of Audiogenic Seizure Effects" section.

Comparison of CMR Structures

Convulsant Drug Effects

As discussed in this chapter, stimulant drugs, including $GABA_A$ receptor antagonists, significantly enhance the responsiveness of BRF neurons. These same agents also enhance the responses of other CMR neurons, including those in the amygdala when simultaneous neuronal recordings were done in BRF and amygdala neurons.[128] The mean firing increase was >250% above predrug control levels in BRF neurons, while the mean increase in amygdala neurons was ~180% in this series of studies. Increases greater than 10% were seen in 57% of IC neurons and 85% of BRF neurons in the same experimental series. By contrast, simultaneous recordings in a CMR site in the BRF and a non-CMR site in primary sensory network nuclei indicate that only minor changes were seen in these non-CMR sites. For example, as shown in Figure 28.6, neuronal firing and responsiveness were greatly increased in the BRF neurons, but the responses of the simultaneously recorded IC neurons increased very slightly, indicating that non-CMR regions are not greatly affected by these agents.

Kindling of Audiogenic Seizure Effects

Many rodent strains are susceptible to sound-induced AGS[150] (see Chapter 26). When AGS are repeatedly induced in a paradigm called AGS kindling, the neuronal network expands to include an additional CMR region, the amygdala (Chapter 27). The neuronal networks that subserve these seizures involve several CMR regions, including the BRF and PAG[140] (Chapter 26). Evaluation of alterations in neuronal responses to acoustic stimuli at intensities below those that trigger AGS has revealed major changes[140] (Chapter 26). The relative firing changes in several CMR structures have been evaluated and compared. In contrast to the short-term neuroplastic changes induced by $GABA_A$ antagonists, when an external sensory stimulus that induces a generalized seizure is repetitively presented, CMR neurons in the amygdala, PAG, and BRF will show long-term neuroplastic changes in responsiveness.[18,116–118] Thus, in the moderate strain of AGS-susceptible rats (genetically epilepsy-prone rats (GEPR-3s)) AGS kindling resulted in response changes in several network nuclei, including the BRF and amygdala as well as the perirhinal cortex. The perirhinal cortex becomes involved in the AGS network in these animals due to AGS kindling. A comparison of the response changes with increasing stimulus intensity seen in CMR neurons in the BRF (pontine) and perirhinal cortex indicates that the BRF shows very extensive mean increases in firing with intensity increases, while the relative change in the mean perirhinal cortex, although statistically significant, is considerably less. The amygdala neuronal-firing changes in AGS kindling were intermediate between those of the BRF and perirhinal cortex.[117] Thus, it can be seen that CMR regions in the AGS network appear to be affected to different degrees by this paradigm.

Electrical Kindling Susceptibility Differences

Another example of the general difference between CMR regions in the brainstem and those in the amygdala is illustrated by the phenomenon known as electrical kindling. Focal repetitive electrical stimulation in CMR sites in the limbic system such as the amygdala readily induces a long-term (kindling) model of seizures.[151] However, it requires considerably more intense stimulation in brainstem sites, including BRF and ventrolateral PAG, which are resistant to the electrical kindling paradigm as compared to limbic sites, including the amygdala.[152] These data further support the greater susceptibility to long-term plasticity in amygdala versus BRF seen in other approaches noted in this chapter.

INTERACTION OF CMR REGIONS

Interactions between CMR regions are highly complex, extensive, redundant, and often reciprocal, which is true of the three exemplar regions that we have been discussing here. Evidence of reciprocal anatomical and neurochemical pathways between BRF, PAG, and the amygdala has been observed anatomically.[153–155] Thus, the BRF, which has massive interconnections within the nuclei that constitute it, also sends projections to and receives input from the PAG and amygdala.[156–159] The amygdala has reciprocal physiologically active connections with the PAG, which are proposed to be very important in pain, mood disorders, and epilepsy[143,160,161] (Chapters 23, 24, and 27). The network interactions between CMR regions have also been implicated in vocalizations and pain in both animals and humans. fMRI studies in humans also support evidence for functional connectivity between PAG and the amygdala in patients that increased in both acute and chronic pain.[162,163] fMRI studies of acupuncture indicate that these CMR structures are also affected by this pain-relieving stimulation therapy.[109] In epilepsy models,

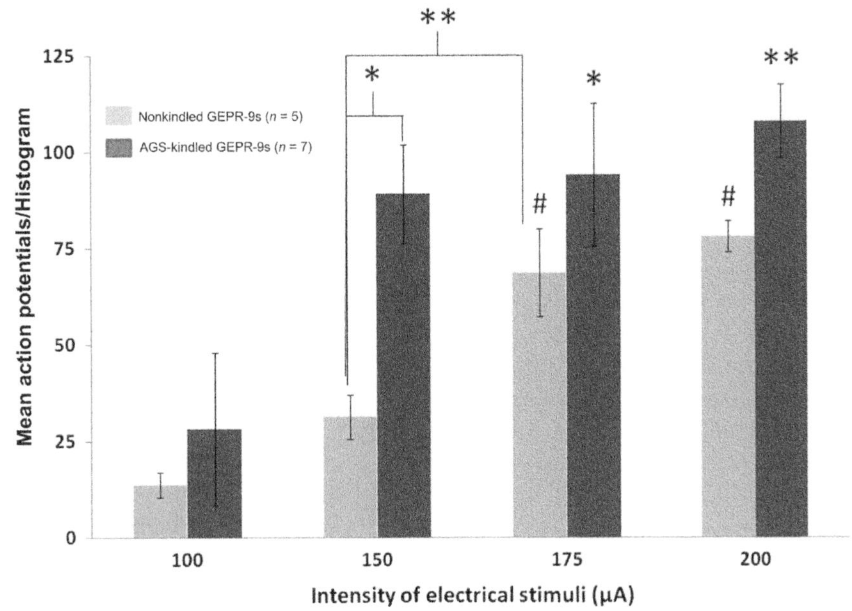

FIGURE 28.7 Effects of increasing the intensity of electrical stimulus in the central nucleus of amygdala on the mean evoked single-unit action potentials (APs) per histogram (post stimulus-time histogram, or PSTH) recorded from the ventrolateral periaqueductal gray (PAG) in AGS-kindled GEPR-9s ($n = 7$ neurons in five rats) (dark bars) as compared with nonkindled GEPR-9s ($n = 5$ neurons in three rats) (lighter bars). There were significant intensity-related firing increases in both groups of rats. The mean differences in the AGS-kindled GEPR-9s, as compared to nonkindled GEPR-9s, were significantly greater and began at a lower stimulus intensity (150 μA) in AGS-kindled rats. The electrical stimulus artifact was seen between 0 and 3 ms, and the evoked single-unit responses appeared within 25 ms following the electrical stimulus. Therefore, the mean of APs and PSTH appearing between 4 and 25 ms of the PSTHs are shown. Statistical comparisons between groups were done using univariate ANOVA followed by independent sample *t*-tests for each electrical stimulus intensity ($^*p < 0.05$), and within-group comparisons were done using one-way ANOVA followed by Tukey HSD ($^{\#}p < 0.001$; $^{**}p < 0.01$; $^*p < 0.05$ (*Source: From Reference 161, with permission.*)) in awake, behaving epileptic rats (GEPR-9) with microwire electrodes. (For color version of this figure, the reader is referred to the online version of this book.)

including AGS kindling, the normal pathway from amygdala to PAG undergoes major neuroplastic changes.[161] As shown in Figure 28.7, mean PAG (ventrolateral) neuronal responses to electrical stimuli in the amygdala (central) are greatly increased as a result of AGS kindling (Chapter 27). Neuroplastic changes in this pathway are implicated in the network expansion, which mediates the additional behavioral phase seen in AGS-kindled seizures.[161] The interactions of these CMR regions have also been shown to become critically involved in several specific learning paradigms.[109,164]

CMR regions can often work together as a CMR network that carries out important physiological functions and may also become involved in CNS disorders. Thus, the three exemplar regions (BRF, PAG, and amygdala) interact with each other in the pain network (Chapter 23). Connections between these CMR regions are implicated in fear-potentiated startle[81,109] (Chapter 13) as well as an epilepsy model in the moderate-seizure strain of GEPR-3s[117] and following AGS kindling in GEPR-9s[18] (Chapters 26 and 27). Thus, interaction of these CMR networks occurs in such exigent conditions, and these CMR networks interact with other primary networks, including the auditory, locomotor, and respiratory networks, as discussed in Chapter 29.

CONCLUSIONS

CMR brain sites, including the BRF, PAG, and amygdala, are highly variable in their firing patterns, which are determined by the circumstances that the organism is experiencing, including conditions that carry salience for the organism. Thus, CMR neurons exhibit response elevation under exigent states and response decrement (habituation) in nonexigent and repetitive conditions. Neurons in CMR regions receive a multitude of inputs. Depending on the conditions being experienced by the organism, these neurons can respond minimally (negatively nonlinear) or become hyperresponsive (positively nonlinear) to these inputs, and, in the latter case, this can result in emergent properties of the networks (see Figure 28.1). The fact that many CMR neurons have numerous connections to other brain sites suggests that these neurons can be considered to exhibit characteristics associated with "hub" neurons in complex network theory.[165] Since many CMR neurons, especially those in the BRF, have connections to motor pathways, these neurons have a major role in sensorimotor integration, including that seen in startle responses. Drugs that act on the CNS, particularly those that enhance the action of inhibitory transmitters, such as GABA, exert major depressant effects on CMR neurons. Therefore, studies of CMR neurons must be performed with unanesthetized animals. Agents that block the action of inhibitory transmitters, especially $GABA_A$ antagonists, induce major nonlinear response enhancement of CMR neurons in several brain regions, in part by blocking the tonic inhibition that is common in CMR neurons. The high degree of neuroplasticity of CMR neurons allows them to play major roles in normal neuronal network function in normal activities, such as learning, but also in CNS disorders. The recent reports that agents that enhance $GABA_A$ receptor activation will enhance cognition may be due to their ability to enhance CMR neuronal responsiveness. This action may allow these agents to potentially enhance cognition in normal aging as well as cognitive declines in CNS disorders, such as Alzheimer's disease, which will need to be evaluated in future studies. Therapeutic measures, including stimulation therapies and drug treatments, also exert major effects on brain regions with large populations of CMR neurons.

Acknowledgments

The authors gratefully acknowledge the technical assistance of Bill Hoffmann and Marc Randall in the experiments from our laboratory. The authors were supported by NIH, NINDS, and NIAAA during the experiments in our lab that are cited. The authors gratefully acknowledge the assistance of Gayle Stauffer and Diana Smith in preparing this manuscript.

References

1. Hayes DJ, Northoff G. Common brain activations for painful and non-painful aversive stimuli. *BMC Neurosci*. 2012;13:60.
2. Shriner AM, Drever FR, Metz GA. The development of skilled walking in the rat. *Behav Brain Res*. 2009;205(2):426–435.
3. Muir GD. Early ontogeny of locomotor behaviour: a comparison between altricial and precocial animals. *Brain Res Bull*. 2000;53(5):719–726.
4. Jackson BE, Segre P, Dial KP. Precocial development of locomotor performance in a ground-dwelling bird (*Alectoris chukar*): negotiating a three-dimensional terrestrial environment. *Proc Biol Sci*. 2009;276(1672):3457–3466.
5. Rossignol S, Frigon A, Barrière G, et al. Chapter 16-Spinal plasticity in the recovery of locomotion. *Prog Brain Res*. 2011;188:229–241.
6. Faingold CL. Electrical stimulation therapies for CNS disorders and pain are mediated by competition between different neuronal networks in the brain. *Med Hypotheses*. 2008;71(5):668–681.
7. Freeman WJ, Kozma R, Werbos PJ. Biocomplexity: adaptive behavior in complex stochastic dynamical systems. *Biosystems*. 2001;59:109–123.
8. Faingold CL. Emergent properties of CNS neuronal networks as targets for pharmacology: application to anticonvulsant drug action. *Prog Neurobiol*. 2004;72(1):55–85.
9. Faingold CL, Caspary DM. Effect of convulsant drugs on the brain-stem. In: Fromm GH, Faingold CL, Browning RA, Burnham WM, eds. *Epilepsy and the Reticular Formation: The Role of the Reticular Core in Convulsive Seizures*. New York, NY: A.R. Liss; 1987:39–80.
10. Faingold CL, Riaz A. Neuronal networks in convulsant drug-induced seizures. In: Faingold CL, Fromm GH, eds. *Drugs for Control of Epilepsy: Actions on Neuronal Networks Involved in Seizure Disorders*. Boca Raton, FL: CRC Press; 1992:213–251.
11. Quirk GJ, Mueller D. Neural mechanisms of extinction learning and retrieval. *Neuropsychopharmacology*. 2008;33(1):56–72.
12. Delgado-García JM, Gruart A. Building new motor responses: eyelid conditioning revisited. *Trends Neurosci*. 2006;29(6):330–338.
13. Maiz J, Karakossian MH, Pakaprot N, Robleto K, Thompson RF, Otis TS. Prolonging the postcomplex spike pause speeds eyeblink conditioning. *Proc Natl Acad Sci USA*. 2012;109(41): 16726–16730.
14. Long JD, Carmena JM. Dynamic changes of rodent somatosensory barrel cortex are correlated with learning a novel conditioned stimulus. *J Neurophysiol*. 2013;109(10):2585–2595.
15. Edlow BL, Takahashi E, Wu O, et al. Neuroanatomic connectivity of the human ascending arousal system critical to consciousness and its disorders. *J Neuropathol Exp Neurol*. 2012;71(6):531–546.
16. Humphries MD, Gurney K, Prescott TJ. The brainstem reticular formation is a small-world, not scale-free, network. *Proc Biol Sci*. 2006;273(1585):503–511.
17. Faingold CL, Randall ME. Pontine reticular formation neurons exhibit a premature and precipitous increase in acoustic responses prior to audiogenic seizures in genetically epilepsy-prone rats. *Brain Res*. 1995;704(2):218–226.
18. Feng HJ, Faingold CL. Repeated generalized audiogenic seizures induce plastic changes on acoustically evoked neuronal firing in the amygdala. *Brain Res*. 2002;932(1–2):61–69.
19. Faingold CL. Anticonvulsant drugs as neuronal network-modifying agents. In: Scjwartzlrpom P, ed. *Encyclopedia of Basic Epilepsy Research*. vol. 1.
20. Jaaskelainen IP, Ahveninen J, Belliveau JW, Raij T, Sams M. Short-term plasticity in auditory cognition. *Trends Neurosci*. 2007;30(12):653–661.
21. Xu J, He L, Wu LG. Role of Ca^{2+} channels in short-term synaptic plasticity. *Curr Opin Neurobiol*. 2007;17(3):352–359.
22. Riedel G, Davies SN. Cannabinoid function in learning, memory and plasticity. *Handb Exp Pharmacol*. 2005;168:445–477.
23. Blair HT, Schafe GE, Bauer EP, Rodrigues SM, LeDoux JE. Synaptic plasticity in the lateral amygdala: a cellular hypothesis of fear conditioning. *Learn Mem*. 2001;8(5):229–242.
24. Olivéras JL, Montagne-Clavel J, Martin G. Drastic changes of ventromedial medulla neuronal properties induced by barbiturate anesthesia. I. Comparison of the single-unit types in the same awake and pentobarbital-treated rats. *Brain Res*. 1991;563(1–2):241–250.
25. Blair RW, Thompson GM. Convergence of multiple sensory inputs onto neurons in the dorsolateral medulla in cats. *Neuroscience*. 1995;67(3):721–729.
26. Ullen F, Deliagina TG, Orlovsky GN, Grillner S. Visual potentiation of vestibular responses in lamprey reticulospinal neurons. *Eur J Neurosci*. 1996;8(11):2298–2307.
27. Martin EM, Pavlides C, Pfaff D. Multimodal sensory responses of nucleus reticularis gigantocellularis and the responses' relation to cortical and motor activation. *J Neurophysiol*. 2010;103(5): 2326–2338.
28. Aravamuthan BR, Angelaki DE. Vestibular responses in the macaque pedunculopontine nucleus and central mesencephalic reticular formation. *Neuroscience*. 2012;223:183–199.
29. Ben Ari Y, Le Gal La Salle G, Champagnat JC. Lateral amygdala unit activity: I. Relationship between spontaneous and evoked activity. *Electroencephalogr Clin Neurophysiol*. 1974;37(5):449–461.
30. Sanghera MK, Rolls ET, Roper-Hall A. Visual responses of neurons in the dorsolateral amygdala of the alert monkey. *Exp Neurol*. 1979;63(3):610–626.

31. Romanski LM, Clugnet MC, Bordi F, LeDoux JE. Somatosensory and auditory convergence in the lateral nucleus of the amygdala. *Behav Neurosci.* 1993;107(3):444–450.
32. Bordi F, LeDoux JE. Response properties of single units in areas of rat auditory thalamus that project to the amygdala. II. Cells receiving convergent auditory and somatosensory inputs and cells antidromically activated by amygdala stimulation. *Exp Brain Res.* 1994;98(2):275–286.
33. Paton JJ, Belova MA, Morrison SE, Salzman CD. The primate amygdala represents the positive and negative value of visual stimuli during learning. *Nature.* 2006;439(7078):865–870.
34. Feng HJ, Faingold CL. The effects of chronic ethanol administration on amygdala neuronal firing and ethanol withdrawal seizures. *Neuropharmacology.* 2008;55(5):648–653.
35. Fenton GE, Spicer CH, Halliday DM, Mason R, Stevenson CW. Basolateral amygdala activity during the retrieval of associative learning under anesthesia. *Neuroscience.* 2013;233:146–156.
36. Hernandez A, Neira S, Soto-Moyano R. Effect of morphine-induced cortical excitation on somatosensory responses evoked in the periaqueductal grey matter. *Eur J Pharmacol.* 1985; 115(2–3):305–308.
37. N'Gouemo P, Faingold CL. Periaqueductal gray neurons exhibit increased responsiveness associated with audiogenic seizures in the genetically epilepsy-prone rat. *Neuroscience.* 1998;84(2):619–625.
38. Derjean D, Moussaddy A, Atallah E, et al. A novel neural substrate for the transformation of olfactory inputs into motor output. *PLoS Biol.* 2010;8(12):e1000567.
39. Zelenin PV. Reticulospinal neurons controlling forward and backward swimming in the lamprey. *J Neurophysiol.* 2011;105(3): 1361–1371.
40. Deliangina TG, Fagerstedt P. Responses of reticulospinal neurons in intact lamprey to vestibular and visual inputs. *J Neurophysiol.* 2000;83(2):864–878.
41. Deliangina TG, Zelenin PV, Fagerstedt P, Grillner S, Orlovsky GN. Activity of reticulospinal neurons during locomotion in the freely behaving lamprey. *J Neurophysiol.* 2000;83(2):853–863.
42. Perreault MC, Glover JC. Glutamatergic reticulospinal neurons in the mouse: developmental origins, axon projections, and functional connectivity. *Ann N Y Acad Sci.* 2013;1279(1):80–89.
43. Hage SR, Jurgens U, Ehret G. Audio-vocal interaction in the pontine brainstem during self-initiated vocalization in the squirrel monkey. *Eur J Neurosci.* 2006;23(12):3297–3308.
44. Jahn K, Deutschlander A, Stephan T, et al. Supraspinal locomotor control in quadrupeds and humans. *Prog Brain Res.* 2008;171:353–362.
45. Jahn K, Zwergal A. Imaging supraspinal locomotor control in balance disorders. *Restor Neurol Neurosci.* 2010;28(1):105–114.
46. Vertes RP, Miller NE. Brain stem neurons that fire selectively to a conditioned stimulus for shock. *Brain Res.* 1976;103(2):229–242.
47. Carlson S, Willott JF. Caudal pontine reticular formation of C57BL/6J mice: responses to startle stimuli, inhibition by tones, and plasticity. *J Neurophysiol.* 1998;79(5):2603–2614.
48. Davis M, Antoniadis EA, Amaral DG, Winslow JT. Acoustic startle reflex in rhesus monkeys: a review. *Rev Neurosci.* 2008;19(2–3):171–185.
49. Gonzalez Andino SL, Grave de Peralta Menendez R. Coding of saliency by ensemble bursting in the amygdala of primates. *Front Behav Neurosci.* 2012;6:38.
50. Bell C, Sierra G, Buendia N, Segundo JP. Sensory properties of neurons in the mesencephalic reticular formation. *J Neurophysiol.* 1964;27:961–987.
51. Lindsley DF, Ranf SK, Sherwood MJ, Preston WG. Habituation and modification of reticular formation neuron responses to peripheral stimulation in cats. *Exp Neurol.* 1973;41(1):174–189.
52. Peterson BW, Franck JI, Daunton NG. Changes in responses of medial pontomedullary reticular neurons during repetitive cutaneous, vestibular, cortical, and tectal stimulation. *J Neurophysiol.* 1976;39(3):564–581.
53. Scheibel ME, Scheibel AB. The response of reticular units to repetitive stimuli. *Arch Ital Biol.* 1965;103:279–299.
54. Ben Ari Y, Le Gal La Salle G. Lateral amygdala unit activity: II. Habituating and non-habituating neurons. *Electroencephalogr Clin Neurophysiol.* 1974;37(5):463–472.
55. Yang L, Long C, Randall ME, Faingold CL. Neurons in the periaqueductal gray are critically involved in the neuronal network for audiogenic seizures during ethanol withdrawal. *Neuropharmacology.* 2003;44(2):275–281.
56. Faingold CL, Hoffmann WE. Effects of bemegride on the sensory responses of neurons in the hippocampus and brain stem reticular formation. *Electroencephalogr Clin Neurophysiol.* 1981;52(4): 316–327.
57. Faingold CL, Gehlbach G, Caspary DM. On the role of GABA as an inhibitory neurotransmitter in inferior colliculus neurons: iontophoretic studies. *Brain Res.* 1989;500(1–2):302–312.
58. Segundo JP, Takenaka T, Encabo H. Somatic sensory properties of bulbar reticular neurons. *J Neurophysiol.* 1967;30(5):1221–1238.
59. Lingenhohl K, Friauf E. Giant neurons in the caudal pontine reticular formation receive short latency acoustic input: an intracellular recording and HRP-study in the rat. *J Comp Neurol.* 1992;325(4):473–492.
60. Weber M, Schnitzler HU, Schmid S. Synaptic plasticity in the acoustic startle pathway: the neuronal basis for short-term habituation? *Eur J Neurosci.* 2002;16(7):1325–1332.
61. Castellucci V, Pinsker H, Kupfermann I, Kandel ER. Neuronal mechanisms of habituation and dishabituation of the gill-withdrawal reflex in Aplysia. *Science.* 1970;167(3926):1745–1748.
62. Farel PB, Glanzman DL, Thompson RF. Habituation of a monosynaptic response in vertebrate central nervous system: lateral column-motoneuron pathway in isolated frog spinal cord. *J Neurophysiol.* 1973;36(6):1117–1130.
63. Heinbockel T, Pape HC. Input-specific long-term depression in the lateral amygdala evoked by theta frequency stimulation. *J Neurosci.* 2000;20(7):RC68.
64. Simons-Weidenmaier NS, Weber M, Plappert CF, Pilz PK, Schmid S. Synaptic depression and short-term habituation are located in the sensory part of the mammalian startle pathway. *BMC Neurosci.* 2006;7:38.
65. Borst JG. The low synaptic release probability in vivo. *Trends Neurosci.* 2010;33(6):259–266.
66. Pompeiano O, Hoshino K. Tonic inhibition of dorsal pontine neurons during the postural atonia produced by an anticholinesterase in the decerebrate cat. *Arch Ital Biol.* 1976;114(3):310–340.
67. Lindquist CE, Birnir B. Graded response to GABA by native extrasynaptic GABA receptors. *J Neurochem.* 2006;97(5):1349–1356.
68. Vanini G, Baghdoyan A. Extrasynaptic $GABA_A$ receptors in rat pontine reticular formation increase wakefulness. *Sleep.* 2013;36(3):337–343.
69. Fritsch B, Qashu F, Figueiredo TH, Aroniadou-anderjaska V, Rogawski MA, Braga MF. Pathological alterations in GABAergic interneurons and reduced tonic inhibition in the basolateral amygdala during epileptogenesis. *Neuroscience.* 2009;163(1): 415–429.
70. Marowsky A, Rudolph U, Fritschy JM, Arand M. Tonic inhibition in principal cells of the amygdala: a central role for alpha3 subunit-containing $GABA_A$ receptors. *J Neurosci.* 2012;32(25): 8611–8619.
71. Stone E, Coote JH, Allard J, Lovick TA. GABAergic control of micturition within the periaqueductal grey matter of the male rat. *J Physiol.* 2011;589(Pt 8):2065–2078.

72. Cope DW, Hughes SW, Crunelli V. $GABA_A$ receptor-mediated tonic inhibition in thalamic neurons. *J Neurosci.* 2005;25(50): 11553–11563.
73. Belelli D, Harrison NL, Maguire J, Macdonald RL, Walker MC, Cope DW. Extrasynaptic $GABA_A$ receptors: form, pharmacology, and function. *J Neurosci.* 2009;29(41):12757–12763.
74. Möhler H. Cognitive enhancement by pharmacological and behavioral interventions: the murine Down syndrome model. *Biochem Pharmacol.* 2012;84(8):994–999.
75. Yeomans JS, Cochrane KA. Collision-like interactions between acoustic and electrical signals that produce startle reflexes in reticular formation sites. *Brain Res.* 1993;617(2):320–328.
76. Davis M, Gendelman DS, Tischler MD, Gendelman PM. A primary acoustic startle circuit: lesion and stimulation studies. *J Neurosci.* 1982;2(6):791–805.
77. Lingenhohl K, Friauf E. Giant neurons in the rat reticular formation: a sensorimotor interface in the elementary acoustic startle circuit? *J Neurosci.* 1994;14(3 Pt 1):1176–1194.
78. Yeomans JS, Li L, Scott BW, Frankland PW. Tactile, acoustic and vestibular systems sum to elicit the startle reflex. *Neurosci Biobehav Rev.* 2002;26(1):1–11.
79. Richardson R, Vishney A. Shock sensitization of startle in the developing rat. *Dev Psychobiol.* 2000;36(4):282–291.
80. Valsamis B, Schmid S. Habituation and prepulse inhibition of acoustic startle in rodents. *J Vis Exp.* 2011;55:e3446.
81. Zhao Z, Davis M. Fear-potentiated startle in rats is mediated by neurons in the deep layers of the superior colliculus/deep mesencephalic nucleus of the rostral midbrain through the glutamate non-NMDA receptors. *J Neurosci.* 2004;24(46): 10326–10334.
82. Reimer AE, de Oliveira AR, Brandão ML. Glutamatergic mechanisms of the dorsal periaqueductal gray matter modulate the expression of conditioned freezing and fear-potentiated startle. *Neuroscience.* 2012;219:72–81.
83. Schmid S, Simons NS, Schnitzler HU. Cellular mechanisms of the trigeminally evoked startle response. *Eur J Neurosci.* 2003; 17(7):1438–1444.
84. Koch M, Schnitzler HU. The acoustic startle response in rats – circuits mediating evocation, inhibition and potentiation. *Behav Brain Res.* 1997;89(1–2):35–49.
85. Heinricher MM, Tavares I, Leith JL, Lumb BM. Descending control of nociception: specificity, recruitment and plasticity. *Brain Res Rev.* 2009;60(1):214–225.
86. Rouwette T, Vanelderen P, Roubos EW, Kozicz T, Vissers K. The amygdala, a relay station for switching on and off pain. *Eur J Pain.* 2012;16(6):782–792.
87. Samineni V, Premkumar L, Faingold CL. Changes in periaqueductal gray neuronal responses to pain induced by barbiturate administration. *Anesthesiology.* submitted for publication.
88. Huttenlocher PR. Evoked and spontaneous activity in single units of medial brain stem during natural sleep and waking. *J Neurophysiol.* 1961;24(5):451–468.
89. Scheibel ME, Scheibel AB. Activity cycles in neurons of the reticular formation. *Recent Adv Biol Psychiatry.* 1965;8:283–293.
90. Reese NB, Garcia-Rill E, Skinner RD. Auditory input to the pedunculopontine nucleus: II. Unit responses. *Brain Res Bull.* 1995;37(3):265–273.
91. Thakkar MM, Strecker RE, McCarley RW. Phasic but not tonic REM-selective discharge of periaqueductal gray neurons in freely behaving animals: relevance to postulates of GABAergic inhibition of monoaminergic neurons. *Brain Res.* 2002; 945(2):276–280.
92. Jha SK, Ross RJ, Morrison AR. Sleep-related neurons in the central nucleus of the amygdala of rats and their modulation by the dorsal raphe nucleus. *Physiol Behav.* 2005;86(4):415–426.
93. Xi M, Fung SJ, Zhang J, Sampogna S, Chase MH. The amygdala and the pedunculopontine tegmental nucleus: interactions controlling active (rapid eye movement) sleep. *Exp Neurol.* 2012;238(1):44–51.
94. Hromádka T, Zador AM, Deweese MR. Up states are rare in awake auditory cortex. *J Neurophysiol.* 2013;109(8):1989–1995.
95. Poskanzer KE, Yuste R. Astrocytic regulation of cortical UP states. *Proc Natl Acad Sci USA.* 2011;108(45):18453–18458.
96. Windels F, Crane JW, Sah P. Inhibition dominates the early phase of up-states in the basolateral amygdala. *J Neurophysiol.* 2010;104(6):3433–3438.
97. Kim SJ, Linden DJ. Ubiquitous plasticity and memory storage. *Neuron.* 2007;56(4):582–592.
98. Marder E, Bucher D. Understanding circuit dynamics using the stomatogastric nervous system of lobsters and crabs. *Annu Rev Physiol.* 2007;69:291–316.
99. Blitz DM, White RS, Saideman SR, et al. A newly identified extrinsic input triggers a distinct gastric mill rhythm via activation of modulatory projection neurons. *J Exp Biol.* 2008;211(Pt 6): 1000–1011.
100. Li W-C, Roberts A, Soffe SR. Specific brainstem neurons switch each other into pacemaker mode to drive movement by activating NMDA receptors. *J Neurosci.* 2010;30(49):16609–16620.
101. Gutierrez GJ, O'Leary T, Marder E. Multiple mechanisms switch an electrically coupled, synaptically inhibited neuron between competing rhythmic oscillators. *Neuron.* 2013;77(5):845–858.
102. Tye KM, Stuber GD, de Ridder B, Bonci A, Janak PH. Rapid strengthening of thalamo-amygdala synapses mediates cue–reward learning. *Nature.* 2008;453(7199):1253–1257.
103. Rosenkranz JA, Venheim ER, Padival M. Chronic stress causes amygdala hyperexcitability in rodents. *Biol Psychiatry.* 2010;67(12):1128–1136.
104. Calu DJ, Roesch MR, Haney RZ, Holland PC, Schoenbaum G. Neural correlates of variations in event processing during learning in central nucleus of amygdala. *Neuron.* 2010;68(5):991–1001.
105. Duvarci S, Popa D, Paré D. Central amygdala activity during fear conditioning. *J Neurosci.* 2011;31(1):289–294.
106. Chang CH, Liang KC, Yen CT. Inhibitory avoidance learning altered ensemble activity of amygdaloid neurons in rats. *Eur J Neurosci.* 2005;21(1):210–218.
107. Rutishauser U, Mamelak AN, Schuman EM. Single-trial learning of novel stimuli by individual neurons of the human hippocampus-amygdala complex. *Neuron.* 2006;49(6):805–813.
108. Rutishauser U, Ross IB, Mamelak AN, Schuman EM. Human memory strength is predicted by theta-frequency phase-locking of single neurons. *Nature.* 2010;464(7290):903–907.
109. Johansen JP, Tarpley JW, LeDoux JE, Blair HT. Neural substrates for expectation-modulated fear learning in the amygdala and periaqueductal gray. *Nat Neurosci.* 2010;13(8):979–986.
110. Walker P, Carrive P. Role of ventrolateral periaqueductal gray neurons in the behavioral and cardiovascular responses to contextual conditioned fear and poststress recovery. *Neuroscience.* 2003;116(3):897–912.
111. Buresova O, Bures J. Classical conditioning and reticular units. *Acta Physiol Acad Sci Hung.* 1965;26:53–57.
112. Desmond JE, Moore JW. Dorsolateral pontine tegmentum and the classically conditioned nictitating membrane response: analysis of CR-related single-unit activity. *Exp Brain Res.* 1986;65(1):59–74.
113. Puryear CB, Mizumori SJ. Reward prediction error signals by reticular formation neurons. *Learn Mem.* 2008;15(12):895–898.
114. Faingold CL, Hoffmann WE, Caspary DM. On the site of pentylenetetrazol-induced enhancement of auditory responses of the reticular formation: localized cooling and electrical stimulation studies. *Neuropharmacology.* 1983;22(8):961–970.

115. Faingold CL, Anderson CA. Loss of intensity-induced inhibition in inferior colliculus neurons leads to audiogenic seizure susceptibility in behaving genetically epilepsy-prone rats. *Exp Neurol*. 1991;113(3):354–363.
116. Raisinghani M, Faingold CL. Pontine reticular formation neurons are implicated in the neuronal network for generalized clonic seizures which is intensified by audiogenic kindling. *Brain Res*. 2005;1064(1–2):90–97.
117. Raisinghani M, Faingold CL. Neurons in the amygdala play an important role in the neuronal network mediating a clonic form of audiogenic seizures both before and after audiogenic kindling. *Brain Res*. 2005;1032(1–2):131–140.
118. Tupal S, Faingold CL. Audiogenic kindling induces plastic changes in the neuronal firing patterns in periaqueductal gray. *Brain Res*. 2011;1377:60–66.
119. Feng HJ, Faingold CL. Ketamine in mood disorders and epilepsy. In: Costa A, Villalba E, eds. *Horizons in Neuroscience Research*. vol. 10. New York: Nova Science Publishers; 2013:103–122.
120. Bibikov NG, Chen QC, Wu FJ. Responses of inferior colliculus neurons to sounds presented at different rates in anesthetized albino mouse. *Hear Res*. 2008;241(1–2):43–51.
121. Moruzzi G, Magoun HW. Brain stem reticular formation and activation of the EEG. *Electroencephalogr Clin Neurophysiol*. 1949;1(4):455–473.
122. Devor M, Zalkind V. Reversible analgesia, atonia, and loss of consciousness on bilateral intracerebral microinjection of pentobarbital. *Pain*. 2001;94(1):101–112.
123. Abulafia R, Zalkind V, Devor M. Cerebral activity during the anesthesia-like state induced by mesopontine microinjection of pentobarbital. *J Neurosci*. 2009;29(21):7053–7064.
124. Cromwell HC, Woodward DJ. Inhibitory gating of single unit activity in amygdala: effects of ketamine, haloperidol, or nicotine. *Biol Psychiatry*. 2007;61(7):880–889.
125. Miller LM, Escabí MA, Read HL, Schreiner CE. Spectrotemporal receptive fields in the lemniscal auditory thalamus and cortex. *J Neurophysiol*. 2002;87(1):516–527.
126. Ticku MK, Maksay G. Convulsant/depressant site of action at the allosteric benzodiazepine-GABA receptor-ionophore complex. *Life Sci*. 1983;33(24):2363–2375.
127. Faingold CL, Hoffmann WE, Caspary DM. Effects of iontophoretic application of convulsants on the sensory responses of neurons in the brain-stem reticular formation. *Electroencephalogr Clin Neurophysiol*. 1984;58(1):55–64.
128. Faingold CL, Hoffmann WE, Caspary DM. Comparative effects of convulsant drugs on the sensory responses of neurons in the amygdala and brainstem reticular formation. *Neuropharmacology*. 1985;24(12):1221–1230.
129. Faingold CL, Stittsworth Jr JD. Comparative effects of pentylenetetrazol on the sensory responsiveness of lateral geniculate and reticular formation neurons. *Electroencephalogr Clin Neurophysiol*. 1980;49(1–2):168–172.
130. Spray KJ, Bernstein IL. Afferent and efferent connections of the parvicellular subdivision of iNTS: defining a circuit involved in taste aversion learning. *Behav Brain Res*. 2004;154(1):85–97.
131. Maren S, Hobin JA. Hippocampal regulation of context-dependent neuronal activity in the lateral amygdala. *Learn Mem*. 2007;14(4):318–324.
132. Chen FJ, Sara SJ. Locus coeruleus activation by foot shock or electrical stimulation inhibits amygdala neurons. *Neuroscience*. 2007;144(2):472–481.
133. Weldon DA, DiNieri JA, Silver MR, Thomas AA, Wright RE. Reward-related neuronal activity in the rat superior colliculus. *Behav Brain Res*. 2007;177(1):160–164.
134. Colas D, Chuluun B, Warrier D, et al. Short-term treatment with the GABAA receptor antagonist pentylenetetrazole produces a sustained pro-cognitive benefit in a mouse model of Down's syndrome. *Br J Pharmacol*. 2013;169(5):963–973.
135. Carp J, Gmeindl L, Reuter-Lorenz PA. Age differences in the neural representation of working memory revealed by multi-voxel pattern analysis. *Front Hum Neurosci*. 2010;4:217.
136. Blisard KS, Fagin K, Falivena P, et al. Experimental seizures in the frog (*Rana pipiens*). *Epilepsy Res*. 1994;17(1):13–22.
137. Popova NK, Lobacheva II, Karmanova IG, Shilling NV. Serotonin in the control of the sleep-like states in frogs. *Pharmacol Biochem Behav*. 1984;20(5):653–657.
138. Eidietis L. The tactile-stimulated startle response of tadpoles: acceleration performance and its relationship to the anatomy of wood frog (*Rana sylvatica*), bullfrog (*Rana catesbeiana*), and American toad (*Bufo americanus*) tadpoles. *J Exp Zool A Comp Exp Biol*. 2006;305(4):348–362.
139. Hamamoto DT, Simone DA. Characterization of cutaneous primary afferent fibers excited by acetic acid in a model of nociception in frogs. *J Neurophysiol*. 2003;90(2):566–577.
140. Faingold CL. Brainstem networks: reticulo-cortical synchronization in generalized convulsive seizures. In: Noebels JL, Avoli M, Rogawski MA, Olsen RW, Delgado-Escueta AV, eds. *Jasper's Basic Mechanisms of the Epilepsies*. 4th ed. New York, NY: Oxford University Press; 2012:257–271.
141. Raisinghani M, Feng HJ, Faingold CL. Glutamatergic activation of the amygdala differentially mimics the effects of audiogenic seizure kindling in two substrains of genetically epilepsy-prone rats. *Exp Neurol*. 2003;183(2):516–522.
142. Marcus G. *Kluge: The Haphazard Evolution of the Human Mind*. Boston, MA: Houghton Mifflin Company; 2008.
143. Behbehani MM. Functional characteristics of the midbrain periaqueductal gray. *Prog Neurobiol*. 1995;46:575–605.
144. Price JL, Drevets WC. Neurocircuitry of mood disorders. *Neuropsychopharmacology*. 2010;35(1):192–216.
145. Luppi PH, Clement O, Sapin E, et al. Brainstem mechanisms of paradoxical (REM) sleep generation. *Pflugers Arch*. 2012;463(1):43–52.
146. Sigurdsson T, Doyère V, Cain CK, LeDoux JE. Long-term potentiation in the amygdala: a cellular mechanism of fear learning and memory. *Neuropharmacology*. 2007;52(1):215–227.
147. Sah P, Westbrook RF, Lüthi A. Fear conditioning and long-term potentiation in the amygdala: what really is the connection? *Ann N Y Acad Sci*. 2008;1129:88–95.
148. Rosenkranz JA. Neuronal activity causes rapid changes of lateral amygdala neuronal membrane properties and reduction of synaptic integration and synaptic plasticity in vivo. *J Neurosci*. 2011;31(16):6108–6120.
149. Tupal S, Faingold CL. Precipitous induction of audiogenic kindling by activation of adenylyl cyclase in the amygdala. *Epilepsia*. 2010;51(3):354–361.
150. Faingold CL. Role of GABA abnormalities in the inferior colliculus pathophysiology – audiogenic seizures. *Hear Res*. 2002;168(1–2):223–237.
151. Bertram E. The relevance of kindling for human epilepsy. *Epilepsia*. 2007;48(Suppl. 2):65–74.
152. Lam A, Whelan N, Corcoran ME. Susceptibility of brainstem to kindling and transfer to the forebrain. *Epilepsia*. 2010;51(9):1736–1744.
153. Thompson RL, Cassell MD. Differential distribution and non-collateralization of central amygdaloid neurons projecting to different medullary regions. *Neurosci Lett*. 1989;97(3):245–251.
154. Takeuchi Y, Satoda T, Tashiro T, Matsushima R, Uemura-Sumi M. Amygdaloid pathway to the trigeminal motor nucleus via the pontine reticular formation in the rat. *Brain Res Bull*. 1988;21(5):829–833.
155. Oka T, Tsumori T, Sokota S, Yasui Y. Neuroanatomical and neurochemical organization of projections from the central

amygdaloid nucleus to the nucleus retroambiguus via the periaqueductal gray in the rat. *Neurosci Res*. 2008;62(4):286–298.

156. Fort P, Luppi PH, Jouvet M. Afferents to the nucleus reticularis parvicellularis of the cat medulla oblongata: a tract-tracing study with cholera toxin B subunit. *J Comp Neurol*. 1994;342(4):603–618.
157. Leite-Almeida H, Valle-Fernandes A, Almeida A. Brain projections from the medullary dorsal reticular nucleus: an anterograde and retrograde tracing study in the rat. *Neuroscience*. 2006;140(2):577–595.
158. Dujardin E, Jurgens U. Afferents of vocalization-controlling periaqueductal regions in the squirrel monkey. *Brain Res*. 2005;1034(1–2):114–131.
159. Viltart O, Sartor DM, Verberne AJ. Chemical stimulation of visceral afferents activates medullary neurones projecting to the central amygdala and periaqueductal grey. *Brain Res Bull*. 2006;71(1–3):51–59.
160. da Costa Gomez TM, Behbehani MM. An electrophysiological characterization of the projection from the central nucleus of the amygdala to the periaqueductal gray of the rat: the role of opioid receptors. *Brain Res*. 1995;689(1):21–31.
161. Tupal S, Faingold CL. The amygdala to periaqueductal gray pathway: plastic changes induced by audiogenic kindling and reversal by gabapentin. *Brain Res*. 2012;1475:71–79.
162. Mainero C, Boshyan J, Hadjikhani N. Altered functional magnetic resonance imaging resting-state connectivity in periaqueductal gray networks in migraine. *Ann Neurol*. 2011;70(5):838–845.
163. Linnman C, Beucke JC, Jensen KB, Gollub RL, Kong J. Sex similarities and differences in pain-related periaqueductal gray connectivity. *Pain*. 2012;153(2):444–454.
164. Pascoe JP, Kapp BS. Electrophysiology of the dorsolateral mesopontine reticular formation during Pavlovian conditioning in the rabbit. *Neuroscience*. 1993;54(3):753–772.
165. Feldt S, Bonifazi P, Cossart R. Dissecting functional connectivity of neuronal microcircuits: experimental and theoretical insights. *Trends Neurosci*. 2011;34(5):225–236.

CHAPTER

29

Neuronal Network Interactions in the Startle Reflex, Learning Mechanisms, and CNS Disorders, Including Sudden Unexpected Death in Epilepsy

Carl L. Faingold[1], *Srinivasan Tupal*[2]

[1]Departments of Pharmacology and Neurology, Division of Neurosurgery, Southern Illinois University School of Medicine, Springfield, IL, USA, [2]Department of Anatomy and Neurobiology, Washington University, St. Louis, MO, USA

INTRODUCTION

As discussed in Chapter 1, neuronal networks exist to carry out important functions for the organism, such as sensory perception in the auditory and visual networks (Chapters 19 and 20). However, these neuronal networks seldom function in isolation. Networks commonly interact with other networks to mediate important physiological functions, and interactions between networks can be magnified in learning paradigms or be intensified by pathological conditions to induce the development of many central nervous system (CNS) disorders (see Chapters 21–27). The types of interactions between networks that can occur include additive (positive) interactions in which one network triggers a second network to carry out a more complex function than "simple" perception of a stimulus (e.g. when the sensory stimulus evokes a response involving a motor movement). More complex positive network interactions between multiple networks are also observed both under natural conditions and in behavioral-conditioning paradigms. The second major category of network interaction is a negative interaction, which occurs when the first network inhibits the action of a second network (e.g. when the sensory stimulus evokes a "freezing" response where the animal ceases any movement). A prototype of these types of interactions is shown in Figure 29.1. Three networks are symbolized by the ovals (Net 1, Net 2, and Net 3). Nets 1 and 2 have exogenous and/or endogenous inputs (Inputs 1 and 2). Each network controls a function or behavior (Functions 1, 2, and 3). Either additive (positive) or negative interactions can occur. Additive network interactions occur when activation of one network leads to activation of a second network, which then may result in feedback activation of each other and/or a third network. For example, Net 1 could be the somatosensory network that is responsible for the organism's ability to perceive touch stimuli, and Net 2 could be the auditory network responsible for the organism's ability to hear. Net 3 could be the limbic network, which is involved in control of the organism's emotional state (Function 3). An example of the interaction of these networks is seen in response to a foot shock stimulus that activates Net 1 and in turn activates Net 3 (to which it projects). A second (acoustic) stimulus that follows closely after the first stimulus activates Net 2, which also projects to Net 3. After a number of repetitions of this stimulus sequence, Net 3 produces fear-potentiated startle, which would be New Function 4. Competitive network interactions can also occur in which two networks compete for dominance over a behavior, such as seen in CNS disorders like epilepsy, chronic pain disorders, and Parkinson's disease; these disorders can be treated with different stimulation therapies, which are proposed to involve competitive network interactions, as discussed in Chapter 31.

Network interactions can result in beneficial outcomes for the organism that enhance survival,[1] but the

Neuronal Networks in Brain Function, CNS Disorders, and Therapeutics
http://dx.doi.org/10.1016/B978-0-12-415804-7.00029-0

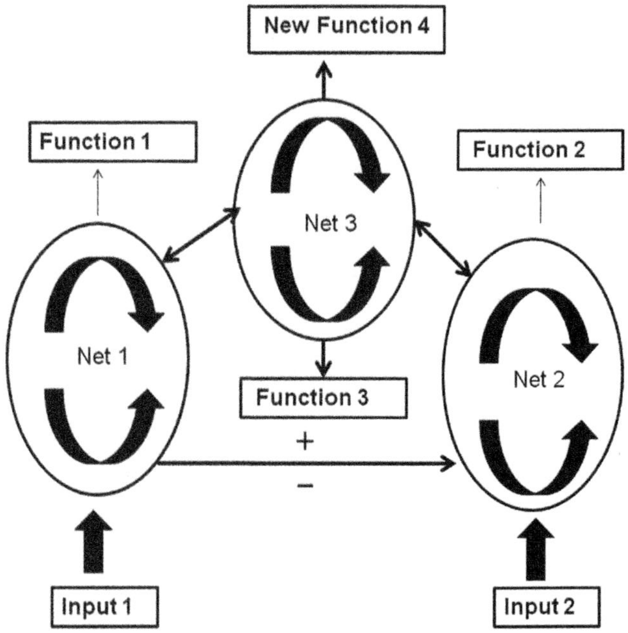

FIGURE 29.1 Diagram of potential multiple network interactions and mechanisms. Both positive (+) and negative (−) interactions can occur, as indicated by the signs above and below the arrow. The three networks are symbolized by the ovals (Net 1, Net 2, and Net 3). Nets 1 and 2 have exogenous and/or endogenous inputs (Inputs 1 and 2). For simplicity, the input to Network 3 is omitted, but it may be spontaneously active. Each network is considered to have a normal function or behavior that it controls (Functions 1, 2, and 3). All nets are shown as undergoing a significant degree of self-organization, as illustrated by the paired semicircular arrows. Positive network interactions can involve the activation of one individual network, which then activates the second network, and they can activate or inhibit each other as well as the third network. For example, Net 1 could be the somatosensory network, which mediates perception of touch stimuli, and Net 2 could be the auditory network responsible for the organism's ability to hear. Net 3 could be the limbic network, which is responsible for the organism's emotional state (Function 3). An example of the interaction of these networks is when a foot shock stimulus activates Net 1 and it projects to Net 3. The second (acoustic) stimulus then occurs, which projects to Net 2 and also projects to Net 3. After a number of repetitions of this stimulus sequence, Net 3 produces fear-potentiated startle, which would be New Function 4.

interactions can also result in deleterious effects on the organism, such as those that have been observed in certain types of epileptic seizures.[2,3] An example of a very serious deleterious network interaction is seen in the sequential interaction of networks that is proposed to occur in human epilepsy, called sudden unexpected death in epilepsy (SUDEP), which is associated with respiratory difficulties in many human cases. In animal models of SUDEP, this phenomenon is proposed to involve the sequential interaction of three networks,[4] as discussed in this chapter. In other situations, networks could be activated by different inputs concurrently, but no interaction between the networks is detectable.

The mechanisms involved in physiologically meaningful interactions between networks are also quite varied. Anatomical connections between the networks that mediate synaptic projections from neurons in one network to those in another network are generally, but not always, required. In accord with the general concepts discussed in Chapter 1, networks can also potentially interact based on neuroactive substances that are released by the activation of one network and carried to another network by synaptic transmission but also by the brain's "circulation system"—that is, by volume conduction (see Chapters 7 and 8).

In many cases, the normal function of the network requires that a second network becomes active to complete some normal "reflex" action, such as the acoustic startle response, which is an innate but usually dormant network interaction. Network interaction could also be induced by several different classes of phenomena, including physiological as well as pathological influences and conditions. Thus, the network interaction could be induced by the animal's experiences in its natural environment, such as the presence of a predator or food source in a particular location in the animal's environment. This interaction can serve important functions for the animal by mediating important learning experiences. A neuronal network interaction can be induced due to a pathological event or events and result in the induction of a CNS disorder, such as chronic pain syndrome induced by repetitive acute pain. Finally, a network interaction could be induced by a therapeutic intervention, including stimulation therapy paradigms, such as acupuncture analgesia or deep-brain stimulation (see Chapter 31). Network interactions can also be acute and short term in nature or long term and chronic. Interactions between neuronal networks may involve sequential or simultaneous network activation or inhibition. The "gate control theory of pain"[5,6] is a prototype of the competitive or negative network interaction. This theory posits that pain perception can be reduced or blocked by peripheral nonpainful stimuli that close the "gate" in the spinal cord and reduce the transmission of pain impulses by a competition between the painful and nonpainful stimuli for transmission to the nociceptive regions of the brain. Thus, as seen in Figure 29.2, it is proposed that both large (Aβ fibers) and small fibers (C fibers) synapse onto the substantia gelatinosa (SG) of the spinal cord and the first central transmission (T) cells. The inhibitory effect exerted by SG cells onto the primary afferent fiber terminals at the T cells is increased by activity in Aβ fibers and decreased by activity in C fibers. The central control trigger is illustrated by the connection from the Aβ fiber system to the central control mechanisms; these mechanisms, in turn, project back to the gate control system (see Chapter 23). Comparisons between the results of network studies in

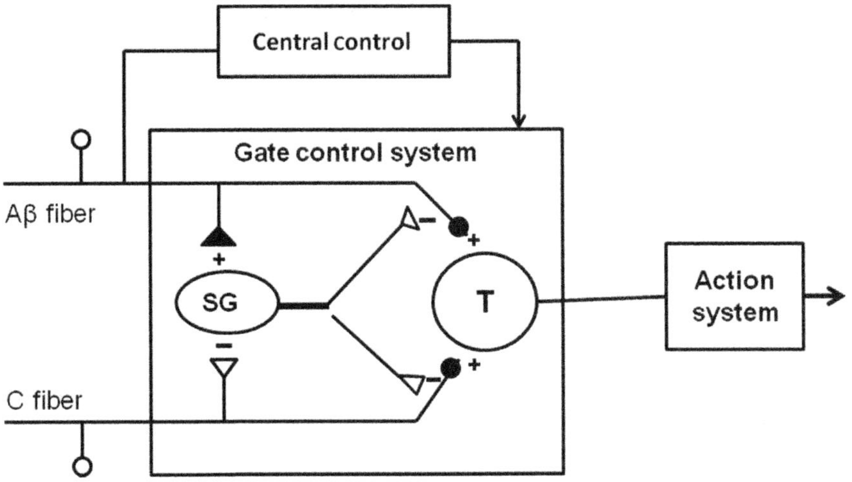

FIGURE 29.2 The gate control theory of pain proposes that both large (Aβ fibers) and small fibers (C fibers) synapse onto cells in the substantia gelatinosa (SG) and the first central transmission (T) cells. The inhibitory effect exerted by SG cells onto the primary afferent fiber terminals at the T cells is increased by activity in Aβ fibers and decreased by activity in C fibers. This network interaction decreases the central perception of pain. The central control trigger is represented by a line running from the Aβ fiber system to the central control mechanisms; these mechanisms, in turn, project back to the gate control system. The T cells project to the entry cells of the action system. +: excitation; −: inhibition. (*Source: From Melzack and Wall*[5] *with permission of* Science.)

human disorders and animal models suggest that there are considerable interspecies network similarities,[7,8] which is vital for being able to apply results in animals to the human conditions being modeled.

Noninvasive approaches to network exploration, especially in humans, include the recording of electrical or magnetic events on various locations on the scalp. These electroencephalography (EEG) and magnetoencephalography (MEG) recordings are widely used as methods of network exploration in humans and are useful clinically (Chapter 6). Thus, brain areas that exhibit synchronized dominant frequencies in EEG or MEG are proposed to be participating in the same network[9] (see Chapter 6). Synchronization of neuronal oscillations may regulate network communication at a systems level based on temporal coordination among anatomically and functionally distributed brain regions. This approach has shown behaviorally significant phenomena that correlate with specific functions related to perception and cognition,[9,10] but the mechanisms that subserve the synchronization are unclear.

The noninvasive technique of functional magnetic resonance imaging, which is used commonly in people and occasionally in animals (Chapters 3 and 6), along with invasive approaches used most commonly in animals (Chapters 1–7) are more direct methods for network exploration. The importance of epilepsy as a prototype network to model CNS disorders (noted in Chapter 1) is exemplified by the fact that certain of these invasive techniques, particularly neuronal recording, can ethically be used in patients with epilepsy but in few other disorders.[11] The results yielded by these techniques in animals are the main basis for the network discussion in the remainder of this chapter.

It is a common finding that primary or "dedicated" sensory networks interact with other primary networks, as well as nonprimary or conditional multireceptive (CMR) networks, as discussed in Chapter 28. Thus, the startle response is a prototypical example of network interaction that is induced by an intense or unexpected stimulus, which is a rapid and extensive interaction of the primary auditory or somatosensory network with the locomotor network, also discussed in detail in Chapter 28.

DUAL NETWORK INTERACTIONS

Many of the primary networks, including the locomotor and respiratory networks, have major interactions with other primary networks, including each other, as discussed in Chapters 17 and 18.

Visual Network Interactions

The primary visual network also has major connections to other networks, which mediate its participation in multisensory interactions and sensorimotor integration. For example, the superior colliculus is part of the dorsal stream of the visual network, which projects to neurons that innervate the muscles that control eye movements (Chapter 19). The visual network also interacts with the auditory network and can magnify the acoustic startle response. Thus, the amplitude of the acoustic startle response is increased when elicited during sustained exposure to bright light (light-enhanced startle), which is subserved by a network that differs from that which mediates the primary acoustic startle response.[12]

Interactions between the visual network and motor network can also occur at the level of the cortex. Thus, locomotion-related activity of neurons in the motor cortex is modified when subjects switch between walking in the darkness and in light. The firing pattern of ~50% of neurons from layer V of the motor cortex was significantly altered by the change in visual input.[13] The visual network at the level of the brainstem also interacts with the olfactory network. Thus, the superior colliculus in the visual system interacts with the olfactory system in rats trained to perform a delayed-response, odor-cued spatial choice task. These visual neurons fired well in advance of movement initiated by the olfactory stimulus.[14] The visual pathway also interacts with epilepsy networks in what is called "reflex epilepsy"—in which a seizure can be induced by visual stimuli, such as a flashing light[15]—but the neuronal network involved has not been established. Visually induced seizures are also observed in epileptic baboons. Network exploration in this model has shown that the epileptic discharges are triggered by the parietal, occipital, and frontocentral cortices, but the subcortical pathway (dorsal or ventral stream) (Chapter 19) that projects to these cortical sites is not yet clear.[16]

Somatosensory Network Interactions

The primary somatosensory network interacts with other networks, including the locomotor network, in the tactile startle response.[17,18] This response involves a direct projection from the principal somatosensory nucleus to the caudal pontine brainstem reticular formation (BRF) neurons, which then projects to motor neurons in the spinal cord.[17] Somatosensory inputs are also important in the function of the locomotor network (Chapter 17). The somatosensory network, including nuclei in the brainstem (cuneate, gracillis, and trigeminal), projects to the auditory network, especially the cochlear nuclei, and has short- and long-term effects on neuronal responses under normal conditions, which are altered in the CNS disorder of tinnitus[19] (Chapter 20).

Pain Network Interactions

The pain network (see Chapter 23) also has significant interactions with other networks involving connections from this pathway to limbic structures, including the amygdala. In addition, the pain network can interact with dormant networks that are or can be activated, especially with stimulation therapies (see Chapter 31). In these cases, competition between networks can exert beneficial effects. Thus, the neuronal network that mediates acupuncture analgesia is proposed to activate structures of the antinociceptive pathway and deactivate limbic structures within the pain-mediating pathway.[20] This appears to involve a dual interaction with and inhibition of the pain network, and a positive interaction with the antinociceptive network.[21]

Auditory Network Interactions

The primary auditory network has been shown to have a number of connections to other networks, which operate during normal brain function, as well as a number of network connections that can be magnified by various kinds of normal experiences and greatly intensified by certain pathological situations. In addition to the locomotor network mentioned in this chapter, the primary auditory network (Chapter 20) can interact with several other networks in differing situations and conditions. These interactions can often occur naturally and can be evoked by repetitive experiences and lead to useful learning, or they can be induced pathologically and contribute to the development of a CNS disorder. Thus, the auditory network is known to interact with the emotional network in the limbic system, particularly the amygdala, which mediates emotional responses. Fear-potentiated startle, discussed in the "Fear-Potentiated Startle" section, and a related conditioning paradigm called fear conditioning (which is covered extensively in Chapter 13) are prominent examples of this normal interaction that are magnified by behavioral-conditioning paradigms. In addition, in a model of the CNS disorder of epilepsy with sound-evoked or audiogenic seizures (AGS), the auditory network interacts with the brainstem locomotor network, and these networks can be induced to interact with the limbic network (amygdala) by a paradigm involving periodic AGS repetition called "AGS kindling" (see Chapter 27). The auditory network can also interact with the cerebellum in the case of pathological conditions such as tinnitus, as discussed in Chapter 20. Tinnitus has also been associated with auditory network interactions with the limbic network (hippocampus).[22]

MULTINETWORK INTERACTIONS

Fear-Potentiated Startle

As discussed in detail in Chapter 28, startle responses involve extensive interactions between a primary sensory (auditory, somatosensory, or visual) pathway and elements of the brainstem locomotor pathway. A phenomenon called "fear-potentiated startle", which is produced by pairing an electric shock to the foot with an acoustic stimulus, results in enhancement of the amplitude of the startle response.[23] This response is a physiological correlate of fear conditioning (Chapter 13). Fear-potentiated startle has been examined in a number of mammalian species, including humans, and it is proposed to be a model of posttraumatic stress disorder.[24,25] As shown in Figure 29.3, fear-potentiated

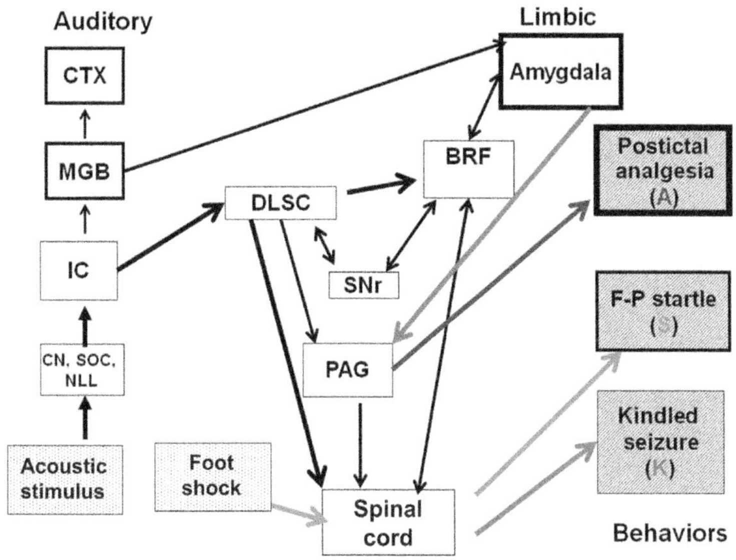

FIGURE 29.3 Specific network interaction diagrams in three related forms of auditory network interactions with other networks, including the somatosensory, pain, and limbic (emotional) networks. (1) Audiogenic seizures (AGS)-induced analgesia (A, blue arrows). The AGS network can also interact with the pain network via a common network nucleus (PAG). (2) The fear-potentiated (F-P) startle network (S, green arrows) involves somatosensory input (foot shock) via the spinal cord, which projects to a common network nucleus (BRF). (3) The AGS-kindling network (K, red arrows) involves the emotional network, including the amygdala. Analgesia is induced after AGS (postictal) and is short term, lasting for >2 h after the seizure. Fear-potentiated startle is induced by repetitive pairing of foot shock with an acoustic stimulus and is long-lasting. AGS kindling consists of daily or twice-daily audiogenic seizure repetition for 14–21 seizures and is long-lasting. The black arrows are pathways that are proposed to be involved in all three networks. BRF = brainstem reticular formation; CN = cochlear nucleus; CTX = cortex; DLSC = deep layers of superior colliculus; IC = inferior colliculus; MGB = medial geniculate body; NLL = nucleus of the lateral lemniscus; PAG = periaqueductal gray; SNr = substantia nigra reticulata; SOC = superior olivary complex. (The figure is reproduced in color section.)

startle initially involves interactions of the auditory network (Chapter 20) with the brainstem locomotor network (Chapter 17), as described in this chapter for the startle response. When the fear-inducing stimulus, the foot shock, is introduced, the network expands to include the amygdala and additional regions of the BRF, which are both CMR structures (Chapter 28). Lesions of the amygdala (central) block fear-potentiated acoustic startle, and electrical stimulation of this structure enhances acoustic startle involving the BRF (the nucleus reticularis pontis caudalis, or PnC), which is a key nucleus in the acoustic startle network (see Chapter 28). The amygdala also projects to other CMR regions, including the periaqueductal gray (PAG), the deep layers of the superior colliculus (DLSC) and deep mesencephalic nucleus (DpMe), and the lateral mesencephalic BRF that also projects to the PnC[23] (Chapter 28). There are both a direct projection between the amygdala and PnC[26] and projections via the DLSC and DpMe that are involved in fear-potentiated startle.[23] Lesions of the PAG prior to and after fear conditioning totally blocked the increase in amplitude of the acoustic startle response, although the baseline amplitude was not affected by the PAG lesions.[27] Similarly, focal blockade of the DLSC–DpMe or the PAG (but not other nearby brainstem sites) blocked fear-potentiated startle when performed before testing but had no effect on baseline startle amplitude. These findings suggest that the DLSC–DpMe pathway is a critical projection pathway in this network between the amygdala and the PnC in mediating fear-potentiated startle.[23,28] Thus, the simple acoustic startle network for the initial response, which involves only a few brainstem nuclei initially (see Chapter 28), undergoes expansion to include limbic and additional brainstem sites due to the introduction of an emotional element (fear) induced by the foot shock. As noted in this section, this interaction of CNS neuronal networks is associated with the occurrence of a major CNS disorder, posttraumatic stress disorder.

AGS Kindling

AGS in rodents involve an interaction between two networks, the brainstem auditory and locomotor networks (see Chapter 26). Repetition of these seizures in an "AGS-kindling" paradigm results in network expansion to involve a third network, the limbic (emotional) network (Chapter 27). As shown in Figure 29.3, in response to the intense acoustic stimulus, the auditory network activates the brainstem locomotor network associated with generalized tonic and/or clonic AGS (see Chapter 26). With frequent repetition of the stimulus, which induces repetitive seizures and results in AGS kindling (see Chapter 27), there is a second input to the locomotor network from the amygdala. The severe seizure strain of genetically epilepsy-prone rats (GEPR-9s) inherits consistent susceptibility to tonic extension AGS in response to intense acoustic stimuli. AGS kindling in GEPR-9s results in prolongation of the seizure and the appearance of an additional seizure behavior (posttonic generalized clonus), which is absent before AGS kindling in these animals.[29] Reversible blockade of the amygdala after AGS kindling temporarily causes the seizure behavior pattern to revert to the behavior pattern seen before AGS kindling.[30] Thus, the input from the amygdala to the locomotor network subserves the additional motor behavior at the end of each kindled AGS seizure. The PAG (ventrolateral) is a requisite nucleus in the nonkindled AGS network in GEPR-9s and several other AGS models.[31–34] The PAG also becomes the critical hub for the AGS-kindled seizure by providing a sequential series of inputs to the locomotor network during the expression of each seizure behavior. Thus, AGS kindling induced significant increases in the acoustic responsiveness of PAG neurons. During AGS in both AGS-kindled and nonkindled GEPR-9s, PAG neurons displayed tonic firing during wild running and tonic extension seizure behaviors. However, the PAG tonic-firing pattern changed to burst firing exclusively after AGS kindling, which was never seen in the PAG of nonkindled rats.[35] Burst firing is a hallmark of neuroplastic changes known to mediate increased synaptic efficiency (Chapter 9), and this firing pattern is also induced in amygdala neurons by AGS kindling.[36] These findings suggest that the amygdala-to-PAG pathway may be a critical element of the expanded seizure network.[35] The pathway between the amygdala (central nucleus) and PAG is implicated in the networks that subserve several other CNS disorders, including pain and anxiety (Chapters 23 and 24), and major input from the amygdala to the PAG is also implicated in the network that mediates AGS kindling in GEPR-9s, as noted here. AGS kindling induces changes in PAG neuronal responses evoked by electrical stimuli in the amygdala (central nucleus). These amygdala stimuli evoked consistent, short-latency PAG neuronal firing, which increased with increasing intensity of the stimulus. After AGS kindling, these PAG neuronal responses exhibited neuroplasticity, as shown by the precipitous increase in firing with increasing stimulus intensity, which was significantly greater than the response pattern in nonkindled GEPR-9s. These findings indicate that neuroplastic changes in the amygdala-to-PAG pathway may be critical in mediating the network expansion that results in the seizure behavior changes in AGS kindling[37] (see Chapter 27). These data indicate that the expansion of the seizure network involves an interaction with the limbic network, which is mediated by reentry from the amygdala back to the PAG that results in the appearance of the final convulsive behavior that is the defining behavior of the AGS-kindled seizure.

Epilepsy and Pain Network Interactions

Generalized seizures induced by electroshock and convulsant drugs as well as AGS can induce analgesia for hours after the seizure.[38–44] Reduced responsiveness to pain also occurs in human epilepsy.[45] GEPR-9s are susceptible to severe AGS, as noted in this chapter and discussed in Chapter 26. The PAG (ventrolateral), as discussed in the "Audiogenic Seizure Kindling" section, is a critical hub in AGS and AGS kindling[32–34] (Chapter 26), but this structure is also known to be a major nucleus in the network that mediates analgesia[46–48] (Chapter 23). The PAG is also an important site for endocannabinoid-mediated analgesia.[49,50] A recent study indicated that seizure-induced analgesia (to radiant heat-induced pain) was observed for at least 120 min after AGS in GEPR-9s.[44] This analgesia was induced by the seizure, since presentation of the same acoustic stimulus in normal rats did not have any significant effect on pain thresholds. Focal blockade of the PAG by microinjection of a cannabinoid (CB1) receptor antagonist in GEPR-9s significantly decreased the seizure-induced (postictal) analgesia. The onset of analgesia was also consistent with the time course of endocannabinoid release after seizure induction observed in previous studies.[51] The nucleus raphe magnus (NRM) is a structure in the rostral ventral medulla that is a major site in the endogenous pain inhibitory system that receives projections from the PAG (Chapter 23). Postictal analgesia induced by a convulsant drug (pentylenetetrazol) is blocked by focal microinjection into the NRM of agents that block acetylcholine receptors, indicating that the NRM is also involved in the network that mediates postictal analgesia.[52] Thus, activation of seizure networks induced by either convulsant drugs or AGS interacts with and activates the antinociceptive network at different nuclei to induce analgesia, which is another example of multinetwork interaction.

SUDEP Network

The final multiple network interaction that we will discuss is potentially the most serious one in animals and people. The phenomenon of SUDEP is a relatively rare but devastating seizure sequela.[53] The most common observed cause of death in SUDEP is respiratory malfunction that occurs after a generalized seizure.[54] Animal models of SUDEP in DBA/2 and DBA/1 strains of mice have been proposed in which interactions occur sequentially among three networks that begin with an additive (positive) interaction and are followed by a negative network interaction. This interaction begins with activation of the auditory network by an intense acoustic stimulus, which leads to activation of the brainstem locomotor network, and this network interaction generates the motor convulsions (AGS) (Chapter 26). This process results in a negative interaction with the respiratory network (Chapter 18), inducing respiratory arrest that leads to cardiac failure and results in sudden death. Death can be prevented by immediate external respiratory support[4,55,56] (see Figure 29.4).

The nature of the network interaction between the seizure network and the respiratory network could be brought about by anatomical and physiological interactions. This network interaction could also be accomplished through volume transmission of neuroactive substances (Chapter 8) such as serotonin (5-HT) and adenosine, that are known to be released as a result of generalized seizures.[59]

The neuromodulatory roles of serotonin and adenosine have been extensively studied in the respiratory network, where they exert important influences on normal respiratory rhythm and pattern generation in these brainstem networks[60–63] (see Chapter 18). Serotonin is known to exert a primarily stimulatory effect, whereas adenosine has a depressant effect on the respiratory network. Recent evidence suggests that agents affecting the action of these substances may

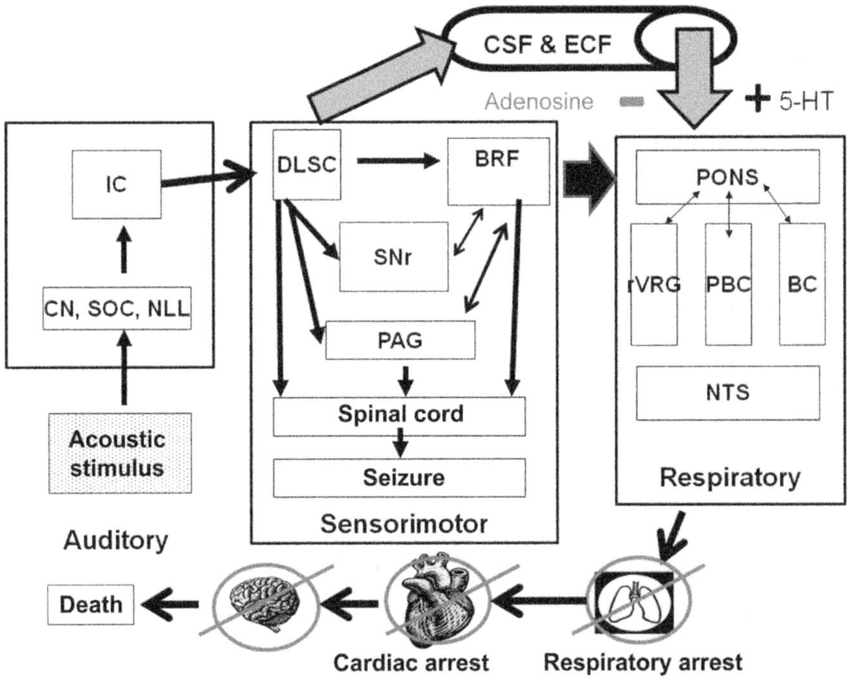

FIGURE 29.4 Diagram of network interactions involved in audiogenic seizures (AGS) that are postulated to occur in the DBA mouse models of human sudden unexpected death in epilepsy (SUDEP), which exhibit AGS, leading to death due to respiratory depression. The diagram of the elements of the normal auditory network needed for AGS induction is shown in the left panel. The diagram of the sensorimotor integration elements is shown in the middle panel. The diagram of the elements of the normal network for respiration is shown in the right panel. High-intensity acoustic stimuli activate the AGS network, which is postulated to involve a network interaction (based on that of GEPR-9s) between the normal brainstem primary auditory network nuclei [the cochlear nucleus (CN) and superior olivary complex (SOC)] up to the level of the inferior colliculus (IC). The IC projects to elements of sensorimotor integration, which project to elements of the normal midbrain locomotion network. This pathway begins with the deep layers of the superior colliculus (DLSC) and proceeds to the periaqueductal gray (PAG), substantia nigra reticulata (SNr), and brainstem (pontine) reticular formation (BRF), which project to the spinal cord. DBA mice that exhibit severe AGS (tonic hind limb extension) exhibit postictal (seizure) depression of consciousness. The depression of consciousness is postulated to involve BRF suppression.[57,58] It is proposed that there is a negative electrophysiological effect from the BRF to areas in the medulla that control respiration. There is also proposed to be a neurochemical-based network interaction between the seizure network and the respiratory network, involving the release of neuroactive substances via volume transmission into the cerebral spinal fluid (CSF) and the extracellular fluid (ECF) that affects the respiratory network. These influences include negative effects, mediated by adenosine and other respiratory depressant neuroactive substances, and positive effects mediated by substances that enhance respiration, such as serotonin (5-HT), and that are released due to the seizure. When the balance of these neuroactive substances is tilted in the negative direction due to diminished 5-HT-mediated activation or excessive adenosine-mediated inhibition, it is proposed to result in respiratory arrest, cerebral shutdown, and sudden death associated with subsequent cardiac failure. The latter events are believed to model a major cause of human SUDEP. The order of events can differ among different SUDEP cases. rVRG = rostral ventral respiratory group; PBC = pre-Bötzinger complex; BC = Bötzinger complex; NTS = nucleus tractus solitarius. (For color version of this figure, the reader is referred to the online version of this book.)

be able to modulate the respiratory network and affect susceptibility to SUDEP in seizure models in animals.

Serotonin in SUDEP

Neurons in the brainstem raphe nuclei are the primary sources of serotonin and include midbrain dorsal and superior central raphe nuclei, pontine raphe and inferior raphe nuclei, and medullary raphe pallidus, magnus, and obscurus nuclei.[64,65] This serotonergic network plays an important role in the maintenance of homeostasis, including thermoregulation and central chemoreception, by mediating ventilator responses to hypoxia, hypercapnia, and acidosis.[66–74] The role of raphe serotonergic neurons as sensors of arterial carbon dioxide and pH is supported by their anatomical contiguity with major blood vessels in the CNS.[75,76] A significant proportion of the broad-ranging influence of serotonergic neurotransmission on behavioral networks occurs through *en passant* or volume neurotransmission (Chapter 8). This involves release of serotonin from the axonal varicosities into the extracellular milieu and diffusion into the cerebrospinal fluid, extracellular fluid, and vasculature. The serotonergic neurons also send long-range projections to cortical, subcortical, and diencephalic areas and play a role in arousal, anxiety, and aggression. Shorter range serotonergic projections from the caudal medullary raphe to other medullary regions include the pre-Bötzinger complex (preBötC), known as the inspiratory central pattern generator, which plays a vital role in modulating respiratory rhythm and pattern generation as well as the ventilatory responses.[72,77,78] The serotonergic neurons in the medullary raphe interact with respiratory motor neurons in the cervical spinal cord and cranial nerve motor nuclei in the brainstem to augment respiratory responses to intermittent hypoxic challenges, which involves long-term plasticity.[60,79] The serotonergic projections, its receptors, and its transporters are expressed in its various brainstem and spinal target regions, including the respiratory network (Chapter 18). The inspiratory preBötC neurons express Gi-coupled 5-HT_{1A} receptors and postsynaptic Gs-coupled 5-HT_4 receptors. Agonists of 5-HT_{1A} and 5-HT_4 receptors can reverse opioid-mediated respiratory depression of preBötC and *N*-methyl-D-aspartate (NMDA) receptor inhibition and barbiturate-mediated apneusis.[80–84] Likewise, Gq-coupled 5-HT_2 receptors and Gs-coupled 5-HT_7 receptors are expressed in cervical spinal phrenic motor nuclei and mediate long-term facilitation.[62,63]

Several studies have observed deficits in serotonergic neurotransmission in DBA mice. The DBA/2 mice carry a single nucleotide polymorphism (homozygous for the G/G allele) in the tryptophan hydroxylase 2 (TPH2) (C1473G) gene, which catalyzes the rate-limiting step in the biosynthesis of 5-HT and results in a reduced rate of synthesis of 5-HT.[85–88] An adaptive propensity for desensitization of 5-HT_{1A} receptors supports maintenance of ambient 5-HT levels in the dorsal raphe nucleus. In addition, the rostral ventral medulla, which contains important nuclei in the respiratory network, exhibits significant deficits in the expression of 5-HT_{2C} and 5-HT_3 receptors in DBA mice.[89,90] These 5-HT-related deficits may contribute to the inability of serotonin to effectively interact with the respiratory network to maintain vital respiratory function during the postictal depression that follows AGS in DBA mice. Selective serotonin reuptake inhibitors (SSRIs), which increase the availability and prolong the effects of 5-HT, when administered prior to seizure induction in DBA mice can prevent seizure-induced respiratory arrest (S-IRA) that follows AGS.[55,91,92] One SSRI (fluoxetine) differed in its effective prophylactic doses between the DBA strains, which may be due, in part, to their differences in 5-HT_{2B} receptor expression in the ventral medulla. Several SSRIs are effective in blocking S-IRA in DBA/1 mice, but only fluoxetine is effective without a partial reduction of the tonic seizure component; one of these SSRIs, paroxetine, has delayed and extremely limited effectiveness.[92] Buspirone, a 5-HT_{1A} receptor partial agonist, is effective against a severe apneustic pattern of breathing in patients[93] and is also effective in reducing S-IRA incidence in DBA/2 mice in our preliminary studies. In contrast, cyproheptadine, a nonselective 5-HT receptor blocker, reversibly induced susceptibility to S-IRA following tonic AGS in those DBA/2 mice ($\sim 15\%$) that exhibit seizures without respiratory arrest.[55] SSRIs have also been shown to reduce the degree of respiratory depression associated with seizures in certain patients.[94] SSRI treatment also has the ability to significantly reduce the number of apneas in patients with sleep apnea[95] and to enhance respiration in rats when administered centrally.[96]

Adenosine in SUDEP

As noted in this chapter, adenosine is well known to be released as a result of seizures. Adenosine has been identified as a transmitter or co-transmitter in many peripheral and CNS sites, including CNS neurons and glia and neuron–glial interactions.[97] Adenosine levels in the brain are known to rise precipitously in human and animal forms of seizure during postictal depression to micromolar levels, which activate all adenosine receptor subtypes.[98,99] Probes implanted in the hippocampus of epileptic patients detected up to a $\sim$30-fold increase of extracellular adenosine during seizure activity.[100] Adenosine released by seizures has been proposed to act as an endogenous anticonvulsant mechanism,[100–102] and it also exerts major neuromodulatory effects on neuronal and glial networks (see Chapter 7). Central control of respiration is mediated by the respiratory network in the brainstem, which includes the pontine respiratory group, ventral respiratory column (VRC), and dorsal respiratory group, including the nucleus of the solitary tract as well as the rostral ventral respiratory group[103,104] (Chapter 18). Adenosine is also implicated in the central control of respiration, and it produces long-lasting inhibition of neurons in this respiratory network, acting at A1 purinergic receptors.[105,106] Adenosine agonists acting at the A1 receptor prolong postictal depression, while A1 antagonists shorten it.[107] Although release of adenosine by seizures is proposed to be a mechanism to limit seizures, the respiratory depressant effect of adenosine may make an important contribution to the respiratory dysfunction commonly seen in association with seizures in epileptic patients.[108] Under normal conditions, adenosine concentrations are kept in the normal range by phosphorylation via adenosine kinase and deamination into inosine by adenosine deaminase.[102] During prolonged seizures or traumatic brain injury, a surge of micromolar levels of adenosine occurs, and at these levels adenosine $A2_BR$ and A3R become activated.[109,110] Likewise, blockade of $A2_AR$ facilitates long-term facilitation of inspiratory motor outputs from phrenic and cranial nerves and is proposed to be a mechanism of the beneficial effect of caffeine against respiratory depression.[111]

A nonselective adenosine antagonist is useful in treating apnea of prematurity (i.e. apnea of a premature infant), acting via a blockade of adenosine receptors A1 and A2, and a block of $A2_A$ receptors may also play an important role.[112] An animal model for SUDEP has been developed that involves the administration of inhibitors of adenosine deaminase and adenosine kinase given prior to induction of acute seizures with kainic acid. This protocol caused more severe seizures than kainic acid alone, and a high incidence of death was seen postseizure, which was not seen with kainic acid alone. They proposed this as a SUDEP model. The nonselective adenosine receptor antagonist (caffeine) blocked the deaths in these mice, and the authors suggest that the action of this agent may have been primarily by actions on $A2_A$ receptors.[101] We performed preliminary studies evaluating the effects of agents that act to block adenosine breakdown in DBA/2 mice and GEPR-9s. The DBA/2 mice were from the minority of these animals that exhibit AGS but not S-IRA,[55] and GEPR-9s seldom if ever exhibit S-IRA after AGS. Our findings indicate that antagonists that blocked the metabolism of adenosine significantly increased the incidence of S-IRA in this group of DBA/2 mice. These agents also significantly depressed respiration in GEPR-9s and caused a significant incidence of postseizure deaths in preliminary studies.[113] Thus, adenosine released by the seizure network, mediated in part by volume transmission, interacted with the respiratory network to produce failure of respiration.

In these animal models of SUDEP, these endogenously released neuroactive substances (5-HT and adenosine) mediate the interactions of the seizure network (brainstem auditory and locomotor nuclei) with the respiratory network. These neuroactive substances appear to play major roles in determining whether the animals will exhibit seizure-induced death. This additive interaction of the auditory network with the locomotor network, which leads to seizure-induced death due to a negative interaction with the respiratory network, is prevented by enhancing the availability of 5-HT but is augmented by agents that enhance the availability of adenosine. If these findings are applicable to human epilepsy, an understanding of network interactions and their mediators has the potential to prevent a fatal outcome (i.e. SUDEP) of this CNS disorder for which there is currently no established therapy.

CONCLUSIONS

Interactions between networks that are dedicated, for example, to a specific sensory modality are very common. These interactions can be additive (positive), where the first network causes the second network to become active, as seen in sensorimotor integration, which is vital to the normal function of an organism in its environment. Network interactions can also be negative, where the initially active network causes another network to become less active. Networks that are not dedicated to a specific function, called CMR networks (Chapter 28), also interact with dedicated networks very commonly. The interaction of dedicated networks with CMR networks is involved in many of the experience-based changes in brain function, including normal learning. However, many CNS disorders involve network interactions that have been subjected to pathological intensification due to a variety of influences, especially those involving repetitive experiences often coupled with conditions that are salient or exigent for the organism, such as rewarding, fearful, or painful conditions (Chapter 28). This network interaction approach provides a testable hypothesis for how therapeutic stimulation protocols exert therapeutic effects and provide potential network sites for therapeutic agents to target.

Acknowledgments

The authors gratefully acknowledge the assistance of Marcus Randall and Srinivasa P. Kommajosyula in the experiments from our lab that are discussed in this chapter. The authors were supported by NINDS, CURE, and The Epilepsy Foundation during these experiments and gratefully acknowledge the assistance of Gayle Stauffer and Diana Smith in preparing this manuscript.

References

1. Neves G, Cooke SF, Bliss TV. Synaptic plasticity, memory and the hippocampus: a neural network approach to causality. *Nat Rev Neurosci.* 2008;9(1):65–75.
2. Dudek FE, Sutula TP. Epileptogenesis in the dentate gyrus: a critical perspective. *Prog Brain Res.* 2007;163:755–773.
3. Hester MS, Danzer SC. Accumulation of abnormal adult-generated hippocampal granule cells predicts seizure frequency and severity. *J Neurosci.* 2013;33(21):8926–8936.
4. Faingold CL. Brainstem networks: reticulo-cortical synchronization in generalized convulsive seizures. In: Noebels JL, Avoli M, Rogawski MA, Olsen RW, Delgado-Escueta AV, eds. *Jasper's Basic Mechanisms of the Epilepsies.* 4th ed. New York, NY: Oxford University Press; 2012:257–271.
5. Melzack R, Wall PD. Pain mechanisms: a new theory. *Science.* 1965;150(3699):971–979.
6. Moayedi M, Davis KD. Theories of pain: from specificity to gate control. *J Neurophysiol.* 2013;109(1):5–12.
7. Lythgoe MF, Sibson NR, Harris NG. Neuroimaging of animal models of brain disease. *Brit Med Bull.* 2003;65:235–257.
8. Blumenfeld H. Functional MRI studies of animal models in epilepsy. *Epilepsia.* 2007;48(Suppl. 4):18–26.
9. Palva S, Palva JM. Discovering oscillatory interaction networks with M/EEG: challenges and breakthroughs. *Trends Cogn Sci.* 2012;16(4):219–230.
10. Melloni L, Molina C, Pena M, Torres D, Siner W, Rodriguez E. Synchronization of neural activity across cortical areas correlates with conscious perception. *J Neurosci.* 2007;27(11):2858–2865.
11. Truccolo W, Donoghue JA, Hochberg LR, et al. Single-neuron dynamics in human focal epilepsy. *Nat Neurosci.* 2011;14: 635–641.
12. Walker D, Yang Y, Ratti E, Corsi M, Trist D, Davis M. Differential effects of the CRF-R1 antagonist GSK876008 on fear-potentiated, light- and CRF-enhanced startle suggest preferential involvement in sustained vs phasic threat responses. *Neuropsychopharmacology.* 2009;34(6):1533–1542.
13. Armer MC, Nilaweera WU, Rivers TJ, Dasgupta NM, Beloozerova IN. Effect of light on the activity of motor cortex neurons during locomotion. *Behav Brain Res.* 2013; May 13. pii: S0166-4328(13)00265-9. [Epub ahead of print].
14. Felsen G, Mainen ZF. Midbrain contributions to sensorimotor decision making. *J Neurophysiol.* 2012;108(1):135–147.
15. Lopes da Silva FH, Harding GF. Transition to seizure in photosensitive epilepsy. *Epilepsy Res.* 2011;97(3):278–282.
16. Szabo CA, Salinas FS, Leland MM, et al. Baboon model of generalized epilepsy: continuous intracranial video-EEG monitoring with subdural electrodes. *Epilepsy Res.* 2012;101(1–2): 46–55.
17. Schmid S, Simons NS, Schnitzler HU. Cellular mechanisms of the trigeminally evoked startle response. *Eur J Neurosci.* 2003;17(7): 1438–1444.
18. Vogel EH, Wagner AR. Stimulus specificity in the habituation of the startle response in the rat. *Physiol Behav.* 2005;86(4):516–525.
19. Shore SE. Plasticity of somatosensory inputs to the cochlear nucleus – implications for tinnitus. *Hear Res.* 2011;281(1–2): 38–46.
20. Campbell A. Point specificity of acupuncture in the light of recent clinical and imaging studies. *Acupunct Med.* 2006;24(3):118–122.
21. Zhao ZQ. Neural mechanism underlying acupuncture analgesia. *Prog Neurobiol.* 2008;85(4):355–375.
22. Kraus KS, Canlon B. Neuronal connectivity and interactions between the auditory and limbic systems – effects of noise and tinnitus. *Hear Res.* 2012;288(1–2):34–46.
23. Zhao Z, Davis M. Fear-potentiated startle in rats is mediated by neurons in the deep layers of the superior colliculus/deep mesencephalic nucleus of the rostral midbrain through the glutamate non-NMDA receptors. *J Neurosci.* 2004;24(46): 10326–10334.
24. Norrholm SD, Jovanovic T, Olin IW, et al. Fear extinction in traumatized civilians with posttraumatic stress disorder: relation to symptom severity. *Biol Psychiatry.* 2011;69(6):556–563.
25. van Well S, Visser RM, Scholte HS, Kindt M. Neural substrates of individual differences in human fear learning: evidence from concurrent fMRI, fear-potentiated startle, and US-expectancy data. *Cogn Affect Behav Neurosci.* 2012;12(3):499–512.
26. Rosen JB, Hitchcock JM, Sananes CB, Miserendino MJ, Davis M. A direct projection from the central nucleus of the amygdala to the acoustic startle pathway: anterograde and retrograde tracing studies. *Behav Neurosci.* 1991;105(6):817–825.
27. Fendt M, Koch M, Schnitzler HU. Lesions of the central gray block conditioned fear as measured with the potentiated startle paradigm. *Behav Brain Res.* 1996;74(1–2):127–134.
28. Reimer AE, de Oliveira AR, Brandão ML. Glutamatergic mechanisms of the dorsal periaqueductal gray matter modulate the expression of conditioned freezing and fear-potentiated startle. *Neuroscience.* 2012;219:72–81.
29. Jobe PC, Browning RA. From brainstem to forebrain in generalized animal models of seizures and epilepsies. In: Hirsch E, Andermann F, Chauvel P, Engel J, Lopes da Silva F, Luders H, eds. *Progress in Epileptic Disorders: Generalized Seizures: From Clinical Phenomenology to Underlying Systems and Networks.* Montrouge, France: John Libbey Eurotext; 2006:33–52.
30. Feng HJ, Naritoku DK, Randall ME, Faingold CL. Modulation of audiogenically kindled seizures by gamma-aminobutyric acid--related mechanisms in the amygdala. *Exp Neurol.* 2001;172(2): 477–481.
31. N'Gouemo P, Faingold CL. Periaqueductal gray neurons exhibit increased responsiveness associated with audiogenic seizures in the genetically epilepsy-prone rat. *Neuroscience.* 1998;84(2): 619–625.
32. N'Gouemo P, Faingold CL. The periaqueductal grey is a critical site in the neuronal network for audiogenic seizures: modulation by $GABA_A$, NMDA and opioid receptors. *Epilepsy Res.* 1999;35(1): 39–46.
33. Raisinghani M, Faingold CL. Identification of the requisite brain sites in the neuronal network subserving generalized clonic audiogenic seizures. *Brain Res.* 2003;967(1–2):113–122.
34. Yang L, Long C, Randall ME, Faingold CL. Neurons in the periaqueductal gray are critically involved in the neuronal network for audiogenic seizures during ethanol withdrawal. *Neuropharmacology.* 2003;44(2):275–281.
35. Tupal S, Faingold CL. Audiogenic kindling induces plastic changes in the neuronal firing patterns in periaqueductal gray. *Brain Res.* 2011;1377:60–66.
36. Feng HJ, Faingold CL. Repeated generalized audiogenic seizures induce plastic changes on acoustically evoked neuronal firing in the amygdala. *Brain Res.* 2002;932(1–2):61–69.
37. Tupal S, Faingold CL. The amygdala to periaqueductal gray pathway: plastic changes induced by audiogenic kindling and reversal by gabapentin. *Brain Res.* 2012;1475:71–79.
38. Coimbra NC, Freitas RL, Savoldi M, et al. Opioid neurotransmission in the post-ictal analgesia: involvement of μ_1-opioid receptor. *Brain Res.* 2001;903(1–2):216–221.
39. De Oliveira RC, de Oliveira R, Ferreira CM, Coimbra NC. Involvement of $5\text{-}HT_2$ serotonergic receptors of the nucleus raphe

magnus and nucleus reticularis gigantocellularis/paragigantocellularis complex neural networks in the antinociceptive phenomenon that follows the post-ictal immobility syndrome. *Exp Neurol*. 2006;201(1):144–153.

40. Portugal-Santana P, Doretto MC, Tatsuo MA, Duarte ID. Involvement of prolactin, vasopressin and opioids in post-ictal antinociception induced by electroshock in rats. *Brain Res*. 2004;1003(1–2):1–8.
41. Urca G, Yitzhaky J, Frenk H. Different opioid systems may participate in post-electro-convulsive shock (ECS) analgesia and catalepsy. *Brain Res*. 1981;219(2):385–396.
42. Freitas RL, Bassi GS, de Oliveira AM, Coimbra NC. Serotonergic neurotransmission in the dorsal raphe nucleus recruits in situ $5\text{-HT}_{2A/2C}$ receptors to modulate the post-ictal antinociception. *Exp Neurol*. 2008;213(2):410–418.
43. Freitas RL, Ferreira CM, Urbina MA, et al. $5\text{-HT}_{1A/1B}$, 5-HT_6, and 5-HT_7 serotonergic receptors recruitment in tonic-clonic seizure-induced antinociception: role of dorsal raphe nucleus. *Exp Neurol*. 2009;217(1):16–24.
44. Samineni VK, Premkumar LS, Faingold CL. Post-ictal analgesia in genetically epilepsy-prone rats is induced by audiogenic seizures and involves cannabinoid receptors in the periaqueductal gray. *Brain Res*. 2011;1389:177–182.
45. Guieu R, Mesdjian E, Roger J, Dano P, Pouget J, Serratrice G. Nociceptive threshold in patients with epilepsy. *Epilepsy Res*. 1992;12(1):57–61.
46. Arvidsson U, Riedl M, Chakrabarti S, et al. Distribution and targeting of a mu-opioid receptor (MOR1) in brain and spinal cord. *J Neurosci*. 1995;15(5 Pt 1):3328–3341.
47. Mayer DJ. Analgesia produced by electrical stimulation of the brain. *Prog Neuropsychopharmacol Biol Psychiatry*. 1984;8(4–6):557–564.
48. Reynolds DV. Surgery in the rat during electrical analgesia induced by focal brain stimulation. *Science*. 1969;164(878):444–445.
49. Hohmann AG, Suplita RL, Bolton NM, et al. An endocannabinoid mechanism for stress-induced analgesia. *Nature*. 2005;435(7045):1108–1112.
50. Maione S, Bisogno T, de Novellis V, et al. Elevation of endocannabinoid levels in the ventrolateral periaqueductal grey through inhibition of fatty acid amide hydrolase affects descending nociceptive pathways via both cannabinoid receptor type 1 and transient receptor potential vanilloid type-1 receptors. *J Pharmacol Exp Ther*. 2006;316(3):969–982.
51. Wallace MJ, Blair RE, Falenski KW, Martin BR, DeLorenzo RJ. The endogenous cannabinoid system regulates seizure frequency and duration in a model of temporal lobe epilepsy. *J Pharmacol Exp Ther*. 2003;307(1):129–137.
52. De Oliveira RC, de Oliveira PC, Zanandrea T, Paschoalin-Maurin T, Coimbra NC. Acetylcholine-mediated neurotransmission within the nucleus raphe magnus exerts a key role in the organization of both interictal and postictal antinociception. *Epilepsy Behav*. 2011;22(2):178–185.
53. Sowers LP, Massey CA, Gehlbach BK, Granner MA, Richerson GB. Sudden unexpected death in epilepsy: fatal post-ictal respiratory and arousal mechanisms. *Respir Physiol Neurobiol*. 2013. pii: S1569-9048(13)00150-X. doi: 10.1016/j.resp.2013.05.010. [Epub ahead of print].
54. Blum AS. Respiratory physiology of seizures. *J Clin Neurophysiol*. 2009;26(5):309–315.
55. Tupal S, Faingold CL. Evidence supporting a role of serotonin in modulation of sudden death induced by seizures in DBA/2 mice. *Epilepsia*. 2006;47(1):21–26.
56. Faingold CL, Randall M, Tupal S. DBA/1 mice exhibit chronic susceptibility to audiogenic seizures followed by sudden death associated with respiratory arrest. *Epilepsy Behav*. 2010;17(4):436–440.
57. Englot DJ, Modi B, Mishra AM, DeSalvo M, Hyder F, Blumenfeld H. Cortical deactivation induced by subcortical network dysfunction in limbic seizures. *J Neurosci*. 2009;29(41):13006–13018. [NIHMSID#158072].
58. Englot DJ, Blumenfeld H. Consciousness and epilepsy: why are complex-partial seizures complex? *Prog Brain Res*. 2009;177:147–170.
59. Fisher RS, Schachter SC. The postictal state: a neglected entity in the management of epilepsy. *Epilepsy Behav*. 2000;1(1):52–59.
60. Feldman JL, Mitchell GS, Nattie EE. Breathing: rhythmicity, plasticity, chemosensitivity. *Annu Rev Neurosci*. 2003;26:239–266.
61. Feldman JL, Del Negro CA, Gray PA. Understanding the rhythm of breathing: so near, yet so far. *Annu Rev Physiol*. 2013;75:423–452.
62. Devinney MJ, Huxtable AG, Nichols NL, Mitchell GS. Hypoxia-induced phrenic long-term facilitation: emergent properties. *Ann N Y Acad Sci*. 2013;1279:143–153.
63. Dale-Nagle EA, Hoffman MS, MacFarlane PM, Mitchell GS. Multiple pathways to long-lasting phrenic motor facilitation. *Adv Exp Med Biol*. 2010;669:225–230.
64. Richerson GB. Serotonergic neurons as carbon dioxide sensors that maintain pH homeostasis. *Nat Rev Neurosci*. 2004;5(6):449–461.
65. Hilaire G, Voituron N, Menuet C, Ichiyama RM, Subramanian HH, Dutschmann M. The role of serotonin in respiratory function and dysfunction. *Respir Physiol Neurobiol*. 2010;174(1–2):76–88.
66. Wang W, Bradley SR, Richerson GB. Quantification of the response of rat medullary raphe neurones to independent changes in pH(o) and P(CO_2). *J Physiol*. 2002;540(Pt 3):951–970.
67. Severson CA, Wang W, Pieribone VA, Dohle CI, Richerson GB. Midbrain serotonergic neurons are central pH chemoreceptors. *Nat Neurosci*. 2003;6(11):1139–1140.
68. Cao Y, Fujito Y, Maatsuyama K, Aoki M. Effects of electrical stimulation of the medullary raphe nuclei on respiratory movement in rats. *J Comp Physiol A Neuroethol Sens Neural Behav Physiol*. 2006;192(5):497–505.
69. Cao Y, Matsuyama K, Fujito Y, Aoki M. Involvement of medullary GABAergic and serotonergic raphe neurons in respiratory control: electrophysiological and immunohistochemical studies in rats. *Neurosci Res*. 2006;56(3):322–331.
70. Besnard S, Denise P, Cappelin B, Dutschmann M, Gestreau C. Stimulation of the rat medullary raphe nuclei induces differential responses in respiratory muscle activity. *Respir Physiol Neurobiol*. 2009;165(2–3):208–214.
71. Buchanan GF, Richerson GB. Central serotonin neurons are required for arousal to CO_2. *Proc Natl Acad Sci USA*. 2010;107(37):16354–16359.
72. DePuy SD, Kanbar R, Coates MB, Stornetta RL, Guyenet PG. Control of breathing by raphe obscurus serotonergic neurons in mice. *J Neurosci*. 2011;31(6):1981–1990.
73. Hodges MR, Best S, Richerson GB. Altered ventilatory and thermoregulatory control in male and female adult Pet-1 null mice. *Respir Physiol Neurobiol*. 2011;177(2):133–140.
74. Corcoran AE, Richerson GB, Hams MB. Serotonergic mechanisms are necessary for central respiratory chemoresponsiveness in situ. *Respir Physiol Neurobiol*. 2013;186(2):214–220.
75. Kinney HC, Broadbelt KG, Haynes RL, Rognum IJ, Paterson DS. The serotonergic anatomy of the developing human medulla oblongata: implications for pediatric disorders of homeostasis. *J Chem Neuroanat*. 2011;41(4):182–199.

76. Takeuchi Y, Sano Y. Serotonin distribution in the circumventricular organs of the rat. An immunohistochemical study. *Anat Embryol (Berl)*. 1983;167(3):311–319.
77. Ptak K, Yamanishi T, Aungst J, et al. Raphé neurons stimulate respiratory circuit activity by multiple mechanisms via endogenously released serotonin and substance P. *J Neurosci*. 2009;29(12): 3720–3737.
78. Kobayashi S, Fujito Y, Matsuyama K, Aoki M. Raphe modulation of the pre-Bötzinger complex respiratory bursts in in vitro medullary half-slice preparations of neonatal mice. *J Comp Physiol A Neuroethol Sens Neural Behav Physiol*. 2010;196(8):519–528.
79. Baker-Herman TL, Mitchell GS. Phrenic long-term facilitation requires spinal serotonin receptor activation and protein synthesis. *J Neurosci*. 2002;22(14):6239–6246.
80. Feldman JL, Windhorst U, Anders K, Richter DW. Synaptic interaction between medullary respiratory neurones during apneusis induced by NMDA-receptor blockade in cat. *J Physiol*. 1992;450:303–323.
81. Lalley PM, Bischoff AM, Richter DW. Serotonin 1A-receptor activation suppresses respiratory apneusis in the cat. *Neurosci Lett*. 1994;172(1–2):59–62.
82. Manzke T, Guenther EG, Ponimaskin EG, et al. 5-HT4(a) receptors avert opioid-induced breathing depression without loss of analgesia. *Science*. 2003;301(5630):226–229.
83. Manzke T, Dutschmann M, Schlaf G, et al. Serotonin targets inhibitory synapses to induce modulation of network functions. *Philos Trans R Soc Lond B Biol Sci*. 2009;364(1529):2589–2602.
84. Dutschmann M, Waki H, Manzke T, et al. The potency of different serotonergic agonists in counteracting opioid evoked cardiorespiratory disturbances. *Philos Trans R Soc Lond B Biol Sci*. 2009;364(1529):2611–2623.
85. Berger SM, Weber T, Perreau-Lenz S, et al. A functional Tph2 C1473G polymorphism causes an anxiety phenotype via compensatory changes in the serotonergic system. *Neuropsychopharmacology*. 2012;37(9):1986–1998.
86. Tenner K, Qadri F, Bert B, Voigt JP, Bader M. The mTPH2 C1473G single nucleotide polymorphism is not responsible for behavioural differences between mouse strains. *Neurosci Lett*. 2008;431(1):21–25.
87. Sakowski SA, Geddes TJ, Kuhn DM. Mouse tryptophan hydroxylase isoform 2 and the role of proline 447 in enzyme function. *J Neurochem*. 2006;96(3):758–765.
88. Zhang X, Beaulieu JM, Sotnikova TD, Gainetdinova RR, Caron MG. Tryptophan hydroxylase-2 controls brain serotonin synthesis. *Science*. 2004;305(5681):217.
89. Uteshev VV, Tupal S, Mhaskar Y, Faingold CL. Abnormal serotonin receptor expression in DBA/2 mice associated with susceptibility to sudden death due to respiratory arrest. *Epilepsy Res*. 2010;88(2–3):183–188.
90. Faingold CL, Randall M, Mhaskar Y, Uteshev VV. Differences in serotonin receptor expression in the brainstem may explain the differential ability of a serotonin agonist to block seizure-induced sudden death in DBA/2 vs. DBA/1 mice. *Brain Res*. 2011;1418: 104–110.
91. Faingold CL, Tupal S, Randall M. Prevention of seizure-induced sudden death in a chronic SUDEP model by semichronic administration of a selective serotonin reuptake inhibitor. *Epilepsy Behav*. 2011;22:186–190.
92. Faingold CL, Randall M. Effects of age, sex and sertraline administration on seizure-induced respiratory arrest in the DBA/1 mouse model of sudden unexpected death in epilepsy (SUDEP). *Epilepsy Behav*. 2013;28:78–82.
93. O'Sullivan RJ, Brown IG, Pender MP. Apneusis responding to buspirone in multiple sclerosis. *Mult Scler*. 2008;14(5):705–707.
94. Bateman LM, Li CS, Lin TC, Seyal M. Serotonin reuptake inhibitors are associated with reduced severity of ictal hypoxemia in medically refractory partial epilepsy. *Epilepsia*. 2010;51(10): 2211–2214.
95. Kraiczi H, Hedner J, Dahlöf P, Ejnell H, Carlson J. Effect of serotonin uptake inhibition on breathing during sleep and daytime symptoms in obstructive sleep apnea. *Sleep*. 1999;22(1):61–67.
96. Annerbrink K, Olsson M, Hedner J, Eriksson E. Acute and chronic treatment with serotonin reuptake inhibitors exert opposite effects on respiration in rats: possible implications for panic disorder. *J Psychopharmacol*. 2010;24(12):1793–1801.
97. Burnstock G. Introduction to purinergic signalling in the brain. *Adv Exp Med Biol*. 2013;986:1–12.
98. Berman RF, Fredholm BB, Aden U, O'Connor WT. Evidence for increased dorsal hippocampal adenosine release and metabolism during pharmacologically induced seizures in rats. *Brain Res*. 2000;872(1–2):44–53.
99. Pedata F, Corsi C, Melani A, Bordoni F, Latini S. Adenosine extracellular brain concentrations and role of A_{2A} receptors in ischemia. *Ann N Y Acad Sci*. 2001;939:74–84.
100. During MJ, Spencer DD. Adenosine: a potential mediator of seizure arrest and postictal refractoriness. *Ann Neurol*. 1992;32(5): 618–624.
101. Shen HY, Li T, Boison D. A novel mouse model for sudden unexpected death in epilepsy (SUDEP): role of impaired adenosine clearance. *Epilepsia*. 2010;51(3):465–468.
102. Boison D. Adenosine dysfunction in epilepsy. *Glia*. 2012;60(8): 1234–1243.
103. Feldman JL, Del Negro CA. Looking for inspiration: new perspectives on respiratory rhythm. *Nat Rev Neurosci*. 2006;7(3): 232–242.
104. Garcia III AJ, Zanella S, Koch H, Doi A, Ramirez JM. Chapter 3—Networks within networks: the neuronal control of breathing. *Prog Brain Res*. 2011;188:31–50.
105. Huxtable AG, Zwicker JD, Poon BY, et al. Tripartite purinergic modulation of central respiratory networks during perinatal development: the influence of ATP, ectonucleotidases, and ATP metabolites. *J Neurosci*. 2009;29(47):14713–14725.
106. Del Negro CA. Disparate purinergic modulation of respiration in rats and mice. *J Physiol*. 2011;589(Pt 18):4409–4410.
107. Kostopoulos G, Drapeau C, Avoli M, Olivier A, Villemeure JG. Endogenous adenosine can reduce epileptiform activity in the human epileptogenic cortex maintained in vitro. *Neurosci Lett*. 1989;106(1–2):119–124.
108. Bateman LM, Li CS, Seyal M. Ictal hypoxemia in localization-related epilepsy: analysis of incidence, severity and risk factors. *Brain*. 2008;131(Pt 12):3239–3245.
109. Lopes LV, Sebastiao AM, Ribeiro JA. Adenosine and related drugs in brain diseases: present and future in clinical trials. *Curr Top Med Chem*. 2011;11(8):1087–1101.
110. Paul S, Elsinga PH, Ishiwata K, Dierckx RA, van Waarde A. Adenosine A(1) receptors in the central nervous system: their functions in health and disease, and possible elucidation by PET imaging. *Curr Med Chem*. 2011;18(31):4820–4835.
111. Hoffman MS, Golder FJ, Mahamed S, Mitchell GS. Spinal adenosine A_{2A} receptor inhibition enhances phrenic long term facilitation following acute intermittent hypoxia. *J Physiol*. 2010; 588(Pt 1):255–266.
112. Mathew OP. Apnea of prematurity: pathogenesis and management strategies. *J Perinatol*. 2011;31(5):302–310.
113. Faingold CL, Randall R, Kommajosyula SP. Role of adenosine in seizure-induced death in DBA/2 mice and genetically epilepsy-prone rats (GEPRs): potential relevance to SUDEP. *Amer Epil Soc Abs*. 2013.

CHAPTER

30

Emergent Properties of Neuronal Networks

Carl L. Faingold

Departments of Pharmacology and Neurology and Division of Neurosurgery, Southern Illinois University School of Medicine, Springfield, IL, USA

EMERGENT PROPERTIES OF NEURONAL NETWORKS

Emergent properties of neuronal networks have been widely observed and are an important feature of normal brain physiology as well as pathophysiology. Emergent properties of the brain are defined as nonlinear events that occur unexpectedly as a result of self-organization within the neuronal network(s) involved. As shown in Figure 30.1 in the top panel, two inputs X and Y impinge on Net 1, which is not subject to self-organization (a single semicircular arrow), and the result of these two inputs only results in linear summation. The output (Z) is the sum of the inputs to this network and is the expected outcome or property of the network. In the bottom panel in Figure 30.1, Net 2, which is subject to a considerable degree of self-organization (dual semicircular arrows), also receives two inputs (X and Y), but this network is subject to nonlinear dynamics, and the output (Z^4) is an emergent property and is unexpectedly much larger than the input due to the confluence of the variety of mechanisms that affect neurons in the intact brain network (see Chapter 1), which are discussed in detail in this chapter. The potential practical value of defining specific emergent properties of central nervous system (CNS) neuronal networks lies in developing a more realistic understanding of the mechanisms governing the normal function of these networks and the changes in network function that occur in CNS diseases that affect specific networks. Knowledge of the emergent properties of neuronal networks that mediate specific CNS disorders has the potential to lead to improved therapy of these brain disorders with CNS drugs that act selectively on these emergent properties on neurons in the critical network "hubs" when therapeutic doses are administered (see Chapter 32).

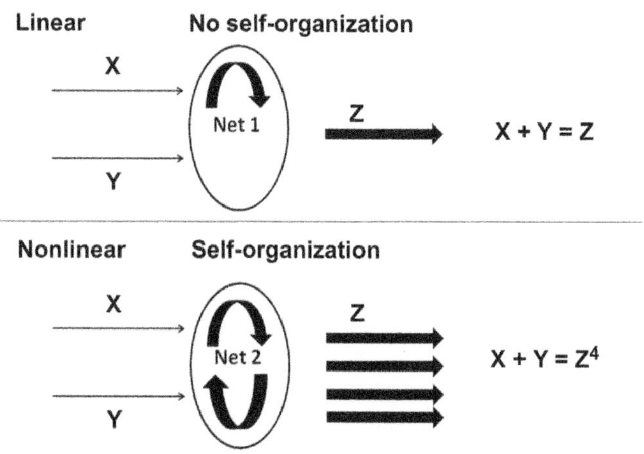

FIGURE 30.1 General principle behind the emergent properties of networks in the CNS. In the top panel, two inputs, X and Y, impinge on Net 1; the result of these two inputs does not cause Net 1 to undergo self-organization (a single semicircular arrow), and the output is limited to linear summation. The output (Z) of Net 1 is simply the sum of the inputs and is the expected outcome or property (nonemergent) of this network. In the bottom panel, Net 2 also receives two inputs (X and Y), but this network is subject to nonlinear dynamics, and the network elements undergo self-organization (dual semicircular arrows), resulting in a much larger than expected output (Z^4), which is an emergent property of this network.

The proposed usefulness of the emergent-property approach is that it attempts to deal with the immense complexity of the brain, which contains an estimated 80–100 billion neurons with trillions of synapses connecting them. This almost unimaginable degree of functional complexity of the brain gave rise to the use of reductionist approaches in isolated neurons or receptor systems in vitro to allow closer examination of neuronal function. These reductionist methods have been rewarding approaches for studying brain mechanisms at the cellular and subcellular level (see Chapter 5). However, these cellular and subcellular mechanisms often are not directly applicable to the same neurons when evaluated in the intact functioning brain due to

Neuronal Networks in Brain Function, CNS Disorders, and Therapeutics
http://dx.doi.org/10.1016/B978-0-12-415804-7.00030-7

the loss of many of the normal influences exerted on these neurons when most of the brain is eliminated in ex vivo or in vitro preparations.[2] A major reason for this is that neurons in the brain exist in neuronal networks with other brain cells, including glia, and are subject to a myriad of controlling mechanisms that are eliminated in the ex vivo and in vitro approaches (see Chapter 1). Neurons in the CNS are organized into networks, initially confined to a brain nucleus (or portion of a nucleus), and those networks are further organized into larger networks that carry out various specific functions, such as sensory processing or locomotion (see, e.g. Chapters 17, 19, and 20). In addition, these networks often do not work in isolation but commonly work in concert with or in competition with networks that subserve an entirely different function (see Chapter 29). Network interactions can produce important complex behaviors, as in the acoustic startle network (an auditory and locomotor network interaction), and they also can work together to mediate brain dysfunctions, such as psychiatric disorders and epilepsy.

When a functional network is active in an awake brain, there are many network control mechanisms, including cellular properties, endogenous neuroactive substances, and the many other influences detailed in Chapters 7–17, which together determine the actual properties (emergent properties) of those neurons that exert major control of network function in this nucleus. As discussed in this chapter, the influences that a brain network is subject to can become highly complex. However, starting simply, we can consider the effect of one influence, such as the action of a neurotransmitter that is released during normal synaptic neurotransmission. In the example in Figure 30.2, the idealized diagram shows the effect of a synaptically released neurotransmitter on neurons in a specific nucleus within a neuronal network in the intact organism that results in the expression of an emergent property. For simplicity, these neurons are shown as having one type of neurotransmitter influence and one cellular property. This neuron is illustrative of the many similar neurons (N) in this network nucleus. In this simplified example, the neurons possess an intrinsic property that is not expressed under basal conditions, and the neurons are relatively quiescent. An example of this would be the propensity to show pacemaker activity. The neurons also possess ligand-gated receptors at which a synaptically released neurotransmitter can exert its effect. When this specific transmitter is synaptically released onto these neurons, it binds to the receptors and causes the group of neurons in this nucleus to exhibit their pacemaker activity to be expressed as emergent property. An example of this is seen in the respiratory network in the medulla, where an excitatory amino acid is released onto the neurons in this respiratory network site and causes respiratory rhythm generation as an emergent property.[1] This emergent property may be a unique property of the neurons in this network nucleus under these conditions.

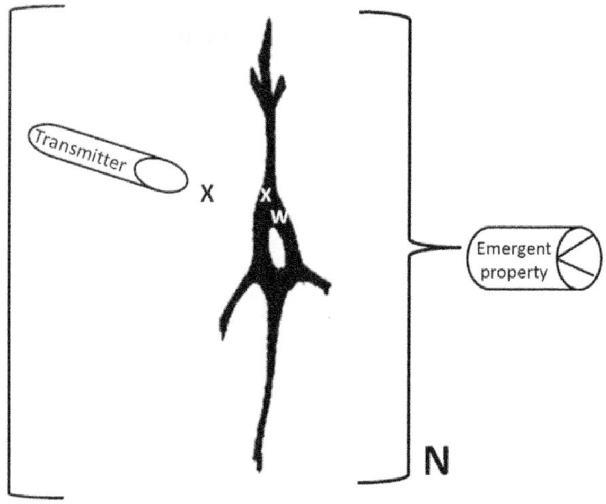

FIGURE 30.2 Idealized diagram of the effect of a synaptically released neurotransmitter on neurons in a specific nucleus within a neuronal network in the intact organism. For simplicity, these neurons are shown as having one type of influence and one cellular property. This neuron is illustrative of the many similar neurons (N) in this nucleus. The neurons possess an intrinsic property (W), which is not expressed under basal conditions, so the neurons are relatively quiescent. An example of this would be the propensity to show pacemaker activity. The neurons also possess ligand-gated receptors (X) at which a synaptically released neurotransmitter can exert its effect. When this specific transmitter is synaptically released onto these neurons, it binds to the receptors and causes the neurons to exhibit their pacemaker activity as an emergent property of the group of neurons in this nucleus as they become active. An example of this is seen in the respiratory network in the pre-Bötzinger complex when an excitatory amino acid is released upon the neurons in this respiratory network site.[1] This emergent property may be a unique property of the neurons in this network nucleus under these conditions.

An emergent property can also be expressed and alter the function of a network due to the effect of a neuroactive agent, which produces an effect on these neurons via volume transmission. Volume transmission involves diffusion of a neuroactive substance three-dimensionally within extracellular and cerebrospinal fluids of the CNS. By this mechanism the neuroactive substance can exert distant as well as local effects (see Chapter 8).[3] Figure 30.3 is a simplified diagram, illustrating the effect of volume transmission on neurons in a specific nucleus within a neuronal network in the intact organism. This neuron is illustrative of the many similar neurons (N) in this nucleus. The neurons possess certain intrinsic properties. The neurons also possess ligand-gated receptors on which neuroactive substances (neurotransmitters or neuromodulators) act. In this example, the neurons are subject to volume transmission, whereby an endogenous (Endo) neuroactive agent is carried to the neurons from nearby (spillover) or

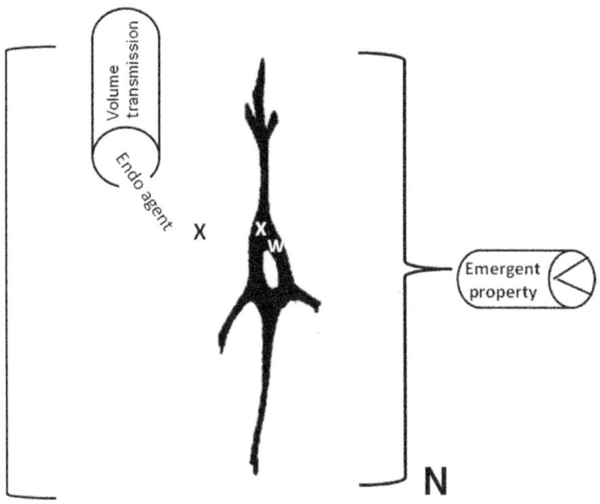

FIGURE 30.3 Simplified diagram illustrating the effect of volume transmission on neurons in a specific nucleus within a neuronal network in the intact organism. This neuron is illustrative of the many similar neurons (N) in this nucleus. The neurons possess certain intrinsic properties (W). The neurons also possess ligand-gated receptors (X) on which neuroactive substances (transmitters or neuromodulators) act. In this example, the neurons are subject to volume transmission, whereby an endogenous (Endo) neuroactive agent is carried to the neurons from nearby (spillover) or distant sites by volume transmission via the extracellular fluid and cerebrospinal fluid and causes the expression of an emergent property, which is postulated to be expressed uniquely in this network nucleus and causes the unique sensitivity of this class of neurons.

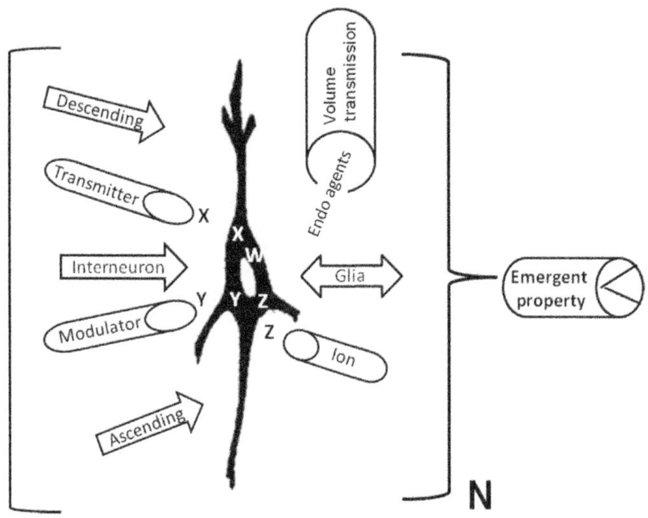

FIGURE 30.4 Idealized diagram of neurons in a specific nucleus within a neuronal network in the intact organism that illustrates many of the influences that affect this "class" (similar neurons) of neurons (N) in this nucleus. The neurons possess certain intrinsic properties (W), such as the propensity to exhibit burst firing. The neurons also possess ligand-gated receptors (X) (e.g. glutamate) (which have specific receptor subunits) on which synaptically released neurotransmitters act as well as other ligand-gated receptors (Y) for neuromodulators (e.g. adenosine). In addition, the neurons possess voltage-gated ion channels (Z) (e.g. sodium channels) at which local ions can act. The neurons receive descending synaptic connections from above and ascending ones from below, which can release neuroactive substances that act at these channels synaptically. Other cellular inputs are received from local interneurons and from glial cells, which may occur by synaptic or volume transmission. Endogenous (Endo) neuroactive agents are carried via volume transmission from nearby (spillover) or distant sites via the extracellular fluid and cerebrospinal fluid to the neurons and also affect the properties of the neurons. An example would be extrasynaptic $GABA_A$ receptors that respond to the low levels of "ambient" GABA[6] in the extracellular fluid. The summation of all these influences determines whether the emergent property is expressed, the actual nature of that property, and its relative sensitivity in that group of neurons. This emergent property is postulated to be expressed uniquely in this network nucleus and causes this class of neurons to respond with unique sensitivity to an endogenous influence. Note: Those influences can also be modified by brain state changes (such as sleep), which can significantly alter the emergent property.

distant sites via the extracellular fluid and cerebrospinal fluid. This neuroactive substance reveals a unique emergent property, which may be expressed solely in this class of neurons in this specific network nucleus. This emergent property causes the neurons in this nucleus to become a pivotal "hub"[4] within the network at which other endogenous or exogenous neuroactive substances can modify network function and render this brain site a critical target for CNS drugs in the intact animal (see Chapter 32).

These emergent properties are an important nexus for understanding network function and dysfunction as well as potential therapeutic interventions[2,5] (see Chapter 32), but, unfortunately, they often go unrecognized. The concept of emergent properties is an outgrowth of complexity theory. Emergent properties can occur at many organizational levels in the brain from the receptor level all the way to the behavioral level due to the phenomenon of self-organization. Emergent properties are commonly seen at the neuronal network (i.e. mesoscopic or intermediate) level in the CNS, and the nature and function of the specific property depend on the particular network's functional role.[2] Networks can be subject to expansion due to repetitive activation (see Chapter 27), and the expanded network possesses additional emergent properties that may be added or superimposed upon the original set of emergent properties. These emergent properties are then conferred on a group of neurons in a specific nucleus within the network, and this nucleus can then become the target for the action of an exogenous substance to which the organism is exposed. This emergent property can simply render those neurons more sensitive than other neurons to this exogenous substance. Therefore, when the intact, unanesthetized organism is exposed to the lowest effective dose of this substance, these neurons become a selective target for that agent.

Figure 30.4 shows an idealized example of a neuron and illustrates a number of the influences that affect it and other similar neurons in this nucleus in the intact organism, which demonstrates the complexity of the milieu affecting neurons in the intact brain. It is the sum of all these influences that determines the emergent property of that group of neurons. The neurons possess certain intrinsic properties (W) and ligand-gated receptors (X) (which have specific receptor subunits) on which synaptically released neurotransmitters act, as well as other ligand-gated receptors (Y) for neuromodulators. In addition, the neurons possess voltage-gated ion channels (Z) at which local ions can act. The neurons receive descending synaptic connections from above and ascending ones from below, which can release substances synaptically. Other cellular inputs are received from local interneurons and from glial cells, which may occur by synaptic or volume transmission. Endogenous neuroactive agents carried via volume transmission in the extracellular fluid and cerebrospinal fluid also affect the properties of the neurons. The summation of all these influences determines whether the emergent property is expressed, the actual nature of that property, and its relative sensitivity to exogenous substances. This emergent property is postulated to be expressed uniquely in this network nucleus and causes this class of neurons to respond with unique sensitivity to an endogenous influence. Note that those influences can also be modified by brain state changes (see Chapters 21 and 22), which can modify this emergent property.

New emergent properties can result from activity-dependent plasticity that occurs in positive processes, such as learning and memory, and disordered processes, such as epilepsy. Combined application of various experimental and computational techniques may be required to fully understand the nature of these changes.[7] In CNS disorders, prevention of the emergence of these different aberrant properties may require agents with different actions, or there may be a concordance of mechanisms acting on emergent properties of multiple networks that many currently effective CNS drugs may possess[2] (see Chapter 32). For example, many anticonvulsant drugs that were developed to treat epilepsy have been found to act on several other CNS disorders, especially chronic pain syndromes, which has led to the idea that these agents may be better classified as "network-modifying" drugs.[8]

As noted here, the key feature of emergent properties is nonlinearity, which means that the output of a system exceeds the input (i.e. "the whole is greater than the sum of its parts"). Complexity theory posits that when a multitude of elements in a complex system interact, new and unexpected properties can emerge because of self-organization. Emergent properties are not predictably based on the properties of the individual network elements and could potentially occur as a unique phenomenon that would not reoccur in a predictable way. For example, in meteorology, where the concept of emergent properties originated,[9] predictability is often lacking (typified by the "butterfly effect"), in part because of the dearth of structural bases for weather. This lack of predictability leads to potential difficulties for studying emergent properties if they can be so unpredictable. However, unlike many other systems where complexity theory is applicable, the brain possesses a structural (anatomical) basis for the network that often allows certain emergent properties to become predictable once they are discovered. Thus, once an emergent property in a brain network has been observed under a given set of circumstances, this property can often reoccur consistently in that network under those same conditions. Thus, it has been postulated that the brain can undergo "mass action", in which the functional neuronal networks expand significantly to encompass numerous neurons and multiple brain networks due to emergent properties.[10,11] Freeman postulates that the functional interconnection of large numbers of otherwise independent neurons in the brain results in the emergence of mesoscopic networks. These networks may exhibit "emergent" properties that are related to but transcend the properties that the neurons would exhibit in isolation.[2,11] Thus, emergent properties have been observed at the mesoscopic level as well as the microscopic and macroscopic (behavioral) levels,[11] as discussed in more detail in this chapter.

Mesoscopic neuronal networks consist of many neurons whose activities are often tightly linked to the network in which they are participating, but experimental studies have shown that this linkage can undergo significant modification under certain circumstances.[12,13] Neurons can actually undergo switching from participation in one network to participation in a different network when the intact organism changes the type of activities in which it is engaged. The capacity of neurons to undergo network switching has been widely seen in invertebrate networks, such as those in the crustacean stomatogastric ganglia. In this network, specific identified neurons in this ganglion participate actively in a network that mediates a specific physiological function. However, when a network that mediates a different function becomes active, this same neuron can change its firing properties to become an integral part of the newly activated network.[14,15] In more evolved species, such as lampreys, the participation of certain reticulospinal neurons changes depending on the mode of locomotion that the network is generating.[16] In mammals, a widespread network oscillation, including fast oscillations (ripples), can greatly alter the discharge pattern of neurons.[17] Thus, hippocampal neurons of the rat switch from a highly variable discharge mode that occurs under one behavioral condition to become highly coordinated under other behavioral conditions, which can impose functionally important emergent properties on these neurons.[18]

As noted here, the emergent properties of neuronal networks have been observed to operate in many forms and levels of complexity of neuronal and brain function. These include central control of respiration, locomotor function, sensory perception (olfaction, vision, audition, touch, and nociception), and sensorimotor integration. In addition, emergent properties occur in brain state transitions (e.g. sleep states), learning and memory (based on neuroplasticity at the synaptic and network levels), cognition, consciousness, and the closely related concept of attention. Emergent properties are also seen in CNS disorders, including neurological disorders (such as epilepsy) and mental disorders (such as bipolar disorder) (see the "Neurological Disorders—Epilepsy" and "Psychiatric Disorders" sections, respectively). An important corollary of emergent-property theory is that these properties can be critical targets of centrally acting therapeutic measures in intact animals[2] (see Chapters 31 and 32).

TYPES OF EMERGENT PROPERTIES

Several different types of emergent properties have been observed, including oscillatory, synchronized, and wave-like network states. For example, traveling electrical waves are observed in olfactory, visual, and visuomotor areas of the cortex in a variety of species in the absence of stimulation; they are subject to phase shifts and are proposed to be an emergent property of these neuronal networks.[19] Other forms of emergent properties have been observed in large networks of neurons, due to self-organization that results in slow rhythmic oscillations of spontaneous activity, including alternating "DOWN" states of generalized neural silence and "UP" states of enhanced excitability.[20] These states have been observed in vivo in the cerebral cortex, striatum, cerebellum, and amygdala and have also been observed in in vitro studies.[20–24] Control of the UP and DOWN states in animals and humans can be exerted by state changes of the brain during the sleep–waking cycle, disrupted by electrical stimulation, or induced pharmacologically by several different agents[20,25,26] (see Chapter 32). Changes in UP and DOWN state duration and recovery are observed in epileptic neuronal networks that may be related to epileptogenicity in animal models.[27]

A very intense emergent property called a "neuronal avalanche" is a form of neuronal network organization that was originally observed in vitro. An avalanche differs in magnitude from other forms of self-organization, such as oscillatory, synchronized, or wave-like network states,[28] and evidence for this phenomenon has also been recently observed in vivo.[29] Unlike most other emergent properties, these avalanches show no characteristic scale and are described by power laws similar to analyses of snow avalanches, earthquakes, and forest fires that all result in a critical state of the system. The resulting networks are suggested to allow extensive information transmission as well as network stability. New computational approaches to analyze the activity seen in networks utilizes nonlinear rate equations similar in structure to the Lotka–Volterra equations used in modeling predator–prey relations and are proposed to model the emergent properties of interacting networks of firing neurons.[30]

LEVELS OF EMERGENT PROPERTIES

Emergent properties have been studied in many fields in addition to neuroscience. These properties have been observed at many levels from the "simplest", such as interactions between individual receptors, to the most complex functions of excitable tissue where different networks interact to produce an emergent behavior. As noted in this chapter, neuronal networks are observed at microscopic, mesoscopic, and macroscopic levels,[11] and emergent properties can also be observed at each level, as discussed here. It also follows that therapeutic interventions can also occur at each of these levels (see Chapters 31 and 32).

Thus, emergent properties have been observed at the receptor level in muscle physiology. Thus, ryanodine receptors (RyRs), which bind and release calcium ions (Ca^{2+}), show a form of emergent property called "calcium sparks".[31] Skeletal and cardiac muscle require Ca^{2+} for excitation–contraction coupling. Specialized regions in the muscle cells (called the sarcoplasmic reticulum) contain ordered arrays of RyRs, which mobilize Ca^{2+} from the cell. During an action potential, the RyRs mediate synchronous release of Ca^{2+} (calcium spark). This release occurs all across the cell due to the summation of small elementary Ca^{2+} release events, arising from the synchronous opening and closing of a group of RyRs. The mechanisms controlling the synchronous RyRs activation and deactivation are currently unknown.[32] However, additional factors, such as L-type Ca^{2+} channel modulators, magnesium ions, and adenosine triphosphate and perhaps other unknown elements, working in combination, may result in an emergent property at the receptor level.[33,34] This emergent property may lead to muscle disorders, such as malignant hyperthermia,[35] and may also represent a novel target for physiological and pharmacological modulation.

Evidence for emergent properties has also been observed in synthetic neuronal networks created by allowing cultured neurons to form networks in vitro. Thus, dissociated rat hippocampal neurons develop into an active network, and this dissociated network exhibited self-organization, resulting in sustained oscillations without input from the sites (cortex or thalamus) that normally provide oscillatory input in the intact brain; networks derived from CNS disorder models, such as epilepsy, express a greater than normal diversity of origin and activation.[36,37] Emergent properties can also be lost in in vitro preparations. Neurons from an invertebrate network exhibit rhythmic emergent properties in vivo due, in part, to intrinsic membrane properties of certain of the neurons. However, when these cells were isolated in culture, a loss of emergent properties was seen, indicating that most features of the functional network in vivo were determined primarily by network interactions.[38] Interestingly, the rhythmic activity in certain of these isolated neurons could be restored in the presence of a specific neuroactive substance. Neuronal networks in the intact mammalian brain show a wide variety of emergent properties that exert major control over relatively fundamental functions, such as respiration or locomotion, as well as more complex functions, such as memory and cognition.

RESPIRATORY NETWORKS OF THE BRAINSTEM

Several examples of emergent properties have been observed in the function of neuronal networks involved in control of respiration. Specific brainstem networks govern mammalian respiration, including several nuclei in the rostral ventrolateral medulla, particularly the pre-Bötzinger complex (Chapter 18). Burst firing (see Chapter 9) in pacemaker neurons in this complex has been shown to contribute importantly to normal respiratory rhythm.[39–44] A major mechanism that has been implicated in control of bursting in these pacemaker neurons is a persistent sodium current. However, when an agent that blocks this sodium current was perfused onto these pacemaker neurons in vitro, the burst firing in the vast majority of these cells was abolished but the actual respiratory-related motor output was not altered, suggesting that this respiratory rhythm is actually an emergent property of the network.[45] Further explorations of the basis of these respiratory-network emergent properties have observed that they involve an interaction of excitatory transmission mediated by alpha-amino-3-hydroxy-5-methyl-4-isoxazole propionic acid (AMPA) receptors interacting with Ca^{2+}-activated nonspecific cation currents mediated, in part, by the action of specific endogenous neuroactive substances, including norepinephrine, and neurokinins interacting with specific ion-gated channels.[1,46–48]

MOTOR CONTROL

Examples of emergent properties have been observed in the function of neuronal networks involved in locomotion. The network that controls the physiology of posture and movement, which involves pathways from the cerebral cortex, cerebellum, and substantia nigra to the pontomedullary reticuloreticular and reticulospinal neurons, exhibits emergent properties that are not encompassed by the sum of the properties of its components.[49] Locomotion rhythms generated in the central-pattern-generator circuit for locomotion in the spinal cord involve pacemaker properties (Chapter 17) that are dependent on *N*-methyl-D-aspartate (NMDA) receptors and other ionic currents, but emergent network properties are also required to give rise to the rhythmic patterns that occur during locomotion.[50]

SENSORY PROCESSING

Several examples of emergent properties have been observed in neuronal networks involved in the processing and perception of sensory stimuli in various sensory modalities. Perception, as well as learning, language, and cognition, are proposed to involve emergent properties of neuronal networks in the human neocortex. Thus, microcolumns and cortical columns act at the mesoscopic level to allow the interaction of neurons and yield emergent behaviors, which have been evaluated using various techniques, including unit recordings, local field potentials, electroencephalography, magnetoencephalography, and functional magnetic resonance imaging (fMRI).[51]

Sensory systems that express emergent properties include the olfactory system. Thus, the cellular interactions among neurons in the olfactory bulb of lizards give rise to additional unpredicted responses or olfactory information coding in this structure that is suggested to be an emergent property of this network.[52] Emergent properties in the somatosensory cortex have also been observed in response to complex tactile stimulation of the vibrissae of rodents, which exhibit nonlinear integration of responses across the entire vibrissal input.[53] In addition, somatosensory neurons in the ventral posterior medial nucleus of the thalamus also exhibit emergent properties in the coding of complex multiwhisker stimulations that were largely independent of corticothalamic feedback connections.[54] Neuronal firing in recurrent laminar visual neocortex neurons cannot fully explain visual perception, but emergent properties, including self-synchronizing gamma oscillations, are proposed to be required to fully explain the dynamics of visual perception.[55] The transformation of spatial and temporal frequency-tuning functions from broad-band and low-pass to narrow-band and -pass profiles is one of the key emergent properties of neurons in the mammalian primary visual cortex based on feedforward and intratelencephalic suppressive mechanisms operating at the network level.[56] fMRI was used to study the emergent properties of populations of neurons in a distributed network of visual areas that process information about the direction of motion, but a discrepancy was observed between the directional signals in certain visual areas, as measured with fMRI, as compared to single-neuron firing. The researchers postulated that neuronal selectivity is a function of the state of adaptation and may be due to feedback from higher areas.[57] Emergent properties that caused increases in nociception have been observed to develop following seizure-induced lesions in several brain structures.[58]

NORMAL BRAIN STATE TRANSITIONS

Examples of emergent properties have been observed in the function of neuronal networks involved in control of the normal brain during the sleep–waking cycle (see Chapters 21 and 22). Thus, for example, thalamic rhythmicity, which is important for sleep state generation, was once thought to be generated by the "pacemaker" properties of thalamic cells and has also been found to be an emergent property of the relay thalamus–nucleus reticularis network.[59] The mechanisms of rhythmicity that govern the synchrony and period of thalamocortical neuronal oscillations involved in sleep spindles are proposed to be an emergent property of interactions between intrinsic and synaptic currents.[60] The global state changes of the sleep–wakefulness cycle are also thought to be governed by emergent properties. Thus, it is proposed that emergent properties of neuronal ensembles subserve the ability of the brain to undergo rapid global state changes, as seen during the sleep–wakefulness cycle. A major source of network control in these cyclic sleep state changes is brought about by changes in specific neuroactive substances that control state transitions in the sleep cycle[61] (Chapters 21 and 22). It has been proposed that the organization of the sleep–waking cycle is an emergent property of forebrain and brainstem local neuronal networks that undergo state transitions, and failure of this organization leads to several different sleep pathologies[62,63] (see Chapters 21 and 22). Circadian rhythm networks also exhibit emergent properties (see Chapter 14).

COGNITION AND MEMORY

Examples of emergent properties have been observed in the function of neuronal networks involved in cognition and emotional behavior. It has been suggested that emotional and cognitive development as well as psychiatric disorders may be the product of emergent properties of brain networks.[64] Attention and cognitive control have been proposed as emergent properties of information representation of neurons in networks of the prefrontal cortex in primates.[65] Brain-imaging studies, including positron emission tomography and fMRI, have provided evidence that learning and memory involve emergent properties of large-scale neural network interactions.[66] Emergent properties of an inhibitory network in area CA3 of the hippocampus are proposed to be key elements in the different forms of long-term plasticity involved in memory observed in this pathway.[67]

Recent theories of conscious versus unconscious information processing in the brain have also emphasized emergent properties of brain networks. Both the integrated information theory of Tononi and colleagues and the global neuronal workspace theory postulated by Dehaene propose that consciousness emerges from network interactions arising from the whole system rather than from individual parts.[68,69]

NEUROLOGICAL DISORDERS—EPILEPSY

Several examples of emergent properties have been observed in the function of neuronal networks involved in epileptic seizures. In experimental epilepsy models, epileptic discharges were characterized as emergent properties of neuronal networks that depend on intrinsic neuronal properties and on the structural and functional organization of the synaptic networks that interconnect them. Fast oscillations are also proposed to be an emergent property of these networks.[70] Entorhinal cortex neurons are reported to exhibit emergent properties, such as delayed firing and enhanced or suppressed responses to repeated stimuli, due to changes in Ca^{2+} levels driven by neuronal firing. These firing changes involve either upregulation or downregulation of currents, depending on whether the Ca^{2+} levels are small or large, respectively, which is mediated, in part, by a specific endogenous neuroactive substance. The authors suggest that these emergent properties may be important in memory as well as the pathophysiology of epilepsy functions of the temporal lobe.[71] Repetitive seizures induce synaptic reorganization of hippocampal and cortical neuronal networks in animals and humans, including mossy fiber sprouting and gliosis; the latter can contribute to recurrent excitation as an emergent property in the epilepsy networks, subserving epileptogenesis.[72,73]

Emergent properties of neuronal ensembles may also subserve the ability of the brain to undergo the major state changes that occur during generalized convulsive seizures.[2,74] Thus, neurons in different nuclei in a network exhibit differential sensitivities to exogenously administered agents, despite the finding that each of these agents significantly diminishes the pathophysiological function of the network.[75] In the case of audiogenic seizures in genetically epilepsy-prone rats, even drugs that act on different components of the same receptor act on emergent properties in different network sites in equivalent therapeutic doses. Thus, doses of competitive NMDA antagonists that block audiogenic seizures act at a totally different site in the audiogenic seizures network from an uncompetitive NMDA antagonist[2] (see Chapter 32). Emergent properties can also result from degenerative processes in CNS disorders, such as stroke and Parkinson's disease[76] (see Chapter 25).

PSYCHIATRIC DISORDERS

Neuronal networks have been proposed for several types of psychiatric disorders, based largely on human imaging data[77–81] (see Chapter 24). Changes in the imaging patterns have also been observed with therapies that effectively control the symptoms of many of these disorders.[82–85] Psychopathology has been proposed to involve self-organizing neuronal interactions at the network level that result in neuroplastic changes that reveal emergent properties at which therapeutics for major psychiatric illnesses can be directed.[64] The stability of neuronal networks of the limbic system involved in emotional behavior is proposed to be influenced by changes in glutamate and gamma-aminobutyric acid (GABA) neurotransmission, resulting in emergent properties and network dysfunction that lead to schizophrenia and obsessive-compulsive disorder.[86] An example of emergent properties observed in the function of neuronal networks involved in psychiatric disorders has been observed in bipolar mood disorders. Thus, neuroimaging of patients suffering from bipolar disorder suggests that this disorder is due to abnormalities within a discrete brain network in the limbic system as an emergent property of these brain networks.[87] Disruptions in network dynamics occur in schizophrenia and several other brain disorders, and alterations in the tonic $GABA_A$ receptors mediated by extrasynaptic $GABA_A$ receptors are proposed to be potential therapeutic targets for the treatment of these diseases.[6] What is needed is identification of animal models of these psychiatric disorders that have similar network nuclei to those identified in these human conditions,[88] and then evaluation of the neuronal activity abnormalities and emergent properties that occur in these network sites can be examined. Once this is accomplished, specific therapies directed at the emergent properties can be developed.

These emergent properties of neurons and networks have potential importance for understanding how networks function, and the evidence is accumulating that emergent properties can actually be important targets for the action of CNS drugs, as discussed in Chapter 32. The action of neuroactive substances, including pharmacological agents, has been widely studied at the microscopic level and at the macroscopic level. However, the actions of drugs at the mesoscopic level is more difficult to evaluate, since it requires prior definition of the network components for a particular function or malfunction, which is only now being developed and only for a few networks, such as those involved in audiogenic seizures (see Chapter 26).

CONCLUSIONS

Emergent properties of neuronal networks serve as an important feature of brain physiology and pathophysiology, which bridge the gap between the properties of single brain neurons and major brain functions, such as perception. The potential heuristic importance of emergent properties lies in improving the understanding of the brain's normal network mechanisms, and network dysfunction in CNS diseases can also be better understood. Improvements in the therapy of these disorders are possible by targeting these emergent properties with CNS drugs that act on these properties in specific network sites. Thus, it is becoming clear that when *therapeutic doses* of drugs are administered to the intact animal, these site-specific emergent properties may be the specific and selective targets of drugs.

Acknowledgments

The author gratefully acknowledges Julio Copello for intellectual input and the assistance of Gayle Stauffer, Diana Smith, and Linda Moss in preparing this manuscript.

References

1. Pace RW, Del Negro CA. AMPA and metabotropic glutamate receptors cooperatively generate inspiratory-like depolarization in mouse respiratory neurons in vitro. *Eur J Neurosci*. 2008;28: 2434–2442.
2. Faingold CL. Emergent properties of CNS neuronal networks as targets for pharmacology: application to anticonvulsant drug action. *Prog Neurobiol*. 2004;72:55–85.
3. Agnati LF, Fuxe K. Volume transmission as a key feature of information handling in the central nervous system possible new interpretative value of the Turing's B-type machine. *Prog Brain Res*. 2000;125:3–19.
4. Bullmore E, Sporns O. Complex brain networks: graph theoretical analysis of structural and functional systems. *Nat Rev Neurosci*. 2009;10:186–198.

5. Faingold CL. Neuronal networks, epilepsy and the action of antiepileptic drugs. In: Faingold CL, Fromm GH, eds. *Drugs for Control of Epilepsy: Actions on Neuronal Networks Involved in Seizure Disorders.* Boca Raton, FL: CRC Press; 1992:1–21.
6. Brickley SG, Mody I. Extrasynaptic $GABA_A$ receptors: their function in the CNS and implications for disease. *Neuron.* 2012; 73:23–34.
7. Garcia-Cairasco N. Learning about brain physiology and complexity from the study of the epilepsies. *Braz J Med Biol Res.* 2009;42:76–86.
8. Faingold CL. Anticonvulsant drugs as neuronal network-modifying agents. In: Schwartzkroin PA, ed. *Encyclopedia of Basic Epilepsy Research.* Vol. 1. Oxford, UK: Academic Press; 2009:50–58.
9. Lorenz EN. *Predictability: Does the Flap of a Butterfly's Wings in Brazil Set off a Tornado in Texas?* American Association for the Advancement of Science; December 29, 1972.
10. Freeman WJ. *Mass Action in the Nervous System.* New York, NY: Academic Press; 1975.
11. Freeman WJ, Kozma R, Werbos PJ. Biocomplexity: adaptive behavior in complex stochastic dynamical systems. *Biosystems.* 2001;59:109–123.
12. Alenda A, Molano-Mazon M, Panzeri S, Maravall Ml. Sensory input drives multiple intracellular information streams in somatosensory cortex. *J Neurosci.* 2010;30:10872–10884.
13. Tsodyks M, Kenet T, Grinvald A, Arieli A. Linking spontaneous activity of single cortical neurons and the underlying functional architecture. *Science.* 1999;286:1943–1946.
14. Blitz DM, White RS, Saideman SR, et al. A newly identified extrinsic input triggers a distinct gastric mill rhythm via activation of modulatory projection neurons. *J Exp Biol.* 2008;211: 1000–1011.
15. Marder E, Bucher D. Understanding circuit dynamics using the stomatogastric nervous system of lobsters and crabs. *Annu Rev Physiol.* 2007;69:291–316.
16. Zelenin PV. Activity of individual reticulospinal neurons during different forms of locomotion in the lamprey. *Eur J Neurosci.* 2005;22:2271–2282.
17. Buzsaki G, Csicsvari J, Dragoi G, Harris K, Henze D, Hirase H. Homeostatic maintenance of neuronal excitability by burst discharges in vivo. *Cereb Cortex.* 2002;12:893–899.
18. Sullivan D, Csicsvari J, Mizuseki K, Montgomery S, Diba K, Buzsaki G. Relationships between hippocampal sharp waves, ripples, and fast gamma oscillation: influence of dentate and entorhinal cortical activity. *J Neurosci.* 2011;31:8605–8616.
19. Ermentrout GB, Kleinfeld D. Traveling electrical waves in cortex: insights from phase dynamics and speculation on a computational role. *Neuron.* 2001;29:33–44.
20. Cowan RL, Wilson CJ. Spontaneous firing patterns and axonal projections of single corticostriatal neurons in the rat medial agranular cortex. *J Neurophysiol.* 1994;71:17–32.
21. Crane JW, Windels F, Sah P. Oscillations in the basolateral amygdala: aversive stimulation is state dependent and resets the oscillatory phase. *J Neurophysiol.* 2009;102:1379–1387.
22. Kerr JN, Plenz D. Action potential timing determines dendritic calcium during striatal up-states. *J Neurosci.* 2004;24:877–885.
23. Oldfield CS, Marty A, Stell BM. Interneurons of the cerebellar cortex toggle Purkinje cells between up and down states. *Proc Natl Acad Sci USA.* 2010;107:13153–13158.
24. Rigas P, Castro-Alamancos MA. Impact of persistent cortical activity (up states) on intracortical and thalamocortical synaptic inputs. *J Neurophysiol.* 2009;102:119–131.
25. Kasanetz F, Riquelme LA, Murer MG. Disruption of the two-state membrane potential of striatal neurones during cortical desynchronisation in anaesthetised rats. *J Physiol.* 2002;543:577–589.
26. Mahon S, Deniau JM, Charpier S. Relationship between EEG potentials and intracellular activity of striatal and cortico-striatal neurons: an in vivo study under different anesthetics. *Cereb Cortex.* 2001;11:360–373.
27. Bragin A, Benassi SK, Engel Jr J. Patterns of the UP–Down state in normal and epileptic mice. *Neuroscience.* 2012;225: 76–87.
28. Beggs JM, Plenz D. Neuronal avalanches in neocortical circuits. *J Neurosci.* 2003;23:11167–11177.
29. Shew WL, Yang H, Yu S, Roy R, Plenz D. Information capacity and transmission are maximized in balanced cortical networks with neuronal avalanches. *J Neurosci.* 2011;31:55–63.
30. Cardanobile S, Rotter S. Emergent properties of interacting populations of spiking neurons. *Front Comput Neurosci.* 2011;5:59.
31. Cheng H, Lederer WJ. Calcium sparks. *Physiol Rev.* 2008;88: 1491–1545.
32. Stern MD, Cheng H. Putting out the fire: what terminates calcium-induced calcium release in cardiac muscle? *Cell Calcium.* 2004;35:591–601.
33. Copello JA, Zima AV, Diaz-Sylvester PL, Fill M, Blatter LA. Ca^{2+} entry-independent effects of L-type Ca^{2+} channel modulators on Ca^{2+} sparks in ventricular myocytes. *Am J Physiol Cell Physiol.* 2007;292:C2129–C2140.
34. Porta M, Diaz-Sylvester PL, Neumann JT, Escobar AL, Fleischer S, Copello JA. Coupled gating of skeletal muscle ryanodine receptors is modulated by Ca^{2+}, Mg^{2+}, and ATP. *Am J Physiol Cell Physiol.* 2012;303:C682–C697.
35. Hopkins PM. Malignant hyperthermia: pharmacology of triggering. *Br J Anaesth.* 2011;107:48–56.
36. Leondopulos SS, Boehler MD, Wheeler BC, Brewer GJ. Chronic stimulation of cultured neuronal networks boosts low-frequency oscillatory activity at theta and gamma with spikes phase-locked to gamma frequencies. *J Neural Eng.* 2012;9: 026015.
37. Raghavan M, Amrutur B, Srinivas KV, Sikdar SK. A study of epileptogenic network structures in rat hippocampal cultures using first spike latencies during synchronization events. *Phys Biol.* 2012;9:056002.
38. Straub VA, Staras K, Kemenes G, Benjamin PR. Endogenous and network properties of Lymnaea feeding central pattern generator interneurons. *J Neurophysiol.* 2002;88:1569–1583.
39. Carroll MS, Ramirez JM. The cycle-by-cycle assembly of respiratory network activity is dynamic and stochastic. *J Neurophysiol.* Sep 19, 2012. [Epub ahead of print].
40. Lindsey BG, Morris KF, Segers LS, Shannon R. Respiratory neuronal assemblies. *Respir Physiol.* 2000;122:183–196.
41. Onimaru H, Homma I. A novel functional neuron group for respiratory rhythm generation in the ventral medulla. *J Neurosci.* 2003;23:1478–1486.
42. Ramirez JM, Zuperku EJ, Alheid GF, Lieske SP, Ptak K, McCrimmon DR. Respiratory rhythm generation: converging concepts from in vitro and in vivo approaches? *Respir Physiol Neurobiol.* 2002;131:43–56.
43. Rekling JC, Feldman JL. PreBotzinger complex and pacemaker neurons: hypothesized site and kernel for respiratory rhythm generation. *Annu Rev Physiol.* 1998;60:385–405.
44. Rybak IA, Shevtsova NA, Paton JF, et al. Modeling the ponto-medullary respiratory network. *Respir Physiol Neurobiol.* 2004;143:307–319.
45. Del Negro CA, Morgado-Valle C, Feldman JL. Respiratory rhythm: an emergent network property? *Neuron.* 2002;34: 821–830.
46. Mironov S. Respiratory circuits: function, mechanisms, topology, and pathology. *Neuroscientist.* 2009;15:194–208.

47. Mutolo D, Bongianni F, Cinelli E, Pantaleo T. Role of neurokinin receptors and ionic mechanisms within the respiratory network of the lamprey. *Neuroscience*. 2010;169:1136–1149.
48. Viemari JC, Ramirez JM. Norepinephrine differentially modulates different types of respiratory pacemaker and nonpacemaker neurons. *J Neurophysiol*. 2006;95:2070–2082.
49. Mori S, Iwakiri H, Homma Y, Yokoyama T, Matsuyama K. Neuroanatomical and neurophysiological bases of postural control. *Adv Neurol*. 1995;67:289–303.
50. Li WC. Generation of locomotion rhythms without inhibition in vertebrates: the search for pacemaker neurons. *Integr Comp Biol*. 2011;51:879–889.
51. Deco G, Jirsa VK, Robinson PA, Breakspear M, Friston K. The dynamic brain: from spiking neurons to neural masses and cortical fields. *PLoS Comput Biol*. 2008;4(8):e1000092.
52. White J, Hamilton KA, Neff SR, Kauer JS. Emergent properties of odor information coding in a representational model of the salamander olfactory bulb. *J Neurosci*. 1992;12:1772–1780.
53. Jacob V, Le Cam J, Ego-Stengel V, Shulz DE. Emergent properties of tactile scenes selectively activate barrel cortex neurons. *Neuron*. 2008;60:1112–1125.
54. Ego-Stengel V, Le Cam J, Shulz DE. Coding of apparent motion in the thalamic nucleus of the rat vibrissal somatosensory system. *J Neurosci*. 2012;32:3339–3351.
55. Leveille J, Versace M, Grossberg S. Running as fast as it can: how spiking dynamics form object groupings in the laminar circuits of visual cortex. *J Comput Neurosci*. 2010;28:323–346.
56. Pinto L, Baron J. Spatiotemporal frequency tuning dynamics of neurons in the owl visual wulst. *J Neurophysiol*. 2010;103: 3424–3436.
57. Tolias AS, Smirnakis SM, Augath MA, Trinath T, Logothetis NK. Motion processing in the macaque: revisited with functional magnetic resonance imaging. *J Neurosci*. 2001;21:8594–8601.
58. Persinger MA, Peredery O, Bureau YR, Cook LL. Emergent properties following brain injury: the claustrum as a major component of a pathway that influences nociceptive thresholds to foot shock in rats. *Percept Mot Skills*. 1997;85:387–398.
59. Buzsaki G. The thalamic clock: emergent network properties. *Neuroscience*. 1991;41:351–364.
60. Sohal VS, Pangratz-Fuehrer S, Rudolph U, Huguenard JR. Intrinsic and synaptic dynamics interact to generate emergent patterns of rhythmic bursting in thalamocortical neurons. *J Neurosci*. 2006;26:4247–4255.
61. Saper CB, Chou TC, Scammell TE. The sleep switch: hypothalamic control of sleep and wakefulness. *Trends Neurosci*. 2001;24:726–731.
62. Clinton JM, Davis CJ, Zielinski MR, Jewett KA, Krueger JM. Biochemical regulation of sleep and sleep biomarkers. *J Clin Sleep Med*. 2011;7:S38–S42.
63. Vetrugno R, Montagna P. From REM sleep behaviour disorder to status dissociatus: insights into the maze of states of being. *Sleep Med*. 2011;12(Suppl. 2):S68–S71.
64. Post RM, Weiss SR. Emergent properties of neural systems: how focal molecular neurobiological alterations can affect behavior. *Dev Psychopathol*. 1997;9:907–929.
65. Courtney SM. Attention and cognitive control as emergent properties of information representation in working memory. *Cogn Affect Behav Neurosci*. 2004;4:501–516.
66. McIntosh AR. Mapping cognition to the brain through neural interactions. *Memory*. 1999;7:523–548.
67. Galvan EJ, Cosgrove KE, Barrionuevo G. Multiple forms of long-term synaptic plasticity at hippocampal mossy fiber synapses on interneurons. *Neuropharmacology*. 2011;60:740–747.
68. Dehaene S, Changeux JP. Experimental and theoretical approaches to conscious processing. *Neuron*. 2011;70(2):200–227.
69. Tononi G. Integrated information theory of consciousness: an updated account. *Arch Ital Biol*. 2012;150(4):293–329.
70. Jefferys JG. Models and mechanisms of experimental epilepsies. *Epilepsia*. 2003;44:44–50.
71. Magistretti J, Ma L, Shalinsky MH, Lin W, Klink R, Alonso A. Spike patterning by Ca^{2+}-dependent regulation of a muscarinic cation current in entorhinal cortex layer II neurons. *J Neurophysiol*. 2004;92:1644–1657.
72. Rakhade SN, Jensen FE. Epileptogenesis in the immature brain: emerging mechanisms. *Nat Rev Neurol*. 2009;5:380–391.
73. Sutula TP, Dudek FE. Unmasking recurrent excitation generated by mossy fiber sprouting in the epileptic dentate gyrus: an emergent property of a complex system. *Prog Brain Res*. 2007; 163:541–563.
74. Faingold CL. Neuronal networks in the genetically epilepsy-prone rat. In: Delgado-Escueta AV, Wilson WA, Olsen RW, Porter RJ, eds. *Jasper's Basic Mechanisms of the Epilepsies*. 3rd ed. Philadelphia, PA: Lippincott Williams and Wilkins; 1999:311–321.
75. Faingold CL. Brainstem networks: reticulo-cortical synchronization in generalized convulsive seizures. In: Noebels JL, Avoli M, Rogawski MA, Olsen RW, Delgado-Escueta AV, eds. *Jasper's Basic Mechanisms of the Epilepsies*. 4th ed. New York, NY: Oxford University Press; 2012:257–271.
76. Qureshi IA, Mehler MF. The emerging role of epigenetics in stroke: III. Neural stem cell biology and regenerative medicine. *Arch Neurol*. 2011;68:294–302.
77. Chen CH, Suckling J, Lennox BR, Ooi C, Bullmore ET. A quantitative meta-analysis of fMRI studies in bipolar disorder. *Bipolar Disord*. 2011;13:1–15.
78. Hughes KC, Shin LM. Functional neuroimaging studies of post-traumatic stress disorder. *Expert Rev Neurother*. 2011;11:275–285.
79. Jones MW. Errant ensembles: dysfunctional neuronal network dynamics in schizophrenia. *Biochem Soc Trans*. 2010;38:516–521.
80. Nakao T, Sanematsu H, Yoshiura T, et al. fMRI of patients with social anxiety disorder during a social situation task. *Neurosci Res*. 2011;69:67–72.
81. Price JL, Drevets WC. Neurocircuitry of mood disorders. *Neuropsychopharmacology*. 2010;35:192–216.
82. Bellani M, Dusi N, Yeh PH, Soares JC, Brambilla P. The effects of antidepressants on human brain as detected by imaging studies. Focus on major depression. *Prog Neuropsychopharmacol Biol Psychiatry*. 2011;35:1544–1552.
83. Patin A, Hurlemann R. Modulating amygdala responses to emotion: evidence from pharmacological fMRI. *Neuropsychologia*. 2011;49:706–717.
84. Rigucci S, Serafini G, Pompili M, Kotzalidis GD, Tatarelli R. Anatomical and functional correlates in major depressive disorder: the contribution of neuroimaging studies. *World J Biol Psychiatry*. 2010;11:165–180.
85. Shaw P, Rabin C. New insights into attention-deficit/hyperactivity disorder using structural neuroimaging. *Curr Psychiatry Rep*. 2009;11:393–398.
86. Deco G, Rolls ET, Albantakis L, Romo R. Brain mechanisms for perceptual and reward-related decision-making. *Prog Neurobiol*. Feb 2, 2012. [Epub ahead of print].
87. Adler CM, DelBello MP, Strakowski SM. Brain network dysfunction in bipolar disorder. *CNS Spectr*. 2006;11:312–320.
88. Berton O, Hahn CG, Thase ME. Are we getting closer to valid translational models for major depression? *Science*. 2012;338: 75–79.

CHAPTER

31

Neuronal Network Involvement in Stimulation Therapies for CNS Disorders

Carl L. Faingold[1], *Hua-Jun Feng*[2]

[1]Departments of Pharmacology and Neurology, Division of Neurosurgery, Southern Illinois University School of Medicine, Springfield, IL, USA, [2]Department of Anesthesia, Critical Care and Pain Medicine, Massachusetts General Hospital and Harvard Medical School, Boston, MA, USA

INTRODUCTION

Stimulation techniques have been widely used to treat a number of different central nervous system (CNS) disorders, with considerable success in some cases, and evidence is developing that neuronal network changes may be a major mechanism mediating the therapeutic effects. Thus, competition between the stimulated network and the disease network and disruption of the disease network are proposed to subserve the therapeutic effects. This competition may center on nuclei that contain a high percentage of conditional multireceptive (CMR) neurons that are activated by both the stimulation process and the CNS disorder network, as discussed in this chapter (also see Chapter 28). The stimulation procedure can be carried out either by invasive techniques where the stimulation device is implanted chronically in the subject or by noninvasive techniques where the stimulation device is applied externally. A number of different noninvasive stimulation techniques, ranging from highly localized acupuncture (which involves placing needles on specific acupoints on the body) to the massive stimulation of electroconvulsive shock, have been used successfully as therapeutic approaches for a wide variety of CNS disorders. Other noninvasive stimulation approaches include transcranial magnetic stimulation (TMS), transcutaneous electrical nerve stimulation (TENS), and trigeminal nerve stimulation (TNS), which are being used therapeutically. Invasive approaches, involving chronically implanted electrodes, include vagus nerve stimulation (VNS) and deep brain stimulation (DBS), which have also been used therapeutically.[1–4] CNS disorders that have been treated with these stimulation techniques include chronic pain syndromes, major depression, Alzheimer's disease, Parkinson's disease, stroke, dystonia, headache, restless legs syndrome, and epilepsy, with at least some degree of success. Most of the techniques discussed in this chapter, with the exception of traditional acupuncture, involve electrical stimulation. Stimulant drugs and light stimulation are stimulation techniques utilized experimentally in animals, but are not yet being utilized therapeutically in patients and are discussed in Chapters 4 and 32.

NONINVASIVE STIMULATION MODALITIES

Acupuncture

Acupuncture is a form of stimulation therapy that involves insertion of fine needles into specific regions of the body, or acupoints, and it has been used in China for over 2000 years. Acupuncture has been used extensively to treat pain of various origins and has been proposed for treatment of many other conditions (see Ref. 5 for a review). Electroacupuncture is a relatively recent variant that employs electrical currents applied to the needles.[6,7] One of the major issues in the investigations of acupuncture is that many different sites for stimulation (acupoints) are used in traditional Chinese medicine to treat various maladies.[8,9]

The effects of stimulation at a number of these acupoints have been evaluated and compared. A large body of literature exists on the modulation of brain activity by acupuncture using imaging techniques.[8,10–12] The studies exhibited significant heterogeneity due to differences in numerous factors, such as manipulation

Neuronal Networks in Brain Function, CNS Disorders, and Therapeutics
http://dx.doi.org/10.1016/B978-0-12-415804-7.00031-9

methods, types of controls, data acquisition approaches, brain regions of interest, and statistical analysis.[8] A meta-analysis of the literature covering English, Chinese, Korean, and Japanese databases evaluated the literature on the response of the brain to acupuncture stimuli using functional magnetic resonance imaging (fMRI).[8] It was shown that acupuncture activates sensorimotor and affective processing brain regions and deactivates the amygdala and the default mode network (DMN) brain regions. Brain responses to acupuncture and sham acupuncture are different in many brain regions.[8] The effects of electroacupuncture in another human fMRI study showed that limbic-prefrontal functional networks were deactivated and that the local functional connectivity was significantly changed during stimulation; the change persisted after the stimulation.[13] An fMRI study of electrical acupuncture examined changes in supraspinal regions excited by thermal pain, including the left amygdala, right raphe nucleus within the reticular formation, bilateral frontal lobes, and right inferior frontal lobe; the study observed that a significant degree of deactivation was induced in these regions depending on the acupoint stimulated.[14]

Significant changes in the activity within brain networks are being revealed using brain-imaging techniques (particularly fMRI) that differ based on which acupoint is being evaluated.[5,15,16] A recent study examined functional connectivity changes and psychophysical responses using fMRI during acupuncture stimulation at three specific acupoints as compared with tactile stimulation or pain induction.[8] Clusters of deactivated regions in the medial prefrontal, medial parietal, and medial temporal lobes, as well as activated regions in the sensorimotor and certain paralimbic structures, were identified, which were virtually identical to the DMN and the anticorrelated task-positive network in response to stimulation (Figure 31.1). fMRI changes in the amygdala and hypothalamus were also frequently observed in acupuncture. When the subjects reported that the acupuncture stimulus induced sharp pain, the deactivation was attenuated or reversed and became activation. Tactile stimulation induced greater activation of the somatosensory network but caused less extensive deactivation of the limbic-related structures. These findings suggest that acupuncture effects are mediated by these deactivated networks and that the effect is dependent on the psychophysical response of the subjects.[8]

Several approaches to evaluating acupuncture fMRI data using computational methods, such as change-point analysis and multivariate Granger causality, as well as techniques that evaluate additional parameters, such as magnetoencephalography, have also been used to better understand network changes induced by acupuncture. In a recent fMRI study, computational evaluation of the effects of acupuncture in healthy humans indicated that the functional networks that were activated exhibited small-world attributes (high

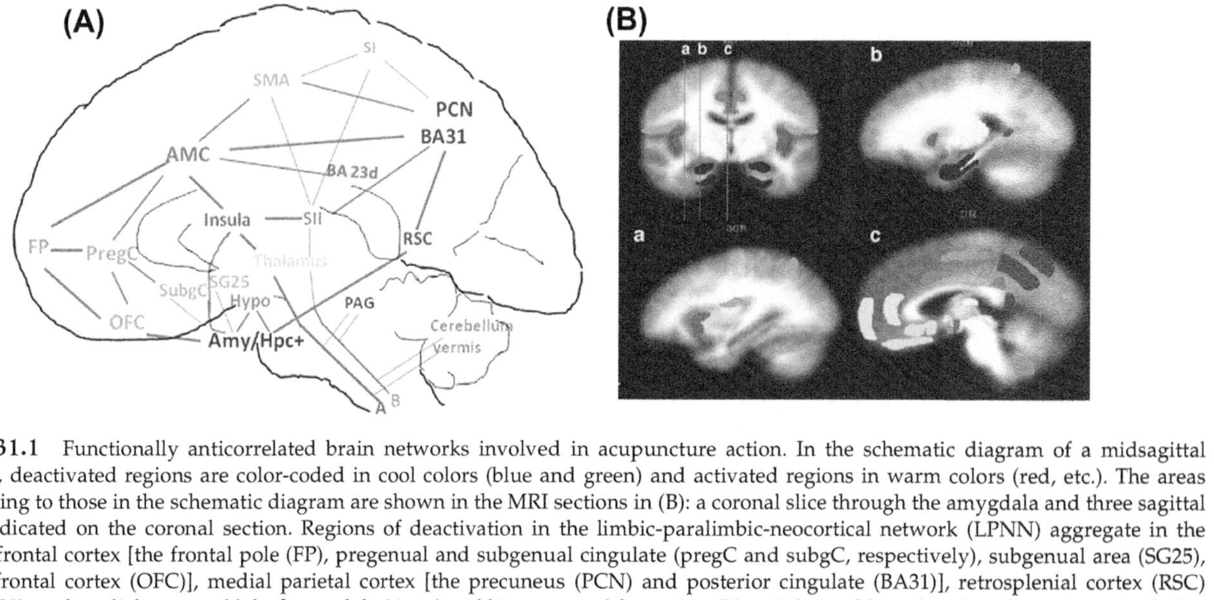

FIGURE 31.1 Functionally anticorrelated brain networks involved in acupuncture action. In the schematic diagram of a midsagittal section (A), deactivated regions are color-coded in cool colors (blue and green) and activated regions in warm colors (red, etc.). The areas corresponding to those in the schematic diagram are shown in the MRI sections in (B): a coronal slice through the amygdala and three sagittal slices as indicated on the coronal section. Regions of deactivation in the limbic-paralimbic-neocortical network (LPNN) aggregate in the medial prefrontal cortex [the frontal pole (FP), pregenual and subgenual cingulate (pregC and subgC, respectively), subgenual area (SG25), and orbitofrontal cortex (OFC)], medial parietal cortex [the precuneus (PCN) and posterior cingulate (BA31)], retrosplenial cortex (RSC) (BA29 and 30), and medial temporal lobe [amygdala (Amy) and hippocampal formation (Hpc+), located lateral to the schematic section]. The hypothalamus, pontine nuclei, and cerebellar vermis also showed deactivation. The secondary somatosensory cortex (SII), right anterior insula, antero-middle cingulate (AMC), supplementary motor area (SMA), posterior cingulate (BA23) dorsal, and sensory divisions of the thalamus comprise the activation network. Several associated cortical areas and the basal ganglia showing activation or deactivation are not shown. (*Source: This figure is adapted from Ref. 16 with permission.*) (The figure is reproduced in color section.)

local and global efficiency) with increased local efficiency as compared to sham acupuncture. Significant changes were observed in the hippocampus, anterior cingulate cortex, and frontal cortex as well as limbic and subcortical brain regions.[17] An application of computational approaches to fMRI data during acupuncture, using graph theory (multivariate Granger causality), investigated causal brain networks that were activated by different acupoints.[18] This study reported that the strength of causal connectivity between the superior temporal gyrus (STG) and anterior insula was enhanced, while the connection strength between the STG and postcentral gyrus was increased following acupuncture at one acupoint. Additionally, the causal influences within the auditory network increased as compared to the executive network following acupuncture stimulation at a different acupoint.[18] Acupuncture effects were also studied, using a nonrepeated event-related fMRI paradigm and control theory (change-point analysis) to evaluate the temporal profile of neural responses. This study observed that the amygdala and perigenual anterior cingulate cortex exhibited increased activities during the initial phase, which decreased gradually. In contrast, the periaqueductal gray and hypothalamus exhibited intermittent activations. The periaqueductal gray is also implicated in pain networks in humans and other animals[19] (see Chapter 23). Persistent activities were also identified in the anterior insula and prefrontal cortices, suggesting that acupuncture induces differential temporal neural responses as a function of time in several brain networks.[20] A magnetoencephalography and structural fMRI study of acupuncture effects at a specific acupoint observed significantly time-varied brain activities with different onset times in the pain inhibition areas (insula and amygdala), but these changes were not seen with stimulation at another (non-acupoint) location.[21] Another functional connectivity fMRI study of electroacupuncture, which allowed the study of continuous-treatment paradigms, found that this treatment increased the connectivity between the periaqueductal gray and several cortical sites, as compared to sham acupuncture.[22]

Although acupuncture has been used primarily for pain treatment, its use in other conditions, such as Parkinson's disease[23] and Alzheimer's disease, has also been evaluated. Thus, the effects of acupuncture, which is being used to treat mild cognitive impairment (MCI) to try to prevent Alzheimer's disease in these patients, were examined using fMRI. In the resting state, the hippocampus, thalamus, and fusiform gyrus of the patients with MCI showed abnormal functional connectivity as compared to healthy patients, but after acupuncture the patterns of these regions were enhanced in the former's resting brain more than in that of the normal individuals.[24] From the foregoing studies, it can also be seen that different acupoints activate different networks, which may be very important for effective acupuncture use in treating different CNS disorders. One possible approach that should be tested involves comparing acupoints that are traditionally thought to affect certain specific points on the body and pairing those with CNS sites known to be associated with activation of those same sites. This would potentially allow therapeutic targeting of specific brain sites that are involved in the neuronal network of a given CNS disorder or that can compete with it (see Chapter 29).

Acupressure, which involves applying continuous pressure over a specific acupoint, has been utilized for reduction of nausea associated with motion sickness, nausea, and vomiting in patients during pregnancy and during chemotherapy.[25]

Mechanisms of Acupuncture Effects

The mechanisms involved in the effects of acupuncture have focused on neurotransmitter changes, involving opioid peptides, glutamate, 5-hydroxytryptamine, and cholecystokinin (see Ref. 26 for a review). Recent evidence indicates that repetitive electroacupuncture causes prolonged increased met-enkephalin expression in a medullary nucleus involved in the pain pathway.[27] The neuronal mechanisms of acupuncture effects were evaluated in rats on neurons in the lateral nucleus (NRL) in the medullary reticular formation, which is reported to play an important role in modulating centrifugal antinociceptive effects.[28] The majority of NRL neurons that project to the nucleus raphe magnus were inhibited, but about one-half of the NRL neurons that project to the spinal cord were excited by electroacupuncture.[28] The brainstem reticular formation (BRF) contains a large percentage of CMR neurons. These neurons are capable of responding to neuronal inputs from many other networks, depending on the conditions that the organism is experiencing, including pain, as discussed in this chapter (see also Chapter 28), and they may also interact with glial cells (see Chapter 12). Competition between the acupuncture input and the pain input for CMR sites may result in reduced activity in the pain-related network and less pain, as discussed in the "General Neuronal Network Mechanisms" section.

Electroconvulsive Shock Stimulation Approaches

One of the oldest electrical stimulation therapies in Western medicine is electroconvulsive shock therapy (ECT), which is a well-established therapy for treatment-resistant depression.[29] The mechanisms involved in the effectiveness of ECT in treating depression are not well understood. Neuronal network analysis of ECT using single photon emission computed tomography showed that specific cortical and subcortical areas were affected by ECT, including the BRF.[30] It has been proposed that the neuroactive substances released as a result of the seizures, which are thought to contribute to the termination of the seizures, exert anticonvulsant effects and also mediate the relatively rapid onset of antidepressant effects that is the major reason for the continued therapeutic use of ECT.[31] The mechanisms involved in the seizure termination include alterations of monoamine neurotransmitter systems, activation of adenosine triphosphate (ATP)-dependent potassium channels, increased release of zinc, increased GABAergic inhibition, and effects on the hypothalamic-pituitary-adrenal axis.[31–33] ECT has also been shown to stimulate neurogenesis,[34] and a possible trophic effect on glial cells has also been proposed.[35] ECT is also associated with increased levels of adenosine and upregulation of adenosine A1 receptors in the brain. Neurotrophic effects evoked by these adenosine receptors, mediated by glial cell networks, have been proposed to contribute importantly to the mechanism of action of ECT.[36,37] Thus, the importance of astrocytic networks in the organization and control of neuronal networks (discussed in Chapters 1 and 12), which is mediated, in part, by adenosine, may play a major role in the ability of ECT to exert its therapeutic effects by modifying or competing with the network that mediates the depressive disorder[31] (Chapter 24).

Other Noninvasive Stimulation Approaches

Other noninvasive stimulation approaches are being utilized, but their use and mechanisms are less well-known and understood. These other noninvasive approaches include TMS, TENS, and TNS.

Transcranial Magnetic Stimulation

TMS involves delivery of brief magnetic pulses by means of a coil placed on the scalp over a given cortical target, which is thought to induce action potentials (activation) in neuronal networks and is often given repetitively in specific paradigms.[38] The most common stimulation site for TMS is the primary motor cortex, and it is thought to preferentially stimulate axons (rather than cell bodies), particularly of interneurons running parallel to the surface of the cortex.[39] Depending on the rate of stimulation, either stimulation or inhibition of corticospinal output can result,[40] but the effects are also proposed to depend on the degree of cortical excitability at the time of the stimulation.[39] TMS is used most commonly in chronic pain syndromes, and the most effective parameter for repetitive stimulation is frequencies $\geq$5 Hz delivered to the motor cortex.[41] TMS has also been utilized with some success in the treatment of stroke, chronic depression, and epilepsy, as well as in rehabilitation from stroke and other disruptions of CNS function.[42–44] The success of TMS in epilepsy may depend on whether the seizure focus is superficial and well localized or deep and not well localized.[42] Repetitive TMS at biologically relevant (theta) frequencies is also being used to improve the symptoms of visuo-spatial deficit in traumatic brain injury.[45,46] TMS over the motor cortex can also activate distant structures, including several other cortical regions, basal ganglia, and the cerebellum as well as structures involved in the sensory and emotional aspects of pain, and involve activation of GABAergic or opioidergic systems, depending on the parameters of stimulation.[39,47] It is proposed that TMS initially excites neurons, which release neurotransmitters into postsynaptic neurons. Repeated TMS produces long-term changes akin to long-term potentiation (LTP) and long-term depression as well as genetic and protein regulation and network oscillation changes.[48] It has recently been proposed that TMS exerts therapeutic effects in epilepsy by a major effect on astrocytic networks.[49] Modulation of astrocytic networks is developing as a potentially important general neuronal network mechanism for several different modes of brain stimulation.

Transcutaneous Electrical Nerve Stimulation

TENS is a noninvasive stimulation therapy that involves delivering low-level electrical currents to the skin. Standard TENS uses high-frequency stimulation (70–100 Hz) at low intensity below the pain threshold, and it causes paresthesia in the painful area. The mechanism of TENS is thought to be based on the gate control theory, wherein stimulation of large-caliber Aβ afferent fibers inhibits the activity of small-caliber Aδ and C fibers at the segmental spinal level (see Chapters 23 and 29).[50] TENS is sometimes combined with acupuncture and is discussed in this chapter as electroacupuncture. The stimulation electrodes are placed on the nerve trunk that innervates the painful region or on a neighboring nerve when allodynia or hyperalgesia is present, and effects develop after 20–60 min and last from 30 min to several hours.[39] A review of TENS controlled therapeutic trials concluded that the analgesic effects of TENS increased with the "dose" of stimulation (the duration of stimulation multiplied by the session frequency multiplied by the total time during which the technique was applied).[51] Since "sham" stimulation cannot be performed because of the induced paresthesia, these trials are only single-blind.

TENS Mechanisms

The effect of TENS has been attributed primarily to a network competition effect in the spinal cord by activation of the gate control theory of pain[50] as well as activation of neurotransmitter systems, particularly endogenous opioid peptide pathways.[52]

Transgeminal Nerve Stimulation and Other Noninvasive Treatments

TNS is a relatively new noninvasive stimulation therapy that involves stimulation of the infraorbital and supraorbital branches of the trigeminal nerve, which is observed to be relatively safe and useful in the therapy of drug-resistant epilepsy as well as depression.[53,54] The trigeminal nerve also projects to structures implicated in depression, such as the nucleus tractus solitarius and locus coeruleus, and these structures could contribute to the effectiveness of this treatment via neuroactive substance release (norepinephrine) and/or network activation of CMR networks in the brainstem[2,55] (see Chapter 28).

Other noninvasive stimulation therapies include transcranial direct current stimulation, which involves passage of a weak direct current via electrodes placed on the scalp over a specific cortical target, which generates membrane potential changes (depolarization or hyperpolarization) in cortical neuronal networks.[38] This technique has been used to treat depression and stroke,[56,57] but this technique will not be discussed in detail here.

INVASIVE STIMULATION MODALITIES

Vagus Nerve Stimulation

Stimulation of the vagus nerve via a chronically implanted stimulator is an effective therapy for epilepsy and major depression.[42,58,59] VNS, which has been utilized in many thousands of patients, involves an electrode surgically implanted in the neck that is connected to a stimulation device implanted near the clavicle.[2] This technique is also being tested for migraine, Alzheimer's disease, and eating disorders.[2] Positron emission tomography scans of the effects of VNS showed increases in blood flow in specific areas of the thalamus and cortex and decreases in blood flow in the limbic system,[60,61] but contradictory results have also been reported.[2]

VNS Mechanisms

Mechanisms involved in the effect of VNS include changes in noradrenergic neurotransmission, and other mechanisms, including attenuation of glutamate-mediated excitotoxicity, enhancement of synaptic plasticity, and anti-inflammatory effects, have been hypothesized.[62,63] It has also recently been proposed that VNS exerts therapeutic effects in epilepsy by a major effect on astrocytes.[49]

Deep Brain Stimulation

DBS involves an invasive chronic implantation of a stimulating electrode into specific regions in the brain. DBS is approved by the US Food and Drug Administration for treatment of several CNS disorders, including essential tremor and Parkinson's disease, and it has a humanitarian device exemption for dystonia and obsessive-compulsive disorder.[64] Thus, localized electrical stimulation of specific sites within the brain has resulted in effective treatments for Parkinson's disease and epilepsy.[64–69] Treatment of the motor manifestations of Parkinson's disease by DBS in the subthalamus has been extensively utilized, and pain, which is also a common symptom of this CNS disorder, has also been observed to be significantly improved by DBS in this brain site.[70] DBS has essentially replaced ablative procedures for Parkinson's disease and other related conditions. DBS in the ventralis intermedius nucleus of the thalamus improves control of tremor in Parkinson's disease and essential tremor, while primary dystonia is controlled by DBS of the globus pallidus internus.[71]

A recent study observed that high-frequency electrical stimulation of the anterior nucleus of the thalamus reduced the number of seizures in patients with medication-resistant epilepsy.[42]

DBS Mechanisms

Although stimulation at low frequencies and intensities increases the activity of a brain area and activates the network, stimulation directly within the disease network, particularly at high frequencies and higher intensities, results in disruptive effects on the network and inhibition of cells in the stimulated site.[65] Most stimulation paradigms employ high frequencies, and network disruption may be a key element in the effectiveness of this approach. In vitro simulation of DBS was done using high-frequency pulses in thalamic slices, and this resulted in increased glutamate release and abolition of spindle oscillations in the reticular nucleus of the thalamus, which may involve the activation of hyperpolarization-activated current (I_h).[72]

A recent experiment, using optogenetic techniques, investigated the network mechanisms for the well-established therapeutic effects of DBS on Parkinson's disease. The roles of different network components in the subthalamic nucleus (STN) site of stimulation were evaluated, and the evidence indicated that the deep layer V neurons in the primary motor cortex were the major source for the therapeutic effect in an animal model of Parkinson's disease. However, neither selective optogenetic stimulation of astroglial cells at the stimulation site nor selective optogenetic stimulation of excitatory neurons in the STN was able to exert the therapeutic effect, suggesting that the cortical-to-STN pathway is the critical network element for the therapeutic effects of DBS in the STN in a Parkinson's disease model.[73] Thus, as seen in the network diagram of the basal ganglia in Parkinson's disease (Figure 31.2), a loss of dopaminergic cells in the substantia nigra pars compacta drives activity changes in two types of dopaminergic-receiving cells in the striatum, D1 and D2 cells, that project to the substantia nigra pars reticulata and globus pallidus, respectively. These changes generate the motor symptoms of Parkinson's disease, which is reversed by DBS of the STN.[74]

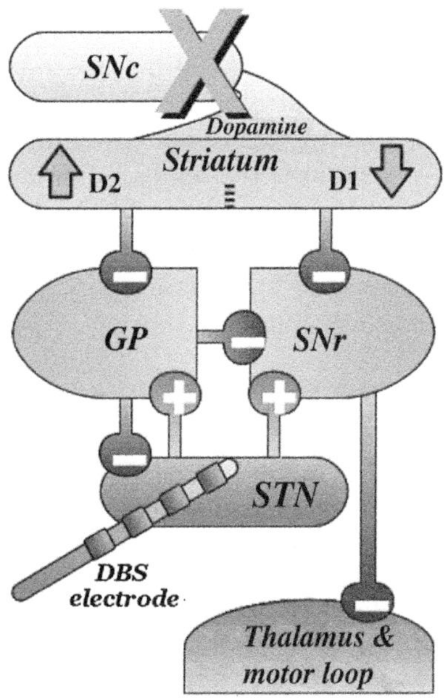

FIGURE 31.2 DBS network diagram. Network diagram of the basal ganglia regions implicated in Parkinsonian disorders. A loss of dopaminergic cells in the substantia nigra pars compacta (SNc) drives activity changes (pink) in two types of dopaminergic-receiving cells in the striatum, D1 and D2 cells, which project to the substantia nigra pars reticulata (SNr) and globus pallidus (GP), respectively. These changes generate the motor symptoms of Parkinsonism, which can be reversed by deep brain stimulation (DBS) of the subthalamic nucleus (STN). The signs of the connections (+ or −) are known, but the detailed network changes driven by Parkinsonism and DBS have yet to be elucidated. (*Source: This figure is adapted from Ref. 74 with permission; see http://brain.utah.edu/research/dorval/mechanisms-of-deep-brain-stimulation.php.*) (For interpretation of the references to color in this figure legend, the reader is referred to the online version of this book.)

GENERAL NEURONAL NETWORK MECHANISMS OF STIMULATION THERAPIES

As discussed in this chapter, CNS neuronal networks are now strongly implicated both in mediating many CNS disorders and in the therapeutic effects of stimulation therapies. Several therapeutic stimulation modalities have been investigated with brain imaging techniques, such as fMRI, as detailed in this chapter. These imaging techniques have led to the identification of the neuronal networks that respond to these treatments.[1,16,75–77] However, it must be remembered that neuronal firing and fMRI changes do not always change in parallel (see Chapter 6). fMRI can identify brain areas that increase or decrease blood flow. However, imaging data do not yield information about the functional operation of the network, in part because of relatively poor temporal resolution and difficulties in differentiating inhibition from excitation. The reasons for this include the observation that active inhibition is also associated with increased blood flow, and excitation can also occur without detectable increases in fMRI signal.[78,79] Thus, after a changing activity pattern in a specific brain area is identified by these imaging techniques, it would be vital to study the change at the neuronal level in the identified area of the intact brain to determine the nature of firing changes in the millisecond range that occur during expression of the disorder, especially if the disorder is episodic (see Chapters 4 and 6). Neuronal recording research must be carried out in unanesthetized organisms, since anesthetics of various kinds, even in subanesthetic doses, significantly alter normal network function in sometimes unpredictable ways[80–86] (see Chapters 23, 28, and 32).

Stimulation-Induced Network Disruption versus Network Competition Mechanisms

One of the most important mechanisms in the therapeutic action of these stimulatory treatments is proposed to involve direct disruption of the function of the neuronal network that mediates the symptoms of the CNS disorder. A simplified view of this process is that it involves "short-circuiting" the network by placing a stimulating electrode directly in a nucleus that is an integral part of the network that mediates the CNS disorder. Direct disruption of the network can occur when a site within the network that mediates the CNS disorder is stimulated at high frequencies. This causes inhibition of network function and reduction or abolition of the symptoms, and it is the proposed mechanism for DBS in Parkinson's disease.[65] Thus, interference of network function by stimulating within the network, particularly by direct brain stimulation, is thought to be an important mechanism of therapeutic stimulation paradigms.

Another major mechanism for the therapeutic effects of stimulation therapies for CNS disorders may involve competition from a different CNS neuronal network, which is activated by the stimulus paradigm, as an emergent property of the CNS (see Chapter 30). The stimulus-activated "emergent" network competes with and diminishes the influence of the CNS disorder network. The stimulus-activated network is proposed to compete with the disease network for prominence within the CNS by "hijacking" those neuronal nuclei that are connected to both the disordered network and the stimulation-activated network.[87] This competition reduces the functional scope of the CNS disorder network and reduces or prevents expression of the symptoms of the disorder[87] (see Chapter 29). This mechanism of network competition may be most prominent in the noninvasive stimulation therapies, such as electroacupuncture, discussed in the "Noninvasive Stimulation Modalities" section. Finally, both network disruption and competition can be evoked by stimulus paradigms with implanted electrodes, such as VNS and DBS, as described in the "Invasive Stimulation Modalities" section. The competition between the disease network and the stimulated network is proposed to involve competition for control of brain regions that contain a high proportion of cells termed "CMR neurons". These sites include the BRF, periaqueductal gray, and amygdala, whose responses vary greatly depending on the behavioral state of the animal (see Chapter 28) (Figure 31.3). The brain regions that contain high proportions of CMR neurons (CMR structures) are postulated to be most recruitable into CNS disorder networks as well as into stimulation-activated networks. This recruitability is due to the fact that the CMR neurons receive relatively weak synaptic inputs from a wide variety of other neuronal networks, allowing them to potentially participate in these "newly" activated neuronal networks (i.e. the networks compete for an overlapping population of CMR neurons). A major mechanism for the recruitment of CMR neurons may be to cause subthreshold synaptic interactions to reach threshold more frequently (see Chapter 28). Neurons in these CMR regions exhibit a high degree of short-term and/or long-term plasticity, depending on the specific CMR site. Thus, network competition for these CMR regions may be a major network mechanism of stimulation therapies (see Chapter 29).

Several primary sensory and motor networks are described in Chapters 17, 19, and 20. Although these networks involve well-defined neuroanatomical pathways, they also send and receive secondary projections with the CMR regions (Chapters 19, 20, and 28). CMR neurons under normal conditions exhibit highly inconsistent and minimal responsiveness to the many inputs that impinge on them "subliminally" from these other neuronal networks. However, under certain conditions, including those that are associated with the development of a CNS disorder (e.g. chronic pain syndrome) or a repetitive stimulation paradigm, these normally subliminal inputs are capable of inducing a major degree of response plasticity in these CMR neurons (see Ref. 87 and Chapter 28). This can be seen with repetitive stimulation, as seen in various CMR sites, associated with LTP (see Chapter 27). Thus, CMR neurons that are minimally or not detectably responsive to a specific stimulus can undergo a major change in responsiveness under certain conditions[84,87,88] (Chapter 28). Another way in which changes in CMR neuronal responsiveness

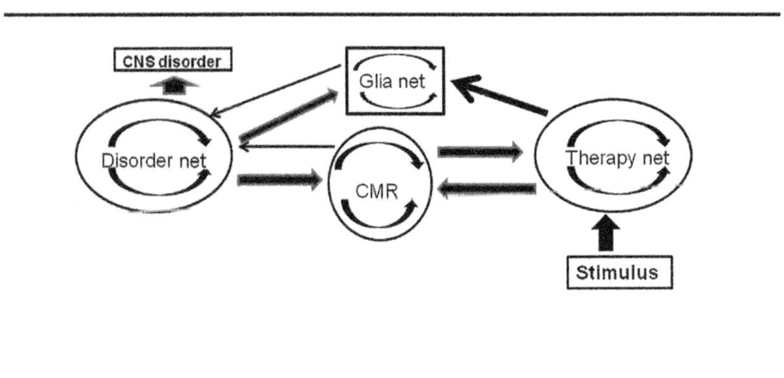

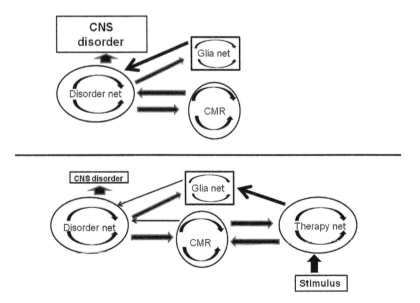

FIGURE 31.3 Theoretical diagram for the network competition mechanism between the network that mediates the CNS disorder (top panel) and the network that mediates the therapeutic effects that result from stimulation paradigms (bottom panel). In the top panel, the CNS disorder network is active and involves one or more conditional multireceptive (CMR) regions and possibly a glial (astrocytic) network. In the bottom panel, the therapeutic network (therapy net) is an emergent property of the brain that mediates the therapeutic effect of the stimulus paradigm (shown on the right). The therapy net exerts major interactive effects on CMR regions and competes with the disorder net for involvement of these neurons, which diminishes the influence of the disorder net and decreases or eliminates the symptoms of the disorder, either acutely or chronically. Either of the networks may interact with the glial network, and interactions of the therapy net with the glial net may also contribute to the effects of the therapy net.

can be demonstrated is with administration of a centrally active drug. The change can proceed in either a positive or negative direction. In the positive direction, the CMR neuron becomes extremely responsive to a stimulus after treatment with a drug that blocks inhibition; the drug is either applied directly onto the neuron or given systemically in an unanesthetized animal. Examples of the ability of CMR neurons in the BRF to undergo major short-term drug-induced neuroplastic changes in response to stimulation are shown in Figure 31.4. Thus, when a $GABA_A$ receptor antagonist is administered systemically to an animal, most BRF neurons undergo a major firing increase in response to the stimulation, as shown by the poststimulus time histograms (PSTHs). Under control conditions (Figure 31.4, left PSTH column) of repeated presentations of a brief peripheral nerve stimulus [Figure 31.4(B)] to a sensory nucleus (the inferior

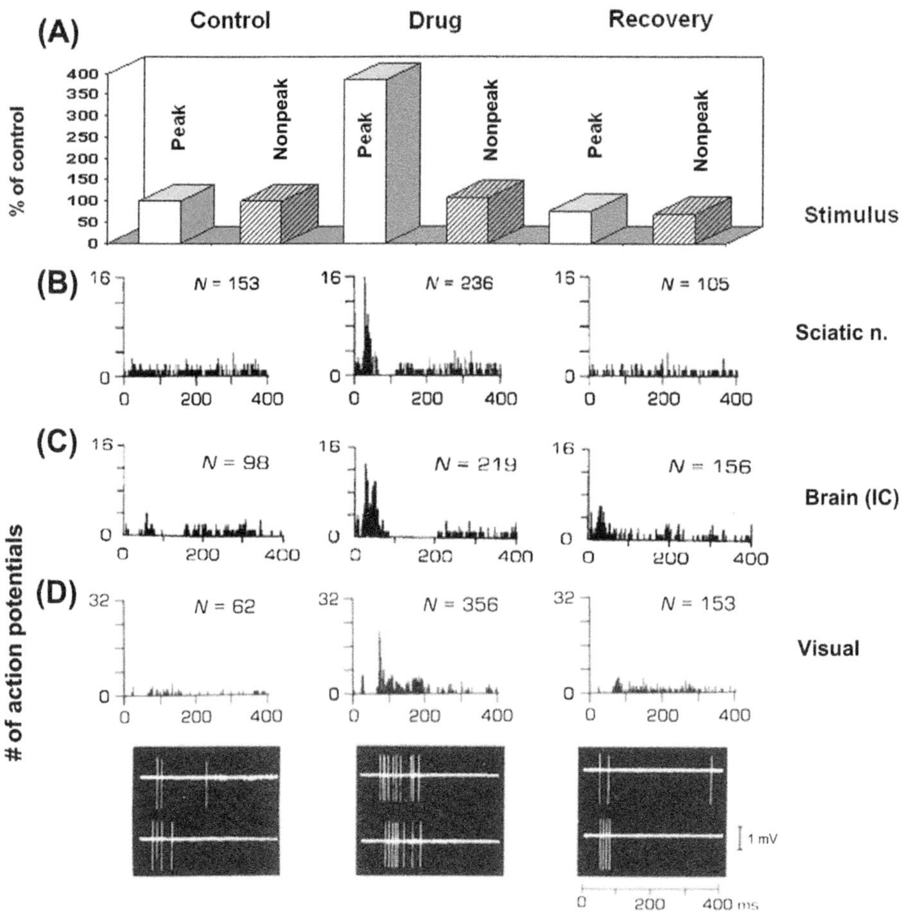

FIGURE 31.4 Changes in responsiveness of conditional multireceptive (CMR) neurons in the brainstem reticular formation to electrical or sensory stimulation after administration of a $GABA_A$ receptor antagonist (pentylenetetrazol in subconvulsant doses). Under control conditions [left column of poststimulus histograms (PSTHs)] of presentations of a brief external stimulus [electrical stimulus to a peripheral (sciatic) nerve (line (B)], to a brainstem sensory nucleus (inferior colliculus, or IC) [line (C)], or to a sensory (visual) stimulus [line (D)], very little evidence of responsiveness is detectable, as shown by the lack of a clear time-locked response peak to the stimulus in the PSTHs (left column). After administration of the $GABA_A$ receptor antagonist, these CMR neuronal responses exhibit major firing increases, which include the induction of a very striking time-locked peak of responsiveness to each stimulus in each PSTH (middle column of PSTHs). These peaks indicate that the drug had induced extensive responsiveness of the CMR neurons to these stimuli. The bar graphs in line (A) compare changes in the PSTH peak period and the rest of the recorded period for the PSTHs in line (B). The peak (the 20–55 ms period after stimulus onset) shows a much greater percentage increase as compared to the rest of the 400 ms sampling period, as shown by the bar graphs for the nonpeak versus peak time points shown above each bar. Note that the neuronal response example in line (D), which showed increased visual responsiveness, also showed major increases of firing in response to auditory stimuli (not shown), emphasizing the multimodality responsiveness of many BRF neurons. The neuroplastic effect is short term, since the firing patterns of these neurons recover to unresponsiveness with time (right column of PSTHs). Examples of raw data (oscilloscope tracings) are shown below each PSTH in line (D). Drug administration: pentylenetetrazol, 15 (B), 10 (C), and 5 (D) mg/kg, intravenously. Recovery times after drug administration: B = 20, C = 22, and D = 23 min. PSTH parameters: 0.5 Hz stimulus rate, 50 stimulus presentations (100 μs single bipolar pulse in (B) and (C), 18.5 lux visual stimulus (strobe) in (D), bin width = 1 ms, scan length = 400 ms). N = number of action potentials per PSTH. This effect was seen in 88% of over 700 bulbar and midbrain RF neurons in unanesthetized cat and rat by systemic or direct (iontophoretic) application of drug (see Refs 84,88).

colliculus, or IC) within the brain [Figure 31.4(C)] or to a sensory (visual) stimulus [Figure 31.4(D)], very little responsiveness is detectable, as illustrated by the lack of a clear time-locked peak in the PSTHs in control of each neuron. However, after administration of a $GABA_A$ receptor antagonist (bicuculline, bemegride, or pentylenetetrazol) in doses below those that induce seizures, these CMR neurons undergo major increases in responsiveness to stimulation and induction of a very striking peak in each PSTH (Figure 31.4, center PSTH column), indicating that these previously unresponsive neurons are now very responsive to the stimuli. The effect of the $GABA_A$ antagonists is concentrated on the response to the stimulus (PSTH peak), while the spontaneous firing (nonpeak period) was not greatly affected, as illustrated in Figure 31.4(A). This neuroplastic effect is short term, since the firing patterns of these neurons return to unresponsiveness over time (Figure 31.4, right PSTH column). Similar changes were observed in other CMR sites, including the pericruciate cortex and the amygdala, following subconvulsant doses of $GABA_A$ receptor antagonists.[88] Other brain sites with lower proportions of CMR neurons, such as primary sensory nuclei (the IC and lateral geniculate body), show only minor changes in responsiveness simultaneous with the major responsiveness changes in CMR-rich sites, such as the BRF (see Ref. 88 and Chapter 28). These $GABA_A$ receptor antagonists and newer related agents have recently been shown to enhance cognition in Down syndrome models.[89,90] It may be worthwhile to consider combining administration of these antagonists with the electrical stimulation paradigms to improve cognition in disorders such as Alzheimer's disease.

Drug effects on neurons in CMR-rich nuclei can also cause responsiveness changes in the negative direction in neurons that are initially responsive to stimuli. These CMR neurons readily lose responsiveness to the stimuli when a drug with depressant or anesthetic properties is administered[84,91] (see Chapter 28). Thus, lateral amygdala neurons can be clearly responsive to a sensory stimulus in an animal's normal (unanesthetized) state, but when a subanesthetic dose of a dissociative anesthetic (ketamine) is given, these neurons become unresponsive to the stimulus. This effect of the drug is short term, and the responsiveness of the amygdala neurons returns with time. The same type of effect on CMR neurons is also seen with depressant anesthetics such as barbiturates (Chapters 28 and 32).[84,86] However, when an external sensory stimulus is repetitively presented, CMR neurons in the amygdala and BRF will also show long-term positive neuroplastic changes in responsiveness.[91–93]

Likewise, the therapeutic effects that result from stimulation paradigms can be short term, long term, or both. Thus, some of the therapeutic stimulation protocols are acutely effective in terminating the symptoms of a CNS disorder that are impending or actively occurring. Examples of the acute effects of stimulation paradigms on the function of neuronal networks that mediate CNS disorders include the data that led to the first stimulus-induced network change that is embodied in the classical gate control theory of pain[50] (see Chapter 29). This theory posits that acute peripheral stimulation of the pathway for touch can compete with the simultaneously activated pain pathway at the level of the spinal cord and reduce the transmission of the painful stimuli up the pain perception pathways to the brain, thereby reducing the sensation of pain.[50] A more recent example of the use of acute stimulation is the use of acute stimulation paradigms to abort seizures. This approach involves a "closed-loop" or responsive stimulation that utilizes an implanted stimulation electrode and an electroencephalogram (EEG) detection circuit. When an epileptiform EEG pattern is detected, the circuit delivers a stimulus to the cortex, and this stimulus aborts the impending seizure.[94] Thus, an ongoing seizure or pain episode may be acutely terminated by an electrical stimulation therapy.

The mechanisms by which each of the stimulation approaches discussed in this chapter are proposed to exert their therapeutic effects include many of the same mechanisms that are known to control the function of neuronal networks (see Chapter 1). Potential mechanisms for the acute effects of stimulation techniques obviously include changes in network input by modifying the properties of local neurons (excitation with lower rates of stimulation and inhibition with higher rates of stimulation) induced by the stimulus itself. Other mechanisms include changes induced in the ionic environment of the neurons in the network, and alterations of the release of neuroactive substances by the affected network neurons and glia, as discussed in Chapters 7, 10, and 12.

As noted here, many of the therapeutic effects that result from stimulation paradigms can also have long-term benefits associated with chronic repetitive stimulation. Most of the therapeutic stimulation methods discussed here require repetitive applications to be effective. The competition between the CNS disorder network and the stimulation-activated network can effectively reduce the scope of the disorder network and result in blockade or diminution of the symptoms of the disorder being mediated by this network. As shown in the diagram in Figure 31.3, a competition between the network that mediates the CNS disorder (top panel) and the network that mediates the therapeutic effect that is induced by the stimulation paradigm is proposed to be a key event in the effectiveness of therapy in certain stimulation paradigms (bottom panel). In the top panel, the CNS disorder network is active and involves one or more CMR regions and possibly a glial (astrocytic) network. In the bottom panel, the therapeutic network (or therapy net) that mediates the therapeutic effect of the stimulus paradigm is shown on the right. The therapy net exerts major interactive effects on the CMR region(s) and competes with the disorder net for involvement of these neurons. This competition diminishes the influence of this network and decreases or eliminates the symptoms of the disorder, either acutely or chronically. Glial networks may interact with either or both of the networks, and the effects of the stimulus paradigm on these glial networks may also contribute to the therapeutic effects of the stimulus paradigm.

Thus, a chronic pain disorder or a chronic epileptic seizure disorder can be prevented by a repetitive stimulation paradigm, as discussed in this chapter for DBS, which can activate a network that competes with the disease network. The need for repetitive stimulation suggests that a cumulative effect is producing a persistent CNS change. Repetitive stimulus paradigms may involve more long-lasting processes that contribute to neuronal network activation and control (see Ref. 87) (Chapter 27). Thus, when the same stimulation protocol is presented continuously or repetitively, it may result in the persistent activation of a preexisting but largely dormant neuronal network, which is in accord with the "theory of conservation of networks".[87] This idea states that there are numerous dormant potential networks that are largely inactive under normal conditions. Stimulus repetition causes these dormant networks to become active on a regular basis, and these formerly dormant networks compete with the CNS disorder network for the CMR regions chronically as described here. Thus, repetitive stimulation of either normal or pathological networks can also cause brain areas that were not participating in the network prior to repetition to become actively involved in the function of the network[82,83,95–97] (see Chapter 27).

Mechanisms for the chronic effects of stimulation techniques include cellular input, the ionic, genetic, and neurotransmitter changes seen in acute stimulation paradigms. With chronic repetitive stimulation paradigms, long-term plasticity mechanisms are elicited. These changes are mediated, in part, by repetitive neuronal firing patterns, which give rise to increased synaptic strengths within the previously dormant therapeutic network. The mechanisms that mediate these changes include induction of burst firing (see Chapter 9), which releases large levels of neuroactive substances. These substances, acting via synaptic transmission and/or volume transmission from the stimulated network, can alter neuronal activity in the CNS disease network (see Chapters 7 and 8). These mechanisms can result in changes in synaptic strength because of mechanisms such as LTP. LTP can lead to longer term changes involving neurotrophic and genetic factors and other elements in the molecular cascade that underlie long-lasting neuronal changes. This can result in synaptic protein synthesis, ultimately yielding anatomical remodeling potentially involving neurogenesis[87,98–100] (see Chapters 7 and 27).

An important example is the release of neuroactive substances, which are proposed to play a major role in the action of the repetitive VNS paradigm. VNS has been shown to increase the firing of serotonin and norepinephrine neurons, induce monoamine receptor changes, and increase extracellular norepinephrine, serotonin, and dopamine levels selectively in specific brain areas.[101] Thus, the VNS stimulation paradigm, which is effective in both epilepsy and mood disorders,[42] may compete with one network and disrupt the other, and this may be accomplished by neurophysiological and/or neurochemical mechanisms.

As noted here, DBS is directed into a critical nucleus within the network that mediates the disorder and disrupts the network (as in Parkinson's disease), or into a site that provides direct inhibitory inputs to that network. However, when DBS is used to treat mood disorders or reduce the pain in Parkinson's disease, this stimulation paradigm may be acting by the network competition mechanism. Likewise, the activation and deactivation of brain sites seen in acupuncture fMRI studies (e.g. Figure 31.1) are evidence that the network affected by this therapeutic stimulation method, although different from that induced by painful stimuli, overlaps and likely competes with the pain network for certain brain areas.[16,102] Thus, some stimulation therapies may induce network disruption and/or network competition to produce the therapeutic effects, depending on the CNS disorder network that is being targeted.

Astrocytic Networks

The foregoing has emphasized the interaction of neuronal networks with each other, but it is also recognized that glial cells are also involved in network interactions. The interaction of neurons with glial cells is recognized as an important element in network control, based on the large number of synaptic contacts for each astrocyte (see Chapters 1 and 12). In addition, recent evidence suggests that networks of astrocytes exist, and the interaction of these networks with neuronal networks, involving glio-transmission, may be an important type of network interaction (see Chapter 12). Thus, astrocytes are also organized into networks, and interactions between astrocytes and neurons (as well as with capillaries) are important in the organization and function of the neuronal networks in the brain. Communication within the astrocyte network involves gap junction channels between astrocytes, which are regulated by extra- and intracellular signals, and these interactions may play an important role in information transfer.[103] These most highly networked astrocytes are proposed to play roles in normal brain function and also in CNS disorders. Recent evidence indicates that astrocytes in different brain regions have functionally different properties that reflect the role of the neurons in those regions. Thus, brainstem astrocytes are very responsive to conditions, such as pH changes, while cortical astrocytes are poorly responsive to the same changes but respond to other changes in conditions.[104] Extensive interactions between neuronal and glial networks are an important potential basis for the effects of stimulation therapies[103,105,106] and may represent another general mechanism of these important therapies.

CONCLUSION

The various therapeutic stimulation methods discussed in this chapter, ranging from noninvasive techniques such as acupuncture to electrodes chronically implanted into the brain, have been successfully utilized to treat a number of conditions, including chronic pain and Parkinson's disease. Many studies on the mechanisms behind the therapeutic effects of these stimulation therapies have shown a number of specific mechanisms, including inhibition or excitation of neurons or glia in specific brain regions. It has recently become clear that network-based mechanisms are very prominently involved in the therapeutic effects of these stimulation paradigms. General mechanisms of stimulation therapies include inhibition when a site in the network is stimulated directly. Another proposed mechanism is based on network competition for neuronal sites that overlap with the CNS disorder network and the network activated by the stimulation. The sites of overlap prominently include CMR regions of the brain, such as the BRF, periaqueductal gray, and amygdala. It is postulated that CMR regions had been recruited into the network that mediates the disorder and are recruited away into the therapeutic network by repetitive stimulation. Such a change in the extent of the disorder network leads to reduction or abolition of the symptoms of the CNS disorder. Stimulation therapies are also being used for rehabilitation in cases of brain damage such as stroke and traumatic brain injury as well as degenerative CNS disorders such as Alzheimer's disease. Recent data suggest the possibility of using $GABA_A$ receptor antagonists, which enhance neuronal responsiveness to various stimuli, in combination with electrical stimulation paradigms to improve cognition. The mechanisms in these cases may involve "rewiring" the damaged network or stimulating the formation of dormant networks to restore function by attempting to "wire around" the damaged brain area. Astrocytic networks can also be activated by stimulation paradigms, and this could lead to inhibition of the network that mediates the disorder and/or competition with this network. Future work on these mechanisms may aid in developing new types of less invasive stimulation therapies, such as TNS or disorder-specific acupoint electrical acupuncture paradigms. These approaches can potentially be utilized to treat many CNS disorders when the networks for these stimulation paradigms are sufficiently established. A novel stimulation approach has been recently suggested, involving the creation of "electroceuticals" to allow nanoscale stimulation to be accomplished via bioengineered molecules that can be incorporated into the body and electrically alter cellular function.[107] Network overlap between the stimulation network and the network mediating the CNS disorder may allow effective competition and provide therapeutic efficacy. If peripheral sites of stimulation can be identified that alter specific CMR brain sites, it may be possible to increase the utility of noninvasive stimulation paradigms as therapeutic modalities in the future. Thus, for example, the recently developed noninvasive TNS approach may potentially replace invasive modalities now being used for epilepsy and mood disorders. This may even be possible with specific acupuncture stimulation sites.

Acknowledgments

The authors gratefully acknowledge the comments of Professor Robert S. Fisher of Stanford University and the assistance of Gayle Stauffer and Diana Smith in preparing this manuscript.

References

1. Been G, Ngo TT, Miller SM, Fitzgerald PB. The use of tDCS and CVS as methods of non-invasive brain stimulation. *Brain Res Rev.* 2007;56(2):346–361.
2. Fanselow EE. Central mechanisms of cranial nerve stimulation for epilepsy. *Surg Neurol Int.* 2012;3(Suppl. 4):247–254.
3. Lee A, Done ML. Stimulation of the wrist acupuncture point P6 for preventing postoperative nausea and vomiting. *Cochrane Database Syst Rev.* 2004;3:CD003281.
4. Thompson A, Morishita T, Okun M. DBS and electrical neuro-network modulation to treat neurological disorders. *Int Rev Neurobiol.* 2012;107:253–282.
5. Huang W, Pach D, Napadow V, et al. Characterizing acupuncture stimuli using brain imaging with fMRI—a systematic review and meta-analysis of the literature. *PLoS One.* 2012;7(4):e32960. http://dx.doi.org/10.1371/journal.pone.0032960. Epub 2012 Apr 9.
6. Meng FG, Chris Kao C, Zhang H, et al. Using electroacupuncture at acupoints to predict the efficacy of hippocampal high-frequency electrical stimulation in pharmacoresistant temporal lobe epilepsy patients. *Med Hypotheses.* 2012; pii:S0306-9877(12)00520-00528.

7. Wang X, Liang XB, Li FQ, et al. Therapeutic strategies for Parkinson's disease: the ancient meets the future—traditional Chinese herbal medicine, electroacupuncture, gene therapy and stem cells. *Neurochem Res*. 2008;33(10):1956–1963.
8. Huang Y, Li TL, Lai XS, et al. Functional brain magnetic resonance imaging in healthy people receiving acupuncture at Waiguan versus Waiguan plus Yanglingquan points: a randomized controlled trial. *Zhong Xi Yi Jie He Xue Bao*. 2009;7(6):527–531.
9. Zhang R, Zou YQ, Huang SQ, et al. MRI cerebral function imaging following acupuncture at Hegu, Zusanli, Neiguan and Sanyinjiao points. *J Clin Rehabil Tissue Eng Res*. 2007;11: 4271–4274.
10. Campbell A. Point specificity of acupuncture in the light of recent clinical and imaging studies. *Acupunct Med*. 2006;24:118–122.
11. Dhond RP, Kettner N, Napadow V. Neuroimaging acupuncture effects in the human brain. *J Altern Complement Med*. 2007;13: 603–616.
12. Lewith GT, White PJ, Pariente J. Investigating acupuncture using brain imaging techniques: the current state of play. *Evid Based Complement Alternat Med*. 2005;2:315–319.
13. Fang J, Wang X, Liu H, et al. The limbic-prefrontal network modulated by electroacupuncture at CV4 and CV12. *Evid Based Complement Alternat Med*. 2012;2012:515893.
14. Shukla S, Torossian A, Duann JR, Leung A. The analgesic effect of electroacupuncture on acute thermal pain perception – a central neural correlate study with fMRI. *Mol Pain*. 2011;7:45.
15. Hui KK, Liu J, Marina O, et al. The integrated response of the human cerebro-cerebellar and limbic systems to acupuncture stimulation at ST 36 as evidenced by fMRI. *Neuroimage*. 2005; 27(3):479–496.
16. Hui KK, Marina O, Claunch JD, et al. Acupuncture mobilizes the brain's default mode and its anti-correlated network in healthy subjects. *Brain Res*. 2009;1287:84–103.
17. Liu B, Chen J, Wang J, et al. Altered small-world efficiency of brain functional networks in acupuncture at ST36: a functional MRI study. *PLoS One*. 2012;7(6):e39342.
18. Zhong C, Bai L, Dai R, et al. Modulatory effects of acupuncture on resting-state networks: a functional MRI study combining independent component analysis and multivariate Granger causality analysis. *J Magn Reson Imaging*. 2012;35(3):572–581.
19. Hayes DJ, Northoff G. Common brain activations for painful and non-painful aversive stimuli. *BMC Neurosci*. 2012;13:60.
20. Bai L, Tian J, Zhong C, et al. Acupuncture modulates temporal neural responses in wide brain networks: evidence from fMRI study. *Mol Pain*. 2010;6:73.
21. Cheng H, Zhang XT, Yan H, et al. Differential temporal neural responses of pain-related regions by acupuncture at acupoint ST36: a magnetoencephalography study. *Chin Med J (Engl)*. 2011;124(8):1229–1234.
22. Zyloney CE, Jensen K, Polich G, et al. Imaging the functional connectivity of the periaqueductal gray during genuine and sham electroacupuncture treatment. *Mol Pain*. 2010;6:80.
23. Joh TH, Park HJ, Kim SN, Lee H. Recent development of acupuncture on Parkinson's disease. *Neurol Res*. 2010;32(Suppl. 1):5–9.
24. Feng Y, Bai L, Ren Y, et al. fMRI connectivity analysis of acupuncture effects on the whole brain network in mild cognitive impairment patients. *Magn Reson Imaging*. 2012;30(5):672–682.
25. Lee EJ, Frazier SK. The efficacy of acupressure for symptom management: a systematic review. *J Pain Symptom Manage*. 2011;42(4):589–603.
26. Zhao ZQ. Neural mechanism underlying acupuncture analgesia. *Prog Neurobiol*. 2008;85(4):355–375. http://dx.doi.org/10.1016/j.pneurobio.2008.05.004. Epub 2008 Jun 5.
27. Li M, Looi A, Tjen SC, Guo ZL, Longhurst JC. Repetitive electroacupuncture causes prolonged increased met-enkephalin expression in the rVLM of conscious rats. *Auton Neurosci*. 2012; 170(1–2):30–35.
28. Moritaka J, Zeredo L, Kimoto M, Nasution H, Hirano T, Toda K. Response properties of nucleus reticularis lateralis neurons after electroacupuncture stimulation in rats. *Am J Chin Med*. 2010; 38(5):869–880.
29. Kennedy SH, Giacobbe P. Treatment resistant depression—advances in somatic therapies. *Ann Clin Psychiatry*. 2007;19(4):279–287.
30. Blumenfeld H, Westerveld M, Ostroff RB, et al. Selective frontal, parietal, and temporal networks in generalized seizures. *Neuroimage*. 2003;19(4):1556–1566.
31. Merkl A, Heuser I, Bajbouj M. Antidepressant electroconvulsive therapy: mechanism of action, recent advances and limitations. *Exp Neurol*. 2009;219(1):20–26.
32. Bolwig TG. How does electroconvulsive therapy work? Theories on its mechanism. *Can J Psychiatry*. 2011;56(1):13–18.
33. Sánchez González R, Alcoverro O, Pagerols J, Rojo JE. Electrophysiological mechanisms of action of electroconvulsive therapy. *Actas Esp Psiquiatr*. 2009;37(6):343–351.
34. Nakamura K, Ito M, Liu Y, Seki T, Suzuki T, Arai H. Effects of single and repeated electroconvulsive stimulation on hippocampal cell proliferation and spontaneous behaviors in the rat. *Brain Res*. 2013;1491:88–97.
35. Ongür D, Heckers S. A role for glia in the action of electroconvulsive therapy. *Harv Rev Psychiatry*. 2004;12(5):253–262.
36. Sadek AR, Knight GE, Burnstock G. Electroconvulsive therapy: a novel hypothesis for the involvement of purinergic signalling. *Purinergic Signal*. 2011;7(4):447–452.
37. van Calker D, Biber K. The role of glial adenosine receptors in neural resilience and the neurobiology of mood disorders. *Neurochem Res*. 2005;30(10):1205–1217.
38. Rosen AC, Ramkumar M, Nguyen T, Hoeft F. Noninvasive transcranial brain stimulation and pain. *Curr Pain Headache Rep*. 2009;13(1):12–17.
39. Nizard J, Lefaucheur JP, Helbert M, de Chauvigny E, Nguyen JP. Non-invasive stimulation therapies for the treatment of refractory pain. *Discov Med*. 2012;14(74):21–31.
40. Pascual-Leone A, Valls-Solé J, Wassermann EM, Hallett M. Responses to rapid-rate transcranial magnetic stimulation of the human motor cortex. *Brain*. 1994;117(Pt 4):847–858.
41. Lefaucheur JP, André-Obadia N, Poulet E, et al. French guidelines on the use of repetitive transcranial magnetic stimulation (rTMS). *Neurophysiol Clin*. 2011;41(5):221–295.
42. Fisher RS. Therapeutic devices for epilepsy. *Ann Neurol*. 2012; 71(2):157–168.
43. Harris-Love M. Transcranial magnetic stimulation for the prediction and enhancement of rehabilitation treatment effects. *J Neurol Phys Ther*. 2012;36(2):87–93.
44. Hoyer EH, Celnik PA. Understanding and enhancing motor recovery after stroke using transcranial magnetic stimulation. *Restor Neurol Neurosci*. 2011;29(6):395–409.
45. Bonnì S, Mastropasqua C, Bozzali M, Caltagirone C, Koch G. Theta burst stimulation improves visuo-spatial attention in a patient with traumatic brain injury. *Neurol Sci*. 2013 Nov;34(11):2053–2056.
46. Villamar MF, Santos Portilla A, Fregni F, Zafonte R. Noninvasive brain stimulation to modulate neuroplasticity in traumatic brain injury. *Neuromodulation*. 2012;15(4):326–338.
47. de Andrade DC, Mahalla A, Adam F, Texeira MJ, Bouhassira D. Neuropharmacological basis of rTMS-induced analgesia: the role of opioids. *Pain*. 2011;152:320–326.
48. Huerta PT, Volpe BT. Transcranial magnetic stimulation, synaptic plasticity and network oscillations. *J Neuroeng Rehabil*. 2009;6:7.
49. Witcher MR, Ellis TL. Astroglial networks and implications for therapeutic neuromodulation of epilepsy. *Front Comput Neurosci*. 2012;6:61.

50. Melzack R, Wall PD. Pain mechanisms: a new theory. *Science.* 1965;150:971–979.
51. McQuay HJ, Moore RA, Eccleston C, Morley S, Williams AC. Systematic review of outpatient services for chronic pain control. *Health Technol Assess.* 1997;1(6):i–iv, 1–135.
52. Bartsch T, Goadsby PJ. Central mechanisms of peripheral nerve stimulation in headache disorders. *Prog Neurol Surg.* 2011; 24:16–26.
53. DeGiorgio CM, Fanselow EE, Schrader LM, Cook IA. Trigeminal nerve stimulation: seminal animal and human studies for epilepsy and depression. *Neurosurg Clin N Am.* 2011;22(4):449–456.
54. Pop J, Murray D, Markovic D, DeGiorgio CM. Acute and long-term safety of external trigeminal nerve stimulation for drug-resistant epilepsy. *Epilepsy Behav.* 2011;22(3):574–576.
55. Schrader LM, Cook IA, Miller PR, Maremont ER, DeGiorgio CM. Trigeminal nerve stimulation in major depressive disorder: first proof of concept in an open pilot trial. *Epilepsy Behav.* 2011;22(3):475–478.
56. Brunoni AR, Ferrucci R, Fregni F, Boggio PS, Priori A. Transcranial direct current stimulation for the treatment of major depressive disorder: a summary of preclinical, clinical and translational findings. *Prog Neuropsychopharmacol Biol Psychiatry.* 2012;39(1):9–16.
57. Madhavan S, Shah BK. Enhancing motor skill learning with transcranial direct current stimulation – a concise review with applications to stroke. *Front Psychiatry.* 2012;3:66.
58. Henry TR. Therapeutic mechanisms of vagus nerve stimulation. *Neurology.* 2002;59(6 Suppl. 4):S3–S14.
59. Milby AH, Halpern CH, Baltuch GH. Vagus nerve stimulation for epilepsy and depression. *Neurotherapeutics.* 2008;5(1):75–85.
60. Chae JH, Nahas Z, Lomarev M, et al. A review of functional neuroimaging studies of vagus nerve stimulation (VNS). *J Psychiatr Res.* 2003;37(6):443–455.
61. Henry TR, Votaw JR, Pennell PB, et al. Acute blood flow changes and efficacy of vagus nerve stimulation in partial epilepsy. *Neurology.* 1999;52:1166–1173.
62. Giorgi FS, Pizzanelli C, Biagioni F, Murri L, Fornai F. The role of norepinephrine in epilepsy: from the bench to the bedside. *Neurosci Biobehav Rev.* 2004;28(5):507–524.
63. Kumaria A, Tolias CM. Is there a role for vagus nerve stimulation therapy as a treatment of traumatic brain injury? *Br J Neurosurg.* 2012;26(3):316–320.
64. Miocinovic S, Somayajula S, Chitnis S, Vitek JL. History, applications, and mechanisms of deep brain stimulation. *JAMA Neurol.* 2013;70(2):163–171.
65. Benabid AL, Wallace B, Mitrofanis J, et al. Therapeutic electrical stimulation of the central nervous system. *C R Biol.* 2005; 328(2):177–186.
66. Fridley J, Thomas JG, Navarro JC, Yoshor D. Brain stimulation for the treatment of epilepsy. *Neurosurg Focus.* 2012;32(3):E13.
67. Pereira EA, Green AL, Bradley KM, et al. Regional cerebral perfusion differences between periventricular grey, thalamic and dual target deep brain stimulation for chronic neuropathic pain. *Stereotact Funct Neurosurg.* 2007;85(4):175–183.
68. Theodore WH, Fisher R. Brain stimulation for epilepsy. *Acta Neurochir Suppl.* 2007;97(Pt 2):261–272.
69. Uc EY, Follett KA. Deep brain stimulation in movement disorders. *Semin Neurol.* 2007;27(2):170–182.
70. Kim HJ, Jeon BS, Paek SH. Effect of deep brain stimulation on pain in Parkinson disease. *J Neurol Sci.* 2011;310(1–2):251–255.
71. Lyons MK. Deep brain stimulation: current and future clinical applications. *Mayo Clin Proc.* 2011;86(7):662–672.
72. Lee KH, Hitti FL, Chang SY, et al. High frequency stimulation abolishes thalamic network oscillations: an electrophysiological and computational analysis. *J Neural Eng.* 2011;8(4):046001.
73. Gradinaru V, Mogri M, Thompson KR, Henderson JM, Deisseroth K. Optical deconstruction of parkinsonian neural circuitry. *Science.* 2009;324(5925):354–359.
74. Dorval C. 2013 with permission; http://brain.utah.edu/research/dorval/mechanisms-of-deep-brain-stimulation.php.
75. Dhond RP, Yeh C, Park K, Ketner N, Napadow V. Acupuncture modulates resting state connectivity in default and sensorimotor brain networks. *Pain.* 2008;136(3):407–418.
76. Enev M, McNally KA, Varghese G, Zubal IG, Ostroff RB, Blumenfeld H. Imaging onset and propagation of ECT-induced seizures. *Epilepsia.* 2007;48(2):238–244.
77. Nahas Z, Teneback C, Chae JH, et al. Serial vagus nerve stimulation functional MRI in treatment-resistant depression. *Neuropsychopharmacology.* 2007;32(8):1649–1660.
78. Buzsaki G, Kaila K, Raichle M. Inhibition and brain work. *Neuron.* 2007;56(5):771–783.
79. Schridde U, Khubchandani M, Motelow JE, Sanganahalali BG, Hyder F, Blumenfeld H. Negative BOLD with large increases in neuronal activity. *Cereb Cortex.* 2008;18(8):1814–1827.
80. Alkire MT, Miller J. General anesthesia and the neural correlates of consciousness. *Prog Brain Res.* 2005;150:229–244.
81. Destexhe A, Contreras D. Neuronal computations with stochastic network states. *Science.* 2006;314(5796):85–90.
82. Faingold CL. Neuronal networks in the genetically epilepsy-prone rat. In: Delgado-Escueta A, Olsen R, Wilson O, eds. *Jasper's Basic Mechanisms of the Epilepsies (Advances in Neurology).* Vol. 79. Philadelphia: Lippincott-Williams and Wilkins; 1999:311–321.
83. Faingold CL. Emergent properties of CNS neuronal networks as targets for pharmacology: application to anticonvulsant drug action. *Prog Neurobiol.* 2004;72(1):55–85.
84. Faingold CL, Caspary DM. Effect of convulsant drugs on the brainstem. In: Fromm GH, Faingold CL, Browning RA, Burnham WM, eds. *Epilepsy and the Reticular Formation: The Role of the Reticular Core in Convulsive Seizures.* New York, NY: AR Liss; 1987:39–80.
85. Maandag NJ, Coman D, Sanganahalli BG, et al. Energetics of neuronal signaling and fMRI activity. *Proc Natl Acad Sci USA.* 2007;104(51):20546–20551.
86. Samineni V, Premkumar L, Faingold CL. Changes in periaqueductal gray neuronal responses to pain induced by barbiturate administration. *Anesthesiology.* submitted for publication.
87. Faingold CL. Electrical stimulation therapies for CNS disorders and pain are mediated by competition between different neuronal networks in the brain. *Med Hypotheses.* 2008;71(5):668–681.
88. Faingold CL, Riaz A. Neuronal networks in convulsant drug-induced seizures. In: Faingold CL, Fromm GH, eds. *Drugs for Control of Epilepsy: Actions on Neuronal Networks Involved in Seizure Disorders.* Boca Raton, FL: CRC Press; 1992:213–251.
89. Colas D, Chuluun B, Warrier D, et al. Short-term treatment with the $GABA_A$ receptor antagonist pentylenetetrazole produces a sustained pro-cognitive benefit in a mouse model of Down's syndrome. *Br J Pharmacol.* 2013;169:963–973.
90. Möhler H. Cognitive enhancement by pharmacological and behavioral interventions: the murine Down syndrome model. *Biochem Pharmacol.* 2012;84(8):994–999.
91. Feng HJ, Faingold CL. Repeated generalized audiogenic seizures induce plastic changes on acoustically evoked neuronal firing in the amygdala. *Brain Res.* 2002;932(1–2):61–69.
92. Raisinghani M, Faingold CL. Pontine reticular formation neurons are implicated in the neuronal network for generalized clonic seizures which is intensified by audiogenic kindling. *Brain Res.* 2005;1064(1–2):90–97.
93. Raisinghani M, Faingold CL. Neurons in the amygdala play an important role in the neuronal network mediating a clonic form of audiogenic seizures both before and after audiogenic kindling. *Brain Res.* 2005;1032(1–2):131–140.

94. Morrell MJ. Responsive cortical stimulation for the treatment of medically intractable partial epilepsy. *Neurology.* 2011;77:1295–1304.
95. Garcia-Cairasco N. A critical review on the participation of inferior colliculus in acoustic-motor and acoustic-limbic networks involved in the expression of acute and kindled audiogenic seizures. *Hear Res.* 2002;168(1–2):208–222.
96. Kilgard MP, Pandya PK, Engineer ND, Moucha R. Cortical network reorganization guided by sensory input features. *Biol Cybern.* 2002;87(5–6):333–343.
97. Wu CW, van Gelderen P, Hanakawa T, Yaseen Z, Cohen LG. Enduring representational plasticity after somatosensory stimulation. *Neuroimage.* 2005;27(4):872–884.
98. Andrews RJ. Neuroprotection trek—the next generation: neuromodulation II. Applications—epilepsy, nerve regeneration, neurotrophins. *Ann N Y Acad Sci.* 2003;993:14–24.
99. Bruel-Jungerman E, Davis S, Laroche S. Brain plasticity mechanisms and memory: a party of four. *Neuroscientist.* 2007;13(5):492–505.
100. Kozisek ME, Middlemas D, Bylund DB. Brain-derived neurotrophic factor and its receptor tropomyosin-related kinase B in the mechanism of action of antidepressant therapies. *Pharmacol Ther.* 2008;117(1):30–51.
101. Manta S, El Mansari M, Debonnel G, Blier P. Electrophysiological and neurochemical effects of long-term vagus nerve stimulation on the rat monoaminergic systems. *Int J Neuropsychopharmacol.* 2013;16(2):459–470.
102. Wager TD, Atlas LY, Lindquist MA, Roy M, Woo MCW, Kross E. An fMRI-based neurologic signature of physical pain. *N Engl J Med.* 2013;368(15):1388–1397.
103. Giaume C, Koulakoff A, Roux L, Holcman D, Rouach N. Astroglial networks: a step further in neuroglial and gliovascular interactions. *Nat Rev Neurosci.* 2010;11(2):87–99.
104. Kasymov V, Larina O, Castaldo C, et al. Differential sensitivity of brainstem versus cortical astrocytes to changes in pH reveals functional regional specialization of astroglia. *J Neurosci.* 2013; 33(2):435–441.
105. Benarroch EE. Neuron-astrocyte interactions: partnership for normal function and disease in the central nervous system. *Mayo Clin Proc.* 2005;80(10):1326–1338.
106. Giaume C, Liu X. From a glial syncytium to a more restricted and specific glial networking. *J Physiol Paris.* 2012;106(1–2):34–39.
107. Famm K, Litt B, Tracey KJ, Boyden ES, Slaoui M. Drug discovery: a jump-start for electroceuticals. *Nature.* 2013;496(7444):159–161.

CHAPTER

32

Neuronal Network Effects of Drug Therapies for CNS Disorders

Carl L. Faingold

Departments of Pharmacology and Neurology, Division of Neurosurgery, Southern Illinois University School of Medicine, Springfield, IL, USA

INTRODUCTION

The first effective and relatively selective central nervous system (CNS) drugs were developed before the concept of neuronal networks of the brain originated. The effects of these CNS drugs on the nervous system have been investigated using the available techniques since the inception of modern pharmacology and neuroscience. However, a true understanding of important details about the mechanisms behind the effects in intact animals has been difficult to obtain, since the brain is subject to an immense degree of complexity, as discussed in Chapters 1, 28, and 30. Therefore, the early CNS drugs came into use largely by trial and error based on drugs purified from traditional, naturally occurring drug sources, such as morphine, caffeine, and reserpine. Once the molecular structure of these effective drugs was determined, new drugs were developed by chemically modifying the established drug molecules. This led to investigations of drug effects on what are now called macroscopic networks—in vivo animal models of CNS disorders. This eventually led to another network level of investigation—the microscopic—which was made possible once techniques were developed in which neurons could be kept viable outside the animal, for example in brain slice (ex vivo) and various types of in vitro preparations (Chapter 5). Thus, the mechanisms of action of CNS drugs that had been identified through macroscopic network investigations in whole animals were then evaluated at the microscopic network level. This paradigm became and remains the main method of determining the mechanisms of action of these CNS drugs—by applying them onto neurons in ex vivo or in vitro preparations and onto isolated receptor systems in vitro[1,2] (see Chapter 5). However, this approach has led to problems of interpretation and even concerns about the therapeutic relevance of the results. These concerns arose because the process of isolating neurons outside of the brain removes many of the important influences that determine how the cell functions in the intact brain (Figure 32.1) and, therefore, potentially alters the neuron's response to the *therapeutic dose* of a given CNS drug significantly.

The macroscopic network level of investigation in animal models was utilized by Merritt and Putnam during the discovery of the first relatively selective anticonvulsant drug, phenytoin.[3] This molecule was a modification of the barbiturate structure, an earlier group of effective anticonvulsants, which depressed consciousness as well as seizures.[3] Subsequently, it was found that barbiturates act to enhance the inhibitory action of an amino acid, gamma-aminobutyric acid (GABA), but phenytoin acts on a different molecular target—the sodium channel.[4] The approach that Merritt and Putnam[3] originally used to evaluate phenytoin involved testing this new drug in animals subjected to treatments (electroshock or convulsant drugs) that induce seizures. The animals could be induced to exhibit seizures that modeled those seen in human epilepsy (see Chapter 30), and new drugs could be tested on these models, which remains the primary method for new anticonvulsant drug screening today. These and many subsequent early studies of the effects of CNS drugs on the activity of the brain were conducted before the concept of neuronal networks was explicitly developed.

Neuronal Networks in Brain Function, CNS Disorders, and Therapeutics
http://dx.doi.org/10.1016/B978-0-12-415804-7.00032-0

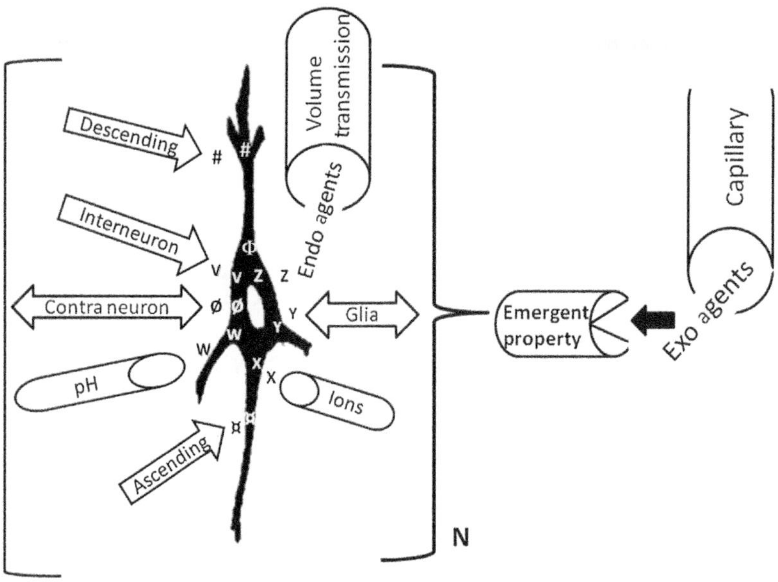

FIGURE 32.1 An idealized diagram of a principal neuron in a specific nucleus within a neuronal network in the brain of an awake, behaving organism; it illustrates many of the influences that affect this "class" of neurons (N) in this nucleus. The neurons possess certain specific intrinsic properties (Φ), such as the propensity to exhibit burst firing or pacemaker activity. These cells also possess specific receptors (#) (metabotropic or ionotropic) onto which descending projections release a specific neuroactive substance. The neurons also possess ligand-gated receptors (V) (e.g. glutamate) (which have specific receptor subunits) onto which interneurons synaptically release a specific neuroactive substance that binds. Projection neurons across the midline for bilaterally connected structures release a neuroactive substance ø, which binds to its specific receptors on contralateral neurons. The principal neurons also possess the property of pH sensitivity (W). Ascending input from neurons in nuclei in the network also release a neuroactive substance (¤) that binds to its specific receptors. The neurons possess voltage-gated ion channels (X) (e.g. K^+ channels) at which local ions can act. The neurons receive input from local glial cells, which release a neuroactive substance (Y) (e.g. adenosine) that acts on specific receptors for this substance. Endogenous (Endo) neuroactive agents (Z) carried via volume transmission from nearby (spillover) or distant sites via the extracellular fluid and cerebrospinal fluid to the neurons also affect the properties of these neurons. An example would be extrasynaptic $GABA_A$ receptors that respond to the low levels of "ambient" GABA in the extracellular fluid. Finally, when an exogenous (Exo) agent, such as a CNS drug, is administered, it is released via the brain blood vessels among other vectors to exert its effects on the emergent property of these principal cells to exert its therapeutic effect on a CNS disorder. Many CNS drugs are postulated to act selectively on a specific nucleus in the neuronal network for this disorder to produce the desired effect when therapeutic doses are given. The summation of all these influences determines whether the emergent property is expressed, the actual nature of that property, and its relative sensitivity in that group of neurons. This emergent property is postulated to be expressed uniquely in this network nucleus and causes this class of neurons to respond with unique sensitivity to a specific exogenous substance. Note that those influences can also be modified by brain state changes (such as sleep), which can significantly alter the emergent property, based on changes in the milieu of the principal neuron. (For color version of this figure, the reader is referred to the online version of this book.)

THE BRAINSTEM RETICULAR FORMATION AROUSAL NETWORK

Almost a dozen years after the pioneering work of Merritt and Putnam,[3] neuronal network theories began to develop when it was proposed that a specific part of the brain, the brainstem reticular formation (BRF), was the brain region responsible for maintaining consciousness. The BRF was proposed by Moruzzi and Magoun[5] (Chapters 21 and 22) to be selectively affected by depressant drugs, such as barbiturates. In recent years, this finding has often been ignored, despite the fact that those early depressant drug studies have been confirmed repeatedly and refined with more modern approaches (Chapters 23 and 28). Thus, many subsequent studies were conducted in animals that were treated with various anesthetic or analgesic drugs, a practice that continues to this day.[6] However, those studies were really unintentional evaluations of drug interactions between the anesthetic drug and the other agent being evaluated.

THE CENTRENCEPHALIC THEORY OF GENERALIZED EPILEPSY

Another early neuronal network theory, which was based on a similar understanding of the organization of the brain, was proposed for generalized epileptic seizures—the centrencephalic theory of Penfield and Jasper,[7] which has proven to be more controversial. The concept was that the BRF (and thalamus) and projections from them to the cortex were the key network elements for the initiation of generalized seizures throughout the brain, which was one of the earliest network attempts to explain CNS disorders. This idea provided an early network basis for evaluating drug effects on these CNS disorders, as discussed in detail in this chapter. Many early experimental studies were done on intact brains using the electroencephalogram (EEG) to evaluate the effects of the CNS drugs. Because the EEG is clinically relevant, this approach remains in use. However, the relationship between EEG activity and neuronal firing, which is the critical element in brain function, has never been established, since EEG changes reflect other, less important phenomena, such as volume conduction, and they lack the temporal and spatial resolution needed for evaluation of the operation of the network.[8]

CNS DRUG DOSAGE

Radioactive ligand binding studies are an important technique for determining the sites in the brain of binding for some CNS drugs. For example, binding studies with opiates were a major breakthrough by Avram Goldstein and coworkers[9] in establishing that CNS drugs were interacting with receptors on brain neurons in specific brain nuclei. However, receptor binding is nearly always done using saturating concentrations, rather than therapeutic concentrations, to allow adequate visualization, and this method has spatial resolution limitations. However, drug binding in specific areas of the brain is not necessarily an indicator that this area is critical for drug action, especially of therapeutic doses. Evaluating drug effects in demonstrably therapeutic doses simultaneous with the evaluation of neuronal effects is critically important, because when CNS drugs are used in patients, the ideal aim is to exert an action on the CNS disorder by selectively affecting only those neurons that mediate the disorder. Higher drug doses cause side effects, such as sedation in many cases, but sedation is often not the desired therapeutic effect, for example, for anticonvulsant drugs in which it is an undesirable side effect. These two effects are separable, since tolerance to the sedative effect of anticonvulsants occurs, while the anticonvulsant effect remains with many of the newer drugs. As noted here, dosage is also a major concern in ex vivo and in vitro studies, since the concentrations needed to observe effects are generally much higher than the therapeutic levels that are achieved when the drug is given to the intact organism to treat a CNS disorder. Therefore, the relevance of the results with these high drug levels may be toxicological at best.

MESOSCOPIC NETWORKS AND CNS DRUGS

These issues have emphasized the importance of investigating networks at the mesoscopic- or middle-level network in vivo as the critical nexus for understanding brain function[10] (see Chapter 1). These middle-level networks, which operate normally only in the intact and unanesthetized animal, can be investigated using techniques that include neuronal recording in awake, behaving animals (Chapter 4). The results from this approach will be the main topic of this chapter. In addition, many studies of drug action are being done in humans using in vivo imaging (Chapter 6) with therapeutic drug levels, and these studies are also discussed in this chapter.

THE BRAIN YOU ANESTHETIZE MAY BE YOUR OWN

The critical importance of avoiding anesthesia when evaluating neuronal-firing changes in mesoscopic networks is due to the fact that even minimal doses of these agents potentially exert important actions on the network (see Chapter 28), which can distort network function in unpredictable ways, as discussed in detail here. These findings have led to the aphorism "The brain you anesthetize may be your own". However, investigations of drug effects on neuronal firing in intact brain networks at the mesoscopic network level, especially in unanesthetized, awake, behaving animals, have lagged behind, in part, because the techniques are less efficient and more time consuming than those of studies at the other levels or in anesthetized animals (Chapter 4). In the end, the reason why mesoscopic network research in awake, behaving animals is needed is because of a basic pharmacological fact—therapeutic doses of the drug being investigated can only be assured when it is demonstrably producing the desired effect and not toxic effects. Thus, study of the ability of an anticonvulsant drug to block seizures at a dose that is not inducing behavioral toxicity, such as ataxia (a common adverse effect of these agents), is vital, because the adverse effect may be due to actions on brain sites that may be different from the site of the anticonvulsant action. This concept is important because the action of the minimally effective dose of a specific drug may be selective for the neurons in one network nucleus, but at higher doses the same drug may also affect neurons in other nuclei. We have demonstrated that this is indeed true for at least one well-established epilepsy network, as discussed here.

As mentioned here, when CNS drugs are evaluated in intact animals, toxicity is also evaluated. So, for the example of anticonvulsant drug screening (macroscopic network effects), the dose of the drug that affects the ability of the animal to cling to a rotating rod estimates the motor impairment dose, which is compared to the anticonvulsant dose to give the therapeutic index, a measure of drug safety.[11] This method remains in use currently, and all potential new drugs for epilepsy are subjected to these macroscopic-level techniques.[12] However, the actual mechanisms and sites of action of these drugs cannot be determined using these macroscopic approaches. This, in turn, has led to a new paradigm, which supplements the older approaches and assures that the effects of therapeutic doses are being evaluated. That is, the drug is administered to animals in vivo in doses that produce the desired therapeutic effect, and changes in neuronal firing in network nuclei are evaluated concurrently (see Chapter 4). As neuronal networks that mediate CNS disorders were being investigated (see Chapters 21–25), the effects of therapeutic levels of the drugs on neurons in these networks could begin to be evaluated. In the cases where this has been done, new insights on how the drugs actually exert their therapeutic effects and where in the network for the CNS disorder they are acting have been observed, which is discussed in detail in the "Drug Effects on Network Emergent Properties" section. Computational analysis of neuronal networks has provided evidence that certain brain nuclei within a network that have a large number of connections and are critical for the function of these brain networks are acting as network "hubs"[13] (see Chapter 1). Experimental evidence indicates that a number of drugs with anticonvulsant effects may alter the function of seizure networks by selectively acting on neurons in specific network hubs. This selectivity is due to emergent properties that are conferred on these neurons by the multitude of influences that these cells are subject to in the intact, unanesthetized animal, as discussed in detail in this chapter.

DRUG EFFECTS ON NETWORK EMERGENT PROPERTIES

Many of these network influences are shown in Figure 32.1, which is an idealized diagram of a principal neuron in a specific nucleus within a neuronal network in the brain of an awake, behaving organism. The diagram illustrates many of the influences that affect this class of principal neurons (N) in this nucleus. These neurons possess certain specific intrinsic properties, such as pacemaker activity, and specific receptors that respond to specific neuroactive substances released by ascending and descending projections. Local interneurons, glia, and projection neurons from the contralateral homonymous nucleus also release neuroactive substances onto these cells. The principal neurons also express pH sensitivity and voltage-gated ion channels at which local ions act. Endogenous (Endo) neuroactive agents are carried via volume transmission from nearby or distant sites via the capillaries, extracellular fluid, and cerebrospinal fluid, and these agents also affect the properties of the principal neurons. The summation of all these influences determines whether the emergent property is expressed, the actual nature of that property, and its relative sensitivity to drug effects. Those influences can also be modified by brain state changes, including those that occur during sleep, which can significantly alter emergent properties based on changes in the milieu of the principal neurons (see Chapter 10). Finally, when an exogenous (Exo) neuroactive agent, such as a CNS drug, is administered, it is carried in the cerebral capillaries and is transferred via volume transmission (see Chapter 8) to act on a specific emergent property of these principal cells (see Chapter 30) to exert its therapeutic effect on the CNS disorder. Thus, many CNS drugs are postulated to act selectively on a specific nucleus in the neuronal network for this disorder to produce the desired effect when therapeutic doses are given. This emergent property is postulated to be expressed uniquely in this network nucleus and causes this class of neurons to respond with unique sensitivity to the lowest effective doses of a specific exogenous substance, including CNS drugs.

A major factor that requires consideration of this complexity (illustrated in Figure 32.1) is the fact that the results of in vitro and in vivo studies on the same drug do not always agree. We have proposed that this occurs because most of the network influences mentioned in Chapter 1, as illustrated in Figure 32.1 and discussed in this chapter and Chapters 7–12, are absent or greatly modified in in vitro preparations. Thus, the confluence of these influences gives rise to emergent properties of those neurons that are conferred by the network, such as increases in receptor sensitivity. This property renders neurons in a particular nucleus of the network as a specific site for the therapeutic action of a drug, but the property may be lost or modified when the neuron is removed from the network, as discussed further in this chapter.

SELECTIVE EFFECTS OF CNS DRUGS: THERAPEUTIC DOSES

It has long been known that certain parts of the brain are relatively selectively affected by CNS drugs. This selectivity, although potentially very important, may be only relative, since doses above the therapeutic range may also be useful for a different therapeutic use. Thus, ketamine in low doses has a selective effect on amygdala neurons,[14,15] and low doses are also used experimentally for relieving depression.[16,17] However, the main use of ketamine is for its anesthetic effect, and this effect requires considerably higher doses and is likely to be less selective. Likewise, for barbiturates relatively low oral doses are used for epilepsy, but relatively higher intravenous (i.v.) doses of ultra-short-acting thiobarbiturates are needed for anesthesia induction, and the highest doses of these agents are toxic, inducing death due to respiratory depression. Similarly, certain benzodiazepines in low doses are useful in treating anxiety disorders, but in higher doses similar agents are used to induce anesthesia or block the repetitive seizures of status epilepticus (see Chapter 26). So a relatively selective effect on specific sites may occur with therapeutic doses of these drugs, but in higher doses the sites that are affected may include additional brain loci and additional mechanisms when the drug induces anesthesia. For example, both enhancement of the inhibitory action of GABA and inhibition of the excitatory action of glutamate are observed with barbiturates.[18] Thus, many earlier in vitro studies of ethanol commonly employed levels that would be toxic to an intact animal (see Ref. 19 for a review). Experiments examining low "cocktail" levels of ethanol in vitro have yielded highly controversial results.[20,21]

Depressant drugs, such as barbiturates, in low doses may affect specific network sites that control epilepsy. However, higher doses will severely depress the CNS and anesthetize the organism, affecting more of the brain's neurons and eventually leading to death in vivo, but this will not occur in vitro unless extremely large toxic amounts are administered. This may be due to the fact that the networks responsible for toxicity and death from these agents, such as the respiratory network (Chapter 18), are not present in vitro, and the function of this absent network is compensated for by supplying high levels of oxygen to the solution bathing the neurons (Chapters 5 and 10). Drugs administered to patients are given systemically, and, if the drug produces the desired effect with little or no side effects, then a priori these doses are therapeutic. It also needs to be kept in mind when comparing doses in vivo with concentrations in vitro that the amount needed to induce an effect in vivo is often considerably lower than that required to achieve an effect in vitro.[22] Finally, another dose issue is how to reconcile doses in animals with those in humans. Although we often use the mg/kg dose, it has been demonstrated that this is not appropriate, since body surface rather than weight is a better determinant of dose consistency; a relative dose ratio between many lab animals and humans has been established.[23]

DRUG EFFECTS ON RHYTHMIC OSCILLATIONS OF THE BRAIN

Networks have been mapped based on a common rhythmic frequency of oscillation of different brain regions, as determined by the EEG and magnetoencephalogram (MEG), which are proposed to synchronize the activity of brain structures to perform cognitive or other functions.[24] Changes in cortical rhythms on EEG have been classified into states of activity. Thus, a macroscopic emergent property characterized by slow rhythmic oscillations of spontaneous activity, involved in the alternating "DOWN" states of generalized neuronal silence and "UP" states of enhanced neuronal excitability, is seen in several brain structures in vivo and in vitro[25] (see Chapters 6, 21, and 30). These state changes are seen during the sleep–waking cycle in unanesthetized animals, but only during non–rapid eye movement (NREM) sleep.[25–28] The rhythmic oscillation of these states is disrupted during episodes of spontaneous cortical desynchronization, which is associated with waking, or by desynchronization induced by stimulation of the BRF.[27] These states are more commonly induced by drug treatment. Thus, UP states and DOWN states in animals and humans can be induced pharmacologically by endogenous neuroactive agents, such as dopamine; general anesthetics, such as urethane; and convulsant drugs, such as picrotoxin, as well as ethanol and hallucinogens.[26,29–32]

PHARMACOLOGICAL MAGNETIC RESONANCE IMAGING STUDIES

As discussed in Chapters 3 and 6, functional magnetic resonance imaging (fMRI) is a well-established technique for studying normal brain networks and network changes in CNS disorders. A very active and important approach to the evaluation of drug effects on neuronal networks related to CNS disorders is using brain imaging (usually fMRI) to study human CNS disorders and examine the changes in these networks induced by drugs that are effective treatments for those disorders—called pharmacological fMRI (phMRI).[33] The importance and usefulness of this approach are considerable, and it has the potential for greatly advancing the understanding and improvement of drug treatment for CNS disorders, as discussed in this chapter. Thus, a wide variety of drug effects on CNS disorder networks has been studied, including networks for neurological disorders, such as epilepsy and chronic pain networks; for psychiatric disorders, such as depressive, bipolar, psychotic, and anxiety disorders;[34–36] and for cognitive disorders, such as Alzheimer disease.[37–39]

However, a number of issues and concerns have arisen about this approach that indicate that the findings of fMRI and phMRI studies need to be confirmed and extended using additional techniques to understand the nature of neuronal events and mechanisms of drug action on the brain. These issues include the use of anesthetics, especially in animal studies, which exert network effects of their own, as discussed here. Intersubject variability of fMRI changes and loss of sensitivity when using group data have raised concerns about the reliability and sensitivity of phMRI.[33] In psychiatric studies, there are concerns about the effects of magnetic stimulation on brain activity during the magnetic resonance imaging (MRI), which have been documented to exert psychometric effects.[40] Other concerns regarding phMRI data include the prolonged, relatively intense acoustic stimulation generated by the MRI device, since neurons in several of the brain regions that have been implicated in important networks, including the amygdala and periaqueductal gray (PAG), are quite responsive to auditory stimuli.[14,41] The most important concern about exploring neuronal networks with fMRI is the fact that decoupling has been observed between electrophysiological events and imaging results from the same brain area[42–44] (see Chapter 6). Certain areas of the brain that are extensively involved in drug effects, including the BRF (discussed extensively in this chapter), are among the areas where results of imaging studies and neuronal firing have been found to disagree (Chapter 6).

DRUG EFFECTS ON INTACT NEURONAL NETWORKS

A direct and critically important method of evaluating the effects of CNS drugs on network activity is neuronal recording in network nuclei in vivo in unanesthetized animals. This method gives a direct readout of what the network neurons are doing as drugs are administered in doses that are in the therapeutic range and below toxic levels, often recording EEG simultaneously.

STIMULANT DRUG EFFECTS ON NEURONAL NETWORK NEURONS

As noted in the introduction of this chapter, the early network theory of seizures of Penfield and Jasper[7] led a number of investigators to examine the role of the BRF in generalized seizures.[45] The studies in the latter volume included examinations of the effects on the BRF of drugs that prevent or induce seizures. Earlier studies employed acutely implanted glass electrodes with micrometer tips in awake but pharmacologically immobilized animals.[46] The drugs with convulsant properties were administered either systemically (i.v.) or directly onto the neurons, using iontophoretic or pneumatic application. As discussed in Chapter 28, these drugs include agents that can induce generalized seizures and act by blocking endogenous inhibitory neuroactive substances, such as GABA, or by enhancing the availability of endogenous excitatory neuroactive substances, such as acetylcholine. These convulsant drugs exert major effects on neuronal networks, particularly in those brain regions that contain high proportions of conditional multireceptive (CMR) neurons, especially the BRF (see Chapter 28). The effects are induced by acute administration and produce short-term neuroplastic changes in neuronal firing at doses that are in most cases considerably below those that would produce seizures. The effects of subconvulsant doses of these convulsant drugs were examined in two regions of the BRF (medulla and midbrain) and six other brain regions: four other CMR regions (the amygdala, substantia nigra, hippocampus, and pericruciate cortex) as well as two primary sensory regions (the lateral geniculate and inferior colliculus).[47] The neuronal responses in the CMR regions greatly increased, while the primary sensory neurons were minimally affected simultaneously with BRF neurons (see Chapter 28).

$GABA_A$ receptor antagonists (pentylenetetrazol, bemegride, and bicuculline) all produced the same major effects on neurons in the BRF (midbrain) and amygdala, often observed simultaneously (Figure 32.2). Simultaneous enhancement of the responses to auditory stimuli of CMR neurons in the amygdala and BRF was induced by administration (i.v.) of convulsant. Examples of the comparative effects on amygdala and BRF neurons are shown by the poststimulus time histograms (PSTHs) in Figure 32.2. Prior to drug administration, the BRF neuron was responsive to the auditory stimulus, as shown by the consistent time-locked response (peak in the PSTH), while the amygdala neuron was not clearly responsive [left columns in Figure 32.2(C) vs. (B), respectively]. After administration of a subconvulsant dose of bemegride, the amygdala neuron became very responsive to the stimulus as indicated by the peak in the PSTH, and the BRF neurons became considerably more responsive. Enhanced sensory responsiveness was also induced in neurons in both sites simultaneously by convulsant drugs that act by enhancing the action of acetylcholine [Figure 32.2(D)] or blocking inhibitory glycine receptors. These plastic changes were short term, and the response patterns of these neurons returned toward the predrug pattern 10–30 min after termination of drug administration.[48] The mean increases of firing from control (predrug) levels were comparable in BRF (>350%) and amygdala (>275%) neurons (Figure 32.2). Increases greater than 10% were seen in 57% of amygdala neurons and 85% of BRF neurons in this experimental series.

STIMULANT DRUG EFFECTS AND COGNITION

Recent reports indicate that agents that reduce $GABA_A$ receptor-mediated inhibition, including pentylenetetrazol, improve cognition in a cognitive disorder model in animals,[49,50] and the enhancement of CMR

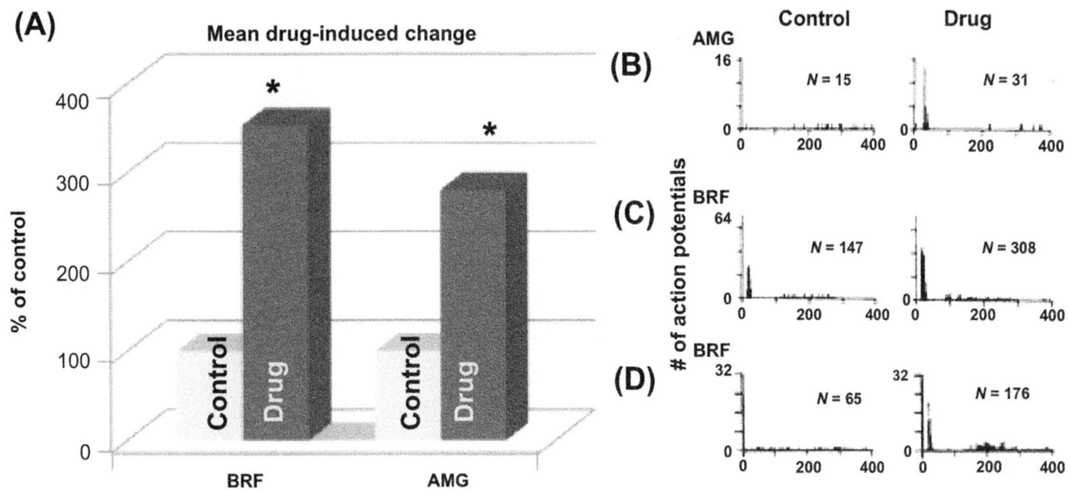

FIGURE 32.2 Effects of convulsant drugs on the responsiveness of neurons in the brainstem reticular formation (BRF) as compared to the amygdala (AMG). The bar graphs in panel (A) show the mean response increase as a percentage of control (predrug) for each brain site for all drugs tested, which was >350% in BRF neurons ($n = 72$ neurons) and >275% in AMG neurons ($n = 65$) in this series of studies. Examples of the comparative effect on neuronal response is the induction of responsiveness in CMR neurons in both brain regions simultaneously by the $GABA_A$ antagonist bemegride on the responses to auditory stimuli of amygdala and brainstem (mesencephalic) reticular formation (BRF) neurons. An example of the comparative effect on amygdala neurons is shown by the poststimulus time histograms (PSTHs) in line (B), while the simultaneously recorded BRF neuron is shown by the PSTHs in line (C). Another BRF neuronal response is shown in (D). The left columns in lines (B), (C), and (D) illustrate the responses of the neurons to the acoustic stimulus in control (prior to drug administration). The BRF in the line (C) neuron was responsive, as shown by the consistent time-locked response (peak in the PSTH), while the amygdala neuron in line (B) and the BRF neuron in line (D) were not clearly responsive. Following administration of bemegride (3.6 mg/kg, i.v.; right column), the amygdala neuron (B) became very responsive to the stimulus, indicated by the peak in the PSTH, and the BRF (C) neuron became considerably more responsive simultaneously. The BRF neuron in line (D) showed the induction of responsiveness after physostigmine (12.5 mg/kg). Increases greater than 10% were seen in 57% of amygdala neurons and 85% of BRF neurons in the same experimental series. Stimuli: 95 dB SPL re 0.002 dyne/cm^2, 0.1 ms clicks with onset at 0 time on each PSTH; PSTH parameters: 50 stimulus presentations, 1 ms bin width, 0.5 Hz rate. Data obtained from unanesthetized cat with glass microelectrodes. N is the total number of action potentials in each PSTH. (*Source: Modified from Faingold et al.,*[48] *with permission.*) (For color version of this figure, the reader is referred to the online version of this book.)

neuronal responsiveness, as discussed in this chapter, could contribute importantly to this effect. In fact, given the finding that aging which results in diminished activation of the primary cortex but which simultaneously increases the activation of CMR areas of the cortex,[51] administration of these stimulant drugs may have potential use for memory improvement in aging. Since responses of neurons in CMR areas of the cortex are also enhanced by $GABA_A$ receptor blockers,[52] the agents that reduce $GABA_A$ receptor-mediated inhibition and enhance CMR responsiveness could potentially improve cognition in normal aging and in disorders of cognition, such as Alzheimer disease. Subconvulsant doses of a cholinesterase inhibitor, physostigmine, also enhance the responses of BRF and amygdala neurons[48] [Figure 32.2(D)]. Physostigmine is the prototype of a centrally acting cholinesterase inhibitor and acts by the same mechanism of most of the drugs that are approved for therapy of Alzheimer disease.[53] The ability to enhance neuronal responsiveness may potentially contribute to the cognitive improvements observed with cholinesterase inhibitors in patients. A recent phMRI study of cholinesterase inhibitor effects in Alzheimer disease patients undergoing an auditory-based memory task showed that suppression of auditory cortical responses was related to success in encoding heard sentences, which is deficient in Alzheimer patients. A centrally active cholinesterase inhibitor (donepezil) partially restored the auditory function in these patients, which was associated with improved memory.[54] Another cholinesterase inhibitor (rivastigmine) was evaluated in Alzheimer disease patients using phMRI, and it showed memory improvements and activation of the prefrontal attention and working memory systems in treated patients as compared to placebo-treated patients.[39]

In animal studies, the response enhancement induced by $GABA_A$ antagonists in BRF neurons could be reversed by drugs that enhance the activation of $GABA_A$ receptors, including iontophoretic application of GABA itself or systemic administration of a benzodiazepine or a barbiturate.[46,55] An example of this is shown in Figure 32.3, which illustrates the effect of systemic administration of an ultra-short-acting barbiturate (thiopental) on the continuing effect of the $GABA_A$ antagonist.[16,47] Thus, the pentylenetetrazol-induced response enhancement in a CMR neuron in the BRF [Figure 32.3(A) and (D)] was temporarily reversed by administration of this ultra-short-acting barbiturate

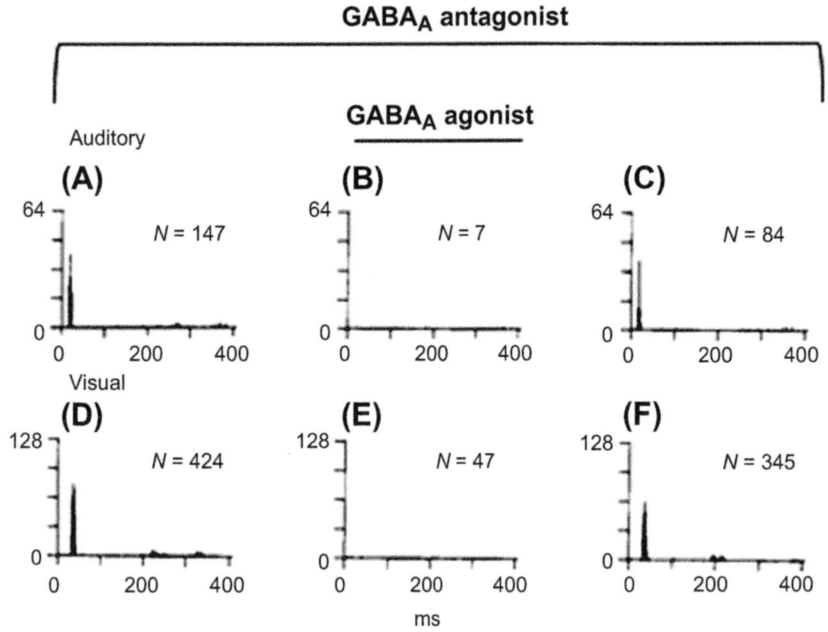

FIGURE 32.3 An example of the effects of a short-acting barbiturate (thiopental) that acts to enhance $GABA_A$ receptor activation on enhanced BRF neuronal response to sensory stimuli induced by the $GABA_A$ antagonist pentylenetetrazol (PTZ). Before thiopental injection, administration of PTZ had induced extensive responsiveness to auditory and visual stimuli (A and D) in this neuron. After thiopental (5 mg/kg, i.v.), the neuron became unresponsive to both stimuli (B and E) despite continued infusion of PTZ at a rate that would normally maintain response enhancement. Responsiveness to both stimuli returned to the enhanced state 26 min after barbiturate administration (C and F). PSTH parameters: 50 stimulus presentations, 1 ms bin width, 0.5 Hz rate. Data obtained from unanesthetized cat with glass microelectrodes. *N* is the total number of action potentials in each PSTH. (*Source: Modified from Faingold and Caspary.*[46])

[Figure 32.3(B) and (E)]. However, with continuing administration of the $GABA_A$ antagonist, the enhancement returned [Figure 32.3(C) and (F)]. This block of response enhancement was also observed with benzodiazepines, which enhance the action of GABA allosterically.[46,47]

DEPRESSANT AND ANESTHETIC DRUG EFFECTS ON NEURONAL NETWORKS

Anesthetic drugs and other central depressant agents, such as the barbiturates, which reverse the effects of the convulsant drugs, depress consciousness. The mechanism of action of many of these agents, including barbiturates, as determined in ex vivo and in vitro studies, involves enhanced activation of $GABA_A$ receptors, as discussed in Chapter 28. However, differences were observed in the behavioral effects of two related CNS depressant agents used in anesthesia, propofol and midazolam, which both enhance $GABA_A$-mediated inhibitory postsynaptic potentials. These differences are proposed to be due to differential actions on network function, which can be assessed only in the intact brain.[56] These agents depress consciousness by acting on the macroscopic level of emergent properties of the neuronal networks underlying consciousness.[56–58] The BRF, which is critically involved in generalized seizures, also plays a critical role in the neuronal network that mediates consciousness. As discussed here, the BRF has long been proposed to be a critical site for the action of depressant drug–induced loss of consciousness (also see Chapters 21 and 22). Thus, the BRF is the site within the brain that is proposed to be most sensitive to the effects of these drugs, including the barbiturates. Most BRF neurons are highly sensitive to low doses of barbiturates and several other drugs used for general anesthesia.[46,59,60] BRF (medullary) neuronal postsynaptic potentials in vitro are also very sensitive to superfusion with barbiturates and other anesthetics.[61] Iontophoretic application of pentobarbital at low currents depressed the spontaneous activity of >80% of the BRF neurons tested, while excitation was not seen.[62] Likewise, when a barbiturate was focally microinjected into a specific area of the midbrain BRF, but not in many other nearby sites, very low doses of the agent selectively produced reversible analgesia, atonia, and loss of consciousness[63] (see Chapter 23). Taken together, these findings are highly supportive of the early hypothesis that the BRF is a critical brain site in the neuronal network that maintains consciousness (see Chapters 21 and 22). The depressant effects of anesthetics are not limited to the BRF, and neurons in other CMR regions, including the PAG (see Chapter 28) and the amygdala, are also quite sensitive to the effects of these agents. The effects of these agents and other types of anesthetic drugs have been evaluated in awake and behaving animals. This involved a more physiological but more technically difficult method of evaluating the effects of CNS drugs on network activity: neuronal recording with chronically implanted electrodes in network nuclei in vivo (Chapter 4). Thus, in chronically implanted awake, behaving rats, most PAG (ventrolateral) neurons respond to nociceptive stimuli, and over 50% of these responses are excitatory (see Chapter 28). However, when a low dose of pentobarbital is administered systemically, the spontaneous firing and nociceptive responses of these PAG neurons is greatly reduced[64] (see Chapter 28).

Brain blood oxygenation, which is an important factor in the blood oxygenation level–dependent (BOLD) fMRI technique, is altered by anesthetic agents, which are commonly used in animal fMRI studies. Thus, fMRI changes in rats treated with isoflurane, ketamine–xylazine, or medetomidine were different from each other and from those of rats in the unanesthetized state, in the absence of systemic blood oxygenation changes and of any neural stimulation.[65] A related sedative agent, the α_2-adrenergic receptor agonist (dexmedetomidine), is often utilized in fMRI studies in experimental animals. However, a recent study observed that this agent altered the response pattern of the somatosensory cortex to peripheral stimulation.[66] The drug constricts cerebral blood vessels and affects epileptic neuronal activity, but the latter change could be antagonized by the administration of inhalation anesthetics. It is unclear what effects the interaction of these CNS drugs would have on neurons in subcortical structures of the somatosensory neuronal network, creating concerns about the applicability of the imaging results to the awake, behaving animal. Thus, many phMRI studies in animals use these anesthetics, which have the potential to obfuscate the effects of other drugs in these studies.[65] The phMRI evaluation of other agents can also be complicated by other drugs with vasoactive properties, since BOLD fMRI relies on neurovascular coupling. Thus, phMRI effects of drugs (including ethanol, which induces hemodynamic changes) can be erroneously interpreted as changes in neuronal activation.[67]

In neuronal studies in animals when a low (subanesthetic) dose of the dissociative anesthetic ketamine, which is an uncompetitive *N*-methyl-D-aspartate (NMDA) receptor antagonist, is administered systemically to awake, behaving rats, neuronal responses in the amygdala to auditory stimuli are greatly depressed.[14,15,68] As shown in Figure 32.4, amygdala (lateral) neurons are clearly responsive to sensory stimuli in the unanesthetized state, as shown by the mean number of action potentials per PSTH in Figure 32.4(A) (control) and the example PSTH in Figure 32.4(B) (top). After administration of a subanesthetic dose of ketamine [30 mg/kg, intraperitoneal (i.p.)], amygdala neurons became unresponsive to the stimulus [Figure 32.4(A) and (B), middle row]. Again, the neuroplastic effect of the drug was short term, and the responsiveness of the amygdala neuron returned with time [Figure 32.4(B), bottom row]. However, amygdala neuronal responses to electrical stimuli in the medial geniculate body (MGB) were not affected by even anesthetic doses of ketamine,[14] and auditory neurons in the MGB, which is the major auditory input to

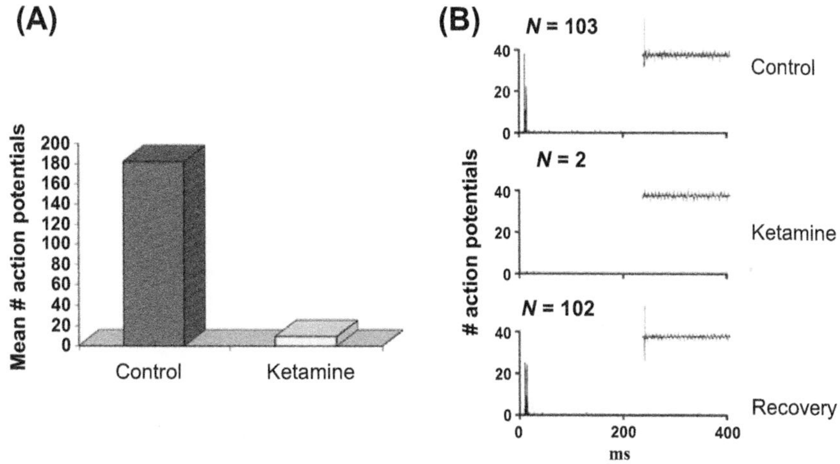

FIGURE 32.4 The action of an uncompetitive NMDA antagonist (ketamine) in a sub-anesthetic dose to reversibly block the responsiveness of neurons in a conditional multireceptive (CMR) brain region in the lateral amygdala. Panel (A) shows a bar graph of the mean effect in eight different lateral amygdala neurons in eight rats. The mean number of action potentials and poststimulus time histogram (PSTH) in control was 182.1 ± 42.0 (SEM) versus 9.6 ± 2.0 after ketamine (30 mg/kg, i.p.). Panel (B) shows a typical example of the effect of ketamine on the firing of lateral amygdala neurons. The lateral amygdala neuron exhibited an onset response before ketamine treatment [panel (B), top row]. The neuronal firing was significantly reduced ($p < 0.01$, paired t-test) and almost completely suppressed 15 min after ketamine treatment [panel (B), middle panel]. Four hours after ketamine treatment, the lateral amygdala neuronal response was comparable to that prior to ketamine treatment [panel (B), bottom row]. The insets [in each row of panel (B)] show examples of the digital oscilloscope tracings for each PSTH. Action potential amplitude: 300 μV. N = number of action potentials in the PSTH. Treatment was given in previously unanesthetized, awake, behaving rats with a microwire recording electrode. Acoustic stimulus parameters: 12 kHz tone burst, 100 ms duration, 5 ms rise–fall, 100 dB SPL, 0.5 Hz rate; PSTH parameters: 50 stimulus presentations, 1 ms bin width. (*Source: Based on data from Feng and Faingold,*[14] *with permission.*) (For color version of this figure, the reader is referred to the online version of this book.)

the amygdala, responded well to acoustic stimuli following anesthetic doses of ketamine.[69]

The selective effect of ketamine on the responses to physiological (auditory) stimuli of amygdala neurons may contribute to the proposed usefulness of this agent to rapidly overcome depression in patients, since the amygdala is proposed to be a key element in the network for this disorder[15,70] (see Chapter 24). Human phMRI studies of ketamine observed increases in the signal in several brain areas, including in the frontal and thalamic regions that were proposed to be associated with glutamate release. This effect could be reduced by drugs thought to block glutamate release (lamotrigine and risperidone).[71] A relatively low dose of ketamine (i.v.) in human volunteers increased the connectivity in the cerebellum and visual cortex relative to the medial visual network, based on fMRI studies. A decrease in connectivity was observed in the auditory and somatosensory network sites involved in pain and emotional networks, which include the amygdala. Connectivity changes due to fluctuations in pain scores were observed in the other pathways, including those of the brainstem, which are involved in descending inhibition of pain.[72] The phMRI response to ketamine in rats treated with two anesthetics with different mechanisms of action resulted in very different profiles of activity.[73] Given the effects of various anesthetics and other CNS depressants on specific brain regions, illustrated by both phMRI and neuronal recordings, it is clearly problematic to evaluate neuronal network mechanisms in anesthetic-treated subjects, whatever their mechanism of action (see Chapter 28).

EFFECTS OF ETHANOL ON NEURONS IN NEURONAL NETWORKS

Other drugs with depressant properties may also exert relatively selective network effects, including the oldest known and most widely used CNS depressant drug—ethanol. The depressant effects of ethanol have been known since antiquity; as characterized by Shakespeare in the play *Othello*, "I would not put a thief in my mouth to steal my brains." How does ethanol steal your brains? Many studies have evaluated the mechanisms of action of ethanol, and two main hypotheses have emerged: enhancement of GABA-mediated inhibition and blockade of glutamate excitatory effects on NMDA receptors.[74,75] However, the dose issue with ethanol is a critical problem, especially with in vitro studies.[20,21] These mechanisms have been determined mostly from in vitro studies where network issues cannot be adequately addressed. However, selectivity of effect may occur only when these neurons are embedded in a neuronal network. If the cells are isolated from the network, certain potentially important influences that confer the selectivity of drug action may be lost. Thus, ethanol has been widely reported to exert different effects on $GABA_A$ receptor function, depending on the brain site and even the cell type within the site.[19,76–78]

Ethanol withdrawal after repetitive administration can induce a seizure-prone state, which can be triggered by acoustic stimuli and result in audiogenic seizures (AGS) in rodents (see Chapter 26). Therefore, the network sites that had been established in the genetic audiogenic seizure models were evaluated in a series of experiments, using the binge protocol method of Majchrowicz.[79] These experiments began with a single dose of ethanol, and the effects on neurons of this dose were evaluated in awake, behaving rats in the network proposed to subserve ethanol withdrawal seizures[80] (see Chapter 26). One hour after a stupor-inducing dose (5 g/kg) of ethanol (via gastric lavage), major reductions in spontaneous and auditory-evoked neuronal firing were observed. Spontaneous neuronal firing was reduced in all five structures examined, ranging from 34% of pre-ethanol control in a primary midbrain auditory nucleus (the inferior colliculus, or IC) to the greatest inhibition (10.8% of control) in the pontine BRF. The reduction of auditory-evoked neuronal firing in the IC to 55% of pre-ethanol control was the smallest change and was significant only at the highest stimulus intensity (100 dB). Neurons in the PAG, lateral amygdala, BRF, and deep layers of the superior colliculus (DLSC) all exhibited significant reductions of auditory responsiveness to 18, 24, 27, and 29%, of pre-ethanol control values, respectively, and the reductions were significant at all intensities tested (85–100 dB).[81–85] As noted in this chapter, enhancement of the action of GABA is a major mechanism of action proposed for ethanol, and the reduction of firing at only high-stimulus intensities in the IC is consistent with the GABA-mediated intensity-induced inhibition seen in the IC[86] (see Chapter 7). The major reductions by ethanol of BRF neuronal firing are consistent with the ability of this agent to depress consciousness (in which this brain region is strongly implicated, as discussed in this chapter). However, acute ethanol exposure excites a type of cerebellar GABAergic interneuron in freely moving animals, resulting in cerebellar granule cell inhibition, which could make a major contribution to the ataxia induced by ethanol in higher doses.[87]

ETHANOL AND EMERGENT PROPERTIES OF NEURONS

The regional differences in the effects of ethanol observed in vivo are not simply due to a differential action of ethanol on inherent cellular properties of neurons in these sites, because the differential effects of this agent often do not persist when these neurons are acutely dissociated from the various brain sites.[88] Thus, differential effects of ethanol were observed in the same lab when in vivo[89] and in vitro effects[88] were compared.[90] The ability of ethanol to block the effects of NMDA was examined on neurons in several brain sites in acutely dissociated neurons in structures, including the lateral septum and hippocampus. The blockade of NMDA excitation by ethanol in the hippocampus was seen in vivo and in vitro, but the effect of ethanol on lateral septal neurons seen in vivo was absent in vitro. This indicates that the properties of the septal neurons in the intact network differed considerably from the properties observed in isolated neurons. This emergent property, which prevented the ethanol from affecting the excitatory amino acid responses of these neurons, would appear to be important in the selective effects on different brain neurons of ethanol in vivo. However, this selectivity may occur only when these neurons are embedded in their network, and, if the cells are isolated from the network, certain potentially important influences that confer the selectivity of drug action may be lost (as discussed here). Thus, ethanol has been widely reported to exert different effects on $GABA_A$ receptor function, depending on the brain site and even the cell type within the site.[19,76–78] These findings imply that a large part of the regional differences in response to drugs may be due, at least in part, to selective drug actions on emergent properties (Chapter 30) conferred on the neurons because of their membership in the network rather than being solely due to the intrinsic properties of neurons in a specific site. The opposite dichotomy between in vivo and in vitro effects is also seen with an uncompetitive NMDA antagonist in another brain site,[90] as discussed in this chapter.

EFFECTS OF ANTICONVULSANT DRUGS ON INTACT NEURONAL NETWORKS FOR SEIZURES

A few phMRI studies of anticonvulsant drug effects in epilepsy patients have been conducted, which correlated drug effects with cognitive and imaging changes.[91] A study on the effects of the anticonvulsant carbamazepine on temporal lobe epilepsy observed temporal lobe imaging changes during memory retrieval with this drug.[92] Another anticonvulsant, topiramate, which has major cognitive side effects, decreased activation of the prefrontal cortex on fMRI in response to a verbal task.[93] One study, which used phMRI of another anticonvulsant drug, valproate, in absence (petit mal) epilepsy patients along with EEG changes, observed abnormal patterns of activity in the midline thalamus, frontal cortex regions, and temporal lobes, which were normalized in patients who were effectively treated with this anticonvulsant drug.[94]

Earlier network neuronal firing studies indicated that the ability to depress reticular formation pathways, involving the PAG and BRF, is an important characteristic of antiepileptic drugs,[45,95] supporting the centrencephalic theory of generalized seizures that was discussed in the "The Centrencephalic Theory of Generalized Epilepsy" section.[7] Neuronal network investigations of the action of different anticonvulsants on neuronal firing have also been carried out in a naturally occurring animal model of generalized seizures: AGS in the genetically epilepsy-prone rat, severe seizure strain (GEPR-9s). Thus, the neuronal network subserving AGS in GEPR-9s has been thoroughly identified (Chapter 26), and the effects of anticonvulsants on neuronal firing in the network have been examined.

The principle behind this series of anticonvulsant drug studies is the hierarchical organization of the AGS network, which is confined to the brainstem, based on the temporal changes in neuronal firing patterns in each network site during AGS. Previous studies established the site of seizure initiation as being in the IC, and the propagation pathway involves specific brainstem nuclei projecting to the spinal cord (see Chapter 26 and Figures 26.1 and 26.2). As discussed in Chapter 26, in the plethora of naturally occurring rodent seizure models that are triggered by intense acoustic stimulation, the seizure initiation site is the IC, based on a multitude of experimental approaches.[86] Therefore, when the lowest effective therapeutic dose of any anticonvulsant drug that reduces seizure severity also reduces IC neuronal responses to the acoustic stimuli that trigger AGS, we conclude that the IC site (and/or the lower brainstem auditory nuclei; see Chapter 20) is (or are, if more than one site is involved) the most important target for that drug's effect. This conclusion is based on the experimentally well-justified premise that reduced firing in the IC will prevent propagation to the remainder of the network and block the seizures. However, if the therapeutic dose of the anticonvulsant does not act on IC neurons but does affect neurons in a different requisite network site in the network hierarchy, neurons in that nucleus are likely to be the major site of action for that drug's therapeutic effects. Certain drugs with anticonvulsant properties act on the initiation site in the IC. However, several others, including drugs with very similar mechanisms of action, do not act on the IC in therapeutic doses but do act elsewhere in the network, providing direct evidence for this concept, as discussed in this chapter. A key element in this approach is that AGS are seizures that are triggered by intense auditory stimuli. Therefore, the neurons in the requisite network nuclei can be probed with the same auditory stimuli at intensities below the seizure-inducing level. The results of this approach indicate that the neurons in all the established network nuclei exhibit elevated responsiveness to the stimulus (see Chapter 26). Therefore, when an anticonvulsant drug reduced this excessive neuronal response to the acoustic stimulus, it was indicative that this site was being affected. The effects of several anticonvulsant drugs were evaluated on the AGS network in awake, behaving GEPR-9s. The data indicate that neurons in specific network nuclei are affected differentially by these anticonvulsants. As shown by the diagram of the neuronal network for AGS in Figure 32.5, this network is organized as a hierarchy. The acoustic stimulus input into the auditory pathway nuclei neurons triggers the seizure by projections to the brainstem locomotion network nuclei (see Chapter 17), which project to the spinal cord. This process produces a sequence of neuronal activations in each network nucleus during each of the behaviors of AGS (see Chapter 26, Fig. 26.2). The emergent properties in each site in the network, which are the targets of systemically administered anticonvulsant drugs, are illustrated in Fig. 32.5.

ANTICONVULSANT ACTIONS ON IC NEURONS

Competitive NMDA antagonists are quite effective anticonvulsant drugs against many forms of experimental seizures, including AGS in GEPR-9s. Systemic

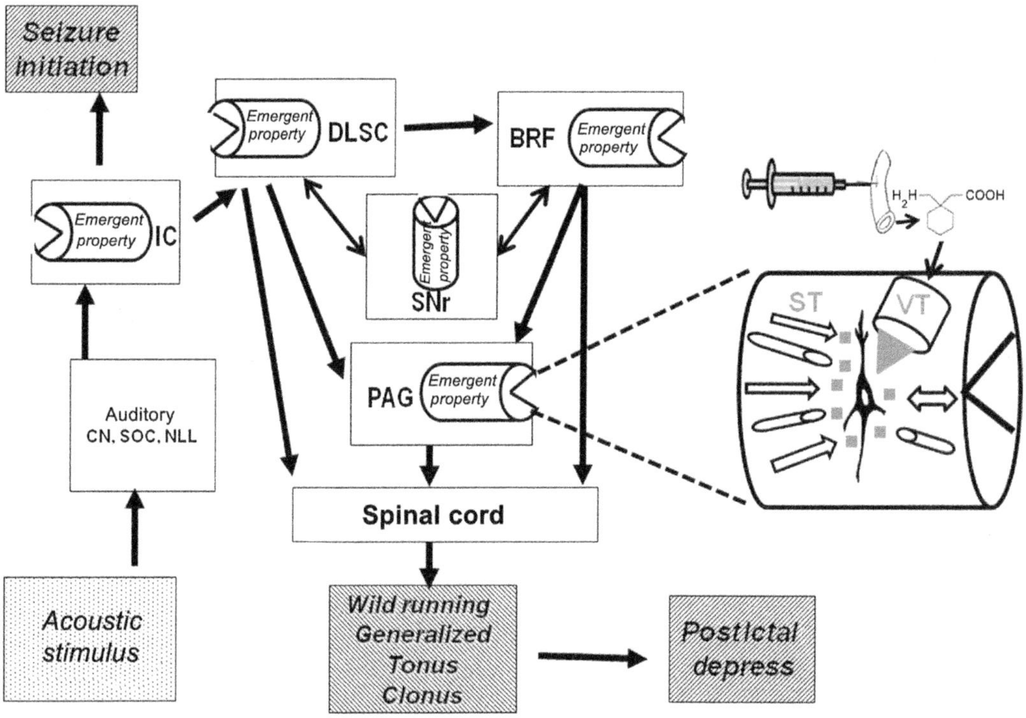

FIGURE 32.5 Diagram of the neuronal network for audiogenic seizures (AGS) with possible emergent properties in each site at which systemically administered drugs that block these seizures may act at therapeutic doses. The network is organized as a hierarchy beginning with the acoustic stimulus input into the auditory pathway nuclei neurons up to the level of the inferior colliculus (IC), and then to the brainstem locomotion network nuclei to the spinal cord, to produce a sequence of neuronal activations in each nucleus during the behaviors of AGS (see Chapter 26, Fig. 26.2). Several drugs with anticonvulsant properties act on neurons in the IC, including competitive NMDA antagonists (such as 2-amino-7-phosphonoheptanoate) and a GABA uptake inhibitor (tiagabine) (note that ethanol also acts there). Other drugs that are effectively anticonvulsant exert no effect on IC neurons, including an uncompetitive NMDA antagonist (MK-801), lamotrigine, and phenytoin. Other effective anticonvulsant drugs act to reduce periaqueductal gray (PAG) neuronal firing such as phenytoin and lamotrigine, but MK-801 does not act on the PAG. Lower doses of phenytoin selectively act on neurons in the brainstem reticular formation (BRF) of the pons, but MK-801 is ineffective there. The substantia nigra reticulata (SNr) is the target of MK-801, but the effect is to increase neuronal firing. No drugs have been observed to act directly on neurons in the deep layers of the superior colliculus (DLSC). The emergent property of each nucleus is seen as a confluence of influences onto the neurons in each nucleus, including neuroactive substances (squares) released onto the neurons via synaptic transmission (ST) and from the blood vessels, and cerebrospinal and extracellular fluids via volume transmission (VT), which is also how the drugs reach each site, as shown in the diagram of an emergent property on the right of the network. CN: cochlear nucleus; SOC: superior olivary complex; NLL: nuclei of the lateral lemniscus. (For color version of this figure the reader is referred to the online version of this book.)

administration of effective anticonvulsant doses of these agents resulted in significant reductions of IC neuronal responses to acoustic stimuli at all stimulus intensities, concomitant with the anticonvulsant effect[96] (see Figure 32.5). These data suggest that competitive NMDA antagonists act in the AGS network at or afferent to the IC,[96] which is consistent with the role of glutamate as the excitatory neurotransmitter in brainstem auditory nuclei, including the IC.[97–99] However, an uncompetitive NMDA antagonist, MK-801 (dizocilpine), did not alter the responses of IC neurons, despite the finding that it blocked AGS at very low doses. Eventually, it was discovered that this agent acted primarily on a totally different site in the seizure network, as discussed in this chapter. Tiagabine is a clinically useful anticonvulsant that blocks uptake of GABA, prolonging its action[100,101] (Figure 32.5). Tiagabine administration produced a nearly complete blockade of seizures in GEPR-9s and reduced the acoustically evoked responses of IC neurons, but, unlike the competitive NMDA antagonists, significant IC neuronal firing reduction was seen only at high acoustic intensities.[102] Ethanol also enhances the action of GABA, as noted in this chapter,[19] and this agent also reduced IC neuronal firing at high intensities only,[82] suggesting that both ethanol and tiagabine enhanced that form of $GABA_A$ receptor-mediated inhibition in IC neurons that is prominent at high acoustic intensities[103,103a] (see Chapter 26). However, several other anticonvulsant drugs, including phenytoin, lamotrigine, and MK-801, blocked AGS without exerting any consistent effect on IC neuronal firing, indicating that their actions are exerted at network sites efferent to the IC, as discussed here.

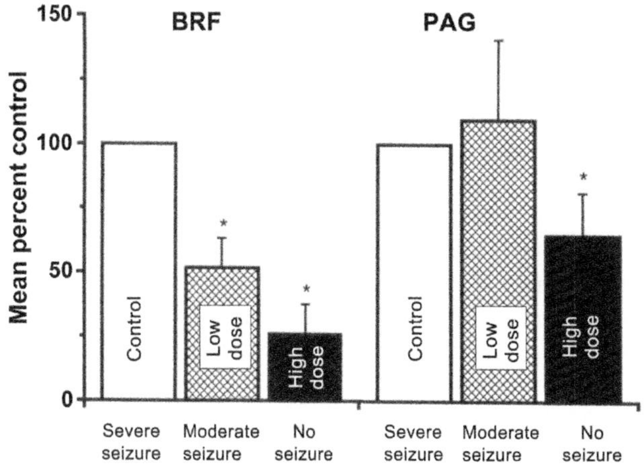

FIGURE 32.6 Effect of a systemically administered anticonvulsant (phenytoin) on neuronal firing in the (pontine) brainstem reticular formation (BRF) and in the periaqueductal gray (PAG) shows a relatively selective effect on the BRF in low doses that reduce seizure severity. Graph of the mean (±SEM) acoustically evoked neuronal firing as a percentage of vehicle control (open bars) on audiogenic seizures (AGS) in genetically epilepsy-prone rats (GEPR-9s) in doses of phenytoin, which significantly reduced seizure severity (low dose) or blocked seizures (high dose). Mean neuronal firing changes are shown after a phenytoin dose (mean: 6.3 mg/kg) that reduced AGS severity (i.e. blocked tonic hind limb extension) (hatched bars) and phenytoin in doses (mean: 8.3 mg/kg) that completely blocked AGS (solid bars). A significant reduction was observed in BRF neuronal firing when seizure severity was reduced (moderate seizure), which was even more greatly reduced when AGS were blocked (no seizure). However, no significant change was observed in PAG firing when the severity of AGS was reduced by phenytoin. At the higher phenytoin dose, PAG neuronal firing was also significantly reduced. These data suggest that a relatively selective effect was exerted by phenytoin on BRF neurons, as compared to the PAG, which generalized to the PAG when the dose was raised. No effect of the seizure blocking dose was seen in other neurons in the AGS network, even at the high dose. Stimulus: 12 kHz 100 ms duration tone bursts. *(Source: Based on N'Gouemo and Faingold,[106] with permission.)*

ANTICONVULSANT ACTIONS ON PAG AND BRF NEURONS

The ventrolateral PAG and BRF are requisite AGS network nuclei that are implicated in the generation of tonic convulsive behaviors (see Chapter 26). AGS in GEPR-9s culminate in tonic hind limb extension, and the elevated acoustically evoked neuronal firing in PAG and BRF neurons changes to tonic firing immediately before the tonic hind limb extension (see Chapter 26, Fig. 26.2).[41,84,104] Phenytoin has long been known to block AGS completely, but lower doses of this agent can block the tonic hind limb extension phase of AGS selectively[105] (Figure 32.5). As noted in this chapter, phenytoin did not exert any effects on IC neuronal firing, but this agent induced consistent changes in PAG and BRF (pontine) auditory-evoked neuronal firing and reduced the severity or blocked AGS in GEPR-9s, depending on the dose (Figure 32.6).[106] Phenytoin in doses that selectively suppressed tonic hind limb extension did not consistently alter PAG neuronal firing, but the same doses of phenytoin resulted in significant (~50%) suppression of BRF neuronal firing. Doses of phenytoin, which completely blocked AGS, significantly (>60%) reduced PAG auditory-evoked neuronal firing and more greatly (~75%) suppressed auditory-evoked BRF firing (Figure 32.6). These results are consistent with a critical role for BRF but not PAG neurons in the generation of tonic convulsive behaviors of AGS. However, the suppression of PAG and BRF neuronal firing induced by phenytoin with complete seizure blockade is consistent with vital roles for both structures in the action of this drug on this seizure network. The differential effects of phenytoin on BRF as compared to PAG (and IC) indicate that this experimental approach is able to identify the most sensitive therapeutic target for anticonvulsant drug action in the seizure network of this model, and it also indicates that this approach may be applicable to various other neuronal networks that exhibit tonic convulsions. Phenytoin is well established to act by blocking sodium channels,[4] which are a fundamental property of essentially all neurons, but the finding that *therapeutic doses* of this agent act selectively on neurons in some network sites but not others vividly illustrates the network selectivity concept. Lamotrigine, which also acts, in part, by blocking sodium channels, also reduced PAG neuronal responses in doses that did not affect IC neuronal firing. However, examination of the effects of MK-801 on BRF and PAG neurons indicated that, despite successful blockade of AGS in GEPR-9s, no consistent change in auditory-evoked neuronal firing in these sites was induced. MK-801 did not consistently affect neuronal firing in DLSC, either. The finding that neurons in none of these established AGS network sites were affected by MK-801 was enigmatic, since this NMDA receptor channel blocker exerted a highly potent anticonvulsant effect on AGS.

ANTICONVULSANT ACTIONS ON THE SUBSTANTIA NIGRA RETICULATA (SNr)

The SNr has long been implicated in the seizure network for several types of seizures, including AGS[107–110] (see Chapter 26). However, reports of the role of the SNr in seizure control have often yielded inconsistent results.[108,111,112] Neuronal recordings, lesion, focal microinjection, and microdialysis data implicate SNr as a site important to the actions of several anticonvulsants, although contrasting effects were seen with the same drugs using different experimental methods.[100,113–117] Regional and developmental differences are reported in the distribution of anticonvulsant effects within the SNr[118] (see Chapter 11). Important age, sex, and regional differences in neurotransmitter actions within the SNr may be a major factor in the inconsistent effects observed in this structure (Chapter 11).

SNr neurons play a major role in control of AGS, based on in vivo neuronal recording studies.[119] MK-801 exerted a prominent effect on SNr neurons concomitant with its suppression of AGS in GEPR-9s and ETX rats. As noted above, MK-801 is the most potent anticonvulsant drug tested against AGS in GEPR-9s, but no consistent changes in auditory-evoked neuronal firing were induced by this agent in the IC, BRF, PAG, or DLSC despite complete AGS blockade.[90] However, MK-801 does exert a prominent and unexpected effect on SNr neurons. MK-801 in anticonvulsant doses (0.01–0.05 mg/kg, i.p.) consistently *increased* the acoustically evoked firing of SNr neurons (Figure 32.7). MK-801 (0.05 mg/kg), which blocked seizures, caused SNr neurons to increase their mean firing rate significantly above control levels (Figure 32.7).

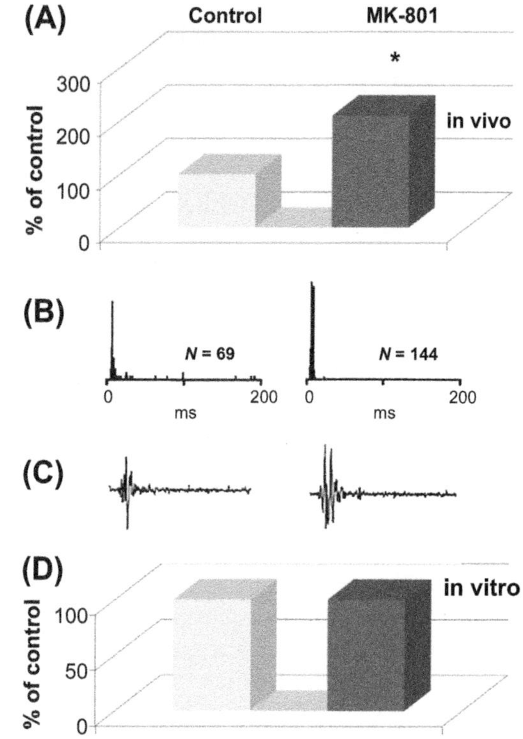

FIGURE 32.7 An uncompetitive NMDA antagonist (dizocilpine, MK-801) blocked audiogenic seizures (AGS) in genetically epilepsy-prone rats (GEPR-9s) and in ethanol withdrawn (ETX) rats and induced significantly increased mean evoked (acoustic) neuronal responses in the substantia nigra reticulata (SNr) in vivo, as shown in (A). However, the mean effect on SNr neurons was absent in vitro (brain slices), as shown in (D). (B) An example of the effect of systemic administration of MK-801 on acoustically evoked SNr neuronal responses in a behaving epileptic rat is shown. In control, this SNr neuron exhibited a consistent response, as shown by the example in the left panel. However, 30 min after MK-801 (0.05 mg/kg, i.p.), the firing was more than doubled, as seen in the right panel, and AGS was blocked. Recovery from the effect occurred by 24 h. (D) No change was induced in SNr neurons ($N = 6$) in vitro. The effect of MK-801 in concentrations up to 200 μM on the mean firing of SNr neurons when depolarized was 12.8 ± 2.6 (SEM) during MK-801 perfusion, as compared to 14.2 ± 1.3 action potentials before MK-801, which was not significant. Post-stimulus time histograms (PSTHs) are shown in (B), and examples of digital oscilloscope tracings of the extracellular action potentials are shown in (C). The increased firing of the SNr neuron is illustrated in the right panel. Amplitude of the action potential is 430 μV, 50 ms scan length. PSTH parameters: peak amplitude (right PSTH) axis is 32 action potentials/bin, 200 ms scan length, 1 ms bin width, 50 stimulus presentations; N = number of action potentials per PSTH. (*Source: Based on data in Faingold,[90] with permission.*) (For color version of this figure, the reader is referred to the online version of this book.)

Thus, the ability of MK-801 to block AGS is correlated with the ability to increase firing of SNr neurons. We then examined the effect of MK-801 on SNr neuronal firing in vitro in the brainstem slice. Concentrations of MK-801 (up to 200 nm) in vitro induced no consistent change in neuronal firing, and the predominant effect observed was a small, nonsignificant reduction of SNr firing.[90] These findings suggest that the significantly increased SNr neuronal firing induced by systemically administered MK-801 is an effect of this agent on the emergent properties of the AGS network but only in the SNr.[90]

EMERGENT PROPERTIES: DIFFERENCES BETWEEN IN VIVO AND IN VITRO STUDIES

How can a drug produce a major effect on specific neurons in vivo, but not produce this effect on the same neurons in vitro? As noted throughout this chapter (see Figure 32.1), there are a number of mechanisms and influences that affect neurons in a neuronal network. In the intact unanesthetized brain in vivo, all of these mechanisms are present. However, when the neurons are removed from the intact brain in ex vivo or in vitro preparations, many of these mechanisms are absent. Thus, SNr neurons in the intact network are tonically inhibited, in part, through GABAergic input from the striatum and globus pallidus.[120] MK-801 may inhibit firing of neurons in those sites that are responsible for tonic inhibition of SNr neurons. Therefore, an inhibitory action of MK-801 on these basal ganglia sites would likely result in a disinhibitory effect on the SNr and contribute to MK-801-induced SNr firing increases seen in vivo, which is supported by binding data of this agent.[121–123] Thus, such an indirect effect of MK-801 on this circuit may contribute importantly to the anticonvulsant effects in vivo.

The dichotomy between the blockade of NMDA-mediated excitation by ethanol in vivo versus in vitro, as discussed in this chapter,[88,89] also supports the differential expression of an emergent property in the microscopic versus the mesoscopic network. Thus, in vivo versus in vitro differences in drug actions reflect the fact that the emergent property of the neurons on which the drug acts in the intact organism (Chapter 30) can change dramatically in either direction in the in vitro condition. These findings are a strong indicator that effects of drugs on neurons in vitro are not a reliable indicator of the true mechanism responsible for the therapeutic effect of a drug in the intact organism. This is likely due to the fact that there are a large number of influences exerted on neurons in an intact neuronal network nucleus (many of which are shown in the example in Chapter 1) that are absent or modified in vitro. Since functioning brain networks possess emergent properties (Chapter 30), we proposed that these properties are critical targets for the action of CNS drugs,[90] and when neurons are isolated from their network, the regional selectivity of drug action can be significantly altered. In addition, as noted in this chapter, achieving an appropriate concentration of the drug in vitro is highly problematic. An "amplification" phenomenon occurs in vivo, so that much smaller concentrations of drugs affecting seizures are needed in vivo as compared to in vitro to obtain the same effect, as demonstrated by Narahashi.[22] Thus, many CNS drugs at therapeutic concentrations exert selective actions on neurons in a specific site within the brain. However, this selectivity is due not only to the intrinsic properties of those neurons but also to a compilation of all the actions exerted on the target neurons by the various influences that impinge on these neurons, as well as their intrinsic properties. This selectivity of drug action may change when the neuron is isolated from the network and the emergent properties are subject to major changes (either loss or gain).

UNDERSTANDING EMERGENT PROPERTIES AS CRITICAL DRUG TARGETS

From the foregoing discussion, it can be seen that in the intact behaving animal, therapeutic doses of these network-modifying anticonvulsant drugs can exert selective effects on specific neuronal network nuclei. As has been discussed in Chapter 30,[90] neuronal networks in awake, behaving animals express emergent properties in neurons in a particular network nucleus because of the many influences on those neurons (see Table 1.1 in Chapter 1). These emergent properties are specific targets of therapeutic doses of CNS drugs in the intact, unanesthetized brain. However, these properties may be greatly altered when the neurons are removed from the network (in vitro) because many of the influences that were present in vivo have been removed, as discussed throughout this chapter. It is not clear how an emergent property actually emerges; that is, how does this multitude of influences "create" the target for specific actions of drugs in therapeutic doses? Several possible mechanisms can be hypothesized. A simple explanation is that a preexisting property (e.g. a receptor or ion channel) undergoes an increase in affinity due to the confluence of these network influences, causing the receptors to undergo an allosteric-type change that increases sensitivity to the drug. For example, anticonvulsant drugs that act in vitro on $GABA_A$ receptors or N-type Ca^{2+} channels may exert differential effects in therapeutic doses on neurons in a specific network nucleus, because the receptors or channels in that nucleus have a relatively higher affinity than other sites for the drug due to the confluence of influences in vivo. Another possible mechanism may involve pH or ion concentration differences caused by a CNS disorder that occur dynamically in vivo and induce changes in ion channel or receptor affinity that are not readily modeled in vitro. Other explanations include the possibility that neurons in CMR brain regions (see Chapter 28) are highly sensitive in vivo, because of their normally tenuous responsiveness to inputs (see Chapter 28). Therefore, relatively small changes in excitability induced by low (therapeutic) drug doses can greatly increase or decrease neuronal responsiveness. This may be the case with CMR neurons, such as those in the BRF (discussed in this chapter), which are highly susceptible to the effects of low doses of both stimulant and depressant drugs. Another possibility is that the drug is affecting an emergent property that is seen only in vivo and is "created" by the confluence of all the in vivo influences detailed in Chapters 1 and 7–12. Thus, emergent properties may follow a similar pattern to the Heisenberg uncertainty principle governing electrons. When you take the neuron out of the intact brain, you alter its properties; that is, by observing it too closely (in vitro), you can greatly alter the influences that contribute to the emergent property. To add to the complexity of the understanding of emergent properties of neuronal networks, these properties are dynamic, and changes in these properties can occur that alter the action of drugs on the network. Understanding drug actions on neuronal networks is further complicated by the fact that drugs that were developed for use in one class of CNS disorder, such as epilepsy, have been found to be effective in different classes of CNS disorders, such as chronic pain.

"ANTICONVULSANT" DRUG EFFECTS ON NETWORKS FOR MULTIPLE CNS DISORDERS

A number of drugs that were developed as anticonvulsants have proven effective for treating chronic pain as well as several psychiatric disorders, leading to the idea that these drugs should be considered "network-modifying agents".[124] This phenomenon of multiplicity of effects was actually observed with one of the earliest selective anticonvulsants—phenytoin. Phenytoin has also long been used for treating chronic pain syndromes, including trigeminal neuralgia,[125] and recently this agent has been utilized in combination with acupuncture to produce an additive therapeutic effect in this syndrome.[126] Anticonvulsants, such as gabapentin and its newer derivative, pregabalin, are approved for treatment of neuropathic pain syndromes as well as epilepsy.[127] These different classes of CNS disorder are mediated by different neuronal networks in the brain, but these networks also have certain brain regions in common.[128] Thus, human and animal phMRI studies have shown that a number of brain areas, including the PAG, are strongly implicated in pain networks, and changes in these pathways are induced by several drugs that possess analgesic properties.[129,130] As mentioned in this chapter, the brainstem and the PAG, in particular, are among the areas that show significant phMRI changes when gabapentin and other drugs that exert analgesic properties are administered in humans and animals.[131–133]

In chronic CNS disorders, such as chronic pain syndromes and progressive epilepsy, additional emergent properties of neurons may develop that are targets for the action of anticonvulsants, such as gabapentin. Recent evidence suggests that the PAG may be a major nexus for both epileptic and chronic pain neuronal networks that is the target of anticonvulsant drugs, such as gabapentin, and may explain why these drugs are effective in these different classes of CNS disorders. Gabapentin exerts effects on PAG neurons in AGS in a somewhat different manner from phenytoin. Repeated, periodic induction of AGS results in AGS kindling, which increases seizure duration and, in GEPR-9s, induces an additional generalized clonus phase [post-tonic clonus (PTC)] (see Chapter 27). Systemic administration of gabapentin in AGS-kindled GEPR-9s blocks this PTC behavior, and the seizures temporarily revert to the unkindled pattern of behaviors that end in tonic hind limb extension.[134] In AGS kindling, the brainstem network expands to include the amygdala (lateral) (Chapter 27), and focal blockade of the amygdala will also cause the AGS-kindled seizure to revert to the unkindled pattern.[135] The pathway between the amygdala (central) and PAG (ventrolateral) is implicated in production of PTC, and AGS kindling-induced changes in this pathway were evaluated by recording PAG neuronal responses evoked by stimulating the amygdala.[134] Electrical stimuli in the amygdala evoked consistent, short-latency, and intensity-dependent PAG neuronal responses that were significantly greater than those seen in unkindled GEPR-9s (see Chapter 27). As mentioned here, gabapentin (50 mg/kg, i.p.) blocked PTC in AGS-kindled GEPR-9s, but the other convulsive behaviors (wild running and tonic hind limb extension), which constitute the AGS behaviors present before AGS kindling, were not affected by this dose of the drug. Simultaneous with the block of PTC, gabapentin significantly reduced PAG neuronal responses to amygdala stimulation (Figure 32.8). These neuronal responses returned to levels similar to those seen prior to AGS kindling.[134] These data suggest that the amygdala-to-PAG pathway may be critical in mediating the emergence of PTC during AGS kindling. The ability of gabapentin to suppress this pathway to the PAG may be important for its anticonvulsant effects in AGS-kindled GEPR-9s. In addition, an effect on PAG neurons may contribute to gabapentin's effectiveness in anxiety and chronic pain, since the networks that mediate these CNS disorders also involve the amygdala-to-PAG pathway, as discussed here. Recent

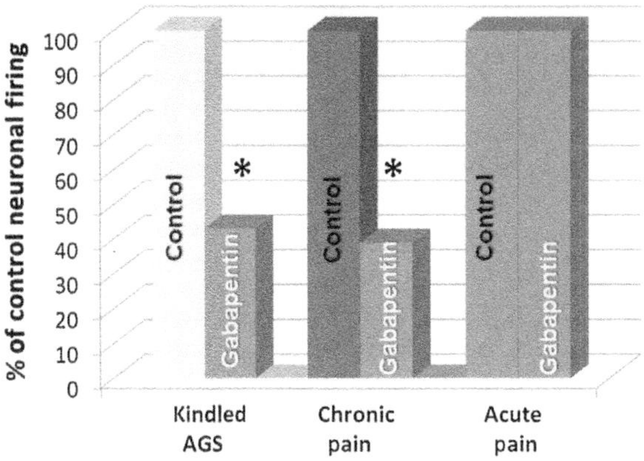

FIGURE 32.8 A network-modifying drug (gabapentin, 50 mg/kg i.p.) significantly reduced periaqueductal gray (PAG) neuronal firing and seizure severity in a repetitive epilepsy model of kindled audiogenic seizures (AGS) in GEPR-9s 60 min after administration. The same dose of this drug significantly reduced PAG neuronal firing and thermal pain in a chronic pain model (paclitaxel), but this dose had no effect on PAG neuronal firing in acute (thermal) pain. In the left pair of bars, a significantly reduced mean PAG (ventrolateral) neuronal responsiveness to amygdala (central) electrical stimulation was induced by gabapentin at all stimulus intensities tested (repeated measures ANOVA and post-hoc paired *t*-test). The middle set of bars shows mean thermal-evoked PAG neuronal responses in rats treated with a chronic pain-inducing protocol (paclitaxel protocol[136]), and a significant reduction in PAG neuronal responses was also observed 60 min after gabapentin (50 mg/kg i.p.) in normal rats. However, in an acute pain protocol (radiant heat to the paw at 53 °C), the same dose of gabapentin induced no significant change in PAG neuronal firing. Data in the left pair of bars are from awake, behaving GEPR-9s subjected to AGS kindling,[134] and data in the middle and right pairs of bars are from normal rats. *Significance at $p < 0.01$ (repeated measures ANOVA). (*Source: Based on data from Tupal and Faingold*[134] *and Samineni et al.*[137]) (For color version of this figure, the reader is referred to the online version of this book.)

data from our lab support this possibility for chronic pain disorders.[137] Chronic pain syndromes are common and are often seen as an adverse effect of cancer chemotherapeutic drugs, such as paclitaxel.[138] As discussed in Chapter 23, the PAG is also strongly implicated in the neuronal networks involved in pain. fMRI data suggest that gabapentin may act on the PAG, as noted in this chapter, and we recently evaluated the effect of this agent on the firing patterns and responses to noxious stimuli of PAG neurons in awake, behaving rats. Gabapentin was administered to normal rats previously treated with a paclitaxel paradigm that induces a chronic pain syndrome,[136] and the changes in pain threshold and PAG neuronal firing were examined. The effects of gabapentin on pain threshold and PAG neuronal responses in rats prior to and after chronic pain induction were evaluated (Figure 32.8). The avoidance response of the animals to a thermal nociceptive stimulus in this chronic pain model was elevated as compared to untreated rats. The nociceptive response in the chronic pain model was significantly reduced by gabapentin (50 mg/kg). However, gabapentin in the same dose did not affect the nociceptive response in rats prior to paclitaxel treatment (acute pain). Neuronal firing patterns in PAG paralleled these behavioral changes. Thus, the same dose of gabapentin significantly reduced the firing of PAG neurons to nociceptive stimuli in the chronic pain model. However, the same dose of gabapentin did not affect PAG neuronal firing or responses to the nociceptive stimuli in the control rats that were not experiencing chronic pain.[137] These data, along with the effects of gabapentin in the AGS-kindling paradigm discussed here, suggest that a similar change in responsiveness of PAG neurons appears to emerge in both of these chronic conditions. This change causes the PAG to become a critical target for therapeutic doses of gabapentin in both pain and epilepsy, which is consistent with the important role of the PAG in the neuronal networks for both disorders (Chapters 26 and 27). In both cases, the therapeutic doses are the same, and in each case this effect is seen only after a chronic expansion of the network is induced. Based on the concept of emergent properties (Chapter 30), we propose that an additional property has emerged in the PAG after either chronic protocol that causes PAG neurons to become highly sensitive to gabapentin, but this sensitivity was absent prior to these network expansion-inducing experiences (Chapter 27).

Gabapentin, which is proposed to act primarily by binding to alpha(2) delta Ca^{2+} channels (N-type) in vitro,[139] may act on the PAG because the network influences at work in chronic pain or epilepsy cause that channel to exhibit an increased affinity for this drug. Alternatively, gabapentin has also been reported to increase the concentration of GABA in the brains of experimental animals,[140] and recent imaging studies of the visual cortex in humans, using proton magnetic resonance spectroscopy, also indicate significant increases in GABA after gabapentin administration.[141] This GABAergic mechanism may become more sensitive to this agent in the intact network due to the chronic conditions. It could also be that the emergent property is occurring because both of these mechanisms are activated. It is also possible that the mechanisms responsible for the drug's effectiveness in the chronic conditions may involve secondary events triggered by the receptor. Thus, the receptor subunits may undergo switching due to the chronicity of the conditions, and these subunits may become a drug target because of the increased sensitivity of this particular subunit.[142] Another possible effect of chronic CNS disorders is that intracellular mechanisms, such as NMDA receptor-mediated increases in Ca^{2+} entry into neurons, cause altered network function and expansion due to chronic network activations caused by seizure repetition or chronic pain[143] (see Chapters 7 and 27).

There are several other mechanisms that are proposed for the action of gabapentin.[144,145] The changes induced by chronic activation of the network may cause these previously reported "minor" mechanisms to become expressed in specific network nuclei to a greater extent. Resolving these possibilities will require extensive further investigation. Thus, these emergent properties may be selective for the specific network sites in which they are observed, or the same emergent property may also occur in networks in related disorders, such as different forms of epilepsy. They may also occur in the neuronal networks for different classes of CNS disorders. Evidence for the idea that the same emergent properties occur in more than one class of CNS disorder is provided by the recent experiments done with the anticonvulsant drug gabapentin in chronic pain and epilepsy, as discussed in this chapter.

CNS DRUGS AND LONG-LASTING NETWORK CHANGES

Long-lasting changes in neuronal networks can occur, and these changes may also interact with the effects of drugs administered chronically. Thus, network properties may be modified due to repetition-induced expansion of the network (see Chapter 27), causing the addition of other sites to the network that possess additional drug targets. Drugs can also prevent long-term changes in neuronal networks, including certain anticonvulsant drugs and agents with neuroprotective properties, which are able to reduce or prevent the network changes induced by repetitive seizures.[146,147]

Drugs can also induce long-lasting network changes, such as neurogenesis, which can be induced by chronic treatment with antidepressants, phosphodiesterase inhibitors, atypical neuroleptics, and agents used in bipolar disorder.[148–151] Several other types of change can occur when a CNS drug is administered chronically, and they may occur in certain parts of the network differentially.[152,153] Chronic CNS disorders may be more prone to changes in neuronal properties with drug administration, including epilepsy and mood disorders, since drug therapy for these conditions is required over extended time periods.

Another acute versus chronic difference in drug effects is that the initial or acute action of a given drug may reflect only the mechanism that acts to abort ongoing seizures, while the ability to act prophylactically to prevent future seizures may involve additional mechanisms that may be only minimally expressed during acute treatment. A case in point is phenobarbital, which is thought to act primarily on $GABA_A$ receptors to enhance the activation of these receptors. This agent is useful prophylactically in epilepsy, and the chronic use of phenobarbital is not precluded by the development of tolerance. A number of explanations have been put forward for this, including the fact that barbiturates possess additional effects, including actions on voltage-gated calcium channels as well as on excitatory amino acid receptors,[154] which may become more prominent with chronic treatment. A related class of anticonvulsant drugs, the benzodiazepines, which also act to enhance $GABA_A$ receptor activation, albeit by a different mechanism, are useful acutely in terminating repetitive seizures (status epilepticus).[155] However, most benzodiazepines are not clinically useful for seizure prophylaxis because of the relatively rapid development of tolerance to their effects and the lack of other actions of these drugs, in contrast to phenobarbital. Chronic administration of certain CNS drugs may also cause receptor downregulation, leading to tolerance and resulting in pharmacoresistance with a loss of effectiveness, a major problem with anticonvulsants. Other types of compensatory mechanisms within the network may lead to tolerance to drug action or to additional chronic effects of the drug that may also contribute to the drug's action.[156,157] In addition to receptor-based tolerance, other mechanisms underlying pharmacoresistance include changes in transporter activity and a neuronal network hypothesis, based on seizure-induced alterations of brain plasticity,[158] which alters the emergent properties of the seizure network.

CONCLUSION

Many CNS drugs exert their effects on specific neuronal networks of the brain, including one of the earliest proposed neuronal networks, the BRF arousal network, and neurons in this network are a major target of CNS depressant drugs. Although mechanisms of CNS drug action on neurons have been widely studied in vitro, concerns have arisen about the applicability of these findings to the intact CNS, since many of the network influences that control neuronal function in vivo are absent in these microscopic networks. Another critical concern is the issue of therapeutic drug doses, which are difficult to evaluate accurately outside the intact animal. This concern has led to the study of midsized (mesoscopic) networks to evaluate the neuronal action of therapeutic doses of depressant and stimulant drugs. It is vital that this be done in awake, unanesthetized animals, since even small doses of anesthetic drugs can profoundly alter network function. PhMRI studies in animals and humans have also provided important insights for understanding the network effects of CNS drugs. Although these methods are a vital link in the study of CNS effects on neuronal networks for CNS disorders, caution about the results of this approach is necessary. The reasons for this caution include the use of anesthetics, intersubject variability, loss of sensitivity with group data, psychometric effects of the magnetic field, and the intense acoustic stimulation generated by the MRI device. The most important caution about phMRI data is, the decoupling between electrophysiological events and imaging results from the same brain area, particularly in subcortical regions. Therefore, determining the effects of appropriate doses of CNS drugs on neuronal firing in network hubs in unanesthetized, awake, behaving animals is critically important for evaluating the therapeutically relevant actions of these agents. In these studies, small doses of CNS stimulants and depressants have been observed to cause major response changes, particularly on neurons in subcortical CMR brain areas, including the BRF, PAG, and amygdala. Neurons in these CMR areas are greatly affected by low subconvulsant doses of $GABA_A$ receptor antagonists or cholinesterase inhibitors, which cause the responsiveness of many of these neurons to increase dramatically. Recent reports indicate that agents that reduce $GABA_A$ receptor-mediated inhibition enhance cognition in animals, and the ability of the same agents to enhance CMR neuronal responsiveness could contribute importantly to this effect. Since aging results in diminished activation of the primary cortex but simultaneous increases in the activation of cortical association areas, administration of these stimulant drugs is potentially useful in slowing normal aging and treating cognitive disorders. Coupling administration of stimulant drugs with therapeutic stimulation paradigms (see Chapter 31) may provide further therapeutic enhancement. Neuronal responsiveness is greatly diminished in CMR brain regions by CNS depressants, including $GABA_A$ receptor-activating agents, NMDA antagonists, and ethanol, in doses that induce minor effects on primary sensory neurons. Neurons in specific nuclei of a well-established brainstem network in an epilepsy model (AGS) are affected differentially by anticonvulsants, which illuminates the importance of emergent properties of neurons embedded in an intact neuronal network. An example of this is seen with an uncompetitive NMDA antagonist, which affects SNr neurons selectively in vivo but not in vitro. The opposite dichotomy of in vivo and in vitro effects is seen with ethanol, supporting the idea that the emergent properties of neurons can change dramatically when removed from the normal influences of the intact network. These findings emphasize the importance of understanding emergent properties of neurons in intact networks as a critical drug target. A number of anticonvulsant agents are also effective for therapy of other CNS disorders, including chronic pain syndromes. Recent studies indicate that an anticonvulsant, gabapentin, exerts selective network effects in both epilepsy and chronic pain by acting on neurons in the same site, the PAG, reinforcing the concept that anticonvulsants are network-modifying agents. Coupling administration of anticonvulsant drugs with therapeutic stimulation paradigms may also provide therapeutic enhancement (see Chapters 31 and 33). Thus, the anticonvulsant phenytoin, which is also used for chronic pain syndromes, when combined with acupuncture resulted in additive effects in treating chronic pain. This combination of a drug with a therapeutic stimulation paradigm may be a promising approach to improvements in therapy, especially if it is coupled with imaging studies that identify the neuronal network that mediates the particular CNS disorder to be treated.

Acknowledgments

The authors gratefully acknowledge the involvement of Vijaya Samineni, Sri Tupal, Marcus Randall, Li Yang, Jim Stittsworth, and Bill Hoffmann in the experiments from our laboratory discussed in this chapter. The author was supported by NINDS and NIAAA during the experiments from our lab, and we gratefully acknowledge the assistance of Gayle Stauffer and Diana Smith in preparing this manuscript.

References

1. Maati H, Mohaou R, Peyronnet C, et al. A human TREK-1/HEK cell line: a highly efficient screening tool for drug development in neurological diseases. *PLoS One*. 2011;6(10):e25602.
2. Porter RJ, Dhir A, Macdonald RL, Rogawski MA. Mechanisms of action of antiseizure drugs. *Handb Clin Neurol*. 2012;108:663–681.
3. Merritt HH, Putnam TJ. A new series of anticonvulsant drugs tested by experiments on animals. *Arch Neurol Psychiatry*. 1938; 39:1001–1015.
4. Mantegazza M, Curia G, Biagini G, Ragsdale DS, Avoli M. Voltage-gated sodium channels as therapeutic targets in epilepsy and other neurological disorders. *Lancet Neurol*. 2010;9(4): 413–424.
5. Moruzzi G, Magoun HW. Brain stem reticular formation and activation of the EEG. *Electroencephalogr Clin Neurophysiol*. 1949; 1(4):455–473.
6. Escobar W, Ramirez K, Avila C, Limongi R, Vanegas H, Vazquez E. Metamizol, a non-opioid analgesic, acts via endocannabinoids in the PAG-RVM axis during inflammation in rats. *Eur J Pain*. 2012;16(5):676–689.
7. Penfield W, Jasper HH. *Epilepsy and the Functional Anatomy of the Human Brain*. Little, Brown; 1954.
8. Buzsáki G, Anastassiou CA, Koch C. The origin of extracellular fields and currents—EEG, ECoG, LFP and spikes. *Nat Rev Neurosci*. May 18, 2012;13(6):407–420.
9. Goldstein A, Lowney LI, Pal BK. Stereospecific and nonspecific interactions of the morphine congener levorphanol in subcellular fractions of mouse brain. *Proc Natl Acad Sci USA*. 1971;68(8): 1742–1747.
10. Freeman WJ, Kozma R, Werbos PJ. Biocomplexity: adaptive behavior in complex stochastic dynamical systems. *Biosystems*. 2001;59:109–123.

11. Klitgaard H, Matagne A, Lamberty Y. Use of epileptic animals for adverse effect testing. *Epilepsy Res.* 2002;50(1–2):55–65.
12. Bialer M, White HS. Key factors in the discovery and development of new antiepileptic drugs. *Nat Rev Drug Discov.* 2010; 9(1):68–82.
13. Bullmore E, Sporns O. Complex brain networks: graph theoretical analysis of structural and functional systems. *Nat Rev Neurosci.* 2009;10(3):186–198.
14. Feng HJ, Faingold CL. Repeated generalized audiogenic seizures induce plastic changes on acoustically evoked neuronal firing in the amygdala. *Brain Res.* 2002;932(1–2):61–69.
15. Feng HJ, Faingold CL. Ketamine in mood disorders and epilepsy. In: Costa A, Villalba E, eds. *Horizons in Neuroscience Research.* Vol. 10. New York: Nova Science Publishers; 2013:103–122.
16. Berman RM, Cappiello A, Anand A, Oren DA, Heninger GR, Charney DS. Antidepressant effects of ketamine in depressed patients. *Biol Psychiatry.* 2000;47:351–354.
17. Aan Het Rot M, Zarate Jr CA, Charney DS, Mathew SJ. Ketamine for depression: where do we go from here? *Biol Psychiatry.* 2012; 72(7):537–547.
18. Solt K, Forman SA. Correlating the clinical actions and molecular mechanisms of general anesthetics. *Curr Opin Anaesthesiol.* 2007; 20(4):300–306.
19. Faingold CL, N'Gouemo P, Riaz A. Ethanol and neurotransmitter interactions—from molecular to integrative effects. *Prog Neurobiol.* 1998;55(5):509–535.
20. Olsen RW, Hanchar HJ, Meera P, Wallner M. $GABA_A$ receptor subtypes: the "one glass of wine" receptors. *Alcohol.* 2007;41(3): 201–209.
21. Yamashita M, Marszalec W, Yeh JZ, Narahashi T. Effects of ethanol on tonic GABA currents in cerebellar granule cells and mammalian cells recombinantly expressing $GABA_A$ receptors. *J Pharmacol Exp Ther.* 2006;319(1):431–438.
22. Narahashi T. Chemical modulation of sodium channels and $GABA_A$ receptor channel. *Adv Neurol.* 1999;79:457–480.
23. Reagan-Shaw S, Nihal M, Ahmad N. Dose translation from animal to human studies revisited. *FASEB J.* 2008;22(3):659–661.
24. Womelsdorf T, Schoffelen J, Oostenveld R, et al. Modulation of neuronal interactions through neuronal synchronization. *Science.* 2007;316:1609–1612.
25. Cowan R, Wilson CJ. Spontaneous firing patterns and axonal projections of single corticostriatal neurons in the rat medial agranular cortex. *J Neurophysiol.* 1994;71(1):17–32.
26. Mahon S, Deniau JM, Charpier S. Relationship between EEG potentials and intracellular activity of striatal and cortico-striatal neurons: an in vivo study under different anesthetics. *Cereb Cortex.* 2001;11(4):360–373.
27. Kasanetz F, Riquelme LA, Murer MG. Disruption of the two-state membrane potential of striatal neurones during cortical desynchronisation in anaesthetised rats. *J Physiol.* 2002;543(Pt 2): 577–589.
28. Mölle M, Born J. Slow oscillations orchestrating fast oscillations and memory consolidation. *Prog Brain Res.* 2011;193:93–110.
29. O'Donnell P. Dopamine gating of forebrain neural ensembles. *Eur J Neurosci.* 2003;17(3):429–435.
30. Gerkin RC, Clem RL, Shruti S, Kass RE, Barth AL. Cortical up state activity is enhanced after seizures: a quantitative analysis. *J Clin Neurophysiol.* 2010;27(6):425–432.
31. Weitlauf C, Woodward JJ. Ethanol selectively attenuates NMDAR-mediated synaptic transmission in the prefrontal cortex. *Alcohol Clin Exp Res.* 2008;32(4):690–698.
32. Lambe EK, Aghajanian GK. Hallucinogen-induced UP states in the brain slice of rat prefrontal cortex: role of glutamate spillover and NR2B-NMDA receptors. *Neuropsychopharmacology.* 2006; 31(8):1682–1689.
33. Mitsis GD, Iannetti GD, Smart TS, Tracey I, Wise RG. Regions of interest analysis in pharmacological fMRI: how do the definition criteria influence the inferred result? *Neuroimage.* 2008; 40(1):121–132.
34. Bouet V, Klomp A, Freret T, et al. Age-dependent effects of chronic fluoxetine treatment on the serotonergic system one week following treatment. *Psychopharmacology (Berl).* 2012;221(2):329–339.
35. Hafeman DM, Chang KD, Garrett AS, Sanders EM, Phillips ML. Effects of medication on neuroimaging findings in bipolar disorder: an updated review. *Bipolar Disord.* 2012;14(4):375–410.
36. Wolf DH, Satterthwaite TD, Loughead J, et al. Amygdala abnormalities in first-degree relatives of individuals with schizophrenia unmasked by benzodiazepine challenge. *Psychopharmacology (Berl).* 2011;218(3):503–512.
37. Zaidel L, Allen G, Cullum CM, et al. Donepezil effects on hippocampal and prefrontal functional connectivity in Alzheimer's disease: preliminary report. *J Alzheimers Dis.* 2012;31(Suppl. 3): S221–S226.
38. Li W, Antuono PG, Xie C, et al. Changes in regional cerebral blood flow and functional connectivity in the cholinergic pathway associated with cognitive performance in subjects with mild Alzheimer's disease after 12-week donepezil treatment. *Neuroimage.* 2012;60(2):1083–1091.
39. Miettinen PS, Pihlajamaki M, Jauhiainen AM, et al. Effect of cholinergic stimulation in early Alzheimer's disease – functional imaging during a recognition memory task. *Curr Alzheimer Res.* 2011;8(7):753–764.
40. Dichter GS, Sikich L, Song A, Voyvodic J, Bodfish JW. Functional neuroimaging of treatment effects in psychiatry: methodological challenges and recommendations. *Int J Neurosci.* 2012;122(9): 483–493.
41. N'Gouemo P, Faingold CL. Periaqueductal gray neurons exhibit increased responsiveness associated with audiogenic seizures in the genetically epilepsy-prone rat. *Neuroscience.* 1998;84(2): 619–625.
42. Devonshire IM, Papadakis NG, Port M, et al. Neurovascular coupling is brain region-dependent. *Neuroimage.* 2012;59:1997–2006.
43. Mishra A, Ellens D, Schridde U, et al. Where fMRI and electrophysiology agree to disagree: corticothalamic and striatal activity patterns in the WAG/Rij rat. *J Neurosci.* 2012;31:15053–15064.
44. Airaksinen AM, Hekmatyar SK, Jerome N, et al. Simultaneous BOLD fMRI and local field potential measurements during kainic acid-induced seizures. *Epilepsia.* 2012;53(7):1245–1253.
45. Fromm GH, Faingold CL, Browning RA, Burnham WM. *Epilepsy and the Reticular Formation: The Role of the Reticular Core in Convulsive Seizures.* A.R. Liss; 1987.
46. Faingold CL, Caspary DM. Effect of convulsant drugs on the brain-stem. In: Fromm GH, Faingold CL, Browning RA, Burnham WM, eds. *Epilepsy and the Reticular Formation: The Role of the Reticular Core in Convulsive Seizures.* New York, NY: A.R. Liss; 1987:39–80.
47. Faingold CL, Riaz A. Neuronal networks in convulsant drug-induced seizures. In: Faingold CL, Fromm GH, eds. *Drugs for Control of Epilepsy: Actions on Neuronal Networks Involved in Seizure Disorders.* Boca Raton, FL: CRC Press; 1992:213–251.
48. Faingold CL, Hoffmann WE, Caspary DM. Comparative effects of convulsant drugs on the sensory responses of neurons in the amygdala and brainstem reticular formation. *Neuropharmacology.* 1985;24(12):1221–1230.
49. Möhler H. Cognitive enhancement by pharmacological and behavioral interventions: the murine Down syndrome model. *Biochem Pharmacol.* 2012;84(8):994–999.
50. Colas D, Chuluun B, Warrier D, et al. Short-term treatment with the $GABA_A$ receptor antagonist pentylenetetrazole produces a

sustained pro-cognitive benefit in a mouse model of Down's syndrome. *Br J Pharmacol.* 2013;169(5):963–973.
51. Carp J, Park J, Polk TA, Park DC. Age differences in neural distinctiveness revealed by multi-voxel pattern analysis. *Neuroimage.* 2011;56(2):736–743.
52. Faingold CL, Hoffmann WE, Caspary DM. Bicuculline-induced enhancement of sensory responses and cross-correlations between reticular formation and cortical neurons. *Electroencephalogr Clin Neurophysiol.* 1983;55(3):301–313.
53. Corbett A, Smith J, Ballard C. New and emerging treatments for Alzheimer's disease. *Expert Rev Neurother.* 2012;12(5):535–543.
54. Dhanjal NS, Warren JE, Patel MC, Wise RJ. Auditory cortical function during verbal episodic memory encoding in Alzheimer's disease. *Ann Neurol.* 2013;73(2):294–302.
55. Faingold CL, Hoffmann WE, Caspary DM. Effects of iontophoretic application of convulsants on the sensory responses of neurons in the brain-stem reticular formation. *Electroencephalogr Clin Neurophysiol.* 1984;58(1):55–64.
56. Baker PM, Pennefather PS, Orser BA, Skinner FK. Disruption of coherent oscillations in inhibitory networks with anesthetics: role of $GABA_A$ receptor desensitization. *J Neurophysiol.* 2002;88(5):2821–2833.
57. Tannenbaum AS. The sense of consciousness. *J Theor Biol.* 2001; 211(4):377–391.
58. Urban BW, Friederich P. Anesthetic mechanisms in-vitro and in general anesthesia. *Toxicol Lett.* 1998;100–101:9–16.
59. Syka J, Popelár J, Radil-Weiss T. Comparison of spontaneous activity of mesencephalic reticular neurones in the waking state and during pentobarbital anaesthesia. *Physiol Bohemoslov.* 1977;26(1):21–30.
60. Shimoji K, Fujioka H, Fukazawa T, Hashiba M, Maruyama Y. Anesthetics and excitatory/inhibitory responses of midbrain reticular neurons. *Anesthesiology.* 1984;61(2):151–155.
61. Cullen KD, Martin RJ. Effects of injectable anaesthetics on responses to L-glutamate and on spontaneous synaptic activity in lamprey reticulo-spinal neurones. *Br J Pharmacol.* 1984;82(3):659–666.
62. Pavlasek J, Hricovini M. Effect of pentobarbital on neurones in the reticular formation of the brain stem: ionophoretic study in the rat. *Gen Physiol Biophys.* 1984;3(6):463–473.
63. Devor M, Zalkind V. Reversible analgesia, atonia, and loss of consciousness on bilateral intracerebral microinjection of pentobarbital. *Pain.* 2001;94(1):101–112.
64. Samineni V, Premkumar L, Faingold CL. Changes in periaqueductal gray neuronal responses to pain induced by barbiturate administration. *Anesthesiology.* submitted for publication.
65. Ciobanu L, Reynaud O, Uhrig L, Jarraya B, Le Bihan D. Effects of anesthetic agents on brain blood oxygenation level revealed with ultra-high field MRI. *PLoS One.* 2012;7(3):e32645.
66. Fukuda M, Vazquez AL, Zong X, Kim SG. Effects of the α_2-adrenergic receptor agonist dexmedetomidine on neural, vascular and BOLD fMRI responses in the somatosensory cortex. *Eur J Neurosci.* 2013;37(1):80–95.
67. Luchtmann M, Jachau K, Tempelmann C, Bernarding J. Alcohol induced region-dependent alterations of hemodynamic response: implications for the statistical interpretation of pharmacological fMRI studies. *Exp Brain Res.* 2010;204(1):1–10.
68. Cromwell HC, Woodward DJ. Inhibitory gating of single unit activity in amygdala: effects of ketamine, haloperidol, or nicotine. *Biol Psychiatry.* 2007;61(7):880–889.
69. Miller LM, Escabi MA, Read HL, Schreiner CE. Spectrotemporal receptive fields in the lemniscal auditory thalamus and cortex. *J Neurophysiol.* 2002;87(1):516–527.
70. Machado-Vieira R, Salvadore G, Diazgranados N, Zarate Jr CA. Ketamine and the next generation of antidepressants with a rapid onset of action. *Pharmacol Ther.* 2009;123:143–150.
71. Doyle OM, De Simoni S, Schwarz AJ, et al. Quantifying the attenuation of the ketamine pharmacological magnetic resonance imaging response in humans: a validation using antipsychotic and glutamatergic agents. *J Pharmacol Exp Ther.* 2013;345(1):151–160.
72. Niesters M, Khalili-Mahani N, Martini C, et al. Effect of subanesthetic ketamine on intrinsic functional brain connectivity: a placebo-controlled functional magnetic resonance imaging study in healthy male volunteers. *Anesthesiology.* 2012;117(4):868–877.
73. Hodkinson DJ, de Groote C, McKie S, Deakin JF, Williams SR. Differential effects of anaesthesia on the phMRI response to acute ketamine challenge. *Br J Med Med Res.* 2012;2(3):373–385.
74. Kumar S, Porcu P, Werner DF, et al. The role of $GABA_A$ receptors in the acute and chronic effects of ethanol: a decade of progress. *Psychopharmacology (Berl).* 2009;205(4):529–564.
75. Chandrasekar R. Alcohol and NMDA receptor: current research and future direction. *Front Mol Neurosci.* 2013;6:14.
76. Aguayo LG, Peoples RW, Yeh HH, Yevenes GE. $GABA_A$ receptors as molecular sites of ethanol action. Direct or indirect actions? *Curr Top Med Chem.* 2002;2(8):869–885.
77. Akk G, Steinbach JH. Low doses of ethanol and a neuroactive steroid positively interact to modulate rat $GABA_A$ receptor function. *J Physiol.* 2003;546(Pt 3):641–646.
78. Kumar S, Sieghart W, Morrow AL. Association of protein kinase C with $GABA_A$ receptors containing $\alpha1$ and $\alpha4$ subunits in the cerebral cortex: selective effects of chronic ethanol consumption. *J Neurochem.* 2002;82(1):110–117.
79. Faingold CL. The Majchrowicz binge alcohol protocol: an intubation technique to study alcohol dependence in rats. *Curr Protoc Neurosci.* 2008 Chapter 9:Unit 9.28.
80. Faingold CL, Knapp DJ, Chester JA, Gonzalez LP. Integrative neurobiology of the alcohol withdrawal syndrome—from anxiety to seizures. *Alcohol Clin Exp Res.* 2004;28(2):268–278.
81. Faingold CL, Riaz A. Increased responsiveness of pontine reticular formation neurons associated with audiogenic seizure susceptibility during ethanol withdrawal. *Brain Res.* 1994;663(1): 69–76.
82. Faingold CL, Riaz A. Ethanol withdrawal induces increased firing in inferior colliculus neurons associated with audiogenic seizure susceptibility. *Exp Neurol.* 1995;132(1):91–98.
83. Yang L, Long C, Faingold CL. Neurons in the deep layers of superior colliculus are a requisite component of the neuronal network for seizures during ethanol withdrawal. *Brain Res.* 2001; 920(1–2):134–141.
84. Yang L, Long C, Randall ME, Faingold CL. Neurons in the periaqueductal gray are critically involved in the neuronal network for audiogenic seizures during ethanol withdrawal. *Neuropharmacology.* 2003;44(2):275–281.
85. Feng HJ, Yang L, Faingold CL. Role of the amygdala in ethanol withdrawal seizures. *Brain Res.* 2007;1141:65–73.
86. Faingold CL. Role of GABA abnormalities in the inferior colliculus pathophysiology – audiogenic seizures. *Hear Res.* 2002; 168(1–2):223–237.
87. Huang JJ, Yet CT, Tsai ML, Valenzuela CF, Huang C. Acute ethanol exposure increases firing and induces oscillations in cerebellar Golgi cells of freely moving rats. *Alcohol Clin Exp Res.* 2012;36(12):2110–2116.
88. Criswell HE, Ming Z, Griffith BL, Breese GR. Comparison of effect of ethanol on N-methyl-D-aspartate- and GABA-gated currents from acutely dissociated neurons: absence of regional differences in sensitivity to ethanol. *J Pharmacol Exp Ther.* 2003;304(1):192–199.
89. Simson PE, Criswell HE, Breese GR. Inhibition of NMDA-evoked electrophysiological activity by ethanol in selected brain regions: evidence for ethanol-sensitive and ethanol-insensitive NMDA-evoked responses. *Brain Res.* 1993;607(1–2):9–16.
90. Faingold CL. Emergent properties of CNS neuronal networks as targets for pharmacology: application to anticonvulsant drug action. *Prog Neurobiol.* 2004;72:55–85.

91. Koepp MJ. Gender and drug effects on neuroimaging in epilepsy. *Epilepsia*. 2011;52(Suppl. 4):35–37.
92. Jokeit H, Okujava M, Woermann FG. Carbamazepine reduces memory induced activation of mesial temporal lobe structures: a pharmacological fMRI-study. *BMC Neurol*. 2001;1:6.
93. Jansen JF, Aldenkamp AP, Marian Majoie HJ, et al. Functional MRI reveals declined prefrontal cortex activation in patients with epilepsy on topiramate therapy. *Epilepsy Behav.* 2006;9(1):181–185.
94. Szaflarski JP, Kay B, Gotman J, Privitera MD, Holland SK. The relationship between the localization of the generalized spike and wave discharge generators and the response to valproate. *Epilepsia*. 2013;54(3):471–480.
95. Fromm GH, Terrence CF, Chattha AS. Differential effect of antiepileptic and non-antiepileptic drugs on the reticular formation. *Life Sci*. 1984;35(26):2665–2673.
96. Faingold CL, Randall ME, Naritoku DK, Boersma Anderson CA. Noncompetitive and competitive NMDA antagonists exert anticonvulsant effects by actions on different sites within the neuronal network for audiogenic seizures. *Exp Neurol*. 1993;119(2):198–204.
97. Faingold CL, Hoffmann WE, Caspary DM. Effects of excitant amino acids on acoustic responses of inferior colliculus neurons. *Hear Res*. 1989;40(1–2):127–136.
98. Zhang H, Kelly JB. Glutamatergic and GABAergic regulation of neural responses in inferior colliculus to amplitude-modulated sounds. *J Neurophysiol*. 2003;90(1):477–490.
99. Parks TN. The AMPA receptors of auditory neurons. *Hear Res*. 2000;147(1–2):77–91.
100. Fink-Jensen A, Suzdak PD, Swedberg MD, Judge ME, Hansen L, Nielsen PG. The gamma-aminobutyric acid (GABA) uptake inhibitor, tiagabine, increases extracellular brain levels of GABA in awake rats. *Eur J Pharmacol*. 1992;220(2–3):197–201.
101. Schousboe A, Madsen KK, White HS. GABA transport inhibitors and seizure protection: the past and future. *Future Med Chem*. 2011;3(2):183–187.
102. Faingold CL, Randall ME, Boersma Anderson CA. Blockade of GABA uptake with tiagabine inhibits audiogenic seizures and reduces neuronal firing in the inferior colliculus of the genetically epilepsy-prone rat. *Exp Neurol*. 1994;126:225–232.
103. Faingold CL, Boersma Anderson CA, Caspary DM. Involvement of GABA in acoustically-evoked inhibition in inferior colliculus neurons. *Hear Res*. 1991;52:201–216.
a. Faingold CL, Gehlbach G, Caspary DM. On the role of GABA as an inhibitory neurotransmitter in inferior colliculus neurons: iontophoretic studies. *Brain Res*. 1989;500(1–2):302–312.
104. Faingold CL, Randall ME. Pontine reticular formation neurons exhibit a premature and precipitous increase in acoustic responses prior to audiogenic seizures in genetically epilepsy-prone rats. *Brain Res*. 1995;704:218–226.
105. Dailey JW, Jobe PC. Anticonvulsant drugs and the genetically epilepsy-prone rat. *Fed Proc*. 1985;44(10):2640–2644.
106. N'Gouemo P, Faingold CL. Phenytoin administration reveals a differential role of pontine reticular formation and periaqueductal gray neurons in generation of the convulsive behaviors of audiogenic seizures. *Brain Res*. 2000;859(2):311–317.
107. Gale K. Mechanisms of seizure control mediated by gamma-aminobutyric acid: role of the substantia nigra. *Fed Proc*. 1985;44(8):2414–2424.
108. Millan MH, Meldrum BS, Boersma CA, Faingold CL. Excitant amino acids and audiogenic seizures in the genetically epilepsy-prone rat. II. Efferent seizure propagating pathway. *Exp Neurol*. 1988;99(3):687–698.
109. Applegate CD, Pretel S, Piekut DT. The substantia nigra pars reticulata, seizures and Fos expression. *Epilepsy Res*. 1995;20(1):31–39.
110. Deransart C, Le Pham BT, Hirsch E, Marescaux C, Depaulis A. Inhibition of the substantia nigra suppresses absences and clonic seizures in audiogenic rats, but not tonic seizures: evidence for seizure specificity of the nigral control. *Neuroscience*. 2001; 105(1):203–211.
111. Gonzalez LP, Hettinger MK. Intranigral muscimol suppresses ethanol withdrawal seizures. *Brain Res*. 1984;298(1):163–166.
112. Frye GD, McCown TJ, Breese GR. Characterization of susceptibility to audiogenic seizures in ethanol-dependent rats after microinjection of gamma-aminobutyric acid (GABA) agonists into the inferior colliculus, substantia nigra or medial septum. *J Pharmacol Exp Ther*. 1983;227(3):663–670.
113. Dalby NO. GABA-level increasing and anticonvulsant effects of three different GABA uptake inhibitors. *Neuropharmacology*. 2000; 39:2399–2407.
114. Bloms-Funke P, Loscher W. The anticonvulsant gabapentin decreases firing rates of substantia nigra pars reticulata neurons. *Eur J Pharmacol*. 1996;316(2–3):211–218.
115. Loscher W, Honack D, Bloms-Funke P. The novel antiepileptic drug levetiracetam (ucb L059) induces alterations in GABA metabolism and turnover in discrete areas of rat brain and reduces neuronal activity in substantia nigra pars reticulata. *Brain Res*. 1996;735(2):208–216.
116. Waszczak BL, Lee EK, Walters JR. Effects of anticonvulsant drugs on substantia nigra pars reticulata neurons. *J Pharmacol Exp Ther*. 1986;239(2):606–611.
117. Wolf R, Tscherne U. Valproate effect on gamma-aminobutyric acid release in pars reticulata of substantia nigra: combination of push-pull perfusion and fluorescence histochemistry. *Epilepsia*. 1994;35(1):226–233.
118. Moshe SL, Garant DS. Substantia nigra GABA receptors can mediate anticonvulsant or proconvulsant effects. *Epilepsy Res Suppl*. 1996; 12:247–256.
119. Faingold CL. Brainstem networks: reticulo-cortical synchronization in generalized convulsive seizures. In: Noebels JL, Avoli M, Rogawski MA, Olsen RW, Delgado-Escueta AV, eds. *Jasper's Basic Mechanisms of the Epilepsies*. 4th ed. New York, NY: Oxford University Press; 2012:257–271.
120. Rick CE, Lacey MG. Rat substantia nigra pars reticulata neurones are tonically inhibited via $GABA_A$, but not $GABA_B$, receptors in vitro. *Brain Res*. 1994;659(1–2):133–137.
121. Bowery NG, Wong EH, Hudson AL. Quantitative autoradiography of [^{3}H]-MK-801 binding sites in mammalian brain. *Br J Pharmacol*. 1988;93(4):944–954.
122. Kornhuber J, Mack-Burkhardt F, Kornhuber ME, Riederer P. [^{3}H] MK-801 binding sites in post-mortem human frontal cortex. *Eur J Pharmacol*. 1989;162(3):483–490.
123. He L, Di Monte DA, Langston JW, Quik M. Autoradiographic analysis of *N*-methyl-D-aspartate receptor binding in monkey brain: effects of 1-methyl-4-phenyl-1,2,3, 6-tetrahydropyridine and levodopa treatment. *Neuroscience*. 2000;99(4):697–704.
124. Faingold CL. Anticonvulsant drugs as neuronal network-modifying agents. In: Schwartzkroin PA, ed. *Encyclopedia of Basic Epilepsy Research*. Vol. 1, Academic Press; 2009:50–58.
125. Cheshire WP. Trigeminal neuralgia: for one nerve a multitude of treatments. *Expert Rev Neurother*. 2007;7(11):1565–1579.
126. Lu DP, Lu WI, Lu GP. Phenytoin (Dilantin) and acupuncture therapy in the treatment of intractable oral and facial pain. *Acupunct Electrother Res*. 2011;36(1–2):65–84.
127. Bialer M. Why are antiepileptic drugs used for nonepileptic conditions? *Epilepsia*. 2012;53(Suppl. 7):26–33.
128. Linnman C, Moulton EA, Barmettler G, Becerra L, Borsook D. Neuroimaging of the periaqueductal gray: state of the field. *Neuroimage*. 2012;60(1):505–522.
129. Wager TD, Atlas LY, Lindquist MA, Roy M, Woo CW, Kross E. An fMRI-based neurologic signature of physical pain. *N Engl J Med*. 2013;368(15):1388–1397.

130. Becerra L, Upadhyay J, Chang PC, et al. Parallel buprenorphine phMRI responses in conscious rodents and healthy human subjects. *J Pharmacol Exp Ther.* 2013;345(1):41–51.
131. Iannetti GD, Zambreanu L, Wise RG, et al. Pharmacological modulation of pain-related brain activity during normal and central sensitization states in humans. *Proc Natl Acad Sci USA.* 2005;102(50):18195–18200.
132. Governo RJ, Morris PG, Marsden CA, Chapman V. Gabapentin evoked changes in functional activity in nociceptive regions in the brain of the anaesthetized rat: an fMRI study. *Br J Pharmacol.* 2008;153(7):1558–1567.
133. Takemura Y, Yamashita A, Horiuchi H, et al. Effects of gabapentin on brain hyperactivity related to pain and sleep disturbance under a neuropathic pain-like state using fMRI and brain wave analysis. *Synapse.* 2011;65(7):668–676.
134. Tupal S, Faingold CL. The amygdala to periaqueductal gray pathway: plastic changes induced by audiogenic kindling and reversal by gabapentin. *Brain Res.* 2012;1475:71–79.
135. Feng HJ, Naritoku DK, Randall ME, Faingold CL. Modulation of audiogenically kindled seizures by gamma-aminobutyric acid--related mechanisms in the amygdala. *Exp Neurol.* 2001;172(2): 477–481.
136. Flatters SJ, Bennett GJ. Ethosuximide reverses paclitaxel- and vincristine-induced painful peripheral neuropathy. *Pain.* 2004; 109(1–2):150–161.
137. Samineni V, Premkumar L, Faingold CL. Chronic pain induces neuroplastic changes in periaqueductal gray neuronal firing: blockade by gabapentin. *Soc Neurosci Abs.* 2012, 178.11/GG2.
138. Yared JA, Tkaczuk KH. Update on taxane development: new analogs and new formulations. *Drug Des Devel Ther.* 2012;6:371–384.
139. Rogawski MA, Bazil CW. New molecular targets for antiepileptic drugs: $\alpha_2\delta$, SV2A, and K_v7/KCNQ/M potassium channels. *Curr Neurol Neurosci Rep.* 2008;8(4):345–352.
140. Richerson GB, Wu Y. Role of the GABA transporter in epilepsy. *Adv Exp Med Biol.* 2004;548:76–91.
141. Cai K, Nanga RP, Lamprou L, et al. The impact of gabapentin administration on brain GABA and glutamate concentrations: a 7T ^{1}H-MRS study. *Neuropsychopharmacology.* 2012;37(13):2764–2771.
142. Ueda H. Molecular mechanisms of neuropathic pain-phenotypic switch and initiation mechanisms. *Pharmacol Ther.* 2006; 109(1–2):57–77.
143. Grabenstatter HL, Russek SJ, Brooks-Kayal AR. Molecular pathways controlling inhibitory receptor expression. *Epilepsia.* 2012; 53(Suppl. 9):71–78.
144. Zhang JL, Yang JP, Zhang JR, et al. Gabapentin reduces allodynia and hyperalgesia in painful diabetic neuropathy rats by decreasing expression level of Nav1.7 and p-ERK1/2 in DRG neurons. *Brain Res.* 2013;1493:13–18.
145. Kumar P, Kalonia H, Kumar A. Possible GABAergic mechanism in the neuroprotective effect of gabapentin and lamotrigine against 3-nitropropionic acid induced neurotoxicity. *Eur J Pharmacol.* 2012;674(2–3):265–274.
146. Hanaya R, Kiura Y, Serikawa T, Kurisu K, Arita K, Sasa M. Modulation of abnormal synaptic transmission in hippocampal CA3 neurons of spontaneously epileptic rats (SERs) by levetiracetam. *Brain Res Bull.* 2011;86(5–6):334–339.
147. Tang H, Long H, Zeng C, et al. Rapamycin suppresses the recurrent excitatory circuits of dentate gyrus in a mouse model of temporal lobe epilepsy. *Biochem Biophys Res Commun.* 2012; 420(1):199–204.
148. Newton SS, Duman RS. Neurogenic actions of atypical antipsychotic drugs and therapeutic implications. *CNS Drugs.* 2007; 21(9):715–725.
149. Longo FM, Yang T, Xie Y, Massa SM. Small molecule approaches for promoting neurogenesis. *Curr Alzheimer Res.* 2006;3(1):5–10.
150. David DJ, Wang J, Samuels BA, et al. Implications of the functional integration of adult-born hippocampal neurons in anxiety-depression disorders. *Neuroscientist.* 2010;16(5): 578–591.
151. Chiu CT, Wang Z, Hunsberger JG, Chuang DM. Therapeutic potential of mood stabilizers lithium and valproic acid: beyond bipolar disorder. *Pharmacol Rev.* 2013;65(1):105–142.
152. Ohno Y. New insight into the therapeutic role of 5-HT_{1A} receptors in central nervous system disorders. *Cent Nerv Syst Agents Med Chem.* 2010;10(2):148–157.
153. Mostert JP, Koch MW, Heerings M, Heersema DJ, De Keyser J. Therapeutic potential of fluoxetine in neurological disorders. *CNS Neurosci Ther.* 2008;14(2):153–164.
154. Loscher W, Rogawski MA. How theories evolved concerning the mechanism of action of barbiturates. *Epilepsia.* 2012;53(Suppl. 8): 12–25.
155. Shorvon S. Clinical trials in acute repetitive seizures and status epilepticus. *Epileptic Disord.* 2012;14(2):138–147.
156. Kobow K, El-Osta A, Blümcke I. The methylation hypothesis of pharmacoresistance in epilepsy. *Epilepsia.* 2013;54(Suppl. 2): 41–47.
157. Rogawski MA. The intrinsic severity hypothesis of pharmacoresistance to antiepileptic drugs. *Epilepsia.* 2013;54(Suppl. 2):33–40.
158. Fang M, Xi ZQ, Wu Y, Wang XF. A new hypothesis of drug refractory epilepsy: neural network hypothesis. *Med Hypotheses.* 2011;76(6):871–876.

CHAPTER

33

Future Trends in Neuronal Networks—Selective and Combined Targeting of Network Hubs

Carl L. Faingold[1], *Hal Blumenfeld*[2]

[1]Departments of Pharmacology and Neurology, Division of Neurosurgery, Southern Illinois University School of Medicine, Springfield, IL, USA, [2]Departments of Neurology, Neurobiology, and Neurosurgery, Yale University School of Medicine, New Haven, CT, USA

INTRODUCTION

One thing that seems crystal clear is that we will never understand brain function by attempting to comprehensively evaluate and combine the information on the activities of each of the estimated 80–100 million neurons in the human brain, integrate this with their multiple synaptic contacts, and factor in the myriad of neuroactive influences on each of these neurons. As chapters throughout this book have illustrated, brain function is carried out by mesoscopic networks of neurons.[1] Many of these networks are organized to perform specific vital functions like breathing or hearing, but others have more complicated functions such as mediating emotional states. These networks often interact with one another in even more complex arrangements that can also mediate central nervous system (CNS) disorders, as discussed in Chapter 29. It is clear that much more needs to be known about these brain mechanisms, and innovative approaches will be needed to ferret out these many mysteries. Our current situation is a bit like the proverbial blind men and the elephant, but the further complexity is that our creature is capable of "shape-shifting" over time as well. We have only isolated pieces of information, which we are trying to fit together into a multidimensional puzzle. For example, we know that these neurons interact in neuronal populations or networks, but we have only a rudimentary idea of the rules that govern these processes. In addition, the brain and its networks can change in response to experience (i.e. they undergo neuroplasticity, as discussed in several chapters of this book). A major class of changes in network function can be considered network expansion ("gain of function") (Chapter 27), but these changes can often be pathological in nature. Thus, certain CNS disorders, such as epilepsy, are subject to gain-of-function neuroplastic changes, even though the "gain" in this case may exacerbate the condition. Networks in other CNS disorders are subject to contraction or "loss of function", which is most commonly seen in neurodegenerative diseases such as Parkinson's disease (Chapter 25) and Alzheimer's disease (AD) (this chapter). An improved understanding of normal networks and how they change in CNS disorders is a critical future goal. Improved approaches to treating these CNS disorders will need to capitalize on our current knowledge to develop drugs with novel mechanisms of action as well as innovative stimulation therapies. It could be argued that our knowledge is too fragmented to accomplish this in an intelligent way. However, because patients are suffering the consequences of CNS disorders now, we need to translate what we already know into better, more targeted approaches to therapy now. Some partially effective drugs might become more effective by better targeting of specific network hubs where they can act selectively on the emergent properties of the neurons in that site (Chapter 30). In addition, improved therapies could also be developed if we had better integration of approaches by combining drugs with targeted stimulation therapies of various kinds, as discussed in this chapter (also see Chapters 31 and 32).

It is generally agreed that the intermediate or mesoscopic neuronal network is the functional unit of the

Neuronal Networks in Brain Function, CNS Disorders, and Therapeutics
http://dx.doi.org/10.1016/B978-0-12-415804-7.00033-2

brain (Chapter 1). Therefore, exploration of the mechanisms involved in the operation of normal mesoscopic networks is critical for improving the understanding of brain function. These advances will proceed initially from the techniques we currently utilize in this research, many of which are described in Chapters 2–6. Newer, not-yet-developed techniques will undoubtedly be added to these approaches, such as improved neuroimaging in awake animals[2] (see Chapter 3) to yield a better understanding of network function. Other approaches include new types of drugs that target networks, including agents that act genetically[3] or epigenetically,[4] and electroceuticals.[5]

GENERAL APPROACH TO NEURONAL NETWORK EXPLORATION

As noted in the introduction, we expect that the future of neuronal network research will involve advances in our understanding of the normal function of these networks, which will allow improvements in the treatment of disorders that affect these networks. Thus, an improved understanding of normal sensory networks will lead to better approaches for treating people who have developed abnormal functions of these systems. So, for example, continuing auditory network research, as discussed in Chapter 20, is likely to lead to improvements in the treatment of disorders that affect this network, such as age-related hearing loss and tinnitus. In locomotor networks, discussed in Chapter 17, improved knowledge of normal function should lead to better treatments for damage to the network, such as spinal cord injuries that prevent normal motor movements.

Research focusing on the nature and mechanisms that are operative in the networks that subserve other CNS disorders is also proceeding and can be expected to yield improved characterization of the causes for these disorders, such as those discussed in Chapters 21–26. Research thus far has indicated that many of these disorders involve the interaction of normal networks with each other; this can be additive in nature, as when one network triggers the activity of a second or even a third network. Alternatively, the interaction can be negative wherein the first network induces a decrease in the function of a second network (see Chapter 29). The study of network interactions is actually in its infancy and requires much more intensive investigation. These research trends can be expected to lead eventually to major improvements in the therapy of these CNS disorders. Better network definition in human disorders is obviously an important need in future research. Our proposal for a potential blueprint for future exploration of CNS neuronal networks and the development of improved drug and stimulation therapies for these disorders is discussed in the "Mechanistic Studies of Drug Actions on Networks" section.

Based on our current understanding of the normal neuronal network mechanisms, we can then evaluate the changes that occur in CNS disorders initially by more extensive use and improved methods of neuroimaging, such as combining positron emission tomography (PET) with magnetic resonance imaging (MRI).[6] We also need to continue to develop animal models that faithfully recreate critical elements of the human disorder. This will likely require the use of more than one model for a given disorder, because each model may not exhibit all the features of the human condition. This may be due, in part, to the fact that animal brains are considerably smaller in neuronal number and synaptic connections and lack much of the sophisticated connectivity of the cerebral cortex that is characteristic of human brains. Also, animal models of behavior, especially for psychiatric conditions, are difficult to develop, because we cannot directly assess the mental state of an animal. Therefore, there is a major inferential element in models of psychiatric disease that exceeds that in models of neurological diseases such as Parkinson's disease and epilepsy, as these diseases in animals exhibit overt, clearly observable similarities (tremors or convulsions) compared to their human counterparts. However, it is more than likely that there are multiple brain networks that can produce similar behaviors, which reinforces the need for multiple models. In many neuronal networks, certain brain structures are requisite (i.e. required) for the CNS disorder to become manifest, but other structures are only ancillary. These ancillary structures receive projections from the requisite network nuclei and may become activated, but their activation is not required for the disorder to occur. However, the ancillary sites may become more involved in the disorder as the network expands due to repetitive episodes of the disorder (Chapter 27). The animal models may or may not show involvement of the ancillary structures, but they do model the many important features of the disorder nonetheless (see Chapters 26 and 27). Once useful models are developed, new therapies, including stimulation paradigms and new and repurposed drugs, can be tested for effectiveness as compared to toxicity (see Chapters 31 and 32).

As useful models have been and continue to be developed, the mechanisms that subserve the function of those networks can be evaluated. The evaluation includes, most importantly, the neuronal firing patterns in the requisite network nuclei that lead to the expression of the disorder, since neurons are the ultimate operational elements in expression of the symptoms. Finally, we can evaluate how therapies, including drugs and therapeutic stimulation paradigms, alter these abnormal network functions in the animal models. These observations will allow a better understanding of how current therapies work and suggest ways to improve them.

As noted in this chapter, a key element in future network exploration is improved neuroimaging of human disorders. Functional MRI (fMRI) is a breakthrough technique for exploring networks, as discussed in Chapters 3 and 6, but there are significant caveats regarding the interpretation of fMRI findings, as discussed in these chapters. The most important concern about fMRI is the decoupling of neuronal firing activity from neuroimaging results for certain important brain areas,[7,8] which clearly indicates that other techniques are needed to supplement fMRI. There may be technical methods for improving this limitation of fMRI.[9] Comparisons between the results of network studies in human disorders and animal models suggest that there are considerable interspecies network similarities[10,11] (see Chapters 3 and 6). It is critically important to have good animal models in which requisite brain sites in the network that subserves the CNS disorder can be identified. This will allow invasive techniques, such as neuronal recording studies, to be performed. Neuronal firing data are critical in order to obtain important mechanistic information that may not be available from neuroimaging data. Although many CNS disorders are stable and/or subject to pathological expansion, many CNS disorders are degenerative (see Chapter 25). The networks in these degenerative disorders undergo degradation, requiring the strategies for therapy to be quite different, as discussed here.

A proposed list of the steps in the future exploration of CNS neuronal networks is shown in Table 33.1. Ideally, future research should start with human neuroimaging of normal network function and evaluation of the changes in these networks in patients with each CNS disorder. It is also extremely important to assess changes in neuroimaging patterns in the network that are induced when effective stimulation or drug therapies are administered. An example of this approach is the abnormal fMRI findings observed in patients with major depression, which can be reversed with successful antidepressant therapies.[12] Once the neuroimaging pattern in the human CNS disorder is developed, animal models need to be identified that mimic the behaviors of the CNS disorder and that show similar neuroimaging patterns to the human condition. An example of this may be the absence (petit mal) form of epilepsy in which neuroimaging of human and animal models exhibits similar patterns, as discussed in this chapter. The action of a drug or stimulation therapy that is effective in the human disorder can then be evaluated using both human and animal neuroimaging. However, it is critically important that the neuroimaging be done in awake, behaving animals, because even low doses of every

TABLE 33.1 Steps in Network Studies for Targeted Therapy of CNS Disorders

1. Network identification, human neuroimaging, and CNS disorders (Chapter 6)
   a. Examined in untreated patients
   b. Evaluate changes with effective therapies (drugs and stimulation paradigms) (Chapters 31 and 32)
2. Network modeling: animal neuroimaging disorder model[a] (Chapter 3)
3. Network operation: model
   a. Identify critical hubs[b]: focal blockade (Chapter 4)
   b. Identify neuron-firing abnormalities in hubs[c] (Chapters 4, 13, 22, and 26–32)
4. Animal model: therapeutics (Chapters 3 and 32)
   a. Determine effective therapies in model: current, new, and repurposed drugs and stimulation paradigms—animal neuroimaging changes
   b. Administer therapeutic doses of drugs and evaluate hub neuron-firing changes based on emergent properties (Chapter 32)
   c. Evaluate stimulation therapies' effects on hub neurons
   d. Examine combination therapies' actions on hub neurons
5. Animal model: mechanistic studies
   a. Evaluate the emergent property action of drugs by local application onto neurons in vivo
   b. Evaluate intracellular mechanisms in vitro (Chapters 5 and 10)
6. Human trials with new and repurposed therapies
7. Human neuroimaging of effective new therapies

[a]*Without anesthesia.*
[b]*It is crucial to differentiate requisite from ancillary sites, because requisite hubs are critical future targets of therapy.*
[c]*It is critical to identify abnormal neuronal firing patterns that the therapy is targeted to normalize.*

sedative, analgesic, and anesthetic drug that has been tested induce major network changes (see Chapters 3, 28, and 32). Thus, in Chapter 3, the differences in the neuroimaging of an animal model of absence epilepsy in the anesthetized as compared to the unanesthetized animal are extensive.

However, we cannot expect neuroimaging results in the animal models to perfectly model those in the human conditions, because of the greater complexity of the human brain, as noted here. We suggest that the approach to this problem should also consider the likelihood that all areas in the human brain that are affected by the CNS disorder are not all necessarily requisite hubs involved in generating the major symptoms of the disorder, which is based on animal studies. Thus, as discussed in several chapters of this volume, it can be seen that certain brain structures are requisite hubs (i.e. required) for the CNS disorder to occur, but a number of other structures may be ancillary. That is, the ancillary structures are connected to and affected by the requisite structures. These ancillary structures may contribute to additional elements or comorbidities of the CNS disorder, but these sites are *not* required for the initiation and expression of the disorder. However, there is no clear way to determine which sites are requisite sites using neuroimaging techniques, and invasive studies of the networks are required. It is also important to administer therapies (drug and stimulation paradigms) in the animal models that are effective in the human condition to verify that these therapies are effective in the models. New potential therapies and repurposed drugs can also be evaluated for effectiveness in the models.

Once the candidates for the sites involved in the neuronal network for a specific CNS disorder are identified, then invasive studies can begin in the animal models. Identification of the requisite brain structures that function as critical network hubs in the animal models can be determined by focal microinjection into the putative network sites identified by the neuroimaging data. To determine whether the identified sites are requisite hubs or ancillary sites, focal inactivation of the sites (see Chapter 4) can determine if this prevents the behavioral characteristic of the CNS disorder in the model. It is important to focally microinject small volumes of agents to localize the effect, and agents such as gamma-aminobutyric acid (GABA) receptor agonists or *N*-methyl-D-aspartate (NMDA) receptor antagonists are preferred since they exert minimal effects on fibers of passage. This approach is necessary to verify that only the neurons in the candidate site are being blocked. The amount of agent microinjected is critical, since microinjection of excessive amounts can exert effects at distant sites by volume transmission (Chapter 8). We propose the use of only reversible inactivation techniques, so recovery from the block can be verified. Thus, if blockade of a putative requisite site does not prevent or greatly modify the expression of the CNS disorder, the site is considered to be ancillary. *This is a very important distinction, since identification of requisite sites is critical for selective targeting of future therapies*. An example of this distinction is the role of the amygdala, which functions as an ancillary site in the audiogenic seizure model of epilepsy, as discussed in this chapter.

Among the requisite structures, there may be critical network hubs that can be targeted to "short-circuit" the rest of the network. An example of this is the periaqueductal gray (PAG) in both epilepsy and pain networks, as described in Chapter 32. Identifying the neuronal firing patterns in the requisite hubs in animal models during expression of the symptoms of the CNS disorder is critical to understanding how the network operates (see Chapter 26). Once a requisite site has been identified, neuronal firing patterns in the site need to be evaluated in awake, behaving animals to observe the changes that are occurring during each episode of the CNS disorder to determine if specific phases of the disorder are associated with specific firing changes as the symptoms begin, proceed, recede, and end (see Chapter 26). *These data are critical for the development of the most effective and selective future therapies by identifying the neuronal firing abnormalities that will be targeted in order to normalize them with the therapeutic intervention*. Neuronal firing information is needed, because this activity is a direct measure in real time of network operation. This contrasts with neuroimaging and field potential recording data, such as the electroencephalogram (EEG), which have much poorer temporal (neuroimaging) and spatial (field potentials) resolution[13] (see Chapter 6) and are only surrogates for the actual operational neuronal mechanisms that mediate expression of the disorder. However, as noted here, the neuronal activity may be abnormal in a putative requisite network, but if blockade of the site does not affect the appearance of the CNS disorder, the site is ancillary. This principle is exemplified by the role of the amygdala in an audiogenic seizure model of epilepsy, which clearly functions as an ancillary site despite exhibiting abnormal firing patterns during the seizure[14,15] (see Chapter 26). The neuronal actions of therapies that have been shown to be effective in the human condition and the model, as well as new potential therapies and repurposed drugs that were effective in the model, should be evaluated. Therapy-induced changes in neuronal firing patterns in requisite network hubs in the animal models are an important step in evaluating the mechanism of these effects. However, this must be limited to therapeutic doses (levels) of effective drugs (or stimulation paradigms), because this allows the search for specific sites of action on emergent properties in specific hubs in the animal model (see Chapter 32). An example of a drug that acts selectively on an emergent property in a requisite hub occurs with therapeutic doses of gabapentin on PAG neurons, which may be sufficient to alleviate the symptoms of both chronic pain and progressive epilepsy disorders, as observed in recent experiments[16–19] (see Chapter 32). A more difficult process to model is the effect of chronic therapies that are often required to treat certain CNS disorders, as this requires longitudinal studies that are not as easily done with invasive techniques. In addition, it must also be recognized that no known drug is a "magic bullet", and the selective effect of any agent on a single brain site is likely to occur only in the therapeutic dose range. It must also be understood that all drugs have potentially important adverse effects and toxicities. In fact, many recent therapeutic improvements involve drugs that may be no more effective than the older drugs, but they are more useful because they produce less severe adverse effects (e.g. newer antidepressant and anticonvulsant drugs). Repurposed drugs that affect one of the requisite sites could be brought back from the bench to the bedside, which could occur relatively quickly since the drugs are already approved by the US Food and Drug

Administration (FDA) for another use, and toxicity and tolerability studies in humans have already been performed. An example of a drug that has been suggested for repurposing is furosemide, which is a nonselective inhibitor of cation–chloride co-transporters (expressed in neurons and glia) and is widely used currently as an antihypertensive drug. Furosemide may have clinically relevant antiepileptic actions, especially in combination with GABA-mimetic drugs such as phenobarbital.[20] Clinical testing of any new or repurposed drugs would need to be done, but this may be problematic financially, especially if the drug patent has expired. Publically supported resources may need to be recruited for these clinical studies. New agents that prove clinically effective should be subject to fMRI studies to evaluate details about the nature of drug-induced changes in network operation. If novel changes are observed, this can lead to an iterative process requiring new studies in the animal models.

The potential application of several aspects of these approaches to therapy of CNS disorders in a prototypical network is shown in Figure 33.1. The network consists of an input, several network nuclei (Sites 1–4) with pathways between the sites, and output via the spinal cord (for example) of the symptom(s) of the CNS disorder. Specific drug therapies for this disorder can act at an emergent property of one or more specific network sites to affect neuronal firing there, reducing network activity and alleviating the symptoms of the disorder. The target for each brain site is illustrated as potentially involving a selective emergent property in a specific network site upon which certain drugs act in therapeutic doses. In gain-of-function CNS disorders, repeated episodes of the disorder can cause the network to expand to an additional nucleus (Site Ω). This often involves neuroplastic changes in the projection pathways, increasing network output, and results in more increased severity and/or additional symptoms of the disorder. Stimulation therapy potentially inactivates network sites or activates dormant pathways that compete with the CNS disorder network for control of the network sites, diminishing its involvement in the CNS disorder. Combined drug and stimulation therapies can potentially exert additive or even synergistic effects.

In loss-of-function CNS disorders, as seen in neurodegenerative disorders, the pathway between two sites of a normal network may degenerate, causing a loss of normal function, which leads to the symptoms of the disorder. Drug and/or therapeutic stimulation paradigms can be directed at a specific nucleus (Site Δ) or pathways to activate a dormant pathway via a previously uninvolved site, such as a conditional multireceptive brain region, or inactivate an overly active site (see Chapter 28). The activation process would bypass the damaged pathway and restore normal function. In

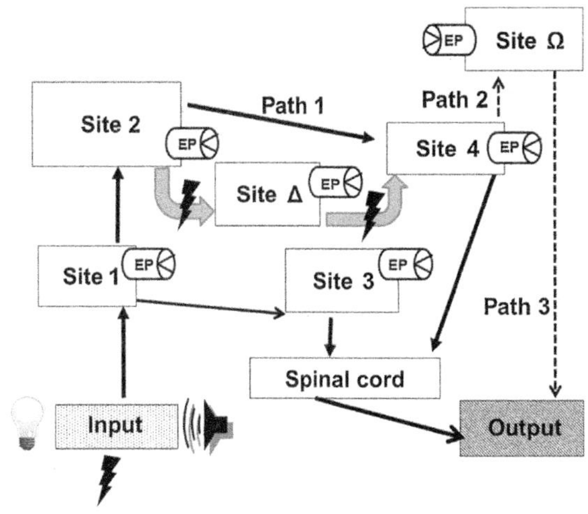

FIGURE 33.1 Prototypical network that subserves a CNS disorder that consists of an input, several network nuclei (Sites 1–4) with pathways between the sites, and output symptoms. The diagram also illustrates potential targets for therapy, including an emergent property (EP) of neurons in each brain site. In "gain-of-function" CNS disorders, such as many cases of epilepsy, after repeated episodes of the disorder the network may expand to additional nuclei (Site Ω) carried by enhanced projections via Path 2, which may result in increased severity of the disorder and/or additional symptoms due to increased output via Path 3. Potential specific drug therapies of this CNS disorder can act at the EP of one or more specific network sites to reduce or block neuronal firing there, reduce activity of the network, and reduce or prevent symptoms of the disorder. Stimulation therapy in the periphery or within the brain can inactivate one or more of the network sites or activate a dormant pathway that competes with the CNS disorder network for control of one or more of the network sites, diminishing its involvement in the CNS disorder. Combined drug and stimulation therapies can potentially exert additive or even superadditive effects. In "loss-of-function" CNS disorders, as seen in neurodegenerative disorders, the pathway (Path 1) between Site 2 and Site 4 may degenerate, causing a loss of normal function and symptoms of the disorder. Drug and/or therapeutic stimulation paradigms can be directed at specific nuclei or pathways to activate a dormant pathway via Site Δ to bypass the damaged pathway and restore normal function. In loss-of-function disorders, a therapeutically useful drug could act on the EP of a network site to increase neuronal firing activity or in a dormant site to restore the normal function of the network, which may also be induced by a therapeutic stimulation paradigm. Again, combined drug and stimulation therapies may exert additive or superadditive effects. (For color version of this figure, the reader is referred to the online version of this book.)

these loss-of-function disorders, a useful drug could act on the emergent property of a network site to increase neuronal firing activity or, in a dormant site, to restore the normal function of the network. Such effects may also be induced by a therapeutic stimulation paradigm, as discussed in this chapter for stroke and AD. Again, combined drug and stimulation therapies may exert additive or synergistic effects.

Emergent properties of neurons in mesoscopic networks are dealt with in detail in Chapter 30 and can really be investigated only in awake, behaving, and drug-free animals. Investigation of the exact nature of the action of drugs on emergent properties needs to be done in vivo beginning with the lowest effective therapeutic dose to assure that it is acting on the emergent property of neurons in a specific brain nucleus in the specific CNS disorder model. It is possible that a general action of a given drug on an emergent property of neurons in a specific brain site can occur in more than one type of disorder, as seen with gabapentin in chronic pain and progressive epilepsy (see Chapter 32). Combinations of drugs and therapeutic stimulation paradigms could also be tested (Chapter 31), such as that which has been utilized in chronic pain therapy.[21,22] Several approaches to evaluating the mechanisms that mediate emergent properties can be envisaged.

MECHANISTIC STUDIES OF DRUG ACTIONS ON NETWORKS

Once experimental evidence indicates that an emergent property is occurring in neurons in a specific network hub, the mechanisms involved in that emergent property need to be investigated, but this process has not been well utilized as yet. Evaluation of the mechanisms that mediate emergent properties in CNS disorder models should involve several of the following approaches in intact, behaving animals. The drug should be administered systemically in the model, and an agent that potentially blocks the putative action of that agent could be applied onto the neurons in the network hub where the emergent property is being expressed. Ideally, this could be applied while recording the activity of the neuron simultaneously. In addition, the agent itself could be directly applied onto the neurons in that network hub to see if it produces the same effect that is seen with systemic administration. An illustrative example of the use of these approaches on the effects of $GABA_A$ receptor antagonists using an iontophoretic or pneumatic application of agents directly onto recorded neurons, as discussed in this chapter, or by microinjection of an antagonist into the site to observe if it blocked the effect of the agent when administered systemically.

Electrical or chemical stimulation of sites within the network can help determine the nature of the relationship between two structures and determine if this relationship undergoes changes from normal animals in the model of the disorder. This could include evaluation of the relationship change of a structure within network ancillary structures to determine neuronal firing changes involved in network expansion (see Chapter 27). For example, network expansion in a repetitive seizure protocol called audiogenic seizure (AGS) kindling results in recruitment of the amygdala as an important (but not requisite) network hub (Chapter 27). The amygdala is known to project to the PAG, which is a requisite hub in the AGS network (see Chapter 26). The amygdala-to-PAG pathway is also implicated in other CNS disorders, including chronic pain, depression, and anxiety (see Chapters 23 and 24). Thus, the amygdala is known to be a key element in the neuronal network for depression, which is a common comorbidity in epileptic patients,[23] and evidence of depression has also been observed in AGS-susceptible rats.[24] Electrical stimulation in the amygdala consistently evokes neuronal responses in PAG,[25] and AGS kindling causes major increases in PAG responsiveness to amygdala stimulation. These findings indicate that a major neuroplastic change has occurred in this pathway.[19] As noted here, once a network hub is characterized in vivo, further studies in vitro may be obtained using brain slices that allow some of the major anatomical pathways to remain intact, which allows intracellular mechanisms to be explored. For example, studies of network mechanisms have examined changes in the properties of PAG neurons associated with AGS susceptibility in PAG brain slices. In these studies, glutamate-mediated excitatory postsynaptic potentials were greatly enhanced in PAG neurons of AGS-susceptible rats as compared to normal rats.[26] These data indicate the nature of a major mechanism of AGS susceptibility in the PAG.

An important point that we will emphasize throughout this chapter is that improved approaches to the treatment of CNS disorders may require employing combined drug treatment with a therapeutic stimulation paradigm (Chapters 31 and 32) (see Refs 21,22). Ideally, such combined therapies would involve a drug that selectively affects neuronal activity in a critical requisite network hub, along with a stimulation paradigm that also selectively affects that site or another critical network nucleus to exert an additive or potentiating effect on this target site. This could involve either neuronal excitation or inhibition or both, depending on the approach needed to control the symptoms of the specific CNS disorder. In neuronal networks for CNS disorders that involve gain-of-function changes, as seen in certain forms of epilepsy, this would involve therapies directed to inhibit neurons in critical network hubs and short-circuit the disordered network. In addition, a stimulation paradigm that enhances firing could be combined with a drug treatment that inhibits that same site to cause a desensitization effect on the network. However, in neuronal networks for CNS disorders that involve loss of function, as seen in degenerative disorders such as Parkinson's disease and AD, the network has undergone deterioration. The approach to therapy in these cases would involve methods of reactivating the damaged pathways or activating alternative pathways to "patch" the network. This would allow normal function to return, as discussed in Chapters 25 and 31 for Parkinson's disease and here for AD.

SPECIFIC APPROACHES TO NEURONAL NETWORK MECHANISMS

Certain elements of the general approach described in Table 33.1 have been applied to neuronal networks in humans and animal models of CNS disorders. This section will illustrate some examples of experiments that involved several of the steps in Table 33.1. However, no comprehensive application of such a systematic approach has been performed as yet. It may not have been possible earlier, because only now have we amassed sufficient information on neuronal networks to employ such a systematic targeted approach. Elements of this comprehensive approach have been employed for various purposes in many animal models. Additional approaches for evaluating whether a specific requisite site is the target of the lowest effective dose of the drug include focal microinjection of the drug into that site to determine if this exerts the same action as systemic administration (see Chapters 4 and 32). If this occurs, it would be an indication that a property of these specific neurons in that site is a critical target of that drug. This property could be an emergent property of those neurons (Chapters 28 and 30). Therefore, to investigate the mechanisms behind the effect, we could evaluate it by combined focal drug administration and neuronal firing experiments using microapplication directly onto the target neurons (e.g. using iontophoresis, which is difficult in awake animals) or with combined electrode cannula implants.[27]

NETWORK EFFECTS OF COMPETITIVE NMDA RECEPTOR ANTAGONISTS

Several steps in the comprehensive approach in Table 33.1 have been performed in research on the effects of agents that antagonize the action of glutamate at NMDA receptors. Note, however, that the experiments in this example and the other examples discussed here were not carried out with this paradigm in mind. These experiments effectively performed several of the steps of this paradigm and are only meant to illustrate that it is practical to accomplish specific steps in this systematic approach. In the following case, the studies began at the model stage. Competitive NMDA antagonists are very effective anticonvulsants in a wide variety of experimental models of epilepsy, including AGS[28–30] (see Chapters 26 and 32). The neuronal effects of these NMDA receptor antagonists were evaluated in the AGS neuronal network. It was observed that these agents were very effective in reducing auditory-evoked neuronal firing in the AGS initiation site in the inferior colliculus (IC) in therapeutic doses that blocked AGS.[29] In addition, when these agents were focally microinjected into the IC, they blocked seizures in the lowest dose of any site in the AGS network (Chapter 26). Iontophoretic application of NMDA receptor antagonists directly onto IC neurons in the intact animal was very effective in reducing neuronal responses to sound and inhibited the effect of applied glutamate. NMDA antagonists were also effective in blocking IC neuronal responses to glutamate in IC brain slices (see Chapter 32). Thus, this effect of NMDA antagonists on IC neurons can be seen as being a major contributor to the anticonvulsant effect of therapeutic doses of these agents in AGS. This extensive series of experiments fulfilled many of the steps in animal models enumerated in the comprehensive paradigm in Table 33.1. However, in this example the data are necessary but not sufficient, because this finding may not be applicable to many seizure types that do not involve the IC, and because we cannot be sure that these agents are not affecting neurons in other sites in the network. The foregoing data illustrate that elements of the recommended paradigm can be accomplished, but important elements were not possible to accomplish at the time these studies were performed. Unfortunately, these NMDA receptor antagonists have not reached the stage of treatment of human CNS disorders thus far, because of highly undesirable psychiatric adverse effects.[31] It may be possible to repurpose the competitive NMDA antagonists in the future, possibly as neuroprotective agents in acute stages of neurodegenerative conditions. In contrast, an uncompetitive NMDA antagonist has been approved for the treatment of AD, and another is used clinically as an anesthetic and experimentally in mood disorders.[32–34] However, anticonvulsant doses of an uncompetitive NMDA antagonist do not affect IC neurons in AGS models and act elsewhere in the network (see Chapter 32).

GENERALIZED CONVULSIVE SEIZURE NETWORK

Another example of the application of elements of the comprehensive paradigm in Table 33.1 involves evaluations of the network basis of generalized tonic-clonic seizures. The brainstem reticular formation (BRF) has long been implicated as a requisite neuronal network hub in the neuronal networks for generalized tonic-clonic seizures (see Chapter 32). Neuroimaging studies in human seizures and animal models have supported this idea.[35–37] Lesion and focal microinjection studies in the BRF have also supported this concept in several animal models.[38–43] BRF neuronal firing changes in several seizure models show major firing increases preceding and in association with tonic seizures.[44–51] Systemic treatment with an anticonvulsant drug selectively blocked BRF neuronal firing simultaneously with the blockade of tonic seizures in an animal model.[52] One of the models in which BRF neurons were shown to exhibit major firing increases was that induced by systemic administration of convulsant drugs.[46,47] Thus, administration of these agents, particularly those that block $GABA_A$-mediated inhibition, such as pentylenetetrazol (PTZ), induces profound nonlinear increases in neuronal response in the BRF to various sensory and electrical stimuli in the brain (see Chapters 28, 31, and 32). In order to establish that the effect of these $GABA_A$ antagonists was exerted on BRF neurons, the effects of direct application of PTZ on the sensory responses of BRF neurons were evaluated in unanesthetized animals.[53] PTZ application directly onto neurons in the BRF was able to induce major increases in neuronal responses to sensory stimuli that were similar to those seen with systemic administration [Figure 33.2(D)−(F)], and the response enhancement induced by systemic administration of PTZ could be reversed by application of GABA directly onto the BRF neurons [Figure 33.2(A)−(C)]. The effect of PTZ could also be blocked by systemic administration of a drug that enhances GABA-mediated inhibition (Chapter 32). These findings exemplify the ability of a drug to exert the same effect on neurons in the same brain site when given systemically or directly applied onto the neurons in vivo, as well as the ability to directly block it by competitively antagonizing the mechanism of action ($GABA_A$ receptor blockade). However, the effect of systemic administration of these agents is not selective only for the BRF, and some, but not all, other brain sites are also affected (see Chapter 32). Therefore, further work is needed to determine the relative importance of this site in generalized tonic-clonic seizure induction using other techniques, such as focal microinjection of a $GABA_A$ antagonist into the BRF on seizure induction by the $GABA_A$ antagonists, which has not yet been done.

ABSENCE EPILEPSY NETWORKS

Many important elements of the network exploration paradigm have been accomplished in the absence (petit mal) form of epilepsy, examining the effects of the anticonvulsant drug ethosuximide. Absence seizures are brief lapses of consciousness in which the thalamus (reticular nucleus) and specific areas of the cortex are the critical neuronal network hubs, based on evidence from a variety of techniques.[54] This conclusion is based, in part, on fMRI studies in patients and in several genetic and induced animal models of absence epilepsy[54] (see Chapter 3). Earlier animal models of absence epilepsy included the feline generalized penicillin model, but more recent studies have been done mainly in genetic

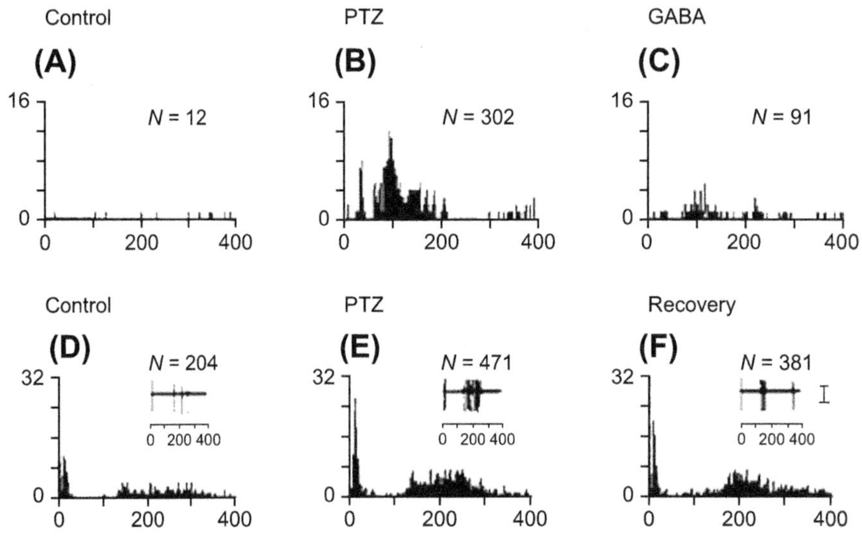

FIGURE 33.2 The effects of a $GABA_A$ antagonist on brainstem reticular formation (BRF) neurons, using systemic administration or iontophoretic application. (A) The poststimulus time histogram (PSTH) of the responses of a BRF (mesencephalon) in the predrug control period shows no evidence of sensory responsiveness to visual stimuli (light flashes) and minimal firing. (B) The responses of the same neuron are shown after administration of the $GABA_A$ antagonist pentylenetetrazol (PTZ; 10 mg/kg i.v.), and they show extensive firing and considerable responsiveness to the same stimuli, as indicated by the time-locked peaks in the PSTH. (C) During the 1 min application of GABA (185 nA) directly onto this neuron, the effect of PTZ was almost completely reversed, and complete recovery from the PTZ occurred rapidly thereafter (not shown). Another BRF neuron showed some response to auditory stimuli, as shown in (D). (E) Iontophoretic application of PTZ (175 nA) greatly enhanced the responsiveness of this neuron; and (F) partial recovery from the effect. The insets above (D−F) are three superimposed oscilloscope trace examples for each PSTH. Data were obtained from unanesthetized cats. (*Source: Modified from Ref. 53 with permission.*)

rodent models, including the WAG/Rij (Wistar albino Glaxo rats of Rijswik) and GAERS (genetic absence epilepsy rats of Strasbourg). Neuroimaging with fMRI in these models during seizures has shown increases in bilateral regions of the somatosensory cortex and thalamus, which may be crucial for triggering seizures in the rodent models.[55–58] In addition, evidence of marked increases in connectivity between cortical areas involved in seizure generation is also seen (even between seizures in the interictal period), suggesting enhanced synchrony and excitability in this network.[58] Many of these changes are prevented by ethosuximide, which is among the most therapeutically effective drugs for this condition[54] (see Chapter 3). Among other potential molecular changes, a T-type calcium channelopathy is implicated as a major epileptogenic mechanism in absence seizures, and ethosuximide is thought to exert its primary action by blocking these channels (see Ref. 54 for a review). Simultaneous in vivo electrocorticographic and intracellular recordings from the cortical region implicated in the network of the GAERS model were evaluated, and systemic injection of therapeutic doses of ethosuximide interrupted the EEG seizures and converted the hyperactive neuronal firing into a normal firing pattern in paralyzed and anesthetized GAERS.[59] Chronic ethosuximide treatment significantly reduced seizures in both the WAG/Rij and GAERS models, which was maintained during the 3-month posttreatment period.[60,61] The anxiety-like comorbid behaviors in these models were also reduced, and these therapeutic effects were associated with increased expression of DNA methyltransferase enzyme messenger RNA in the cortex.[61,62] In slice studies of thalamic reticular neurons from GAERS, ethosuximide and newer agents with a similar mechanism of action attenuated burst firing of these neurons.[63] In GAERS and WAG/Rij rats, focal microinjection of ethosuximide into the cortical areas implicated in the absence seizure network produced an immediate cessation of seizure activity like that seen with systemic administration. However, there was a delayed onset, with microinjection of this agent into the thalamic nuclei areas implicated in the seizure network.[64,65] These data all agree that the thalamus and cortex are the key elements in this neuronal network, but some controversy remains regarding the primacy of these sites as the principal site of action of ethosuximide within the network. Taken together these studies on the effect of this drug on absence seizures constitute one of the closest to fulfilling the suggested paradigm in Table 33.1. However, recent MRI studies indicate that an additional structure, the BRF, may also be involved in the absence network.[66,67] Although many of the recommended approaches in Table 33.1 have been carried out in this example, more work needs to be done.

TEMPORAL LOBE COMPLEX PARTIAL SEIZURE NETWORKS

Network approaches have greatly enhanced the understanding of temporal lobe seizures. Here, we will focus on a specific network that illustrates the principles of requisite hub interactions with other secondary sites, which can also have important involvement in CNS disorders. In temporal lobe seizures, high-frequency neuronal firing occurs in the medial temporal lobe. A puzzling aspect of temporal lobe seizures is that although they are not generalized, they often cause loss of consciousness. Partial seizures with loss of consciousness are referred to as complex partial seizures, in contrast to simple partial seizures in which consciousness is spared. Neuroimaging from human temporal lobe complex partial seizures has revealed abnormally increased activity in the medial temporal lobe. In addition, network effects are observed, including abnormal activity increases in the thalamus, hypothalamus, and upper brainstem, combined with abnormal *decreased* activity in the bilateral fronto-parietal association cortex.[68] Intracranial EEG from patients with temporal lobe seizures shows slow wave activity resembling coma or sleep in the same fronto-parietal regions exhibiting single photon emission computed tomography (SPECT) decreases in association with impaired consciousness, whereas seizures without impaired consciousness do not show changes outside the mesial temporal lobe.[69,70] An animal model has greatly added to the network understanding of impaired consciousness in temporal lobe complex partial seizures.[71–73] Neuroimaging of focal hippocampal seizures in the rat demonstrated increases in the hippocampus and decreases in the fronto-parietal association cortex, similar to the human condition. In addition, electrophysiological recordings from specific nodes confirmed the presence of seizure activity in the hippocampus and pathological slow wave activity in the frontal cortex.[71,73] Based on these findings, the network inhibition hypothesis[36,37] was proposed to explain how focal seizure activity in requisite nodes such as the hippocampus can produce slow wave activity in the cortex through remote network effects (Figure 33.3). According to this view, temporal lobe seizures propagate to subcortical structures that inhibit the brainstem, diencephalic, and basal forebrain arousal systems, which in turn leads to a depressed state of cortical function and loss of consciousness (Figure 33.3). In support of the network inhibition hypothesis, additional recording and disconnection experiments from a rat model have shown the following during hippocampal seizures: (1) increased activity in subcortical regions, including the lateral septum and anterior hypothalamus, which may provide GABAergic inhibition to the arousal areas; (2) cutting

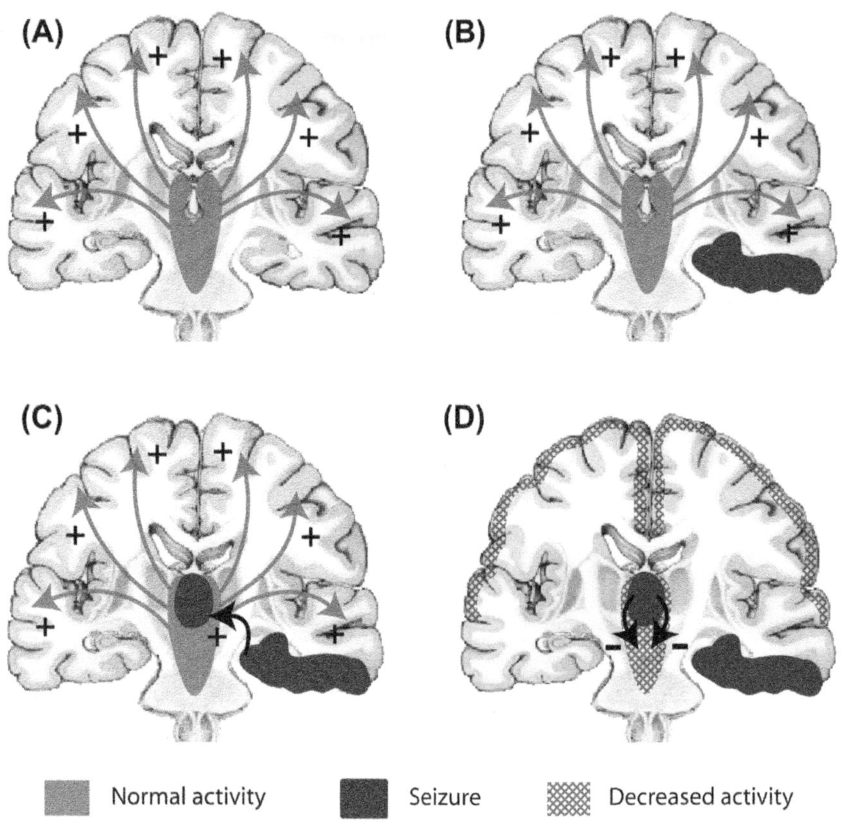

FIGURE 33.3 The network inhibition hypothesis for impaired consciousness in temporal lobe complex partial seizures. (A) Under normal conditions, the upper brainstem–diencephalic activating systems interact with the cerebral cortex to maintain normal consciousness. (B) A focal seizure involving the mesial temporal lobe. If the seizure remains confined, then a simple-partial seizure will occur without impairment of consciousness. (C) Spread of seizure activity from the temporal lobe to midline subcortical structures. Propagation often occurs to the contralateral mesial temporal lobe as well (not shown). (D) Inhibition of subcortical activating systems leads to depressed activity in the bilateral frontoparietal association cortex, and to loss of consciousness. (*Source: Modified with permission from Ref. 74.*)

the fornix prevents propagation of seizures to subcortical structures, and also prevents cortical slow wave activity and behavioral arrest in rats; (3) stimulation of the lateral septum can reproduce the slow wave activity and behavioral arrest seen in seizures; (4) recordings from brainstem cholinergic pedunculopontine tegmental neurons show decreased firing during seizures; and (5) amperometric measurements show decreased cholinergic neurotransmission in the intralaminar thalamus and in the cortex during seizures with cortical slow wave activity.[71,73,75] In summary, these findings suggest that focal temporal lobe seizures inhibit subcortical arousal systems, leading to a cortical sleep-like state and impaired consciousness. Although the main goal of epilepsy therapy is to stop seizures, for patients with medically and surgically refractory epilepsy, it would greatly enhance quality of life to at least prevent loss of consciousness during seizures and the accompanying practical and psychosocial consequences. Depressed arousal during and following seizures might also contribute to respiratory depression and sudden unexpected death in epilepsy (SUDEP), which are discussed in Chapter 29. A network understanding of these phenomena may lead to new therapies, including targeted drug treatment and neurostimulation, to improve arousal and preserve consciousness during seizures.

EXAMPLES OF POTENTIAL FUTURE APPLICATIONS

Based on the principles of network exploration discussed throughout this volume and the paradigm for network evaluation of therapies that is contained in Table 33.1, we propose several potential future applications of network knowledge to the treatment of certain CNS disorders. Chapter 31 discusses the network implications of invasive and noninvasive stimulation paradigms that have proven useful for treating CNS disorders and have revealed important information about the neuronal networks for these disorders. Thus, therapies for chronic pain may activate networks of their own that overlap with and may compete with the chronic pain network, according to the postulated network competition mechanism, described here and in Chapter 29. In future fMRI studies, it would be useful to identify peripheral sites that, when stimulated noninvasively, such as with trigeminal nerve stimulation, may also affect sites that are involved in the neuronal networks for a CNS disorder. This would allow such noninvasive techniques to replace the invasive ones. This may even be possible with specific acupuncture stimulation sites, using a transcutaneous electrical nerve stimulation (TENS) unit (Chapter 31).

Thus, relatively long-duration electrical acupoint stimulation, which is effective in chronic pain and other disorders, was recently shown in an fMRI study to alter the activation of specific neuronal networks by acting on several brain areas, including the frontal gyrus, orbitofrontal cortex, anterior cingulate gyrus, and hippocampus.[76] The extension of fMRI mapping studies to the other acupoints in the Chinese acupuncture meridians would potentially allow the targeting of other brain regions that could be important sites for neuronal networks to facilitate the treatment of different CNS disorders.

The drug therapies discussed in this chapter and Chapter 32 can improve the symptoms of many CNS disorders, and therapeutic doses of a number of drugs have been identified that have potentially selective effects on the emergent properties of neurons in critical hubs of the network. Other existing drugs need to be tested for repurposing, as noted here. The new types of drugs discussed here, including gene-based therapies, may provide important new therapeutic potential for treatment of CNS disorders by targeting them to specific regions of the neuronal network for the disorder. Inserting genes that enhance inhibition into specific areas showing abnormal activity, based on neuroimaging of the network, has the potential for improving therapy. Thus, some success has been achieved with long-term transgene expression in certain chronic neurological diseases, including Parkinson's disease, using genetic vectors to increase dopamine or GABA synthesis in specific nuclei of the neuronal network[77] (see Chapter 25).

More effective therapy could involve targeted combinations of stimulation (Chapter 31) and drug therapies (discussed in Chapter 32). Once we have identified the requisite network hubs for the disorder that are affected by effective stimulation paradigms (e.g. with a TENS unit), a specific drug that targets an emergent property in a network site selectively could be combined with stimulation to produce additive effects. Alternatively, the drug may actually target a different requisite site, which would also reduce the expression of the disorder by acting on multiple network hubs to provide additive effects. Several other combinations of stimulation and/or inhibition within network nuclei could also be useful in improving therapy. Based on our current knowledge, combination stimulation and drug therapies may be the best way to improve targeting of future therapies for CNS disorders. Thus, because of the incomplete effectiveness of many CNS drugs and stimulation therapies that are currently available to treat CNS disorders, we propose that combined treatments may have the potential to exert additive effects if targeting is based on well-researched network-based approaches. The therapeutic effect of the genetically based treatments mentioned in this chapter may be enhanced by stimulation paradigms that are targeted to the region of interest to provide the "nurture" for the change in "nature" that the genetic therapy is attempting to accomplish. Thus, the stimulation paradigm might enhance the expression of the genetic therapy. There are recent examples of additive effects of drug and stimulation paradigms that are used in chronic pain disorders in which anticonvulsant drugs combined with stimulation therapies provide additive therapeutic effects in several types of neuralgia.[21,22] The ability and extensive use of anticonvulsant drugs to effectively treat many other CNS disorders have led to the idea that these agents should be more properly termed "network-modifying agents"[78] (see Chapter 32). Such combined drug and stimulation approaches would likely need to be individualized for each patient based on potential neuronal network differences among patients with similar symptoms. If a therapy is only partially effective in a given patient, adding another therapy that is also partially effective may provide overall better therapeutic effects. Rather than the current non-network-based trial-and-error approaches, we may be able to combine previously identified paradigms that target specific brain sites, such as content-specific visual stimuli that activate the amygdala,[79] to be given in concert with drugs that target the amygdala in major depressive disorders, as discussed here.

In major depression, fMRI changes in amygdala and cingulate and insular cortex activity are observed, which can be normalized with effective antidepressant therapies, as noted in this chapter.[12] However, current therapies for depression are not completely effective in patients who do improve, and in many patients they are not effective at all, indicating the need for better therapies. Several additional approaches have been explored, including uncompetitive NMDA antagonists, such as ketamine,[34] and new noninvasive stimulation techniques, including trigeminal nerve stimulation, which have also been shown to be useful in the therapy of depression.[80–82] fMRI studies in patients indicate that the amygdala is activated by the presentation of angry facial stimuli,[83] and ketamine has been shown to selectively inhibit amygdala neuronal responses to sensory stimuli in animals.[15,84] The targeted combination of drug administration of a nonselective NMDA channel blocker, simultaneously with an amygdala-selective stimulus paradigm, such as angry face presentation, could potentially have additive effects in depression therapy. If this was done with a repetitive protocol, it has the potential to produce enhanced antidepressant effects through a long-lasting deconditioning-like effect, reducing the activity of the neuronal network that mediates the depression. A new nonselective NMDA channel blocker (AZD6765) acts like ketamine but shows a lower level than ketamine of "trapping" at NMDA channels. This property permits agonist dissociation and channel closure, while the antagonist is bound to its site in the channel. This lower trapping is reported to reduce the risk of psychotomimetic effects induced by ketamine and has an improved therapeutic safety profile in initial patient studies, as well as displaying antidepressant-like properties in animal models.[85] Therefore, combining this new drug simultaneously with an amygdala-selective stimulus paradigm might increase the effectiveness of treatment. Another potentially useful combined approach could involve the administration of uncompetitive NMDA antagonists along with new noninvasive electrical stimulation paradigms, such as trigeminal nerve stimulation (mentioned in this section), which may affect brainstem elements of the depression neuronal network,[81] which would target two different elements of the neuronal network for depression. The efficacy of such approaches would likely be enhanced if further neuronal recording studies in the neuronal networks of animal models of depression were available for testing new potential therapeutic modalities. A number of animal models for major depression have been developed, including the flinders sensitive line (FSL) rat.[86] FSL rats exhibited greater than normal activation in the amygdala and hypoactivation in the prefrontal cortex in response to a fear stimulus (odor),[87] which shares some similarities with the depression networks observed in human studies. Neurophysiological recordings in mice engineered to express a human loss-of-function depression allele associated with major depression show increased intranetwork synchrony within the medial prefrontal cortex and amygdala and increased internetwork synchrony between these two brain regions, based on neuronal recordings, which were reversed with an antidepressant drug.[88] Since the antidepressants currently available are not completely effective, it might be useful to determine whether combined therapy with a drug that acts on another mechanism, such as ketamine, or an antidepressant stimulation paradigm[89] would normalize the neuronal firing changes seen in this model.

In chronic pain syndromes, some success has been achieved with combined therapies, and there could be future improvements by extending this approach. Combined stimulation and drug administration approaches may be an important way of using current knowledge to lead to important improvements in chronic pain therapy. Thus, pregabalin combined with TENS stimulation and phenytoin combined with electroacupuncture exerted improved therapeutic effects compared to a single type of therapy for several forms of neuralgia.[21,22] As shown in Figure 33.4, patients suffering from glossopharyngeal neuralgia showed "great improvement" to a significantly elevated degree when treated with electroacupuncture and phenytoin than that seen with electroacupuncture alone.[22] Although there are many

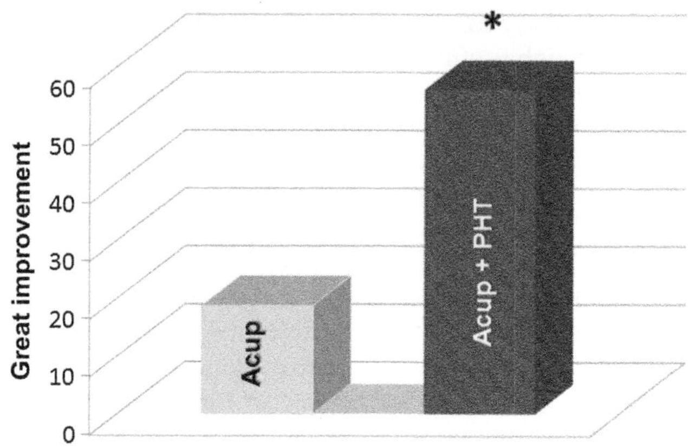

FIGURE 33.4 Effects of combined stimulation and drug therapies on a chronic pain syndrome. Electroacupuncture (Acup) stimulation in patients with glossopharyngeal neuralgia showed great improvement in pain in a limited number of patients, but with the addition of phenytoin (PHT), a significantly greater incidence of great improvement was seen (*$p < 0.05$, Mann–Whitney U test). (*Source: Based on data from Ref. 22 with permission.*) (For color version of this figure, the reader is referred to the online version of this book.)

varieties of chronic pain syndromes, the neuroimaging results of many chronic pain disorders indicate that certain network hubs may be critical network nuclei involved in the majority of them. These include several cortical areas and subcortical areas, including the PAG, as mentioned in this chapter. The PAG has also been found to be a critical element in pain networks in humans and animal models.[90,91] By targeting one of these structures, such as the PAG, that is contained in the neuronal networks of both human and animal models of a CNS disorder, such as chronic pain, therapy can potentially be directed toward that structure. This has the potential to short-circuit the rest of the pain network and alleviate the symptoms, as seen with PAG electrical stimulation.[90] Alternatively, if there are sites in the therapeutic network for stimulation paradigms that compete with the pain network, drugs that selectively enhance neuronal responses in those competing sites might enhance the effectiveness of the stimulation paradigm.

In stroke patients, electrical stimulation approaches, including acupuncture, are reported to significantly improve overall health and quality of life.[92] Repetitive transcranial magnetic stimulation, transcranial direct-current stimulation, and AD drugs, including cholinesterase inhibitors and memantine, have shown some effectiveness in treating stroke-induced aphasia.[93] fMRI studies indicate that certain brain regions promote improvement of language deficits, while others may hinder recovery through maladaptive reorganization of neuronal networks (see Ref. 94). Rehabilitation treatments for stroke have successfully used musical elements of speech (melody and rhythm) to improve expressive language; these capitalize on preserved function (singing) and engage language-capable regions associated with remodeling and plasticity increases in projection pathways.[95,96] The target for stroke treatment involves identifying the specific pathways in the networks that are damaged using neuroimaging and employing strategies that activate dormant networks, which can transfer the information over an alternative pathway, to reconnect the circuit and restore function to the network.[97] A combination of the stimulation techniques with the drugs that have demonstrated some effectiveness has the potential to provide targeted improvements in the therapy of stroke. Thus, cholinesterase inhibitors, which enhance conditional multireceptive (CMR) neuronal responsiveness (see Chapters 28 and 32) if added to a targeted stimulation therapy method, may be a useful future approach. A number of animal models have been developed for modeling ischemic stroke, including the middle cerebral artery occlusion model.[98] Neuroimaging in this model has identified the brain regions that are damaged in the model, which resemble those in patients.[99] By utilizing these models in appropriately aged animals and utilizing the methods described in Table 33.1, it may be possible to improve therapy using electrical stimulation paradigms in combination with drug treatments that enhance the activity in the damaged pathways or in potential alternative pathways to compensate for the pathway damage.

Future improvements in treating drug abuse, based on neuronal network approaches, may also be feasible. Electroacupuncture combined with drugs that target specific sites in the neuronal networks that mediate the rewarding effects of (and withdrawal from) drugs of abuse, including alcohol, may also have promise for targeted improvement in treating drug abuse. Thus, extensive research has delineated the neuronal network underlying reward, which is associated with drugs of abuse, including ethanol, and key elements in the mesolimbic reward network have been defined using various techniques.[100,101] A number of drugs that act on the major receptors in the network modulate the effects of abuse-prone agents, blocking the rewarding effects and/or preventing withdrawal syndromes of the specific agents. Thus, the administration of specific agents has had some degree of success in the prevention, treatment, and withdrawal amelioration of abusable agents, including ethanol, opiates, and stimulants.[102–104] However, the success of these drug-based therapeutic approaches is variable and limited. Stimulation-based therapies have also been utilized, including electroacupuncture, and some success has been achieved in human and animal models of drug abuse. Reduction of self-administration of abused agents has been observed with various (but not all) protocols and sites of electroacupuncture; amelioration of withdrawal symptoms and reduced drug-seeking behavior have also been observed with these stimulus paradigms.[105–110] Combined electroacupuncture and antagonist therapy have shown improved treatment for opiate withdrawal,[111] suggesting that such combined approaches may be an important future trend. There may be additional improvements in these combined therapies if agents that enhance the activation of specific structures in the neuronal network evoked by the effective stimulation protocols, as shown by neuroimaging studies,[112,113] are targeted for enhancement by drugs that selectively affect neurons in critical hubs in this network.

Posttraumatic stress disorder (PTSD) is a common psychiatric disorder that occurs after an intense experience that elicited fear, helplessness, and/or horror. The syndrome consists of three symptom clusters: re-experiencing the traumatic event, avoidance symptoms, and psychophysiological reactivity in response to trauma-related stimuli. The neuronal network that subserves PTSD has been proposed.[114] Interestingly, a major component of this network includes the pathway between the amygdala and the PAG, as discussed in this chapter, which is also implicated in networks for chronic pain and in animal models of seizures (see Chapter 32). Fear conditioning and fear-potentiated startle are proposed as models for PTSD (Chapters 13 and 29). Approaches to treating PTSD have involved methods to induce extinction of fear responses by repeated presentations of a symptom-triggering stimulus under non-fearful conditions, which involve similar network nuclei, including the amygdala in rat and human studies.[114] It has been widely observed in human fMRI studies that amygdala activity is consistently activated by the presentation of fearful stimuli, such as fearful faces, as mentioned here, and this occurs to an abnormal degree in people with PTSD and other fear disorders.[79,115] Gabapentinoids (gabapentin and pregabalin)[116] and other anticonvulsant drugs, as well as certain antianxiety drugs, have been observed to reduce the symptoms of PTSD in patients.[117–122] Successful therapy has also been carried out in PTSD with pregabalin and antianxiety drugs. A combined treatment of presenting the fearful face stimuli that activate the amygdala and treating with pregabalin, which reduces amygdala and insula activation but increases medial prefrontal cortex activation in healthy volunteers,[83] suggests the potential usefulness of combined therapies in PTSD. Similarly, animal studies using behavioral extinction paradigms combined with antidepressant drugs were able to increase fear extinction.[123] Administration of a partial NMDA receptor agonist (D-cycloserine) in combination with a stimulation paradigm that simulated the fear-inducing condition resulted in greater improvement of the symptoms in PTSD and related anxiety disorders.[124] The improved success of combined drug and stimulation therapy in PTSD treatment may provide better treatment of this disabling CNS disorder. The inhibitory effect of gabapentin on PAG neuronal responses to electrical stimulation of the amygdala may indicate an important locus within the PTSD network at which these gabapentinoids are acting.[19] The action of other effective and potential drug therapies for PTSD on the emergent properties of neurons in this pathway will need to be examined to determine if this network effect is a general action or if the other agents target the emergent properties in the other requisite hubs in the neuronal network for PTSD. The combination of drugs and appropriately targeted forms of stimulation therapy for PTSD, which may need to be patient specific, can be expected to improve clinical outcomes.

AD is a common form of dementia in the elderly that involves progressive cognitive decline mediated by neurodegenerative changes in the brain that include amyloid plaques and neurofibrillary tangles as well as reactive microgliosis, dystrophic neurites, and loss of neurons and synapses.[125–127] Neuroimaging studies of AD have demonstrated the location of atrophic changes affecting the brain in AD and allow evaluation of the progression of this disorder.[128,129] Animal models of AD include transgenic mice that develop pathological changes that are age dependent. Neurofibrillatory tangles, which are seen in human AD, occur in other transgenic mice models of AD that express additional gene alterations such as mutated human tau or nitric oxide synthase deletion. These AD models are largely based on inducing genetic mutations that are associated with familial AD, which is an uncommon variant of AD. However, the models have generated insights into the molecular mechanisms of AD and have allowed testing of potential therapies.[130] Recent neuroimaging studies in certain of these models show patterns and progressive changes that are analogous to those seen in patients.[131] Currently approved therapies for AD include centrally active cholinesterase inhibitors and an uncompetitive NMDA receptor antagonist (memantine), but the effectiveness of these agents has been modest, and combined therapy with both types of drugs has the potential to be additive.[132,133] Stimulation therapies have also been utilized experimentally to treat AD, and acupuncture has been reported to successfully treat mild cognitive impairment in an effort to prevent AD progression in these patients. fMRI indications of abnormal functional connectivity were improved after acupuncture treatments.[134] Vagus nerve stimulation or deep brain stimulation with in-dwelling electrodes in the nucleus basalis, a key network nucleus in AD, induces improvement of the symptoms of this disorder, suggesting its potential usefulness in AD.[135,136] Even studies in cognitively intact aging human brain observe diminished activation of the primary cortex, but widespread increases in activation of nonprimary areas of the cortex were observed simultaneously.[137] These fMRI data led to the idea that cognitively successful aging involves a transition from the activation of faster and smaller cortical networks to that of larger but slower networks. This transition may be facilitated by stimulation paradigms that have the ability to enhance this process.

Stimulant drugs, including GABA antagonists and cholinesterase inhibitors, similar to the agents approved to treat AD, may have the potential for use in memory improvement in aging. As noted in this chapter, the responses of neurons in nonprimary cortical areas are enhanced by administration of these agents (see Chapter 32), which could potentially improve cognition in normal aging and in CNS disorders of cognition, such as AD. Cholinesterase inhibitors enhance neuronal responsiveness in animals,[46,47] which may contribute to the therapeutic effects of these agents in AD patients to successfully correct deficiencies in encoding auditory input and improve memory in these patients.[138,139] Thus, these cholinesterase inhibitors and $GABA_A$ antagonists, such as PTZ, enhance neuronal responses in the BRF and also in amygdala and nonprimary cortical neurons. Since the latter areas generally exhibit a higher degree of long-term plasticity (Chapter 28), an effect in these sites could potentially subserve therapeutic improvement in cognitive disorders. Recent reports indicate that agents that block $GABA_A$ receptor-mediated inhibition, including PTZ, improve cognition in a cognitive disorder model in animals.[140,141] The enhancement of CMR neuronal responsiveness induced by these agents could contribute importantly to this effect. PTZ was used clinically at one time as a diagnostic agent to provoke abnormal EEG changes in patients who were suspected of having epilepsy,[142] but the toxic dose of PTZ may be too close to its diagnostic dose. However, other agents, including a partial inverse agonist that acts on $\alpha(5)$ $GABA_A$ receptors[141] and a $GABA_B$ antagonist that, like PTZ, induces cognitive enhancement in an animal model of cognitive disorders,[141,143] may be safer alternatives for treating impaired cognition. As noted here, certain stimulus paradigms have also been reported to enhance cognition in AD patients. Therefore, combinations of drug and stimulation therapies may well be advantageous in this disorder as well. Other potentially therapeutic stimuli include cognitive-stimulating computer programs or olfactory stimulation, which might target an important abnormal network node in this disorder, since the loss of the sense of smell is a common finding in AD patients.[144] Combining these stimulus approaches with GABA antagonists or cholinesterase inhibitors, which induce similar sensory response-enhancing effects in animals, could be beneficial. There may also be patterns of sensory stimulation that could be utilized with current AD drugs, such as cholinesterase inhibitors or even the mild stimulant caffeine, which also mildly enhances sensory responses and is reported to ameliorate AD.[145] These combinations of drugs and stimulation procedures may potentially foster increases in synaptic strength and other changes that can prevent or compensate for the network degeneration occurring in this disorder (Chapters 7, 15, and 16). The choice of drugs and stimulation paradigms might need to be personalized for each patient based on cognitive and neuroimaging changes in that individual.

As noted in this chapter, some of these combined approaches have achieved some degree of success in chronic pain syndromes.[21,22] There are obviously many details to developing the best strategies for these combined drug and therapeutic approaches that will require much future research. However, if informed and organized efforts are made to apply what we know now based on neuronal network concepts in an integrated way, it is likely that it could lead to major improvements in the treatment of many of these disabling and debilitating CNS disorders.

CONCLUSION

As stated in Chapter 1, many current investigators of specific neuronal network function may consider this book, with its emphasis on network interactions, to be premature. However, the exploration of these networks is not only to gain new knowledge on how the brain works, as important as that is. It is our contention that the main driving force behind neuronal networks research is and should be improved therapy of CNS disorders in human patients. One of us (CF) has been subject to a neurological disease for nearly all of his adult life, and the other (HB) has spent a long career treating patients with these disorders. We know the pain, suffering, and debilitation that can accompany these disorders, and we strongly believe that the information the field already possesses, some of which is detailed in this volume, can be utilized more effectively now to devise more effective treatment of these disorders and improve the lives of these patients. We believe that this possibility is not premature but timely. It is imperative to move forward despite our incomplete knowledge because serious CNS disorders are not currently treatable (e.g. amyotrophic lateral sclerosis), are poorly treated (e.g. AD), or often are not well controlled (e.g. epilepsy), and therapy improvements are needed now. With the current state of knowledge, we are admittedly working from "rough drafts" of how the brain and its networks function. However, a relatively primitive state of knowledge plus guided serendipity[146] and a prepared mind have often led to breakthroughs in the past, some of which are detailed in this book and have proven effective in cases that have failed standard therapies. Finally, the field is really in its infancy of understanding how therapeutic measures, including stimulation and drug treatments, actually work to treat CNS disorders, and yet these treatments are nonetheless effective. Obviously, much more research on every one of these network research "silos" is currently ongoing and still needs to be carried forward vigorously.

By envisioning ways in which some of the principles of network research can be brought together, we hope to accelerate our knowledge—and, by combining established information in one research silo with information in other silos, this process may be able to accelerate. Thus, network information obtained from physiological and pathological (neurological disorders, psychiatric disorders, and chronic pain) research has the potential to reveal general network mechanisms, accelerating knowledge and application of this knowledge to the therapy of CNS disorders of varying types. Bringing together techniques from these research paradigms has the potential to do this. For example, combining knowledge obtained from the dominant network approach in human CNS disorders, fMRI, with neuronal recording studies that are most commonly done in animal models (e.g. Ref. 9) has the potential to evaluate the mechanisms that subserve the neuroimaging changes. The alteration of these mechanisms by treatments that are effective in the disorder will allow the observation of neuronal mechanisms by which the drug or stimulation protocol alters network function in the animal model. Application of this knowledge should lead to the establishment of important approaches for the testing of potential future therapeutic measures.

Acknowledgments

The authors gratefully acknowledge the assistance of Gayle Stauffer and Diana Smith in preparing this manuscript.

References

1. Freeman WJ, Kozma R, Werbos PJ. Biocomplexity: adaptive behavior in complex stochastic dynamical systems. *Biosystems.* 2001;59:109–123.
2. Thanos PK, Robison L, Nestler EJ, et al. Mapping brain metabolic connectivity in awake rats with μPET and optogenetic stimulation. *J Neurosci.* 2013;33(15):6343–6349.
3. Salta E, De strooper B. Non-coding RNAs with essential roles in neurodegenerative disorders. *Lancet Neurol.* 2012;11(2):189–200.
4. Gray SG. Epigenetic treatment of neurological disease. *Epigenomic.* 2011;3(4):431–450.
5. Famm K, Litt B, Tracey KJ, Boyden ES, Slaoui M. Drug discovery: a jump-start for electroceuticals. *Nature.* 2013;496(7444):159–161.

6. Garibotto V, Heinzer S, Vulliemoz S, et al. Clinical applications of hybrid PET/MRI in neuroimaging. *Clin Nucl Med.* 2013;38(1): e13–e18.
7. Schridde U, Khuchandani M, Motelow JE, Sanganahalli BG, Hyder F, Blumenfeld H. Negative BOLD with large increases in neuronal activity. *Cereb Cortex.* 2008;18(8):1814–1827.
8. Mishra AM, Ellens DJ, Schridde U, et al. Where fMRI and electrophysiology agree to disagree: corticothalamic and striatal activity patterns in the WAG/Rij rat. *J Neurosci.* 2011;31(42): 15053–15064.
9. Hyder F, Herman P, Sanganahalli BG, Coman D, Blumenfeld H, Rothman DL. Role of ongoing, intrinsic activity of neuronal populations for quantitative neuroimaging of functional magnetic resonance imaging-based networks. *Brain Connect.* 2011;1(3):185–193.
10. Lythgoe MF, Sibson NR, Harris NG. Neuroimaging of animal models of brain disease. *Br Med Bull.* 2003;65:235–257.
11. Blumenfeld H. Functional MRI studies of animal models in epilepsy. *Epilepsia.* 2007;48(Suppl. 4):18–26.
12. Bellani M, Dusi N, Yeh PH, Soares JC, Brambilla P. The effects of antidepressants on human brain as detected by imaging studies. Focus on major depression. *Prog Neuropsychopharmacol Biol Psychiatry.* 2011;35(7):1544–1552.
13. Buzsáki G, Anastassiou CA, Koch C. The origin of extracellular fields and currents—EEG, ECoG, LFP and spikes. *Nat Rev Neurosci.* 2012;13(6):407–420.
14. Chakravarty DN, Faingold CL. Differential roles in the neuronal network for audiogenic seizures are observed among the inferior colliculus subnuclei and the amygdala. *Exp Neurol.* 1999;157(1): 135–141.
15. Feng HJ, Faingold CL. Repeated generalized audiogenic seizures induce plastic changes on acoustically evoked neuronal firing in the amygdala. *Brain Res.* 2002;932(1–2):61–69.
16. Samineni VK, Premkumar LS, Faingold CL. Post-ictal analgesia in genetically epilepsy-prone rats is induced by audiogenic seizures and involves cannabinoid receptors in the periaqueductal gray. *Brain Res.* 2011;1389:177–182.
17. Samineni V, Premkumar L, Faingold CL. Chronic pain induces neuroplastic changes in periaqueductal gray neuronal firing: blockade by gabapentin. *Soc Neurosci Abs.* 2012, 178.11/GG2.
18. Samineni V, Premkumar L, Faingold CL. Changes in periaqueductal gray neuronal responses to pain induced by barbiturate administration. *Anesthesiology.* submitted for publication.
19. Tupal S, Faingold CL. The amygdala to periaqueductal gray pathway: plastic changes induced by audiogenic kindling and reversal by gabapentin. *Brain Res.* 2012;1475:71–79.
20. Loscher W, Puskarjov M, Kaila K. Cation-chloride cotransporters NKCC1 and KCC2 as potential targets for novel antiepileptic and antiepileptogenic treatments. *Neuropharmacology.* 2013;69:62–74.
21. Barbarisi M, Pace MC, Passavanti MB, et al. Pregabalin and transcutaneous electrical nerve stimulation for postherpetic neuralgia treatment. *Clin J Pain.* 2010;26(7):567–572.
22. Lu DP, Lu WI, Lu GP. Phenytoin (Dilantin) and acupuncture therapy in the treatment of intractable oral and facial pain. *Acupunct Electrother Res.* 2011;36(1–2):65–84.
23. Kanner AM. The treatment of depressive disorders in epilepsy: what all neurologists should know. *Epilepsia.* 2013;54(Suppl. 1):3–12.
24. Jobe PC. Affective disorder and epilepsy comorbidity in the genetically epilepsy prone-rat (GEPR). In: Gilliam F, Kanner AM, Sheline YI, eds. *Depression and Brain Dysfunction.* London: Taylor & Francis; 2006:121–157.
25. Behbehani MM. Functional characteristics of the midbrain periaqueductal gray. *Prog Neurobiol.* 1995;46:575–605.
26. Long C, Yang L, Faingold CL, Evans MS. Excitatory amino acid receptor-mediated responses in periaqueductal gray neurons are increased during ethanol withdrawal. *Neuropharmacology.* 2007;52(3):802–811.
27. Lehew G, Nicolelis MA. State-of-the-art microwire array design for chronic neural recordings in behaving animals. In: Nicolelis MA, ed. *Methods for Neuronal Ensemble Recordings.* Boca Raton, FL: CRC Press; 2008.
28. Croucher MJ, Collins JF, Meldrum BS. Anticonvulsant action of excitatory amino acid antagonists. *Science.* 1982;216(4548): 899–901.
29. Faingold CL, Randall ME, Naritoku DK, Boersma Anderson CA. Noncompetitive and competitive NMDA antagonists exert anticonvulsant effects by actions on different sites within the neuronal network for audiogenic seizures. *Exp Neurol.* 1993;119(2):198–204.
30. Mares P, Folbergrová J, Kubová H. Excitatory aminoacids and epileptic seizures in immature brain. *Physiol Res.* 2004; 53(Suppl. 1):S115–S124.
31. Gunduz-Bruce H. The acute effects of NMDA antagonism: from the rodent to the human brain. *Brain Res Rev.* 2009;60(2):279–286.
32. Hyde C, Peters J, Bond M, et al. Evolution of the evidence on the effectiveness and cost-effectiveness of acetylcholinesterase inhibitors and memantine for Alzheimer's disease: systematic review and economic model. *Age Ageing.* 2013;42(1):14–20.
33. Bowles ED, Gold ME. Rethinking the paradigm: evaluation of ketamine as a neurosurgical anesthetic. *AANA J.* 2012;80(6): 445–452.
34. Aan Het Rot M, Zarate Jr CA, Charney DS, Mathew SJ. Ketamine for depression: where do we go from here? *Biol Psychiatry.* 2012;72(7):537–547.
35. DeSalvo MN, Schridde U, Mishra AM, et al. Focal BOLD fMRI changes in bicuculline-induced tonic-clonic seizures in the rat. *Neuroimage.* 2010;50(3):902–909.
36. Norden AD, Blumenfeld H. The role of subcortical structures in human epilepsy. *Epilepsy Behav.* 2002;3(3):219–231.
37. Blumenfeld H. Impaired consciousness in epilepsy. *Lancet Neurol.* 2012;11(9):814–826.
38. Browning RA. Role of the brain-stem reticular formation in tonic-clonic seizures: lesion and pharmacological studies. *Fed Proc.* 1985;44(8):2425–2431.
39. Millan MH, Meldrum BS, Boersma CA, Faingold CL. Excitant amino acids and audiogenic seizures in the genetically epilepsy-prone rat. II. Efferent seizure propagating pathway. *Exp Neurol.* 1988;99(3):687–698.
40. Riaz A, Faingold CL. Seizures during ethanol withdrawal are blocked by focal microinjection of excitant amino acid antagonists into the inferior colliculus and pontine reticular formation. *Alcohol Clin Exp Res.* 1994;18(6):1456–1462.
41. Ishimoto T, Omori N, Mutoh F, Chiba S. Convulsive seizures induced by *N*-methyl-D-aspartate microinjection into the mesencephalic reticular formation in rats. *Brain Res.* 2000;881(2): 152–158.
42. Frye CA, Manjarrez J, Camacho-Arroyo I. Infusion of 3α,5α-THP to the pontine reticular formation attenuates PTZ-induced seizures. *Brain Res.* 2000;881(1):98–102.
43. Raisinghani M, Faingold CL. Identification of the requisite brain sites in the neuronal network subserving generalized clonic audiogenic seizures. *Brain Res.* 2003;967(1–2):113–122.
44. Faingold CL, Caspary DM. Changes in reticular formation unit response patterns associated with pentylenetetrazol-induced enhancement of sensory evoked responses. *Neuropharmacology.* 1977;16(2):143–147.
45. Faingold CL. Pentylenetetrazol-induced enhancement of responses of mesencephalic reticular neurons to visual stimuli. *Brain Res.* 1978;150(2):418–423.

46. Faingold CL, Hoffmann WE, Caspary DM. Comparative effects of convulsant drugs on the sensory responses of neurons in the amygdala and brainstem reticular formation. *Neuropharmacology.* 1985;24(12):1221–1230.
47. Faingold CL, Hoffmann WE, Caspary DM. Mechanisms of sensory seizures: brain-stem neuronal response changes and convulsant drugs. *Fed Proc.* 1985;44(8):2436–2441.
48. Faingold CL, Riaz A. Increased responsiveness of pontine reticular formation neurons associated with audiogenic seizure susceptibility during ethanol withdrawal. *Brain Res.* 1994;663(1): 69–76.
49. Faingold CL, Randall M. Pontine reticular formation neurons exhibit a premature and precipitous increase in acoustic responses prior to audiogenic seizures in genetically epilepsy-prone rats. *Brain Res.* 1995;704(2):218–226.
50. Raisinghani M, Faingold CL. Pontine reticular formation neurons are implicated in the neuronal network for generalized clonic seizures which is intensified by audiogenic kindling. *Brain Res.* 2005;1064(1–2):90–99.
51. Faingold CL. Brainstem networks: reticulo-cortical synchronization in generalized convulsive seizures. In: Noebels JL, Avoli M, Rogawski MA, Olsen RW, Delgado-Escueta AV, eds. *Jasper's Basic Mechanisms of the Epilepsies.* 4th ed. Bethesda, MD: National Center for Biotechnology Information (US); 2012.
52. N'Gouemo P, Faingold CL. Phenytoin administration reveals a differential role of pontine reticular formation and periaqueductal gray neurons in generation of the convulsive behaviors of audiogenic seizures. *Brain Res.* 2000;859(2):311–317.
53. Faingold CL, Hoffmann WE, Caspary DM. Effects of iontophoretic application of convulsants on the sensory responses of neurons in the brain-stem reticular formation. *Electroencephalogr Clin Neurophysiol.* 1984;58(1):55–64.
54. Hughes JR. Absence seizures: a review of recent reports with new concepts. *Epilepsy Behav.* 2009;15(4):404–412.
55. Nersesyan H, Hyder F, Rothman D, Blumenfeld H. Dynamic fMRI and EEG recordings during spike-wave seizures and generalized tonic-clonic seizures in WAG/Rij rats. *J Cerebral Blood Flow Metab.* 2004;24:589–599.
56. Tenney JR, Duong TQ, King JA, Ferris CF. fMRI of brain activation in a genetic rat model of absence seizures. *Epilepsia.* 2004;45:576–582.
57. David O, Guillemain I, Saillet S, et al. Identifying neural drivers with functional MRI: an electrophysiological validation. *PLoS Biol.* 2008;6(12):2683–2697.
58. Mishra AM, Bai X, Motelow JE, et al. Increased resting functional connectivity in spike-wave epilepsy in WAG/Rij rats. *Epilepsia.* 2013;54(7):1214–1222.
59. Polack PO, Charpier S. Ethosuximide converts ictogenic neurons initiating absence seizures into normal neurons in a genetic model. *Epilepsia.* 2009;50(7):1816–1820.
60. Blumenfeld H, Klein JP, Schridde U, et al. Early treatment suppresses the development of spike-wave epilepsy in a rat model. *Epilepsia.* 2008;49(3):400–409.
61. Dezsi G, Ozturk E, Stanic D, et al. Ethosuximide reduces epileptogenesis and behavioral comorbidity in the GAERS model of genetic generalized epilepsy. *Epilepsia.* 2013;54(4):635–643.
62. Sarkisova KY, Kuznetsova GD, Kulikov MA, van Luijtelaar G. Spike-wave discharges are necessary for the expression of behavioral depression-like symptoms. *Epilepsia.* 2010;51(1):146–160.
63. Tringham E, Powell KL, Cain SM, et al. T-type calcium channel blockers that attenuate thalamic burst firing and suppress absence seizures. *Sci Transl Med.* 2012;4(121):121ra19.
64. Danober L, Deransart C, Depaulis A, Vergnes M, Marescaux C. Pathophysiological mechanisms of genetic absence epilepsy in the rat. *Prog Neurobiol.* 1998;55:27–57.
65. Manning JP, Richards DA, Leresche N, Crunelli V, Bowery NG. Cortical-area specific block of genetically determined absence seizures by ethosuximide. *Neuroscience.* 2004;123(1):5–9.
66. Berman R, Negishi M, Vestal M, et al. Simultaneous EEG, fMRI, and behavioral testing in typical childhood absence seizures. *Epilepsia.* 2010;51(10):2011–2022.
67. Carney PW, Masterton RA, Harvey AS, Scheffer IE, Berkovic SF, Jackson GD. The core network in absence epilepsy. Differences in cortical and thalamic BOLD response. *Neurology.* 2010;75(10): 904–911.
68. Blumenfeld H, McNally KA, Vanderhill SD, et al. Positive and negative network correlations in temporal lobe epilepsy. *Cereb Cortex.* 2004;14:892–902.
69. Blumenfeld H, Rivera M, McNally KA, Davis K, Spencer DD, Spencer SS. Ictal neocortical slowing in temporal lobe epilepsy. *Neurology.* 2004;63:1015–1021.
70. Englot DJ, Yang L, Hamid H, et al. Impaired consciousness in temporal lobe seizures: role of cortical slow activity. *Brain.* 2010;133(Pt 12):3764–3777.
71. Englot DJ, Mishra AM, Mansuripur PK, Herman P, Hyder F, Blumenfeld H. Remote effects of focal hippocampal seizures on the rat neocortex. *J Neurosci.* 2008;28(36):9066–9081.
72. Englot DJ, Blumenfeld H. Consciousness and epilepsy: why are complex-partial seizures complex? *Prog Brain Res.* 2009;177:147–170.
73. Englot DJ, Modi B, Mishra AM, DeSalvo M, Hyder F, Blumenfeld H. Cortical deactivation induced by subcortical network dysfunction in limbic seizures. *J Neurosci.* 2009; 29(41):13006–13018.
74. Blumenfeld H, Taylor J. Why do seizures cause loss of consciousness? *Neuroscientist.* Oct 2003;9(5):301–310.
75. Motelow JE, Gummadavelli A, Zayyad Z, et al. Brainstem cholinergic and thalamic dysfunction during limbic seizures: possible mechanism for cortical slow oscillations and impaired consciousness. *Soc Neurosci Abs*; 2012. Online at: http://websfnorg/.
76. Zhang Y, Jiang Y, Glielmi CB, et al. Long-duration transcutaneous electric acupoint stimulation alters small-world brain functional networks. *Magn Reson Imaging.* 2013 pii: S0730-725X(13)00033-7.
77. Chtarto A, Bockstael O, Tshibangu T, Dewitte O, Levivier M, Tenenbaum L. A next step in adeno-associated virus (AAV)-mediated gene therapy for neurological diseases: regulation and targeting. *Br J Clin Pharmacol.* 2013;76(2):217–232. http://dx.doi.org/10.1111/bcp.12065.
78. Faingold CL. Anticonvulsant drugs as neuronal network-modifying agents. In: Schwartzkroin PA, ed. *Encyclopedia of Basic Epilepsy Research.* Vol. 1. Academic Press; 2009:50–58.
79. van der Zwaag W, Da Costa SE, Zurcher NR, Adams Jr RB, Hadjikhani N. A 7 tesla fMRI study of amygdala responses to fearful faces. *Brain Topogr.* 2012;25(2):125–128.
80. DeGiorgio CM, Fanselow EE, Schrader LM, Cook IA. Trigeminal nerve stimulation: seminal animal and human studies for epilepsy and depression. *Neurosurg Clin N Am.* 2011;22(4):449–456.
81. Schrader LM, Cook IA, Miller PR, Maremont ER, DeGiorgio CM. Trigeminal nerve stimulation in major depressive disorder: first proof of concept in an open pilot trial. *Epilepsy Behav.* 2011;22(3):475–478.
82. Fanselow EE. Central mechanisms of cranial nerve stimulation for epilepsy. *Surg Neurol Int.* 2012;3(Suppl. 4):247–254.
83. Aupperle RL, Tankersley D, Ravindran LN, et al. Pregabalin effects on neural response to emotional faces. *Front Hum Neurosci.* 2012;6:42.
84. Feng HJ, Faingold CL. Ketamine in mood disorders and epilepsy. In: Costa A, Villalba E, eds. *Horizons in Neuroscience Research.* Vol. 10. New York: Nova Science Publishers; 2013:103–122.

85. Zarate CA, Mathews D, Ibrahim L, et al. A randomized trial of a low-trapping nonselective *N*-methyl-D-aspartate channel blocker in major depression. *Biol Psychiatry;* 2012 pii: S0006-3223(12) 00941-9. http://dx.doi.org/10.1016/j.biopsych.2012.10.019.
86. Overstreet DH, Wegener G. The flinders sensitive line rat model of depression—25 years and still producing. *Pharmacol Rev.* 2013;65(1):143–155.
87. Huang W, Heffernan ME, Li Z, Zhang N, Overstreet DH, King JA. Fear induced neuronal alterations in a genetic model of depression: an fMRI study on awake animals. *Neurosci Lett.* 2011;489(2):74–78.
88. Dzirasa K, Kumar S, Sachs BD, Caron MG, Nicolelis MA. Cortical-amygdalar circuit dysfunction in a genetic mouse model of serotonin deficiency. *J Neurosci.* 2013;33(10):4505–4513.
89. Hamani C, Nobrega JN. Preclinical studies modeling deep brain stimulation for depression. *Biol Psychiatry.* 2012;72(11):916–923.
90. Pereira EA, Lu G, Wang S, et al. Ventral periaqueductal grey stimulation alters heart rate variability in humans with chronic pain. *Exp Neurol.* 2010;223(2):574–581.
91. Hayes DJ, Northoff G. Common brain activations for painful and non-painful aversive stimuli. *BMC Neurosci.* 2012;13:60.
92. Pulman J, Buckley E. Assessing the efficacy of different upper limb hemiparesis interventions on improving health-related quality of life in stroke patients: a systematic review. *Top Stroke Rehabil.* 2013;20(2):171–188.
93. Allen L, Mehta S, McClure JA, Teasell R. Therapeutic interventions for aphasia initiated more than six months post stroke: a review of the evidence. *Top Stroke Rehabil.* 2012;19(6):523–535.
94. Berthier ML, García-Casares N, Walsh SF, et al. Recovery from post-stroke aphasia: lessons from brain imaging and implications for rehabilitation and biological treatments. *Discov Med.* 2011;12(65):275–289.
95. Schlaug G, Marchina S, Norton A. Evidence for plasticity in white-matter tracts of patients with chronic Broca's aphasia undergoing intense intonation-based speech therapy. *Ann N Y Acad Sci.* 2009;1169:385–394.
96. Schlaug G, Marchina S, Wan CY. The use of non-invasive brain stimulation techniques to facilitate recovery from post-stroke aphasia. *Neuropsychol Rev.* 2011;21(3):288–301.
97. Deller T, Haas CA, Freiman TM, Phinney A, Jucker M, Frotscher M. Lesion-induced axonal sprouting in the central nervous system. *Adv Exp Med Biol.* 2006;557:101–121.
98. Liu F, McCullough LD. Middle cerebral artery occlusion model in rodents: methods and potential pitfalls. *J Biomed Biotechnol.* 2011:464701.
99. Hoehn M, Nicolay K, Franke C, Van Sanden BD. Application of magnetic resonance to animal models of cerebral ischemia. *J Magn Reson Imaging.* 2001;14(5):491–509.
100. O'Connell LA, Hofmann HA. The vertebrate mesolimbic reward system and social behavior network: a comparative synthesis. *J Comp Neurol.* 2011;519(18):3599–3639.
101. Söderpalm B, Ericson M. Neurocircuitry involved in the development of alcohol addiction: the dopamine system and its access points. *Curr Top Behav Neurosci.* 2013;13:127–161.
102. Amato L, Davoli M, Minozzi S, Ferroni E, Ali R, Ferri M. Methadone at tapered doses for the management of opioid withdrawal. *Cochrane Database Syst Rev.* 2013;2:CD003409.
103. Clapp P. Current progress in pharmacologic treatment strategies for alcohol dependence. *Expert Rev Clin Pharmacol.* 2012;5(4): 427–435.
104. Haile CN, Mahoney 3rd JJ, Newton TF, De La Garza 2nd R. Pharmacotherapeutics directed at deficiencies associated with cocaine dependence: focus on dopamine, norepinephrine and glutamate. *Pharmacol Ther.* 2012;134(2):260–277.
105. Janssen PA, Demorest LC, Kelly A, Thiessen P, Abrahams R. Auricular acupuncture for chemically dependent pregnant women: a randomized controlled trial of the NADA protocol. *Subst Abuse Treat Prev Policy.* 2012;7:48.
106. Li J, Sun Y, Ye JH. Electroacupuncture decreases excessive alcohol consumption involving reduction of FosB/ΔFosB levels in reward-related brain regions. *PLoS One.* 2012;7(7):e40347.
107. Lee BH, Ma JH, In S, et al. Acupuncture at SI5 attenuates morphine seeking behavior after extinction. *Neurosci Lett.* 2012;529(1):23–27.
108. Li J, Zou Y, Ye JH. Low frequency electroacupuncture selectively decreases voluntarily ethanol intake in rats. *Brain Res Bull.* 2011;86(5–6):428–434.
109. Wang GB, Wu LZ, Yu P, Li YJ, Ping XJ, Cui CL. Multiple 100 Hz electroacupuncture treatments produced cumulative effect on the suppression of morphine withdrawal syndrome: central preprodynorphin mRNA and p-CREB implicated. *Peptides.* 2011; 32(4):713–721.
110. Meade CS, Lukas SE, McDonald LJ, et al. A randomized trial of transcutaneous electric acupoint stimulation as adjunctive treatment for opioid detoxification. *J Subst Abuse Treat.* 2010;38(1):12–21.
111. Lee JH, Kim HY, Jang EY, et al. Effect of acupuncture on naloxone-precipitated withdrawal syndrome in morphine-experienced rats: the mediation of GABA receptors. *Neurosci Lett.* 2011;504(3):301–305.
112. Huang W, Pach D, Napadow V, et al. Characterizing acupuncture stimuli using brain imaging with fMRI—a systematic review and meta-analysis of the literature. *PLoS One.* 2012;7(4):e32960.
113. Yang ES, Li PW, Nilius B, Li G. Ancient Chinese medicine and mechanistic evidence of acupuncture physiology. *Pflugers Arch.* 2011;462(5):645–653.
114. Parsons RG, Ressler KJ. Implications of memory modulation for post-traumatic stress and fear disorders. *Nat Neurosci.* 2013;16(2): 146–153.
115. Bremner JD. Neuroimaging in posttraumatic stress disorder and other stress-related disorders. *Neuroimaging Clin N Am.* 2007;17: 523–538.
116. Rogawski MA, Bazil CW. New molecular targets for antiepileptic drugs: $\alpha_2\delta$, SV2A, and K_V7/KCNQ/M potassium channels. *Curr Neurol Neurosci Rep.* 2008;8(4):345–352.
117. Hamner MB, Brodrick PS, Labbate LA. Gabapentin in PTSD: a retrospective, clinical series of adjunctive therapy. *Ann Clin Psychiatry.* 2001;13(3):141–146.
118. Berlin HA. Antiepileptic drugs for the treatment of post-traumatic stress disorder. *Curr Psychiatry Rep.* 2007;9(4):291–300.
119. Fowler M, Garza TH, Slater TM, Maani CV, McGhee LL. The relationship between gabapentin and pregabalin and post-traumatic stress disorder in burned service members. *J Burn Care Res.* 2012;33(5):612–618.
120. Pena DF, Engineer ND, McIntyre CK. Rapid remission of conditioned fear expression with extinction training paired with vagus nerve stimulation. *Biol Psychiatry.* 2013;73(11):1071–1077.
121. Nonaka A, Masuda F, Nomura H, Matsuki N. Impairment of fear memory consolidation and expression by antihistamines. *Brain Res.* 2013;1493:19–26.
122. Deschaux O, Zheng X, Lavigne J, et al. Post-extinction fluoxetine treatment prevents stress-induced reemergence of extinguished fear. *Psychopharmacology (Berl).* 2013;225(1):209–216.
123. Karpova NN, Pickenhaben A, Lindholm J, et al. Fear erasure in mice requires synergy between antidepressant drugs and extinction training. *Science.* 2011;334(6063):1731–1734.
124. de Kleine RA, Hendriks GJ, Kusters WJ, Broekman TG, van Minnen A. A randomized placebo-controlled trial of D-cycloserine to enhance exposure therapy for posttraumatic stress disorder. *Biol Psychiatry.* 2012;71:962–968.

125. Mayeux R, Stern Y. Epidemiology of Alzheimer disease. *Cold Spring Harb Perspect Med.* 2012;2(8) pii: a006239. http://dx.doi.org/10.1101/cshperspect.a006239.
126. Krstic D, Knuesel I. Deciphering the mechanism underlying late-onset Alzheimer disease. *Nat Rev Neurol.* 2013;9(1):25–34.
127. Holtzman DM, Mandelkow E, Selkoe DJ. Alzheimer disease in 2020. *Cold Spring Harb Perspect Med.* 2012;2(11) pii: a011585. http://dx.doi.org/10.1101/cshperspect.a011585.
128. Roman G, Pascual B. Contribution of neuroimaging to the diagnosis of Alzheimer's disease and vascular dementia. *Arch Med Res.* 2012;43(8):671–676.
129. Teipel SJ, Grothe M, Lista S, Toschi N, Garaci FG, Hampel H. Relevance of magnetic resonance imaging for early detection and diagnosis of Alzheimer disease. *Med Clin North Am.* 2013;97(3):399–424.
130. LaFerla FM, Green KN. Animal models of Alzheimer disease. *Cold Spring Harb Perspect Med.* 2012;2(11) pii: a006320. http://dx.doi.org/10.1101/cshperspect.a006320.
131. Teng E, Kepe V, Frautschy SA, et al. [F-18]FDDNP microPET imaging correlates with brain Aβ burden in a transgenic rat model of Alzheimer disease: effects of aging, in vivo blockade, and anti-Aβ antibody treatment. *Neurobiol Dis.* 2011;43(3):565–575.
132. Martinez A, Lahiri DK, Giacobini E, Greig NH. Advances in Alzheimer therapy: understanding pharmacological approaches to the disease. *Curr Alzheimer Res.* 2009;6(2):83–85.
133. Giacobini E. Cholinesterases in human brain: the effect of cholinesterase inhibitors on Alzheimer's disease and related disorders. In: Giacobini E, Pepeu G, eds. *The Brain Cholinergic System in Health and Disease.* Oxon, UK: Informa Healthcare; 2006:235–264.
134. Feng Y, Bai L, Ren Y, et al. fMRI connectivity analysis of acupuncture effects on the whole brain network in mild cognitive impairment patients. *Magn Reson Imaging.* 2012;30(5):672–682.
135. Laxton AW, Lozano AM. Deep brain stimulation for the treatment of Alzheimer disease and dementias. *World Neurosurg.* 2013;80 (3-4):S28. e1-S28.e8 http://dx.doi.org/10.1016/j.wneu.2012.06.028.
136. Merrill CA, Jonsson MA, Minthon L, et al. Vagus nerve stimulation in patients with Alzheimer's disease: additional follow-up results of a pilot study through 1 year. *J Clin Psychiatry.* 2006;67(8):1171–1178.
137. Carp J, Park J, Polk TA, Park DC. Age differences in neural distinctiveness revealed by multi-voxel pattern analysis. *Neuroimage.* 2011;56(2):736–743.
138. Dhanjal NS, Warren JE, Patel MC, Wise RJ. Auditory cortical function during verbal episodic memory encoding in Alzheimer's disease. *Ann Neurol.* 2013;73(2):294–302.
139. Miettinen PS, Pihlajamaki M, Jauhiainen AM, et al. Effect of cholinergic stimulation in early Alzheimer's disease—functional imaging during a recognition memory task. *Curr Alzheimer Res.* 2011;8(7):753–764.
140. Colas D, Chuluun B, Warrier D, et al. Short-term treatment with the $GABA_A$ receptor antagonist pentylenetetrazole produces a sustained pro-cognitive benefit in a mouse model of Down's syndrome. *Br J Pharmacol.* 2013;169(5):963–973.
141. Möhler H. Cognitive enhancement by pharmacological and behavioral interventions: the murine Down syndrome model. *Biochem Pharmacol.* 2012;84(8):994–999.
142. Ghazy A, Lundervold A, Veger T. Combined activation of the EEG with brietal and pentetrazol. *Clin Electroencephalogr.* 1978;9(2):60–68.
143. Kleschevnikova AM, Belichenko PV, Faizi M, et al. Deficits in cognition and synaptic plasticity in a mouse model of Down syndrome ameliorated by $GABA_B$ receptor antagonists. *J Neurosci.* 2012;32(27):9217–9227.
144. Segura B, Baggio HC, Solana E, et al. Neuroanatomical correlates of olfactory loss in normal aged subjects. *Behav Brain Res.* 2013;246:148–153.
145. Wostyn P, Van Dam D, Audenaert K, De Deyn PP. Increased cerebrospinal fluid production as a possible mechanism underlying caffeine's protective effect against Alzheimer's disease. *Int J Alzheimers Dis.* 2011:617420.
146. Benabid AL, Torres N. New targets for DBS. *Parkinsonism Relat Disord.* 2012;18(Suppl. 1):S21–S23.

Index

Note: Page numbers with "*f*" denote figures; "*t*" tables.

B

C

N

O

P

R

S

Color Plates

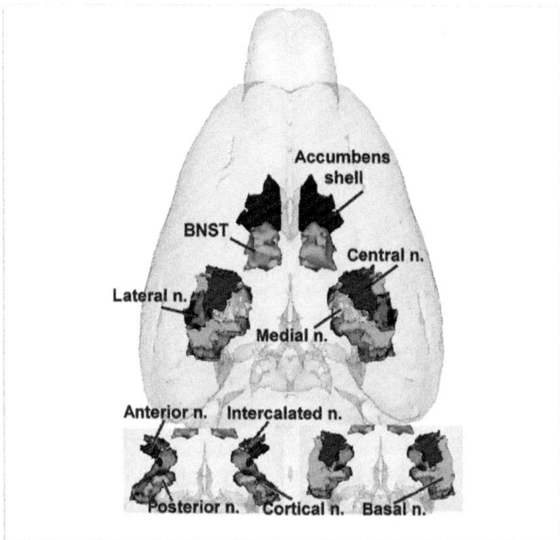

FIGURE 3.8 **Amygdala in 3D**. The image shows a translucent shell of the brain with the location of different subregions of the amygdala depicted in color as 3D volumes.

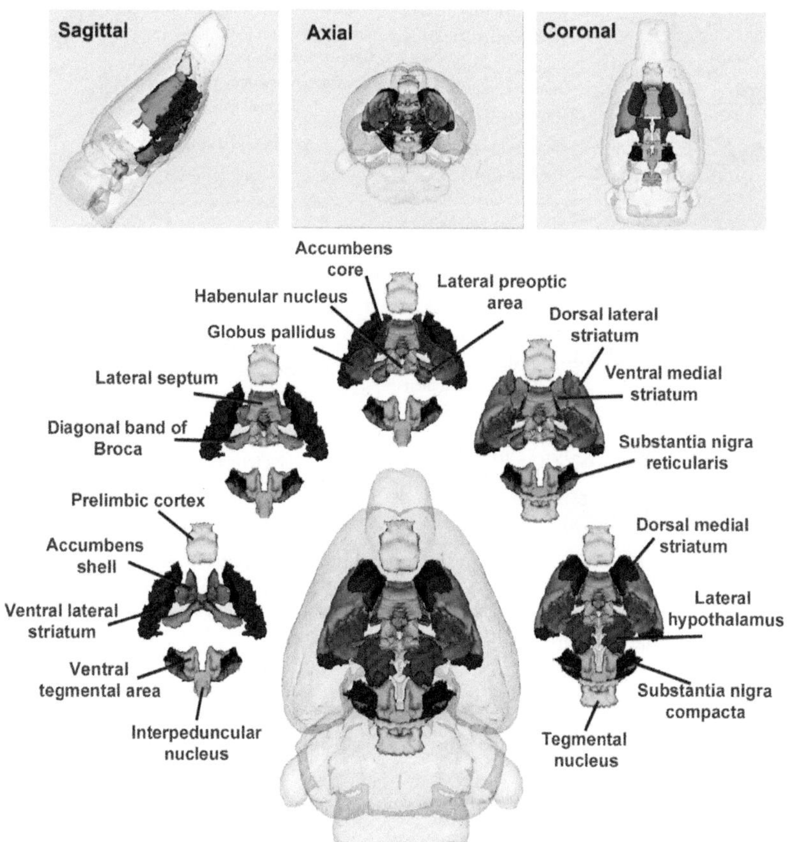

FIGURE 3.9 **Habenular system**. The central image is a coronal view of a translucent shell of the brain, showing the total composite and location of different subregions of the habenular system depicted in color as 3D volumes. Surrounding this are different layers of the habenular system showing a caudal (deepest)-to-dorsal perspective to enable identification of all subregions. The panels on the top show the habenular system in different orthogonal directions.

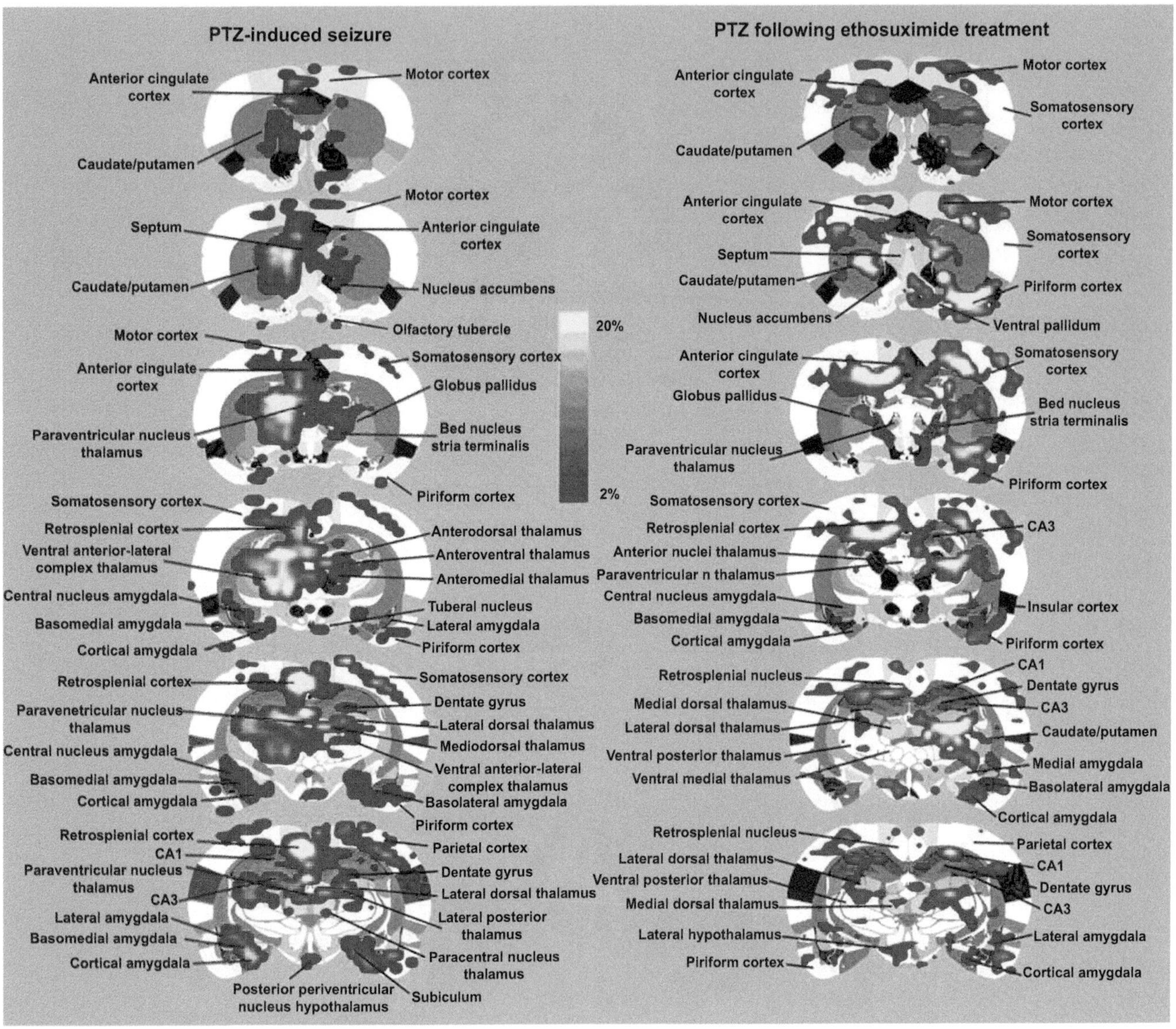

FIGURE 3.11 Pentylenetetrazol-induced seizure. Shown in the left column is the pattern of PTZ-induced changes in BOLD signal before seizure onset (first 30 s after PTZ injection). The right column is the pattern of PTZ-induced activity in the presence of ethosuximide (ESM). The composite map of all subjects ($n = 5$ in each group) is shown registered to six contiguous coronal sections of the segmented atlas. The scale bar shows the percentage change in BOLD signal intensity. *Source: Adapted from Ref. 43.*

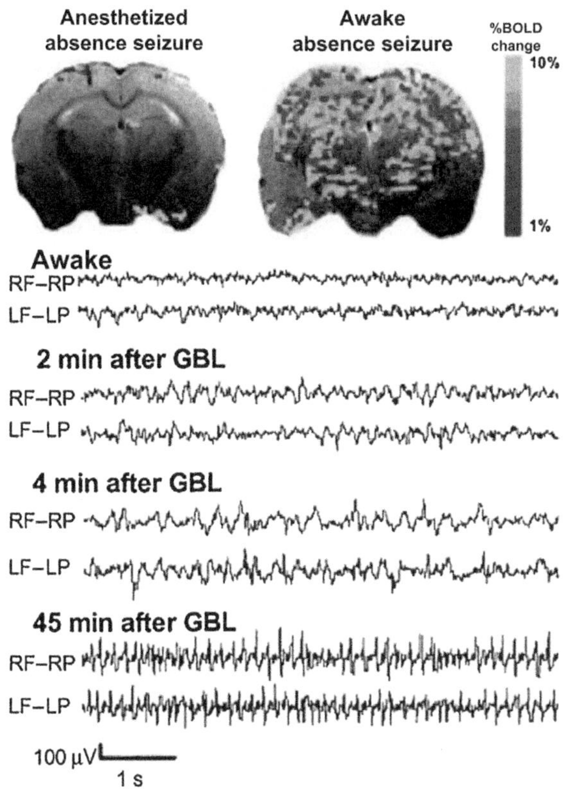

FIGURE 3.12 γ-**Butyrolactone-induced seizure in rats**. The top left image shows BOLD signal changes in a rat experiencing an absence seizure while continuously anesthetized with 2% isoflurane. The top right image shows BOLD signal changes in a rat experiencing an absence seizure but not anesthetized. The bottom traces show representative data from an EEG recording collected during the functional magnetic resonance imaging experiment. Nonmagnetic epidural electrodes were placed in the frontal and parietal cortices to monitor seizure activity during the imaging session. Placement of electrode leads is labeled. RF: right frontal cortex; RP: right parietal cortex; LF: left frontal cortex; LP: left parietal cortex. *Source: Adapted from Ref. 11.*

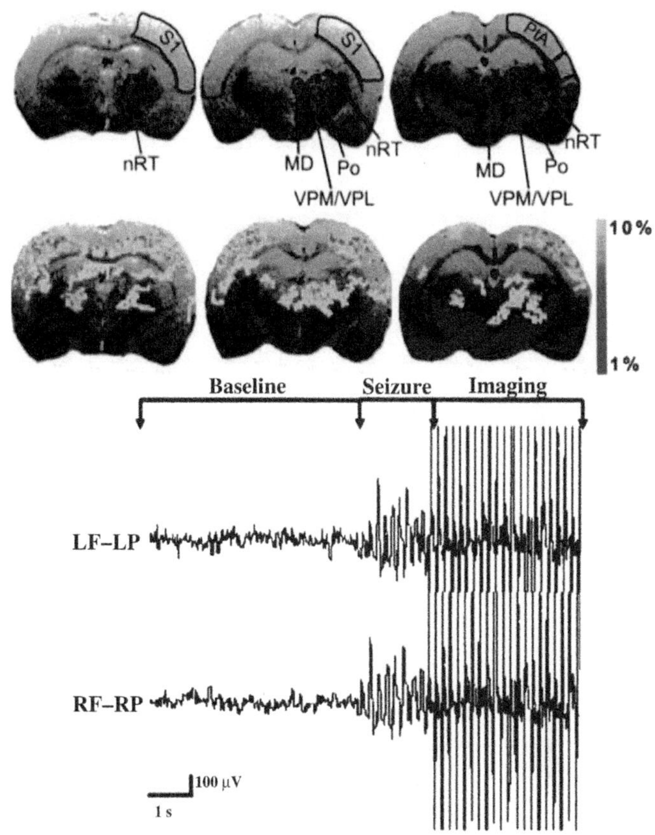

FIGURE 3.13 **Genetic model of absence seizure**. Shown at top are representative BOLD activation maps of three consecutive axial sections of the rat brain during spontaneous spike-and-wave discharges from a single subject. The top row shows the regions of interest used for analysis. MD: mediodorsal thalamic nuclei; nRT: nucleus reticularis thalami; Po: posterior thalamic nuclear group; PtA: parietal association cortex; S1: sensory cortex; Te: temporal cortex; VPM and VPL: ventral posteromedial and posterolateral thalamic nucleus. At the bottom are representative EEG recordings collected during the imaging session. Nonmagnetic epidural electrodes were placed in the frontal and parietal cortices to monitor seizure activity during the imaging session. Normal, awake EEG was present during baseline imaging. Imaging was triggered after the formation of epileptiform activity similar to that shown during the seizure period. Artifact due to image acquisition can be seen with a delay of ~2 s after seizure activity. RF: right frontal cortex; RP: right parietal cortex; LF: left frontal cortex; LP: left parietal cortex. *Source: Adapted from Ref. 10.*

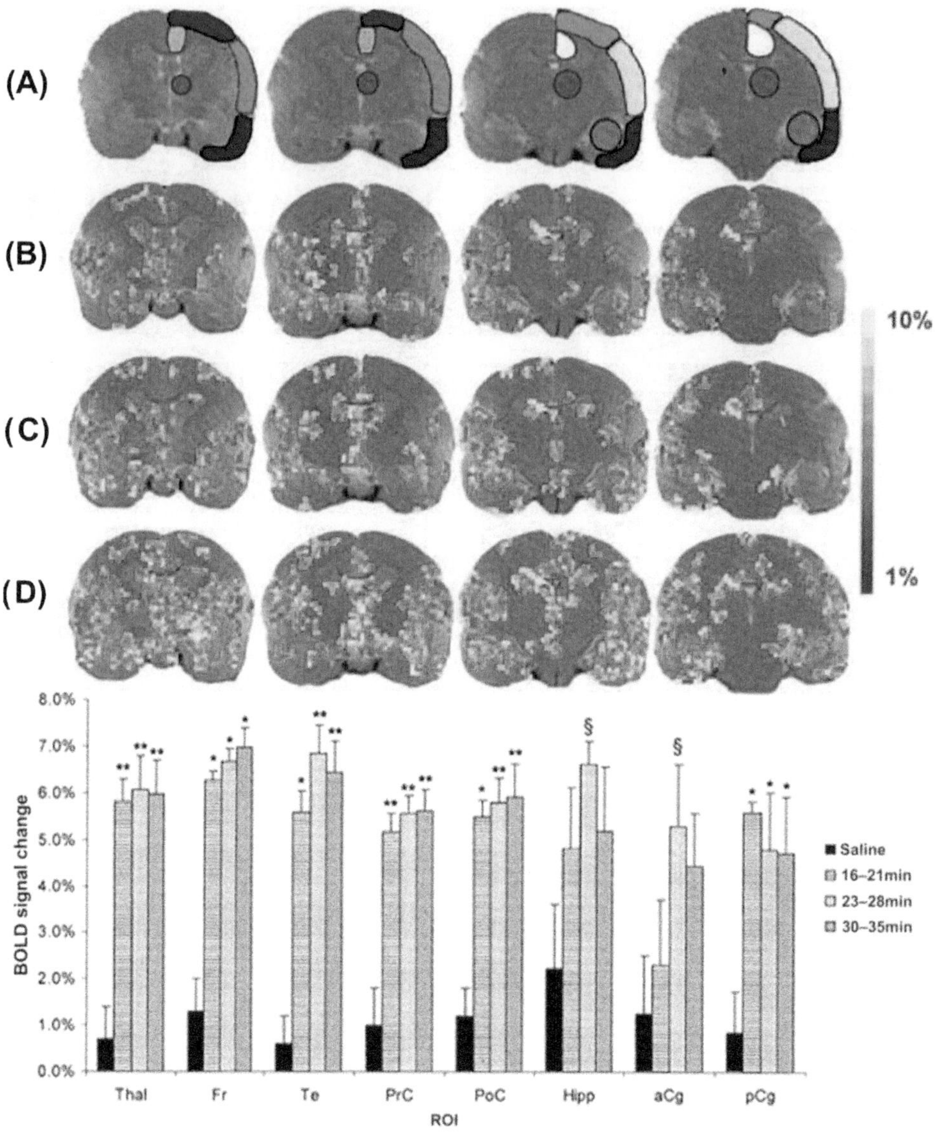

FIGURE 3.15 **γ-Butyrolactone-induced seizure activity in monkeys.** Activation maps of blood oxygenation level–dependent (BOLD) signal responses during absence seizure. The colored pixels indicate the statistically significant ($p < 0.05$) pixels, which are determined by t test analysis and overlaid onto the corresponding anatomy. Four consecutive slices through the brain are shown for an individual marmoset. (A) Anatomic images, with regions of interest used for analysis outlined according to the following color code: thalamus (blue), hippocampus (orange), frontal cortex (red), temporal cortex (purple), precentral cortex (green), postcentral cortex (yellow), anterior cingulate cortex (light blue), and posterior cingulate cortex (white). (B–D) Activation corresponding to images collected 16–21 min, 23–28 min, and 30–35 min after γ-butyrolactone injection, respectively. Change in blood-oxygen-level–dependent (BOLD) signal intensity for each region of interest (ROI). The BOLD signal intensity change during 3 Hz spike-wave discharges is shown for cortical and subcortical ROIs (mean ± SEM, $N = 5$ marmosets). Signal changes after the control injection of saline are shown, along with signal changes occurring 16–21 min, 23–28 min, and 30–35 min after the γ-butyrolactone injection. Time blocks with significantly different signal changes from the control injection are noted (§$p < 0.05$, *$p < 0.01$, **$p < 0.001$). All ROIs are bilateral structures, so the signal changes from each hemisphere were combined. Thal: thalamus; Fr: frontal cortex; Te: temporal cortex; PrC: precentral cortex; PoC: postcentral cortex; Hipp: hippocampus; aCg: anterior cingulate cortex; pCg: posterior cingulate cortex. *Source: Adapted from Ref. 12.*

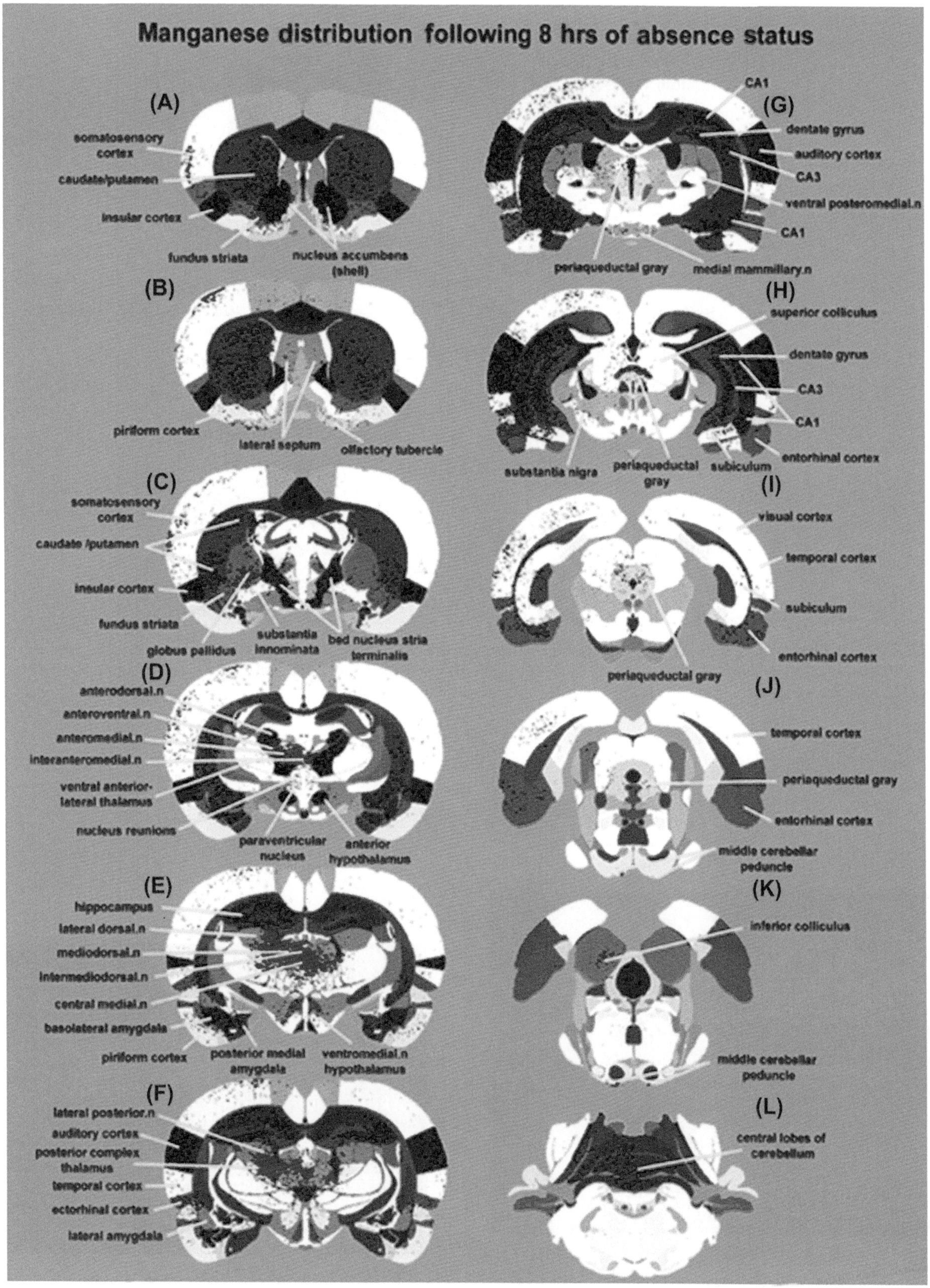

FIGURE 3.16 **Manganese distribution with absence status epilepticus.** Areas with increased signal intensity due to the presence of manganese are shown above as red dots. The serial brain sections are taken from a single rat and are representative of the distribution pattern observed in all animals studied.

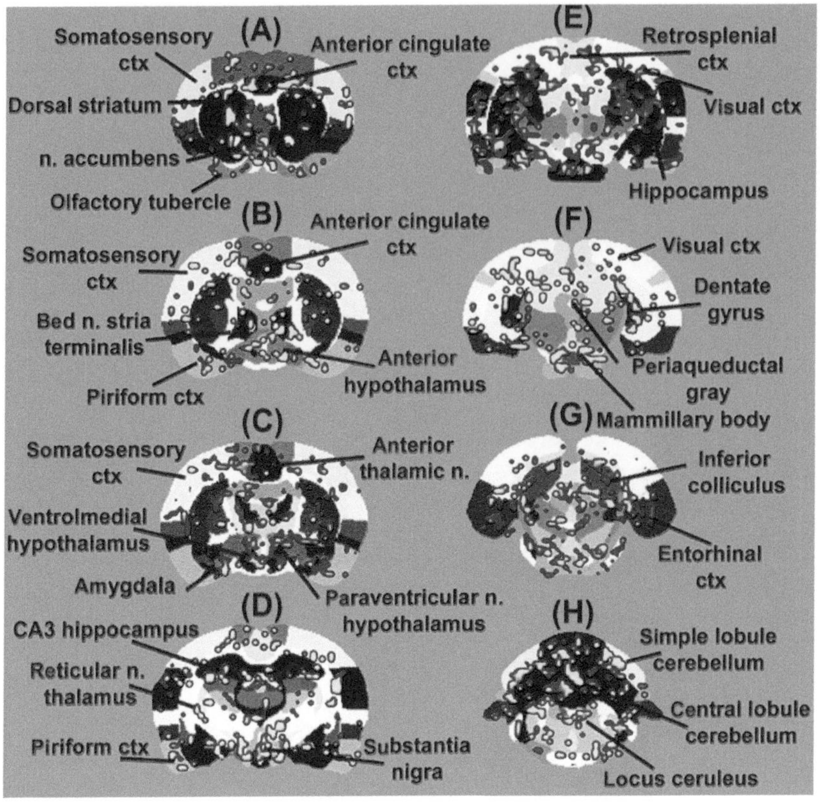

FIGURE 3.17 **BOLD imaging following γ-butyrolactone**. Shown are activation maps of positive BOLD signal registered to axial sections of the 3D MRI rat atlas. The red-yellow depicts the localization of significantly activated and interpolated voxels that exceed a 2% threshold above baseline. The data are the significant change over baseline as an average of five animals.

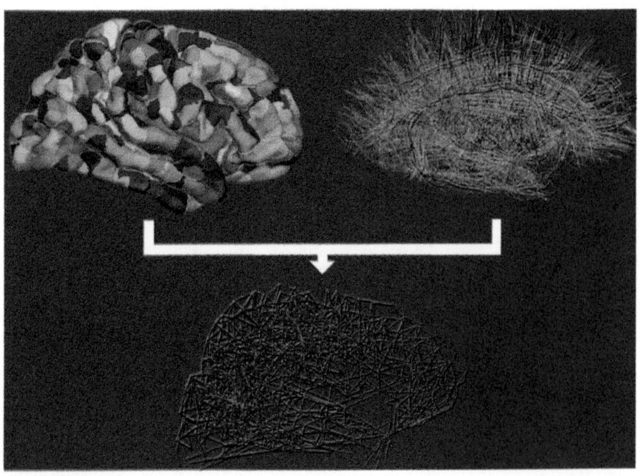

FIGURE 6.1 Identification of networks in the human brain by anatomical parcellation into 1000 regions (top left) and tractography using diffusion spectrum imaging (top right). The two methods are combined to form a whole-brain anatomical network composed of neural regions and their white matter connections (bottom). *Source: Reproduced with permission from Ref. 13.*

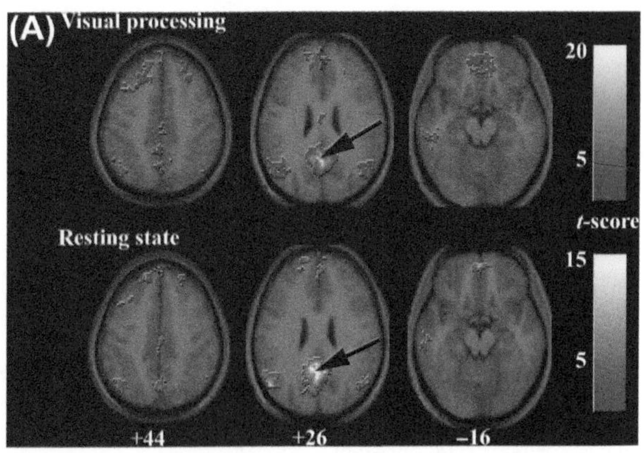

FIGURE 6.3 Resting state networks recapitulate task-based networks. (A) Connectivity maps for the posterior cingulate cortex. Networks found during a visual processing task (top) and resting state (bottom) are similar. *Source: Reproduced with permission from Ref. 45. Copyright © 2003 National Academy of Sciences USA.*

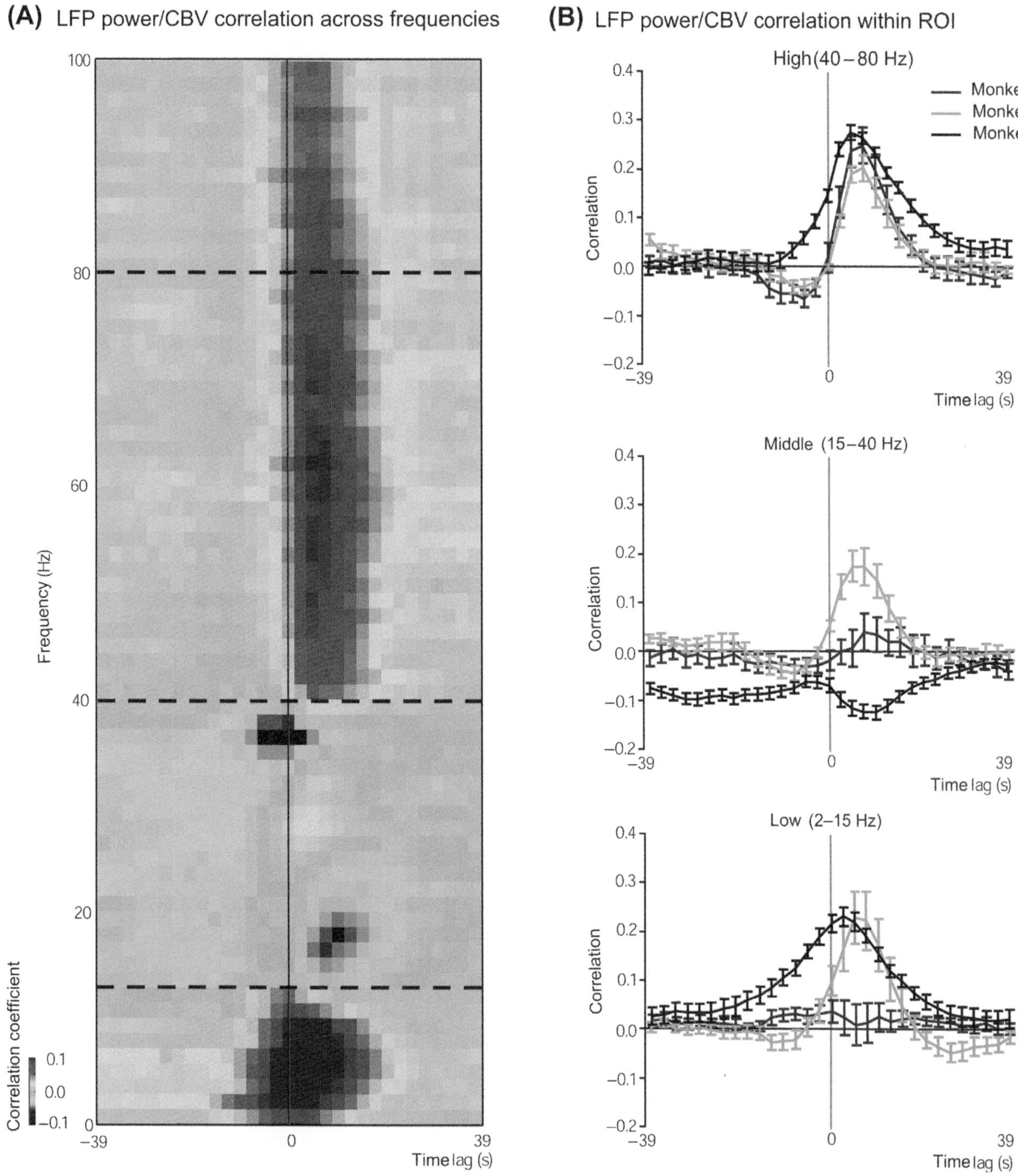

FIGURE 6.4 In simultaneous fMRI and electrophysiological recordings in macaque V1, resting state fMRI signals are related to local field potentials. (A) Correlations between fMRI and LFP power during the resting state show distinct relationships across frequency bands. (B) For three monkeys, correlation is consistently positive in the 40–80 Hz range, has a variable and slightly negative correlation in the 15–40 Hz range, and is generally positive in the 2–15 Hz range. *Source: Reproduced with permission from Ref. 76.*

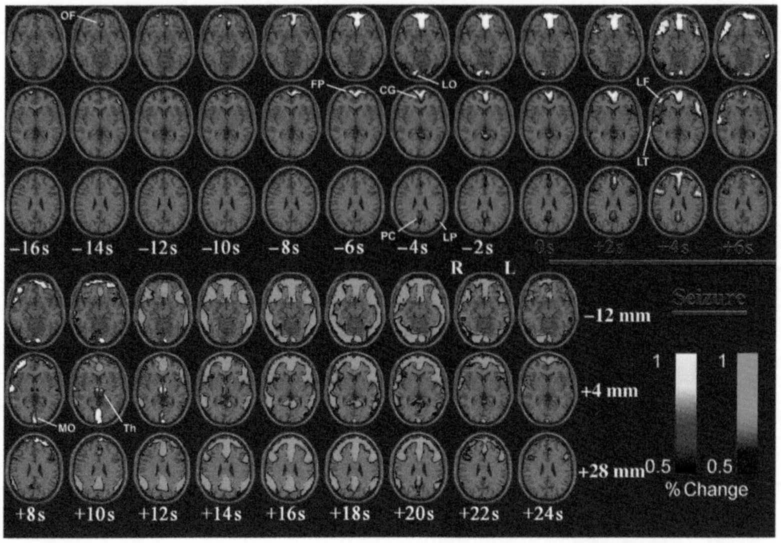

FIGURE 6.5 Dynamic changes in network activation before, during, and after absence seizures. Time course maps of percentage change from baseline show early increases (red) even before seizure onset in the frontal cortex, then progress to include a frontoparietal network and the thalamus. Profound widespread decreases (blue) are seen after end of seizure. *Source: Reproduced with permission from Ref. 41.*

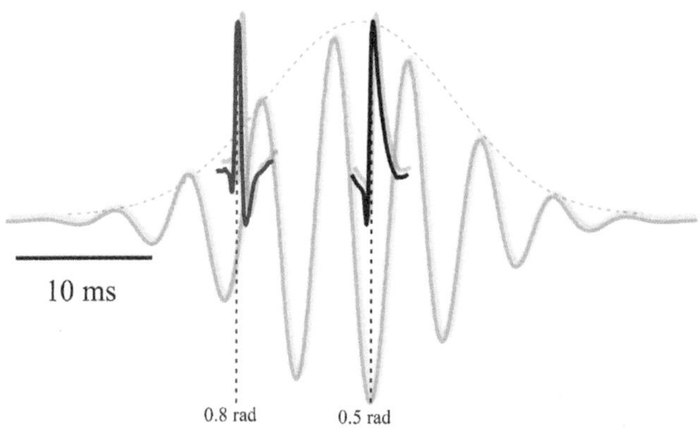

FIGURE 9.2 **Temporal relationship of putative interneurons and pyramidal cells to ripples recorded from the human hippocampus**. This figure summarizes the findings from Ref. 25 that reported the spiking relationship of putative interneurons (red) and pyramidal cells (blue) to ripple oscillations (green). This schematic highlights the burst-like appearance of ripples, which are temporally limited and have a clear peak in amplitude (the gray dotted line represents the amplitude envelope of the ripple). The peak in amplitude corresponds to the time when pyramidal cells are most likely to fire, whereas the interneurons are more like to fire before pyramidal cells earlier in the ripple cycle. In relation to when in the cycle cells will fire, pyramidal cells are more likely to discharge at the trough of the ripple, whereas interneurons discharge approximately 0.5 ms later. The spikes are not on the same time base as the ripple, to demonstrate their waveforms.

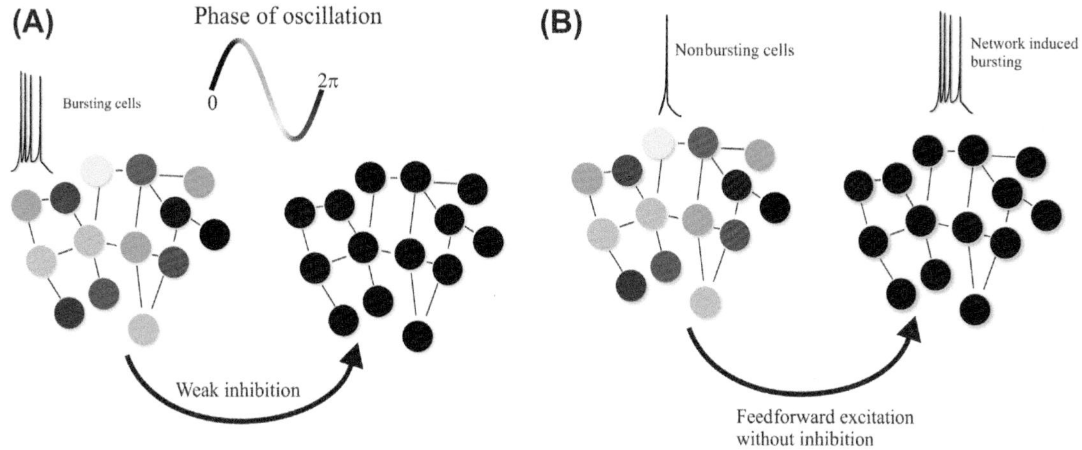

FIGURE 9.5 **Network manifestations of bursting phenomena.** (A) In a population of interconnected but asynchronous cells (the colors depict the phase of the cell's oscillation), a small amount of inhibition can strongly synchronize the population, not unlike that which is seen in the thalamus. The weak inhibition results in de-inactivation of voltage-dependent currents, and thus it provides a synchronizing force to an active population of neurons. From a systems perspective, the fact that the cells are already bursting creates homogeneity in the system, and the inhibition then provides the strong coupling. This can result in a critical state transition[94] from asynchrony to synchrony. Such a mechanism may also underlie how information can be rerouted on a fixed architecture.[95] (B) The organization of a network connection can transform a population of inherently nonbursting cells to bursting through network dynamics. This may be particularly important in the context of epilepsy, where aberrant network interactions could render the population bursting. Invoking the mechanism of (B), preserved inhibition could then strongly synchronize the population if the excitatory interactions are not sufficient to achieve this, resulting in seizures.

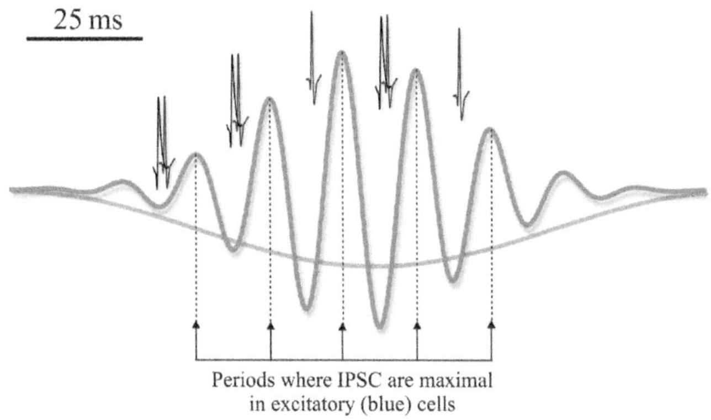

FIGURE 9.6 **A feedforward mechanism for bursting and cross-frequency coupling (nesting).** A theta oscillation (gray) and associated gamma oscillation (green), with associated spiking of interneurons (red) and excitatory cells (blue). The gamma oscillation is expanded in amplitude to highlight its features relative to the theta oscillation. Within the theta cycle, excitatory cells generate action potentials that excite interneurons. The interneurons feedback onto the excitatory cells, generating inhibitory postsynaptic potentials (IPSPs) in the excitatory cells. These precisely timed IPSPs summate across the population of excitatory cells to generate large sources and hence the strong temporal correlation to the positive-going component of the gamma oscillation. During periods of strong inhibitory cell drive, excitatory cell activity is suppressed. What is not immediately apparent is that each excitatory cell may not discharge on every gamma cycle. However, among a population of excitatory cells, the probability of any one cell discharging is highest at the trough of the theta oscillation, and thus as a population a highly stereotypical envelope of gamma oscillation is generated through this feedback mechanism. The "clock-like" precision of the nested gamma oscillation thus is a population event that is tightly controlled in time by the intrinsic circuitry and temporal organization of cellular discharge. *(Source: This schema has been adapted from Ref. 117.)* Such a "chronocircuit" has been described in the hippocampus as well.[118] This figure also highlights that oscillatory activity; here in this case, the theta oscillation generates periods of increased excitability. Such periods of excitability increase the probability of cells firing at specific times. In the context of the communication through coherence (CTC) hypothesis, such rhythmic gain control is associated with elevated period of neuronal discharge, hence burst generation. Such burst generation, however, need not manifest in individual cells. The burst in fact may be generated by the increased probability of a population of cells increasing their firing rates during specific time windows, and thus the burst in fact may be a population phenomenon.

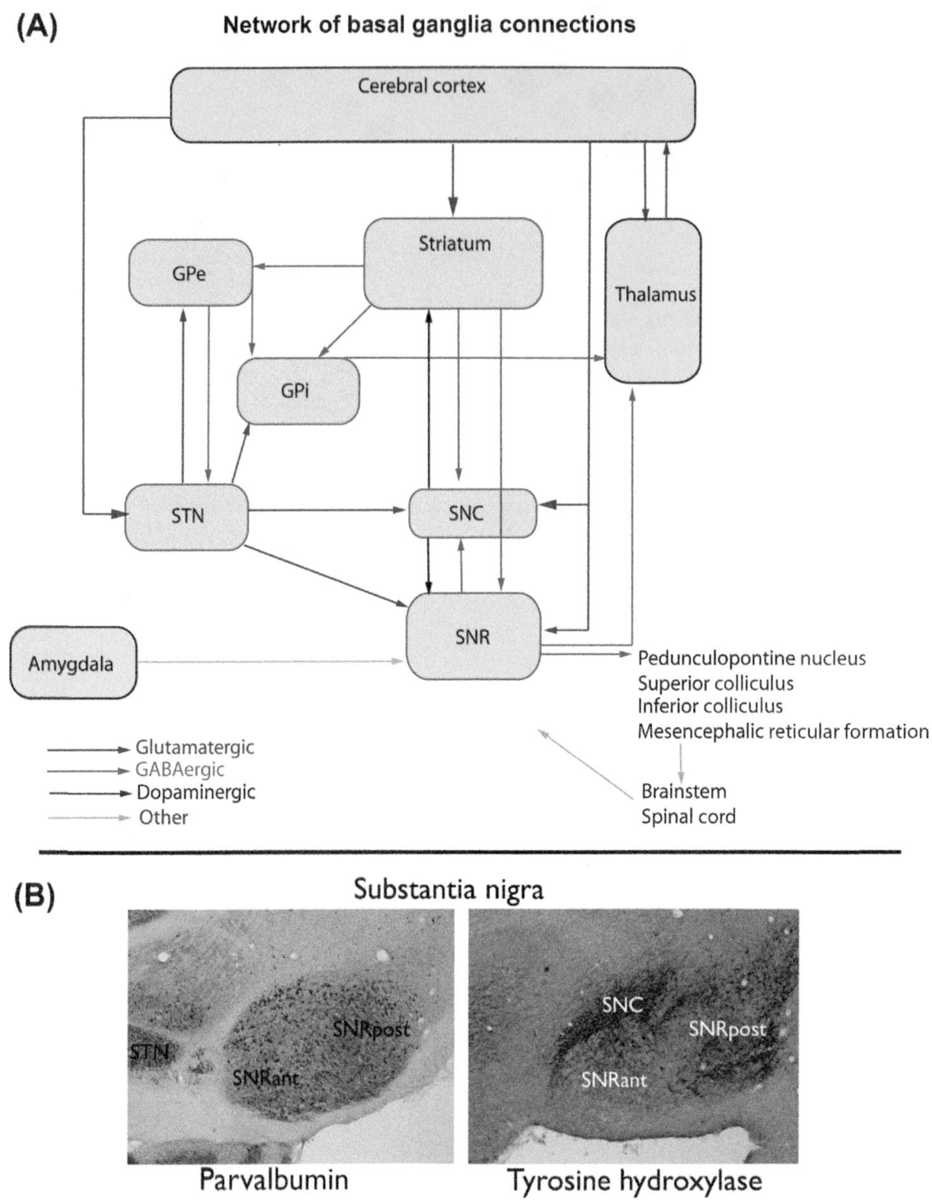

FIGURE 11.1 The circuitry of connections within and beyond the basal ganglia and substantia nigra regional organization. (A): The basal ganglia nuclei are shown here with the yellow boxes. The direct pathway involves striatal projections to the GPi–SNR and subsequently to the thalamus. The indirect pathway traverses through the striatum toward the GPe and STN, which then activates the SNR. (B): The SN consists of two distinct regions with different functions in seizure control. Sagittal sections of a PN30 rat SN are shown here, stained either with antiparvalbumin antibody (left panel) to indicate the majority of GABAergic neurons or with antityrosine hydroxylase antibody to label dopaminergic neurons in the SNC or SNRpost. The SNRant consists of almost exclusively GABAergic neurons (parvalbumin-positive). Regional differences in the connectivity of the two regions have been reported, but these have not yet been fully described.[10,11] GPe: globus pallidum externa; GPi: globus pallidum interna; STN: subthalamic nucleus; SNR: substantia nigra pars reticulata; SNC: substantia nigra pars compacta.

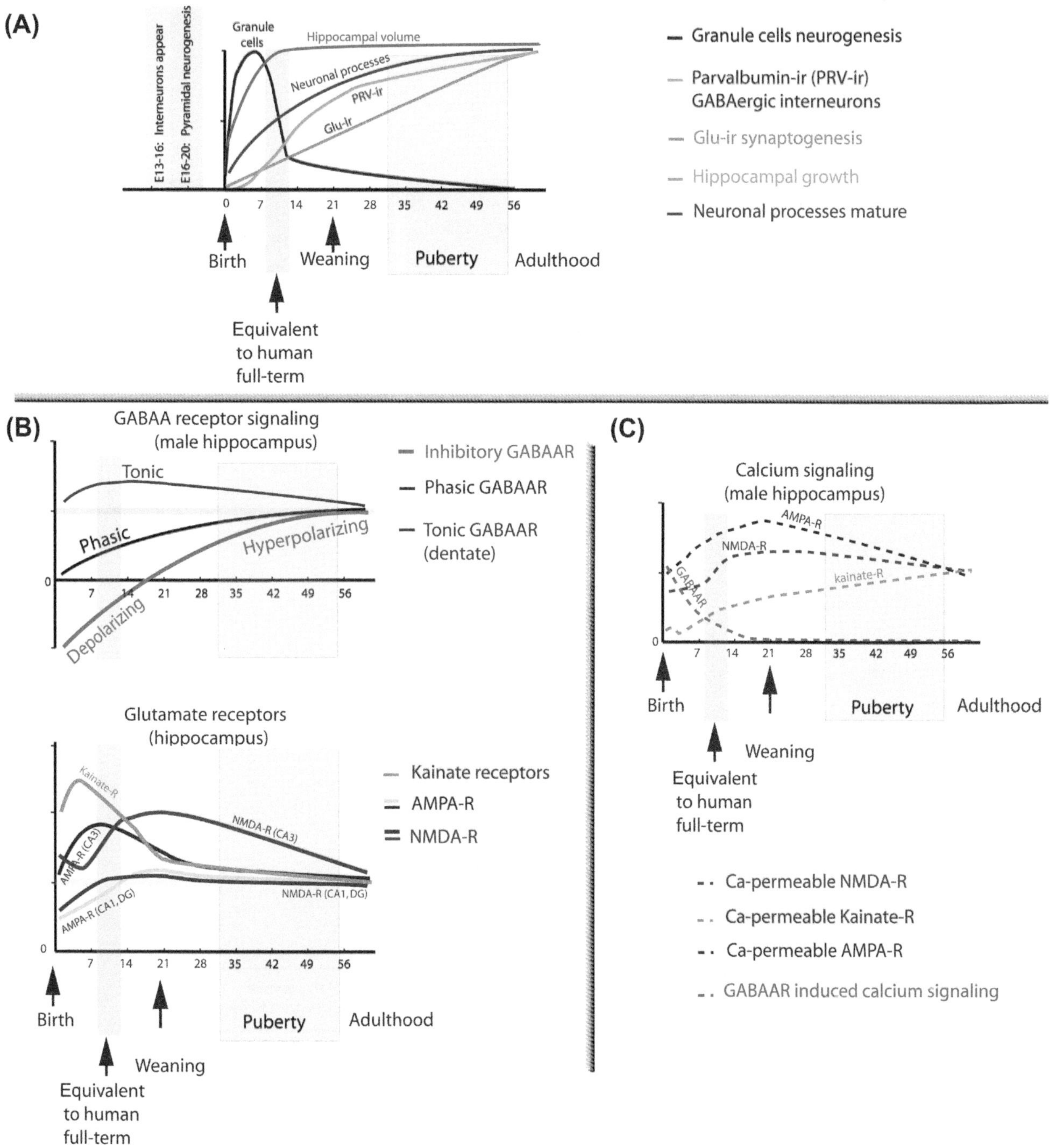

FIGURE 11.3 Developmental changes in the hippocampus of male rodents. (A) Developmental changes in neurogenesis, excitatory (glutamatergic: Glu-ir) and GABAergic synaptogenesis, and hippocampal growth in rodents.[69] *(Source: Modified from Ref. 69 with permission from John Wiley and Sons.)* (B) Developmental changes in tonic, phasic, and depolarizing versus hyperpolarizing $GABA_A$ receptor responses[65,67,70,71] (upper panel) and of kainic acid,[72] NMDA, and AMPA receptor expression in the rat male hippocampus[71,73] (lower panel). Region, sex, and cell type differences are also reported. (C) Developmental changes in $GABA_A$ or glutamate receptor–induced increases in intracellular calcium in the male rat hippocampus, based on E-gaba studies, and the relative expression of calcium-permeable glutamatergic receptors.[67,72,74,75]

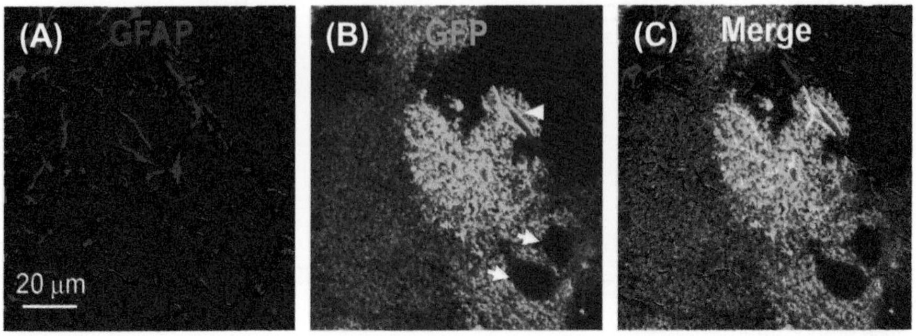

FIGURE 12.1 **Astrocytic morphology and structural relationship with neurons.** (A) Immunostaining against the glial-specific protein GFAP reveals only a limited portion of the astrocytic structure, composed mainly of primary processes. (B) When the fluorescent marker GFP is specifically expressed in a subpopulation of astrocytes, fine higher order processes become visible, revealing the complexity of the astrocytic morphology. Astrocytes contact neuronal cell bodies (arrows in B) and blood vessels (arrowhead in B). Images in A−B are merged in (C). *Source: Reproduced with permission from Ref. 10.*

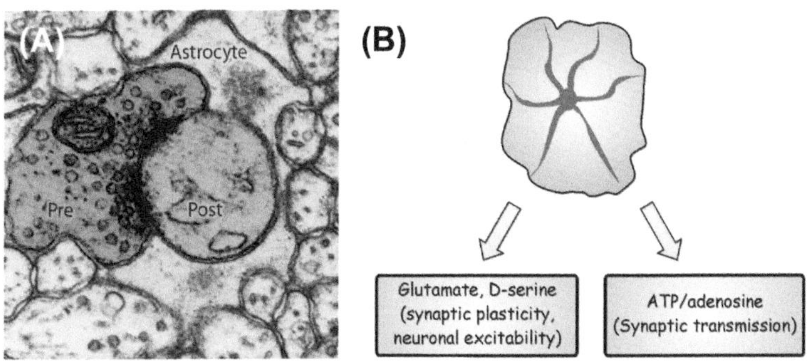

FIGURE 12.2 **Astrocytes modulate neuronal function by releasing different chemical transmitters.** (A) The structural basis of the concept of the tripartite synapse is shown in this electron microscopy image. The astrocytic process (green) enwraps both the presynaptic (red) and postsynaptic (orange) terminals. *(Source: Reproduced with permission from Ref. 12.)* (B) Astrocytes release glutamate and D-serine that, by activating NMDA receptors, modulate synaptic plasticity, neuronal excitability, and synchrony. Astrocytes also release ATP, which is degraded to adenosine and strongly suppresses synaptic transmission by activating adenosine A1 receptors. *Source: Modified from Ref. 13.*

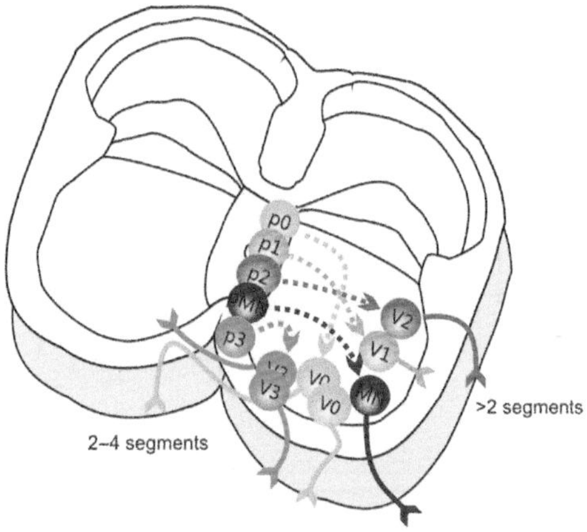

	Progenitors	Postmitotic		Transmitter	Axonal projection	
V0	Dbx1/2	?	V0d	GABA/Glycine 70%	Commissural	MN ?
		Evx1/2	V0v	Glutamate 25%	Commissural	MN ?
		Pitx2	V0c	Acetylcholine 5%	Ipsilateral/Bilateral	MN IaIN ?
V1	Dbx2	En1	RC	GABA/Glycine	Ipsilateral	MN IaIN
			IaIN			MN IaIN
			75% ?			?
V2	Lhx3/4	Lhx3, Chx10 (EphA4)	V2a	Glutamate	Ipsilateral	MN V0
		GATA2/3	V2b	GABA/Glycine		?
pMN	Nkx6-1	Hb9	MN	Acetylcholine	Perhipheral	Muscles
V3	Nkx2-2, Nkx6-1	Sim1	V3s	Glutamate	Commissural 85%	MN RC IaIN V2
			V3r		Ipsilateral 15%	
?	?	Hb9	?	Glutamate	Ipsilateral	MN ?

FIGURE 17.4 Diagram representing the progenitor domains (p0–p3) that give rise to ventral spinal interneuron groups (V0–V3). The transcription factors that characterize the progenitor domains and the postmitotic interneuron subgroups are illustrated. Where possible the transmitter phenotypes of the interneuron subgroups are given, along with their known sites of termination. Motoneuron progenitors and their associated transcription factors are also illustrated. Interneurons that express Hb9 (similar to motoneurons) are also illustrated, although the cardinal progenitor group that produces them is not known. V0d: dorsal V0 interneurons; V0v: ventral V0 interneurons; V0c: cholinergic V0 interneurons; RCs: Renshaw cells; IaIN: Ia inhibitory interneurons; V2a: excitatory V2 interneurons; V2b: inhibitory V2 interneurons; MN: motoneurons; V3s: V3 interneurons producing synchrony; V3r: V3 interneurons with connections expected of rhythm-generating layer neurons.

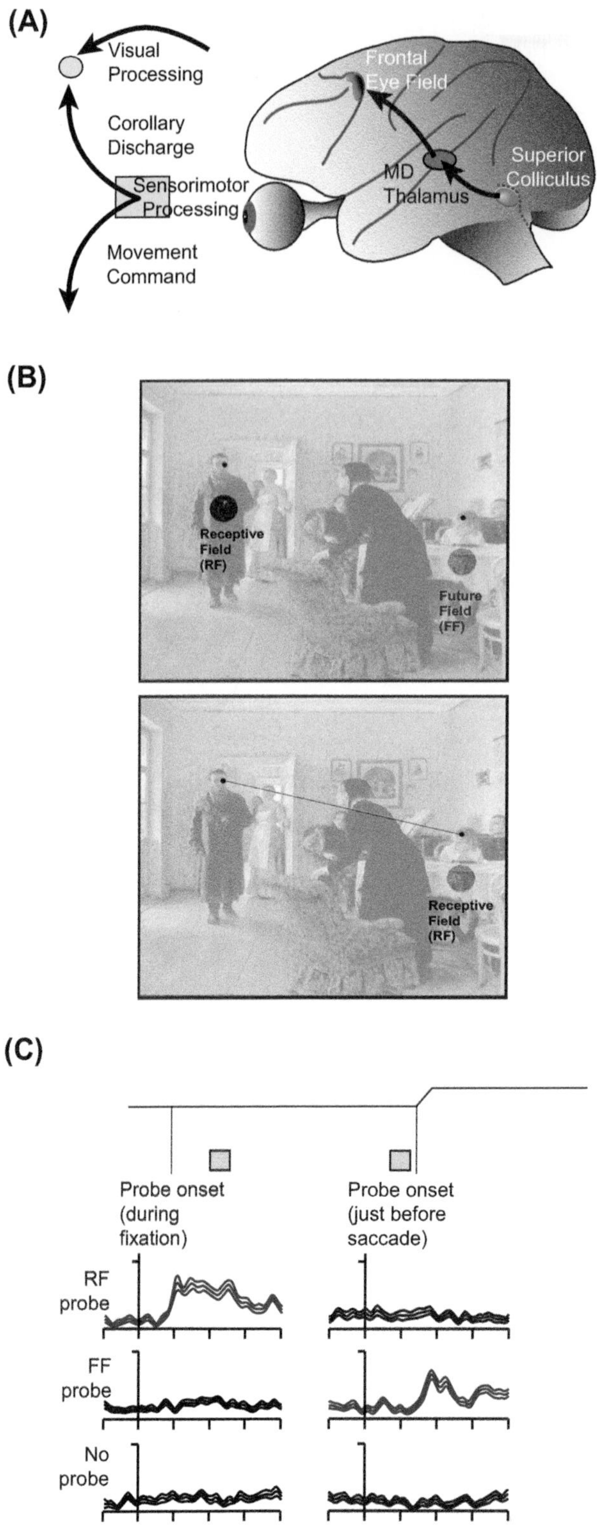

FIGURE 19.6 Spatial stability during eye movements is achieved through integration of visual and motor signals. During eye movements, the visual system "compensates" for shifts in the location of the retinal image, to generate visual representations in externally based coordinates ("spatial stability"). Whereas early visual areas, such as V1, encode information in purely retinal coordinates, higher association areas of the cortex, such as the LIP in the parietal lobe and the FEF in the frontal lobe, adjust their responses during eye movements to compensate for the shift in the retinal image. Perception correlates with neural representations in higher association areas but does not correlate with retinal representations in the early visual areas. Eye movement compensation is achieved by integrating visual signals, and a motor signal that is a copy ("corollary discharge") of the movement command is sent to the eyes (A, left). The superior colliculus, for instance, sends motor commands to generate eye movements, and at the same time it projects through the medial dorsal nucleus of the thalamus (MD) to the FEF (A, right). During saccadic eye movements, neurons in the FEF exhibit "shifting receptive fields" (B, C). To probe the responses properties of these neurons, visual stimuli are presented before and after an eye movement in their receptive field (RF), as well as in their "future field" (FF), which corresponds to the RF after the eye movement (B). Notably, shortly prior to the eye movement, these neurons become nonresponsive to stimuli in the RF but respond robustly to stimuli in the FF (C). *Source: Reproduced, with permission, from Wurtz RH. Neuronal mechanisms of visual stability.* Vision Res. *2008;48:2070–2089.*

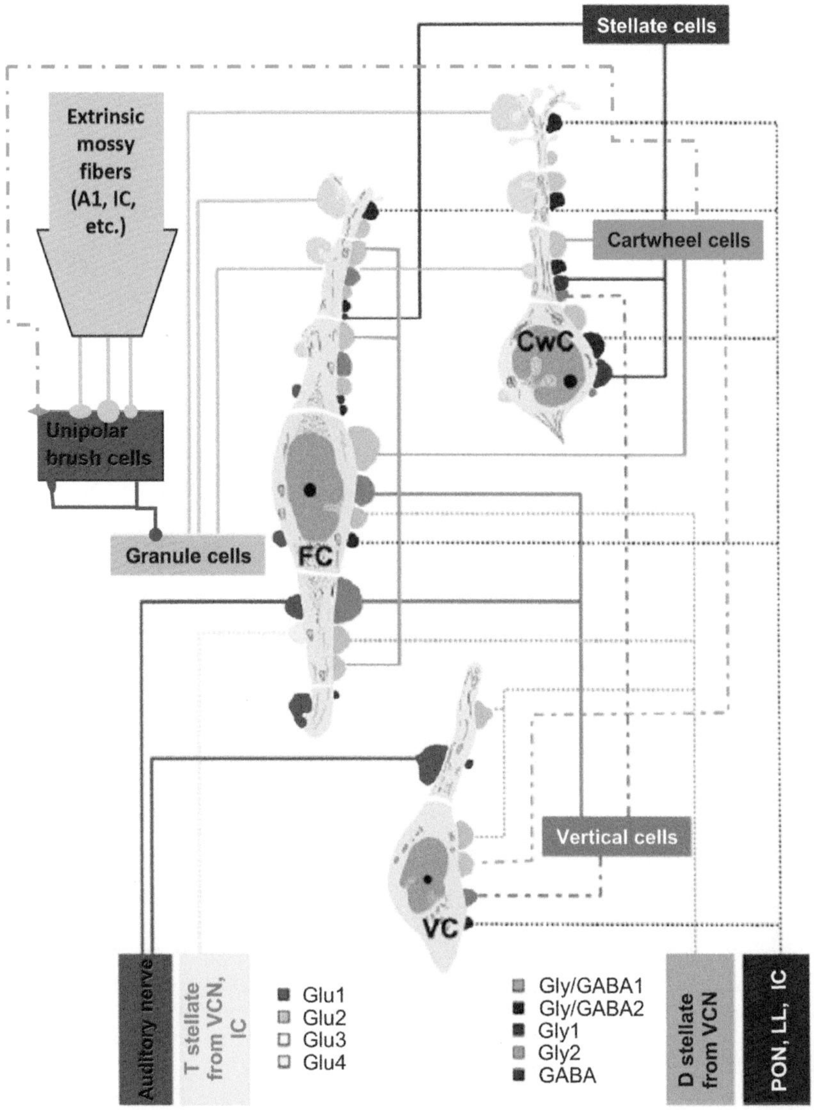

FIGURE 20.2 A summary of the neurotransmitter connections in the dorsal cochlear nucleus of the rat, adapted from Rubio.[26] It has been hypothesized that, following damage to the auditory periphery, there is a compensatory downregulation of inhibitory interneurons, particularly vertical cells, and an upregulation of excitatory interneurons, particularly unipolar brush cells. Also note that unipolar brush cells, via their descending mossy fiber inputs, comprise an excitatory positive feedback loop. *Source: Reprinted with permission Ref. 26.*

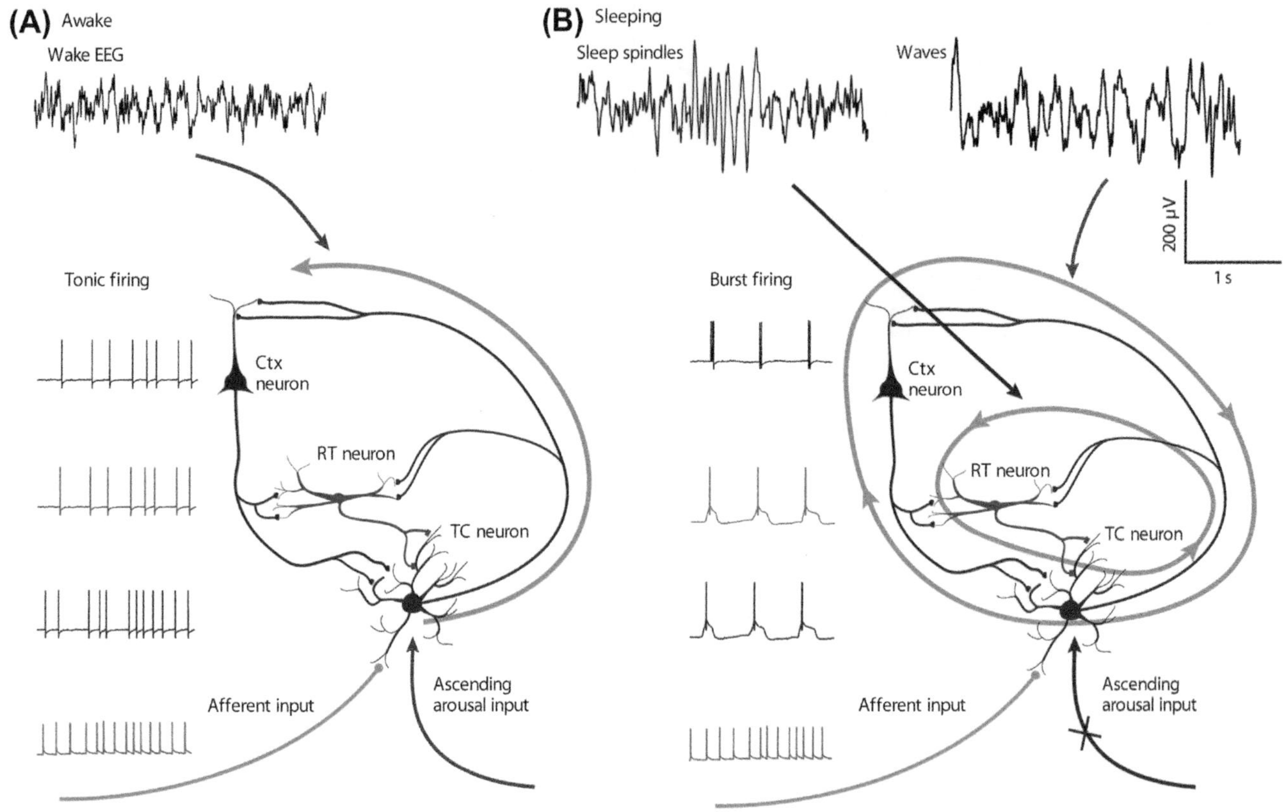

FIGURE 21.4 **Neuromodulators alter thalamic firing.** (A) During wakefulness, excitatory ascending input to the thalamus depolarizes thalamic intralaminar and relay neurons. This allows a tonic firing mode and faithful transmission of afferent sensory input. (B) During sleep, the thalamus is hyperpolarized due to withdrawal of excitatory ascending input. As a result, the tonic fires in bursts and does not relay afferent sensory input. *Source: Reproduced with permission from Ref. 11.*

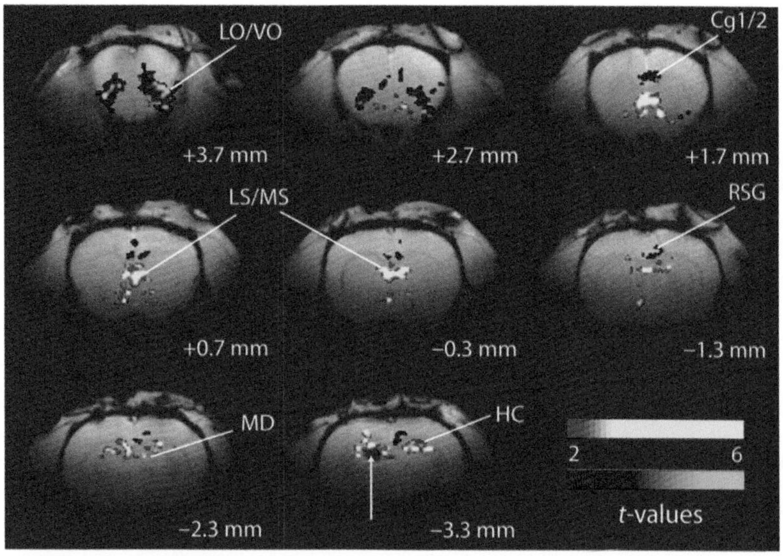

FIGURE 21.6 **Neuroimaging reveals consciousness networks.** Blood oxygen level dependent (BOLD) fMRI during a rodent model of complex partial seizures demonstrates coordinated cortical and subcortical changes. Seizures are induced by hippocampal stimulation (arrow indicates electrode), which leads to seizure activity (and an increased BOLD signal) in the hippocampus and septal nuclei, which causes slow oscillations (and a decreased BOLD signal) in the orbital frontal cortex. Limbic seizures of this kind are associated with behavioral arrest and decreased responsiveness in both animal models and human patients with temporal lobe epilepsy. Cg1/2: anterior cingulate cortex; HC: hippocampus; LO/VO: lateral and ventral orbital frontal cortex; LS/MS: lateral and medial septal nuclei; MD: mediodorsal thalamus; RSG: retrosplenial granular cortex. *Source: Reproduced with permission from Ref. 345.*

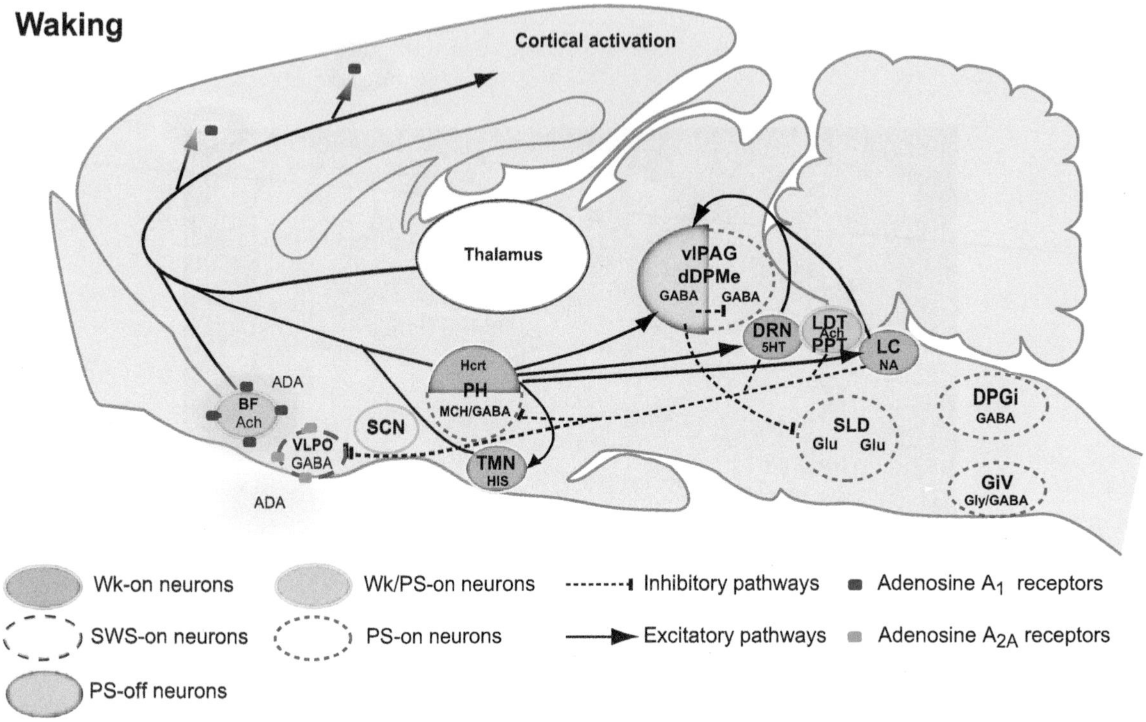

FIGURE 22.1 **Neuronal networks responsible for waking.** At sleep–wake transitions, the hypocretin neurons would be the first to start firing, exciting all the other waking systems (histaminergic, monoaminergic, and cholinergic). In turn, these waking systems activate the thalamus and/or the cortex, leading to cortical activation and, importantly, inhibiting the GABAergic SWS (non-REM, or NREM, sleep)-active neurons of the VLPO and MnPn. Abbreviations: 5HT, 5-hydroxytryptamine (serotonin); Ach, acetylcholine; ADA, adenosine; BF, basal forebrain; DPGi, dorsal paragigantocellular reticular nucleus; dDPMe, deep mesencephalic reticular nucleus; DRN, dorsal raphe nucleus; GABA, gamma-aminobutyric acid; GiV, ventral gigantocellular reticular nucleus; Gly, glycine; Hcrt, hypocretin (orexin)-containing neurons; His, histamine; LC, locus coeruleus; LDT, laterodorsal tegmental nucleus; MCH, neurons containing melanin-concentrating hormone; NA, noradrenaline; PH, posterior hypothalamus; PPT, pedunculopontine tegmental nucleus; PS, paradoxical sleep; RT, reticular thalamic neurons; SCN, suprachiasmatic nucleus; SLD, sublaterodorsal nucleus; SWS, slow-wave sleep; TMN, tuberomamillary nucleus; vlPAG, ventrolateral periaqueductal gray; VLPO, ventrolateral preoptic nucleus; W, waking.

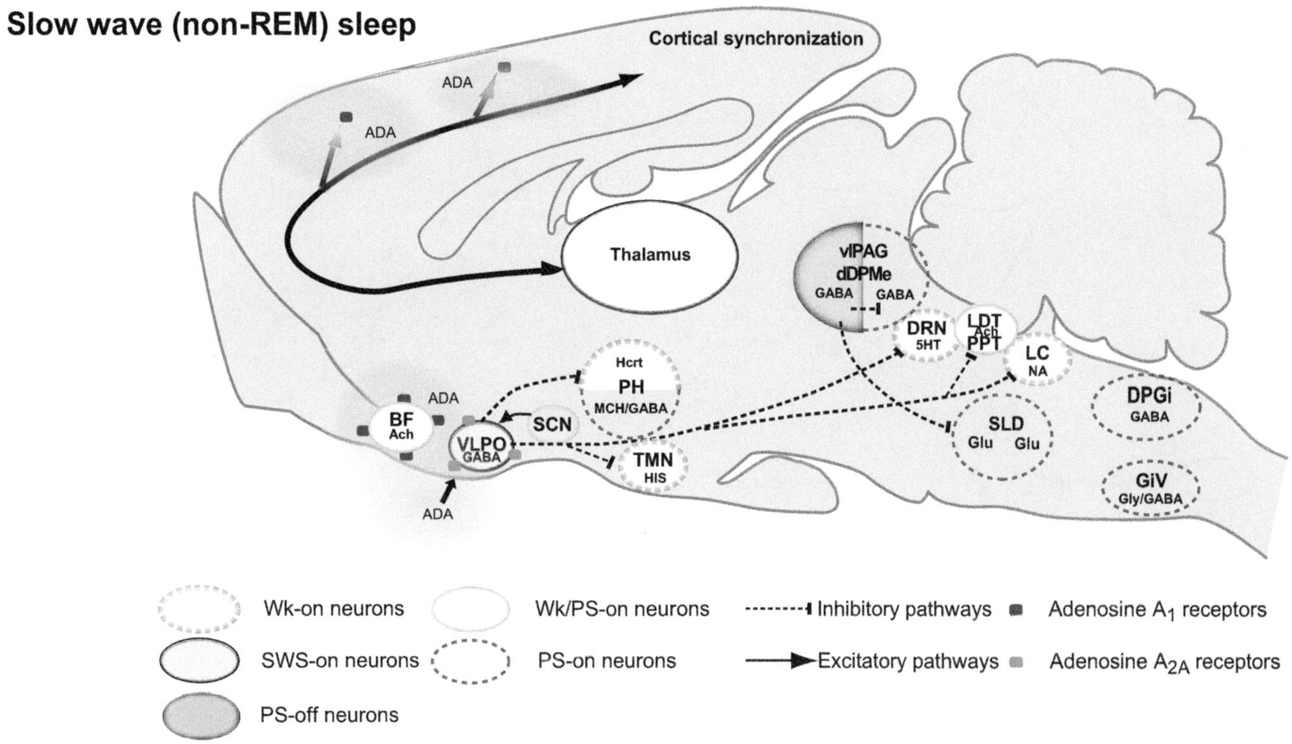

FIGURE 22.2 **Neuronal networks responsible for slow-wave (NREM) sleep.** VLPO and MnPo GABAergic neurons would be inhibited by noradrenergic and cholinergic inputs during waking. The majority of them would start firing at sleep onset (drowsiness) in response to excitatory, homeostatic (adenosine), and circadian drives (suprachiasmatic input). These activated neurons, through the reciprocal GABAergic inhibition of all wake-promoting systems, would be in a position to suddenly unbalance the "flip-flop" network, as required for switching from W (drowsiness) to a consolidation of SWS sleep. Conversely, the slow removal of excitatory influences would result in a progressive firing decrease in VLPO neurons and therefore an activation of wake-promoting systems leading to the awakening event.

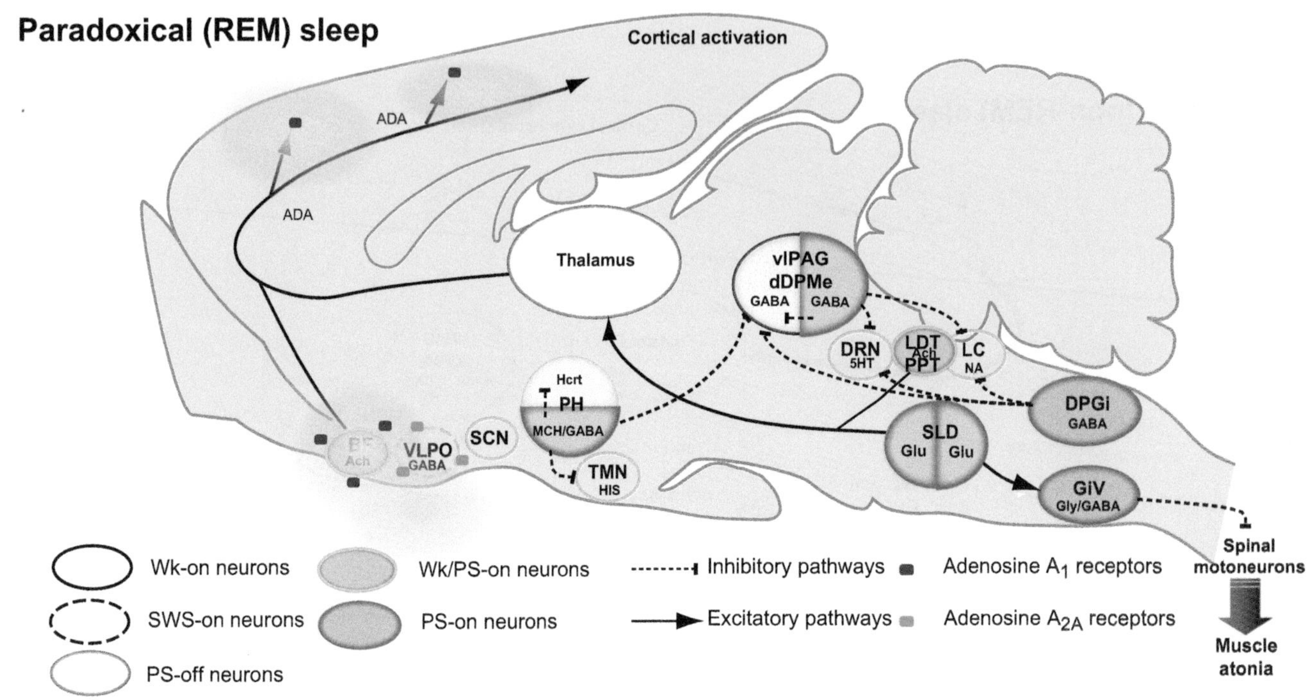

FIGURE 22.3 **Neuronal networks responsible for paradoxical (PS; also called REM) sleep.** PS onset would be due to the activation of glutamatergic PS-on neurons localized in the sublaterodorsal tegmental nucleus (SLD). During waking (W) and SWS (NREM) sleep, these PS-on neurons would be inhibited by a tonic inhibitory GABAergic tone originating from PS-off neurons localized in the ventrolateral periaqueductal gray (vlPAG) and the dorsal deep mesencephalic nucleus (dDPMe). These neurons would be activated during W by the hypocretin (Hcrt) neurons and the monoaminergic neurons. The onset of PS would be due to the activation by intrinsic mechanisms of PS-on GABAergic neurons localized in the posterior lateral hypothalamic area, the dorsal paragigantocellular reticular nucleus (DPGi), and the vlPAG. These neurons would also inactivate the PS-off monoaminergic neurons during PS. The disinhibited ascending SLD PS-on neurons would in turn induce cortical activation via their projections to intralaminar thalamic relay neurons in collaboration with W/PS-on cholinergic and glutamatergic neurons from the LDT and PPT, mesencephalic and pontine reticular nuclei, and basal forebrain. Descending PS-on SLD neurons would induce muscle atonia via their excitatory projections to glycinergic premotoneurons localized in the alpha and ventral gigantocellular reticular nuclei (GiA and GiV, respectively). The exit from PS would be due to the activation of waking systems since PS episodes are almost always terminated by an arousal. The waking systems would inhibit the GABAergic PS-on neurons localized in the DPGi and vlPAG. Since the duration of PS is negatively coupled with the metabolic rate, we propose that the activity of the waking systems is triggered to end PS to restore competing physiological parameters like thermoregulation.

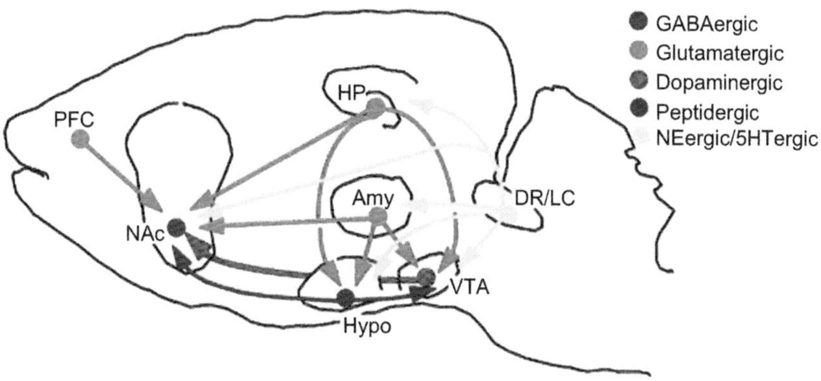

FIGURE 24.2 The figure offers a simplified model of neural circuits involved in processing mood. While the hippocampus (HP) and the amygdala (Amy) play a central role in processing emotion, they are regulated by the prefrontal cortex (PFC). The nucleus accumbens (NAc) and hypothalamus (Hypo) play a large role in reward, fear, and motivation. Not discussed extensively in this chapter, but alluded to here, is the role of neurotransmitters in these networks. The ventral tegmental area (VTA) provides dopaminergic input to the NAc; inputs to most of the other brain areas are not shown in the figure. Norepinephrine (NE, from the locus coeruleus or LC) and serotonin (5HT from the dorsal raphe and other raphe nuclei) innervate all of the regions shown in the figure. In addition, strong connections between the hypothalamus and VTA-NAc pathway have been established in recent years. GABA, gamma-aminobutyric acid; DR, dorsal raphe. (*Source: Reprinted from Nestler EJ & Carlezon WA. Mesolimbic Dopamine Reward Circuit in Depression; Biological Psychiatry, 2008; 59 (12) 111–1159 with permission from Elsevier.*)

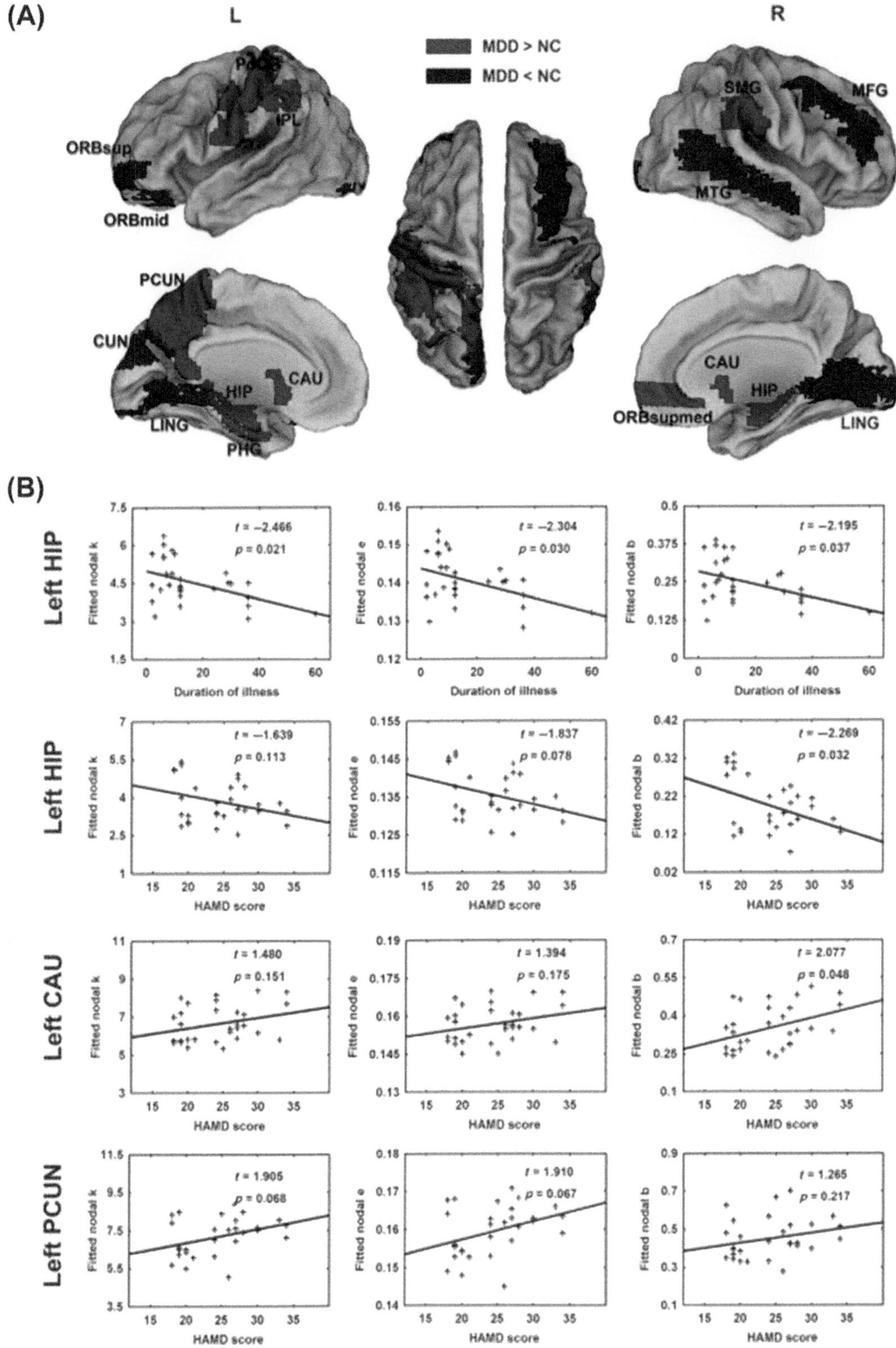

FIGURE 24.3 This study demonstrates the multiple cortical regions associated with depressed mood in medication naïve, first episode of Major Mood Disorder (MDD). Brain regions showing abnormal nodes in brain functional networks and their relationships with clinical variables in MDD patients. (A) Regions with abnormal nodes in MDD patients include: CAL, calcarine fissure and surrounding cortex; CAU, caudate nucleus; CUN, cuneus; HIP, hippocampus; MFG, middle frontal gyrus; ORBmid, middle frontal gyrus, orbital part; ORBsup, superior frontal gyrus, orbital part; ORBsupmed, superior frontal gyrus, medial orbital; PCUN, precuneus; PHG, parahippocampal gyrus; PoCG, postcentral gyrus; R, right hemisphere; SMG, supramarginal gyrus.MTG, middle temporal gyrus; IPL, inferior parietal, but supramarginal and angular gyri; L, left hemisphere; LING, lingual gyrus. (B) Scatter plots of nodal metrics against disease duration and HAMD scores which rate depressive symptoms (the higher the score the greater the depression). HAMD, Hamilton Depression Rating Scale; MDD, major depressive disorder; NC, normal control subjects. (*Source: Reprinted from Zhang J et al. Disrupted Brain Connectivity Networks in Drug-Naïve, First Episode Major Depressive Disorder; 2011, 70 (4) 334–342 with permission from Elsevier.*)

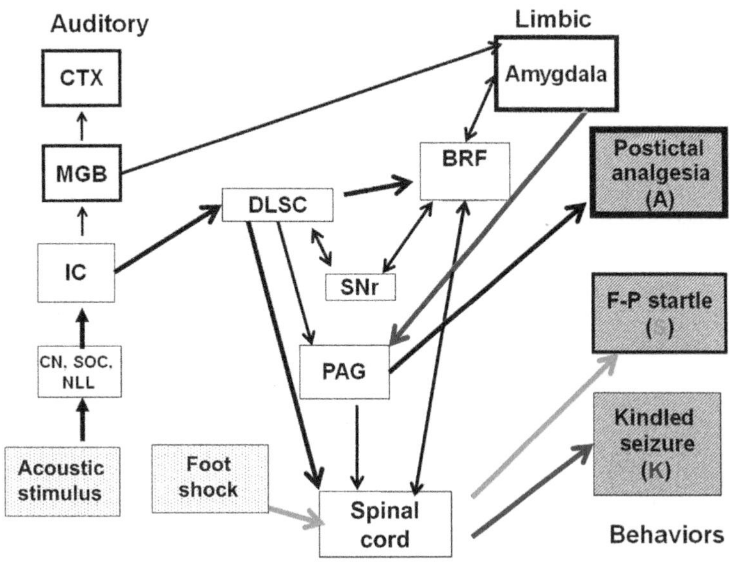

FIGURE 29.3 Specific network interaction diagrams in three related forms of auditory network interactions with other networks, including the somatosensory, pain, and limbic (emotional) networks. (1) Audiogenic seizures (AGS)-induced analgesia (A, blue arrows). The AGS network can also interact with the pain network via a common network nucleus (PAG). (2) The fear-potentiated (F-P) startle network (S, green arrows) involves somatosensory input (foot shock) via the spinal cord, which projects to a common network nucleus (BRF). (3) The AGS-kindling network (K, red arrows) involves the emotional network, including the amygdala. Analgesia is induced after AGS (postictal) and is short term, lasting for >2 h after the seizure. Fear-potentiated startle is induced by repetitive pairing of foot shock with an acoustic stimulus and is long-lasting. AGS kindling consists of daily or twice-daily audiogenic seizure repetition for 14–21 seizures and is long-lasting. The black arrows are pathways that are proposed to be involved in all three networks. BRF = brainstem reticular formation; CN = cochlear nucleus; CTX = cortex; DLSC = deep layers of superior colliculus; IC = inferior colliculus; MGB = medial geniculate body; NLL = nucleus of the lateral lemniscus; PAG = periaqueductal gray; SNr = substantia nigra reticulata; SOC = superior olivary complex.

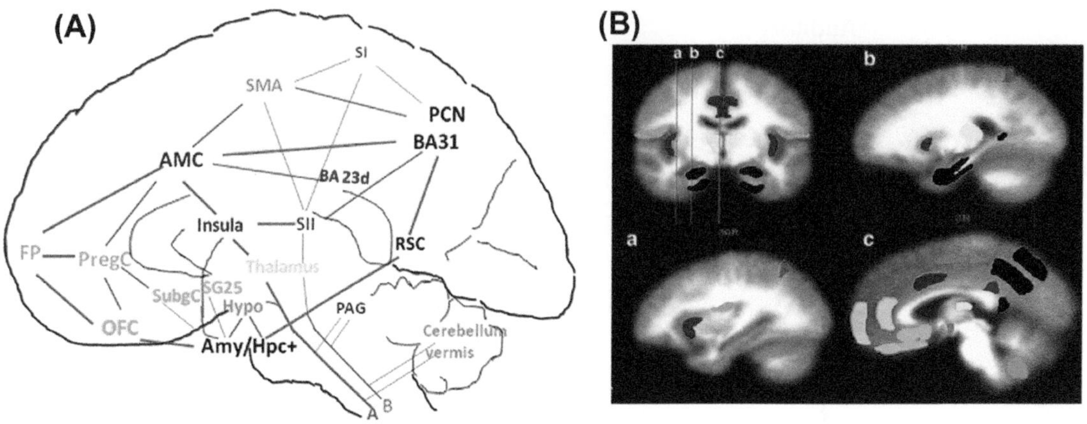

FIGURE 31.1 Functionally anticorrelated brain networks involved in acupuncture action. In the schematic diagram of a midsagittal section (A), deactivated regions are color-coded in cool colors (blue and green) and activated regions in warm colors (red, etc.). The areas corresponding to those in the schematic diagram are shown in the MRI sections in (B): a coronal slice through the amygdala and three sagittal slices as indicated on the coronal section. Regions of deactivation in the limbic-paralimbic-neocortical network (LPNN) aggregate in the medial prefrontal cortex [the frontal pole (FP), pregenual and subgenual cingulate (pregC and subgC, respectively), subgenual area (SG25), and orbitofrontal cortex (OFC)], medial parietal cortex [the precuneus (PCN) and posterior cingulate (BA31)], retrosplenial cortex (RSC) (BA29 and 30), and medial temporal lobe [amygdala (Amy) and hippocampal formation (Hpc+), located lateral to the schematic section]. The hypothalamus, pontine nuclei, and cerebellar vermis also showed deactivation. The secondary somatosensory cortex (SII), right anterior insula, antero-middle cingulate (AMC), supplementary motor area (SMA), posterior cingulate (BA23) dorsal, and sensory divisions of the thalamus comprise the activation network. Several associated cortical areas and the basal ganglia showing activation or deactivation are not shown. *Source: This figure is adapted from Ref. 16 with permission.*

Printed and bound by CPI Group (UK) Ltd, Croydon, CR0 4YY
08/05/2025
01865034-0006